Slatter's Fundamentals of

Veterinary Ophthalmology

Slatter's Fundamentals of
Veterinary
Ophthalmology

Fourth Edition

David J. Maggs, BVSc (Hons)
Diplomate, American College of Veterinary
 Ophthalmology;
Associate Professor
Veterinary Medical Teaching Hospital
University of California–Davis
Davis, California

Paul E. Miller, DVM
Diplomate, American College of Veterinary
 Ophthalmology;
Clinical Professor of Comparative
 Ophthalmology
School of Veterinary Medicine
Veterinary Medical Teaching Hospital
University of Wisconsin–Madison
Madison, Wisconsin

Ron Ofri, DVM, PhD
Diplomate, European College of Veterinary
 Ophthalmology;
Senior Lecturer, Veterinary Ophthalmology
Koret School of Veterinary Medicine
Hebrew University of Jerusalem
Rehovot, Israel

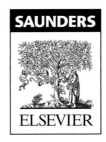

SAUNDERS

ELSEVIER

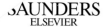

11830 Westline Industrial Drive
St. Louis, Missouri 63146

SLATTER'S FUNDAMENTALS OF VETERINARY OPHTHALMOLOGY,
EDITION 4   ISBN: 978-0-7216-0561-6

Notice

Knowledge and best practice in this field are constantly changing. As new research and experience broaden our knowledge, changes in practice, treatment and drug therapy may become necessary or appropriate. Readers are advised to check the most current information provided (i) on procedures featured or (ii) by the manufacturer of each product to be administered, to verify the recommended dose or formula, the method and duration of administration, and contraindications. It is the responsibility of the practitioner, relying on his or her own experience and knowledge of the patient, to make diagnoses, to determine dosages and the best treatment for each individual patient, and to take all appropriate safety precautions. To the fullest extent of the law, neither the Publisher nor the Authors assume any liability for any injury and/or damage to persons or property arising out or related to any use of the material contained in this book.

The Publisher

Library of Congress Control Number 2007924244

Publishing Director: Linda Duncan
Acquisitions Editor: Anthony Winkel
Developmental Editor: Maureen Slaten
Publishing Services Manager: Patricia Tannian
Senior Project Manager: Kristine Feeherty
Design Direction: Amy Buxton

Printed in China

Last digit is the print number: 9 8 7 6 5 4 3 2 1

CONTRIBUTORS

Itamar Aroch, DVM, DECVIM-CA
Senior Lecturer, Small Animal Medicine
Koret School of Veterinary Medicine
Hebrew University of Jerusalem
Rehovot, Israel

Bradford J. Holmberg, DVM, MS, PhD, DACVO
Veterinary Referral Centre
Little Falls, New Jersey

Gila A. Sutton, DVM, MSc, DACVIM-LA
Clinical Instructor, Equine Internal Medicine
Koret School of Veterinary Medicine
Hebrew University of Jerusalem
Rehovot, Israel

Brian P. Wilcock, DVM, MS, PhD, DACVP
Department of Pathobiology
Ontario Veterinary College
University of Guelph
Ontario, Canada

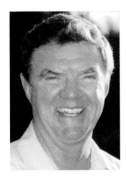

Dr. Douglas H. Slatter was an important and unique individual. As a student he excelled, graduating from the veterinary school at the University of Queensland in 1970. He was immediately accepted into a graduate program at Washington State University and completed a Master of Science degree. During this time Dr. Slatter learned considerable clinical ophthalmology under the tutelage of Dr. Gary Bryan, DACVO. Next, Dr. Slatter attended Colorado State University (CSU) in a Doctorate of Philosophy Degree program at the Surgical Metabolic Laboratory directed by Dr. William Lumb. Dr. Slatter excelled in this diverse academic environment. He had special interests in cardiac surgery and ophthalmology. While at CSU, he spent time with Dr. Glenn Severin, DACVO, DACVIM, furthering Dr. Slatter's clinical knowledge of veterinary ophthalmology.

An important friend at CSU was Mrs. Mary Fischer, BS, MS. Mrs. Fischer had been the chief laboratory technician in the ophthalmology section of the Armed Forces Institute of Pathology. She had been hired in the CSU Department of Pathology to bring her expertise to the Specialty Pathology Laboratory directed by Dr. Stuart Young, DACVP, Hon DACVO. Dr. Slatter worked diligently with Dr. Young and Mrs. Fischer in developing retinal digesting techniques to advance the study of retinal vascular disease in dogs. His doctoral thesis, "Effects of Hyperproteinemia and Aging on Canine Eyes" (1975), was the culmination of this collaboration.

Dr. Slatter was a perfect student. He accomplished an amazing feat by sitting for his board certification in veterinary surgery and veterinary ophthalmology in the same year, passing both examinations with high marks. Furthermore, Dr. Slatter completed his doctoral research project and earned his PhD degree in the same year. During this busy year he completed rough-draft preparations for the soon-to-be-published first edition of this textbook: *Fundamentals of Veterinary Ophthalmology*.

After graduate school, Dr. Slatter returned to Australia and taught ophthalmology and small animal surgery at Murdoch University, Western Australia. He married Dr. Elizabeth Chambers, and Dr. Chambers proved to be his soul mate, best friend, and fellow collaborator throughout the remainder of their lives.

In 1984, Drs. Slatter and Chambers returned to the United States. Dr. Slatter had been a visiting Professor of Ophthalmology at the Scheie Eye Institute, University of Pennsylvania. Drs. Slatter and Chambers eventually acquired the Animal Eye Clinic in La Habra, California, from retiring Dr. Ralph Vierheller, DAVCO, DACVS. Dr. Slatter and Dr. Vierheller had the distinction of being board certified in both ophthalmology and surgery. Dr. Slatter continued with academic pursuits while in private practice. He was an adjunct professor of veterinary ophthalmology at the Southern California College of Optometry in Fullerton, California. Drs. Slatter and Chambers practiced in La Habra, California, for the remainder of their lives. In addition, they operated ophthalmology clinics throughout the Los Angeles basin; in Bakersfield, California; and in Incline Village, Nevada. Despite his busy practice schedule, Dr. Slatter traveled throughout the world lecturing about ophthalmology and surgery. He made it a priority to vacation in his homeland of Australia at least twice each year. During these working vacations, he managed to operate a land development company and a small airplane import business. His passion and skill as a private pilot were well respected in both Australia and the United States. He was also a licensed Justice of the Peace in Australia.

Throughout his years in private practice, Dr. Slatter continued to pursue academic excellence. He published revisions to his original ophthalmology text, and he organized and edited the two-volume *Textbook of Veterinary Surgery* and the pocket companion to that book. Each of his textbooks and their revisions were translated into several foreign languages. Dr. Slatter also contributed more than 60 peer-reviewed scientific manuscripts during his career.

In addition to being a Diplomate in both the American Colleges of Veterinary Ophthalmology and Surgery, Dr. Slatter was a Diplomate of European College of Veterinary Surgeons, a Fellow of the Royal College of Veterinary Surgeons, a Member of the Australian College of Veterinary Scientists, and one of four founding members of the International Society of Veterinary Ophthalmology.

Dr. Douglas H. Slatter and Dr. Elizabeth D. Chambers were popular speakers, educators, and clinicians who devoted their lives to improving veterinary ophthalmology and veterinary surgery. They will be missed.

J. Daniel Lavach, DVM, DACVO
Reno, Nevada

CONTENTS

1 STRUCTURE AND FUNCTION OF THE EYE, *1*
Paul E. Miller

2 DEVELOPMENT AND CONGENITAL ABNORMALITIES, *20*
Ron Ofri

3 OCULAR PHARMACOLOGY AND THERAPEUTICS, *33*
David J. Maggs

4 GENERAL PATHOLOGY OF THE EYE, *62*
Brian P. Wilcock

5 BASIC DIAGNOSTIC TECHNIQUES, *81*
David J. Maggs

6 EYELIDS, *107*
David J. Maggs

7 CONJUNCTIVA, *135*
David J. Maggs

8 THIRD EYELID, *151*
David J. Maggs

9 LACRIMAL SYSTEM, *157*
Paul E. Miller

10 CORNEA AND SCLERA, *175*
David J. Maggs

11 UVEA, *203*
Paul E. Miller

12 THE GLAUCOMAS, *230*
Paul E. Miller

13 LENS, *258*
Ron Ofri

14 VITREOUS, *277*
Ron Ofri

15 RETINA, *285*
Ron Ofri

16 NEUROOPHTHALMOLOGY, *318*
Ron Ofri

17 ORBIT, *352*
Paul E. Miller

18 OCULAR MANIFESTATIONS OF SYSTEMIC DISEASES, *374*
Itamar Aroch, Ron Ofri, and Gila A. Sutton

19 OCULAR EMERGENCIES, *419*
Paul E. Miller

20 OPHTHALMOLOGY OF EXOTIC PETS, *427*
Bradford J. Holmberg

APPENDIX: BREED PREDISPOSITION TO EYE DISORDERS, *442*
Paul E. Miller

GLOSSARY, *455*

STRUCTURE AND FUNCTION OF THE EYE

Paul E. Miller

FUNDAMENTALS OF VISION
CENTRAL VISUAL PATHWAYS

VASCULAR ANATOMY AND PERIPHERAL
NEUROANATOMY

OCULAR REFLEXES
PHYSIOLOGY OF THE AQUEOUS

Vision is a complex phenomenon in which light emanating from objects in the environment is captured by the eye and focused onto the retinal photoreceptors (Figures 1-1 and 1-2). Electrical signals originating from these cells pass through a number of cell types in the retina and throughout the central nervous system (CNS) before arriving at the visual cortex, where the sensation of vision occurs. Numerous species variations exist on this basic theme, each allowing the animal to exploit a particular ecologic niche. The basic similarities among all vertebrate eyes and how they respond to insult allow the comparative ophthalmologist to confidently treat a wide range of ocular conditions in a diverse array of species.

FUNDAMENTALS OF VISION

The act of "seeing" is a complex process that depends on (1) light from the outside world falling onto the eye, (2) the eye efficiently transmitting and properly focusing the images of these objects on the retina, (3) the retina detecting these light rays, (4) transmission of this information via the visual pathways to the brain, and (5) the brain processing this information so as to make it useful. Differentiating between objects (e.g., a predator versus its surroundings) is one of the most critical aspects of vision, and because this distinction is so important for survival, normal animals can "see" an object if it differs sufficiently from its surroundings in any *one* of five different aspects: luminance ("brightness"), motion, texture, binocular disparity (depth), and color. In general, objects are differentiated on the basis of their motion, texture, depth, and luminance roughly equally well, but separations based on color are less easily made. Although the individual components of vision can be divided into the ability to detect light and motion, visual perspective, visual field of view, depth perception, visual acuity, and the perception of color and form, the complete visual experience is a synthesis of these parts into a unified perception of the world.

Sensitivity to Light

The visual system of most domestic mammals has evolved to improve performance under a wide range of lighting conditions so that they may exploit specific ecologic niches. Of domestic mammals, cats are probably the most efficiently adapted for nocturnal vision, with a minimum light detection threshold up to seven times lower than that in humans. Other adaptations that permit cats to function well in nocturnal conditions are a tapetum lucidum, which reflects 130 times more light than the human fundus; a vertical slit pupil, which produces a smaller aperture in bright light than what is possible with a circular pupil but also allows the pupil to dilate 6 mm more than the human pupil; a large cornea, which permits more light to enter the eye; a relatively posteriorly located lens, which produces a smaller but brighter image on the fundus; and a retina rich in light-sensitive rod photoreceptors (Figure 1-3). Many of the other domestic mammals have similar but fewer extreme adaptations for vision in dim light, allowing them to exploit a photic environment that is not strictly diurnal or nocturnal.

The tapetum is cellular in dogs and cats and collagenous in horses and ruminants, suggesting that the visual advantages this structure offers are of sufficient magnitude that it has evolved separately at least twice in mammals (Figure 1-4). In both cases, the variety of tapetal colors seen during ophthalmoscopy results from the differential interaction of light with the tapetum's physical structure rather than from the inherent spectral composition, or color, of its pigments. The dorsal location of the tapetum may enhance the view of the usually darker ground, and the ventrally located, usually darkly pigmented nontapetal region may reduce light scattering originating from the brighter sky. In cats, the tapetum may also absorb light in the shorter wavelengths and, via fluorescence, shift it to a longer wavelength that more closely approximates the maximal sensitivity of the photopigment, rhodopsin. This shift may brighten the appearance of a blue-black evening or night sky and enhance the contrast between other objects in the environment and the background sky.

The rhodopsin photopigment of dogs and cats is tuned to a slightly different wavelength of light from that in humans and, as is typical of species adapted to function well in dim light, takes longer to completely regenerate after extensive exposure to bright light. The ranges of wavelengths to which rhodopsin in dogs, cats, and humans is sensitive are similar, however, indicating that vision in dim light is not enhanced by expanding the range of detectable wavelengths. The slight wavelength shifts in the maximal sensitivity of rhodopsin across species

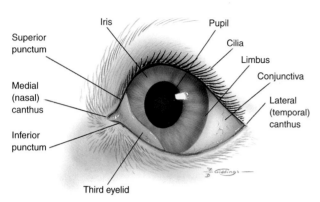

Figure 1-1. Frontal view of the external structures of the canine eye.

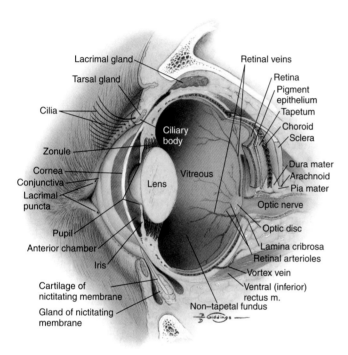

A

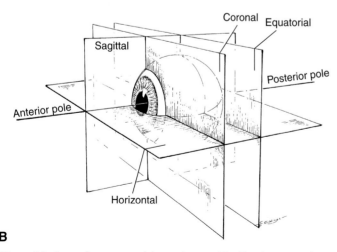

B

Figure 1-2. Internal structures of the canine eye **(A)**. Also shown are the standard reference planes **(B)**.

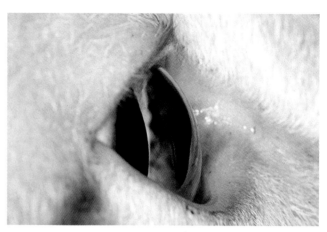

Figure 1-3. External view of the eye of a normal cat. Nocturnal adaptations that allow more light to enter the eye include a large cornea, a deep anterior chamber, and a relatively posteriorly located lens. (From Czederpiltz JMC, et al. [2005]: Putative aqueous humor misdirection syndrome as a cause of glaucoma in cats: 32 cases. J Am Vet Med Assoc 227:1476.)

suggests that domestic mammals and humans do not perceive the world in exactly the same way.

Sensitivity to Motion

Although little work has been done on the motion-detecting abilities of most domestic animals, it is probable that the perception of movement is a critical aspect of their vision and that they, like people, are much more sensitive to moving objects than stationary ones. Rod photoreceptors, which dominate the retinas of domestic mammals, are particularly well suited for detecting motion and shapes, and it follows that the motion-detecting abilities of domestic mammals—especially in dim light—would be well developed. In a study of the visual performance of police dogs, the most sensitive dogs could recognize a moving object up to 900 m away but could recognize the same object, when stationary, at only 585 m or less. Because of the superior visual acuity of the human fovea, the minimum threshold for motion detection in bright light for cats is approximately 10 to 12 times greater than that for humans. Although humans may be better equipped to detect motion when directly viewing an object in bright light, it is possible that the vision of domestic mammals may be superior in dim light, when an object is viewed peripherally, or if it is moving at a certain speed to which the retina is particularly attuned.

The ability to detect motion may help explain certain behavior—much of the very large peripheral visual field of the horse probably supports only the detection of brightness and motion. When combined with a "prey mentality," this may cause the horse to treat every moving object in its peripheral field of view as dangerous and to be avoided. Similarly, many dogs and cats ignore static objects, but when these objects move, chase behavior is elicited, suggesting that the visual system has preferences for objects moving at certain speeds.

Sensitivity to Flickering Lights

Although not related to motion detection, the point at which rapidly flickering light fuses into a constantly illuminated light (flicker fusion) provides insight into the functional charac-

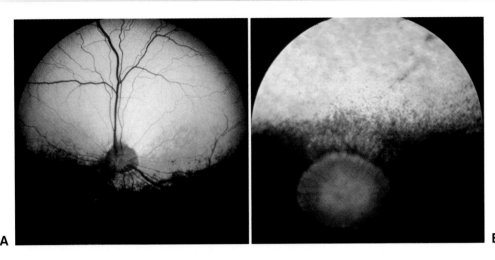

Figure 1-4. Cellular tapetum of a dog (**A**) and fibrous tapetum of a horse (**B**). (**B** from Gilger B [2005]: Equine Ophthalmology. Saunders, St. Louis. **A** and **B** courtesy Dr. Christopher J. Murphy.)

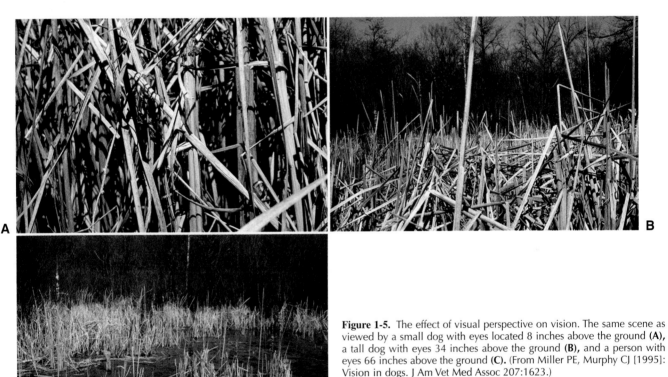

Figure 1-5. The effect of visual perspective on vision. The same scene as viewed by a small dog with eyes located 8 inches above the ground (**A**), a tall dog with eyes 34 inches above the ground (**B**), and a person with eyes 66 inches above the ground (**C**). (From Miller PE, Murphy CJ [1995]: Vision in dogs. J Am Vet Med Assoc 207:1623.)

teristics of rod and cone photoreceptors. The flicker frequency at which fusion occurs varies with the intensity and wavelength of the stimulating light. Because dogs can detect flicker at 70 to more than 80 Hz, a television program in which the screen is updated 60 times/sec and appears to people as a fluidly moving story line may appear to dogs as rapidly flickering.

Visual Field of View

The extent of the visual field (i.e., the area that can be seen by an eye when it is fixed on one point) and the height of the eyes above the ground may vary greatly among breeds and species

and has a major impact on the perception an animal has of its environment (Figure 1-5). For example, when the visual fields of its two eyes are combined, the horse has a total horizontal visual field of up to 350 degrees, with 55 to 65 degrees of binocular overlap and a virtually complete sphere of vision around its body (Figure 1-6). The length of the horse's nose interferes with binocular vision, and so a horse views an object binocularly until it is about 1 m away, at which point the horse must turn its head and observe with only one eye. In comparison, humans have a visual field of approximately 180 degrees (140 degrees of overlap), cats have a 200-degree field of view (140-degree overlap), and depending on breed, dogs have 250

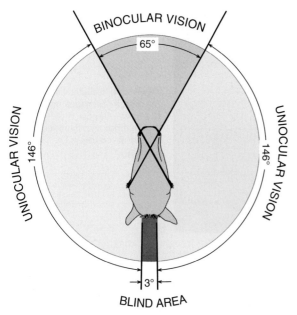

Figure 1-6. The visual field of the horse showing a binocular field (65 degrees) comparable to that of a dog but with much larger panoramic monocular fields (146 degrees), and a very small blind area (3 degrees).

degrees (30 to 60 degrees of binocular overlap) (Figure 1-7). The horse has only a few minor "blind spots," which are located superior and perpendicular to the forehead, directly below the nose, in a small oval region in the superior visual field where light strikes the optic nerve itself, and the width of the head directly behind. Clearly, this extensive visual field makes it very difficult for a person or potential predator to "sneak up" on a horse.

Depth Perception

Depth perception is enhanced in those regions in which the visual fields of the two eyes overlap. Merely viewing an object

with both eyes simultaneously does not guarantee improved perception of depth. *Stereopsis* (binocular depth perception) results when the two eyes view the object from slightly different vantage points and the resulting image is blended or fused into a single image. If the two images are not fused, double vision may result. (Such an alteration in vision may occur in animals with orbital diseases.) Although binocular depth perception is superior if the images can be blended into one, monocular depth perception is also possible. Horses make distance judgments on the basis of static monocular clues; these clues include relative brightness, contour, areas of light and shadows, object overlay, linear and aerial perspective, and density of optical texture. In addition, movement of the head results in an apparent change in the relative positions of the objects viewed (a phenomenon known as *parallax*) and produces the sensation that objects are moving at different speeds, allowing depth to be estimated (Figure 1-8).

Visual Acuity

Visual acuity refers to the ability to see details of an object separately and in focus. It depends on the optical properties of the eye (i.e., the ability of the eye to generate a precisely focused image), the retina's ability to detect and process images, and the ability of higher visual pathways to interpret images sent to them. In general, visual acuity in most domestic mammals is limited by the retina and not by the optical properties of the eyes or by postretinal neural processing in the brain. The latter two factors can limit visual discrimination in a variety of disease states, such as when the lens is removed or when higher CNS visual pathways are impaired.

Optical Factors in Visual Acuity

The optical media of the eye, namely the cornea, aqueous humor, lens, and vitreous humor, are responsible for creating a properly focused image on the retina. The cornea and, to a lesser extent,

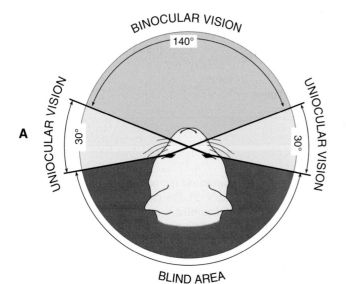

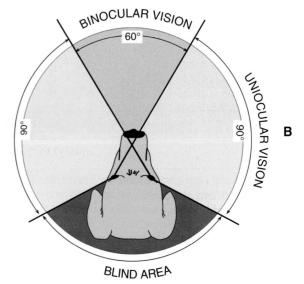

Figure 1-7. A, Visual field of a cat showing a large binocular field (140 degrees) with a relatively small monocular field (30 degrees) and a relatively large posterior blind area (160 degrees). **B,** Monocular and binocular visual fields in a typical mesocephalic dog. The dog has a modest binocular visual field (60 degrees) with relatively large monocular visual fields (90 degrees) and a posterior blind area of approximately 120 degrees.

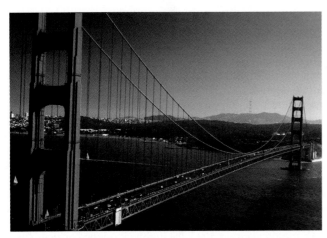

Figure 1-8. A number of cues allow depth to be perceived with one eye or in a two-dimensional photograph. These cues include apparent size (the left tower appears closer because it is larger than the right), looming (cars moving toward the viewer appear to become progressively larger), interposition (near objects such as the bridge overlay the more distant hills), aerial perspective (water vapor and dust in the air make the more distant hills less distinct and relatively color-desaturated), shading (shadows on the tower suggest depth), perspective (the parallel roadways appear to converge toward the horizon), relative velocity (the nearer cars appear to move faster than more distant ones), and motion parallax (if the eye is fixed on the center of the bridge, the images of near objects appear to move opposite to the direction the observer moves the head, whereas distant objects move in the same direction as the head). (From Gilger B [2005]: Equine Ophthalmology. Saunders, St. Louis.)

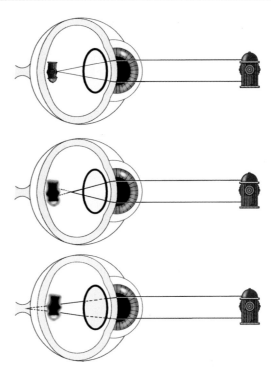

Figure 1-9. *Top,* The image is properly focused on the retina (emmetropia). *Middle,* The image is focused in front of the retina, making the eye nearsighted (myopia). *Bottom,* The image is in focus at a plane that is behind the retina, making the eye farsighted (hyperopia). (Modified from Miller PE, Murphy CJ [1995]: Vision in dogs. J Am Vet Med Assoc 207:1623.)

the lens are the principal refracting surfaces of the eye, and their ability to bend (refract) light is determined by their radii of curvature and the differences between their refractive index and that of the adjacent air or fluid. If the focal length of the focusing structures of the eye does not equal the length of the eye, a *refractive error* is present. In a normally focused *(emmetropic)* eye, parallel rays of light (effectively anything 20 feet or more away from the eye) are accurately focused on the retina. If parallel rays of light are focused in front the retina, *myopia* (nearsightedness) results. If they are focused behind the retina, *hyperopia* (farsightedness) results (Figure 1-9). Such errors in refraction are usually expressed in units of optical power called *diopters* (D). The extent of the error can be expressed by the formula $D = 1/f$, where f equals the focal length (in meters) of either the lens or the optical system as a whole. Therefore if an eye is 2 D myopic at rest, it is focused at a plane located 0.5 m in front of the eye. Similarly, an eye that is emmetropic at rest but can accommodate (change focus) 3 D is capable of clearly imaging objects on the retina that range from as far away as the visual horizon (infinity) to as near as 0.33 m in front of the eye.

The average resting refractive state of the dog is within 0.25 D of emmetropia. There are individuals, however, that are significantly myopic, and breed predispositions to myopia are found in German shepherds and Rottweilers. In one study, 53% of German shepherds were myopic by –0.5 D or more in a veteri-nary clinic population, but only 15% of German shepherds in a guide dog program were myopic, suggesting that dogs with visual disturbances such as nearsightedness do not perform as well as normally sighted dogs. It may be reasonable to screen dogs that will be expected to perform visually demanding tasks, or those on which human life relies for refractive errors, before embarking on extensive training programs. Although studies of the refractive

errors of cats and horses are somewhat conflicting, it appears that the average refraction for these species approximates emmetropia, although deviations of 1 to 2 D do regularly occur.

In addition to myopia and hyperopia, other optical aberrations (e.g., astigmatism) may result from imperfections in the refractive media such as the cornea or lens and lead to degradation of the image formed on the retina. Astigmatism occurs when different regions of the optical system (especially cornea or lens) do not focus light in a uniform fashion, resulting in warping of the image, an extreme example of which can be found in the irregular mirrors found at carnivals. Spontaneous astigmatism is generally uncommon in dogs but has been observed in a variety of breeds. Astigmatism commonly accompanies corneal diseases that result in scarring and distortion of the corneal curvature (Figure 1-10).

Although visual acuity requires that optical portions of the eye be transparent and that optical blur from refractive errors or astigmatism be limited, an adjustable focusing (accommodative) mechanism is needed if objects at different distances are to be seen with equal clarity. Accommodation in dogs and cats may be brought about by altering the curvature of the lens surface or, more likely, by moving the lens anteriorly (Figure 1-11). The accommodative range for most domestic animals is quite limited and does not generally exceed 2 to 3 D for dogs, 4 D for cats, and less than 2 D for horses. This finding suggests that dogs are capable of accurately imaging objects on the retina that are within 50 to 33 cm of their eyes but that objects nearer than this will be blurred. Hence, dogs use other senses, such as smell or taste, to augment vision in the investigation of very near objects. For comparison, young children are capable of accommodating approximately 14 D, or to about 7 cm.

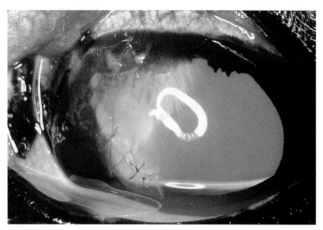

Figure 1-10. Corneal astigmatism after a corneal laceration with subsequent scarring. Note the irregular flash artifact on the cornea indicating that light is being unevenly focused on the retina. (From Gilger B [2005]: Equine Ophthalmology. Saunders, Philadelphia. Courtesy Dr. Ellison Bentley.)

Loss of the lens, as occurs after cataract surgery, results in severe hyperopia (farsightedness), with objects being focused approximately 14 D behind infinity, and a reduction in visual acuity to 20/800 or worse. This means that aphakic eyes are unable to image *any* object clearly, whether near or far away, and are unable to accommodate. Although the aphakic dog is extremely "farsighted," it must be kept in mind that, for objects of similar size, objects that are closer to the dog will create a much larger image on the retina than objects that are located far away. Therefore the aphakic dog may be able to better visually orient to near objects despite being "farsighted." Surprisingly, although this degree of hyperopia is markedly debilitating to some dogs, most dogs are still able to visually orient adequately in their environment without correction.

Retinal Factors in Visual Acuity

The retina may be the limiting factor in visual acuity for normal domestic animals, and its architecture may provide clues to the potential visual abilities of the eye. Enhanced vision in dim light as occurs in dogs typically requires that a greater number of photoreceptors (primarily rods) synaptically converge on a single ganglion cell. This results in reduced visual acuity, just as high-speed photographic film produces a "grainy" image in bright daylight. Additionally, the tapetum also scatters light and further degrades visual acuity in bright light. Retinas with excellent resolving power have a high ratio of ganglion cells to photoreceptors, a large number of ganglion cells and optic nerve fibers, and a high density of photoreceptors and usually lack a tapetum. In primates, the fovea has one ganglion cell per cone, whereas in cats, the peak ratio is one ganglion cell for every four cones. In all species, there are fewer ganglion cells in the periphery of the retina than in the center, and the ratio may decline to 1:16 in primates and 1:20 in cats, explaining the reduced visual acuity of their peripheral visual fields.

Domestic mammals lack the highly developed primate fovea but, instead, have a generally oval visual streak that contains the greatest density of photoreceptors, ganglion cells, and rhodopsin and thereby affords the greatest visual acuity. The visual streak, located in the tapetal region slightly superior and temporal to the optic nerve, has approximately linear, short temporal and longer nasal extensions (Figure 1-12). The oval temporal part of the visual streak is relatively free of blood vessels larger than capillaries, and nerve fibers take a curved course to the optic disc dorsal and ventral to the visual streak, presumably to avoid interfering with light reaching the photoreceptors. The temporal, oval portion of the streak may facilitate binocular vision, whereas the nasal, linear portion may be used to scan the horizon and better use the wider field of view available to the domestic mammals.

Wolves, presumably the ancestors of modern-day dogs, have a pronounced visual streak with a dense central area and extensions far into the temporal and nasal portions of the retina. In contrast, domesticated dogs, even of the same breed, have either a similar pronounced visual streak or a smaller, less densely packed, moderately pronounced visual streak. Wolves also generally have a greater maximum density of ganglion cells (12,000 to 14,000/mm^2) than do most dogs (6,400 to 14,400/mm^2). This difference implies that the visual acuity of wolves may be better than that of some dogs, and that the constancy of the form of the visual streak in wolves may be a

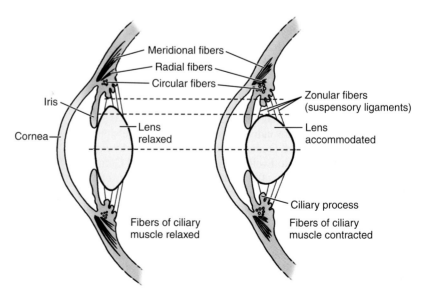

Figure 1-11. Classic accommodation in primates. *Left,* Distant vision. Relaxation of the ciliary muscle increases tension on the lens zonules, which flattens the lens and brings distant objects into focus. *Right,* Near vision. Contraction of the ciliary muscle reduces tension on the zonules, which allows the elastic lens capsule to assume a more spheric shape. The resulting increase in lens power allows near objects to be brought into focus on the retina. The importance of this mechanism of accommodation in most domestic mammals is debated. (Modified From Getty R [1975]: Sisson and Grossman's The Anatomy of the Domestic Animals, 5th ed. Saunders, Philadelphia.)

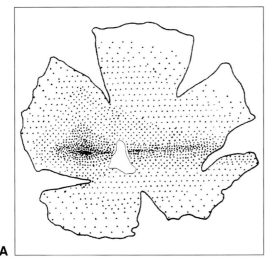
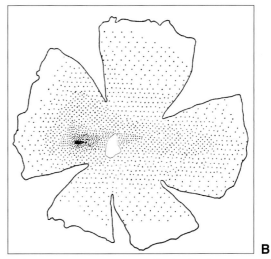

A   B

Figure 1-12. Diagram of retinal ganglion cell densities from the right retinas of a German shepherd with a very pronounced wolflike visual streak **(A)** and a beagle with a moderately pronounced visual streak **(B).** Retinas were cut radially to flatten them and are displayed at the same magnification. The intensity of the dots reflects varying ganglion cell densities. The irregular shape in the center of each retina is the region of the optic nerve head. Ganglion cells could not be seen in this area because of thick, overlying nerve fiber layer. (From Miller PE, Murphy CJ [1995]: Vision in dogs. J Am Vet Med Assoc 207:1623.)

result of environmental selective pressures that were altered by domestication. It is unclear whether there are differences in the visual acuity of dog breeds that have been developed to hunt by sight (sight hounds) and breeds that have been developed to hunt by smell (scent hounds), although the finding of a large number of beagles (a scent hound) with a pronounced visual streak suggests that there are insignificant differences between these two groups of dogs, despite their uses.

Estimates of Visual Acuity

The most familiar indicator of visual acuity for the human eye is the *Snellen fraction,* which relates the ability of a subject to distinguish between letters or objects at a fixed distance (usually 20 feet, or 6 m) with a standard response. Snellen fractions of 20/20, 20/40, and 20/100 mean that the test subject needs to be 20 feet away from a test image to discern the details that the average person with normal vision could resolve from 20, 40, and 100 feet away, respectively. This test actually measures the ability of the area of greatest visual acuity (the fovea) to discriminate between objects of high contrast. Peripheral visual acuity in humans is typically quite poor (i.e., 20/100, 20/200, or worse), presumably because the photoreceptor density is lower and the ratio of photoreceptors to ganglion cells is higher in these regions of the retina than in the fovea. The visual acuity of the normal dog ranges between 20/50 and 20/140, with 20/75 or so being the likely average. Feline visual acuity has been estimated to be between 20/100 and 20/200, whereas the larger eye of the horse (hence a greater numbers of photoreceptors) may result in a visual acuity of 20/30. The visual acuity of cattle, however, is unclear, because the size of their eyes and density of ganglion cells would suggest they possess a visual acuity comparable to that of horses but behavioral studies that depend on the cooperation of the animal have documented a visual acuity of only 20/240 to 20/440.

Most commonly used procedures to determine vision in animals (e.g., determination of menace responses by moving a hand across the visual field or having the animal's eyes follow

a moving cotton ball) test the motion sensitivity of virtually the entire retina, and positive responses are still present even though visual acuity may be very poor (up to 20/20,000). Visually distinguishing the fine details in objects is less important for most domestic mammals (even working animals) than it is for most people. The trade-off of improved vision in dim light for less acute vision in bright light allows such animals to exploit ecologic niches inaccessible to people and aids in both seeking prey and avoiding predators.

Color Vision

Color vision in domestic mammals has been the subject of numerous studies with conflicting results. More recent, well-controlled studies suggest that most domestic mammals possess, and use, color vision.

The presence of cone photoreceptors in domestic mammals suggests the potential for color vision, although the numbers and types of cones are smaller than those in humans. Cones constitute less than 10% of the visual streak in the dog, whereas they occupy almost 100% of the human fovea. Additionally, instead of three types of cones ("red," "green," and "blue") found in humans with normal color vision, dogs have only two functional cone types. One type of canine cone is maximally sensitive to light at 429 to 435 nm ("violet" to normal humans and corresponding to the "blue" cone), and another type has maximal sensitivity to light at 555 nm ("yellow-green" to normal humans) with extension into the red end of the color spectrum (corresponding to the "red" cone). Dogs lack, or do not use, "green" cones and appear to confuse red and green colors (red-green color blindness, or *deuteranopia*). This means that dogs are unable to differentiate middle to long wavelengths of light, which appear to people as green, yellow-green, yellow, orange, or red.

Although it is not known whether the dog's "blue" and "red" cones perceive colors in the same way as those of humans, the canine visible spectrum may be divided into two hues: one in the human violet and blue-violet range (430 to 475 nm), which is probably seen as blue by dogs, and a second in the human greenish-yellow, yellow, and red range (500 to 620 nm), which is probably seen as yellow by dogs. Dogs also appear to have a narrow region (475 to 485 nm, blue-green to humans) that appears colorless. Light in this spectral neutral point probably appears to be white or a shade of gray to dogs. In people with deuteranopia, however, the neutral point is in a greener (505-nm) region of the spectrum, so dogs are not exactly the same as red-green color blind humans. Wavelengths at the two ends of the spectrum (blue at one end and yellow at the other) probably provide the most saturated colors. Intermediate wavelengths are less intensely colored, appearing as if they were blends with white or gray.

The cat has a limited but detectable capacity for color vision and can distinguish between two stimuli if they differ greatly in spectral content, especially if the stimuli are also large. Cats appear to have the physical capacity (based on the presence of three types of cones) for *trichromacy* like humans, although behavioral studies have not demonstrated this ability and it is, at best, a pale copy of human trichromacy. Horses appear to have both a short-wavelength-sensitive (blue) cone with a peak sensitivity of approximately 428 nm, and a second cone with a peak sensitivity between the human red and green cones (539 nm, and called a middle–long-wavelength-sensitive cone). Therefore although horses have only two cones like dogs, orange and blue colors appear similar (shades of gray) to horses, whereas red and green appear similar (as shades of gray) to dogs (Figures 1-13 and 1-14). Cattle and swine also appear to have two functional cone pigments. The yellow tint to the equine lens probably filters out blue wavelengths, diminishing certain optical aberrations as well as glare and increasing the contrast of certain objects on select backgrounds.

Restrictions in color vision are probably of limited consequence to domestic mammals, as it is likely that they react only to colors of biologic importance to them. Problems may arise when one is teaching hunting and working dogs to

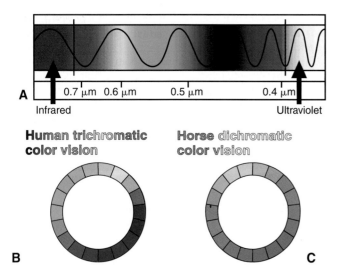

Figure 1-13. A, The color spectrum and corresponding wavelengths of light. **B** and **C,** Difference between dichromatic color vision of the horse and normal human color vision. **B,** Color wheel representing the spectrum of colors perceived by the trichromatic human visual system. **C,** Reducing the number of types of cone from three to two results in dichromatic color vision and an enormous reduction in the number of different colors seen. (**A** from Gilger B [2005]: Equine Ophthalmology. Saunders, Philadelphia. **B** and **C** from Carrol J, et al. [2001]: Photopigment basis for dichromatic color vision in the horse. J Vis Sci 1:80.)

distinguish red, orange, yellow, and green objects solely on the basis of color. In these cases, other visual clues, such as relative brightness and contrast, or the other senses—smell, sound, taste, and touch—are required to differentiate objects that appear similar in color. Additionally, dogs, and probably most other domestic mammals, are able to differentiate perfectly between closely related shades of gray indistinguishable to the human eye. This ability is far more valuable in exploiting their ecologic niche than color vision, because it increases visual discrimination when insufficient light may be present to effectively stimulate cones.

CENTRAL VISUAL PATHWAYS

The eye is only the first step in "seeing" (Figure 1-15). Vision is not simply a recording of each pixel in a scene, as a camera would make, because that would quickly overwhelm the visual system with massive amounts of information that may not be pertinent to the animal's survival or lifestyle. The brain does not, and cannot, consciously pay attention to the flood of information it receives from the eyes, but instead categorizes the information into specific "topics" that are channeled to specific areas of the brain for further processing. These "topics" are "internal" features such as texture and contrast, the direction and velocity of the object's movement, its overall orientation as represented on the retinal surface, its shape, its color, and many other aspects. Additionally, unlike a camera, the brain compares the current image with previous images, images from the other eye, and input from other senses such as hearing, smell, and touch. Once this comparison is completed, only the information that is relevant for the task at hand, or the animal's survival, rises to the level of conscious attention. Therefore the act of seeing depends not only on the function and health of the eye but also on the cognitive processes in the brain that decide what information merits conscious attention and what is to remain subconscious or ignored.

The central visual pathway begins with the retina, which is in effect an extension of the brain. In this tissue, information is processed in three functional stages. The first stage occurs in the *rod and cone photoreceptors*. These cells have varying sensitivity to different wavelengths of light and require different numbers of photons to strike them in order to elicit a response. The second stage of retinal processing occurs in the *outer plexiform layer*. At this level the photoreceptors, bipolar cells, and horizontal cells synaptically interact, and the responses of some photoreceptors are modulated by what is happening to other photoreceptors (so-called "on" and "off" or "center" and "surround" responses). These responses are associated with the static and spatial aspects of an object and serve to better define an object's brightness and borders by altering its contrast with surrounding objects. The third stage occurs in the synaptic interactions in the *inner plexiform layer*, which is more concerned with the dynamic and temporal aspects of vision. At this stage, transient responses that may underlie motion and direction sensitivity may occur in the amacrine and retinal ganglion cells. The amount of retinal processing of an image before it gets to the brain varies greatly by species.

Retinal ganglion cell nerve fibers then form the *nerve fiber layer* of the retina, converge at the *optic disc*, turn posteriorly, gain a myelin sheath, and pass through the sievelike opening in the sclera, the *lamina cribrosa*. The fibers pass via the *optic*

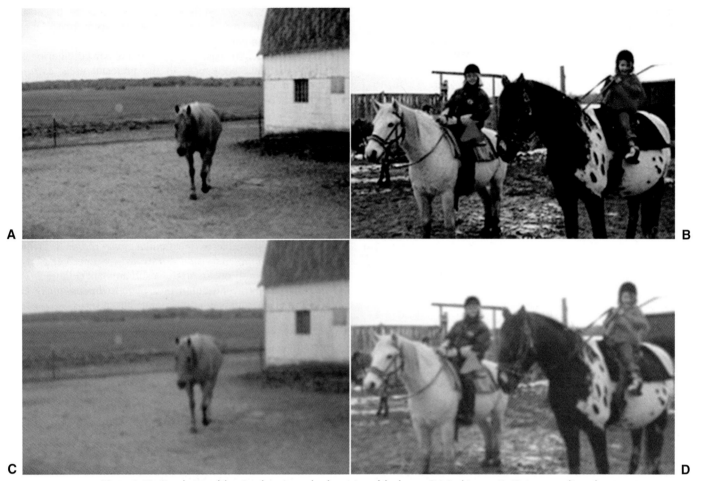

Figure 1-14. Simulation of the visual acuity and color vision of the horse. Original image **(A, B)**. Images adjusted to reflect the visual acuity and color vision abilities of the horse **(C, D)**. (From Carrol J, et al. [2001]: Photopigment basis for dichromatic color vision in the horse. J Vis Sci 1:80.)

nerve to the *optic chiasm* (see Figures 1-2, 1-15, and 1-16). Fibers coming from different parts of the retina maintain definite positions within the optic nerve and throughout the path to the visual cortex. Fibers from both optic nerves enter the optic chiasm, where partial decussation, or "crossing over" of fibers from one side to the other, may occur (see Figure 1-15).

The proportion of optic nerve fibers that decussate in the chiasm is related to the relative laterofrontal positioning of the orbit and eye in the skull and degree of binocular overlap. Animals with laterally directed eyes and no overlap between the *visual fields* of the two eyes exhibit complete decussation at the chiasm, and the information from the right (or left) visual field is processed entirely by the opposite visual cortex. As the eyes become more frontally directed in different species, however, it becomes possible for an object to be seen with both eyes. For example, an object in the animal's right visual field (on its right side) falls on the nasal area of the right retina and the temporal area of the left retina. In order for the same side of the brain (the left side in this example) to continue to process all the information from the right visual field, some optic nerve fibers must remain ipsilateral and must not decussate at the chiasm. This percentage varies by species, but in horses and cattle, which have relatively laterally directed eyes, 83% to 87% of the optic nerve fibers cross, whereas the percentage decreases—75% for dogs, 67% for cats, and 50% for

humans—as the eyes become more frontally directed. This finding is clinically relevant because species with extensive binocular overlap will not necessarily bump into objects if only one eye is blind or there is a lesion on only one side of the brain.

The optic chiasm receives the optic nerves as they enter the cranial vault via the *optic foramen and canals* (Figure 1-17). The chiasm lies at the base of the brain adjacent and anterior to the *hypophysis,* which sits in the *pituitary fossa* of the *postsphenoid bone.* This relationship between the pituitary and the chiasm and optic tracts is important in considering the potential effect of space-occupying masses of the pituitary on vision.

From the optic chiasm, fibers enter the *left and right optic tracts,* which then pass laterally from the chiasm, anterior to the hypophysis, and beneath the ventral surface of the *cerebral peduncle.* The tracts then curve dorsally and posteriorly, between the cerebral peduncle to which they are attached laterally and the *pyriform lobe.* The tracts thus pass to the *lateral geniculate body.* Before reaching the lateral geniculate body, some 20% to 30% of the fibers leave the tracts and enter the *pretectal area.* Some of these fibers enter the *superior colliculus* directly, and others pass via the tracts and lateral geniculate body to the colliculus indirectly. The majority of fibers entering the lateral geniculate body synapse here with the third ascending neuron in the visual

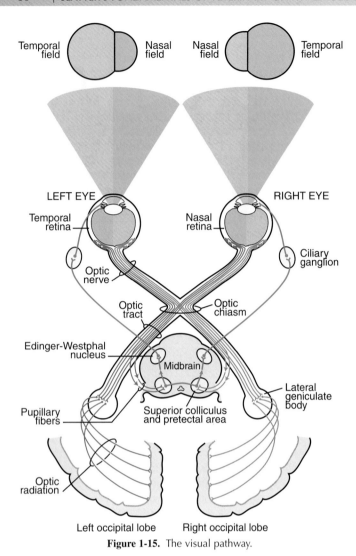

Figure 1-15. The visual pathway.

system, which passes without further synapse to the visual cortex. The first two synapses are the photoreceptor-bipolar and bipolar-ganglion cell interfaces.

Those fibers that leave the optic tracts before entering the lateral geniculate body pass to the pretectal area, carrying afferent impulses of the *pupillary light reflex.* In the pretectal area much decussation occurs, and the fibers pass to the midline *Edinger-Westphal nuclei* of the *oculomotor nerve* (see Figure 1-15). Efferent impulses pass from these nuclei to the *pupillary sphincter muscle* in each iris.

A positive pupillary light reflex does not mean that the eye can see. Fibers that mediate the reflex arc leave the optic tracts before the tracts enter the lateral geniculate body.

From the lateral geniculate body, fibers pass forward and lateral to the lateral ventricle as the fanlike *optic radiation,* which enters the *occipital or visual cortex,* where interpretation of some visual stimuli occurs in domestic animals (Figure 1-18). Increases in intraventricular pressure *(hydrocephalus)* can affect the visual pathway at this point.

In dogs and cats the visual cortex is not the sole center of interpretation of visual stimuli. If the cortex is removed, light perception and discrimination of light intensity are retained, but familiarity of surroundings is lost. Subcortical integration is believed to occur in the superior colliculus.

VASCULAR ANATOMY AND PERIPHERAL NEUROANATOMY

Further details of orbital anatomy may be found in Chapter 17.

Arterial Supply

The major arterial supply of the eye is from the *external ophthalmic artery,* a branch of the *internal maxillary artery,*

Figure 1-16. Ventral view of the brain and cranial nerves in the dog. Structures important to the visual system are highlighted. (From Done SH, et al. [1996]: Color Atlas of Veterinary Anatomy, Volume 3. Mosby, St. Louis.)

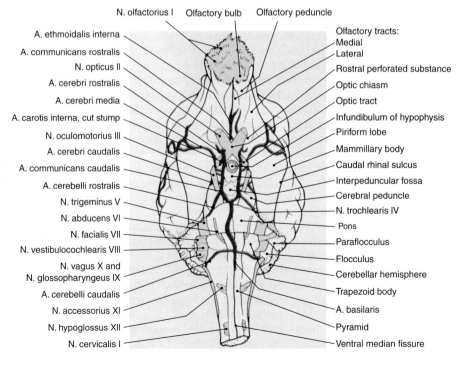

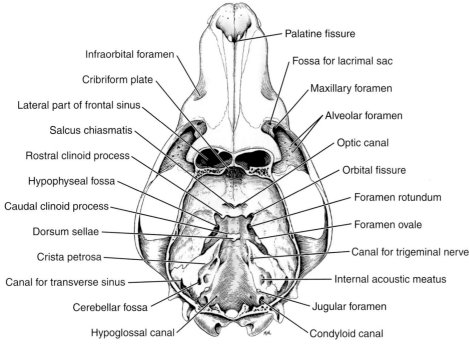

Figure 1-17. Skull of the dog with calvaria removed, dorsal aspect. Structures important to the visual system are highlighted. (Modified from Evans HE [1993]: Miller's Anatomy of the Dog, 3rd ed. Saunders, Philadelphia. © Cornell University 1964.)

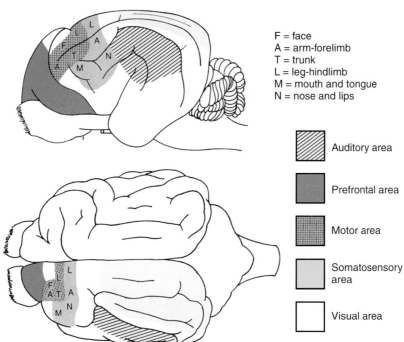

F = face
A = arm-forelimb
T = trunk
L = leg-hindlimb
M = mouth and tongue
N = nose and lips

Auditory area

Prefrontal area

Motor area

Somatosensory area

Visual area

Figure 1-18. Motor and sensory areas of the cerebral cortex of the dog. (Modified from Hoerlein BF [1978]: Canine Neurology, 3rd ed. Saunders, Philadelphia.)

which arises from the *external carotid artery* (Figure 1-19). The contribution from the internal carotid artery is small, unlike the situation in primates, and is via an *internal ophthalmic artery,* which arises from the *circle of Willis.* The internal ophthalmic artery enters the orbit through the optic canal with the optic nerve. From the external ophthalmic artery, numerous *short posterior ciliary arteries* arise (Figure 1-20) and penetrate the sclera around the optic nerve head. These arteries supply the retina and choroid.

There is no central retinal artery in domestic species. Single *medial and lateral long posterior ciliary arteries* pass around the globe horizontally, within the sclera, to supply the ciliary body. Muscular branches of the orbital artery, which supplies the extraocular muscles, also enter the globe near the insertions of these muscles. These *anterior ciliary arteries* anastomose with the long posterior ciliary arteries to form the ciliary arterial supply. When the globe is prolapsed, these muscular branches may be destroyed, decreasing the available supply to

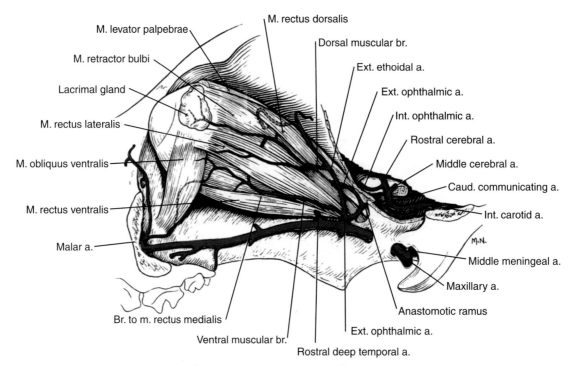

Figure 1-19. Arteries of the orbit and extrinsic ocular muscles in the dog, lateral aspect. (From Evans HE [1993]: Miller's Anatomy of the Dog, 3rd ed. Saunders, Philadelphia.)

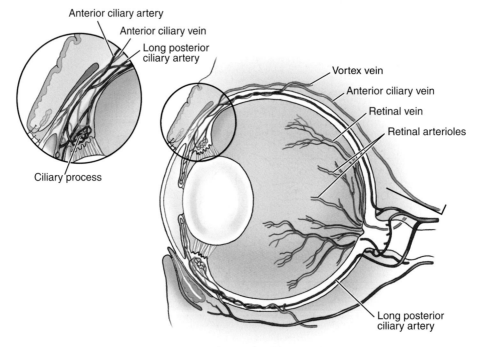

Figure 1-20. Vascular supply of the canine eye.

the anterior segment of the eye. Branches from the ciliary arterial network form the *major arterial circle of the iris.* The deep conjunctival arterioles at the limbus anastomose with the anterior ciliary arteries before they enter the sclera, and also with arterioles in the ciliary body. Vascular events of clinical importance (e.g., inflammation in one area of this network of anastomosing vessels) can often be seen in other parts, and their origin must be distinguished clinically if possible (see Figure 1-20).

The eyelids are supplied by the superficial temporal artery, a branch of the external carotid artery, and by the malar artery, a branch of the infraorbital artery.

Venous Drainage

The retina is drained by the retinal veins and venules, which run from the peripheral retina toward the optic nerve head (see

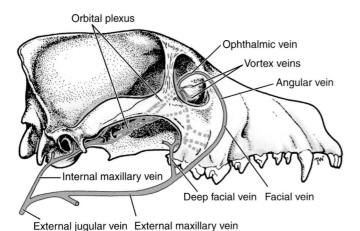

Figure 1-21. The venous drainage of the eye and orbit of the dog. (Modified from Startup FG [1969]: Diseases of the Canine Eye. Williams & Wilkins, Baltimore.)

Figures 1-20 and 1-21). The venous circle they form at the optic disc may be complete or incomplete in the dog. The venous circle drains posteriorly through the sclera via the *posterior ciliary veins* to a dilation in the orbital vein, the *superior (dorsal) ophthalmic vein.*

The choroid is drained by approximately four *vortex veins,* which leave the globe near the equator and join the *superior* and *inferior ophthalmic veins.* The ciliary body is drained by the anterior ciliary veins to the same superior and inferior ophthalmic veins that drain to the *orbital venous plexus* at the apex of the orbit. This plexus drains to the cavernous venous sinus within the cranial vault. The cavernous sinus drains via

the *vertebral sinuses, external jugular vein,* and *internal maxillary vein.* Venous blood thus passes posteriorly from the orbit via this route. It may also pass anteriorly via anastomoses between the ophthalmic veins and the *malar, angularis oculi,* and *facial veins* to the *external maxillary* and *external jugular veins.*

Considerable species variation exists in the vascular supply and drainage of the eye and orbit.

Nerve Supply of the Eye and Adnexa

The general plan of nerve supply to the eye is shown in Figure 1-22. For further details, see Chapter 16.

Optic Nerve (Cranial Nerve II)

The *optic nerve* and meninges pass from the globe, through the cone formed by the *retractor bulbi muscles,* via the *optic canal* to the *optic chiasm.* The dura covering the nerve is continuous with the outer layers of the sclera. The optic nerve consists of ganglion cells, whose cell bodies lie in the ganglion cell layer of the retina. It is a tract of the CNS, not a peripheral nerve.

Oculomotor Nerve (Cranial Nerve III)

The nucleus of the oculomotor nerve lies in the brainstem and has several components serving different extraocular muscles, the *ventral rectus, dorsal rectus, medial rectus, inferior oblique,* and *levator palpebrae superioris muscles.* The nerve also carries parasympathetic fibers originating from the Edinger-Westphal nucleus, which lies near the other nuclei of the oculomotor nerve, and serves the *sphincter pupillae* and *ciliary muscles.* The oculomotor nerve thus contains efferent

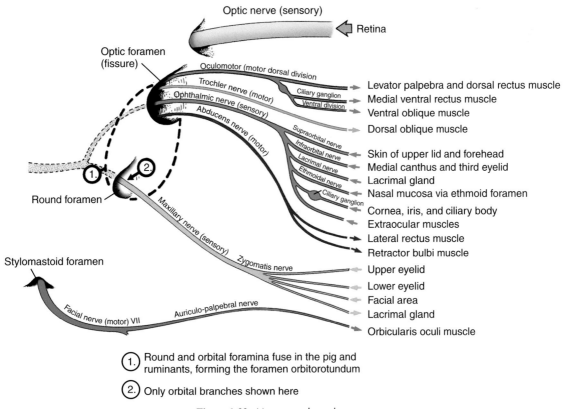

Figure 1-22. Nerve supply to the eye.

motor fibers to the striated extraocular muscles, of mesodermal origin, and parasympathetic fibers to the smooth muscles of the iris and ciliary body, of neuroectodermal origin.

The oculomotor nerve leaves the brainstem on its ventromedial surface (see Figure 1-16), and passes ventral to the optic tracts, through the cavernous sinus, and enters the orbit via the *orbital fissure (foramen orbitorotundum* in cattle, sheep, and pigs). In the orbit, the nerve divides into dorsal and ventral rami. A branch from the ventral ramus passes to the *ciliary ganglion*, where the preganglionic parasympathetic fibers synapse. For more details on the fibers leaving the ciliary ganglion, see Figures 1-23 and 1-24.

Trochlear Nerve (Cranial Nerve IV)

The trochlear nerve leaves the brainstem on the dorsal surface and runs lateral to the tentorium cerebelli to the orbital fissure. It passes through the fissure with the oculomotor nerve and the ophthalmic branch of the trigeminal nerve. The trochlear nerve innervates the *dorsal oblique muscle* only.

Trigeminal Nerve (Cranial Nerve V)

The sensory branches of the trigeminal nerve receive the majority of the input from the orbit and periocular area. The nerve has both motor and sensory roots (see Figure 1-16), which pass in a common sheath through the *petrous temporal bone* to the *trigeminal ganglion*. The three branches of the nerve—*ophthalmic, maxillary,* and *mandibular*—arise from the *trigeminal ganglion*. The ophthalmic nerve leaves the cranial cavity via the orbital fissure, and the maxillary nerve via the round foramen (see Figure 1-22).

Once in the orbit, the ophthalmic nerve divides into *supraorbital (frontal), lacrimal,* and *nasociliary nerves*. The supraorbital nerve is sensory to the middle of the upper eyelid and adjacent skin (Figure 1-25). In horses, cattle, sheep, and pigs, the nerve reaches the upper lid via the *supraorbital foramen,* but in dogs and cats, it passes beneath the orbital ligament.

The *lacrimal nerve* supplies the lacrimal gland. The nasociliary nerve, the major continuation of the ophthalmic nerve in the orbit, gives rise to the *ethmoidal* and *infratrochlear nerves*. The ethmoidal nerve passes through the *ethmoidal foramen* to supply the mucous membranes of the nasal cavity. The infratrochlear nerve passes beneath the trochlear, penetrates the *septum orbitale*, and innervates the medial canthus, third eyelid, and adjacent lacrimal system (see Figure 1-25). Within the orbit, the nasociliary nerve gives off the *long ciliary nerve,* which enters the globe near the optic nerve to provide sensory innervation to the globe itself.

The *maxillary nerve* passes through the round foramen and via the *alar canal* to the *pterygopalatine fossa*. It gives rise to the *zygomatic nerve,* which divides into *zygomaticotemporal* and *zygomaticofacial* branches within the orbit. The zygomaticotemporal branch supplies sensory innervation to the lateral upper lid and rostral temporal area. The zygomaticofacial branch emerges from the periorbita ventral to the lateral canthus and supplies the lateral lower lid and surrounding skin. Postganglionic sympathetic fibers from the *cranial cervical ganglion* may also be distributed to the orbit via the branches of the maxillary nerve, which has no other branches of ophthalmic significance.

Abducent Nerve (Cranial Nerve VI)

The abducent nerve leaves the ventral surface of the medulla oblongata (see Figure 1-16) and passes through the wall of the cavernous sinus, forward via the orbital fissure (see Figure 1-22), to enter the orbit and supply the *retractor bulbi* and *lateral rectus muscles.*

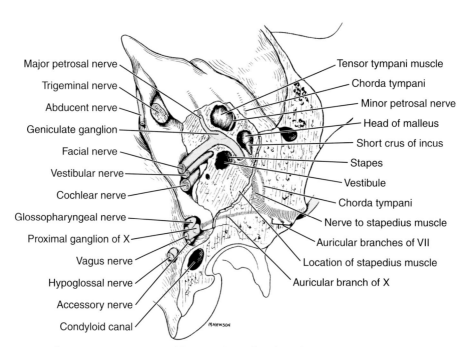

Figure 1-23. The canine petrous temporal bone, sculptured to show the path of the facial nerve, dorsal aspect. (Modified from Evans HE [1993]: Miller's Anatomy of the Dog, 3rd ed. Saunders, Philadelphia. © Cornell University 1964.)

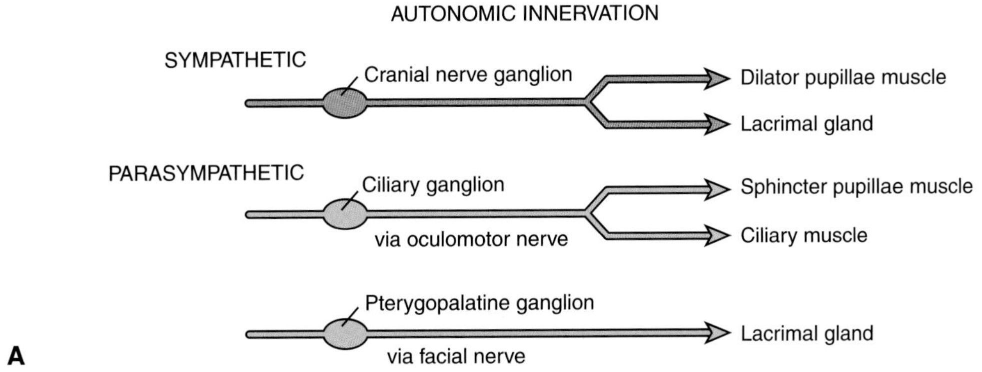

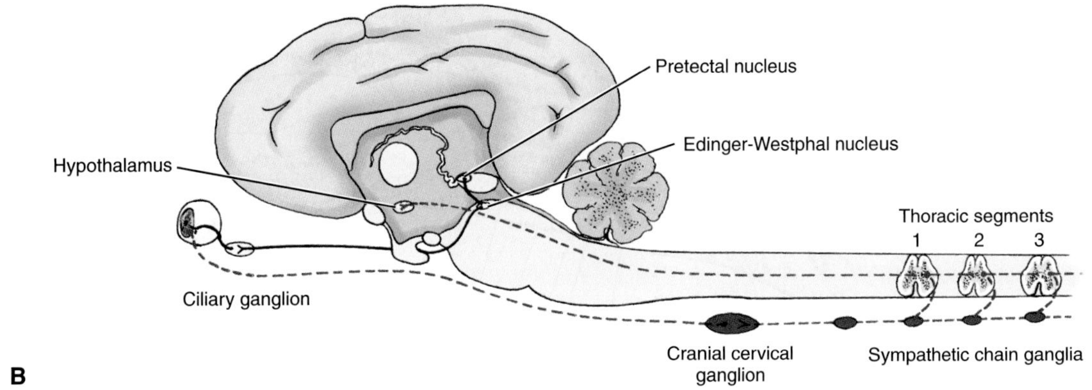

AUTONOMIC INNERVATION

Figure 1-24. A, Autonomic innervation of the eye. **B,** The motor pathways to the iris: parasympathetic constrictor and sympathetic dilator. (**B** modified from Hoerlein BF [1978]: Canine Neurology, 3rd ed. Saunders, Philadelphia.)

Facial Nerve (Cranial Nerve VII)

The mixed facial nerve contains somatic motor and parasympathetic fibers, innervating the *orbicularis oculi* and *retractor anguli muscles* and the *lacrimal gland*. Cell bodies of the motor fibers are found in the *facial nucleus* in the medulla oblongata. The parasympathetic cell bodies are located in the *rostral salivatory nucleus* in the medulla. The nerve leaves the brainstem lateral to the origin of the abducent nerve (see Figure 1-16) and, with the *vestibulocochlear nerve,* enters the *petrous temporal bone* near the acoustic meatus (see Figure 1-23), a point of clinical significance to be discussed later with hemifacial spasm (see Chapter 16). The facial nerve enters the facial canal of the temporal bone, where the *geniculate ganglion* is situated.

From the ganglion arises the *major petrosal nerve.* Joined by the *deep petrosal (sympathetic) nerve,* the *nerve of the pterygoid canal* is formed and passes via the pterygoid canal to the *pterygopalatine fossa,* ending as the *pterygopalatine ganglion.* The parasympathetic fibers synapse here, and some pass to the lacrimal gland.

The facial nerve passes from the geniculate ganglion and emerges from the *stylomastoid foramen* to give numerous branches. The facial trunk terminates as the *auriculopalpebral nerve,* which crosses the temporal region and *zygomatic arch* (see Figure 1-25). The *palpebral branch* supplies the *orbicularis oculi* and *retractor anguli oculi muscles.*

Autonomic Innervation

Action of the Ocular Muscles with Autonomic Innervation (Table 1-1)

The *pupillary dilator and sphincter muscles* are antagonistic to each other and control the size of the pupil. As one muscle contracts, the other relaxes. If either muscle fails to function, the effects of the remaining muscle predominate; for example, paralysis of the dilator muscle alone results in a small pupil *(miosis)* because of the unbalanced action of the sphincter muscle.

The *ciliary muscle* varies in size and orientation among species but in general is composed of one set of smooth muscle fibers arranged so as control tension on the lens zonules and the refractive power of the lens and another set that controls the relative width of the iridocorneal angle, through which aqueous humor exits the eye. *Müller's muscle* elevates the upper eyelid together with the *levator palpebrae superioris muscle.* If either muscle is defective or denervated, the upper eyelid droops *(ptosis).*

Table 1-1 | **Actions of the Ocular Muscles with Autonomic Innervation**

SYMPATHETIC	PARASYMPATHETIC
M. dilator pupillae	M. sphincter pupillae
Müller's muscle	Ciliary muscle

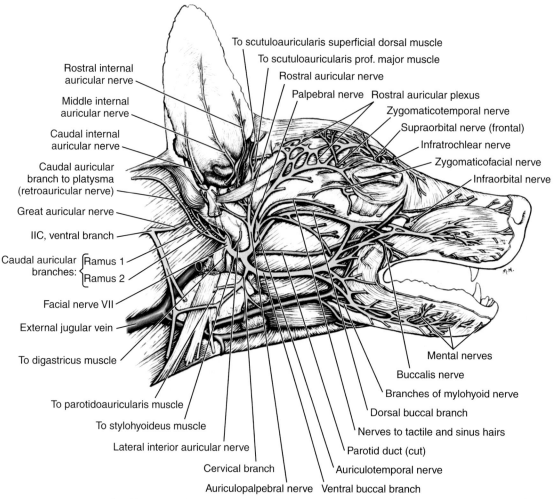

Figure 1-25. Superficial branches of the facial and trigeminal nerves in the dog, lateral aspect. (Modified from Evans HE [1993]: Miller's Anatomy of the Dog, 3rd ed. Saunders, Philadelphia. © Cornell University 1964.)

Parasympathetic Supply

Parasympathetic fibers arise from the Edinger-Westphal nucleus of the oculomotor nerve and pass via the nerve to synapse in the ciliary ganglion (see Figures 1-24 and 1-26).

Other fibers that pass into the ciliary ganglion but do not synapse in it are as follows:

• Postganglionic sympathetic fibers from the cranial cervical ganglion
• Sensory fibers from the ophthalmic branch of the trigeminal nerve (V)

Sympathetic Supply

Sympathetic fibers from the brain pass down the cervical spinal cord and leave via spinal nerves of segments T1 and T2 (see Figures 1-24 and 1-26). The fibers leave the nerves, pass to the sympathetic trunk, and pass cranially with it, in its common sheath with the vagus nerve. The sympathetic trunk terminates cranially at the *cranial cervical ganglion,* where many of the fibers synapse. Postganglionic fibers pass via a variety of pathways to the pupillary dilator muscle and to Müller's muscle.

OCULAR REFLEXES

All ocular reflexes and responses may be thought of as having five parts: (1) a receptor, (2) an afferent neuron, (3) interneuronal connections, (4) an efferent neuron, and (5) an effector. Knowledge of the pathways involved in each of the reflexes and responses is invaluable for the localization of neuroophthalmic lesions. Table 1-2 summarizes these reflexes and responses.

Pupillary Light Reflex (See Figures 1-24 and 1-27)

Constriction of the pupil on the same *(ipsilateral)* side as the stimulus is termed the *direct pupillary reflex,* whereas pupillary constriction on the opposite *(contralateral)* side is called the *consensual light reflex.* In order to obtain reliable reflexes, a bright penlight or transilluminator must be used. Both direct and consensual responses are present in normal animals, although considerable differences exist in the speed of the reflexes between small and large animal species.

Palpebral/Corneal Reflex

The palpebral/corneal reflex is elicited by touching either the periocular skin (palpebral) or the cornea (corneal). This reflex

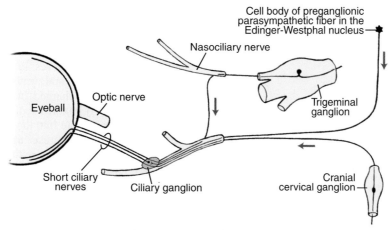

Figure 1-26. Autonomic innervation of the eye. (Modified from Getty R [1975]: Sisson and Grossman's The Anatomy of the Domestic Animals, 5th ed. Saunders, Philadelphia.)

Table 1-2 | **Neuroophthalmic Reflexes and Responses**

REFLEX	STIMULUS	RECEPTOR	AFFERENT NEURON	INTERNEURON	EFFERENT NEURON	EFFECTOR	RESPONSE
PLR	Light	Photoreceptors	II	Subcortical	III	Iris Sphincter	Constrict pupil
Menace response	Hand motion	Photoreceptors	II	Cortical Cerebellum	VII	OOM	Blink
					VI	RBM	Retract globe
					XI	BCM	Turn head/neck
Dazzle	Bright light	Photoreceptors	II	Subcortical	VII	OOM	Blink
Palpebral	Touch lids	Touch receptors skin	V (Ophth)	Subcortical	VII	OOM	Blink
Corneal	Touch cornea	Touch receptors cornea	V (Ophth)	Subcortical	VII	OOM	Blink
					VI	RBM	Retract globe
Doll's eye (VOR)	Head motion	Semicircular canals	VIII	Subcortical Cerebellum	III	Extraocular muscles	Maintain line of sight

BCM, Brachiocephalic muscles; *OOM,* orbicularis oculi muscle; *PLR,* pupillary light reflex; *RBM,* retractor bulbi muscles; *VOR,* vestibuloocular reflex.

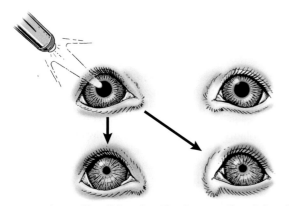

Figure 1-27. The pupillary light reflex. The direct pupillary light reflex is the response shown by the eye being illuminated. The consensual pupillary light reflex is the response shown by the contralateral eye, which is not being illuminated.

is important to protecting the eye, and interference with it (e.g., facial paralysis, trigeminal palsy, local anesthesia) often results in severe ocular damage. Closure of the lids of the stimulated eye is referred to as the *direct corneal reflex,* and closure of the contralateral lids is termed the *consensual corneal reflex.* In normal animals, the direct reflex is typically more pronounced than the consensual reflex.

Menace Response

The menace response is a learned response rather than a true reflex, and as such, it may be absent in normal young, naïve, or stoic animals. Therefore lack of this response in such animals should not be taken as definitive proof that they are blind. The stimulus is hand movement across the animal's visual field, and care must be taken to prevent air currents from stimulating a corneal or palpebral reflex and causing a false-positive response. Motion parallel to the ocular surface (as opposed to directly toward the eye) or application of the stimulus behind a sheet of glass or plastic may prevent air currents from stimulating the corneal reflex and causing a false-positive response. Such false-positive and false-negative responses are often misinterpreted by owners as evidence of sight or blindness in an animal.

PHYSIOLOGY OF THE AQUEOUS

Aqueous humor fills the *aqueous compartment,* which consists of the *anterior chamber* between the iris and cornea, and the *posterior chamber,* between the posterior iris surface and the anterior lens surface. The posterior chamber should not be confused with the *vitreous compartment,* which is located posterior to the lens (Figure 1-28).

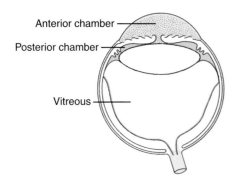

Figure 1-28. The chambers of the eye. The aqueous compartment is subdivided into two chambers by the iris diaphragm. The anterior chamber is anterior to the plane of the iris and pupil (blue), whereas the posterior chamber (green) is posterior to the iris-pupil plane but anterior to the vitreous (white). The retina and optic nerve are in yellow. (Modified from Fine S, Yanoff M [1972]: Ocular Histology: A Text and Atlas. Harper & Row, New York.)

Formation and Composition

In order to maintain the optical clarity of the eye, a series of *blood-ocular barriers* are present in the normal eye. The *blood-aqueous barrier* reduces aqueous humor protein concentrations to about 0.5% of plasma concentrations and also prevents many substances, including drugs, from entering the aqueous. Most large molecules, including proteins, are unable to pass through or between cells in the two layers of the ciliary epithelium overlying the ciliary processes because of tight intercellular junctions between cells. Similarly, a *blood-retinal barrier* formed by the retinal capillary endothelial cells and their basement membrane also limits passage of substances into the retina so as to prevent distortion of the photoreceptors. The exact anatomic location of the barrier, however, is probably different for different substances (e.g., capillary endothelial cells, endothelial basement membrane, or intercellular junctions). Inflammation and certain diseases frequently disrupt the blood-ocular barrier and allow higher amounts of proteins, including immunoglobulins and fibrinogen, to enter the eye.

Aqueous is produced in the *ciliary body,* by *passive (diffusion and ultrafiltration)* and *active (selective transport against a concentration gradient) processes.* Fluid from ciliary capillaries passes into the stroma of the *ciliary processes,* through the ciliary epithelium, and into the posterior chamber. An *energy-dependent transport mechanism* similar to that in the renal epithelium is present in the ciliary body and results in higher concentrations of certain substances (e.g., ascorbic acid) in the aqueous than in the plasma. Sodium and chloride ions are actively pumped into the aqueous and draw water passively along a concentration gradient. Na-K–activated ATPase is present in the inner layer of the unpigmented ciliary epithelium and may be associated with the "sodium pump" that probably accounts for the majority of actively formed aqueous.

Aqueous humor is also produced via the enzyme *carbonic anhydrase,* which catalyzes the formation of carbonic acid from carbon dioxide and water. Carbonic acid dissociates, allowing negatively charged bicarbonate ions to pass to the aqueous. Positively charged sodium ions, and eventually water, then follow bicarbonate into the posterior chamber. Drugs that inhibit carbonic anhydrase therefore result in decreased aqueous production and a reduction in intraocular pressure (IOP; see later). Aqueous carries nutrients for the tissues it bathes (i.e., iris, cornea) and receives constant contributions of waste products of metabolism. Thus the composition changes as it passes from the ciliary body to the drainage angle.

Aqueous may then leave the eye via several routes. In the *conventional* or *traditional outflow route,* aqueous humor passes through the pupil into the anterior chamber, and from there it enters the *trabecular meshwork* in the *drainage (iridocorneal) angle,* the blood-free venous angular aqueous plexus, and eventually the systemic venous circulation through a plexus of small veins in the sclera, the *scleral venous plexus.* Contraction of smooth muscle fibers of the ciliary muscle that insert into the trabecular meshwork are probably capable of increasing drainage of aqueous from the eye by increasing the size of the spaces in the trabecular meshwork. The vast majority of aqueous humor leaves the eye via the traditional outflow route.

An alternative route of drainage—the *uveoscleral route*—normally accounts for about 3% to 15% of aqueous outflow in most species, and probably more in the horse. Aqueous passes through the ciliary body and choroid via the supraciliary and suprachoroidal spaces, and from there it passes through the sclera into the orbit. Outflow via this route may be substantially increased in certain disease states and in response to some antiglaucoma drugs, such as the prostaglandin derivatives.

Pressure Dynamics

Equilibrium between formation (production) and drainage (outflow) of aqueous results in a relatively constant *intraocular pressure* (IOP) (Table 1-3). IOP is affected by factors such as age, species, mean arterial pressure, central venous pressure, blood osmolality, and episcleral venous pressure. IOP typically exceeds the pressure in the draining venous system (the episcleral veins) because aqueous humor is actively produced and the trabecular meshwork slows its departure (provides *resistance*) from the eye. The ease with which aqueous humor leaves the eye is called the *facility of outflow (C).* The various

Table 1-3 | **Aqueous Humor Statistics**

SPECIES	RATE OF FORMATION (μL/min)	FACILITY OF OUTFLOW (μL/min/mm Hg)	UVEOSCLERAL OUTFLOW (%)	EPISCLERAL VENOUS PRESSURE (mm Hg)
Dog	2.5	0.25 (normal) 0.13 (glaucoma)	15 (normal) 3 (glaucoma)	10-12
Cat	15.0	0.19	3	8
Rabbit	4.0	0.23	13-25	9
Human	2.0	0.28 (normal) 0.18 (glaucoma)	4-14	5-15

Modified from Gum G (1991): Physiology of the eye, in Gelatt KN (editor): Veterinary Ophthalmology, 2nd ed. Lea & Febiger, Philadelphia.

features of IOP dynamics may be related to each other with the following equation:

$$IOP = \frac{\text{Aqueous secretion}}{\text{Outflow facility}} + \text{Episcleral venous pressure}$$

or

$$P_o = (F/C) + P_e$$

where IOP (P_o) is expressed in mm Hg, F is the rate of aqueous formation in μL/min, C is the facility of aqueous outflow in μL/min/mm Hg via both the conventional and uveoscleral outflow routes, and P_e is the episcleral venous pressure in mm Hg. These relationships make it clear that there are multiple avenues for decreasing IOP, including decreasing aqueous humor secretion, increasing conventional or uveoscleral outflow, and potentially lowering episcleral venous pressure. They also suggest that (1) IOP can be reduced only to 8 to 9 mm Hg (episcleral venous pressure) by methods that improve outflow via the conventional pathways but that (2) in theory, improving outflow via the uveoscleral pathway can achieve very low IOPs because this route drains into the orbit, which has a pressure of only 1 to 3 mm Hg.

BIBLIOGRAPHY

Budras KD, et al. (2002): Anatomy of the Dog: An Illustrated Text. Schlütersche, Hannover, Germany.

Duke-Elder S (1958, 1968): System of Ophthalmology: Vol. 1: The Eye in Evolution, and Vol. IV: Physiology of the Eye and of Vision. Henry Kimpton, London, pp. 605-706.

Evans HE (1993): Miller's Anatomy of the Dog, 3rd ed. Saunders, Philadelphia.

Jacobs GH (1993): The distribution and nature of color vision among the mammals. Biol Rev 68:413.

Kaufman PL, Alm A (2003): Adler's Physiology of the Eye, 10th ed. Mosby, St. Louis.

Miller PE, Murphy CJ (1995): Vision in dogs. J Am Vet Med Assoc 207:1623.

Miller PE, Murphy CJ (2005): Equine vision: normal and abnormal, in Gilger BC (editor): Equine Ophthalmology. Saunders, St. Louis, pp. 371-408.

Neitz J, et al. (1989): Color vision in the dog. Vis Neurosci 3:119.

Peichl L (1992): Topography of ganglion cells in the dog and wolf retina. J Comp Neurol 324:603.

Prince JH, et al. (1960): Anatomy and Histology of the Eye and Orbit of Domestic Animals. Charles C. Thomas, Springfield, IL.

Samuelson D, et al. (1989): Morphologic features of the aqueous humor drainage pathways in horses. Am J Vet Res 50:720.

Walls GL (1963): The Vertebrate Eye and Its Adaptive Radiation. Hafner, New York.

DEVELOPMENT AND CONGENITAL ABNORMALITIES*

Ron Ofri

DEVELOPMENT
Formation of Optic Primordia

Broadly speaking, the embryonic and fetal development of the eye occurs in three stages:

- *Embryogenesis:* Segregation of the primary layers of the developing embryo. The period begins with fertilization and ends with differentiation of the primary germ layers.
- *Organogenesis:* Separation into the general pattern of various organs.
- *Differentiation:* Detailed development of the characteristic structure of each organ.

It is assumed that the embryonic development of the eye is similar in sequence for all mammalian species and that inter-species differences pertain mostly to the duration of gestation and the age of the various anatomic end points—for example, regression of embryonic vasculature or eyelid opening.

The *optic primordia* (rudimentary eye) develops from that portion of the embryo that later forms the anterior part of the central nervous system (CNS). The first step in the *embryogenesis* of the future eye takes place at the embryonic plate stage, when the ectoderm invaginates along the posterior-anterior axis to form the *neural groove.* The two neural lips of the groove subsequently fuse, thus turning the groove into the *neural tube* (Figures 2-1 and 2-2). At the site of fusion, between the ectoderm and the neuroepithelium (the epithelium of the neural tube), neuroepithelial cells proliferate to form the *neural crest* cells and migrate sideways into the paraxial and lateral mesoderm. These neural crest cells mix with mesodermal cells and form the secondary mesenchyme; this secondary mesenchyme forms the main mesodermal structures of the eye. Therefore the eye develops from the neural ectoderm, neural crest, and surface ectoderm, with minor contributions from the mesoderm.

The anterior end of the neural tube enlarges and bends down to form the primordia of the CNS. On its outer surface, on both sides, appear two small pits called the *optic grooves* or *optic pits.* These pits, which appear on day 13 of gestation in the dog, are the anlage of the eyes (see Figure 2-2, *G*).

With the closure of the anterior end of the neural tube, intratubular fluid accumulates and its pressure causes the evagination of the optic grooves and their transformation into the two *optic vesicles* (Figures 2-3 and 2-4). This marks the beginning of *organogenesis.* In the dog this event occurs on the fifteenth day of gestation. The lumen of the neural tube remains connected to the cavities of the optic vesicles by two *optic stalks* (see Figure 2-4, *D*). Under the pressure of the intratubular (intraventricular) fluid, the optic vesicles continue to enlarge and bulge, eventually coming in contact with the surface ectoderm. At the site of contact with the optic vesicle the surface ectoderm thickens and forms the *lens placode* (Figures 2-3; 2-4, *C*; and 2-5). The contact of the optic vesicle with the surface ectoderm serves as an induction for the optic vesicle to start invaginating, thus forming the double-layered *optic cup* (see Figures 2-3 and 2-4, *E* and *F*).

The invagination of the vesicle progresses from inferior to superior but is not completed on the ventral side of the optic cup, where a fissure, called the *embryonic optic fissure,* remains. The double layers of the optic cup are aligned on both sides of the fissure, which extends posteriorly under the optic stalk. This fissure allows the secondary mesenchyme present around the cup to penetrate into the cavity of the optic cup to form the *hyaloid vascular system* (twenty-fifth day of gestation in the dog) (see Figure 2-4, *G* and *H*). This fissure gradually closes leaving a small aperture at the anterior end of the optic stalk, through which the *hyaloid artery* passes (Figure 2-6). The hyaloid artery supplies the inner layers of the optic cup and developing lens vesicle. The two lips of the optic fissure fuse anteriorly to the optic stalk. The fusion process progresses anteriorly and posteriorly, eventually causing closure of the optic cup and allowing intraocular pressure to build up (see Figure 2-6).

The lens placode thickens to become the *lens vesicle.* Following the invagination of the optic vesicle, the lens vesicle finds itself embedded inside the cavity of the cup (see Figure 2-4, *F* and *H*). Anteriorly, the hyaloid artery gives branches, the *tunica vasculosa lentis,* which cover the posterior and lateral faces of the lens. This vascular network supplies the metabolic requirements of the lens during development. The hyaloid vascular system disappears at advanced stages of the development or during the postnatal period. In dogs remnants of the hyaloid system might remain visible until the fourth postnatal

*The author wishes to acknowledge the contribution of Dr. Robert Barishak, and to thank him for his input throughout the years and to this chapter.

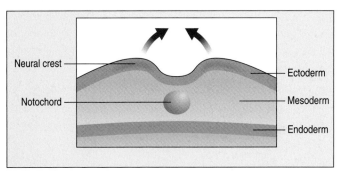

Figure 2-1. Developing embryo at the start of neural tube formation. (From Yanoff M, Duker J [2004]: Ophthalmology, 2nd ed. Mosby, St. Louis.)

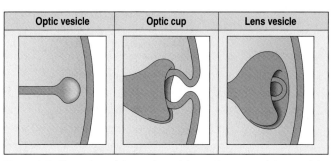

Figure 2-3. Formation of the optic vesicle, optic cup, and lens vesicle. (From Yanoff M, Duker J [2004]: Ophthalmology, 2nd ed. Mosby, St. Louis.)

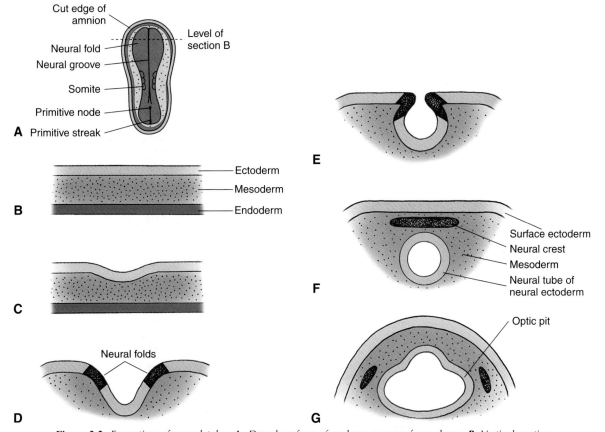

Figure 2-2. Formation of neural tube. **A,** Dorsal surface of embryo as seen from above. **B,** Vertical section through three-layered embryonic disc. **C,** Neural groove forms in neural plate area of ectoderm. **D,** Neural groove invaginates and neural folds are formed. **E,** Neural folds continue to grow toward each other. **F,** Neural crest cells separate from ectoderm of neural folds as the folds fuse; neural tube is formed (of neural ectoderm); and surface ectoderm is again continuous. **G,** Evaginations in area of forebrain form the optic pits. (From Remington LA [2005]: Clinical Anatomy of the Visual System, 2nd ed. Butterworth-Heinemann, St. Louis.)

month, whereas in cattle they may persist until 12 months of age. In humans, but not in domestic animals, the caudal portions of the hyaloid artery and vein transform themselves into the central retinal artery and vein.

At this stage of development, organogenesis has been completed and the general structure of the eye has been determined. It is followed by a period of *differentiation* as the specific structures of the eye begin to form. Their development

is reviewed in the following sections, beginning with the posterior parts of the eye and progressing anteriorly.

Retina

The optic cup is lined by two layers of epithelium of neuroectodermal origin (see Figure 2-4, *H*). The inner layer, facing the vitreous, is nonpigmented, but the outer layer, facing the

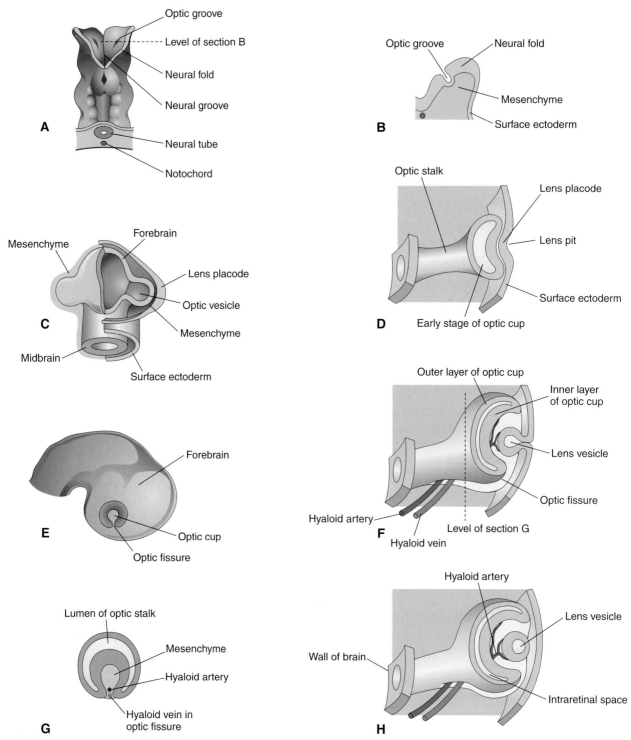

Figure 2-4. Early eye development. **A,** Dorsal view of the cranial end of 22-day embryo, showing the first indication of eye development. **B,** Transverse section through neural fold, showing an optic groove. **C,** Forebrain and its covering layers of mesenchyme and the surface ectoderm from an embryo of about 28 days. **D, F,** and **H,** Sections of the developing eye, illustrating early stage in the development of the optic cup and lens vesicle. **E,** Lateral view of the brain of an embryo at about 32 days, showing the external appearance of the optic cup. **G,** Transverse section through the optic stalk, showing the optic fissure and its contents. (From Remington LA [2005]: Clinical Anatomy of the Visual System, 2nd ed. Butterworth-Heinemann, St. Louis.)

(future) sclera, is pigmented. The anterior rim of the cup will form the anterior uvea (ciliary body and iris), and the posterior part of the cup will form the retina. The two epithelial layers of the optic cup will form the two epithelial layers of the retina and the anterior uvea.

The outer epithelial layer of the posterior optic cup forms the *pigment epithelium of the retina*. The inner epithelial layer forms the *sensory retina* (Figure 2-7). The two layers of the posterior optic cup are separated by the intraretinal space representing the cavity of the optic vesicle, which has gradually

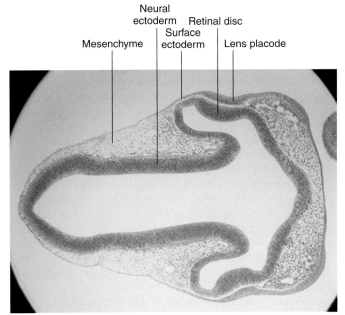

Mesenchyme — Neural ectoderm — Surface ectoderm — Retinal disc — Lens placode

Figure 2-5. Light micrograph of 6-mm pig embryo showing thickening of lens placode. (From Remington LA [2005]: Clinical Anatomy of the Visual System, 2nd ed. Butterworth-Heinemann, St. Louis.)

been obliterated during the invagination of the optic vesicle. Diseases of the posterior segment of the eye cause retinal detachment in this space as the sensory retina separates from the pigment epithelium.

The *common neuroblastic layer,* which is the nuclear portion of the sensory retina, divides into an *outer neuroblastic layer*

and an *inner neuroblastic layer* (see Figure 2-7). These outer and inner neuroblastic layers are separated by the fiber layer of Chievitz. The cells of the outer neuroblastic layer differentiate into *cones* and *rods* externally and *horizontal cells* internally. The cells of the inner neuroblastic layer differentiate into *ganglion cells, amacrine cells, bipolar cells,* and *Müller's cells.* The rods and cones (i.e., the *photoreceptors*) form the *outer retina* and are adjacent to the choroid and sclera (Figure 2-8). The ganglion cell layer, which originated in the inner neuroblastic layer, is called the *inner retina* because it is adjacent to the vitreous. The resulting retina is called an *inverted retina* because the photoreceptors are close to the outer layers of the eye and light must pass through all of the retinal layers to reach the photoreceptors. The reason for this arrangement is to place the photoreceptors next to the choroid, thus giving these cells, which have very high metabolic requirements, their own "private" blood supply.

There is species variation in the degree of retinal development present at birth. In dogs it is possible to record electrophysiologic activity of the photoreceptors during the first postnatal week; signals reach adult amplitude by 5 to 8 weeks of age. Similarly, differentiation of the rod and cone inner and outer segments is evident histologically during the first 8 weeks of life.

Optic Nerve

Axons from the ganglion cells grow toward the optic stalk, thus forming the *nerve fiber layer,* the innermost layer of the retina (see Figures 2-6, *B* and *D*; and 2-8). Axons from throughout the entire retina converge on the optic disc, where they form into bundles collectively known as the *optic nerve* (cranial nerve II)

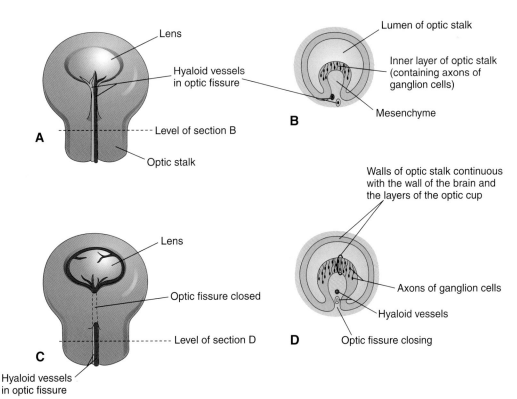

Figure 2-6. Closure of optic fissure. **A** and **C,** Views of inferior surface of optic cup and stalk, showing progressive stages in closure of optic fissure. **B** and **D,** Transverse sections through optic stalk, showing successive stages in closure of optic fissure. Note that the lumen of optic stalk is obliterated gradually. (From Remington LA [2005]: Clinical Anatomy of the Visual System, 2nd ed. Butterworth-Heinemann, St. Louis.)

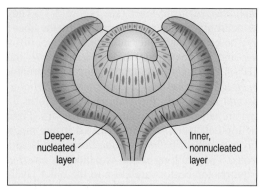

Figure 2-7. The two retinal walls. The inner retinal wall shows two zones—an inner, nonnucleated layer and a deeper, nucleated layer. (From Yanoff M, Duker J [2004]: Ophthalmology, 2nd ed. Mosby, St. Louis.)

(Figure 2-9). The axons of optic nerve extend posteriorly to form the optic chiasm and optic tracts before making their first synapse at the lateral geniculate nucleus.

As the ganglion cell axons collect at the optic disc they displace primitive neuroectodermal cells forward, into the vitreous cavity. These displaced cells form a glial sheath around the hyaloid artery. At the disc, the same cells may form an agglomeration called *Bergmeister's papilla*, which protrudes into the vitreous. The papilla may persist into adult life (especially in ruminants), or it may atrophy, thus forming a depression, known as the *physiologic optic cup*, in the optic disc (Figure 2-10). In newborns this physiologic optic cup may be confused with a coloboma of the optic disc. In patients with glaucoma the physiologic optic cup may enlarge owing to the forces of the increased intraocular pressure on this region of the eye.

Vitreous

The embryonic vitreous consists of the primary, secondary, and tertiary vitreous (Figure 2-11). The *primary vitreous* develops with the hyaloid vasculature (Figure 2-12). It has mesenchymal, neuroectodermal, and ectodermal components. The mesenchymal elements enter posteriorly with the hyaloid vessels, and anteriorly through the space between the anterior rim of the optic cup and the lens vesicle. The ectodermal elements are the fibrils produced by the posterior face of the lens. The primary vitreous also contains neuroectodermal elements, which consist of the fibrils produced by the inner limiting membrane of the retina. The *secondary vitreous* is the "definitive" vitreous that will persist into adulthood. It is denser, is more homogeneous and avascular, and is laid down around the primary vitreous (see Figures 2-11, *B*, and 2-13). It is also secreted by the inner limiting membrane of the retina. The *tertiary vitreous* is secreted by the ciliary epithelium. Bundles of fibers extend from the ciliary epithelium toward the lens equator, covering the secondary vitreous anteriorly (see Figure 2-11, *C*). In the adult they persist as *lens zonules* (suspensory ligament of the lens).

Lens

As noted earlier, thickening of the lens placode (on the seventeenth day of gestation in the dog) occurs as a result of induction by the optic vesicle. The placode then invaginates, and by day 25 it forms the *lens vesicle* (see Figures 2-3 and 2-4, *D*, *F*, and *H*). This vesicle is lined by surface ectodermal cells, the apex of which is directed toward the center of the lens vesicle cavity (Figures 2-14 and 2-15). The base of the cells forms the primitive lens capsule. The anterior cells of the lens

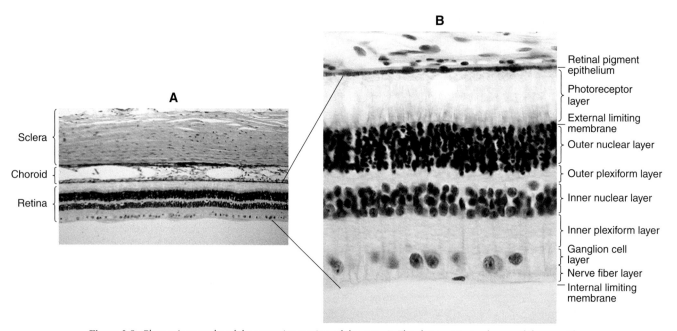

Figure 2-8. Photomicrographs of the posterior section of the eye. **A,** The three posterior layers of the eye. The sclera is the outermost layer, whereas the retina faces the vitreous. **B,** An enlargement of the 10 layers of the retina. The retinal pigment epithelium and the photoreceptors are the outermost layer of the retina, facing the choroid. The ganglion cell layer and nerve fiber layer are the innermost layers of the retina, facing the vitreous. (From Remington LA [2005]: Clinical Anatomy of the Visual System, 2nd ed. Butterworth-Heinemann, St Louis.)

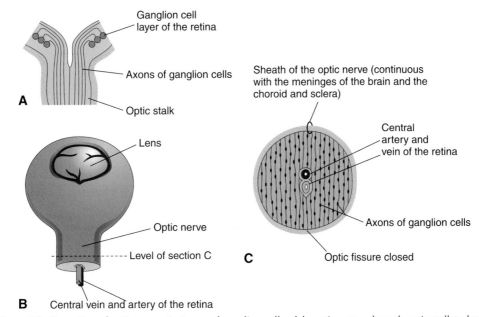

Figure 2-9. Formation of optic nerve. **A,** Axons of ganglion cells of the retina grow through optic stalk to brain. **B,** Transverse section through the optic stalk, showing the formation of the optic nerve. The optic nerve is formed after closure of the optic fissure (this stage follows the stage shown in Figure 2-6, *C*). **C,** The lumen of the optic stalk is obliterated as axons of ganglion cells accumulate in the inner layer of the stalk. (From Remington LA [2005]: Clinical Anatomy of the Visual System, 2nd ed. Butterworth-Heinemann, St. Louis.)

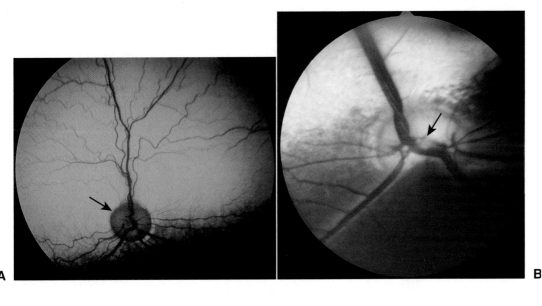

Figure 2-10. Optic nerve heads of a dog **(A)** and a sheep **(B)**. The dark spot in the center of the canine optic nerve head is the physiologic optic cup *(arrow)*. The pink tuft in the center of the sheep optic nerve head is the ovine Bergmeister's papilla *(arrow)*. (Courtesy University of California, Davis, Veterinary Ophthalmology Service Collection.)

vesicle remain cuboidal, but the posterior cells elongate, become columnar, and form the *primary lens fibers* (Figure 2-16). These fibers extend anteriorly, thus filling the cavity of the vesicle with lens fibers (see Figures 2-14, *D* and *E*; and 2-16, *C* and *D*). Their nuclei disappear, and these fibers constitute the *embryonal nucleus* of the lens. As a result, the posterior aspect of the adult lens is devoid of cells and is composed only of a lens capsule. The anterior cuboidal cells, on the other hand, remain as the adult *lens epithelium*.

The junction between the anterior lens epithelium and the primary lens fibers extends along the equator of the lens and forms the *equatorial zone*. Epithelial cells in this area form the *secondary lens fibers*; these fibers extend anteriorly along the lens epithelium and posteriorly along the lens capsule. Secondary lens fibers continue to form throughout

life from those equatorial epithelial cells that maintain their lifelong mitotic activity. Successive layers of fibers are deposited on top of preexisting fibers, like the layers of an onion. As a result the embryonal nucleus is surrounded by the fetal nucleus, which in turn is surrounded by the adult nucleus and cortex (Figure 2-17).

Because none of the lens fibers is quite long enough to reach fully from pole to pole, and because the cells are too thick at the ends for all to meet in a single point, they meet in a Y-shaped structure known as the *lens suture*. The anterior lens suture is an upright Y, and the posterior suture is inverted (Figures 2-16, *F* and *G;* and 2-18).

The *lens capsule* is secreted anteriorly by the anterior lens epithelium. Its formation continues throughout life, and therefore its thickness increases with age. The posterior lens capsule,

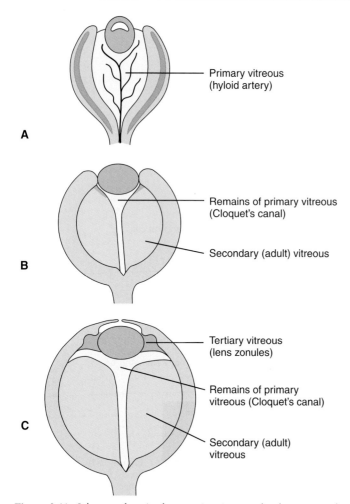

Primary vitreous
(hyloid artery)

Remains of primary vitreous
(Cloquet's canal)

Secondary (adult) vitreous

Tertiary vitreous
(lens zonules)

Remains of primary
vitreous (Cloquet's canal)

Secondary (adult)
vitreous

Figure 2-11. Scheme of main features in vitreous development and regression of hyaloid system, shown in drawings of sagittal sections. **A,** Hyaloid vessels and branches occupy much of the space between lens and neural ectoderm, forming the primary vitreous. **B,** An avascular secondary vitreous of fine fibrillar composition fills the posterior part of the eye. The primary vitreous shown in **A** is condensed into Cloquet's canal as the hyaloid vessels atrophy. **C,** Vessels of hyaloid system atrophy progressively. Zonular fibers (tertiary vitreous) begin to stretch from growing ciliary region toward lens capsule. (Modified from Duke-Elder S [editor] [1963]: System of Ophthalmology. Vol III: Normal and Abnormal Development, Part 1. Embryology. Henry Kimpton, London.)

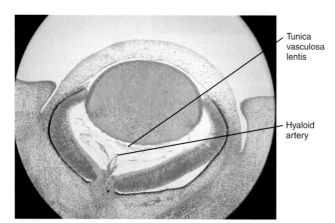

Tunica vasculosa lentis

Hyaloid artery

Figure 2-12. Light micrograph of 25-mm pig embryo showing the hyaloid arterial system filling future vitreal cavity. Vessels are evident extending through the optic stalk, and the vascular network attached to posterior lens is evident. (Modified from Remington LA [2005]: Clinical Anatomy of the Visual System, 2nd ed. Butterworth-Heinemann, St. Louis.)

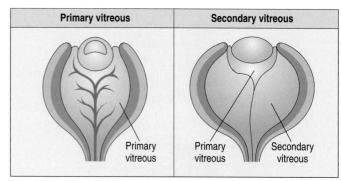

Primary vitreous	Secondary vitreous

Primary vitreous

Primary vitreous

Secondary vitreous

Figure 2-13. Vitreous development. The primary vitreous and hyaloid artery fill the optic cup. The primary vitreous retracts and the hyaloid artery regresses, while the secondary avascular vitreous develops. (From Yanoff M, Duker J [2004]: Ophthalmology, 2nd ed. Mosby, St. Louis.)

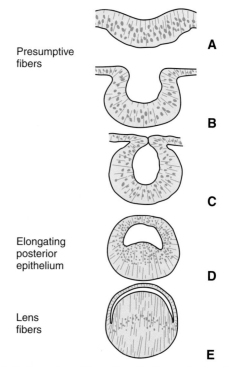

Presumptive fibers

Elongating posterior epithelium

Lens fibers

Figure 2-14. A, Formation of lens placode. **B,** Invagination forming lens vesicle. **C to E,** Development of embryonic nucleus. **C,** Hollow lens vesicle is lined with epithelium. **D,** Posterior cells elongate, becoming primary lens fibers. **E,** Primary lens fibers fill lumen, forming embryonic nucleus. Curved line formed by cell nuclei is called the lens bow. Anterior epithelium remains in place. (From Remington LA [2005]: Clinical Anatomy of the Visual System, 2nd ed. Butterworth-Heinemann, St. Louis.)

which is much thinner, is formed by the basal membrane of the elongating primary lens fibers.

Primitive Vascular System

The hyaloid artery, a branch of the internal ophthalmic artery, enters the optic cup through the embryonal optic fissure (see Figure 2-6, *A*). Its branches continue forward, reach the anterior margin of the optic cup, and anastomose with the *annular vessel* (see Figure 2-6, *C*) formed by the *choriocapillaris*, which is the capillary plexus that surrounds the optic cup. The hyaloid artery is called *vasa hyaloidea propria*; its anterior dividing branches form a net around the lens called the *lateral* and

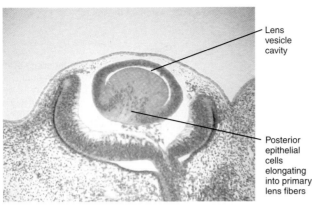

Figure 2-15. Light micrograph of 15-mm pig embryo showing lens vesicle filling with primary lens fibers; lens bow configuration is evident. (Modified from Remington LA [2005]: Clinical Anatomy of the Visual System, 2nd ed. Butterworth-Heinemann, St. Louis.)

Lens vesicle cavity

Posterior epithelial cells elongating into primary lens fibers

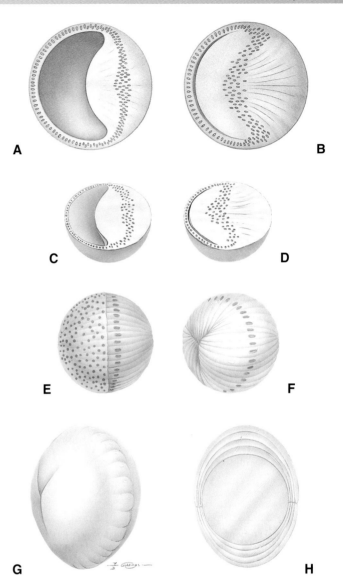

Figure 2-16. Stages of development of the lens. **A,** Elongation and anterior growth of posterior cuboidal epithelial cells to form primary lens fibers. **B,** Elongation of primary lens fibers to fill the cavity in the lens vesicle, and formation of the lens bow of cuboidal cell nuclei. **C** and **D,** Secondary lens fibers proliferate from the equatorial region of the lens, covering the primary lens fibers and scattered cuboidal cell nuclei. **E,** The adult lens. **F** and **G,** Appearance of the Y sutures. **H,** New layers of secondary lens fibers are laid down around the central primary lens fibers. Growth continues throughout life. (**A** modified from Severin GA [2000]: Severin's Veterinary Ophthalmology Notes, 3rd ed. Severin, Ft. Collins, CO.)

posterior tunica vasculosa lentis (Figure 2-19). The *anterior tunica vasculosa lentis* is formed by branches from the annular vessel. These tunicas are responsible for vascular supply to the lens during embryonic development. During the last stages of embryologic development or soon after birth, as the aqueous humor takes over this metabolic function, the hyaloid vasculature atrophies, regresses, and is replaced by the *pupillary membrane* (see also next section, Ciliary Body and Iris).

The mesenchyme around the optic cup forms the *choroid,* which surrounds the choriocapillaris. The *nasal* and *temporal long posterior ciliary arteries* branch off the ophthalmic artery and advance forward in the horizontal plane through the choroid to supply the future ciliary body. At the level of the ciliary body they anastomose to form the *major vascular circle of the iris.* Posteriorly, the *short ciliary arteries* arrange themselves around the entrance of the optic nerve into the globe (Figure 2-20). The vessels form an anastomosing plexus, called the *Haller-Zinn vascular circle,* which plays a role in the vascular supply of the optic nerve head.

Ciliary Body and Iris

The adult *ciliary body* is lined with two layers of epithelium of neuroectodermal origin. The inner layer, close to the vitreous, is unpigmented. This layer is the anterior extension of the sensory neuroretina, though it contains no neural elements. The outer layer is pigmented and is the anterior continuation of the retinal pigment epithelium. The ciliary epithelium forms folds called *ciliary processes* (Figure 2-21). These processes are the production site of the aqueous humor; they also serve as the anchoring site of the lens zonules, which suspend the lens in the eye. The underlying *ciliary muscle* and stroma of the ciliary body originate from the neural crest–derived secondary mesenchyme; the power of the muscle's contraction and relaxation is transferred through the ciliary processes and zonules to the lens, changing its refraction and the focusing of the eye.

The anterior rim of the optic cup forms the *iris,* which has two pigmented epithelial layers on its posterior face. These epithelial layers are continuous with the two layers of the epithelium of the ciliary body. The sphincter and dilator smooth muscles of the mammalian iris, which control the constriction and dilation of the pupil through their antagonistic actions, are derived from the neuroectoderm of the anterior rim of the optic cup. The iris stroma originates from the neural crest–derived secondary mesenchyme (see Figure 2-21). This mesenchyme continues to grow over the anterior part of the lens, covering the hole that will be the future pupil with a membrana pupillaris, which replaces the anterior tunica vasculosa lentis at the same location (see Figures 2-19 and 2-22). This membrane contains branches from the major arterial circle of the iris that form a vascular net over the iris and the pupil. However, strands of the membrana pupillaris may remain attached to the anterior surface of the iris. These strands, known as *persistent pupillary membranes,* are inherited as a homozygous recessive trait in the basenji.

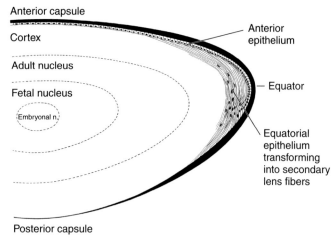

Figure 2-17. Adult lens showing the successive layers of the lens that are laid around the embryonal nucleus throughout life. (From Remington LA [2005]: Clinical Anatomy of the Visual System, 2nd ed. Butterworth-Heinemann, St. Louis.)

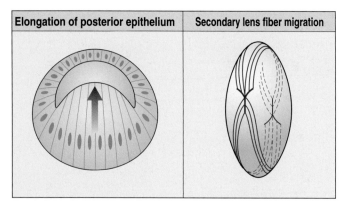

Figure 2-18. Lens embryogenesis. *Left,* Elongation of the posterior epithelium results in obliteration of the lens lumen. *Right,* Secondary lens fiber migration leads to the formation of the Y sutures. (From Yanoff M, Duker J [2004]: Ophthalmology, 2nd ed. Mosby, St. Louis.)

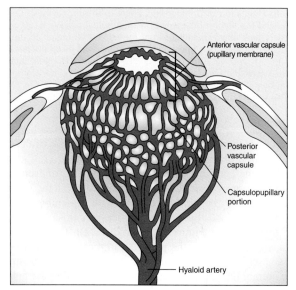

Figure 2-19. Hyaloid vasculature and primary vitreous during embryologic ocular development. (From Yanoff M, Duker J [2004]: Ophthalmology, 2nd ed. Mosby, St. Louis.)

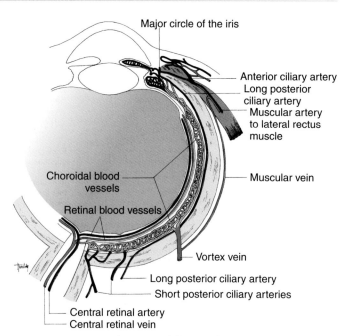

Figure 2-20. Horizontal section of the eye showing ciliary circulation. (From Remington LA [2005]: Clinical Anatomy of the Visual System, 2nd ed. Butterworth-Heinemann, St. Louis.)

Cornea and Anterior Chamber

The outer *corneal epithelium* derives from the surface ectoderm, but the inner layers, which include the *corneal stroma* and *corneal endothelium,* derive from the secondary mesenchyme. *Descemet's membrane* is secreted by the endothelial cells (see Figure 2-22). Further ingrowth of secondary mesenchyme occurs between the epithelium and endothelium, forming the corneal stroma.

Between the cornea and the lens two spaces develop: the *posterior chamber* between the iris and the lens, and the *anterior chamber* between the iris and the cornea (Figure 2-23). After the regression of the pupillary membrane, aqueous may flow from the posterior chamber to the anterior chamber through the pupil.

Sclera and Extraocular Muscles

Neural crest–derived mesenchyme surrounds the optic cup and forms two layers. The inner layer, which is adjacent to the retina, is the *choroid,* and the outer layer is the *sclera.* Condensation of the sclera begins anteriorly, near the ciliary body, and proceeds posteriorly to the optic nerve, where it is continuous with the dura mater of the optic nerve. Extraocular muscles form in the neural crest–derived secondary mesenchyme of the orbit.

Eyelids and Third Eyelid

The lower eyelid and the third eyelid are formed by the maxillary process. The upper eyelid is formed by the paraxial mesoderm. During development the upper and lower eyelids are fused (Figure 2-24). With time, these fused eyelids separate, although the age at which separation occurs varies among species. In horses, cattle, sheep, and pigs, lids open at 7 to 10 days postpartum. During the formation of the eyelids their inner surface

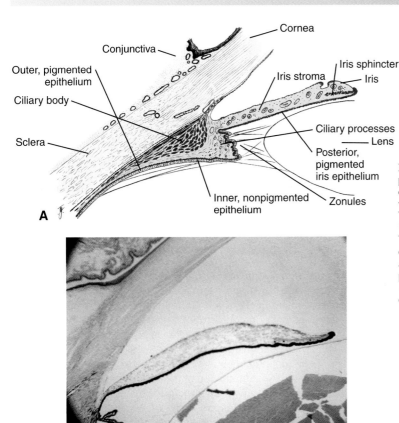

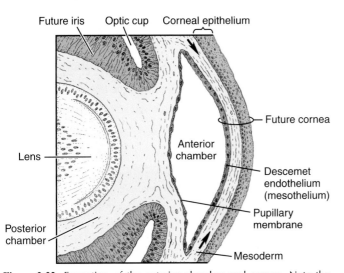

Figure 2-21. A diagram **(A)** and a photomicrograph **(B)** of the periphery of the anterior segment of the eye. The nonpigmented epithelium is the innermost layer of the ciliary body, facing the vitreous, and is continuous with the sensory retina (not shown). The pigmented epithelium is the outer layer, facing the sclera, and is continuous with the retinal pigment epithelium (not shown). These two epithelial layers continue anteriorly as the pigmented epithelium on the posterior aspect of the iris. The zonules (which are the tertiary vitreous) suspend the lens from the ciliary processes, and their remnants can be seen in **B.** (Modified from Remington LA [2005]: Clinical Anatomy of the Visual System, 2nd ed. Butterworth-Heinemann, St. Louis.)

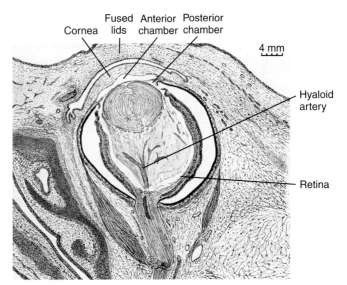

Figure 2-22. Formation of the anterior chamber and cornea. Note the pupillary membrane, which replaced the anterior tunica vasculosa lentis, covering the future pupil.

Figure 2-23. Section through eye and orbit of 48-mm human embryo (approximately 9.5 weeks). (Modified from Remington LA [2005]: Clinical Anatomy of the Visual System, 2nd ed. Butterworth-Heinemann, St. Louis.)

(and the anterior sclera) is lined with *palpebral conjunctiva* derived from the surface ectoderm. This ectoderm also contributes to the formation of lid epidermis, cilia, and a number of glands: the lacrimal and nictitating glands, which produce the aqueous portion of the tear film; the tarsal meibomian glands, which produce the lipid component of the tear film; and Zeiss (sebaceous) and Moll (sweat) glands. Neural crest–derived secondary mesenchyme contributes to the development of the

tarsus and dermis of the lids, but mesoderm contributes to the formation of eyelid muscles.

Nasolacrimal System

The *nasolacrimal groove* separates the *lateral nasal fold* from the *maxillary processes*. At the bottom of the groove a solid cord of ectodermal cells forms and gets buried as the maxillary

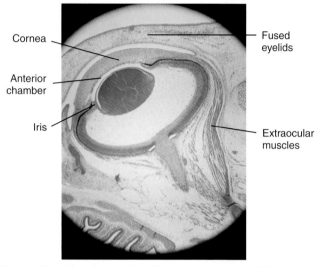

Figure 2-24. Light micrograph of 45-mm pig embryo. Eyelids are fused, extraocular muscle is evident, and axons are evident in optic nerve. (Modified from Remington LA [2005]: Clinical Anatomy of the Visual System, 2nd ed. Butterworth-Heinemann, St. Louis.)

process grows over it to fuse to the lateral nasal fold. Two ectodermal buds grow from the proximal end of the buried cord toward the upper and lower lid folds near the nasal canthus. These buds form the superior and inferior *lacrimal puncta*. The distal end of the cord enters the ventral nasal meatus. The entire cord becomes the *nasolacrimal duct* by a process of canalization. Incomplete canalization is common in domestic animals, resulting in obstruction of the tear drainage. In dogs the puncta and the upper half of the nasolacrimal duct are most commonly affected. In horses the nasal meatus of the duct may be imperforate.

CONGENITAL ABNORMALITIES

Teratology is the branch of embryology that deals with abnormal development and congenital malformations. It is important to remember that not all congenital abnormalities are necessarily inherited, as some may result from toxicity or disease during development. Conversely, not every inherited abnormality is necessarily congenital. Many inherited disorders (e.g., cataract, progressive rod cone degeneration) may be manifested later in life.

The most important determining aspect of the character of a deformity is the stage of development at which the etiologic agent acts. Factors acting during the early period of *embryogenesis* are generally lethal. Those occurring during *organogenesis* result in gross deformities affecting the whole eye (e.g., anophthalmia, microphthalmia, and cyclopia). If the factor acts during the *fetal* period, when the most fundamental and active stage has been completed, minor defects of individual parts of the eye caused by arrests in development and associated deformities due to aberrant growth may occur. Because much of the development and differentiation of the eye occurs very early in gestation (during the first 2 weeks in the dog), events initiated during this time may result in malformations in structures that do not fully mature until much later. Studies of the effect of exposure to teratogens on ocular development have identified narrow, critical periods for induction of malformations; for example, exposure during gastrulation (formation of the mesodermal germ layer) results in a spectrum of malformations

including microphthalmia, cataract, retinal dysplasia, anterior segment dysgenesis, and optic nerve hypoplasia. It is only by detailed study of anomalies that etiology and pathogenesis of the lesions are understood, and subsequent diagnosis and evaluation simplified.

The stage of development (e.g., embryogenesis, organogenesis, or fetal period) at which a teratogenic factor acts is most important in determining the final effects on the eye.

In this section common congenital abnormalities of the whole eye of domestic animals are considered. Abnormalities of the individual parts of the eye are discussed in the relevant chapters.

Anophthalmos and Microphthalmos

Anophthalmos means the total absence of an eye. It may be caused by the suppression of the optic primordia during the development of the forebrain, may be caused by the abnormal development of the forebrain, or may be due to the degeneration of the optic vesicles after they have already formed as a result of a teratogenic insult.

True anophthalmos is very rare, and its diagnosis is made after histologic examination of the orbital contents has not shown the presence of any ocular structure. Most instances of presumed clinical anophthalmos are cases of extreme microphthalmos, because some histologic evidence of a rudimentary eye can usually be found.

Microphthalmos is an eye that is smaller than normal (Figure 2-25). Microphthalmos is most frequent in pigs and

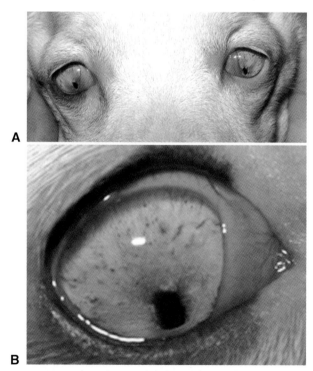

Figure 2-25. A, Bilateral microphthalmia as part of a multiple ocular defects syndrome, which also includes developmental defects in the iris, lens, retina and embryonic hyaloid apparatus. **B,** Close-up of the right eye of the same dog, highlighting the microphthalmia and iris abnormalities. (Courtesy University of California, Davis, Veterinary Ophthalmology Service Collection.)

Table 2-1 | **Anomalies Associated with Microphthalmos in Dogs**

ANOMALY	DOG
Anterior segment dysgenesis	Saint Bernard
	Doberman
Cataract	Old English sheepdog
	Miniature schnauzer
	Cavalier King Charles spaniel
Persistent hyperplastic primary vitreous	Irish wolfhound
Retinal dysplasia	Saint Bernard
	Doberman

Modified from Cook C (1995): Embryogenesis of congenital eye malformations. Vet Comp Ophthal 5:110.

dogs. In pigs, vitamin A deficiency in the dam is the most common cause. In dogs, microphthalmos occurs frequently as part of the collie eye anomaly. Administration of griseofulvin to pregnant cats for treatment of dermatomycosis has resulted in anophthalmos or microphthalmos in their kittens. In white shorthorn cattle hereditary microphthalmos is associated with large lids and third eyelid, resulting in entropion because the small globe does not support the elongated lids.

Microphthalmos may occur in eyes that are otherwise (functionally) normal, if all the internal eye structures remain proportional in size. It may also occur in eyes with multiple ocular anomalies, including cataract, retinal dysplasia, and anterior segment dysgenesis (Table 2-1). In Jersey calves, an autosomal recessive condition causes congenital blindness with microphthalmos, *aniridia* (lack of iris), *microphakia* (small lens), *ectopia lentis* (malpositioned lens), and cataract. Lambs grazing on seleniferous pasture in Wyoming were afflicted with microphthalmos, ectopia lentis or aphakia, optic nerve hypoplasia, persistent pupillary membrane, uveal coloboma, and nonattachment of the retina. In Hereford cattle an encephalopathy-microphthalmos syndrome is inherited as a simple autosomal recessive hereditary trait. Animals present with a domed skull, degeneration of skeletal muscles, small palpebral fissures, small orbits, retinal dysplasia, vitreous syneresis, microphakia, and bilateral microphthalmos.

Cyclopia and Synophthalmus

In *cyclopia* there is a single eye. In *synophthalmus* the eyes are fused in the midline (Figure 2-26). These conditions are incompatible with life.

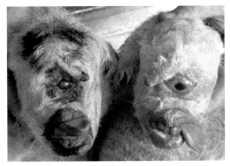

Figure 2-26. Cyclopia in lambs whose dam grazed on *Veratrum californicum*. (Courtesy University of Wisconsin–Madison Veterinary Ophthalmology Service Collection.)

In cyclopia the prosencephalon does not show cleavage; there is one midbrain, one dorsal cyst, and a single optic nerve and optic canal. The frontonasal process presents a proboscis (displaced nose) above the single orbit. The lids of the two eyes are fused around the single orbit. Cyclopia has been reported, in Idaho and Utah, in lambs born to ewes that grazed on *Veratrum californicum* on the fourteenth day of gestation and, in Western Australia, in lambs born to ewes that grazed on unknown toxic plants.

Coloboma

Coloboma is a condition in which a portion of the eye, usually a portion of the uvea, is lacking. Most colobomas (*typical colobomas*) are due to an incomplete closure of the embryonic optic fissure (Figure 2-27). These colobomas are usually situated in the inferonasal portion of the eye. The extent of the coloboma may vary. Severe colobomas are associated with the formation of an orbital cyst (microphthalmos with orbital cyst), because the optic fissure failed to close and form a vesicle. Moderate colobomas may involve numerous ocular structures, whereas mild cases may manifest as only a simple notch in the lower nasal quadrant of the pupil.

Atypical colobomas are not associated with the incomplete closure of the embryonic fissure and are not located in the lower nasal quadrant. They are usually due to lack of induction of one tissue by another. For example, lack of induction by retinal pigment epithelium may cause colobomas in the choroid and sclera, whereas lack of induction by the anterior rim of the optic cup may result in aniridia, or lack of iris.

Colobomas of the optic nerve head may be seen in dogs affected with collie eye anomaly (Figure 2-28) and in basenjis that present with persistent pupillary membranes. In cats,

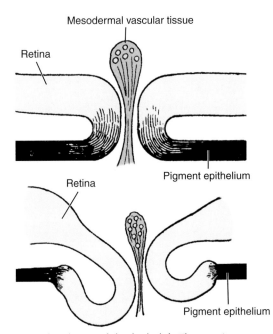

Figure 2-27. The closure of the fetal cleft. The margins come together accurately *(top)*, but subsequently an excessive growth of the inner (retinal) layer leads to its eversion *(bottom)*, causing a coloboma of the retina and posterior uvea. (Modified from Duke-Elder S [editor] [1963]: System of Ophthalmology, Vol III: Normal and Abnormal Development. Part 2: Congenital Deformities. Henry Kimpton, London.)

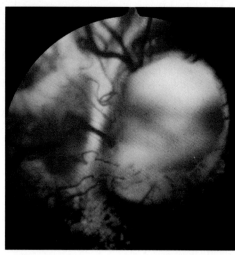

Figure 2-28. A coloboma of the optic nerve head and sclera as part of the collie eye anomaly syndrome.

colobomas in the lateral segments of the upper eyelids are common. These must be surgically corrected, because they allow facial hair to irritate the cornea and conjunctiva.

BIBLIOGRAPHY

Achiron R, et al. (2000): Axial growth of the fetal eye and evaluation of the hyaloid artery: in utero ultrasonographic study. Prenat Diagn 20:894.

Aguirre G, et al. (1972): The development of the canine eye. Am J Vet Res 33:2399.

Bailey TJ, et al. (2004): Regulation of vertebrate eye development by Rx genes. Int J Dev Biol 48:761.

Baker CV, Bronner-Fraser M (2001): Vertebrate cranial placodes I: embryonic induction. Dev Biol 232:1.

Barishak RY (2001): Embryology of the Eye and Its Adnexa. S. Karger, Basel, Switzerland.

Bistner SI, et al. (1973): Development of the bovine eye. Am J Vet Red 34:7.

Boroffka SA (2005): Ultrasonographic evaluation of pre- and postnatal development of the eyes in beagles. Vet Radiol Ultrasound 46:72.

Collinson JM, et al. (2004): Analysis of mouse eye development with chimeras and mosaics. Int J Dev Biol 48:793.

Cook C (1995): Embryogenesis of congenital eye malformations. Vet Comp Ophthal 5:110.

Cook C, et al. (1993): Prenatal development of the eye and its adnexa, in Tasman Jaeger W (editor): Duane's Foundations of Clinical Ophthalmology. JB Lippincott, Phildelphia, p. 1.

Cook CS (1989): Experimental models of anterior segment dysgenesis. Ophthalmic Paediatr Genet 10:33.

Cvekl A, Tamm ER (2004): Anterior eye development and ocular mesenchyme: new insights from mouse models and human diseases. Bioessays 26:374.

Duddy JA, et al. (1983): Hyaloid artery patency in neonatal beagles. Am J Vet Res 44:2344.

Gould DB, et al. (2004): Anterior segment development relevant to glaucoma. Int J Dev Biol 48:1015.

Gum GG, et al. (1984): Maturation of the retina of the canine neonate as determined by electroretinography and histology. Am J Vet Res 45:1166.

Jubb KF, Kennedy PC (1993): Pathology of the Domestic Animals, 4th ed, Vol II. Academic Press, New York.

McAvoy JW, et al. (1999): Lens development. Eye 13:425.

Mey J, Thanos S (2000): Development of the visual system of the chick: I. Cell differentiation and histogenesis. Brain Res Brain Res Rev 32:343.

Pichaud F, Desplan C (2002): Pax genes and eye organogenesis. Curr Opin Genet Dev 12:430.

Provis JM (2001): Development of the primate retinal vasculature. Prog Retin Eye Res 20:799.

Reza HM, Yasuda K (2004): Lens differentiation and crystallin regulation: a chick model. Int J Dev Biol 48:805.

Rutledge JC (1997): Developmental toxicity induced during early stages of mammalian embryogenesis. Mutat Res 12:113.

Sengpiel F, Kind PC (2002): The role of activity in development of the visual system. Curr Biol 12:R818.

Spencer WH (1996): Ophthalmic Pathology, 4th ed. Saunders, Philadelphia.

Stromland K, et al. (1991): Ocular teratology. Surv Ophthalmol 35:429.

Zieske JD (2004): Corneal development associated with eyelid opening. Int J Dev Biol 48:903.

OCULAR PHARMACOLOGY AND THERAPEUTICS

David J. Maggs

THERAPEUTIC FORMULATIONS
ROUTES OF ADMINISTRATION
ANTIBACTERIAL DRUGS
ANTIFUNGAL DRUGS
ANTIVIRAL DRUGS
CORTICOSTEROIDS
NONSTEROIDAL ANTIINFLAMMATORY
  DRUGS

IMMUNOMODULATING THERAPY
  (IMMUNOSUPPRESSANTS AND
  IMMUNOSTIMULANTS)
MAST CELL STABILIZERS AND
  ANTIHISTAMINES
HYPEROSMOTIC AGENTS
AUTONOMIC DRUGS
CARBONIC ANHYDRASE INHIBITORS

PROSTAGLANDIN ANALOGUES
LOCAL ANESTHETICS
ENZYMES AND ENZYME INHIBITORS
TEAR REPLACEMENT PREPARATIONS
  ("ARTIFICIAL TEARS")
MISCELLANEOUS THERAPEUTIC AGENTS
PHYSICAL THERAPY

THERAPEUTIC FORMULATIONS

Although topical application of solutions, suspensions, and ointments is most common in ocular medicine, parenteral methods of administration via a systemic (i.e., intravenous, intramuscular, subcutaneous) or local (i.e., subconjunctival, intraorbital, intracameral, intravitreous) route are also used. Drugs for ocular administration are prepared in various ways. The topical use of powders for ocular treatment is detrimental to the eye and outmoded. Solutions, suspensions, and ointments for topical application must have physical characteristics within a relative narrow range to be well tolerated. Of these the most important characteristics are tonicity and pH. These parameters must also be considered by compounding pharmacists when formulating drugs for topical ophthalmic use.

Ophthalmic preparations must be sterile, especially if they enter the interior of the eye. Bacterial filtering and the addition of preservatives such as benzalkonium chloride are used to limit contamination of multidose containers. However, these preservatives are also toxic to mammalian cells. This fact has a number of important clinical implications:

- Topical drug use is *not* benign and should always be limited to the lowest effective concentration, frequency, and duration.
- Drugs designed for topical use should not be used intraocularly or injected, especially subconjunctivally.
- Preservatives in ophthalmic drugs and diagnostic agents may interfere with diagnostic attempts to isolate and grow microbes from the ocular surface.

Although topical application of drugs provides excellent drug concentrations at the ocular surface, there are two critical barriers to penetration of drugs into the eye. These are the blood-ocular barrier (which, like the blood-brain barrier, is impermeable to most drugs unless there is significant intraocular inflammation) and the cornea (which becomes more permeable when ulcerated).

ROUTES OF ADMINISTRATION

The main factors governing choice of the route of administration are as follows:

- Inherent properties of the drug
- Site of desired action (surface or intraocular structures)
- Frequency of administration possible
- Drug concentration required at target tissue
- Vascularity of the target tissue

Some drugs, because of their properties, are restricted as to the routes by which they can be given. For example, polymyxin B cannot be given systemically because of nephrotoxicity or by subconjunctival injection because of local irritation. Drugs required in high concentration in the cornea or conjunctiva are usually administered by frequent topical application or subconjunctival injection. If high concentrations are required in the anterior uveal tract (i.e., iris or ciliary body), subconjunctival injection, systemic administration, or frequent topical application of drugs that will pass through the intact cornea are used. Drugs that do not pass through the blood-ocular barrier still reach high concentrations in the highly vascular anterior uvea (iris and ciliary body), posterior uvea (choroid), and sclera. With inflammation the blood-ocular barrier may be reduced, and drugs that cannot normally enter the aqueous or vitreous humor may do so. If high concentrations are required within orbital tissues, systemic administration is usually used. Choice of route is summarized in Figure 3-1.

The cornea may be considered a trilaminar (lipid-water-lipid) "sandwich," in which the epithelium and endothelium are relatively lipophilic and hydrophobic, whereas the stroma is relatively hydrophilic and lipophobic. Lipid-soluble drugs (e.g., chloramphenicol) penetrate more readily, whereas electrolytes and water-soluble drugs (e.g., neomycin, bacitracin, and penicillin) penetrate poorly if at all after topical application. The lipophilic properties of the epithelium may be partially bypassed by subconjunctival injection, provided that other properties of the drug are suitable for administration by this route.

Figure 3-1. Sites of drug administration. **A,** Topically applied ointments, suspensions, and solutions achieve high drug concentrations on the corneal and conjunctival surface. Not all penetrate through the cornea and so are not uniformly useful for treating intraocular disease. Penetration to the posterior segment is extremely limited for all topical medications. **B,** Subconjunctival injections facilitate high drug concentrations at the ocular surface and provide a variable-duration depot effect. Not all drugs are tolerated at this site. Intraocular penetration varies with drug type. **C,** Intraocular (intracameral or intravitreal) injection of drugs is used rarely because general anesthesia is needed, serious ocular risks are associated with this route of therapy, and alternative routes often provide equivalent intraocular drug concentrations. **D,** Systemically administered drugs (oral or parenteral) reach all *vascular* ocular structures but are not delivered in useful concentrations to the avascular structures, such as the cornea and lens. Intraocular penetration of systemically administered drugs depends on the patency of the blood-ocular barrier and the lipophilicity of the drug.

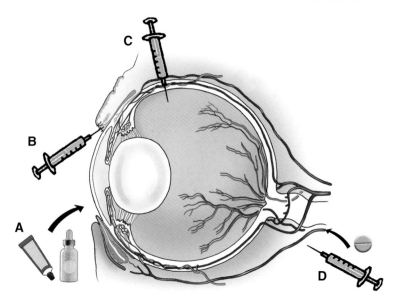

Higher or more prolonged drug concentrations and therapeutic effects may be achieved with the following approaches:

- Increasing drug concentration in the topical preparation; for example, 1% prednisolone suspension results in higher intraocular concentrations than does 0.5% suspension (Figure 3-2).
- Increasing the frequency of application; for example, topical administration every 10 minutes for an hour results in higher concentrations than does a single application.
- Slowing absorption. Drugs released over a long period can be used to maintain drug concentrations. This is one mechanism whereby subconjunctival administration leads to higher topical concentrations of drug because of delayed release ("leakage") of drug back along the injection tract. Penetration of topically administered drugs can also be enhanced through the use of preparations that maintain longer contact with the eye before being washed away by the tears (e.g., ointments, suspensions, or more viscous solutions).
- Facilitation of passage of drug between epithelial cells by limited and controlled damage of the intercellular adhesions of the epithelium with a surface-active preservative such as benzalkonium chloride (an additive in some drugs).

Solutions and Suspensions ("Drops")

Ophthalmic solutions and suspensions (or "drops") are commonly used for topical treatment of ocular disease. They are usually easily instilled in dogs and cats but not in large animals. The correct method for instilling eyedrops is shown in Figure 3-3. Drops permit the delivered dose to be controlled and varied easily, and they are alleged to interfere less with repair of corneal epithelium than ointments, although this last feature is unlikely to be clinically significant. Drops are quickly diluted and eliminated from the eye by tears, so greater frequency of application or drug concentration may be required, especially with increased lacrimation. It is important to note that systemic absorption of drugs from the conjunctival sac after topical application is rapid and may result in notable blood concentrations. This may be of clinical significance with use of phenylephrine (producing systemic hypertension) and long-term corticosteroid use (inducing iatrogenic hyperadrenocorticism).

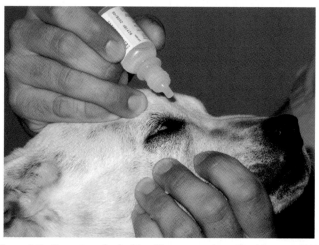

Figure 3-3. Correct method of instilling an eyedrop. The lower eyelid is held open with the hand being used to restrain the patient's head. The upper eyelid is retracted with the hand holding the medication. The medication container is held 1 to 2 cm from the eye, and a single drop is instilled. Care must be taken to avoid the bottle touching the eye because this may injure the ocular surface or cause contamination of the drug remaining in the bottle.

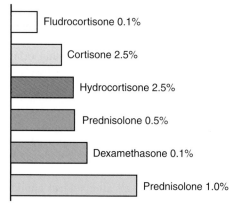

Fludrocortisone 0.1%

Cortisone 2.5%

Hydrocortisone 2.5%

Prednisolone 0.5%

Dexamethasone 0.1%

Prednisolone 1.0%

Figure 3-2. Relative antiinflammatory action of various corticosteroid preparations. Note that prednisolone (1.0%) and dexamethasone are relatively more potent than hydrocortisone. (Modified from Havener WH [1994]: Ocular Pharmacology, 6th ed. Mosby, St. Louis.)

Continuous or Intermittent Ocular Surface Lavage Systems

With frequent treatment or in horses with painful eyes, a lavage system allows medications to be conveniently, safely, and frequently delivered into the conjunctival sac. Originally, such systems were placed within the nasolacrimal duct and medications were instilled in a retrograde fashion. More recently subpalpebral lavage systems have been described that are simply placed and avoid nasal irritation and risk of dislodgement. A two-hole technique through the skin of the upper eyelid has now been replaced by single-hole systems, owing to the commercial availability of lavage systems with footplates to prevent inadvertent removal. The original one-hole system was placed in the central upper lid but is associated with a relatively high risk of complications, most notably corneal ulceration due to rubbing of the footplate on the cornea. Placement of the subpalpebral lavage system in the ventromedial conjunctival fornix may be preferred because of the natural corneal protection provided by the third eyelid at that point (Figure 3-4).

Subpalpebral lavage systems placed in the medial aspect of the lower lid are associated with less common and less severe ocular complications than those placed centrally and dorsally, even when left in place and used by owners for up to 55 days after discharge from hospital. The lavage tube leads back to the shoulder, where it is secured at the mane and where drugs can be administered with less risk of injury to the eye or the operator. Drugs are injected into the tube and either slowly propelled to the eye with a gently administered bolus of air from a syringe or continuously propelled by a gravity-fed bottle or small mechanical infusion pump connected to the tube. This method of therapy is usually reserved for horses with severe corneal or uveal disease. A protective eyecup can be applied over the lavage tube for protection of the eye and apparatus. Ointments (and some more viscous suspensions) cannot be applied through lavage systems.

Ointments

In horses the orbicularis oculi muscle is very powerful, and it is impossible to tilt the head to allow a drop of solution to

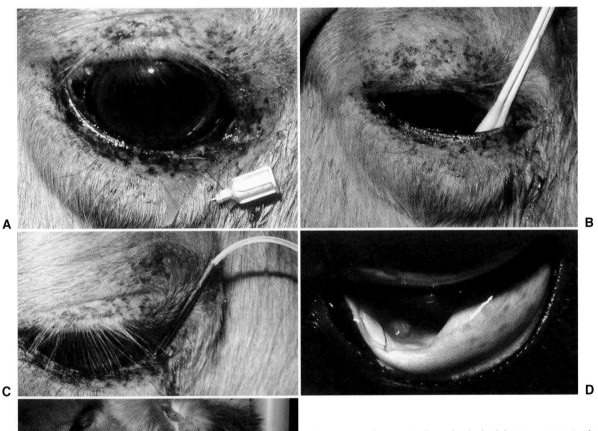

Figure 3-4. Placement of a subpalpebral lavage system in the medial aspect of a horse's lower eyelid. **A,** A local (subcutaneous) injection of lidocaine is administered. **B,** The palpebral and fornicial conjunctival surfaces are anesthetized with proparacaine-soaked cotton-tipped applicators held in place for 1 or 2 minutes. **C,** A trocar is used to penetrate the lower lid from the conjunctival fornix, and the lavage tube is threaded through it. **D,** The trocar is removed, and the lavage tube is pulled down until it lies snugly in the ventral conjunctival fornix between the third eyelid and lower lid. **E,** The lavage tube is sutured in place with adhesive tape tabs, and an injection port is placed at its terminus near the mane on the same side as the affected eye.

enter without contaminating the bottle. Ointments are preferred in such patients. Ointments also allow longer contact between the drug and surface tissues. Finally, less drug enters the nasolacrimal apparatus. Therefore ointments achieve higher tissue concentrations than solutions or suspensions do. A soothing effect occurs on instillation, they are a more stable medium for labile antibiotics and drugs, and they also provide physical lubrication and protect against desiccation better than solutions do. However, because oily ointment bases cause severe intraocular inflammation, and because application of ointments may result in ocular trauma from the tube itself, ointments are not recommended when globe perforation has occurred or is likely. Because they make tissue handling difficult and cause granulomatous inflammation if they penetrate ocular surface structures, ointments should also not be used before ocular or adnexal surgery. Finally, owners tend to overmedicate when using ointments, resulting in loss of medication, higher cost, and lower compliance with treatment regimens. As little as 0.5 cm of ointment from a fine nozzle is sufficient to medicate an eye.

Subconjunctival, Subtenons, and Retrobulbar Injection

Subconjunctival injection permits a portion of the administered drug to bypass the barrier of the corneal epithelium and penetrate transsclerally. However, a notable proportion of the injected drug leaks back out the injection tract and is absorbed as if it had been administered topically. Subconjunctival administration is used to facilitate high drug concentrations in anterior regions of the eye, whereas deeper injections beneath Tenon's capsule allow greater diffusion of drugs through the sclera and into the eye. Mydriatics (for pupillary dilation), antibiotics, and corticosteroids are the main groups of drugs administered by this route. Some irritating drugs (e.g., polymyxin B) or any topical drug containing a preservative cannot be given subconjunctivally. Drugs with potent systemic sympathomimetic or vasopressor effects also should not be given in this manner.

In cooperative patients, subconjunctival injections can be given using topical anesthesia only. Handheld lid retractors may be helpful in all species (Figure 3-5). For horses and cattle, one should also consider tranquilization, appropriate restraint (a twitch for horses and nose grips for cattle), and an

auriculopalpebral nerve block to produce akinesia of the upper lid (see Chapter 5). A few drops of topical ophthalmic anesthetic (e.g., proparacaine) are instilled into the conjunctival sac. Conjunctival anesthesia is facilitated by a cotton-tipped applicator soaked in topical anesthesia and placed against the conjunctiva at the planned injection site for about 30 seconds. The solution for subconjunctival injection then is administered through a 25- to 27-gauge needle with a 1-mL tuberculin or insulin syringe under the bulbar conjunctiva as close as possible to the lesion being treated (Figure 3-6). Injection under the palpebral conjunctiva is not effective. The needle is rotated on withdrawal to limit leakage through the needle tract. Up to 1 mL of drug can be given beneath the bulbar conjunctiva, but most injections do not exceed 0.5 mL. Slight hemorrhage into the injection site occasionally occurs but is absorbed within 7 to 10 days. Injections of depot preparations should be avoided at this site because they often lead to granuloma formation.

Supplies for subconjunctival injection are topical anesthetic, a cotton-tipped applicator, a 1-mL syringe (tuberculin or insulin), a 25- to 27-gauge needle, and solution for injection.

Retrobulbar injection is used rarely and only for treatment of disease processes in the orbit or posterior half of the globe. These areas can usually be treated adequately with safer and simpler systemic routes of treatment. Therefore this route of therapy is now generally limited to the injection of local anesthetic into the muscle cone behind the globe for removal of the bovine eye.

Systemic Drug Administration

Although there are rare exceptions, systemically administered drugs should be considered to reach only the vascular tissues of the eye and surrounding structures—that is, *not* the cornea, the lens, or (in the presence of an intact blood-ocular barrier) the aqueous or vitreous humor. This knowledge may be used to the clinician's advantage. For example, systemic administration of a corticosteroid for control of uveitis in the presence of corneal ulceration is safe and effective, because the target tissue (the uvea) is vascular, but the drug will not reach the avascular cornea in quantities sufficient to retard healing. Equally, the systemic administration of an antibiotic for treatment of

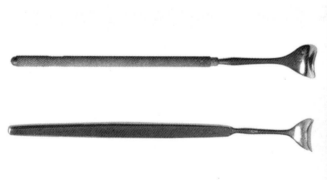

A

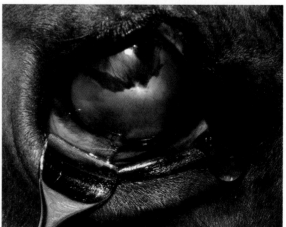

B

Figure 3-5. A, Handheld lid retractors. **B,** Retractor in use.

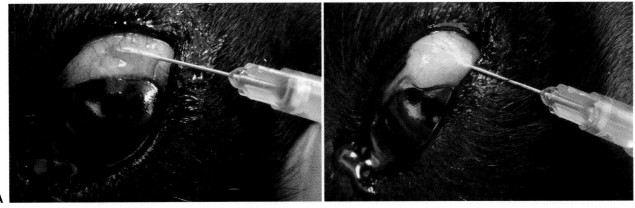

Figure 3-6. Subconjunctival injection technique. **A,** After application of a topical anesthestic, a 25- to 27-gauge needle is inserted beneath the bulbar conjunctiva. Care must be taken not to penetrate the globe. **B,** The medication injected forms a noticeable bleb that reduces in size over the next few minutes to hours. (Courtesy Dr. David Ramsey.)

an ulcer in a nonvascularized cornea is of little value, and topical administration is most effective. Therefore systemically administered drugs should be reserved for treatment of diseases of the eyelids, conjunctiva, sclera, uvea (iris, ciliary body, choroid), retina, optic nerve, extraocular muscles, and orbital contents.

As with other body systems, intravenous, subcutaneous, and intramuscular injections provide relatively high plasma concentrations of a drug to the vascular components of the eye. However, because continuous treatment is necessary for many ocular disorders, oral drug administration by owners is used most frequently, particularly in dogs and cats. Continuous intramuscular administration is used occasionally in large animals. Intravenous therapy is rarely used for ocular disease, with the important exception of the administration of mannitol for reduction of intraocular pressure (IOP) and vitreous volume in acute glaucoma.

Intraocular drug concentrations attainable by systemic routes depend on the following three important factors:

- Absorption of the drug from the injection site or gastrointestinal tract, and the plasma concentrations reached
- Vascularity of the target tissue
- Properties of the drug with respect to the blood-ocular barrier. Systemically administered drugs will not reach those areas of the eye "protected" by an intact blood-ocular barrier (the vitreous, aqueous humor, and retina). In inflamed eyes, this barrier is usually much less effective.

Some examples reinforce these general points. Although penicillin is readily absorbed by intramuscular injection, penicillin G is poorly absorbed orally because it is destroyed by gastric acid. Even when adequate plasma concentrations are achieved, it penetrates the blood-ocular barrier poorly. By contrast, chloramphenicol is well absorbed by dogs after oral administration and, once in the plasma, passes the blood-aqueous barrier well. From these examples, it follows that the clinician must understand the properties of the individual drugs used in order to predict their applicability for ophthalmic use.

ANTIBACTERIAL DRUGS

Antibacterial drugs act by altering cell wall synthesis, protein synthesis, or cell wall permeability in bacteria but may also have undesirable effects on the cells of the patient. Although not strictly accurate, the terms *antibiotics* and *antibacterials*

often are used interchangeably. Antibacterial agents may be classified as bactericidal (destroying bacteria) or bacteriostatic (inhibiting bacterial growth and reproduction; Box 3-1). Some antibiotics may act in either manner, depending on concentration. Combining bactericidal and bacteriostatic antibiotics may result in antagonism between the agents, although the clinical importance of this effect is debated. In particular, combinations of bactericidal drugs infrequently used elsewhere in the body are commonly employed in topical treatment of the eye. This practice allows a wider spectrum of activity than with single drugs and reduces the chance of drug resistance. The combination of neomycin, polymyxin B, and bacitracin (or gramicidin) as so-called triple antibiotic is very useful. For resistant infections combinations of agents with differing mechanisms are sometimes used—for example, a penicillin or cephalosporin (which inhibits cell wall synthesis) with an aminoglycoside (which inhibits intracellular protein synthesis).

Selection and Administration of Antibiotics

The following factors must be considered in the selection of an antibiotic:

- The offending organism and its sensitivity
- Location of the organism
- Penetration of available drugs to that site
- Pharmacokinetics of the available drugs
- Spectrum of activity of available drugs

Box 3-1	**Classification of common ophthalmic antibiotics**
Bactericidal	**Bacteriostatic**
Aminoglycosides	Chloramphenicol
Bacitracin	Cephalosporins
Erythromycin*	Erythromycin*
Fluoroquinolones	Tetracyclines
Potentiated sulfonamides	
Neomycin	
Penicillins	
Polymyxins	
Vancomycin	

*Depending on concentration and organism.

- Toxicity of available drugs
- Owner compliance

The ideal basis for selection of an ocular antibiotic consists of identification of the responsible organism and its antibiotic sensitivity. However, obtaining this information often cannot be justified because of expense or because treatment must be instituted before the results of such testing are available. Therefore knowledge of the most likely organisms, their sensitivity, and the most likely effective antibiotics is necessary. Treating infections on such an empirical basis, although practical and often unavoidable, does not always lead to a satisfactory result. A more rational choice of therapeutic agent can be made after examination of the staining and morphologic characteristics of organisms seen on a Gram-stained or Diff-Quik–stained sample of the affected tissue and is essential in severe or nonresponsive infections. In more severe infections (e.g., stromal corneal ulcers or endophthalmitis), the organism should be identified, and a combination of routes of administration and synergistic drugs should be considered. If ocular infections persist or recur despite treatment with the appropriate antibiotic (based on results of culture and sensitivity testing), the infection may be secondary to an underlying disorder or pathologic process. Alternatively, a fastidious bacterium or nonbacterial microbe not originally cultured (*Chlamydophila* spp., *Mycoplasma* spp., fungus, virus, etc.) may be present.

Organisms commonly isolated from the conjunctival sacs of normal and diseased animals are given in Tables 3-1 through 3-9. These tables highlight a number of important general points about ocular surface flora that are relevant when interpreting these data in an individual patient:

- There are marked species, individual, geographic, and seasonal variations in the normal ocular surface flora.
- The normal conjunctival sac often contains potential pathogens.
- Because of the variety of organisms present, empirical treatment with standard antibiotics may be unsuccessful.
- Care is advisable in interpretation of frequency and sensitivity data from different geographic areas.
- In vitro sensitivity data may not necessarily reflect in vivo experience when one is using topically applied antibiotics, because high surface concentrations can be achieved.
- Previously untreated infections seen in general practice may have a different spectrum of sensitivity from those reported in referral hospital populations.

The following sections provide a summary of some important properties of antibiotics used commonly in veterinary ophthalmology, and Table 3-10 lists the typical Gram-staining characteristics of, and the antibiotics of choice for, common organisms.

Penicillins

The penicillins form a large family of natural and synthetic derivatives of 6-aminopenicillanic acid that range considerably in stability, solubility, spectrum of activity, ocular penetration, and resistance to β-lactamase.

Penicillin G

Penicillin G is soluble in water, attains high concentrations in blood, and is excreted in urine in 4 to 6 hours. Penicillin G is available in crystalline, procaine, and benzathine forms.

Table 3-1 | **Normal Flora of the Canine Conjunctival Sac**

AREA AND FLORA	PERCENTAGE OF CASES WITH POSITIVE CULTURES
WESTERN UNITED STATES*	
Diphtheroids	75.0
Staphylococcus epidermidis	46.0
Staphylococcus aureus	24.0
Bacillus spp.	12.0
Gram-negative organisms (*Acinetobacter, Neisseria, Moraxella,* and *Pseudomonas* spp.)	7.0
Streptococcus spp. (α-hemolytic)	4.0
Streptococcus spp. (β-hemolytic)	2.0
MIDWESTERN UNITED STATES†	
S. epidermidis	55.0
S. aureus	45.0
Streptococcus spp. (α-hemolytic)	34.0
Diphtheroids	30.0
Neisseria spp.	26.0
Pseudomonas spp.	14.0
Streptococcus spp. (β-hemolytic)	7.3
EASTERN AUSTRALIA‡	
S. aureus	39.0
Bacillus spp.	29.0
Corynebacterium spp.	19.0
S. epidermidis	16.0
Yeasts	5.0
Streptococcus spp. (α-hemolytic)	3.0
Streptococcus spp. (nonhemolytic)	3.0
Micrococcus spp.	3.0
Neisseria spp.	2.0
Streptococcus spp. (β-hemolytic)	1.0
Pseudomonas spp.	1.0
Nocardia spp.	1.0
Escherichia coli	1.0
Clostridium spp.	1.0
Enterobacter spp.	1.0
Flavobacterium spp.	1.0
Branhamella catarrhalis	1.0

*Data from Bistner SI, et al. (1969): Conjunctival bacteria: clinical appearances can be deceiving. Mod Vet Pract 50:45.
†Data from Urban W, et al. (1972): Conjunctival flora of clinically normal dogs. Am J Vet Med Assoc 161:201.
‡Data from McDonald PJ, Watson ADJ (1976): Microbial flora of normal canine conjunctivae. J Small Anim Pract 17:809.

Because it is unstable at low pH, oral administration is not possible, so the agent is administered by injection. Because of its high water solubility, penicillin G does not penetrate the intact cornea when applied topically and does not pass through the intact blood-ocular barrier. It is most effective against gram-positive organisms, but it is susceptible to β-lactamase. For all of these reasons penicillin G does not have a great number of uses in veterinary ophthalmology, with perhaps the exception of subconjunctival injection for treatment of susceptible infections and in situations in which frequent applications of medication are inconvenient (e.g., infectious bovine keratoconjunctivitis).

Sodium Methicillin

Methicillin is resistant to β-lactamase and is used by intravenous infusion for resistant staphylococci. Renal excretion is rapid. Because the drug is unstable in solution, it should be dissolved just before use. Methicillin can be used topically or by subconjunctival injection for corneal infections. Methicillin

Table 3-2 | Organisms Cultured from Dogs with External Ocular Disease

AREA AND FLORA	PERCENTAGE OF CASES WITH POSITIVE CULTURES
THE NETHERLANDS*	
Streptococcus canis	20.3
No growth	18.7
Staphylococcus epidermidis	14.0
Staphylococcus aureus	7.8
Other nonpathogenic *Streptococcus* spp.	7.8
Nocardia spp.	7.8
Absidia ramosa (fungus)	7.8
Pseudomonas aeruginosa	6.1
Corynebacterium spp.	4.6
Other pathogenic *S. canis* spp.	3.1
Proteus vulgaris	3.1
Clostridium perfringens	1.5
Candida spp.	1.5
COLORADO†	
S. aureus	68.0
S. epidermidis	27.0
Streptococcus spp. (β-hemolytic)	19.0
Streptococcus spp. (α-hemolytic)	17.0
Proteus mirabilis	11.0
Escherichia coli	10.0
Bacillus spp.	5.0
Corynebacterium spp.	3.0
P. aeruginosa	2.0
Klebsiella spp.	1.0
ILLINOIS‡	
Staphylococcus spp.	39.4
Coagulase positive	29.0
Staphylococcus intermedius	17.0
S. epidermis	11.0
Streptococcus spp.	25.2
β-Hemolytic streptococci	17.0
Pseudomonas spp.	9.4

*Data from Verwer MAJ, Gunnick JW (1968): The occurrence of bacteria in chronic purulent eye discharge. J Small Anim Pract 9:33.
†Data from Murphy JM, et al. (1978): Survey of conjunctival flora in dogs with clinical signs of external eye disease. J Am Vet Med Assoc 172:66.
‡Data from Gerding PA, et al. (1988): Pathogenic bacteria and fungi associated with external ocular diseases in dogs: 131 cases (1981-1986). J Am Vet Med Assoc 193:242.

Table 3-3 | Normal Flora of the Feline Conjunctival Sac

AREA AND FLORA	PERCENTAGE OF CASES WITH POSITIVE CULTURES	
	CONJUNCTIVA	LIDS
WESTERN UNITED STATES		
Staphylococcus epidermidis	16.3	13.3
Staphylococcus aureus	10.4	8.8
Mycoplasma spp.	5.0	—
Bacillus spp.	2.9	1.7
Streptococcus spp. (α-hemolytic)	2.5	1.7
Corynebacterium spp.	1.3	—
Escherichia coli	—	0.4

Data from Campbell L (1973): Ocular bacteria and mycoplasma of the clinically normal cat. Feline Pract Nov-Dec:10.

Table 3-4 | Fungal Flora from Normal Horses (50 Horses)

ORGANISM	PERCENTAGE OF CASES WITH POSITIVE CULTURES
Aspergillus spp.	36.0
Cladosporium spp.	34.0

Positive but no quantitative data given: *Alternaria, Fusarium, Monotospira, Paecilomyces, Phoma, Pullularia, Scopulariopsis, Streptomyces, Trichoderma, Verticullium* spp.

Modified from Smith PJ, et al. (1997): Identification of sclerotomy sites for posterior segment surgery in the dog. Vet Comp Ophthalmol 7:180.

Table 3-5 | Organisms Cultured from Horses with External Ocular Disease (123 Eyes)

ORGANISM	PERCENTAGE OF CASES WITH POSITIVE CULTURES
Streptococcus spp. (total)	43.9
β-Hemolytic	26.0
Other hemolytic	17.9
Staphylococcus spp.	24.4
Pseudomonas spp.	13.8
Bacillus spp.	10.6
Enterobacter spp.	6.5
Escherichia coli	4.0
Corynebacterium spp.	3.2
Proteus spp.	3.2
Aspergillus spp.	2.4
Klebsiella spp.	2.4
Moraxella spp.	2.4
Pasteurella spp.	2.4
Mima spp.	1.6
Diplococcus spp.	0.8
Flavobacterium spp.	0.8
Fusarium spp.	0.8
Neisseria spp.	0.8
Nocardia spp.	0.8
Penicillium spp.	0.8
Rhizopus spp.	0.8
Trichosporon spp.	0.8

Data from McLaughlin SA, et al. (1983): Pathogenic bacteria and fungi associated with extraocular disease in the horse. J Am Vet Med Assoc 182:241.

Table 3-6 | Normal Flora of the Bovine Conjunctival Sac

AREA AND FLORA	PERCENTAGE OF CASES WITH POSITIVE CULTURES
NORTHEASTERN AUSTRALIA	
Unidentified gram-positive cocci	54.4
Corynebacterium spp.	27.4
Moraxella nonliquefaciens	26.9
Streptococcus faecalis	20.0
No growth	13.4
Neisseria (Branhamella) catarrhalis (nonhemolytic)	10.5
Unidentified gram-negative rods	8.5
Acinetobacter spp.	8.0
Moraxella bovis	6.5
Coliforms	6.5
Staphylococcus aureus	4.1
Moraxella liquefaciens	2.2
Bacillus spp.	1.3
Unclassified *Moraxella*	1.0
Actinobacillus spp.	0.7
Proteus spp.	0.0

Data from Wilcox G (1970): Bacterial flora of the bovine eye with special reference to *Moraxella* and *Neisseria*. Aust Vet J 46:253.

Table 3-7 | **Normal Flora of the Ovine Conjunctival Sac**

AREA AND FLORA	PERCENTAGE OF CASES WITH POSITIVE CULTURES
EASTERN AUSTRALIA	
No growth	60.0
Neisseria ovis	24.0
Micrococcus spp.	NQD
Streptococcus spp.	NQD
Corynebacterium spp.	NQD
Achromobacter spp.	NQD
Bacillus spp.	NQD
Moraxella spp.	NQD

Data from Spradbrow P (1968): The bacterial flora of the ovine conjunctival sac. Aust Vet J 44:117.
NQD, No quantitative data (present in small numbers, but NQD given).

Table 3-8 | **Normal Bacterial Flora of South American Camelid Eyes (88 Animals)**

ORGANISM	PERCENTAGE OF CASES WITH POSITIVE CULTURES
GRAM-POSITIVE	
Staphylococcus spp.	58
Bacillus spp.	28
Streptomyces spp.	18
α-Hemolytic *Streptococcus* spp.	13
Corynebacterium spp.	8
Micrococcus/Planococcus spp.	7
GRAM-NEGATIVE	
Pseudomonas spp.	41
Pasteurella ureae	9
Klebsiella spp.	2
Escherichia coli	2

Data include llama, alpaca, and guanaco eyes and are from Gionfriddo JR, et al. (1991): Bacterial and mycoplasmal flora of the healthy camelid conjunctival sac. Am J Vet Res 52:1061.

Table 3-9 | **Normal Fungal Flora of South American Camelid Eyes (127 Animals)**

ORGANISM	PERCENTAGE OF CASES WITH POSITIVE CULTURES*
Aspergillus spp.	20-43
Fusarium spp.	2-30
Rhinocladiella spp.	8-35
Penicillium spp.	3-33
Mucor spp.	5-14
Dematiaceous fungi	12-33

Data include llama, alpaca, and guanaco eyes and are from Gionfriddo JR, et al. (1992): Fungal flora of the healthy camelid conjunctival sac. Am J Vet Res 53:643.
*Percentages varied according to season and camelid species.

may be expected to enter the aqueous humor in therapeutic concentrations when the blood-ocular barrier is disrupted by inflammation.

Sodium Oxacillin

Oxacillin is resistant to β-lactamase; it is also acid-stable and may be used orally. Unfortunately, much of it is bound to plasma protein in the circulation and cannot enter the aqueous humor, even in an inflamed eye. Oxacillin is useful in orbital and adnexal infections when given orally.

Amoxicillin and Ampicillin

Ampicillin is a broad-spectrum penicillin that is often effective against *Escherichia coli* and *Proteus* spp. and may be given orally, intramuscularly, or subconjunctivally. Although it enters the aqueous humor to some extent, ampicillin is not the agent of first choice for gram-negative infections, because the high inhibitory concentrations necessary are not always reached in the aqueous humor. Amoxicillin has a spectrum of activity similar to that of ampicillin but is better absorbed from the gastrointestinal tract than ampicillin. Both ampicillin and amoxicillin are susceptible to β-lactamase. Amoxicillin reaches blood concentrations two to three times higher than those of ampicillin after oral administration, but both drugs enter the uninflamed eye to about the same degree. Because it inhibits β-lactamases, clavulanic acid is added to preparations of amoxicillin. This preparation is useful in initial treatment of chronic staphylococcal blepharitis—in which the staphylococci are often β-lactamase producers—and orbital cellulitis, which may involve anaerobic bacteria implanted from the oral cavity.

Cephalosporins

A range of cephalosporins is available. They are generally similar to the penicillins in mechanism of action and pharmacology but are less susceptible to staphylococcal β-lactamases. A type of β-lactamase (cephalosporinase) produced by some gram-negative organisms may inactivate them. Cephalosporins have had excellent results when administered subconjunctivally or topically via lavage tube to horses with corneal ulceration, particularly those infected with *Streptococcus* spp. They are also very useful for bacterial blepharitis. Cefazolin is the antibiotic of choice for perioperative antimicrobial prophylaxis in small animal surgery.

Chloramphenicol

Chloramphenicol is a broad-spectrum bacteriostatic antibiotic effective against a wide range of gram-positive and gram-negative organisms, *Rickettsia*, spirochetes, and *Chlamydophila* spp. However, *Pseudomonas aeruginosa* is often resistant. Because of its lipid solubility, chloramphenicol passes the blood-ocular barrier and through corneal epithelium better than most water-soluble antibiotics. Chloramphenicol may be administered orally, intramuscularly, subcutaneously, intravenously, subconjunctivally, or topically. Because absorption after oral administration results in high blood concentrations, this is the route of choice for infections in the posterior globe and orbit. Despite controversial toxicity studies in cats, the drug has been used clinically over many years with few ill effects except anorexia and occasional pyrexia in some cats after systemic administration, provided that administration is not prolonged. Because of its wide spectrum of activity and intraocular penetration, chloramphenicol as an ointment or drops was widely used in veterinary practice for ocular surface injuries and infections, but its use is declining in favor of bactericidal antibiotics. Polymyxin B is often added to aid in control of gram-negative organisms, especially *Pseudomonas* spp. It is still useful in the topical treatment of suspected *Chlamydophila* infections in cats, although systemically administered drugs are preferable (see Chapter 7).

Table 3-10 | **Antibiotics of Choice for Common Organisms**

ORGANISM	DRUG OF CHOICE	ORGANISM	DRUG OF CHOICE
GRAM-POSITIVE COCCI		**FUNGI AND YEASTS**	
Staphylococcus spp.	Neomycin	*Fusarium* spp.	Natamycin
	Bacitracin		Thiabendazole
	Amoxicillin	*Aspergillus* spp.	Amphotericin B
	Cephalosporins		Ketoconazole
	Erythromycin		Itraconazole
	Fluoroquinolones		Flucytosine
Staphylococcus aureus	Gentamicin		Nystatin
	Oxacillin	*Candida* spp.	Nystatin
	Methicillin		Amphotericin B
	Cephalosporins		Flucytosine
	Fluoroquinolones		Ketoconazole
Staphyococcus epidermidis	Neomycin		Itraconazole
	Gentamicin	*Cryptococcus* spp.	Ketoconazole
	Erythromycin		Itraconazole
	Fluoroquinolones		Flucytosine
Streptococcus spp.	Penicillin	*Penicillium* spp.	Natamycin
	Chloramphenicol	*Blastomyces* and *Histoplasma* spp.	Ketoconazole
	Amoxicillin		Itraconazole
	Cephalosporins		Amphotericin B
		Microsporon spp.	Ketaconazole
GRAM-NEGATIVE COCCI		*Trichophyton* spp.	Itraconazole
Neisseria spp.	Penicillin	*Epidermophyton* spp.	Griseofulvin
	Tetracyclines		
	Sulfonamides (± trimethoprim)	**ACTINOMYCETES**	
		Actinomyces spp.	Penicillin
GRAM-POSITIVE RODS			Tetracyclines
Corynebacterium spp.	Penicillin	*Nocardia* spp.	Chloramphenicol
	Tetracyclines		(± streptomycin)
	Sulfonamides (± trimethoprim)		(± isoniazid)
GRAM-NEGATIVE RODS		**CHLAMYDIA**	
Pseudomonas aeruginosa	Polymixin B	*Chlamydia* and *Chlamydophila* spp.	Azithromycin
	Gentamicin		Doxycycline
	Tobramycin		Tetracyclines
	Amikacin		Chloramphenicol
	Fluoroquinolones		
Escherichia coli	Chloramphenicol	**MYCOPLASMA**	
	Tetracyclines	*Mycoplasma* spp.	Tetracyclines
	Gentamicin		Erythromycin
	Fluoroquinolones		Chloramphenicol
Enterobacter spp.	Amoxicillin (± streptomycin)		
Proteus spp.	Gentamicin		
	Fluoroquinolones		
	Tobramycin		
	Amikacin		
	Chloramphenicol		
Hemophilus spp.	Amoxicillin		
	Tetracyclines		
Moraxella spp.	Penicillin		
	Tetracyclines		

Aminoglycosides

Neomycin

Neomycin is a particularly useful bactericidal agent for ocular use and is active against gram-positive and gram-negative bacteria, including *Staphylococcus aureus*. Bacterial resistance develops less readily to neomycin than to streptomycin, and neomycin is more effective against *Proteus vulgaris* than is polymyxin B. Because of nephrotoxicity and ototoxicity, neomycin is administered only topically or by subconjunctival injection. Topical hypersensitivity to neomycin occasionally develops.

Gentamicin

Gentamicin (perhaps only because of its relatively low cost) has unfortunately been used frequently and indiscriminately as a topical agent of first choice for bacterial prophylaxis. Given its relatively narrow effective spectrum, and because this spectrum encompasses gram-negative organisms, which are not commonly found as part of the ocular surface flora, such use is questionable. As a result of this over-use, the value of gentamicin for treatment of more resistant organisms is now markedly diminished. Gentamicin is variably effective against many strains of *S. aureus, Pseudomonas* spp., *E. coli, Aerobacter, Klebsiella* spp., and *Proteus* spp. Topical application does not result in high intraocular concentrations, and although some drug enters the eye after subconjunctival or intravenous injection, vitreous penetration is poor regardless of route of administration. Long-term systemic therapy is limited by ototoxicity and nephrotoxicity. Gentamicin (like other aminoglycosides) causes cataract and severe retinal degeneration when injected intraocularly.

Tobramycin

Similar to gentamicin, tobramycin is effective against β-lactamase–producing staphylococci and is synergistic with carbenicillin in the treatment of resistant *Pseudomonas* infections. Resistance to tobramycin is less frequent, probably because of its more recent introduction. It is also ototoxic and nephrotoxic when given systemically but may be administered topically. The injectable form (but not the topical drug) may also be administered via subconjunctival injection.

Amikacin

Organisms that are resistant to gentamicin, neomycin, and tobramycin may be susceptible to amikacin. However, when other aminoglycosides are effective, amikacin has no advantage over them. Amikacin is ototoxic and nephrotoxic but may be administered topically and subconjunctivally. Its use should be restricted to *Pseudomonas* spp. and other bacteria resistant to alternate aminoglycosides. For *Pseudomonas* infections, a proposed order of choice for usage is neomycin, gentamicin, tobramycin, and amikacin.

Bacitracin

Bacitracin is effective against gram-positive organisms and is not inactivated by inflammatory exudates; bacterial resistance to it develops rarely. Bacitracin is used very frequently in combination with one or more agents effective against gram-negative organisms for surface infections of the lids, conjunctiva, and cornea and is particularly useful for staphylococcal blepharoconjunctivitis in dogs. Intraocular penetration after topical application is poor, and because of nephrotoxicity, bacitracin is not used systemically.

Polymyxin B

Polymyxin B is used largely because of its activity against *Pseudomonas* spp., which may cause rapid and devastating infections of the cornea in dogs, horses, and cats because of antibiotic resistance and protease production. Polymyxin B is also effective against *E. coli* but not against *Proteus* spp. Although this agent does not penetrate intact corneal epithelium significantly, corneal ulcers will allow therapeutic concentrations to be achieved in the stroma. Polymyxin B causes severe chemosis and necrosis after subconjunctival injection and should not be used via this route.

Tetracyclines

Tetracyclines are broad-spectrum bacteriostatic antibiotics; however, *Staphylococcus*, *Pseudomonas*, and *Proteus* spp. are usually resistant. Intraocular penetration is very poor regardless of route of administration. To avoid permanent dental discoloration, tetracyclines should not be administered systemically to young animals. Tetracyclines are useful in treatment of infections with *Chlamydophila* and *Mycoplasma* spp. in cats. Systemic administration to dogs affected with periocular staining from pigments in the tears results in a decrease in staining while the drug is being administered. Long-acting parenteral tetracycline preparations are effective for treatment of *Moraxella bovis* infection in cattle.

Azithromycin

Azithromycin is the first of a subclass of macrolide antibiotics termed *azalides*. It is characterized by high and prolonged tissue concentrations after oral administration and has been used for *Chlamydophila felis* infections in cats. However, results of a recent experimental study in specific pathogen-free cats suggest that although azithromycin and doxycycline both reduce chlamydophilal shedding and signs of infection in a similar manner, the duration of this effect on shedding is temporary with azithromycin. Azithromycin has also been suggested as a therapeutic agent for *Toxoplasma gondii*.

Sulfonamides

Although sulfonamides are bacteriostatic and act by blocking utilization of para-aminobenzoic acid (PABA) by bacteria, potential sulfonamides in more common use are bactericidal. Sulfonamides inhibit many gram-positive and some gram-negative organisms, including *Pseudomonas* spp. As a class, sulfonamides tend to have the same range of therapeutic action and exhibit mutual cross-resistance. Drugs that are esters of PABA (e.g., procaine, tetracaine) and purulent exudates that contain PABA interfere with the action of sulfonamides. The action of gentamicin against *Pseudomonas* spp. is inhibited by sulfacetamide. For all of these reasons, topically administered sulfonamides have largely been replaced by other topical antibiotics. Because other antibiotics are more effective for intraocular infection, systemic sulfonamides also are rarely indicated in ophthalmic therapy, with the possible exception of treatment of ocular toxoplasmosis. Several sulfonamides are confirmed causes of keratoconjunctivitis sicca in dogs, but tear production in horses is unaffected by these agents.

Fluoroquinolones

Fluoroquinolones are potent, bactericidal agents active against a broad range of bacterial pathogens. They exert their action by inhibiting DNA gyrase. Plasmids capable of transferring resistance to quinolone activity are now known, and resistance to fluoroquinolones by mutation has been demonstrated in numerous bacterial species. Fluoroquinolones are generally rapidly absorbed after oral administration, with peak serum concentrations reached in 30 to 60 minutes. Typical minimum inhibitory concentrations for commonly encountered organisms are presented in Table 3-11.

Enrofloxacin and Orbifloxacin

Enrofloxacin and orbifloxacin are similar agents. Enrofloxacin is metabolized to ciprofloxacin. Enrofloxacin enters the tears in inhibitory concentrations for most common pathogens. It is eliminated by glomerular filtration and biliary secretion. Both agents are useful for staphylococcal infections of the eyelids and orbital area but have limited effect against anaerobic bacteria often found in orbital cellulitis and abscesses. Because they disrupt cartilage synthesis, enrofloxacin and orbifloxacin are not typically recommended in dogs of the smaller breeds between 2 and 8 months of age, in larger breeds until 12 months of age, and in giant breeds until 18 months of age.

Retinal degeneration has been demonstrated after the clinical and experimental use of enrofloxacin in cats. Typically,

Table 3-11 | **Minimum Inhibitory Concentrations of Fluoroquinolones for Common Organisms**

	ENROFLOXACIN (µg/mL)	ORBIFLOXACIN (µg/mL)	CIPROFLOXACIN (µg/mL)
Staphylococcus spp.	0.125	0.195->25	3.13-50.0
Pseudomonas aeruginosa	0.5-8.0	0.39->25	2.0-4.0
Escherichia coli	0.016-0.031	0.012-6.25	>2.0
Proteus mirabilis	0.062-0.125	0.39-1.56	0.5-2.0

affected cats are presented for rapid vision loss with widely dilated pupils. No age, breed, or sex predilection has been determined, and no consistent underlying condition for which the enrofloxacin was prescribed has been identified. The single and cumulative doses of enrofloxacin incriminated and the duration of therapy before onset of blindness vary; however, in a published retrospective series, only one cat believed to be affected received less than 5 mg/kg once daily. Mydriasis is an early sign of toxicity in some animals. A striking feature of this toxicity is the rapidity with which funduscopic evidence of retinal degeneration (tapetal hyperreflectivity and retinal vascular attenuation, sometimes with mottling of the nontapetal fundus) appears to occur. In some cases retinal degeneration is advanced at presentation, sometimes within days of starting the drug. No evidence of pain or inflammation is noted, and no treatment is possible other than cessation of the drug. The extent to which vision is regained is variable but usually minimal. Histopathology of affected retinas has revealed outer retinal degeneration, with diffuse loss of the outer nuclear and photoreceptor layers, and hypertrophy and proliferation of the retinal pigment epithelium. Electro-retinographic abnormalities have also been demonstrated. At present, enrofloxacin dosage in cats should not exceed 5 mg/kg daily, and this dose may be best divided. It is important to note that enrofloxacin is not licensed in the United States for parenteral use in cats.

Ciprofloxacin, Ofloxacin, and Others

An increasing array of topical ophthalmic fluoroquinolone solutions is becoming available. Some recent additions are ciprofloxacin, ofloxacin, norfloxacin, levofloxacin, gatifloxacin, and moxifloxacin. These drugs are especially valuable in mixed or virulent surface infections, especially deep or rapidly progressive corneal ulcers. They should be used only until bacterial sensitivity results are available, and definitely not for general prophylaxis against surface infection. All of these topical fluoroquinolones penetrate through the cornea, even when the epithelium is intact, and are found in the aqueous humor after topical instillation of drops.

ANTIFUNGAL DRUGS

Important ophthalmic fungal infections may be considered in the following three categories:

- Infections of the eyelids and surrounding skin
- Intraocular infection (usually endophthalmitis) associated with penetrating foreign bodies or systemic mycoses, such as cryptococcosis, blastomycosis, histoplasmosis, and coccidioidomycosis
- Mycotic keratitis following corneal penetration or ulceration

Fungal infections of the eyelids and surrounding skin are treated with the same therapeutic agents as used for dermato-mycoses; the reader should refer to Chapter 6 of this text and a dermatology text for current diagnostic and therapeutic approaches. Table 3-12 lists the major antifungal drugs used in the treatment of the systemic mycoses in veterinary medicine, along with their predicted spectra and penetration of various tissues. The following section discusses some of these agents commonly used for treatment of patients with fungal endophthalmitis or keratitis.

Natamycin

Natamycin is the only commercially available antifungal agent formulated and licensed in the United States for topical ophthalmic use, although it is expensive. It is available as a 5% ophthalmic suspension, which is viscous but will pass through ocular lavage systems in the horse without causing obstruction. It is effective against a broad variety of fungi, including *Candida, Aspergillus, Cephalosporium, Fusarium,* and *Penicillium* spp.

Azoles

Itraconazole, ketoconazole, fluconazole, voriconazole, clotrimazole, and miconazole are members of the azole group. They are especially useful for the treatment of systemic and ocular *Cryptococcus* spp. and *Coccidioides immitis* infections. Side effects in dogs include inappetence, pruritus, alopecia, and reversible lightening of the hair coat. In cats, anorexia, fever, depression, and diarrhea may occur. Long-term therapy, up to 6 months or longer, may be necessary because the drugs are fungistatic. Most azoles do not cross the blood-ocular barriers well. The exceptions are fluconazole and voriconazole. In horses administered an oral loading dose of fluconazole (14 mg/kg) followed by a daily maintenance dose (5 mg/kg) for 10 days, drug concentrations in the aqueous humor exceeded the minimum inhibitory concentration (MIC) for many fungi (although some studies suggest that *Aspergillus* spp. are relatively resistant to fluconazole). By contrast, itraconazole was not detected in the aqueous humor after oral or intravenous administration in horses.

The intravenous forms of miconazole and fluconazole have been administered topically in some horses, and some practitioners choose vaginal miconazole preparations (without alcohol) for topical corneal use. A compounded formulation of itraconazole with dimethyl sulfoxide ointment has been shown to penetrate the cornea well and was effective in resolving keratomycosis in 80% of horses treated in the northeastern United States. Finally, there are recent data showing that topically applied voriconazole (1%) is well tolerated, penetrates the cornea very well, and achieves therapeutic concentrations in the aqueous humor.

Flucytosine

Flucytosine has activity against *Cryptococcus, Aspergillus,* and *Candida* spp. and is known to cross the blood-brain barrier in

Table 3-12 | **Antifungal Agents Used in the Treatment of Systemic Mycoses**

CLASS	DRUG NAME/FORMULATION/ MANUFACTURER	PHARMACOLOGY	INDICATIONS
Echinocandins	Caspofungin/intravenous/Merck	Metab: liver Elim: bile/feces RF*: No change CNS[†]: <10% Abs: none	Patients refractory to or intolerant of amphotericin B or Itraconazole B or Itraconazole
Pyrimidines	Flucytosine/oral/ICN	Metab: none Elim: renal RF*: reduce dose CNS[†]: 75% Abs: 90%	Azole resistance, infections caused by *Candida* spp. or *Cryptococcus* spp.
Azoles	Fluconazole/oral or intravenous/generic	Metab: liver Elim: renal RF*: reduce dose CNS[†]: >60% Abs: 90%	Infections caused by *Candida* spp. or *Cryptococcus* spp.,[‡] with CNS involvement
	Itraconazole/oral or intravenous/Janssen	Metab: GI/liver Elim: feces/bile RF*: reduce dose CNS[†]: <10% Abs: 10%-20% capsules 50% oral solution	*Coccidioides,*[‡] *Aspergillus,* nonmeningeal *Blastomyces* or *Histoplasma,*[‡] intolerance to amphotericin B
	Ketoconazole/oral/generic	Metab: GI/liver Elim: bile/feces RF*: none CNS[†]: <10% Abs: 75%	*Candida, Blastomyces, Histoplasma, Chromomyces* spp.
	Voriconazole/oral or intravenous/Pfizer	Metab: GI/liver Elim: bile/feces RF*: none CNS[†]: 75% Abs: 96%	Acute or refractory *Aspergillus,*[‡] *Candida krusei, Candida glabrata,*[‡] *Scedosporium,* and *Fusarium*
Polyenes	Amphotericin B deoxycholate/ intravenous/Geneva	Metab: none Elim: bile/feces RF*: reduce dose CNS[†]: <10% Abs: none	Life-threatening infections due to *Aspergillus, Blastomyces, Candida, Coccidioides, Cryptococcus, Histoplasma, Sporotrix, Zygomyces*
	Amphotericin B colloidal dispersion/ intravenous/Intermune	Metab: none Elim: bile/feces RF*: reduce dose CNS[†]: <10% Abs: none	As above. Use in patients with RF or toxicity to amphotericin B deoxycholate.
	Amphotericin B lipid complex/ intravenous/Elan	Metab: none Elim: bile/feces RF*: reduce dose CNS[†]: <10% Abs: none	As above
	Liposomal amphotericin B/ intravenous/Fujisawa	Metab: none Elim: bile/feces RF*: reduce dose CNS[†]: <10% *(CNS penetration may be greater than others)* Abs: none	As above. Use in those patients with refractory disease, with intolerance to above, or with CNS involvement.

From Wiebe V, Karriker M (2005): Therapy of systemic fungal infections: a pharmacologic perspective. Clin Tech Small Anim Pract 20:250.
Abs, Oral bioavailability; *CNS,* central nervous system; *Elim,* elimination; *GI,* gastrointestinal; *Metab,* metabolism; *RF,* renal failure.
*Dose adjustment required in RF.
[†]Percent of plasma concentration in CNS.
[‡]Fungal disease in which the listed agent is the drug of choice.

reasonable concentrations. It likely does cross the blood-ocular barriers as well. It has been used in combination with ketoconazole for treatment of feline endophthalmitis and meningitis due to *Cryptococcus* spp.

Amphotericin B

Amphotericin B may be used topically, subconjunctivally, or parenterally. It has a wide range of activity against fungi but is also toxic to host cells. Because of systemic toxicity and the serious nature of lesions for which it is used, amphotericin B should be used only in institutions in which adequate supportive care and laboratory monitoring are available. More recently lipid-complex formulations have been developed that reduce toxicity. Amphotericin is used for treatment of systemic infections with *Histoplasma, Blastomyces, Cryptococcus,* and *Coccidioides* spp.

ANTIVIRAL DRUGS

The use of antiviral drugs in veterinary ophthalmology is restricted to treatment of herpetic keratoconjunctivitis due to feline herpesvirus (FHV-1) in cats or, occasionally, equine herpesvirus (EHV-2) in horses. Systemically administered antiviral agents can be associated with significant toxicity and must be used with caution. In addition, all currently available antiviral agents are virostatic, and most penetrate the cornea poorly. Therefore all currently available antiviral agents require frequent topical application to be effective. Therapeutic effects are best achieved by applying solutions every 2 hours. Clearly this frequency is impossible in many veterinary situations; however, very frequent application of ointments or solutions (at least 5 or 6 times daily) should be the goal. Therapy is continued until active inflammation and ulceration disappear. Herpetic keratitis is resistant to cure in some individuals, and no antiviral agent has been proven to act against latent FHV-1 in the trigeminal ganglia. Recurrences are therefore common and should be expected in susceptible animals. A number of agents have been tested in vitro against FHV-1 and have shown marked variability in potency (Table 3-13). Idoxuridine and vidarabine are often preferred in feline herpetic keratitis because of cost and efficacy and because they are well tolerated by most cats. None of the agents has proven activity against other feline viruses.

Table 3-13 | **Relative In Vitro Potency of Select Antiviral Agents against Feline Herpesvirus**

ANTIVIRAL DRUG	ED_{50} (mm)
Trifluridine	0.67
Ganciclovir	5.2
Idoxuridine	4.3-6.8
Cidofovir	11.0
Penciclovir	13.9
Vidarabine	21.4
Acyclovir	57.9-85.6
Foscarnet	232.9

Data from Nasisse MP, et al. (1989): In vitro susceptibility of feline herpesvirus-1 to vidarabine, idoxuridine, trifluridine, acyclovir, or bromovinyldeoxyuridine. Am J Vet Res 50:158; and Maggs DJ, Clarke HE (2004): In vitro efficacy of ganciclovir, cidofovir, penciclovir, foscarnet, idoxuridine, and acyclovir against feline herpesvirus type-1. Am J Vet Res 65:399.
ED_{50}, Effective dose$_{50}$ (or the in vitro concentration that is associated with suppression of viral growth to 50% of that seen without drug).

Idoxuridine

Idoxuridine is chemically similar to thymidine, one of the constituents of nucleic acids, which it replaces during DNA synthesis, thereby inhibiting viral replication. Idoxuridine is no longer commercially available in North America but can be compounded as a 0.1% solution or 0.5% ointment. It penetrates the intact cornea poorly after topical application but is generally well tolerated by cats. It must be applied at least 5 times daily.

Trifluridine (Trifluorothymidine)

Trifluridine inhibits DNA polymerase and thymidine synthetase and is the most active agent against feline herpesvirus in vitro. In humans with herpetic keratitis the dosage recommended is 1 drop applied every 2 hours until reepithelialization occurs, then every 4 hours for another 7 days. An effect should be seen within 7 days. Obviously this dosage is often impractical in animals. Like other antiviral agents, though, trifluridine should be used at least 5 times daily. Trifluridine may be extremely irritating to cats, and it tends to be the most expensive agent when purchased in its commercial form. These factors make it a less viable choice despite its antiviral efficacy.

Vidarabine

Vidarabine interferes with viral DNA synthesis, and is moderately active against FHV-1 replication in vitro. It is usually well tolerated when applied topically as an ointment.

Acyclovir and Valacyclovir

Acyclovir is widely available as a systemic drug but in some countries is also available in a topical (ophthalmic) preparation. The in vitro efficacy of acyclovir against FHV-1 is low. This feature is compounded by relatively low bioavailability after oral dosing in cats. Finally, cats receiving acyclovir sometimes show toxic adverse effects. Taken together, this combination of features makes acyclovir an unsatisfactory drug for the treatment of FHV-1 in cats. Doses as high as 100 mg/kg in cats failed to achieve plasma acyclovir concentrations that approximated those shown to be effective against FHV-1 in vitro, and yet produced clinical evidence of toxicity in some cats. The principal toxic effects seen in cats are leukopenia and anemia. Although normalization of complete blood count (CBC) values usually accompanies withdrawal of acyclovir therapy and appropriate supportive care, toxicity significantly limits use of this drug for treatment of FHV-1 in cats.

Valacyclovir is absorbed more readily than is acyclovir and then is metabolized to acyclovir. Unfortunately, this enhanced bioavailability is associated with fatal hepatic and renal necrosis in cats, and valacyclovir must not be used in cats.

Idoxuridine and vidarabine are the preferred topical antiviral agents for cats infected with FHV-1. Acyclovir is ineffective, and valacyclovir is toxic.

CORTICOSTEROIDS

Although frequently misused with disastrous results, corticosteroids are among the clinician's most useful and powerful drugs, with specific properties, indications, and contra-indications that must be understood.

The following are good general rules to help govern ophthalmic use of corticosteroids:

- Corticosteroids must not be used topically or subconjunctivally when fluorescein indicates a corneal epithelial defect.
- Corticosteroids should not be used unless a diagnosis has been made and a specific immunologic or inflammatory response is to be inhibited.
- Every "red" eye should be stained with fluorescein and its IOP should be measured before indiscriminate therapy with corticosteroids is initiated.
- For nonulcerative corneal disease or intraocular disease, a penetrating topical corticosteroid such as prednisolone or dexamethasone must be administered. Hydrocortisone does not penetrate the cornea.
- For inflammatory disorders of the eyelids, posterior segment, optic nerve, or orbit, corticosteroids must be administered systemically, not topically.

Properties of Corticosteroids

Prostaglandins are formed from arachidonic acid via the cyclo-oxygenase and lipoxygenase pathways in response to irritating or immunologic stimuli (Figure 3-7). When prostaglandins are released intraocularly, they cause miosis, a rise in aqueous humor protein concentration, vasodilation within the conjunctiva and iris, and a very transient rise in IOP, followed by a more lasting lowering of IOP. Corticosteroids induce production of an inhibitor of phospholipase A_2 and therefore act on both the cyclooxygenase and lipoxygenase pathways, whereas nonsteroidal antiinflammatory drugs (NSAIDs) inhibit just the cyclooxygenase pathway (see Figure 3-7). At a physiologic level corticosteroids decrease cellular and fibrinous exudation, inhibit degranulation of mast cells, decrease release of inflammatory mediators including prostaglandins, inhibit fibroblastic and collagen-forming activity, retard epithelial and endothelial regeneration and repair, diminish postinflammatory neovascularization, inhibit humoral and cell-mediated immune responses, and tend to restore normal permeability to inflamed capillaries. As such, they can cause devastating progression of some ocular diseases, especially those with an infectious component. However, they are particularly useful in treating ocular disease when correctly used, because severe or chronic inflammation that would be desirable in other organs and tissues (e.g., fibrous tissue formation and contraction, neovascularization, infiltration with inflammatory cells) may be particularly damaging in the eye if allowed to proceed unchecked.

Perhaps the most important ocular indication for corticosteroids is the control of inflammation that accompanies immune-mediated ocular diseases, such as lens-induced uveitis, chronic superficial keratitis ("pannus"), nodular granulomatous episcleritis (NGE), and uveodermatologic (Vogt-Koyanagi-Harada–like [VKH-like]) syndrome. It is essential to appreciate that these ocular diseases are like immune-mediated disease elsewhere—that is, they tend to have a waxing-waning course and are often recurrent, with each episode doing more permanent

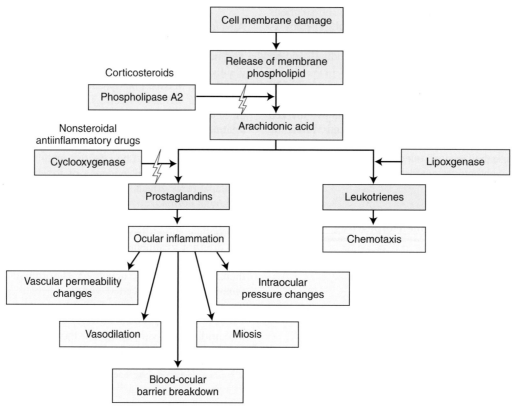

Figure 3-7. The arachidonic acid cascade and effects on ocular structures. Corticosteroids inhibit phospholipase A_2 and therefore both arms of the inflammatory cascade. Nonsteroidal antiinflammatory drugs inhibit the cyclooxygenase pathway only. (Modified from Giuliano EA [2004]: Nonsteroidal anti-inflammatory drugs in veterinary ophthalmology. Vet Clin North Am Small Anim Pract 34:708.)

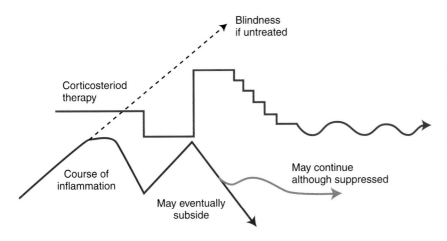

Figure 3-8. The course of chronic/recurrent intraocular or ocular surface inflammation can be modified by antiinflammatory therapy. The diagram illustrates control by treatment, relapse with tapering of treatment, control by more intense treatment, and, finally, quiescence. (Modified from Gordon D [1959]: The treatment of chronic uveitis: preliminary comments on chronic degenerative diseases. Arch Ophthalmol 62:400.)

damage to the globe (Figure 3-8). Severe ophthalmic inflammation, no matter how brief, or chronic inflammation, even if mild, often results in loss of vision and must be treated vigorously if irreparable damage is to be averted. In these diseases a rapid diagnosis must be made, corticosteroid therapy begun early, clinical signs of inflammation monitored closely, and therapy tapered slowly to avoid progression. If the clinical effect is less than desired, it is often better to increase the frequency of dosage rather than changing the concentration of the drug.

Corticosteroids reduce resistance to many microorganisms and should not be used in their presence without coincident use of an effective antimicrobial agent. Accurate differential diagnosis is essential whenever steroids are used. In addition to potentiating microbial infection corticosteroids increase the activity of proteases present in corneal ulcers by up to 13 times, often resulting in rapid collagenolysis ("melting") of the cornea with rupture of the globe and prolapse of the ocular contents. Likewise, although inhibition of collagen formation and fibroblastic activity by corticosteroids is useful in reducing corneal scarring, it may be detrimental to the healing of surgical wounds, requiring that suture removal be delayed. Ocular discharge or pain in any patient undergoing corticosteroid treatment requires immediate cessation of the corticosteroid and a prompt and complete ophthalmic examination.

Topically administered corticosteroids also are known to elevate IOP. This issue has been most closely investigated in humans, in whom a familial susceptibility to ocular hypertension from topical dexamethasone use is noted. Small increases in IOP also have been recorded experimentally in beagles with inherited open-angle glaucoma and in cats in response to topical corticosteroids, but clinically significant complications resulting from such pressure elevations have not been reported.

Ocular Penetration of Corticosteroids

Dexamethasone, betamethasone, prednisolone, prednisone, triamcinolone, and hydrocortisone are used commonly in veterinary ocular therapy. A variety of other corticosteroids used in human ophthalmic therapy because they are less likely to raise IOP are not widely used in veterinary ophthalmology. Corticosteroids penetrate the cornea to varying extents when applied topically. Factors affecting the penetration and effect of a corticosteroid are as follows:

- The salt used: Acetates are more lipid-soluble and penetrate the cornea better than succinates or phosphates.
- Frequency of application: More frequent application results in higher intraocular concentration.
- Concentration of the drug: Low concentrations of a highly potent steroid may have less antiinflammatory effect than a high concentration of a less potent steroid; for instance, topical 1.0% prednisolone has an antiinflammatory effect similar to that of 0.1% dexamethasone, although dexamethasone has a greater ocular antiinflammatory potency than prednisolone (see Figure 3-2).
- Proximity to the site of inflammation: The route of administration is chosen in relation to the intended site of action (see Figure 3-1). Inflammation of the cornea, conjunctiva, or anterior uvea is usually treated topically with a penetrating corticosteroid, or occasionally with subconjunctival injection. Systemic therapy is required if involvement of adnexal, posterior uveal, retinal, optic nerve, or orbital tissues is suspected. The retrobulbar route is also effective for disorders of the choroid, retina, optic nerve, and orbit but is rarely used.

For most ocular disorders topical administration of 1.0% prednisolone or 0.1% dexamethasone is advised. Hydrocortisone, a low-potency corticosteroid, does not penetrate the cornea in any meaningful quantities. This feature renders it useless for intraocular or deep corneal disease. Its availability only in combination with three antibiotics in commercial preparations makes it an even less appropriate choice for most surface eye disease of dogs, cats, and horses.

Most injectable steroids are suitable for subconjunctival use, with periods of activity varying from 7 to 10 days (triamcinolone, dexamethasone) to 2 to 4 weeks (methylprednisolone). Care must be taken with repository forms given subconjunctivally because they may leave unsightly and sometimes inflamed subconjunctival plaques requiring surgical removal. Repository corticosteroids also have the distinct disadvantage that they cannot be removed if the disease process changes.

Long-Term Therapy

Unlike with the human eye, long-term topical therapy with corticosteroids does not predispose the canine eye to glaucoma or cataract. Occasional statements that such treatment results in fungal superinfection (infection with unusual organisms) are not supported by research evidence. However, long-term topical usage in dogs may cause increases in liver enzymes and, especially in smaller dogs, adrenal suppression, and these effects should be taken into account in interpretation of laboratory tests and in management of patients with hepatic or endocrine disorders. Perhaps the most common clinical scenario in which the systemic effects of a topically applied corticosteroid may be important is the treatment of lens-induced uveitis due to cataracts in diabetic dogs. Although serious clinical disturbances due to such treatment occur infrequently, the lowest concentration and frequency that produce the desired clinical effect should be used, or an NSAID considered. In particularly susceptible animals on continuous therapy, occasional laboratory evaluation should be considered.

Long-term use of topical corticosteroids may cause reversible adrenocortical suppression or may disrupt management of diabetes mellitus. Clinical consequences in otherwise healthy patients are rare.

General Indications for Corticosteroid Use

General indications for use of corticosteroids are as follows:

- Immune-mediated ocular disorders (seasonal allergic conjunctivitis, drug and contact allergies, chronic superficial keratitis or "pannus," eosinophilic keratoconjunctivitis, episcleritis, some cases of keratoconjunctivitis sicca, lens-induced uveitis, uveodermatologic (VKH-like) syndrome, etc.)
- Traumatic conditions resulting in severe inflammation (proptosis of the globe, contusion with hyphema)
- Anterior uveitis
- Postoperative immunomodulation (e.g., after corneal transplant or cataract extraction)
- Reduction of postoperative swelling and inflammation after cryosurgery (e.g., cyclocryotherapy or cryoepilation for distichiasis or eyelid tumors)

NONSTEROIDAL ANTIINFLAMMATORY DRUGS

Numerous NSAIDs have an important place in ophthalmology because of their potency, the destructive ocular effects of uncontrolled inflammation, and the sometimes undesirable effects of corticosteroids. NSAIDs inhibit the cyclooxygenase pathway but not the lipoxygenase pathway; therefore they tend to be less potent than corticosteroids. Carprofen, which inhibits cyclooxygenase-2, represents the newer class of more selective cyclooxygenase inhibitors that are claimed to have fewer and lesser deleterious effects on prostaglandin synthesis in the gastrointestinal tract and kidneys. The original systemic agents used for ocular disorders in animals were acetylsalicylic acid (aspirin), and flunixin meglumine. Although flunixin is not approved by the U.S. Food and Drug Administration (FDA) for use in dogs, there are a number of studies describing its use in this species.

Many NSAIDs are available for human use, but, because of severe side effects, caution must be used in extrapolating their systemic use to animals. For example, ibuprofen, naproxen, and indomethacin should not be used systemically. Recently carprofen, ketoprofen, piroxicam, meloxicam, deracoxib, and etodolac have become available for veterinary use, typically for uveitis or postoperative analgesia. Systemic nonsteroidal drugs inhibit disruption of the blood-ocular barriers (aspirin and flunixin, 70% to 80%; dexamethasone and flunixin, 61%; aspirin, 50%; carprofen, 71%). Etodolac has similar ophthalmic uses but also causes keratoconjunctivitis sicca in some dogs. When given orally these drugs sometimes result in gastric ulceration and hemorrhage. This effect is not related to hydrochloric acid production per se, and cimetidine has not been proven to have a protective effect in dogs. However, the ulcerogenic effects of orally administered NSAIDs may be reduced by the concomitant oral administration of misoprostol. All drugs in the NSAID class should be used with caution and never in association with systemic corticosteroids.

Topical NSAIDs, including indomethacin, flurbiprofen, suprofen, diclofenac, and ketorolac, are available and may be used in place of topical corticosteroids, compared with which they appear to be slightly less potent but also less likely to inhibit would healing. They are used for the same conditions that corticosteroids would be but may be preferred in diabetic or cushingoid patients owing to their lack of systemic adrenocortical effects. Topical NSAIDs inhibit breakdown of the blood-aqueous barrier by 80% to 99% in research studies. Clinical use of NSAIDs is summarized in Table 3-14.

IMMUNOMODULATING THERAPY (IMMUNOSUPPRESSANTS AND IMMUNOSTIMULANTS)

Various drugs are used to modulate (upregulate or downregulate) the host immune response. A complete discussion of these agents is beyond the scope of this book, and only those currently used for specific ocular disorders in animals are referred to.

Azathioprine

Azathioprine is an antimetabolite and T-cell suppressor used to treat severe immune-mediated diseases of dogs in which an infectious organism is not suspected, such as uveodermatologic syndrome (VKH-like syndrome), serous retinal detachments, nodular granulomatous episcleritis, and optic neuritis. It may be used alone or in combination with corticosteroids if they have failed when used alone. The immunosuppressive effects of azathioprine may not be evident or complete until 3 to 5 weeks after initiation of therapy, and additional agents may be necessary during this period. The recommended initial dose for most immune-mediated disorders in dogs is 2 mg/kg daily. This should be tapered at about 1 week to 0.5 to 1 mg/kg every second day, and reduced again to 1 mg/kg once weekly as soon as clinical signs permit it. Lower doses and shorter durations may be used if responses are rapid. Plasma hepatic enzyme concentrations, total white blood cell count, and platelet count should be monitored every 2 weeks for the first 8 weeks, then at least monthly during therapy. Elevations of liver enzymes may occur, especially if corticosteroids are used concurrently. This drug is less safe in cats, for which alternatives should be sought.

Cyclosporine

Cyclosporine suppresses production of the lymphokine interleukin-2 by helper T lymphocytes and enhances function

Table 3-14 | **Clinical Use of Nonsteroidal Antiinflammatory Drugs**

DRUG	SPECIES	INDICATION	DOSE, ROUTE, FREQUENCY
Carprofen	Dog	Surgical	≤ 4.0 mg/kg IV, SC, IM once at induction
		Antiinflammatory	≤ 2.2 mg/kg PO q12-24h PRN
	Cat	Surgical	≤ 4.0 mg/kg SC lean weight once at induction
	Horse	Antiinflammatory	0.7 mg/kg IV, PO q12-24h PRN
Flunixin meglumine	Dog	Surgical	0.25-1.0 mg/kg IV, SC, IM q12-24h for 1-2 treatments
	Cat	Surgical	0.25 mg/kg SC q12-24h for 1-2 treatments
	Horse	Antiinflammatory	1.1 mg/kg IV, IM, PO q12-24 h
Meloxicam	Dog	Surgical	≤ 0.2 mg/kg IV, SC once
			≤ 0.1 mg/kg IV, SC, PO q12-24h thereafter
		Antiinflammatory	≤ 0.2 mg/kg PO once
			≤ 0.1 mg/kg PO q24h thereafter
	Cat	Surgical	≤ 0.2 mg/kg SC, PO once
			≤ 0.1 mg/kg SC, PO lean body weight q2-3d
		Antiinflammatory	≤ 0.2 mg/kg SC, PO once
			≤ 0.1 mg/kg SC, PO lean body weight q2-3d
	Horse	Antiinflammatory	0.6 mg/kg IV q12-24h
Ketoprofen	Dog	Surgical	≤ 2.0 mg/kg IV, IM, SC, PO once
			≤ 1.0 mg/kg q24h thereafter
		Antiinflammatory	≤ 2.0 mg/kg PO once
			≤ 1.0 mg/kg q24h thereafter
	Cat	Surgical	≤ 2.0 mg/kg SC once
			≤ 1.0 mg/kg PO q24h thereafter
		Antiinflammatory	≤ 2.0 mg/kg PO once
			≤ 1.0 mg/kg PO q24h thereafter
	Horse	Antiinflammatory	2.2 mg/kg IV, IM q12-24h
Phenylbutazone	Dog	Antiinflammatory	10-14 mg/kg PO q8-12h
	Horse	Antiinflammatory	2.2-4.4 mg/kg IV, PO q12-24h
Aspirin	Dog	Antiinflammatory, antithrombotic	10 mg/kg q12h PO
	Cat	Antiinflammatory, antithrombotic	10-20 mg/kg q48-72h PO
	Horse	Antiinflammatory, antithrombotic	17 mg/kg q48h PO
Ketorolac	Dog	Surgical	0.3-0.5 mg/kg IV, IM
	Cat	Surgical	0.25 mg/kg IM q12h for 1-2 treatments
Etodolac	Dog	Antiinflammatory	≤ 15 mg/kg PO q24h
Deracoxib	Dog	Antiinflammatory	≤ 4 mg/kg PO q24h

Data from Davidson G (1999): Etodolac. Compend Contin Educ Pract Vet 21:494; Fox SM, Johnson SA (1997): Use of carprofen for the treatment of pain and inflammation in dogs. J Am Vet Med Assoc 210:1493; Hulse D (1998): Treatment methods for pain in the osteoarthritic patient. Vet Clin North Am Small Anim Pract 28:361; Mathews KA (2002): Non-steroidal anti-inflammatory analgesics: a review of current practice. J Vet Emerg Crit Care 12:89; Moses VS, Bertone AL (2002): Nonsteroidal anti-inflammatory drugs. Vet Clin North Am Equine Pract 18:21; and Smith SA (2003): Deracoxib. Compend Contin Educ Pract Vet 25:419.

This information is compiled without regard to regulatory approval for use of these drugs, which varies by country. It is the individual clinician's responsibility to determine the conditions for appropriate use in a particular patient. Because of the incidence of gastrointestinal and renal side effects with this group of drugs, care is necessary in their use.

of suppressor T lymphocytes. Cyclosporine affects both cell-mediated immunity and, possibly, humoral immunity by inhibition of helper T cells but does not affect epithelial wound healing. When applied topically it penetrates the eye poorly and is not useful via this route for treatment of intraocular inflammation. However, topical application is used for moderating immune responses involving the lacrimal gland, conjunctiva, cornea, and sclera. It is used for treatment of keratoconjunctivitis sicca, corneal graft rejection, autoimmune keratitis (especially "pannus"), and immune-mediated episclerokeratoconjunctivitis. Intraocular concentrations are achieved with the use of intravitreous or suprachoroidal implants. These devices have been used successfully for the treatment of equine recurrent uveitis in selected individuals.

Cyclosporine's most important ophthalmic use is in treatment of canine keratoconjunctivitis sicca. It reduces autoimmune destruction of the lacrimal gland and gland of the third eyelid (with spontaneous regeneration of these glands while treatment is continued) and directly reduces keratoconjunctivitis. The drug is also directly lacrimogenic. Finally, cyclosporine directly stimulates canine conjunctival goblet cells to secrete mucin, possibly accounting for some of its therapeutic effect in canine keratoconjunctivitis sicca and qualitative tear film disturbances. For all of these seasons, it is the most frequently used drug for canine keratoconjunctivitis sicca. Cyclosporine is absorbed systemically after topical administration in dogs, and although depressed cell-mediated immunity can be demonstrated by lymphocyte stimulation indices, clinically relevant immunosuppression has not been reported. The drug is applied as a 1% or 2% solution in corn, canola, or olive oil, or as a 0.2% ointment. An aqueous preparation can be compounded. Cyclosporine is also used orally for the treatment of canine atopic dermatitis, including blepharitis.

Tacrolimus

The mechanism of action of tacrolimus is similar to that of cyclosporine, in that it reduces T-cell activation by inhibiting calcineurin-dependent activation of lymphokine expression, apoptosis, and degranulation. However, the intracellular receptors for tacrolimus and cyclosporine are different, leading some veterinary ophthalmologists to use tacrolimus when cyclosporine is not effective for the treatment of keratoconjunctivitis in dogs. A 0.02% aqueous suspension was recently investigated in a double-masked study of 105 dogs with keratoconjunctivitis sicca. Dogs naïve to tear stimulation therapy, dogs maintained successfully on cyclosporine therapy, and dogs unresponsive to cyclosporine therapy were all included. Twice-daily tacrolimus administration was continued for 6 to 8 weeks. Schirmer tear test results improved by 5 mm/min in more than 85% of dogs never treated before and in 51% of dogs whose disease was unresponsive to cyclosporine.

In March 2005 the FDA issued a public health advisory to inform health care providers and patients about a potential cancer risk (lymphoma and "skin cancer") associated with the commercial topical (dermatologic) preparation of tacrolimus for human use. This issue may be relevant to topical (ophthalmic) veterinary use. The FDA's concern was based on information from animal studies, case reports in a small number of patients, and how drugs of this class work. The FDA estimates that it may take human studies of 10 years or more in duration to determine whether use of tacrolimus is linked to cancer. In the meantime the agency advises that tacrolimus should be used only as labeled and for patients whose disease is unresponsive to or who are intolerant of other treatments. The FDA also recommends avoiding use of tacrolimus in children younger than 2 years, using tacrolimus only for short periods of time rather than continuously, and using the minimum amount needed to control the patient's symptoms. Owners of veterinary patients should be advised of these guidelines and to wear gloves when applying this medication. Additionally, tacrolimus and cyclosporine are currently not recommended for patients with active feline herpesvirus infection.

Immunostimulants

Nonspecific immune stimulants are sometimes used with variable results to treat ocular neoplasia. Perhaps the most widely used is live bacille Calmette-Guérin (BCG) vaccine or cell wall extracts of the same organism for the treatment of periocular equine sarcoid. Extracts of other organisms that stimulate the reticuloendothelial system, nonspecific immunostimulants, and staphylococcal bacterins have also been used on occasions for ophthalmic conditions, but little is published regarding their use.

MAST CELL STABILIZERS AND ANTIHISTAMINES

Medications that stabilize mast cells are used topically to prevent release of histamine and other mediators of inflammation in humans. They have received less use in veterinary patients; however, some veterinarians recommend their use in patients with seasonal allergic conjunctivitis or eosinophilic keratoconjunctivitis, usually in association with topical corticosteroids. Examples of mast cell stabilizers are sodium cromoglycate, olopatadine, and lodoxamide.

Antihistamines are little used in ocular therapy. Systemic antihistamines may be of some use in acute allergic conjunctivitis; however, contact dermatitis and conjunctivitis, especially of the drug-induced variety, are not histamine-mediated. In almost all ocular disorders for which antihistamines have been advocated, corticosteroid or immunosuppressive therapy is more effective.

HYPEROSMOTIC AGENTS

A hyperosmotic agent increases the osmotic concentration of blood perfusing the eye when administered systemically or of the tear film when applied topically. Because of the corneal epithelial and blood-ocular barriers, little or no osmotic agent enters the aqueous humor or vitreous, and the osmotic gradient created causes withdrawal of water from the eye to the vascular system or tears. Systemic administration of osmotic agents therefore causes reduction of vitreous volume. This, in turn, reduces IOP, both directly and via posterior movement of the lens, which reduces pupillary block and increases aqueous humor outflow facility via opening of the iridocorneal angle and ciliary cleft (see Chapter 12). Mannitol is the most commonly used systemic agent. Other osmotic agents, such as urea, glycerol, and isosorbide, were used in the past but are not used now because they lower IOP less effectively, cause tissue necrosis after perivascular leakage (urea), or cause emesis (glycerol). Osmotic drugs are applied topically to clear or reduce corneal edema. Hypertonic (5%) sodium chloride is the commonly used topical agent.

Mannitol

Mannitol is a vegetable sugar that is not metabolized and is excreted in the urine, causing osmotic diuresis. However, diuresis is not the cause of reduced IOP. Mannitol is not absorbed after oral administration and therefore must be administered intravenously. After intravenous administration IOP typically falls within 30 to 60 minutes and remains low for 5 to 6 hours. Mannitol increases serum osmolality and stimulates thirst, but if the ophthalmic effect is to be maintained, water intake must be controlled by providing small amounts of water or ice cubes. Mannitol is not used for long-term treatment of glaucoma and should not be used in animals with chronic renal failure or congestive heart failure. For acute glaucoma 1 to 2 g/kg mannitol should be administered intravenously over 10 to 20 minutes. This can be used in conjunction with an oral or topical carbonic anhydrase inhibitor and a topical miotic agent such as pilocarpine (or, more recently, a synthetic prostaglandin analogue), because these agents are synergistic.

Topical Hyperosmotic Sodium Chloride

Sodium chloride prepared as 5% ointment or solution can be used for reduction of corneal edema as seen in bullous keratopathy, superficial corneal erosion, and endothelial dysfunction. In patients with more advanced corneal edema the goal of therapy should be not clearing of the corneal opacity but rather reduction of epithelial bullae. Responses are somewhat limited by the short time such applications alter tear osmolality. Therefore frequent application is necessary. Because of duration of effect, ointments are usually more successful and appear to be less irritating.

AUTONOMIC DRUGS

Many important diagnostic and therapeutic drugs used in ophthalmology act on ocular structures with autonomic innervation. The autonomic nervous system is divided into parasympathetic and sympathetic components, with antagonistic but not necessarily equal actions. Important features of the parasympathetic and sympathetic innervation of the eye, and the sites of action of commonly used drugs, are summarized in Figures 3-9 and 3-10. In both systems the neurohumoral transmitter at the ganglion is acetylcholine, which passes across the synaptic cleft and depolarizes the postsynaptic membrane. This action of acetylcholine is terminated through its cleavage by acetylcholinesterase. In the parasympathetic system the postganglionic transmitter is also acetylcholine, but in the sympathetic system, it is norepinephrine. Norepinephrine also causes depolarization of the muscle cell, but it is not dissipated as simply as acetylcholine in the parasympathetic system. After release by the postganglionic sympathetic terminal norepinephrine may enter the effector cell, may diffuse into the vascular system, may undergo enzymatic degradation, or may be reabsorbed by the postganglionic terminal (Figure 3-11). After a period of absence, sympathetic or parasympathetic effector cells that are deprived of transmitter substance become very sensitive to the effects of that transmitter if it is applied. This phenomenon, *called denervation hypersensitivity*, is used to pharmacologically localize the site of denervation in Horner's syndrome.

Autonomic drugs may upregulate or downregulate the passage of a nerve impulse in a number of ways (see Figures 3-9 and 3-10). The ocular effects of the autonomic agents commonly used in animals include mydriasis (pupil dilation), miosis (pupil constriction), cycloplegia (paralysis of the ciliary muscle), and ciliary body contraction (opening of the iridocorneal angle); they are summarized in Box 3-2. Note that pharmacologic mydriasis may be caused by paralysis of the iris sphincter muscle or stimulation of the iris dilator muscle, whereas miosis may be caused by stimulation of the iris sphincter muscle or paralysis of the dilator muscle. However, species variation occurs. The iris in birds and reptiles is composed predominantly of striated fibers, and skeletal neuromuscular blocking agents (sometimes in addition to autonomic agents) must be used to produce mydriasis because the parasympatholytic agents used in mammals have little effect (see Chapter 20).

Parasympatholytic (Anticholinergic) Agents

Atropine

Atropine is a parasympatholytic agent used as a mydriatic and a cycloplegic agent principally for treatment of anterior uveitis (iridocyclitis). In patients with anterior uveitis, mydriasis reduces

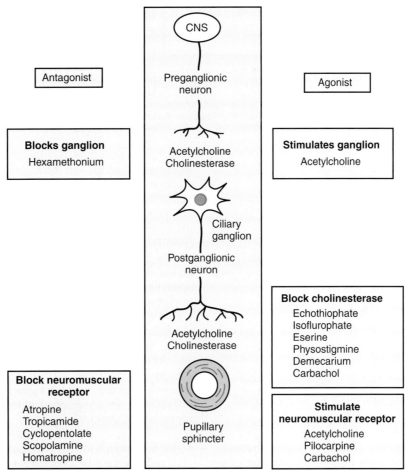

Figure 3-9. Parasympathetic innervation of the eye and sites of action of major drugs. Acetylcholine activity is limited by endogenous acetylcholinesterase. *CNS,* Central nervous system.

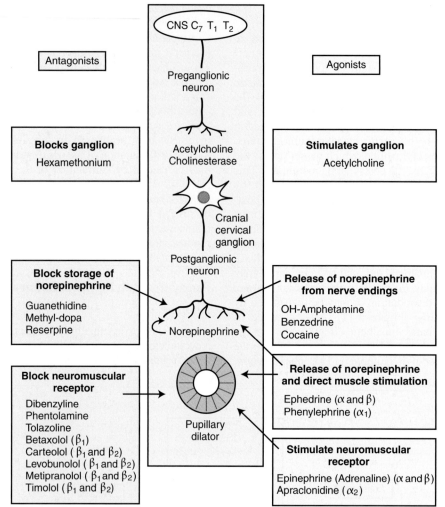

Figure 3-10. Sympathetic innervation of the eye and sites of action of major drugs. Endogenous amine oxidases limit norepinephrine action at the neuromuscular junction. Endogenous catecholomethyl transferase limits norepinephrine action within the muscle cell. *CNS,* Central nervous system; *C₇,* seventh cervical nerve; *T₁, T₂,* first and second thoracic nerves.

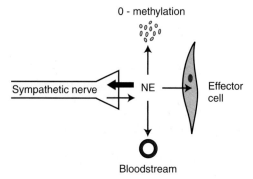

Figure 3-11. Fate of norepinephrine. After release by the postganglionic sympathetic terminal, norepinephrine *(NE)* may enter the effector cell, diffuse into the vascular system, undergo enzymatic degradation, or be reabsorbed by the postganglionic terminal. (Modified from Kramer SG, Potts AM [1969]: Iris uptake of catecholamines in experimental Horner's syndrome. Am J Ophthalmol 67:705.)

the chances of posterior synechia, whereas cycloplegia reduces the pain of ciliary body spasm. Mydriasis induced by atropine may be enhanced by addition of sympathomimetic agents (e.g., phenylephrine); however, the sympathomimetic agents do not augment cycloplegia and therefore are not analgesic. Atropine's duration of action may be many days in some dogs and cats, and longer than 1 week in horses. Therefore atropine (1%) drops and ointment should always be administered therapeutically to effect (i.e., until mydriasis is induced). Initially the frequency may be 2 or 3 times daily, but this can usually be reduced rapidly. The long duration of action also makes atropine an inappropriate mydriatic agent for ophthalmic examination, for which short-acting agents such as tropicamide are preferred. Atropine (and other dilating agents) may induce ocular hypertension and ultimately worsen glaucoma in susceptible breeds of dogs (e.g., basset hound, cocker spaniel). The parasympatholytic properties of atropine also decrease tear flow after conjunctival instillation. Therefore atropine is contraindicated in animals affected with lens luxation, glaucoma, and keratoconjunctivitis sicca.

Following are some important species-specific considerations for the use of atropine:

- Horses in which topical atropine is being used frequently should be carefully observed for signs of colic, including absence of borborygmi, kicking or looking at the abdomen, increased pulse rate, and sweating.

<table>
<tr><td colspan="2">Box 3-2 | Ophthalmic drugs with autonomic actions</td></tr>
</table>

Sympathomimetic

Direct-Acting

Epinephrine
Dipivefrin
Phenylephrine

Indirect-Acting

Hydroxyamphetamine
Cocaine

Sympatholytic (β-Blockers)

Timolol
Betaxolol

Parasympathomimetic

Direct-Acting

Acetylcholine
Carbachol (also acts indirectly)
Pilocarpine

Indirect-Acting

Reversible
    Carbachol (also acts
        directly)
    Demecarium bromide
        (slowly reversible)
    Physostigmine
Irreversible
    Isoflurophate
    Echothiophate

Parasympatholytic

Atropine
Tropicamide

Species and individual variations in response to these drugs exist.

- The presence of serum atropine esterase in some rabbits is alleged to limit the duration of effect and efficacy of atropine in those individuals.
- Paradoxically, atropine solution placed in the oral cavity or reaching it via the nasolacrimal duct acts as a promoter of salivary secretion because of its bitter taste. This effect is more noticeable with atropine solution than with ointment and may be especially troublesome in cats. However, this side effect may be used to test the patency of the parotid salivary duct before or after its translocation for therapy of keratoconjunctivitis sicca.

Tropicamide

Tropicamide is a fast-acting parasympatholytic with short duration of effect that is used to induce mydriasis for intraocular examination. Tropicamide is also used after intraocular surgery (such as cataract removal), when the prolonged mydriasis seen with atropine may unnecessarily increase the risk of glaucoma. When 1% tropicamide is instilled into the conjunctival sac, mydriasis occurs after 15 to 20 minutes (or slightly longer in animals with highly pigmented irides). Onset of mydriasis in normal eyes may be hastened by a second drop 5 minutes after the first. Lack of mydriasis 20 minutes after 2 drops of 1% tropicamide indicates that uveitis or posterior synechia may be present. In most patients, mydriasis and cycloplegia last approximately 2 to 3 hours (12 to 18 hours in some dogs and cats and up to 12 hours in most horses). This duration of effect, along with its lower potency compared with atropine, limits the therapeutic use of tropicamide. There is no evidence that animals that undergo dilation with tropicamide (or atropine) suffer retinal damage from ambient light levels under normal clinical circumstances. Diagnostic mydriasis with tropicamide in breeds of dogs susceptible to

glaucoma (e.g., American cocker spaniel, basset hound) may increase IOP, but because this effect is transient, it is unlikely to precipitate glaucoma.

Tropicamide is the mydriatic agent of choice for diagnostic purposes in common domestic mammals.

Miscellaneous Parasympatholytic Agents

Other parasympatholytic agents are used rarely in veterinary medicine. Homatropine (0.5% to 2%) causes mydriasis and cycloplegia intermediate in duration between atropine and tropicamide. Cyclopentolate is a commonly used diagnostic mydriatic agent in human beings but is used rarely in animals, because its effects last up to 3 days and it may cause pain and chemosis when administered topically.

Sympathomimetic (Adrenergic) Agents

Epinephrine (Adrenaline), Dipivefrin, and Phenylephrine

Epinephrine is the archetypical sympathomimetic agent; however, it penetrates the eye poorly and so has had limited use for intraocular disease when applied topically. It also is rapidly absorbed systemically when applied topically and so exerts some unwanted systemic side effects. It also deteriorates in solution owing to oxidization. For these reasons it has been replaced by phenylephrine or dipivefrin (an epinephrine prodrug). Dipivefrin is converted to epinephrine as it traverses the cornea and so enters the eye in its active form but has limited surface or systemic side effects. Epinephrine is occasionally still used to stimulate contraction of vascular smooth muscle, resulting in vasoconstriction and control of intraoperative hemorrhage. This is achieved by topical application for conjunctival or scleral hemorrhage or intracameral use during intraocular surgery to control hemorrhage and to induce mydriasis. Care must be taken with intraocular use of epinephrine because of the danger of inducing cardiac arrhythmias under general anesthesia. The vasoconstrictive effects of the sympathomimetic drugs may also be used to distinguish deep (episcleral) vessels, which do not blanch rapidly, from superficial (conjunctival) blood vessels, which do blanch rapidly after topical application of these agents in animals with reddened eyes. This practice assists in differentiating "deep" intraocular and potentially blinding disease, such as anterior uveitis, from superficial and less urgent conjunctivitis (see Chapter 7). Epinephrine is also occasionally used to retard absorption of drugs (e.g., penicillin, lidocaine) injected with it, particularly in the retrobulbar space.

The sympathomimetic agents may be used to pharmacologically localize the lesion in patients with Horner's syndrome when sympathetic innervation of the eye is interrupted. This maneuver relies on the phenomenon known as "denervation hypersensitivity" (described previously). Instillation of a dilute solution of a direct-acting sympathomimetic (typically 0.2% to 1.0 % phenylephrine) into the conjunctival sac results in faster mydriasis in the affected eye than in the normal (contralateral) eye if the lesion is postganglionic. Topically applied phenylephrine may also be used in differential diagnosis of protrusion of the third eyelid ("haws") in cats, because it stimulates the sympathetically innervated smooth muscles controlling this membrane.

These drugs may also be used to augment mydriasis, but without coincident paralysis of the sphincter muscle with a parasympatholytic agent, they are weak mydriatic agents and so are not used alone for this purpose. Phenylephrine causes some mydriasis in dogs but is ineffective as a mydriatic in horses and cats. Repeated use of phenylephrine at short intervals and high concentrations can cause systemic hypertension.

Topical application of dipivefrin is also used for treatment of glaucoma. Following conversion to epinephrine this drug acts intraocularly to decrease production of aqueous humor without causing major changes in pupil size. It also stabilizes vascular endothelium. For this reason it has some use in treatment of glaucoma secondary to anterior uveitis in domestic animals.

Parasympathomimetic (Cholinergic) Agents

All commonly used topical parasympathomimetic agents in veterinary ophthalmology (see Box 3-2) induce miosis and/or increase the facility of outflow of aqueous humor in glaucomatous and normal eyes. This effect may be due to stimulation of portions of the ciliary muscle that insert in the area of the iridocorneal angle, resulting in increased drainage via the trabecular meshwork. Contraction of the ciliary muscle may also result in larger trabecular spaces through which fluid may exit. Therefore their clinical indication is for treatment or delaying the onset of glaucoma. It is important to note that ciliary muscle spasm is often painful, especially in patients with preexisting anterior uveitis (iridocyclitis); therefore these drugs may induce intraocular pain.

Direct-Acting Parasympathomimetic Agents

PILOCARPINE. Pilocarpine is the archetypical direct-acting parasympathomimetic agent. It acts directly on the muscle cells of the pupillary sphincter and ciliary body and is effective even in the denervated eye or after retrobulbar anesthesia when release of acetylcholine at the neuromuscular junction is blocked. Pilocarpine also stimulates secretory glands and may be used topically or systemically in patients with keratoconjunctivitis sicca, although the T cell–modulating drugs, such as cyclosporine and tacrolimus, are more effective, have fewer side effects than pilocarpine, and have largely replaced it for treatment of this disease. Overdosage of topically or systemically applied pilocarpine results in salivation, vomiting, and diarrhea, especially in cats. Pilocarpine penetrates the eye after topical instillation, and intraocular concentration depends on frequency of application and concentration of the drops. However, pilocarpine tends to be very irritating and induces breakdown of the blood-ocular barrier (and aqueous flare) when applied topically, especially at higher concentrations. As a result of these side effects and the availability of more potent, better-tolerated hypotensive agents, it is now rarely used for management of glaucoma in veterinary ophthalmology.

Indirect-Acting Parasympathomimetic Agents

Organophosphates are indirect-acting parasympathomimetic agents and may be reversible or irreversible in nature. They act by inhibition of cholinesterase, causing preservation of acetylcholine, and hence have no effect on denervated structures. Combinations of direct- and indirect-acting parasympathomimetic agents do not result in more profound or prolonged miosis, and with some combinations, competitive inhibition occurs. The reversible inhibitors such as physostigmine and carbachol are not used in the control of glaucoma, because the irreversible agents such as demecarium are more effective and require less frequent administration. If treatment with any of the irreversible agents fails, the use of another member of the group is rarely useful. All drugs of this group may cause severe and even fatal systemic toxicity through excessive topical treatment (concentration or frequency of application), especially in cats. Signs of systemic toxicity include vomiting, diarrhea, anorexia, and weakness. Particular care must be taken to avoid additive effects of these drugs with other organophosphates in flea collars, washes, and systemic parasiticides.

DEMECARIUM. Demecarium is stable in aqueous solution and is usually administered once or twice daily. Demecarium bromide, given once daily in conjunction with a topical corticosteroid (also once daily), significantly prolongs the time to onset of primary glaucoma in dogs. Iridocorneal angle closure was delayed for 32 months in dogs treated with this combination, compared with 8 months in untreated dogs. This drug is no longer commercially available but can be compounded as a 0.125% or 0.25% solution.

CARBACHOL. Carbachol is a direct-acting parasympathomimetic agent. However, it is reported to also have some indirect (cholinesterase-inhibiting) action. It causes modest decreases in IOP in beagles with inherited open-angle glaucoma. It has longer duration of action than pilocarpine, requiring administration 2 to 3 times daily, but frequently has systemic side effects in dogs. Despite being a more powerful miotic than pilocarpine, carbachol (3%) is less useful in the treatment of glaucoma than the irreversible cholinesterase inhibitors. It is used intracamerally by some veterinary ophthalmologists immediately after cataract surgery to reduce transient postoperative rises in IOP.

Sympatholytic Agents (Adrenergic Antagonists)

Numerous agents have become available that block, with different selectivity, α- and/or β-receptors. β-Blockers (β-antagonists) are thought to lower IOP by reducing blood flow to the ciliary body. However, sympathetic receptors are found in the iridocorneal angle and drainage pathway and may also play a role in the action of these drugs.

An expanding array of topical sympatholytic agents is used for human glaucoma. Examples are timolol, betaxolol, levobunolol, carteolol, and metipranolol. Those that have been studied in veterinary patients (principally dogs and cats) lower IOP poorly and have limited use in therapy of overt glaucoma in these species. However, these agents may have a role in glaucoma prophylaxis in dogs. A recent study showed that betaxolol given twice daily significantly prolonged the time to onset of primary glaucoma to 32 months, compared with 8 months in untreated dogs. Care must be taken in administering these agents to animals with cardiac or respiratory disease, and therapy should be stopped 3 to 4 days before administration of general anesthesia. Timolol (0.5%) has been studied in normal horses and does lower IOP, but only by about 4 to 5 mm Hg. Its efficacy in horses with glaucoma has not been studied.

CARBONIC ANHYDRASE INHIBITORS

The enzyme carbonic anhydrase is present in ciliary body epithelium, where it is responsible, in part, for aqueous humor production. Carbonic anhydrase inhibitors (CAIs) reduce aqueous humor production by up to 50%, thereby decreasing IOP, and their role in veterinary ophthalmology is in the management of acute glaucomatous crises as well as long-term control of IOP in some patients. When administered systemically these drugs also inhibit carbonic anhydrase in the renal tubular epithelium and may cause mild diuresis. However, just as with osmotic agents, their IOP-lowering effect is not the result of this diuresis. Similarly, other diuretics such as furosemide do not significantly reduce aqueous humor production or IOP and should not be used for this purpose. Although diuresis is usually not clinically significant with this group of agents, systemically administered CAIs may cause other undesirable side effects, such as metabolic acidosis (usually noted as panting), gastrointestinal disturbance, and, in some cases, increased urinary loss of potassium with long-term use. Occasionally, severe skin reactions or disorientation have been reported with some CAIs. If side effects occur in a particular patient, they are rapidly reversible upon discontinuation of the drug, and another CAI may be better tolerated. Topically administered CAIs are not associated with systemic side effects.

Systemic Carbonic Anhydrase Inhibitors

The archetypical CAI was acetazolamide; however, because this drug causes vomiting more frequently than more modern agents in this group, it has now been largely replaced by CAIs such as methazolamide and dichlorphenamide. These drugs are usually administered two to three times daily at 2 to 5 mg/kg. They are typically well tolerated in dogs, but side effects seem more frequent in cats.

Topical Carbonic Anhydrase Inhibitors

Dorzolamide and brinzolamide are topically applied CAIs. They lower IOP in dogs and cats when applied three times daily and are a useful part of a combined regimen to lower IOP. They may be used in patients whose glaucoma occurs secondary to uveitis and have the advantage of lack of systemic side effects. However, they occasionally sting and tend to be expensive. They are usually used to replace rather than supplement systemically administered CAIs.

PROSTAGLANDIN ANALOGUES

Latanoprost, travoprost, bimatoprost, and unoprost are synthetic prostaglandins developed for the treatment of glaucoma in human beings but with some application in canine glaucoma. Latanoprost is potent and effective in reducing IOP in canine glaucoma, and is also important in the emergency treatment of glaucoma in dogs, in which it has largely replaced pilocarpine (see Chapter 12). Travoprost lowers IOP significantly, and to a degree equivalent to that achieved by latanoprost, in normal dogs. Prostaglandin analogues are ineffective in the treatment of glaucoma in cats and horses.

LOCAL ANESTHETICS

Topical (local) anesthetics are used for ocular examinations and minor manipulative and surgical procedures, but *never* for therapeutic purposes. The effect on corneal sensation of a single drop of proparacaine or 2 drops separated by 1 minute

has been studied. Application of 1 drop leads to maximal anesthesia for 15 minutes and statistically (although not necessarily clinically) significant reductions in corneal sensation for 45 minutes. These times increase to 25 minutes (maximal) and 55 minutes (duration) if a second drop is applied 1 minute after the first. In addition, 2 drops applied 1 minute apart caused a significantly greater anesthetic effect than did 1 drop when measured 30 through 55 minutes after application. Again, this difference was statistically significant, but its clinical significance was not explored.

The following cautionary notes should be considered in the use of this group of drugs:

- All topical anesthetics inhibit corneal epithelialization and are toxic to normal corneal epithelium. They produce small punctate ulcerations in normal cornea.
- Some are extremely toxic systemically (5 mL of 2% tetracaine solution is a fatal human dose) and are rapidly absorbed from the conjunctival sac. This fact is of most importance in the treatment of very small (exotic) veterinary patients.
- Some anesthetics are antigenic and may cause sensitization.
- Local anesthetics should not be dispensed to owners for any reason.
- Local anesthetics placed into diseased, painful eyes abolish protective reflexes and increase the chance of further injury (e.g., entropion) in addition to causing corneal lesions themselves.
- Ophthalmic anesthetics (like all other topical drugs) are unsuitable for injection.

Local anesthetics should not be used therapeutically or included in any therapeutic regimen or preparation.

Classically it has been recommended that samples for bacterial analysis should be taken before local anesthetics are placed in the eye, because these agents and the preservatives they contain may be bactericidal. In reality this practice is often too uncomfortable for the patient, raising the risk of patient movement and globe rupture. There is also evidence to suggest that although topical anesthetic agents may alter the bacteria cultured in some circumstances, this feature is not consistent, and the change in bacteria cultured before and after anesthesia is rarely of clinical relevance. However, local anesthesia does reduce Schirmer tear test values by about 50% and should not be used before such tests. Of the many agents available 0.5% proparacaine is generally the most useful. Short-term storage of proparacaine at room temperature does not reduce efficacy, but storage at room temperature for more than 2 weeks results in a decrease in drug effect. Brownish solutions of proparacaine are inactivated and should not be used. Tetracaine may cause sensitivity reactions in dogs.

ENZYMES AND ENZYME INHIBITORS

Enzymes and enzyme inhibitors are used infrequently in veterinary ophthalmology but have a critical role when they are employed. Classically they fall into two broad categories: those agents used to catalyze dissolution of the protein within a blood clot, and those employed to retard the degradation of collagen in a cornea during "melting" or corneal malacia.

Hyaluronidase

Hyaluronidase depolymerizes hyaluronic acid, an important constituent of connective tissue, allowing faster passage of drugs through tissues. Therefore it is sometimes injected into the retrobulbar region to promote dispersion of contrast or anesthetic agents through orbital tissues. The permeability of tissues returns to normal in 1 to 2 days. The enzyme is nontoxic and does not cause inflammation or affect capillary permeability. However, it will not dissolve fibrin or inflammatory exudates.

Tissue Plasminogen Activator

Recombinant tissue plasminogen activator (TPA) is used by intracameral injection to lyse newly formed fibrin deposits and facilitate dispersion of hyphema in uveitis, especially traumatic and postoperative intraocular inflammation. Intracameral injections should be performed only by those trained in this technique. Doses of 15 to 25 µg are typically used. TPA must be kept frozen until used.

Protease Inhibitors

Tear film and corneal proteases are produced by corneal epithelial cells, stromal fibrocytes, inflammatory cells, and certain bacteria, such as *Pseudomonas* spp. They are important for normal wound healing, especially in the cornea. However, in some disease states, their production, activation, and deactivation become unregulated, leading to detrimental effects. One of the most dramatic examples of this is their role in the pathogenesis of melting or malacic corneal ulcers in which there is altered protease homeostasis.

There are at least four categories of proteases, but matrix metalloproteinases and serine proteases appear most important in corneal disease and health. They have been demonstrated in increased amounts in the tear films of dogs, cats, and horses with corneal ulceration, and reduction of tear film proteolytic activity has been demonstrated in horses as ulcers heal. Therefore various protease inhibitors have been explored for the treatment of corneal ulceration. Those used historically and currently include *N*-acetylcysteine, disodium ethylenediamine tetra-acetate (EDTA), tetracycline antibiotics, and autogenous serum. Of these only serum is believed to have broad activity against both serine proteinases and metalloproteinases. Serum also contains numerous growth factors that are believed to be helpful in corneal wound healing. These facts, along with the easy and inexpensive procurement of serum from the patient and because it is predictably well tolerated when topically applied, make autogenous serum the first-choice proteinase inhibitor for ophthalmic use.

Matrix metalloproteinase (collagenase) inhibitors are extremely important agents in the treatment of corneal ulceration. Autogenous serum is the most accessible and most broad in its therapeutic effects and is well tolerated.

TEAR REPLACEMENT PREPARATIONS ("ARTIFICIAL TEARS")

Artificial tear preparations are used when the normal tear quality or quantity is altered or when loss of tears is increased due to evaporation, or, in some cases, primary corneal pathology. These agents are lacrimomimetic and are not to be confused with lacrimogenic agents, such as cyclosporine. The production of endogenous tears is always preferred over the replacement of tears with "artificial" tears. Aqueous solutions such as normal saline are unsuitable for tear replacement because they do not adhere to the lipophilic corneal epithelium and have extremely brief ocular retention times. Additionally they dilute what endogenous tears are present, and the preservatives most contain may cause inflammation or worsening of primary disease. Therefore aqueous solutions must be modified by the addition of agents to bind the solution to the epithelium and/or increase viscosity of the preparation. In the normal precorneal tear film this function is performed by mucopolysaccharide molecules within the mucin layer of the tear film and having both hydrophilic and lipophilic ends. Solutions modified in this way, termed *mucinomimetic,* have longer contact time and better "eye feel," and offer more antidesiccant advantages than traditional saline solutions. The inclusion of a bicarbonate-based buffer to retain pH near that of normal tears also helps corneal epithelium return to normal in the human eye.

Indications for tear replacement preparations are as follows:

- For treatment of keratoconjunctivitis sicca ("dry eye")
- For treatment of exposure keratitis (e.g., facial nerve paralysis, buphthalmos, breed-associated lagophthalmos)
- In patients with abnormal tear film breakup time (qualitative tear film disturbances)
- During and after general anesthesia to prevent corneoconjunctival desiccation
- As a lubricant, refractive/electroconductive, and cushioning solution during gonioscopy and electroretinography
- As a diluent for compounding of some ophthalmic solutions
- In patients with primary corneal disease, such as feline corneal sequestration and canine superficial punctate keratitis

The most commonly used classes of lacrimomimetic preparations, grouped according to the viscosity agent used, are listed in Table 3-15.

MISCELLANEOUS THERAPEUTIC AGENTS

Surgical Adhesives

Tissue adhesive (isobutyl cyanoacrylate) has been advocated for treating some corneal ulcers in dogs, cats, and rabbits; however, it must not be permitted to enter the eye and so should not be used on leaking corneal wounds. Cyanoacrylate is used on a carefully dried corneal surface, where it engenders some inflammatory reaction that may be beneficial in stimulating healing in superficial nonhealing (indolent) corneal ulcers. Large amounts or long-term use of cyanoacrylate, however, results in severe inflammation.

Eye Washes (Collyria)

Sterile eye wash is used for removal of purulent exudates, foreign bodies, and irritants from the eyelids and conjunctival sac but not for long-term therapy. Many commercial formulas are available. Eye washes in examination rooms should be changed regularly to prevent overgrowth with contaminating microbial agents. Boric acid solution was commonly used in the past, but because of its weak germicidal action and systemic toxicity, it is no longer advocated.

Table 3-15 | **Commonly Used Lacrimomimetic Solutions and Ointments**

VISCOSITY AGENT	PRESERVATIVE	PRODUCT NAME	SOURCE
POLYVINYL ALCOHOL			
Polyvinyl alcohol 1.4%	Benzalkonium chloride	AKWA Tears	Akorn
Polyvinyl alcohol 3%	Thimerosal	Liquifilm Forte	Allergan
Polyvinyl alcohol 1.4%	Chlorobutanol	Liquifilm Tears	Allergan
Polyvinyl alcohol 1.4%	Benzalkonium chloride	Dry Eyes	Bausch & Lomb
Polyvinyl alcohol	Benzalkonuim chloride	Hypotears Lubricating Eye Drops	CIBA Vision
Polyvinyl alcohol 1%	None	Hypotears PF Eye Drops	CIBA Vision
Polyvinyl alcohol	None	Ocutears PF	Ocumed
Polyvinyl alcohol	Unknown	Ocutears	Ocumed
Polyvinyl alcohol	None	Tearfair	Pharmafair
CELLULOSE SOLUTIONS			
Carboxymethylcellulose 0.25%	None	Theratears	Advanced Vision Research
Carboxymethylcellulose 1.0%	None	Celluvisc Lubricant	Allergan
Carboxymethylcellulose 0.5%	Purite	Refresh Tears	Allergan
Hydroxypropylmethylcellulose 0.5%	Chlorobutanol	Lacri-Lube	Allergan
Carboxymethylcellulose 1.0%	None	Refresh Plus	Allergan
Carboxymethylcellulose 0.5%	None	Cellufresh	Allergan
Hydroxypropylmethylcellulose 1%	Benzalkonium chloride	Isopto Alkaline	Alcon
Hydroxypropylmethylcellulose 0.5%	Methylparaben, propylparaben	Isopto Tears Plain	Alcon
Hydroxyethylcellulose	Benzalkonium chloride	Comfort Tears	Barnes-Hind
Methylcellulose 1%	None	Murocell	Bausch & Lomb
Hydroxypropylmethylcellulose	Sodium perborate	GenTeal Lubricating Eye Drops	CIBA Vision
Hydroxypropylmethylcellulose 0.5%	Benzalkonuim chloride	Tearisol	Iolab
Hydroxypropylmethylcellulose 0.50%	Sorbic acid	TearGard	Med Tec
Hydroxypropylmethylcellulose and dextran	None	LubriFair	Pharmafair
Hydroxypropylmethylcellulose and glycerine	Sorbic acid	Clear Eyes	Ross Laboratories
POLYMER COMBINATIONS			
Hydroxypropylmethylcellulose and dextran 70	Benzalkonium chloride	Tears Renewed	Akorn
Hydroxymethylcellulose and povidone 1.67%	Thimerosal	Adsorbotear	Alcon
Hydroxypropylmethylcellulose and dextran	None	Bio Tears	Alcon
Hydroxypropylmethylcellulose and dextran	Polyquarternium	Tears Naturale II	Alcon
Hydroxypropylmethylcellulose and dextran	None	Tears Naturale Free	Alcon
Polyvinyl alcohol 1.4% and povidone 0.6%	Chlorobutanol	Tears Plus	Allergan
Polyvinyl alcohol 1.4% and dextran	None	Refresh Tears	Allergan
Hydroxypropylmethylcellulose and dextran	Benzalkonium chloride	Lubri Tears	Bausch & Lomb
Hydroxypropylmethylcellulose, dextran 0.1%, povidone 0.1%, and glycerin 0.2%	Benzalkonium chloride	Moisture Drops	Bausch & Lomb
Polyethylene glycol 0.2%, dextran 0.1%, and polycarbophil	None	Aquasite	CIBA Vision

Continued

Table 3-15 | **Commonly Used Lacrimomimetic Solutions and Ointments—cont'd**

VISCOSITY AGENT	PRESERVATIVE	PRODUCT NAME	SOURCE
Polyvinyl alcohol 1%, hydroxyethylcellulose, and dextran	Benzalkonium chloride	Hypotears	Iolab
Polyvinyl alcohol 1%, hydroxyethylcellulose, and dextran	Benzalkonium chloride	Hypotears PF	Iolab
Hydroxypropylmethylcellulose and dextran	None	LubriFair Solution	Pharmafair
Polyvinyl alcohol 1.4% and povidone 0.60%	Benzalkonium chloride	Murine Eye Lubricant	Ross Laboratories
Hydroxypropylmethylcellulose and dextran	Benzalkonium chloride	Nature's Tears	Rugby
OINTMENTS			
White petroleum and mineral oil	None	AKWA ointment	Akron
White petroleum, mineral oil, and anhydrous liquid lanolin	None	Duratears Naturale Lubricant Eye Ointment	Alcon
White petroleum, mineral oil, and lanolin	Chlorobutanol	Lacri-Lube	Allergan
White petroleum, mineral oil, and lanolin	None	Lacri-Lube NP	Allergan
White petroleum, mineral oil, and lanolin	Chlorobutanol	Lacri-Lube S.O.P.	Allergan
White petroleum, mineral oil, and lanolin	None	Refresh PM	Allergan
White petroleum and mineral oil	None	Dry Eyes	Bausch & Lomb
White petroleum and mineral oil	None	Duolube	Bausch & Lomb
White petroleum and mineral oil	None	Hypotears Ointment	CIBA Vision
White petroleum	None	Lipotears	Coopervision
White petroleum, mineral oil, and lanolin	None	Hypo Tears	Iolab
White petroleum	Methylparaben	Ocutube	Ocumed
White petroleum	None	Petroleum Ointment Sterile	Pharmafair
White petroleum, mineral oil, and lanolin derivatives	None	TearFair Ointment	Pharmafair
White petroleum, mineral oil, and lanolin	None	LubriFair Ointment	Pharmafair
VISCOELASTIC PRODUCTS			
Hylan 0.15%	None	I-Drop Vet	I-Med
Hylan 0.40%	None	I-Drop Vet	I-Med
GLYCERIN PRODUCTS			
Glycerin 0.3%	None	Dry Eye Therapy	Bausch & Lomb
Glycerin 0.4%	Benzalkonium chloride	Eye Lube A	Optoptics

From Grahn BH, Storey ES (2004): Lacrimostimulants and lacrimomimetics. Vet Clin North Am Small Anim Pract 34:739.

Germicides

Germicides are used for disinfection of instruments, for preoperative preparation of the lids and ocular surface, and as preservatives in eyedrops. A number of solutions have been used as topical antiseptics or germicides for the eye. However, many are toxic to the corneal and conjunctival epithelium and should not be used. Povidone-iodine solution is a reliable and nonirritating agent for destruction of bacteria, fungi, and viruses on the ocular surface and periocular skin before surgery, and is the preferred product for this purpose. It is mixed with normal saline to form a 2% solution. Povidone-iodine *solution,* not surgical *scrub,* must be used. Benzalkonium chloride is a wetting agent that enhances corneal penetration of certain drugs as well as acting as a preservative. It is no longer used for surgical preparation of the patient or for sterilization of instruments. Other solutions, such as hexachlorophene, cresol, and mercury- and silver-containing compounds, can be very irritating to the ocular surface, and their use is contraindicated. In particular, silver nitrate applicator sticks (used for hemostasis after nail trimming in dogs) cause severe keratitis and epithelial sloughing in dogs and must not be used near the ocular surface.

Astringents and Cauterants

Astringents are locally acting protein precipitants; cauterants are severe protein-precipitating agents that cause local tissue destruction. Examples are copper sulfate, trichloracetic acid, phenol, iodine, and zinc sulphate. Such agents have historically been used (sometimes indiscriminately) to treat a variety of ocular diseases. However, identification and removal of the cause or more modern medical and surgical approaches usually achieve a better result in a more controlled manner, and astringents and cauterants are no longer recommended for ocular use.

Vitamins

Various vitamins have been advocated for their supposed therapeutic efficacy in the treatment of ocular disorders of animals. In the absence of a specific vitamin deficiency (e.g., vitamin A deficiency causing nyctalopia in cattle or conjunctivitis in turtles) there usually is little to be gained from such local therapy. The exception is systemic and ocular signs of warfarin poisoning, which are treated with vitamin K and its analogues.

Antiparasitic Agents

Ivermectin is now used, almost to the exclusion of all older parasiticides, for treatment of parasitism such as habronemiasis and onchocerciasis in horses and ocular filariasis in small animals. When it is used at excessive doses or at normal doses in a susceptible individual such as a collie, ocular signs of ivermectin toxicity may be seen. They include mydriasis, reduction or absence of pupillary light reflexes, blindness, and retinal folds or edema. These signs are typically temporary.

PHYSICAL THERAPY

Contact Lenses

Therapeutic soft contact lenses (TSCLs) have been used in veterinary patients as bandages to protect the cornea during healing or sometimes as vehicles for delivery of hydrophilic drugs. Degradable collagen shields are also available; however, these typically degrade more rapidly than preferred (usually within 72 hours). Both lens types must be placed behind the leading edge of the third eyelid to reduce the chance of being dislodged. Many ophthalmologists recommend also placing a partial temporary tarsorrhaphy over the TSCL, a maneuver that requires general anesthesia or sedation and regional anesthesia. A temporary tarsorrhaphy will continue to provide a "bandage" effect even if the TSCL is dislodged. Hydrophilic TSCLs may be soaked in a concentrated solution of some drugs before being placed on the eye to afford some depot effect.

Irradiation

Irradiation may be used therapeutically for several ophthalmic diseases but also produces ophthalmic disease if the eye must be placed in the field during irradiation for other diseases such as nasal or orbital neoplasia. Radiation exerts its effect on rapidly dividing cells, which in the eye include lymphocytes, vascular endothelium (uvea, conjunctiva, eyelids, retina), and epithelial (eyelid, lacrimal gland, corneal, conjunctival, ciliary body, iridal, retinal, and lenticular) cells. From this list it is clear that the effects of inadvertent or intentional irradiation of the eye are potentially wide-ranging. Two forms of radiation are commonly used for the treatment of ocular disease—β-irradiation and x- or γ-irradiation. Because of safety precautions, licensing, and expense, treatment tends to be limited to larger veterinary hospitals, and referral of cases requiring such therapy is advocated.

β-Irradiation

β-Rays are low-energy electrons that penetrate tissue to 3 to 4 mm. Therefore they are used to treat superficial lesions only. β-irradiation for ophthalmic use is obtained from a strontium-90 ophthalmic applicator. This therapy is used to control corneal neovascularization and pigmentation seen with chronic superficial keratitis ("pannus") in dogs and to treat malignant ocular neoplasms, including squamous cell carcinoma of the lids, third eyelid, and conjunctiva in cattle, cats, and horses especially. Because of shallow penetration, β-irradiation from an applicator applied to the limbus does not reach the equatorial zone of the lens (Figure 3-12).

γ- and X-Irradiation

γ-Rays and x-rays have similar wavelength, energy, and penetrating properties but differ in origin. γ-rays emanate from the nucleus, and x-rays from the extranuclear portion, of the atom. Both penetrate deeply and are used for lesions inaccessible to β-irradiation. Superficial, orthovoltage, and megavoltage radiotherapy, cobalt 60, cesium-135, and radon and gold implants (brachytherapy) have all been used. Penetrating (x and γ) irradiation may interfere with cell division in the equatorial region of the lens, especially in young animals, resulting in partial or complete "radiation cataract." Higher doses result in keratitis (41%), conjunctivitis (mild,

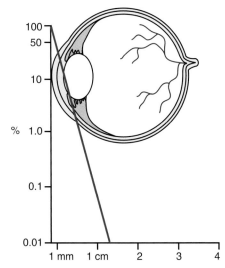

Figure 3-12. Graph indicating the decrease in intensity of β-irradiation emitted from a strontium-90 ophthalmic applicator as a function of tissue depth. By 1-mm tissue penetration, the radiation intensity has decreased to 50%. The diagram of the eye is drawn to scale to show the relationship of decreasing intensity to various structures of the eye. (Modified from Gillette EL [1970]: Veterinary radiotherapy. J Am Vet Med Assoc 157:1707.)

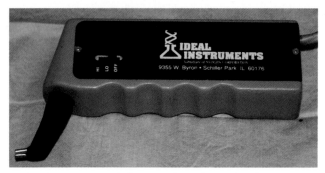

Figure 3-13. Radiofrequency hyperthermia handpiece.

34%; severe, 28%), cataract (28%), and keratoconjunctivitis sicca. In one study, progression to corneal perforation occurred in 24% of patients, and 63% of cases of conjunctivitis and keratitis were refractory to treatment.

Hyperthermia

Hyperthermia (local induction of heat within a tissue) is used to treat squamous cell carcinoma and some other tumors of the eye and adnexa in horses and cattle. The temperature of the tissue is increased to 50° C for 30 sec/cm^2 by the local passage of radiofrequency current through the tissue (Figure 3-13).

Lasers in Veterinary Ophthalmology

Lasers have been described for cyclophotocoagulation (glaucoma), retinopexy (retinal detachment), rupturing of iris cysts, correction of entropion, and ablation of intraocular and adnexal neoplasms. However, their advantages (if any) over standard surgical approaches have not been investigated or proven in most of these diseases. Diode, neodymium:yttrium-aluminum-garnet, and CO$_2$ lasers are used most commonly in veterinary ophthalmology.

BIBLIOGRAPHY

Avunduk AM, et al. (2003): Comparison of efficacy of topical and oral fluconazole treatment in experimental *Aspergillus* keratitis. Curr Eye Res 26:113.

Ball MA, et al. (1997): Corneal concentrations and preliminary toxicological evaluation of an itraconazole/dimethyl sulphoxide ophthalmic ointment. J Vet Pharmacol Ther 20:100.

Ball MA, et al. (1997): Evaluation of itraconazole-dimethyl sulfoxide ointment for treatment of keratomycosis in nine horses. J Am Vet Med Assoc 211:199.

Beale KM (1988): Azathioprine for treatment of immune-mediated diseases of dogs and cats. J Am Vet Med Assoc 192:1316.

Berdoulay A, et al. (2005): Effect of topical 0.02% tacrolimus aqueous suspension on tear production in dogs with keratoconjunctivitis sicca. Vet Ophthalmol 8:225.

Bhattacherjee P, et al. (1999): Pharmacological validation of a feline model of steroid-induced ocular hypertension. Arch Ophthalmol 117:361.

Brightman AH, et al. (1981): Effect of aspirin on aqueous protein values in the dog. J Vet Med Assoc 178:572.

Bromberg NM (2002): Cyanoacrylate tissue adhesive for treatment of refractory corneal ulceration. Vet Ophthalmol 5:55.

Brooks DE, Ollivier FJ (2004): Matrix metalloproteinase inhibition in corneal ulceration. Vet Clin North Am Small Anim Pract 34:611.

Bussieres M, et al. (2005): The use of carbon dioxide laser for the ablation of meibomian fundamental adenomas in dogs. J Am Anim Hosp Assoc 41:227.

Carvalho AB, et al. (2006): Effects of travoprost 0.004% compared with latanoprost 0.005% on the intraocular pressure of normal dogs. Vet Ophthalmol 9:121.

Cawrse MA, et al. (2001): Effects of topical application of a 2% solution of dorzolamide on intraocular pressure and aqueous humor flow rate in clinically normal dogs. Am J Vet Res 62:859.

Clode AB, et al. (2006): Evaluation and concentration of voriconazle in aqueous humor after topical and oral administration in horses. Am J Vet Res 67:296.

Davidson G (1999): Etodolac. Compend Contin Educ Pract Vet 21:494.

Davidson MG (2000): Pharm profile: dorzolamide. Compend Cont Ed Pract Vet 22:340.

Davis JL, et al. (2005): Pharmacokinetics and tissue distribution of itraconazole after oral and intravenous administration to horses. Am J Vet Res 66:1694.

Eichenbaum JD, et al. (1988): Effect in large dogs of ophthalmic prednisolone acetate on adrenal gland and hepatic function. J Am Anim Hosp Assoc 24:705.

Fox SM, Johnston SA (1997): Use of carprofen for the treatment of pain and inflammation in dogs. J Am Vet Med Assoc 210:1493.

Gelatt KN, et al. (2001): Enrofloxacin-associated retinal degeneration in cats. Vet Ophthalmol 4:231.

Gelatt KN, et al. (1995): Evaluation of multiple doses of 4 and 6% timolol, and timolol combined with 2% pilocarpine in clinically normal beagles and beagles with glaucoma. Am J Vet Res 56:1325.

Gelatt KN, et al. (1995): Evaluation of mydriatics in horses. Vet Comp Ophthal 5:104.

Gelatt KN, MacKay EO (2001): Changes in intraocular pressure associated with topical dorzolamide and oral methazolamide in glaucomatous dogs. Vet Ophthalmol 4:61.

Gelatt KN, MacKay EO (1998): The ocular hypertensive effects of topical 0.1% dexamethasone in beagles with inherited glaucoma. J Ocular Pharmacol Ther 14:57.

Gemensky-Metzler A, et al. (2004): The use of semiconductor diode laser for deflation and coagulation of anterior uveal cysts in dogs, cats, and horses: a report of 20 cases. Vet Ophthalmol 7:360.

Gerding PA, et al. (1988): Pathogenic bacteria and fungi associated with external ocular diseases in dogs: 131 cases (1981-1986). J Am Vet Med Assoc 193:242.

Gilger B, et al. (1997): Neodymium:yttrium-aluminum-garnet laser treatment of cystic granula iridica in horses: eight cases (1988-1996). J Vet Med Assoc 211:341.

Gilger BC, et al. (1996): Lymphocyte proliferation and blood drug levels in dogs with keratoconjunctivitis sicca receiving long-term ocular cyclosporine. Vet Comp Ophthalmol 6:125.

Gionfriddo JR, et al. (1992): Fungal flora of the healthy camelid conjunctival sac. Am J Vet Res 53:643.

Gionfriddo JR, et al. (1991): Bacterial and mycoplasmal flora of the healthy camelid conjunctival sac. Am J Vet Res 52:1061.

Giuliano EA (2004): Nonsteroidal anti-inflammatory drugs in veterinary ophthalmology. Vet Clin North Am Small Anim Pract 34:707.

Giuliano EA, et al. (2000): Inferomedial placement of a single-entry subpalpebral lavage tube for treatment of equine eye disease. Vet Ophthalmol 3:153.

Grahn BH, Storey ES (2004): Lacrimostimulants and lacrimomimetics. Vet Clin North Am Small Anim Pract 34:739.

Gum GG, et al. (1993): Effect of topically applied demecarium bromide and echothiophate iodide on intraocular pressure and pupil size in beagles with normotensive eyes and beagles with glaucoma. Am J Vet Res 54:287.

Gum GG, et al. (1993): The tonographic effects of pilocarpine and pilocarpine-epinephrine in normal beagles and beagles with inherited glaucoma. J Small Anim Pract 34:112.

Gum GG, et al. (1991): The effect of topical timolol maleate on intraocular pressure in normal beagles and beagles with inherited glaucoma. Prog Vet Comp Ophthalmol 1:141.

Herring IP, et al. (2005): Duration of effect and effect of multiple doses of topical ophthalmic 0.5% proparacaine hydrochloride in clinically normal dogs. Am J Vet Res 66:77.

Hulse D (1998): Treatment methods for pain in the osteoarthritic patient. Vet Clin North Am Small Anim Pract 28:361.

Hunter RP, et al. (1995): Pharmacokinetics, oral bioavailability and tissue distribution of azithromycin in cats. J Vet Pharmacol 18:38.

Kainer RA, et al. (1980): Hyperthermia for treatment of ocular squamous cell tumors in cattle. J Am Vet Med Assoc 176:356.

Kray KT, et al. (1985): Cromolyn sodium in seasonal allergic conjunctivitis. J Allergy Clin Immunol 76:623.

Krohne SDG (1998): Carprofen inhibition of flare in the dog measured by laser flare photometry. Vet Comp Ophthalmol 1:81.

Krohne SDG, Vestre WA (1987): Effects of flunixin meglumine and dexamethasone on aqueous protein values after intraocular surgery. Am J Vet Res 48:420.

Latimer FG, et al. (2001): Pharmacokinetics of fluconazole following intravenous and oral administration and ocular tissue and body fluid concentrations of fluconazole following repeated oral dosing in horses. Am J Vet Res 62:1606.

Maggs DJ (2005): Update on pathogenesis, diagnosis, and treatment of feline herpesvirus type 1. Clin Tech Small Anim Pract 20:94.

Maggs DJ, Clarke HE (2004): In vitro efficacy of ganciclovir, cidofovir, penciclovir, foscarnet, idoxuridine, and acyclovir against feline herpesvirus type-1. Am J Vet Res 65:399.

Mathews KA (2002): Non-steroidal anti-inflammatory analgesics: a review of current practice. J Vet Emerg Crit Care 12:89.

McLaughlin SA, et al. (1983): Pathogenic bacteria and fungi associated with extraocular disease in the horse. J Am Vet Med Assoc 182:241.

Mison MB, et al. (2003): Comparison of the effects of the CO_2 surgical laser and conventional surgical techniques on healing and wound tensile strength of skin flaps in the dog. Vet Surg 32:153.

Moore CP, et al. (1995): Antibacterial susceptibility patterns for microbial isolates associated with infectious keratitis in horses: 63 cases (1986-1994). J Am Vet Med Assoc 207:928.

Moore CP, et al. (1983): Bacterial and fungal isolates from equids with ulcerative keratitis. J Am Vet Med Assoc 182:600.

Moses VS, Bertone AL (2002): Nonsteroidal anti-inflammatory drugs. Vet Clin North Am Equine Pract 18:21.

Nasisse MP, et al. (1997): Effects of valacyclovir in cats infected with feline herpesvirus 1. Am J Vet Res 58:1141.

Nasisse MP, et al. (1989): In vitro susceptibility of feline herpesvirus-1 to vidarabine, idoxuridine, trifluridine, acyclovir, or bromovinyldeoxyuridine. Am J Vet Res 50:158.

Olivero DK, et al. (1991): Clinical evaluation of 1% cyclosporine for keratoconjunctivitis sicca in dogs. J Am Vet Med Assoc 199:1039.

Ollivier FJ, et al. (2004): Profiles of matrix metalloproteinases in equine tear fluid during corneal healing in 10 horses with ulcerative keratitis. Vet Ophthalmol 7:397.

Owen RA, Jagger DW (1987): Clinical observations on the use of BCG cell wall fraction for treatment of periocular and other equine sarcoids. Vet Rec 120:548.

Owen WMA, et al. (2003): Efficacy of azithromycin for the treatment of chlamydophilosis. J Feline Med Surg 5:305.

Owens JG, et al. (1996): Pharmacokinetics of acyclovir in the cat. J Vet Pharmacol Ther 19:488.

Plummer CE, et al. (2006): Suspected ivermectin toxicosis in a miniature mule foal causing blindness. Vet Ophthalmol 9:29.

Rainbow ME, Dziezyc J (2003): Effects of twice daily application of 2% dorzolamide on intraocular pressure in normal cats. Vet Ophthalmol 6:147.

Roberts SM, et al. (1987): Ophthalmic complications following megavoltage irradiation of the nasal and paranasal cavities in dogs. J Am Vet Med Assoc 190:43.

Roberts SM, et al. (1986): Antibacterial activity of dilute povidone-iodine solutions used for ocular surface disinfection in dogs. Am J Vet Res 47:1207.

Roberts SM, et al. (1984): Effect of ophthalmic prednisolone acetate on the canine adrenal gland and hepatic function. Am J Vet Res 45:1711.

Rothschild CM, et al. (2004): Effects of trimethoprim-sulfadiazine on tear production and the fluctuations of Schirmer tear test values in horses. Vet Ophthalmol 7:385.

Simsek NA, et al. (1996): An experimental study on the effect of collagen shields and therapeutic contact lenses on corneal wound healing. Cornea 15:612.

Smith SA (2003): Deracoxib. Compend Contin Educ Pract Vet 25:419.

Sparks AH, et al. (1999): The clinical efficacy of topical and systemic therapy for the treatment of feline ocular chlamydiosis. J Feline Med Surg 1:31.

Spradbrow P (1968): The bacterial flora of the ovine conjunctival sac. Aust Vet J 44:117.

Stiles J (2004): Warning of an adverse effect of etodolac. J Am Vet Med Assoc 225:503.

Stiles J, et al. (2001): The efficacy of 0.5% proparacaine stored at room temperature. Vet Ophthalmol 4:205.

Studer ME, et al. (2000): Effects of 0.005% latanoprost solution on intraocular pressure in healthy dogs and cats. Am J Vet Res 61:1220.

van der Woerdt A, et al. (2000): Effect of single- and multiple-dose 0.5% timolol maleate on intraocular pressure and pupil size in female horses. Vet Ophthalmol 3:165.

Ward DA (1996): Comparative efficacy of topically applied flurbiprofen, diclofenac, tolmetin, and suprofen for the treatment of experimentally induced blood-aqueous barrier disruption in dogs. Am J Vet Res 57:875.

Wiebe V, Karriker M (2005): Therapy of systemic fungal infections: a pharmacologic perspective. Clin Tech Small Anim Pract 20:250.

Wilcox G (1970): Bacterial flora of the bovine eye with special reference to *Moraxella* and *Neisseria*. Aust Vet J 46:253.

Willis A, et al. (2001): Effects of topical administration of 0.005% latanoprost solution on eyes of clinically normal horses. Am J Vet Res 62:1945.

Willis AM, et al. (2001): Effect of topical administration of 2% dorzolamide hydrochloride or 2% dorzolamide hydrochloride–0.5% timolol maleate on intraocular pressure in clinically normal horses. Am J Vet Res 62:709.

Zhan G, et al. (1992): Steroid glaucoma: corticosteroid-induced ocular hypertension in cats. Exp Eye Res 54:211.

GENERAL PATHOLOGY OF THE EYE

Chapter

4

Brian P. Wilcock

OCULAR INJURY
OCULAR INFLAMMATION

RESTORATION OF HOMEOSTASIS:
   OCULAR WOUND HEALING

OCULAR NEOPLASIA
HISTOLOGIC BASIS FOR COMMON
   CLINICAL LESIONS

Ocular pathology is relevant to those interested in clinical veterinary ophthalmology because examination of the eye is the direct observation of its gross pathology; even the ophthalmoscope is a low-power microscope. There is a strong correlation between the observations made on clinical examination and the results of microscopic examination. Clinicians and pathologists use exactly the same terminology—a welcome accord that is almost unique among medical specialties and is further testimony to the inseparability of clinical ophthalmology and ophthalmic pathology.

The widely held perception that ocular pathology is so complicated and so different from the pathology of other tissues that it must forever remain the realm of the specialist is untrue. The fundamental pathologic events in the eye are identical to those occurring in other tissues. The *outcomes* of these events may be quite different because of the following three important principles of ocular pathology.

First, the globe is a closed, fluid-filled sphere that is relatively impervious to events occurring in other body systems but highly sensitive to events occurring elsewhere within the eye itself. The internal environment of the eye is separated from general body circulation by a series of intercellular tight junctions (the *blood-ocular barrier*). At the same time the fluid aqueous and vitreous allow diffusion of soluble nutrients and growth factors throughout the eye. This fluid environment permits structures like lens, cornea, and (in some species) even retina to exist with a degree of avascularity critical to proper optical function. The disadvantage of this closed system is that potentially injurious chemicals, such as inflammatory mediators, cell breakdown products, and chemical promoters of fibroplasia, are also retained and distributed throughout the globe. In nonocular settings, such chemicals are rapidly diluted, deactivated, or destroyed as they leave the immediate vicinity of their generation.

Second, proper ocular function requires precise anatomic relationships among many constituent parts. Many portions of the eye are uniquely unforgiving of the presence of even minor changes in microanatomy or physiology that occur during inflammation and wound healing. A good example is serous retinal detachment, in which serous inflammation, ordinarily a minor event, causes blindness as it elevates the retina out of visual focus and leads to eventual ischemic retinal necrosis because it separates the retina from its choroidal source of oxygen and other nutrients. Similarly, something that is usually as harmless as edema can, within highly regimented tissues like cornea or lens, critically alter the passage of light to the point of causing blindness.

Third, some of the most important ocular tissues (retina, corneal endothelium, most of the lens) are postmitotic and thus have limited capacity to regenerate after injury. In these optically sensitive tissues the types of repair phenomena (e.g., fibrosis) that might return other organs to acceptable function often do not restore (and might even worsen) ocular function. The repair of a skin wound by fibrous scarring is a familiar and useful phenomenon, but scarring of similar magnitude would be blinding in the cornea. Development of relatively minor amounts of granulation tissue, which would be helpful or inconsequential elsewhere, can create occlusion of the pupil or of the trabecular meshwork, leading to glaucoma.

OCULAR INJURY

The basics of tissue reaction to injury are the same within the eye as within other tissues, and it is not the purpose of this chapter to review what is amply discussed in any textbook of general pathology. Presented here is a brief overview of those responses, with a particular emphasis on those aspects that are different, or have a different significance, within the eye from those in other tissues.

Causes of Ocular Injury

Ocular injury can be attributed to a wider diversity of noxious stimuli than is true of any other tissue. Most organs are injured by only one or two types of agents on a regular basis, and suffer injury only infrequently from other types of processes. The eye is quite commonly injured by such a wide diversity of agents as ultraviolet irradiation, nutritional excesses and deficiencies, toxicities, infectious agents of all types, physical trauma, desiccation, genetic disorders, immune-mediated phenomena, and neoplasia.

Although diseases that initially affect the eye rarely result in disease in other tissue, the converse is not true. The eye may be affected by disease in other tissues when its structural or physiologic barriers (i.e., the blood-ocular barrier, retinal vascular autoregulation) are insufficient to maintain ocular homeostasis. Examples are ocular manifestations of systemic infectious disease, metastatic neoplasia, hypertension and diabetes, and systemic nutritional deficiencies and toxicities.

Consequences of Ocular Injury

At the cellular level the reaction of ocular tissue to injury is the same as elsewhere, and depends on the nature, duration, and severity of the insult. The response to the injurious stimulus is one or more of the following: *resistance, adaptation, injury, containment,* and *repair*.

Like any other tissue, the various ocular tissues are not without intrinsic resiliency and may successfully *resist* mild and transient injury. Alternatively, mild injury may simply be absorbed without any detectable change in ocular homeostasis. More substantial injury, particularly if prolonged, will likely trigger one or more *adaptational changes*, and even more severe/persistent injury may cause cell death *(necrosis)*. In most instances such necrosis is then followed by some form of *inflammatory reaction* intended to neutralize or otherwise contain the injurious agent. Such containment is then followed by tissue repair, ordinarily including varying proportions of *fibrosis* and *parenchymal regeneration*.

The various ocular tissues continuously interact with innumerable internal and external environmental stimuli. The outcome of that ongoing interaction is the dynamic equilibrium that we casually refer to as "normal." The definition of "normal" is always subjective and is greatly influenced by the sensitivity of the techniques we use to detect abnormalities.

When faced with an environmental challenge that exceeds their resistance (yet is not severe enough to cause outright necrosis), the various parts of the eye respond with gradual transformation into one or more *adaptational states*: hypertrophy, hyperplasia, metaplasia, dysplasia, and atrophy. A stimulus that exceeds adaptational capacity triggers degeneration and, if severe, necrosis. The same stimuli, if applied to the globe during its prenatal or postnatal development, can result in various degrees of developmental arrest known as *agenesis, aplasia,* or *hypoplasia*.

Agenesis, Aplasia, Hypoplasia

Agenesis, aplasia, and hypoplasia reflect varying severities of developmental arrest in which the organ primordium is absent *(agenesis),* has failed to develop beyond its most primitive form *(aplasia),* or has failed to complete its development *(hypoplasia)*. Because the eye of some species (notably, dogs and cats) continues to develop for many weeks after birth, there is ample opportunity for hypoplasia to occur in response to postnatally acquired stimuli. In the eye one must therefore always be careful to distinguish truly *congenital* (present at birth) from *developmental* (occurring at any time during development) stimuli.

Hypertrophy

Hypertrophy is defined as an increase in tissue mass because of an increase in cell size. It is most commonly encountered as hypertrophy of the retinal pigment epithelium (RPE) subsequent to retinal detachment of more than a few hours' duration. It is a rapid, reliable, and more or less specific change that allows one to separate genuine detachment from artifact (Figure 4-1). Hypertrophy is also seen in many other ocular tissues as a prelude to replication, such as occurs with hypertrophy of iris endothelium preparatory to the development of a preiridal fibrovascular membrane, hypertrophy of corneal stromal fibroblasts in the early stages of stromal repair, and hypertrophy of lens epithelium at various stages of cataract formation.

Hyperplasia

Hyperplasia is defined as an increase in tissue mass because of an increased number of cells. It may or may not be accompanied

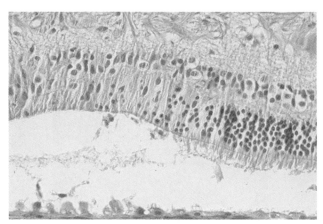

Figure 4-1. Focal hypertrophy of the retinal pigment epithelium at a site of serous retinal detachment. Degeneration of the photoreceptors and of the neurons within the outer nuclear layer indicates that this detachment has been present for at least several weeks.

by hypertrophy of the same cells. In general, hyperplasia is the more efficient response to a need for more tissue mass in all tissues that are capable of mitotic replication. It is seen under many of the same circumstances as hypertrophy, and is relatively less common in the eye than it is in most other tissues because so many of the ocular tissues have limited or no proliferative capability. Many of the most dramatic examples of hyperplasia within the eye are combined with metaplastic changes, as described later. In most instances hyperplasia within the eye is seen as a transient phase of tissue regeneration that precedes eventual normalization of the reparative tissue mass. It is seen in conjunctival and corneal epithelium following any kind of injury and may remain in a permanently excessive state in the form of an epithelial facet (a plaquelike corneal epithelial thickening). Similarly, it may remain as a plaque of hyperplastic lens capsule epithelium in the form of an anterior capsular or subcapsular cataract (Figure 4-2).

Atrophy

Atrophy implies the reduction of tissue mass at some point after the tissue had reached its full development. Causes are as diverse as ischemia, denervation, lack of hormonal or other trophic stimulation, disuse, and loss of mass due to degeneration or necrosis. Within the eye "atrophy" is used most frequently to describe senile *iris atrophy* and pressure-induced *glaucomatous atrophy* of ciliary processes, retina, and optic nerve, and as a relatively imprecise umbrella for a group of so-called retinal atrophies (Figures 4-3 and 4-4).

The retinal atrophies comprise a very mixed group of syndromes that can be called "atrophies" only in the most superficial way. They include several congenital photoreceptor dystrophies, in which the clinical and histologic lesions are delayed in onset, and others in which the mechanism of so-called atrophy is outright necrosis (as with viral retinopathies and those caused by light or toxins).

Metaplasia

Metaplasia is the conversion of one adult tissue type into another, related and more durable, tissue type. The most prevalent examples are conversion of fibrous tissue into bone, or columnar

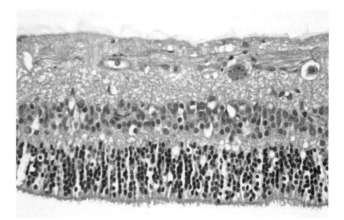

Figure 4-4. Photoreceptor atrophy in a canine retina. Only a clubbed vestige of the photoreceptors remains. This could be either inherited retinal atrophy or retinal atrophy secondary to prolonged detachment.

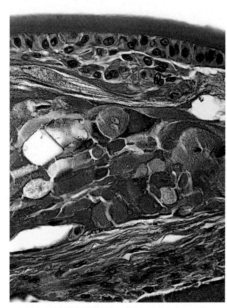

Figure 4-2. Hyperplasia and fibrous metaplasia of lens epithelium creates an anterior polar subcapsular cataract. Hydropic degeneration of regenerating lens fibers creates the so-called bladder cells typical of cataract.

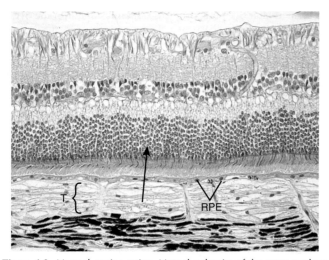

Figure 4-3. Normal canine retina. Note the density of the outer nuclear layer (arrow) and the long, slender photoreceptors that contact the surface of the inconspicuous cuboidal cells that represent the retinal pigment epithelium (RPE). The tapetum (T) and pigmented choroid are shown external to the RPE.

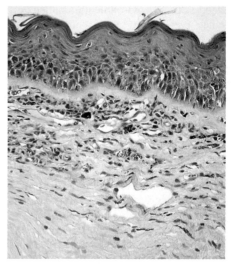

Figure 4-5. Corneal cutaneous metaplasia in a dog with chronic corneal irritation from entropion. Irregular epithelial hyperplasia, keratinization, pigmentation, and superficial stromal fibrosis are present. This is a universal response of cornea to any type of prolonged, mild to moderate injury (e.g., chronic desiccation, any chronic irritation.)

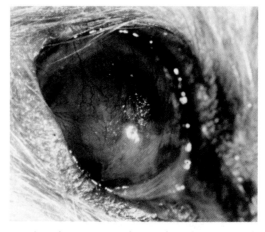

Figure 4-6. Clinical counterpart of corneal cutaneous metaplasia, in a dog with chronic keratoconjunctivitis sicca.

mucosal epithelium into stratified squamous epithelium. The usual stimulus seems to be the need to adapt to a more hostile environment by acquiring a more durable cellular phenotype. Metaplasia is a relatively uncommon reaction in most tissues, but it is a particularly prevalent and clinically important reaction within the eye. Common examples are so-called cutaneous metaplasia of the cornea in cases of chronic keratoconjunctivitis sicca or exposure keratitis, under which circumstances the cornea seems to recall its embryologic origins as skin, and thus undergoes keratinization, pigmentation, and vascularization (Figures 4-5 and 4-6). In this instance metaplasia is a protective adaptation, because the epithelium shifts to a phenotype more able to withstand dryness or chronic abrasion. Similarly, conjunctiva commonly undergoes metaplasia to a stratified squamous (and sometimes keratinized) epithelium in response to chronic irritation.

Other important examples of metaplasia occur inside the eye as fibrous metaplasia of corneal endothelium, lens epithelium, ciliary and iris epithelium, and RPE. All of these tissues are capable of fibrouslike metaplasia and quite substantial proliferation, creating retrocorneal, transpupillary, cyclitic, and retroretinal fibrous membranes. The significance of these membranes varies with location: Those crossing the pupil create the risk of blocking the outflow of aqueous humor and thus can cause glaucoma, whereas in other locations they may impair the passage of light or the diffusion of nutrients.

The most remarkable example of metaplasia is the development of lens fibers within injured bird retina (lentoid bodies). Such dramatic metaplasia defies our current understanding of ocular embryology, in that lens supposedly is of purely epithelial origin and theoretically cannot arise as a metaplastic phenomenon within the neuroectodermal retina.

Dysplasia

Dysplasia means disorderly proliferation. The term can be used in an embryologic context to signify disorderly development of a tissue, in the context of wound healing to imply a transient jumbling of tissue organization that precedes normalization, or in a neoplastic context to describe the state of disordered proliferation that is a prelude to malignant transformation. In ocular pathology we use it in all three contexts. Familiar examples are jumbled retinal development that may be inherited or may follow viral or chemical injury to the developing retina (Figures 4-7 and 4-8), conjunctival or corneal epithelial dysplasia that is a prelude to actinic squamous cell carcinoma, and non-neoplastic jumbling of corneal epithelium in any healing corneal ulcer (see Figure 4-5).

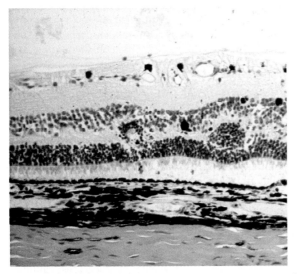

Figure 4-7. Disorderly repair within a neonatal canine retina injured by canine distemper virus infection. Although this is technically a postnecrotic retinal "dysplasia," the appearance is completely different from that of the retinal folds and rosettes seen in the idiopathic inherited dysplasias that occur in many breeds of dogs.

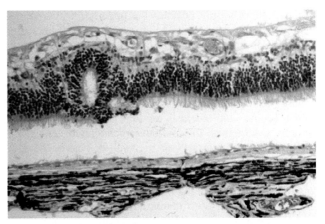

Figure 4-8. Disorganized retinal development in a dog with inherited retinal dysplasia. The rosettelike structures most often represent transverse sections through retinal folds, which in turn probably represent redundant retina in a globe with an imbalance between retinal and choroidal/scleral growth.

Dystrophy

The much-abused term *dystrophy* is strictly defined as degeneration caused by tissue malnutrition, but hardly anyone uses it in that fashion. It tends to be used to describe a variety of juvenile or adult-onset degenerative diseases that have a presumed congenital basis. Ocular examples are several degenerative corneal diseases characterized by adult-onset stromal deposition of lipid or mineral, and unexplained progressive degeneration of corneal endothelium that is clinically observed as progressive diffuse corneal edema (corneal endothelial dystrophy). Using this definition, one should classify many of the inherited photoreceptor atrophies (so-called progressive retinal atrophies) as dystrophies.

Necrosis

Any tissue subjected to an injurious environmental stimulus beyond its adaptational range will undergo lethal injury, termed *necrosis*. Most such injuries affect cell membranes and result in defective regulation of transmembrane ion exchange. Particularly critical is an influx in calcium from the calcium-rich extracellular fluid. When present in excess within the intracellular environment, calcium is a powerful cytotoxic agent that, among many other activities, disrupts oxidative phosphorylation within the mitochondria and triggers hypoxic cell death. The morphologic outcome of the membrane damage and energy paralysis is cellular swelling, hydropic disruption of the cytocavitary network, irreversible mitochondrial swelling, and eventually, irreversible damage to nuclear chromatin that manifests as the familiar histologic hallmarks of necrosis: nuclear pyknosis, karyorrhexis, and karyolysis.

Although necrosis is obviously a significant event because such dead cells lose all function, we are often more able to detect the *sequelae of necrosis* than the actual necrosis itself. These sequelae may relate to the loss of barrier function, electrical activity or secretory function, or to the initiation of inflammation and healing.

LOSS OF BARRIER FUNCTION. Normal ocular function depends on the preservation of numerous critical barriers to maintain ocular clarity. For example, we ordinarily detect corneal epithelial necrosis only because the underlying hydrophobic collagenous stroma osmotically imbibes the water from the tear film, resulting in rapid localized corneal opacity (Figures 4-9 and 4-10). Staining of the defect by fluorescein to facilitate clinical detection operates on exactly the same principle, as this hydroscopic dye binds to the now-exposed collagenous stroma. Similarly, necrosis of corneal endothelium results in deep corneal stromal edema, and necrosis of lens epithelium results in hydropic swelling of the normally dehydrated lens fibers, which we detect as cataract (see Figure 4-2). Loss of the endothelial tight junctions (as in vascular hypertension, infection with such organisms as the rickettsiae of Rocky Mountain spotted fever) within the iris or choroidal blood vessels results in serous effusion or even hemorrhage, which interferes with the clarity of the ocular media, or more serious consequences of retinal ischemia.

LOSS OF ELECTRICAL ACTIVITY. Necrosis within the retina, if extensive, may be detected as alterations in vision or as changes in the electroretinogram. Focal necrosis may be detected

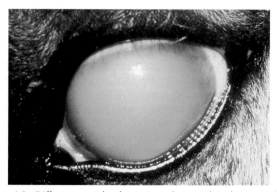

Figure 4-9. Diffuse corneal edema in a horse. The absence of conjunctival vascular reaction suggests that the cause is probably diffuse corneal endothelial disease (lens luxation, glaucoma, or immune-mediated injury).

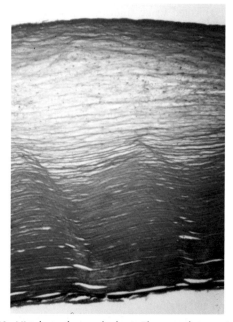

Figure 4-10. Histology of corneal edema. The normal stroma is diluted by the accumulation of fluid, changing the refractive index of the cornea and causing the characteristic gray opacity noted on clinical examination.

only by noting an increase in the tapetal reflex, because the necrosis (especially if it involves the outer nuclear layer and photoreceptors) causes a focal thinning in the light-absorbing retina. Necrosis of the tapetum itself would create a focal fundic black spot as the normally hidden pigmented choroid becomes exposed.

LOSS OF SECRETORY FUNCTION. Damage to the ciliary epithelium results in a profound reduction in the production of aqueous humor. This reduction explains, in part, the routine observation of transient ocular hypotension during uveitis of any cause. We use it to our advantage in the management of glaucoma when we attempt to selectively destroy ciliary epithelium by transscleral application of cold or laser energy to the ciliary body.

INITIATION OF INFLAMMATION: THE FIRST STEP TOWARD NORMALIZATION. It is paradoxical that our first clinical clue that there is something wrong with the eye is often the detection of inflammation because, in fact, inflammation is actually the first step in the repair process. In any tissue, cell death triggers a localized inflammatory reaction intended to ingest and remove the dead tissue. The mechanisms by which cellular injury triggers inflammation are several: release of chemicals from injured cell membrane (particularly prostaglandins) that act as direct inflammatory mediators, release of inflammatory mediators from other cells within the neighborhood (particularly mast cells or platelets), and activation of latent mediators within the plasma that frequently pools in areas vacated by recently destroyed parenchymal cells. In addition to the generation of chemicals intended to trigger the inflammatory response, these same events usually generate locally acting growth factors that stimulate parenchymal regeneration and fibrovascular stromal repair once the hostile events of inflammation have subsided. During the interval between necrosis and eventual repair, the injured tissue is frequently involved in profound inflammation that may be much more obvious, and more significant, than the tissue injury that triggered it. Although it is true that necrosis of any cause will trigger some inflammation, necrosis is not the only trigger. In fact, in most situations it is not the most potent initiator of inflammation (infectious agents and immune phenomena are more prevalent and more potent causes).

Ocular inflammation and subsequent repair are of such importance that they deserve specific consideration as separate topics.

OCULAR INFLAMMATION

Philosophically, inflammation should be considered a transient, controlled vascular and cellular response by living tissue to injury of almost any type. That response should be qualitatively and quantitatively appropriate to the nature of the tissue injury, and it should serve to neutralize and remove the injury's stimulus while also laying the groundwork for parenchymal and stromal repair. In evolution, inflammation probably first appeared as a débridement phenomenon, whereby macrophages or their equivalent would move into injured tissue, clear up the debris, and prepare the way for healing to occur. We now know that this débridement itself consists of at least two simultaneous phenomena, namely, the removal of tissue debris and the production of various growth factors that initiate the subsequent tissue repair. Later in evolution the inflammatory process assumed a more defensive role, tightly integrating with the immune system to recognize and destroy a variety of infectious and noninfectious "foreign" agents.

The major mechanical and chemical events of inflammation do not differ among the various mammalian species. Considered here are those aspects of inflammation that have particularly important consequences for the eye or that are somehow modified by peculiarities of ocular anatomy or physiology.

When it works as it should, the inflammatory reaction is a beneficial physiologic reaction that is limited only to the immediate area of injury. It should persist only as long as is necessary for its defensive and débridement activities, and it should selectively recruit only those body defenses most effective in combating the specific injurious agent. Inflammation should thus exhibit a remarkable degree of moderation and specificity so that there is no undue injury to bystander tissues or to the overall health of the animal. This remarkable balancing act is achieved by the local release of a wide range of *chemical mediators* that reside within normal parenchymal tissue, within leukocytes or platelets, and within the plasma itself. It is not practical to attempt to list all of the inflammatory mediators, their origins, and their physiologic activity. Not only does this list grow almost daily, but such lists tend to reinforce the mistaken view that a given mediator has a specific, invariable biologic activity.

Like letters of the alphabet, each inflammatory mediator is a hormonelike member of a complex biologic alphabet. Each "letter" may thus have many different meanings, depending on the company it keeps and in what sequence the letters occur. These inflammatory mediators are part of a larger group of locally acting hormonelike messengers called *cytokines*, so named because they stimulate some kind of proliferative activity on the part of neighboring cells. These cytokines create the biologic language that carries the instructions for everything from coordinated embryologic development to orderly cell death *(apoptosis)*. One must thus read the supposed activity of any given cytokine with substantial skepticism, because *there is no guarantee that the activity that we have determined by in vitro testing of isolated mediators at arbitrary dosages has anything to do with their in vivo activity at physiologic dosages and in the company of many other members of the cytokine alphabet.*

Although our understanding of the chemical mediation of inflammation and repair is still quite primitive and is largely limited to making lists of the chemicals involved, we know quite a lot about the mechanical events of inflammation. These events represent a stepwise, highly integrated chronologic sequence that involves changes in *microvascular blood flow, endothelial permeability, leukocyte migration, humoral and leukocyte-dependent neutralization of foreign material, and tissue débridement preparatory to parenchymal and stromal repair.*

The initial events of inflammation involve microvascular dilation *(hyperemia)* and endothelial cell contraction to increase the permeability of postcapillary venules to plasma solutes. This creates the redness and serous effusion that typify early inflammation, and that will continue as long as the active phase of inflammation persists. These early events are *stereotypic:* They are identical regardless of the stimulus, and they have no diagnostic specificity in terms of predicting what type of injury might have occurred. They occur in response to the rapid release of preformed chemical mediators such as histamine from mast cells or platelets within the region of initial injury.

These short-acting vasoactive mediators are then reinforced by a wide variety of mediators that are synthesized de novo from parenchymal cells, leukocytes, and other cells at sites of inflammation.

This *serous effusion* that characterizes the very early stages of inflammation is beneficial, because it serves to flood the region with a substantial array of such activated humoral defenses as complement and some broadly acting antibodies as well as to engender the leakage of fibrinogen, which will then create the fibrin scaffold that will enhance both the migration and the phagocytic efficacy of the leukocytes that follow.

Within minutes of the initiation of the preceding changes in vascular permeability, leukocytes begin to settle out of circulation, bind to endothelial cells, migrate through the now-permeable endothelial junctions, and then move through the tissues in search of the cause of tissue injury. We have recognized for many years that the types of leukocytes recruited carry substantial diagnostic value, because certain types of infectious agents or immune responses habitually recruit specific types of leukocytes. As a rule neutrophil-dominated inflammation is equated with bacterial infection, eosinophils predict hypersensitivity reactions, especially to parasites, and macrophage-dominated (granulomatous) inflammation is restricted to cell-mediated immune events and to inflammation initiated by a relatively small group of poorly degradable infectious or noninfectious agents. Only recently, however, has the basis for that sometimes remarkable specificity become apparent.

Part of the answer lies in the mixture of mediators/cytokines that are triggered by certain types of infections, but there was always an inexplicable problem: Most described *chemotactic mediators* have a fairly broad range of activity, so that many of them attract neutrophils, eosinophils, and macrophages with almost equal avidity. How, then, could we explain the empiric observation of almost purely eosinophilic infiltrates in some parasitic diseases, or purely neutrophilic infiltrates in many bacterial infections? The answer seems to lie in a second level of leukocyte "screening" that occurs at the level of the endothelial cells themselves. The locally generated inflammatory mediators rapidly stimulate the expression of leukocyte-specific *adhesion molecules* on the surface of the venular endothelium, which will bind only to complementary receptors on the surface of stimulated leukocytes that have fallen under the influence of these same local mediators. Thus, although the general chemotactic stimulus may attract many different leukocyte types into the permeable venules, only those leukocytes that can pass this second screening test will actually be allowed to enter the tissue to take up the "search-and-destroy" mission.

The leukocytes that thus enter the tissue become intermingled with the serum and fibrin that may already have accumulated because of the previous increase in vascular permeability, and these mixtures form the *inflammatory exudates* that for years have formed the basis for the prediction of disease causation based on histologic or cytologic evaluation of such exudates. These exudates are not static but are constantly changing in amount and in cellular and humoral makeup according to the ever-changing nature of the battle between the injurious agent and the tissue defenses. In its simplest form these changes may be nothing more than a gradual reduction in the intensity of the vascular response and leukocytic recruitment as the humoral and cellular defenses accomplish their task of diluting and destroying the offending agent. On the other hand, the nonspecific humoral and cellular defenses may become modified by the addition of specific immune responses as the battle continues. These immune responses act, in general, to improve both the specificity and the efficacy of what at first are relatively broad and nonselective defensive strategies.

The purpose of these defenses is to confront and destroy the offending agent. In some circumstances this is a messy affair, with spillage of leukocyte contents or excessive diffusion of humoral cytotoxic chemicals (like complement fragments) into the local environment. The resulting *bystander injury* is a substantial and undesirable side effect of inflammation, and it is sometimes a justification for intervening with drugs to dampen the inflammatory response.

Peculiarities of Ocular Inflammation

The eye seems reluctant to become involved in inflammatory disease, and for good reason: The visual function of the eye is easily disturbed and is sometimes destroyed by minor degrees of inflammation that would be considered inconsequential in most other tissues. The blood-ocular barrier, the protective presence of eyelids, the tear film, the bony orbit, and a carefully regulated system of intraocular immune tolerance all seem designed to spare the globe from the need to participate in inflammatory responses (inflammation is a second level of defense to be triggered in any tissue only when the primary structural barriers have failed). When the intraocular tissues do become involved in an inflammatory reaction, the outcome is strongly influenced by the following three unique factors:

- The globe is a closed sphere that prevents the usual dissipation of inflammatory mediators and the clearing of exudates. Intraocular inflammation is thus virtually always diffuse, because inflammatory mediators and injurious agents easily become dispersed throughout the fluid media. Although clinicians distinguish anterior uveitis from posterior uveitis, on a histologic basis virtually all intraocular inflammation is diffuse (i.e., endophthalmitis). The diffusion of inflammatory mediators also probably explains why, for example, inflammation that predominantly affects the iris will also trigger perivascular inflammation within the distant retina, or why corneal stromal inflammation will inevitably cause increased vascular permeability within the iris and ciliary body, resulting in a clinically detectable increase in protein within the aqueous humor.
- The intraocular environment contains virtually no resident defenses. There are virtually no resident granulocytes, macrophages, or lymphocytes. There are no mechanisms for self-cleansing like coughing or peristalsis.
- The function of the eye is easily disturbed by what ordinarily might seem like minor manifestations of inflammation, such as accumulation of fluid, leukocytes, or tissue debris, or even by transient fluctuations in tightly regulated intraocular physiologic processes like production of aqueous humor. Even mild serous effusion can create vision-threatening serous retinal detachment, corneal edema, and cataract, whereas fibrinous effusions threaten to create traction retinal detachment, pupillary block, or occlusion of other parts of the aqueous drainage pathway, culminating in glaucoma (Figure 4-11).

Inflammation can occur in any of the intraocular and periocular tissues, but the periocular tissues—eyelid, conjunctiva, and orbital soft tissue—react exactly like other soft tissues,

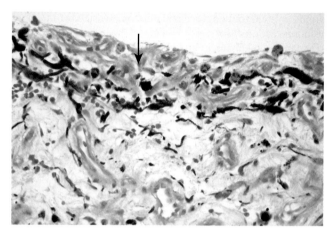

Figure 4-11. A layer of granulation tissue *(arrow)* has formed on the anterior surface of the iris, representing a source fo hyphema and the potential to cause glaucoma via occlusion of the pupil or the filtration angle.

such as skin and muscle. Our discussion here is limited to those ocular tissues that, for one reason or another, undergo rather specific and unusual patterns of inflammation.

Corneal Inflammation

The causes of corneal injury and subsequent inflammation are thoroughly discussed elsewhere in this text, but it is nonetheless useful to remember that the normal cornea is highly resistant to infectious disease. With the possible exception of viral keratitis, almost all inflammatory corneal disease is triggered by some kind of "environmental" injury to the cornea: abnormalities in the quantity or quality of the tear film, mechanical irritation from eyelids, cilia, or foreign bodies, or outright physical trauma. We nonetheless are often guilty of drawing excessively simplistic (and usually erroneous) conclusions about the significance of various bacterial or fungal isolates in the pathogenesis of corneal disease. Such erroneous conclusions often form the basis for ineffective or even harmful antimicrobial therapy.

Because inflammation is fundamentally a vascular event, the avascular cornea cannot undergo true inflammation until it has acquired blood vessels by ingrowth from the limbus. The very acute manifestations of corneal "inflammation" after injury (neutrophilia and corneal edema) are in fact passive events related to corneal ulceration, so that neutrophils and fluid are imbibed from the adjacent tear film. The first genuine inflammatory reaction to corneal injury occurs in the nearest available vascular bed, ordinarily that of the limbus. Depending on the diffusion of inflammatory mediators, vessels within the conjunctiva or even the iris may participate. A peripheral ring of edema (serous effusion) commonly accompanies increased permeability of limbal perivascular venules, and protein effusion from the iris vessels enters the aqueous humor to create *aqueous flare*. Leukocytes (usually neutrophils) migrate through these permeable vessels, and those from the bulbar conjunctiva or limbic sclera migrate into the corneal stroma at a level appropriate to the localization of the stimulus. Shallow injuries/infections thus stimulate only a superficial stromal infiltration.

The corneal stroma may be the victim of *bystander injury* as the intracellular neutrophilic enzymes diffuse into the surrounding tissue while the neutrophils do battle with various infectious agents. The resulting lesion (Figures 4-12 and 4-13) is known as *suppurative keratomalacia* (*malacia* = softening).

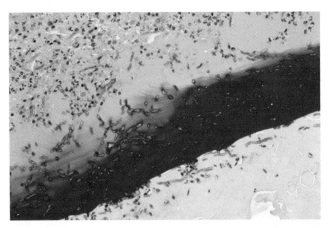

Figure 4-12. Severe deep mycotic keratitis. The deep corneal stroma has been destroyed by the bystander effects of neutrophil accumulation. Descemet's membrane, staining magenta, is heavily infiltrated by fungal hyphae.

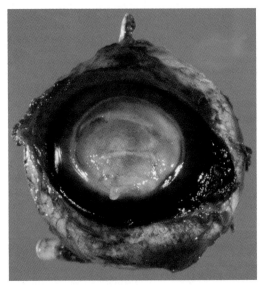

Figure 4-13. Suppurative keratomalacia in an enucleated equine globe. The corneal stroma was destroyed by enzymes released from neutrophils immigrating into the cornea in response to opportunistic bacterial infection.

These leukocytes and the injured cornea itself are the most important sources of the fibroblastic and angioblastic growth factors that, after a delay of 3 or 4 days, initiate the ingrowth of blood vessels and fibroblasts from the limbus. There will also be fibroblastic transformation of the keratocytes themselves, which begin to produce large amounts of extracellular matrix, particularly chondroitin sulphate.

As all clinicians recognize, the transformation of the avascular cornea into a vascularized tissue capable of participating fully in inflammatory responses is a mixed blessing, for the enhanced protective and wound-healing capabilities of this "transformed" cornea are at the same time the events that will lead to some degree of permanent corneal scarring. Incidentally, this 3- to 4-day delay in ingrowth of blood vessels is a "period of grace" during which the cornea (either with or without our assistance) can try to deal with minor injury without running the risk of permanent scarring.

Nomenclature of Intraocular Inflammation

In theory one can have inflammation that is isolated to any of the intraocular compartments. Thus, one can postulate the existence of *iritis, cyclitis* (inflammation of the ciliary body), *choroiditis, retinitis,* and even *hyalitis* (inflammation of the vitreous itself). In reality, however, the interior of the globe almost always acts as a unit when responding to inflammatory stimuli, simply because the fluid ocular media do not allow rigid isolation of inflammatory agents or inflammatory chemical mediators. Thus we habitually use broader terminology, as follows:

- *Anterior uveitis (iridocyclitis):* Inflammation of the iris and ciliary body, with inflammatory exudate accumulating within the aqueous humor as aqueous flare or (if purulent) hypopyon.
- *Posterior uveitis:* Inflammation of the choroid, often with accumulation of inflammatory exudate in the subretinal space to cause retinal detachment.
- *Chorioretinitis:* Inflammation affecting the choroid and adjacent retina, almost always with exudate accumulating within the adjacent vitreous and subretinal space.
- *Endophthalmitis:* Inflammation of the entire uveal tract along with inflammatory effusion into the aqueous and vitreous humors.
- *Panophthalmitis:* Endophthalmitis that has extended to involve even the sclera. Although there are traditional clinical criteria to distinguish anterior from posterior uveitis, or choroiditis from chorioretinitis, almost all substantial intraocular inflammatory disease is histologically classified as *endophthalmitis.* Even when the majority of the inflammation is limited to the iris, there is almost always some inflammation within retina, choroid, and vitreous. *Panophthalmitis* is actually quite rare and is almost entirely limited to being a late complication of uncontrolled bacterial endophthalmitis after penetrating injury.

Common Sequelae of Intraocular Inflammation

Inflammatory Retinal Detachment

Because the retina is not truly attached to the RPE, there is a potential space between the photoreceptors and the RPE that is the remnant of the original optic vesicle. Any increase in permeability within the choroidal blood vessels, such as with hypertension or with acute inflammation, results in accumulation of fluid between the RPE and the photoreceptors, creating a serous retinal detachment (Figure 4-14). Much less common is the so-called traction detachment that results from organization of vitreal fibrinous exudates. Because the outer half of retina is nourished by diffusion from the choroid, any separation has dire consequences in terms of outer retinal viability. The rapidity with which there is microscopically visible photoreceptor injury, and the time at which that injury becomes irreversible, varies with the nature of the subretinal fluid and with the height of the detachment (i.e., the nutrient diffusion distance). Light-microscopic evidence of photoreceptor damage occurs within about 10 days following experimental infusion of saline into the subretinal space. It seems to occur much more quickly if that fluid is laden with leukocytic or other tissue breakdown products (see Figure 4-1).

Cataract

Because lens nutrition depends totally on the controlled flow of normal aqueous humor to deliver nutrients and remove wastes,

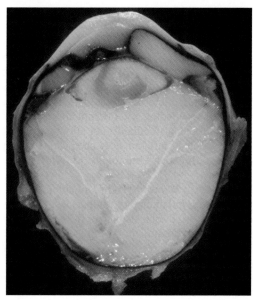

Figure 4-14. Diffuse endophthalmitis has caused serous retinal detachment, posterior synechia, and iris bombé. The fixative has caused coagulation of the markedly increased protein within the aqueous and vitreous humors that represents the inevitable outcome of greater vascular permeability during acute inflammation.

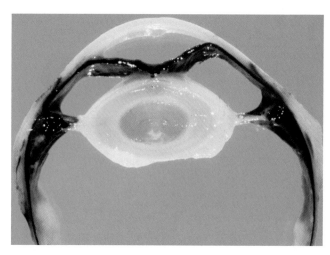

Figure 4-16. Posterior synechia leading to a pupillary block, iris bombé, and secondary peripheral anterior synechia. The pupillary block and the peripheral anterior synechia combined to cause inevitable secondary glaucoma.

inflammation results in cataract because of the reduction in the production of aqueous and the addition of abnormal chemical constituents as by-products of inflammation.

Glaucoma

Most cases of secondary glaucoma are related to consequences of inflammation that, in most other tissues, would have been considered minor inconveniences. Because the iris normally

contacts the anterior face of the lens, the most common of such complications is *posterior synechia*, in which the inflamed iris adheres to the surface of lens and results in pupillary obstruction and iris bombé (Figures 4-14 to 4-17). In contrast, iridocorneal *adhesion (anterior synechia)* is almost always associated with perforating corneal injury, which serves to "suck" the iris up to the corneal defect to facilitate its adhesion at that site (Figure 4-18). In contrast to what is often written, glaucoma caused by accumulation of inflammatory debris within the trabecular meshwork appears to be a very rare event in any of the domestic species. This is hardly surprising, because it is unlikely that exudate will seal a significant proportion of the 360-degree filtration angle. A more important cause of glaucoma is the development of a *preiridal fibrovascular membrane* on the face of the iris and within the trabecular meshwork itself. Such membranes are nothing more than ordinary granulation tissue, the normal response to the need to rebuild tissue scaffolding preparatory to parenchymal regeneration. Within the unforgiving environment of the eye, however, this granulation tissue can be deadly, because

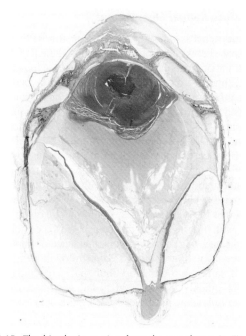

Figure 4-15. The histologic section from the eye shown in Figure 4-14. The endophthalmitis occurred in response to a penetrating corneal injury (cat claw) that could have created traumatic uveitis, lens-induced (phacoclastic) uveitis, and/or bacterial endophthalmitis.

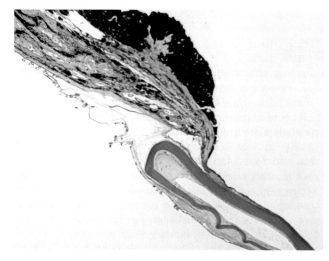

Figure 4-17. The iris adheres to the anterior capsule of a liquefied and collapsed lens, resulting in pupillary block and secondary glaucoma.

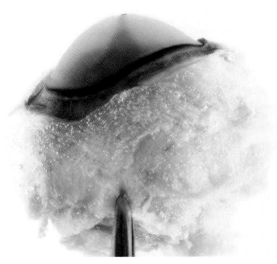

Figure 4-18. Transilluminated bovine globe with anterior synechia. The iris is drawn into a tent as it anchors into the cornea at the site of previous perforating injury.

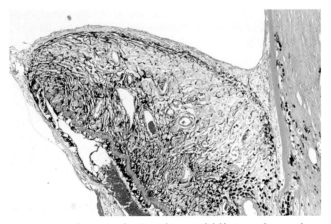

Figure 4-19. Higher magnification of a preiridal fibrovascular membrane. The iris blood vessels are activated in response to angiogenic factors contained within the aqueous humor, and migrate onto the surface of the iris. They may cause pupillary block, peripheral anterior synechia, or hemorrhage.

it may seal the pupillary aperture *(pupillary block)* or impair outflow through the pectinate ligament (Figure 4-19).

Alterations in the Blood-Ocular Barrier and Implications for Immune-Mediated Disease

One of the fundamental events of inflammation, occurring within minutes of the inflammatory stimulus, is the chemically mediated contraction of endothelial cells that creates gaps through which fluid and, later, leukocytes may leave the vascular compartment. This results in rapid dissolution of the blood-ocular barrier at the level of the endothelium of iris vasculature. Disruption of the blood-ocular barrier is not so rapid within ciliary processes, which tend to distend with accumulating inflammatory exudates until, eventually, the tight junctions of the nonpigmented epithelium become disrupted. At this stage these two components of the blood-ocular barrier are temporarily incompetent; restitution of this disrupted barrier takes many months and may never be perfectly restored. As a result of this disruption there is an abnormally vigorous exchange of molecular substances between the intraocular and extraocular environments. In terms of therapy, this disruption of the blood-ocular barrier allows access of a wide range of therapeutic agents to the eye, a positive side effect of the inflammatory process. It also results in interaction between ocular antigens and the systemic immune system, an interaction that ordinarily is tightly regulated to maintain tolerance by the extraocular immune system to small amounts of leaking intraocular antigens.

The concept that most intraocular antigens, particularly those of lens, are totally "foreign" is incorrect, but the amount that normally reaches systemic (splenic) immunocytes is very small. The concept of *anterior chamber–associated immune deviation* presumes that intraocular antigens are somehow processed within the eye (probably by dendritic cells within the trabecular meshwork) before draining from the trabecular meshwork into systemic circulation. These antigens, upon reaching the spleen, initiate a typical humeral immune response but an atypical, muted T-cell response. There is no defect in proliferation of antigen-specific cytotoxic T cells, but there is induction of a population of suppressor T cells, which inhibits any cell-mediated hypersensitivity to the sensitizing antigen. The theoretical result is that any lymphocytes that return to the eye are capable of producing only the most localized and specific types of inflammatory events, and the subsets of T cells that produce a lot of nonspecific "bystander" injury are suppressed.

Following virtually any kind of ocular injury, antigens leaving the eye reach the spleen, stimulate lymphoid proliferation, and result in return of splenic lymphocytes to the eye about 1 week later. Typically these lymphocytes are seen as perivascular aggregates in the iris and ciliary stroma. As in inflammatory reactions anywhere else, only a small proportion of these returning lymphocytes are specifically sensitized to the initiating antigen. The rest carry receptors for a wide variety of unrelated antigens, which may be important to our understanding of the recurrent nature of many cases of uveitis in domestic animals. In brief, it is quite plausible that the recurrent bouts of uveitis are triggered by exposure of these polyclonal lymphocytes to a wide variety of antigens, even vaccinal antigens, that have nothing to do with the events that caused the original bout of uveitis.

The very slow restitution of a blood-ocular barrier and the presence of these polyclonal reactive lymphocytes would seem to guarantee that all uveitis be persistent or cyclical. The presence of active transforming growth factor-beta (TGF-β) in normal aqueous humor has a profound inhibitory effect on lymphocyte (particularly T-cell) proliferation and also on the action of such potent effectors of cell-mediated immunity as interleukin-2 and interleukin-4. What we see is the outcome of a very complex interaction of many interacting and overlapping regulatory systems designed to enhance the specificity of the immune response, and to limit its duration and harmful side effects.

Etiologic Implications of Inflammatory Exudates

The admirable specificity of the acute inflammatory response notwithstanding, it is essential to recognize that inflammation is a dynamic and changing system and that the initial events of inflammation blend with those of immune-mediated events even within a few days. Thus inflammation that is initially suppurative may change into something that looks granulomatous or lymphocytic, and conversely, it is theoretically possible that neutrophilic inflammation may become eosinophilic, or that eosinophilic may become granulomatous. An example is *feline infectious peritonitis,* which is described as being granulomatous or pyogranulomatous but which may be suppurative, fibrinous, lymphocytic-plasmacytic, or granulomatous, depending on the stage of the disease and on complex immunologic interactions that remain undiscovered.

Another example is *phacoclastic uveitis,* which varies from suppurative to lymphocytic to granulomatous, depending on the interval between lens injury and histologic examination. This is a delayed, immune-mediated reaction to the release of large amounts of previously normal lens protein into the intraocular environment. Although that lens protein is certainly not completely "foreign," the sudden release of a large volume of such protein after spontaneous or traumatic lens rupture overwhelms immune tolerance and results in a severe suppurative-to-granulomatous perilenticular uveitis that often destroys the globe. Even if the inflammation can be successfully controlled, its wound-healing sequelae often induce pupillary block and secondary glaucoma. The amount of lens material leaking out of the lens seems to be the most important determinant of whether this fateful reaction is triggered. There are other variables as well, for considerable species differences cannot be explained just on the basis of duration of disease or the size of the lens capsular defect. In rabbits and birds the reaction in phacoclastic uveitis is much more granulomatous than in dogs, cats, or horses (Figures 4-20 and 4-21).

Nonetheless, certain broad principles allow a guess as to the nature of the offending agent until more definitive identification (via culture or other means) is available:

Suppurative exudates imply bacterial infection, particularly when the neutrophils are lytic. Neutrophils also predominate in the early stages of phacoclastic uveitis.

Eosinophilic exudates occur with parasitic migration but are only rarely seen within the globe. They more frequently occur around parasitic migration tracts within the conjunctiva (as with *Habronema* or *Onchocerca* lesions in horses). More commonly, eosinophilic infiltrates are seen with allergic reactions and are particularly frequent in the conjunctiva and cornea of cats affected with eosinophilic keratitis.

Granulomatous inflammation is inflammation that is dominated, from its onset, by macrophages. It is a term that is commonly abused, because how many macrophages are required, or what percentage of the total leukocyte population must be macrophages before such a classification can be properly used, has not been established. Because all inflammation will sooner or later become dominated by mononuclear leukocytes, there is a danger that the somewhat specific term "granulomatous" will be used interchangeably with simple chronic inflammation. There are numerous dramatic examples of granulomatous inflammation in ocular pathology. Leakage of sebaceous secretion from inflamed or neoplastic sebaceous glands results in a pure granulomatous periadnexal inflammation known as *chalazion.* A mixed lymphocytic and granulomatous nodular inflammation of the conjunctiva or adjacent sclera is common in dogs and has variously been called *nodular fasciitis, nodular granulomatous episcleritis,* or even *fibrous histiocytoma.* Various *systemic mycoses* stimulate a granulomatous or mixed neutrophilic-histiocytic (pyogranulomatous) infiltrate, commonly

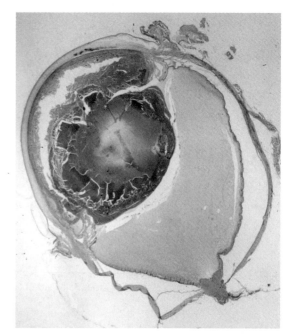

Figure 4-20. Traumatic lens rupture resulting in an intractable, immune-mediated pyogranulomatous perilenticular inflammation known as phacoclastic uveitis.

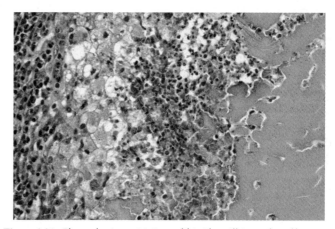

Figure 4-21. Phacoclastic uveitis in a rabbit. The still-intact lens fibers are surrounded by a layer of neutrophils, then foamy macrophages, and then lymphocytes. The character of the reaction varies substantially with time and with the species.

more obvious in the subretinal space and choroid than in the anterior uvea (Figure 4-22). Finally, cell-mediated immune responses frequently culminate in granulomatous inflammation, as occurs in *phacoclastic uveitis* and in the diffuse granulomatous destructive endophthalmitis known as *uveodermatologic syndrome (Vogt-Koyanagi-Harada–like syndrome)* that appears to be an immune response against intraocular (and occasionally epidermal) melanin pigment.

Lymphocytic-plasmacytic inflammation is the most common pattern of inflammation within the globe. It may reflect specific recruitment of lymphocytes and plasma cells in response to viral infection or to other intraocular antigens incapable of inducing the other humoral and cellular types of inflammation. Often, however, lymphocytic-plasmacytic inflammation reflects

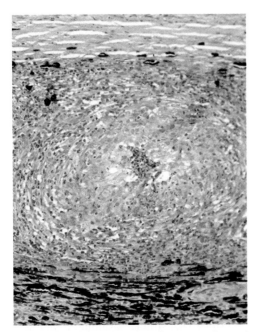

Figure 4-22. Choroidal suppurating granuloma in a dog with systemic blastomycosis. With higher magnification, budding yeast was found in similar granulomas throughout the choroid and subretinal space.

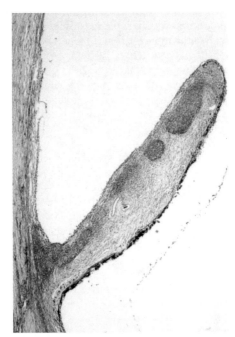

Figure 4-23. Coalescing perivascular lymphoid aggregates create so-called lymphonodular uveitis in a cat. Similar lesions are seen in all species as the common histologic counterpart of persistent or recurrent uveitis. The cause is rarely determined, and such cases are frequently dismissed as "immune-mediated."

nothing more than the normal maturation of the inflammatory response. Virtually all types of inflammation, as they age, recruit growing numbers of long-lived mononuclear leukocytes that eventually predominate within the exudate. Such accumulations may reflect a very specific response to an infectious agent that is now recognized as an antigen, but it is equally possible that these lymphocytes are responding to normal ocular antigens excessively exposed by the inflammatory disruption of the blood-ocular barrier. Lymphocytic anterior uveitis is the usual pattern seen in posttraumatic uveitis even when there has been no penetrating injury. Regardless, lymphocytes and plasma cells may occur as diffuse uveal infiltrates or as discrete perivascular lymphoid aggregates. In all domestic species we see persistent or recurrent lymphocytic-plasmacytic uveitis, and hardly ever do we identify a specific offending agent or antigen (Figures 4-23 and 4-24).

RESTORATION OF HOMEOSTASIS: OCULAR WOUND HEALING

The mechanisms of wound healing within the eye have received a great deal of attention for two reasons. First, healing of ocular injuries is intrinsically important for the well-being of the eye, and even minor defects in this normally well-regulated process may have disastrous consequences for optical clarity, aqueous drainage, or other ocular functions that are exquisitely sensitive to minor changes in anatomic fidelity. Second, the ability to directly visualize the sequelae to injury in such tissues as cornea or even retina has made the eye a much-favored tissue for basic research in the mechanisms and pharmacologic manipulation of wound healing.

Wound healing includes both mitotic parenchymal regeneration and regeneration of the connective tissue scaffolding, sometimes simply referred to as "scarring." They frequently are portrayed as competing or antagonistic activities, but they are

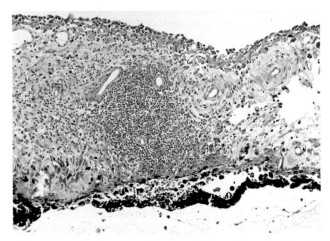

Figure 4-24. A higher magnification of the perivascular lymphoid accumulation within the iris of a cat with lymphonodular uveitis seen in Figure 4-23.

interdependent and even complementary. Following any substantial tissue injury, successful parenchymal regeneration requires the removal of any persisting infection and tissue debris, the preservation or reconstruction of a connective tissue scaffold, the survival of an adequate population of mitotically competent germinal cells, and the presence of an adequate blood supply. If the initial injury has so damaged the original tissue stromal scaffold or vasculature that it cannot perform this supportive role, parenchymal regeneration must wait until a new scaffold and/or vasculature has been recruited from the nearest available source. Although this new scaffolding may seem unsightly or even excessive, it is a deliberate and essential prerequisite to parenchymal rebuilding.

At a molecular level wound healing is regulated by a variety of locally produced cytokines, the most important of which are basic fibroblast growth factor (bFGF), epidermal growth factor (EGF), TGF-β, platelet-derived growth factor (PDGF), and vascular endothelial growth factor (VEGF). As with those cytokines that act as inflammatory mediators, the action of these wound-healing cytokines also is greatly influenced by the *context* in which each occurs (i.e., where, when, how much, and in what company). Although interest in these cytokines has given rise to a huge body of literature, it is wise to remember the four classic "morphologic" prerequisites for regeneration: débridement, stromal scaffold, germinal cells, and blood supply. It is inadequacy in one or more of these traditional prerequisites that most commonly results in a failure of proper healing, and it also is these various phenotypic parameters that we attempt to manipulate by such procedures as mechanical or chemical débridement, suturing, and grafting. Nonetheless, the availability of at least a few of these cytokines as purified therapeutic agents holds great promise in the investigation and treatment of a whole range of conditions typified by apparently defective repair.

Germinal Cells

Tissue regeneration can occur only in those tissues that contain a population of mitotically competent germinal cells. The application of this principle to the eye is obvious when one deals with wound healing in retina. Injuries to the developing retina often result in disorderly reparative proliferation of the retinal neurons, leading to retinal dysplasia. Exactly the same injury to the adult retina results in retinal scarring, because only the glial cells and vasculature are able to proliferate in the mature retina. The age at which the retinal neurons cease mitotic activity varies with the species and results in a different temporal definition of "retinal dysplasia," depending on the species involved. For cattle and horses lesions of retinal dysplasia (rosettes and disordered intermixing of the various retinal layers) is necessarily an in utero event, but in dogs and cats injury to the retina any time up to about week 6 after birth results in retinal dysplasia. Because, in the latter two species, the retina matures first near the optic disc and ceases mitotic activity last near the ora ciliaris, it is sometimes possible to determine the age at which the insult occurred from the topographic distribution of the dysplastic lesions. In those areas of retina that had ceased mitotic activity at the time of the injury, retinal scars rather than dysplastic foci will develop. In at least some species of fish the retina retains mitotic capability throughout life, and thus lesions of retinal dysplasia could develop at any age.

At the opposite end of the regenerative spectrum is the conjunctival and corneal epithelium. The normal corneal epithelium turns over every 7 to 10 days, fed by a population of germinal cells with a limited number of "preprogrammed" mitotic cycles (the *transient amplifying population*). The *permanent replicative population*, with no apparent limit on mitotic capability, is found at the junction of corneal and conjunctival epithelium near the limbus.

After shallow injury to the corneal epithelium, the immediate (after about 1 hour) reaction is one of flattening and sliding by viable adjacent wing cells, and then by basal cells, so that even large (1-cm) defects may be covered in as little as 72 hours if the basal lamina is intact. Within 24 to 36 hours

mitotic figures are seen within the permanent replicative population at the limbus but are inconspicuous in the epithelium adjacent to the ulcer itself. After a single injury mitotic activity becomes maximal at 10 days, dropping rapidly thereafter.

The loss of the hydrophobic epithelial barrier allows for the rapid osmotic absorption of water from the tear film into the superficial stroma. Even in nonseptic shallow ulcers the fluid absorption is usually accompanied by modest numbers of neutrophils (Figures 4-25 and 4-26). In the presence of bacterial or fungal contamination the number of neutrophils is greatly increased. The leakage of neutrophil enzymes into the surrounding stroma may lead to stromal malacia and the risk of corneal perforation and iris prolapse (Figures 4-27 and 4-28).

Persistent or repeated corneal epithelial injury, in the presence of a competent germinal population and an adequate stroma, results in epithelial hyperplasia and even dysplasia. Such stimulated epithelium may acquire rete ridges and even pigmentation, perhaps because the ingrowing cells from the limbus have not entirely abandoned their conjunctival heritage. If the stimulus is chronic desiccation, the epithelium will also undergo adaptive keratinization. In most cases there is accompanying injury to the superficial stroma, resulting in ingrowth of fibroblasts and blood vessels in parallel with the adaptive epithelial changes and leading to so-called corneal cutaneous metaplasia (Figures 4-29 and 4-30).

A variety of ocular tissues, particularly corneal endothelium and lens epithelium, offer interesting adaptations in cellular regeneration. Depending on the species, each of these tissues has relatively little mitotic capability and, under normal circumstances, regenerates poorly. This is true of corneal endothelium, which is claimed not to regenerate at all in adult dogs and cats. Loss of corneal endothelial cells results in sliding of adjacent

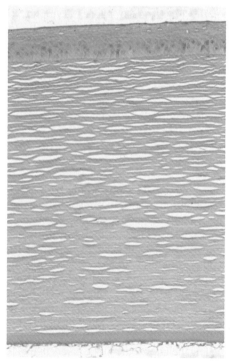

Figure 4-25. Normal canine cornea. The nonkeratinized, nonpigmented, stratified corneal epithelium adheres to the surface of a cell-poor, avascular, and highly regimented fibrous stroma.

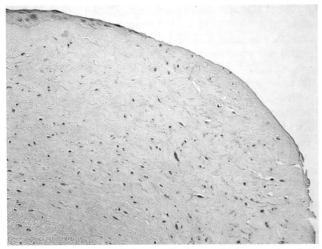

Figure 4-26. Acute corneal ulcer. Within hours of injury causing shallow ulceration, viable epithelial cells adjacent to the defect flatten and slide across the surface of the defect. The denuded corneal stroma rapidly absorbs water and neutrophils from the tear film.

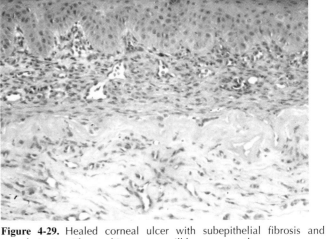

Figure 4-29. Healed corneal ulcer with subepithelial fibrosis and vascularization. The resulting cornea will be permanently opaque.

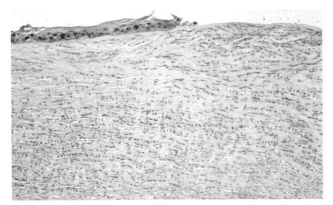

Figure 4-27. Acute corneal ulcer progressing to suppurative keratitis. If the exposed stroma becomes contaminated with bacteria, the recruitment of neutrophils is greatly increased, and the potential for neutrophil-mediated stromal destruction (keratomalacia) is similarly greater.

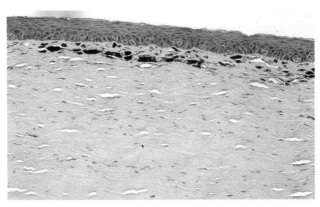

Figure 4-30. Corneal cutaneous metaplasia with subepithelial scarring and pigmentation. This could be a sequel to previous ulceration, or to persistent sublethal corneal irritation to which the cornea must adapt.

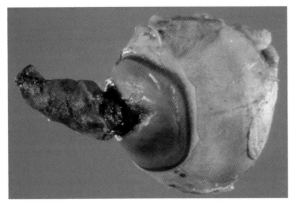

Figure 4-28. Rapidly progressing corneal ulcer leading to perforation and iris prolapse.

viable endothelium to seal the defect and may not cause any permanent functional impairment of the endothelial monolayer. In contrast, some injuries result in fibroblastic metaplasia of the corneal endothelium. In this fibroblastic disguise the epithelium seems to acquire very dramatic proliferative capabilities,

sometimes resulting in so-called retrocorneal fibrous membrane, which can lead to glaucoma. Similarly the mature lens epithelium appears to have very little replicative capability yet responds with fibroblastic metaplasia to a variety of injuries; in this form, it is capable of dramatic proliferation, which can result in drastic consequences in terms of pupillary obstruction. As one "descends" the phylogenetic scale the proliferative capacity of ocular tissues increases, so that adult corneal endothelial cells and even retinal neurons in reptiles, amphibians, and fish may retain mitotic capability.

Tissue Scaffold

To rebuild a functionally significant anatomic unit, epithelial cells require some kind of tissue scaffold as a "road map" for repair. If the initial injury has not left enough of the original scaffold, a new one must be built with contributions from the epithelial cells themselves (i.e., basement membrane) and from proliferation of adjacent stroma. When properly regulated the combination of these two phenomena results in perfect, or almost perfect, restitution of normal structure and function.

The best example is healing of corneal ulcers. A shallow defect heals by sliding, replication, and eventual normalization of the corneal epithelium as described earlier. Adhesion to the denuded stroma is at first via fibronectin and laminin produced by reactive stromal fibroblasts, absorbed leukocytes, and the epithelium itself. In as little as 3 days, the epithelium produces at least some fragments of new basement membrane in amounts great enough to be microscopically detected. It tends to do this even if the original membrane is still present, and this thickening or duplication of basement membrane serves as a reliable marker of previous epithelial injury in cornea and lens. Re-formation of the hemidesmosomes and the ultrastructural collagenous anchoring fibrils that represent the normal, firm adhesion between the epithelium and the stroma may require many weeks.

Those defects that involve a loss of more than the superficial 25% of the stroma often require both stromal and epithelial repair (this figure is arbitrary and just an approximation; numerous exceptions exist). In these instances the epithelial regeneration must await the rebuilding of the stromal scaffold that occurs via a process of fibroplasia and angiogenesis identical to wound healing in the skin. The major difference, of course, is the need for the normally avascular corneal stroma to recruit angioblasts from the limbus, and thus the process of corneal stroma repair is considerably delayed compared with that occurring in normally vascularized collagenous tissues such as the dermis. Under experimental circumstances recruitment of the angioblasts begins by budding from venules at the limbus within as little as 72 hours after corneal injury, and these vessels migrate in a laminar fashion into the stroma, moving approximately 1 mm per day.

The combination of stromal fibroplasia and vascularization (usually termed *granulation tissue*) can be seen migrating all the way from the limbus to the site of stromal injury. Over the bed of granulation tissue, the epithelium slides, proliferates, produces new basement membrane, and adheres. As in wounds elsewhere, the fibroblasts produce a whole sequence of precollagenous and collagenous matrix types that eventually remodel into a stroma that is only slightly less regular than the adjacent normal stroma. The resultant scar never quite matches the normal cornea in terms of histologic architecture or optical clarity, but some cases come very close (see Figure 4-30).

The same phenomena of epithelial proliferation, basement membrane reduplication, and stromal fibroplasia/angiogenesis occur elsewhere in the eye, but in these noncorneal locations they usually seem unwelcome events. For example, injury to lens epithelium via perforation, by adherence of pupillary membranes, or sometimes just through the biochemical events of cataract results in plaquelike proliferation and fibrous metaplasia of capsular epithelium, usually with reduplication of multiple laminae of basement membrane to increase the density and thus the visual significance of the lens opacity. As a more exaggerated example, the devastating consequences of lens rupture (*phacoclastic uveitis*) seem to be the result of escape of the lens epithelium through a rent in the lens capsule, resulting in perilenticular proliferation of this fibroblastic epithelial membrane to cause pupillary block and secondary glaucoma (see later). The important phenomenon of *preiridal fibrovascular membrane* (and rarely, preretinal fibrovascular membrane) is no more than a proliferation of granulation tissue

from the stroma of the iris (or retina) that is "accidentally" exposed to growth factors released at some distant site within the eye (see Figures 4-18 and 4-19). Ciliary body tumors and detached retinas are particularly common and potent initiators of preiridal and, occasionally, preretinal membranes. These membranes are initially fragile and may lead to intractable hyphema or, as they mature, may cause pupillary block, retinal detachment, or sealing of the filtration angle. Trabecular endothelial cells within the filtration angle are also susceptible to the same proliferative stimuli and may contribute to the glaucoma that frequently follows the formation of preiridal membranes.

Adequate Nutrition

Lack of adequate nutrition is an important determinant of wound healing in the cornea and lens, two tissues that normally have a precarious nutritional supply. Cornea is nourished by absorption from the tear film, anterior chamber, and vascular network at the limbus. Of these, the presence of a quantitatively and qualitatively adequate tear film appears to be most important. Ingrowth of blood vessels from the limbus is commonly seen during the healing of any severe corneal injury (see Figures 4-29 and 4-30). Although it may have serious implications for later corneal transparency, this ingrowth is an essential ingredient of the wound-healing process. Such vessels are permanent, although they diminish in size and are no longer filled with blood, because the requirement for this augmented nutritional support fades after reconstruction of the corneal wound.

Various types of conjunctival grafts are nothing more than efforts to speed up the arrival of blood vessels into the injured corneal stroma, therefore augmenting whatever nutrition is arriving via the tear film.

Diseases Resulting from Defective Wound Healing

Although many ocular syndromes could be considered the result of *inappropriate* wound healing—corneal stromal scarring, posterior synechia, traction retinal detachment and postnecrotic retinal dysplasia, which have been mentioned already—the wound healing in those syndromes is perfectly normal and appropriate to the nature of the initial injury. There are, however, a few examples of *improperly regulated or inadequate wound healing* that cause distinct ocular disease syndromes.

The syndromes canine persistent ulcer, feline corneal sequestration, and equine corneal sequestration are probably all reflections of the same fundamental defect. With every significant corneal epithelial injury, there is a transient degeneration of the most superficial corneal stroma, characterized by cellular apoptosis and stromal matrix disintegration. In normal wound healing that superficial stromal degeneration is only transient and does not interfere with subsequent migration and adhesion of the regenerating epithelium. In some individuals, however, the depth and persistence of that stromal degeneration are excessive and it becomes histologically visible as a corneal sequestrum. Because permanent adhesion of the regenerating epithelium depends on the extension of ultrastructural "anchors" from the epithelial cell membranes into the superficial stroma, the inability of the degenerate stroma to secure those anchors results in ineffective epithelial adhesion and recurrent ulceration. In dogs the most obvious clinical manifestation is the recurring ulceration; in cats the absorption of colored breakdown products from the tear film into the area of stromal degeneration (creating the familiar dark brown-to-black lesion of feline corneal sequestration) is more obvious.

Preiridal fibrovascular membrane is an important lesion in all species, reflecting the inappropriate activation of what would otherwise be considered a normal wound-healing response. It is a membrane of highly vascular granulation tissue growing out of the iris stroma onto the anterior surface of the iris (see Figure 4-19). In this location it has the potential to act as a source for persistent hyphema and to cause glaucoma by creating either a peripheral anterior synechia or a pupillary block. This fibrovascular membrane is stimulated in response to angiogenic growth factors originating elsewhere within the globe, most commonly from detached retinas and from intraocular neoplasms. The membrane is considered "inappropriate" because it has nothing to do with wound healing of the iris itself. These angiogenic growth factors are secreted into the aqueous or vitreous and activate the fibrous and vascular stroma of the distant iris seemingly by accident (the iris stroma has no epithelial membrane along its anterior surface, so the iris stroma is always in free communication with whatever chemicals are found within the aqueous humor). Understanding the pathogenesis and significance of preiridal fibrovascular membranes has provided a long-overdue explanation for why detached retinas or even small intraocular tumors can cause persistent hyphema and/or glaucoma.

The understanding of normal wound healing represents an exciting frontier in terms of therapeutic intervention. We now have a whole variety of chemical promoters and inhibitors of many different aspects of wound healing, including epithelial proliferation, fibroplasia, and angiogenesis. The problem is that we still do not understand the complexity of their interactions with one another and with various components of the ocular environment that determine their activity in vivo. As mentioned previously, most of these chemicals can manifest different (and sometimes even contradictory) activities, depending on dosage, the time at which they are introduced, and the presence or absence of other chemical mediators. We are still in the early stages of learning when and how to use these products; it appears that most of the time there is no deficiency in the availability of the naturally occurring chemical mediators of wound healing. In many cases, simply adding more of these mediators is unnecessary and even potentially harmful.

OCULAR NEOPLASIA

The eye is the origin for only a limited variety of neoplasms, and accurate predictions about the type and the prognosis can frequently be made even in the absence of histologic confirmation. Details about clinical appearance, treatment, and prognosis can be found in the appropriate chapters elsewhere in this text. This discussion is limited to fundamental aspects of cancer biology and the common principles that influence the effects of neoplasms on the globe and its adnexa.

There is little point in attempting to summarize here what fills many volumes of oncology textbooks. The following are some principles derived from this huge body of knowledge that are particularly important for ocular neoplasms.

Most types of malignant neoplasia develop stepwise after one or more injuries to replicative cells. The biochemical and structural alterations in malignant cells closely resemble changes in normal cells that are in the process of wound healing.

Ocular examples are numerous. The best known are the various manifestations of sunlight-induced injury to the conjunctiva and eyelid skin. Initial injury is followed by hyperplastic epithelial regeneration, but if the injury persists, progressive dysplasia and, eventually, neoplasia occur. The most common outcome is squamous cell carcinoma, but we suspect that hemangioma/hemangiosarcoma of the third eyelid or temporal bulbar conjunctiva in dogs has a similar pathogenesis. Another striking example is primary feline ocular sarcoma, which most frequently seems to originate as a strong fibroblastic wound-healing response after lens perforation, but which, in some cats, slowly transforms into pleomorphic and very malignant stromal sarcoma as these proliferating fibroblasts somehow escape normal biologic control mechanisms (Figures 4-31 and 4-32).

By the time they are first diagnosed, most neoplasms have already completed most of their theoretical biologic lifespan and have been undergoing continuous biochemical and structural phenotypic variation throughout that interval. Such tumors almost always contain numerous clones that are structurally and biochemically different from their neighbors. This concept of continuous diversification is critical to understanding how tumors can suddenly change in their behavior, and why chemotherapy or radiation therapy is almost never successful in achieving cure. The unstable genome that is inherent in neoplasia continues to become ever more unstable and thus creates an increasing diversity of daughter cells. At least some of these diverse mutants succeed in establishing their own small colonies of progeny, and therefore many large tumors have distinct subpopulations that may differ in behavior and histologic appearance from other portions of the same tumor. No matter how effective the chemotherapy, somewhere there will always be that one clone that is sufficiently "different" that it will escape destruction.

This concept also explains the empirical observation that metastatic foci in different organs may be quite dissimilar from one another and from the parent tissue. As a metastatic embolus of tumor lands in some distant organ, not every member of that diverse cluster will find that distant site to be equally hospitable. One may flourish where the others cannot. This kind of marked diversity is common within feline iris melanomas,

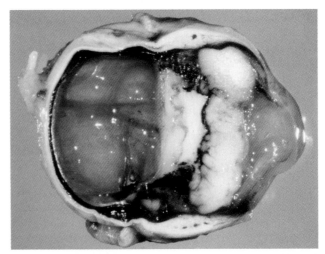

Figure 4-31. Feline primary ocular sarcoma, creating a perilenticular pleomorphic sarcoma derived from fibroblastic metaplasia of injured lens epithelium. Virtually all such cases show histologic evidence of previous lens rupture.

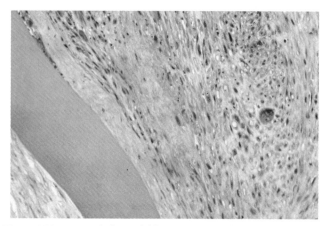

Figure 4-32. Histopathology of feline primary ocular sarcoma, showing pleomorphic malignant stromal cells adjacent to the lens capsule.

which not only change histologic character and clinical behavior over time but also show diverse histologic character within the same tumor at the time of enucleation.

Malignancy (literally meaning "life threatening") requires that the tumor depart significantly from the structure and function of the parent tissue, acquiring the ability to penetrate normal structural barriers, survive in normally inhospitable foreign environments, and ignore the many levels of behavioral control normally exerted by the body's homeostatic mechanisms. The basis for the histologic prediction of tumor behavior is based on the somewhat tenuous hypothesis that the degree to which a neoplasm departs from the microscopic appearance of the parent tissue predicts how much it will depart from the behavior of the parent tissue. This empirical observation seems at odds with the fundamental concept of neoplasia as an unpredictable genetic wild card. Nonetheless, most tumors do seem to follow some loose behavioral rules. There is a general correlation between how primitive a tumor looks and how aggressively it behaves. The underlying principle here is that primitive cells resemble the embryonic tissue that was, during embryogenesis, able to disseminate and colonize throughout the body. Presumably, such primitive cells no longer require the local nutritional/hormonal/environmental factors that define the specific niche occupied by the parent normal tissue.

There is no uniform system by which we can measure the level of primitiveness (anaplasia) of different tumors and therefore predict their behavior. Criteria like mitotic index and degree of nuclear variation cannot be applied with equal success to all tumors. Even more importantly, the *degree of anaplasia* required to confer behavioral malignancy varies among tumors. Presumably, those cell types that are already very much "at home" throughout the body (e.g., endothelial cells, lymphocytes, endocrine cells) will require relatively little anaplasia before the neoplastic cells are able to survive in distant metastatic sites. Conversely, highly specialized and tissue-specific cells such as ciliary epithelial cells would have to become very anaplastic before they would consider anywhere other than the globe to be a hospitable environment. This may explain why most primary intraocular neoplasms, even when histologically quite anaplastic, rarely establish successful metastatic foci.

The traditional insistence that all tumors be classified as either benign or malignant is biologically invalid. Just as all people cannot be classified as young or old, as ugly or beautiful, or as tall or short, so neoplasia represents a biologic continuum

with completely harmless ("benign") and invariably deadly ("malignant") as only the two extremes. The great majority of tumors are somewhere in between, and our job is to properly predict where they belong along that behavioral continuum. Some ocular tumors are invariably benign regardless of histologic appearance (ciliary body tumors), and others are unexpectedly malignant despite a relatively bland histologic appearance (conjunctival melanomas), so it is no easy task to properly predict the behavior of the various ocular neoplasms.

Clinical Signs Associated with Ocular Neoplasia

Hyphema

Spontaneous unilateral intraocular hemorrhage (*hyphema*) has long been cited as a clue to the presence of intraocular neoplasia, even though the explanation was obscure. It now seems that the bleeding originates from the fragile vessels of a preiridal fibrovascular membrane, which is formed as an "accidental" response to the diffusion of growth factors produced by the tumor itself. These growth factors are intended to recruit the blood vessels and fibrous stroma that the tumor needs for its own continued growth. Because epithelial tumors have a much greater need for stromal/vascular support than round cell tumors, melanomas, and various stromal tumors, these preiridal fibrovascular membranes are much more likely to be seen with iridociliary adenomas than anything else.

Glaucoma

Intraocular tumors frequently cause glaucoma. Some (e.g., canine anterior uveal melanomas and feline iris melanomas) do so by direct occlusion of the filtration angle (Figure 4-33). Ciliary epithelial tumors (even very small ones that would otherwise be innocuous) do so by inducing preiridal membranes that occlude the pupil or trabecular meshwork.

Uveitis

It is not clear how much inflammation is actually caused by intraocular neoplasms. In many instances the rise in aqueous protein and the presence of hyperemia or even hemorrhage are interpreted as evidence of uveitis although in fact they reflect

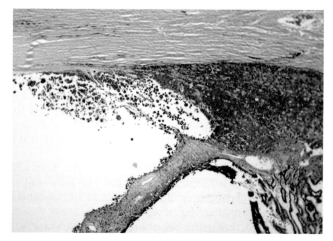

Figure 4-33. Canine anterior uveal melanocytoma. The trabecular meshwork is filled with large, heavily pigmented epithelioid melanocytes, resulting in secondary glaucoma.

proliferation of leaking blood vessels in response to tumor-associated growth factors. Tumor necrosis may trigger inflammation, as may immune response to tumor antigens.

HISTOLOGIC BASIS FOR COMMON CLINICAL LESIONS

The greatest practical benefit to understanding the general pathology of the eye is to bring elucidation to the myriad of clinical disguises worn by some of the most common ocular lesions, some of which do not match one's previous experience nor the pictures in textbooks. Given here are some of the most common of these clinical observations and their histologic basis.

Corneal Edema

The diffuse gray opacity characteristic of corneal edema is explained by histologic and ultrastructural changes within the corneal stroma. The increased binding of water changes the critical spatial relationships among the stromal collagen fibrils, resulting in greatly increased scattering (refraction) of light as it attempts to pass through the edematous stroma. The initial defect that permitted the edema usually is disruption of one or more of the structural barriers that actively and passively limit the presence of water within the stroma: epithelial ulceration, corneal endothelial damage, or ingrowth of leaking blood vessels into the stroma. Loss of surface epithelium (corneal ulcer) results in a zone of edema only slightly larger than the ulcer itself. Loss or functional defect of the corneal endothelium is often quite diffuse and creates diffuse edema, while edema that results from leaking blood vessels occurs as a gray halo surrounding the immature vessels as they grow inward from the limbus.

Corneal Pigmentation

Corneal pigmentation is most commonly the result of ingrowth by pigmented conjunctival epithelial cells in response to persistent corneal epithelial injury that has exceeded the regenerative abilities of the resident corneal epithelial cells. Depending on the severity of the injury, that ingrowth may be accompanied by angiogenesis and fibroplasia, although that is not always the case. The bulbar conjunctiva is the normal home for the permanent replicative reservoir of corneal epithelial cells; under normal circumstances these cells lose their pigment and become true "corneal" cells as they migrate into the cornea itself. It is not known why, under circumstances of persistent irritation, they retain their conjunctival character (or at least their pigment). The common clinical designation "pigmentary keratitis" is firmly entrenched but incorrect, because inflammation is not an intrinsic part of this reaction.

Aqueous Flare

Aqueous flare results from the scattering of light as it hits the higher number of protein molecules that have entered the aqueous humor as a result of increased vascular permeability within the iris or ciliary body. Usually, it is the clinical counterpart of greater vascular permeability due to acute inflammation (serous uveitis). It may also occur in animals with vascular hypertension and as serum leakage from the immature vessels within a preiridal fibrovascular membrane, so aqueous flare is *not* specific for uveitis.

As in other tissues the serous inflammation may progress to fibrinous or suppurative inflammation. Fibrin within the aqueous humor looks like fibrin anywhere else, and ordinarily it is transient because the inflamed anterior chamber also contains abundant fibrinolytic plasmin. Purulent exudate settles by gravity and looks like fluffy or globular yellow-white material in the ventral portion of the anterior chamber. This accumulation is commonly called *hypopyon*.

Keratic Precipitates

Keratic precipitates are small, shimmering, refractile or globular accumulations of leukocytes that adhere to the corneal endothelium (see Figure 4-25). With inflammation, the corneal endothelium expresses *adhesion molecules* that bind with complementary receptors on the surface of neutrophils or macrophages. Those clusters formed by macrophages tend to be larger and to glitter with engulfed lipids, creating so-called mutton fat precipitates. Unlike aqueous flare, keratic precipitates reflect a substantial leukocytic contribution to the inflammation, but not to the point of hypopyon.

Hyphema

Intraocular hemorrhage (*hyphema*) in animals without any history of ocular trauma and with a normal coagulation profile most commonly originates from a preiridal fibrovascular membrane associated with the presence of intraocular epithelial neoplasia or retinal detachment. Such membranes ordinarily cannot be detected by clinical examination. Other less common causes of unexplained intraocular hemorrhage are ocular vascular hypertension and increased vascular fragility associated with severe acute inflammation.

Changes in Pupil Shape

Some changes in pupil shape are due to changes in innervation and have no histologic counterpart. Commonly, irregular or scalloped pupillary margins are due to fibrinous or fibrous adhesions that change the configuration of the pupillary border of the iris (see Figure 4-26). This border may fold forward to adhere to the anterior face of the iris (ectropion uveae) or backward to adhere to the posterior iris epithelium (entropion uveae) or to the lens itself (posterior synechia). Sometimes the adhesion is a fibrinous or fibrous sequel to ocular inflammation, but other examples reflect the formation of *preiridal fibrovascular membranes* driven by the release of angiogenic and fibroblastic growth factors from any one of several intraocular sources. In descending order of prevalence, these sources are detached retinas, intraocular neoplasms, and leukocytes or platelets within chronic inflammatory reactions.

Changes in Iris Color

Change in iris color is perhaps most commonly seen in cats with diffuse iris melanoma, diffuse uveal infiltration by lymphoma, or chronic uveitis, but such changes can be seen in any species. The changes in color are attributable to dilution of iris pigment by infiltrating leukocytes or tumor cells, to changes in optical density associated with inflammatory edema, and/or to increased stromal density due to fibrin accumulation or fibrosis.

Lens Opacity

Most lenticular opacity is the visible counterpart of hydropic degeneration of lens fibers, which is the general definition of *cataract*. This degeneration is seen histologically as swollen fibers (bladder cells), as spherical globules of denatured lens protein (morgagnian globules), or as lakes of free fluid (see Figure 4-2). Much less commonly cataract may be caused by reparative proliferation of lens epithelium or the lens capsule. The gradual central opacification of the lens that occurs as a normal aging change, called *nuclear sclerosis*, is due to the accumulation of compacted, effete lens fibers that have outlived their useful function but that, because of the lens capsule, cannot be shed. It has no easily seen microscopic counterpart.

Retinal Pathology: Hyperreflectivity and Opacity

The endless variations on the theme of hyperreflectivity and opacity seen in various retinal diseases can be directly correlated to histologic changes in retina, tapetum, and choroid. *Atrophy* of any region of retina overlying tapetum results in an increase in the amount of light reflected by the tapetal mirror and is seen by the observer as a bright spot. Conversely, any kind of exudate in front of the tapetum (preretinal, intraretinal, or subretinal) results in increased absorption of light and thus creates a focus of opacity. The exact location of this exudate can be determined by looking at the retinal blood vessels. If the vessels also are cloudy, then the exudate must be preretinal or within the nerve fiber or ganglion cell layers of the retina itself. If the vessels are sharply visualized, but the tapetum is still cloudy, then the exudate exists either within the outer retina or in the subretinal space.

Dark gray or black spots in the tapetal fundus may represent postnecrotic "holes" in the tapetum such that the pigment of the choroid becomes visible. Alternatively, such spots may represent intraretinal clumps of melanin-laden macrophages derived from the RPE. Such *phagocytic metaplasia* is seen as a consequence of chorioretinitis or, presumably, anything else that damages or somehow triggers this phagocytic response within the pluri-potential RPE cells. It is seen in retinas of dogs that have survived canine distemper or in calves surviving in utero bovine viral diarrhea infection (see Figure 4-6).

BIBLIOGRAPHY

Aiello LP (1997): Vascular endothelial growth factor: 20th century mechanisms, 21st century therapies. Invest Ophthalmol Vis Sci 38:1647.

Bentley E, et al. (2002): The effect of chronic corneal débridement on epithelial and stromal morphology in dogs. Invest Ophthalmol Vis Sci 43:2136.

D'Amore PA (1994): Mechanisms of retinal and choroidal vascularization. Invest Ophthalmol Vis Sci 35:3974.

Dubielzig RR, et al. (1994): Morphologic features of feline ocular sarcomas in 10 cats: light microscopy, ultrastructure, and immunohistochemistry. Prog Vet Comp Ophthalmol 4:7.

English RV (1992): Regulation of intraocular immune responses. Progr Vet Comp Ophthalmol 2:41.

Freeman CS (1990): An overview of tumor biology. Cancer Invest 8:71.

Jampel MD, et al. (1990): Transforming growth factor—in human aqueous humor. Curr Eye Res 9:963.

Lu L, et al. (2001): Corneal epithelial wound healing. Exp Biol Med 226:653.

Martin P (1997): Wound healing—aiming for perfect skin regeneration. Science 276:75.

McCracken JS, et al. (1979): Morphologic observations on experimental corneal vascularization in the rat. Lab Invest 41:519.

Montali RJ (1988): Comparative pathology of inflammation in higher vertebrates (reptiles, birds and mammals). J Comp Pathol 99:1.

Pober J, Cotran RS (1991): What can be learned from the expression of endothelial adhesion molecules in tissues? Lab Invest 64:301.

Raphael B, et al. (1993): Enhanced healing of cat corneal endothelial wounds by epidermal growth factor. Invest Ophthalmol Vis Sci 34:2305.

Rosenbaum JT (1993): Cytokines: the good, the bad, and the unknown. Invest Ophthalmol Vis Sci 34:2389.

Streilein JW (1993): Tissue barriers, immunosuppressive microenvironments and privileged sites: the eye's point of view. Reg Immunol 150:1727.

Tripathi RC, et al. (1990): Prospects for epidermal growth factor in the management of corneal disorders. Surv Ophthalmol 34:457.

van der Woerdt A (2000): Lens-induced uveitis. Vet Ophthalmol 3: 227.

Wahl SM, et al. (1989): Role of growth factors in inflammation and repair. J Cell Biochem 40:193.

Wilcock BP, et al. (2002): Histological Classification of Ocular and Otic Tumors of Domestic Animals. WHO International Histologic Classification of Tumors of Domestic Animals, Second Series. AFIP, Washington, DC.

Chapter 5

BASIC DIAGNOSTIC TECHNIQUES

David J. Maggs

MEDICAL HISTORY
EXAMINATION PROCEDURE
SCHIRMER TEAR TEST
MICROBIOLOGIC SAMPLING

ASSESSMENT OF PUPIL SIZE, SHAPE,
  SYMMETRY, AND MOBILITY
EXAMINATION OF THE ANTERIOR
  SEGMENT

OPHTHALMOSCOPY
NORMAL FUNDUS
EXAMINATION OF THE POSTERIOR
  SEGMENT
ADDITIONAL DIAGNOSTIC TESTING

Early and correct diagnosis of ocular disorders, which is essential to a successful clinical result and a satisfied client, relies almost completely on a thorough, orderly, and complete ocular examination. As with all other body systems, investigation of a patient with ocular disease comprises the taking of a thorough and directed history, a complete examination of the ocular and periocular structures, and then, in many cases, some specialized diagnostic testing as directed by the history and examination findings. The aim of this chapter is to help the reader develop a systematic approach to the ocular examination, including the basic principles of some specialized diagnostic methods. As with other body systems, a problem-oriented approach is encouraged. Most of the examination techniques described in this chapter are applicable to exotic or avian species, sometimes with minor modifications. However, the reader is referred to Chapter 20 for more specific description of examination techniques and diagnostic testing in exotic and avian species. Additionally, this chapter introduces many new terms, and the reader is referred to the Glossary for a full definition of these.

MEDICAL HISTORY

A thorough, relevant history is an important part of the diagnostic process. To use the problem-oriented approach, the clinician first determines the major problems that have caused the owner to present the animal for examination. These problems form a temporary problem list and not only will direct the examination but also may suggest further avenues of questioning while the clinician is obtaining the complete history from the owner. Delaying taking the complete history until after the initial problems have been determined saves time and avoids the collection of irrelevant historical data.

Questions that are often helpful during the collection of a history for an ophthalmic patient include the following:

- Where does the animal live, and what is its diet?
- Has the patient had any major diseases or injuries in the past, especially recent and especially ocular? If the animal has already lost one eye, an attempt should be made to determine the cause of loss. This may be of considerable assistance in diagnosing the current problem and assessing client compliance with treatment instructions, and may also

affect the client's understanding of the disease and his or her reactions to proposed treatment.
- Is the animal experiencing visual difficulties? If so, is vision worse at night, during the day, or in familiar or unfamiliar environments? How long has the visual deficit been present? Is the visual problem slowly improving or getting worse? Is the visual deficit worse on one side than the other?
- Has there been any discharge from the eye? If so, what kind?
- Has the affected eye appeared painful?
- Has the eye appeared discolored (e.g., opacity of the cornea due to edema, leukocoria due to cataract, redness due to episcleral or conjunctival injection)?
- Has the eye appeared abnormal in any other way?
- Has the animal shown any behavioral or locomotor disturbances recently?
- Have any of the animal's close relatives or other members of the herd or household been affected with ocular disease?

EXAMINATION PROCEDURE

An ophthalmic examination requires a minimum of equipment (Box 5-1). Ideally the examination is conducted in dim ambient light, preferably in a darkened room or stall, to minimize interfering reflections. Once sedated, a horse can be examined with the examiner's and the horse's heads under a blanket or dark cloth. Although the order in which the examination is conducted is not critical for all components, certain tests either would compromise later parts of the ocular examination or should not be performed until certain conditions have been ruled out because they could exacerbate or complicate those conditions or render them impossible to further examine. The major components of the ocular examination and the order in which each should be completed are described in Figure 5-1. Sometimes this order can be best recalled and examination findings best recorded on a form designed specifically for the ophthalmic examination (Figure 5-2).

SCHIRMER TEAR TEST

The Schirmer tear test (STT) is a semiquantitative method of measuring production of the aqueous portion of the precorneal tear film. It must be performed before application of any topical solutions, because these would artificially but temporarily raise

Box 5-1 | **Basic instruments and supplies**

- Focal light source (e.g., Finoff transilluminator)
- Magnifying loupes (e.g., Optivisor)
- Direct ophthalmoscope
- Indirect funduscopic lens (e.g., 20 D or 2.2 Panretinal lens)
- Schirmer tear test strips
- Fluorescein test strips
- Tonometer (e.g., Tono-Pen)
- Tropicamide (1%)
- Proparacaine (topical anesthetic)
- Sterile eye wash/rinse

the STT value. In addition, some topical solutions exert a more protracted inhibitory effect. For example, topically applied anesthetics or parasympatholytic drugs used to induce mydriasis, and local anesthetics, both will reduce STT values. Finally, manipulative procedures such as corneal or conjunctival scrapings, flushing of the lacrimal apparatus, and potentially even application of bright lights to an inflamed eye will result in artificially elevated STT values. For these reasons, if the STT is to be performed, it should be done as the first component of the ophthalmic examination.

The test is performed with sterile, individually packaged strips of absorbent paper with a notch 5 mm from one end. Each strip is folded at the notch and hooked over the middle to lateral third of the lower lid for 60 seconds (Figure 5-3). The distance from the notch to the end of the moist part of the paper is measured immediately on removal of the strip from the eye. This is the STT 1, which measures basal and reflex tearing, including that due to corneal stimulation provided by the test strip itself. That is why the STT strip should be placed in the middle to lateral region of the lower eyelid, where it can gently contact the corneal surface. If it is placed more medially, the third eyelid can protect the cornea and reduce STT 1 results. In normal dogs, the STT 1 result should exceed 15 mm in 1 minute. Readings of less than 10 mm in 1 minute are considered diagnostic for keratoconjunctivitis sicca. Values between 10 and 15 mm in 1 minute are considered highly suggestive of keratoconjunctivitis sicca, particularly if appropriate clinical signs are present.

The reported range for STT results in normal cats is 3 to 32 mm in 1 minute with a mean of 17 mm in 1 minute. However, experience suggests that lower readings than the reported mean can be expected in a clinical setting. This is probably due to autonomic control of secretion and short-term alterations in tear flow due to stress in the examination room. Values should still be recorded in cats but should be interpreted with caution and always in conjunction with clinical signs. Commercial strips are often unsuitable for horses if left in place for 60 seconds because of greater tear production in this species, which quickly saturates the entire strip. Some recommend broader strips, but these must be prepared in a very uniform manner. Rather, it is probably better to leave a standard strip in place for only 30 seconds in this species. STT results are also published for a number of exotic species (see Chapter 20).

For measurement of the STT 2, corneal sensation is abolished with topical anesthetic, and lower test values result because the afferent limb of the reflex path is blocked and reflex secretion by the lacrimal and nictitans glands is reduced. The STT 2 has not received widespread clinical application in animals but is sometimes referred to in texts and research studies.

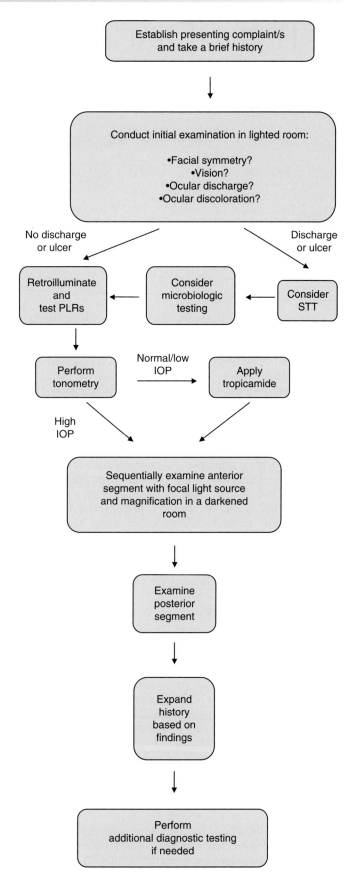

Figure 5-1. Suggested order for the complete ophthalmic examination in all species. *IOP,* Intraocular pressure; *PLRs,* pupillary light reflexes; *STT,* Schirmer tear test.

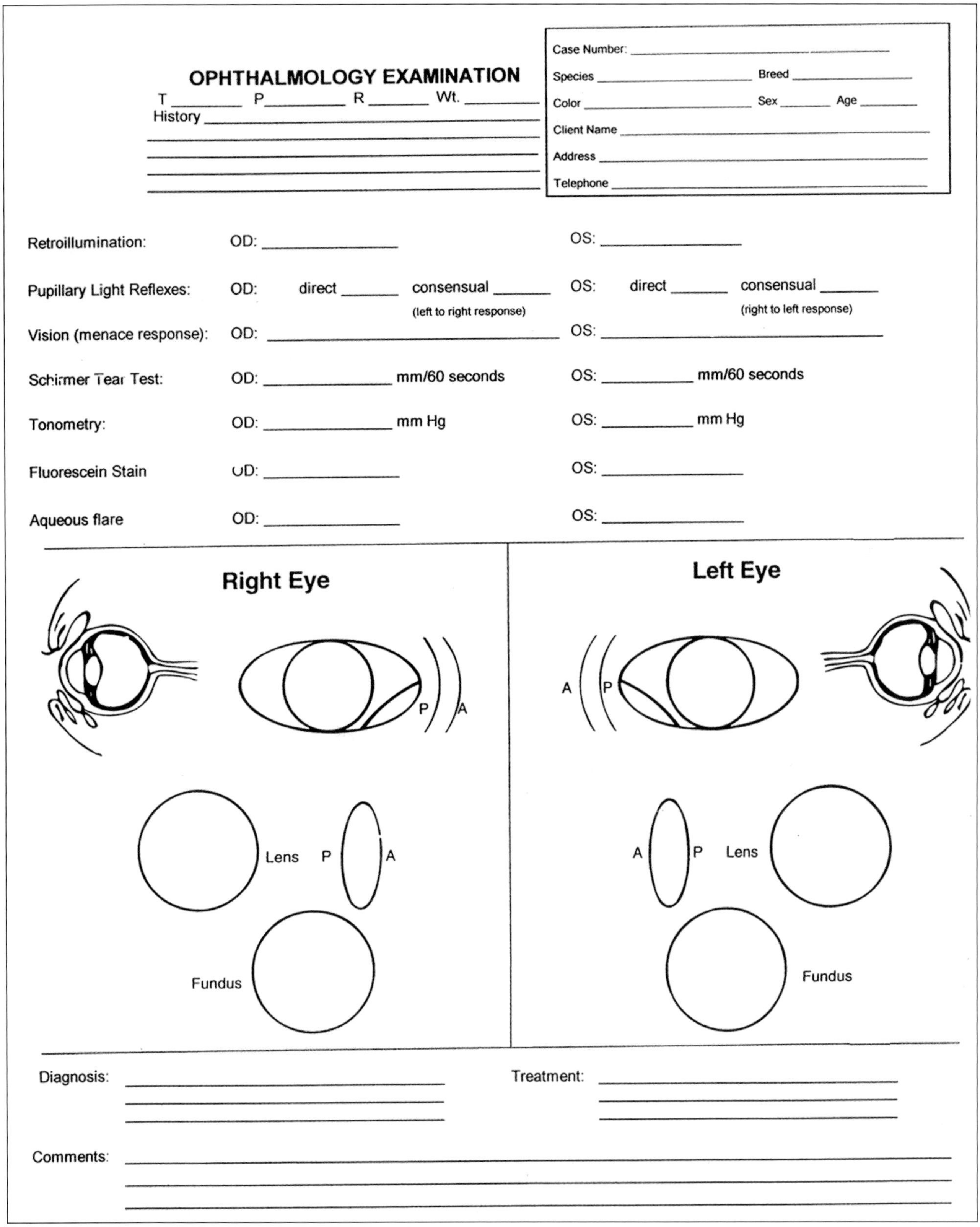

OPHTHALMOLOGY EXAMINATION

T _____ P _____ R _____ Wt. _____

History _____
_____
_____
_____

Case Number: _____
Species _____ Breed _____
Color _____ Sex _____ Age _____
Client Name _____
Address _____
Telephone _____

Retroillumination: OD: _____ OS: _____

Pupillary Light Reflexes: OD: direct _____ consensual _____ OS: direct _____ consensual _____
(left to right response) (right to left response)

Vision (menace response): OD: _____ OS: _____

Schirmer Tear Test: OD: _____ mm/60 seconds OS: _____ mm/60 seconds

Tonometry: OD: _____ mm Hg OS: _____ mm Hg

Fluorescein Stain OD: _____ OS: _____

Aqueous flare OD: _____ OS: _____

Right Eye — Lens P A — Fundus

Left Eye — A P Lens — Fundus

Diagnosis: _____ Treatment: _____

Comments: _____

Figure 5-2. Sample ophthalmic examination sheet. (Courtesy University of Missouri, Columbia, Veterinary Ophthalmology Service Collection.)

MICROBIOLOGIC SAMPLING

Ocular surface samples (typically a swab or scraping) may be assessed for presence of a microbial pathogen by cytologic assessment, culture, polymerase chain reaction, or immuno-fluorescent antibody labeling. Some of these tests, especially microbial culture, may be affected by many of the drugs applied topically to the eye and by the preservatives that accompany them. Although topical anesthetic agents do contain preservatives, application of a topical anesthetic is essential for the safe and

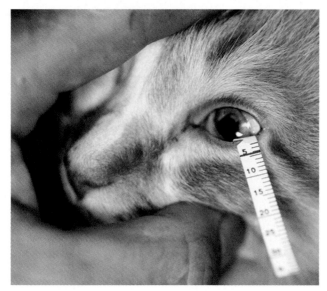

Figure 5-3. Schirmer tear test being performed on a cat. Note that the strip is placed into the lower lateral conjunctival fornix so that it lightly contacts the lateral cornea.

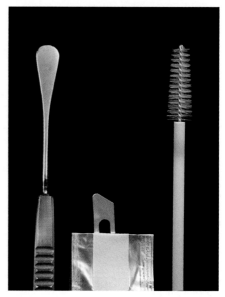

Figure 5-4. Instruments suitable for collecting ocular surface samples for cytologic and microbiologic examination. *Left to right,* Kimura platinum spatula, handle-end of Bard-Parker scalpel blade, cytology brush.

humane collection of samples from the ocular surface. Therefore, if indicated, samples for microbiologic analysis should be collected early in the examination process, immediately after the STT if it is done. The indications for collection of samples for microbiologic assessment include notable purulent inflammation; chronic, unresponsive, or severe corneal or conjunctival lesions; deep corneal ulcers with stromal loss or malacia ("melting"); and severe blepharitis or periocular dermatitis.

Traditionally, microbiologic specimens have been collected with a moist swab. However, some ophthalmologists prefer to collect more cellular specimens from corneal or conjunctival lesions by scraping or with a cytology brush. These samples can be submitted for culture and sensitivity testing, cytologic assessment, and Gram staining. A sterile instrument such as a Kimura spatula, a cytology brush, or the handle-end of a scalpel blade should be used (Figure 5-4). Samples should be placed into or onto media suitable for the organisms being sought, as advised by the laboratory that will receive and interpret the samples, and shipped appropriately and as soon as possible.

ASSESSMENT OF PUPIL SIZE, SHAPE, SYMMETRY, AND MOBILITY

Pupil dilation is essential if a thorough examination of the half of the eye behind the iris (the ciliary body, lens, vitreous, retina, tapetum, optic nerve head, choroid, and posterior sclera) is to be conducted. However, pupil dilation will completely prohibit assessment of pupil size, symmetry, shape, position, and reaction to light. It will also limit examination of the iris itself. Therefore anisocoria, dyscoria, corectopia, or altered pupillary light reflexes (PLRs) will be missed if a patient's pupils are dilated before two straightforward tests are completed. Before application of a topical mydriatic agent, patients should be examined by retroillumination and their direct and consensual PLRs should be assessed. Pupil shape and the speed and magnitude of the PLR differ among species. The feline pupil is a vertical ellipse, the dog's and bird's are circular, and most large herbivores are horizontal slits. Despite these differences in pupil shape, pupils in these species dilate to approximately circular.

Retroillumination

Retroillumination is a simple but extremely useful technique for assessment of pupil size, shape, and symmetry. A focal light source (Finoff transilluminator or direct ophthalmoscope) is held up to the examiner's eye and directed over the bridge of the patient's nose from at least arm's length from the patient so as to equally illuminate the two pupils and elicit the fundic reflection (Figure 5-5). This reflection is usually gold or green in tapetal animals and red in atapetal individuals. With each eye equally illuminated, the fundic reflex is used to assess and compare pupil size, shape, and equality (Figure 5-6). Retroillumination can also be used to judge the clarity of all of the transparent ocular media (tear film, cornea, aqueous humor, lens, and vitreous). Opacities in the ocular media will obstruct the fundic reflection and can be noted for more detailed subsequent examination. Retroillumination is particularly useful for differentiating nuclear sclerosis from cataract (see Chapter 13).

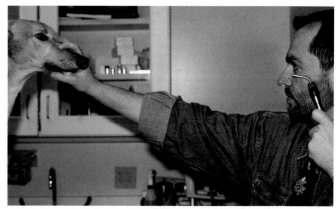

Figure 5-5. Retroillumination is performed with a focal light source held close to the examiner's eye or with the direct ophthalmoscope held up to the examiner's eye. The examiner stands at arm's length from the patient and directs the light over the bridge of the patient's nose so as to illuminate both pupils equally.

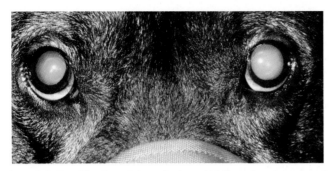

Figure 5-6. Retroilluminated view of a dog with bilateral nuclear sclerosis (visible as a translucent ring inside the pupils of both eyes). The tapetal reflection is used to "backlight" (or retroilluminate) all the clear ocular media (vitreous, lens, anterior chamber, cornea, and tear film).

Pupillary Light Reflexes

Following assessment of resting pupil size, shape, and symmetry, pupil reactivity should be assessed (see also Chapter 16). The reflex constriction of the pupil in response to light striking the retina is termed the *pupillary light reflex*. In most mammals, constriction of the pupil of the illuminated eye (the direct PLR) is slightly greater than that of the pupil of the contralateral or nonilluminated eye (the indirect or consensual PLR). Interpretation of the PLR requires an understanding of the neurologic reflex as well as other potential confounding factors. The neural arc being tested has an afferent arm, which includes the retina, optic nerve, optic chiasm, optic tract, pretectal area, and the parasympathetic nucleus of cranial nerve (CN) III, where there is a synapse with the pupillomotor fibers of CN III (oculomotor nerve), which stimulate the smooth muscles of the iris sphincter muscle to cause pupil contraction. In addition to pathology at any point along this neurologic pathway, the PLR may be decreased or absent if there is iris atrophy (due to age), iris ischemia, (due to acute glaucoma), physical obstruction of the pupil (due to synechia or lens dislocation), prior use of a dilating drug, or high concentrations of circulating epinephrine (i.e., in fearful animals). The effect of these confounding factors is exacerbated if a weak light source is used. Also, it is critical to understand that because the PLR is a subcortical reflex and requires relatively little retinal function, a positive direct PLR is *not* an indicator of vision. However, because it tests many but not all of the same pathways required for vision, it should be tested in all animals in which vision is impaired as it may help with anatomic localization of the defect.

Both the extent and speed of the PLR should be assessed and compared in the two eyes and against what is considered normal for that species. The PLR tends to be fastest and most complete in carnivores, with the cat's being the fastest of all common domestic animals. The normal equine pupil constricts slowly in response to a bright light. The PLR of the cow and sheep is somewhat more rapid. Birds and reptiles do have a PLR, but they can override it because their iris musculature is skeletal rather than smooth (see Chapter 20).

A positive direct pupillary light reflex is not a reliable indicator of vision or normal retinal function.

EXAMINATION OF THE ANTERIOR SEGMENT

Every attempt should be made to avoid sedation or anesthesia before or during the ophthalmic examination in small animals, because its use complicates the examination in many ways. Reflexes and responses, vision, pupil size, globe movement and position, STT value, moistness of the corneoconjunctival surface, palpebral fissure size, and deviations of the visual axes cannot be assessed accurately if anesthesia or sedation has begun. Further, the globe becomes enophthalmic and rolls ventromedially, and the third eyelid covers much of the globe, making a complete eye examination impossible.

The exception to this rule is in the horse, in which sedation and an auriculopalpebral nerve block are essential for a good eye examination and should be performed after the assessment of pupil size, vision, STT (if necessary), and all reflexes and responses. The auriculopalpebral nerve block provides paresis of the orbicularis oculi muscle and limits eyelid closure, which is very forceful in the horse. Without an auriculopalpebral block, it is generally not possible to examine the whole globe of the horse and peripheral lesions will be missed. The auriculopalpebral nerve is found by running a finger up and down over the zygomatic process of the facial bone. The nerve can be palpated as it runs transversely in the subcutaneous space across the lower third of this process (Figure 5-7, *A*). Approximately 2 mL of lidocaine is then injected over the nerve (Figure 5-7, *B*). Sometimes sedation can be avoided in horses if a twitch is used. For food animals, a suitable crush or race/chute and (especially in cows) nose tongs are useful.

In all species and before sedation (if used), the eyes and periocular region should first be examined from a distance and in normal ambient light for gross abnormalities, including asymmetry, palpebral fissure size, ocular or nasal discharge or dryness, periocular alopecia, deviations of the visual axes, redness or other color change, and corneal clarity and moistness (reflectivity). The animal's response to the new environment of the examination room may also be used to judge visual function. Neuroophthalmic and visual testing may then be conducted. Vision testing could include maze testing, tracking of objects that do not emit sound or odor (thrown cotton balls or a laser pointer are excellent). The menace response, if conducted in such a way that air currents and direct contact with the vibrissae are avoided, can also be used. Normal palpebral reflex (a complete blink in reaction to digital stimulation of the eyelid skin) should then be verified for

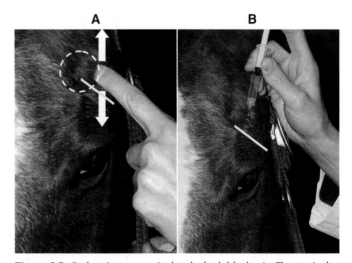

Figure 5-7. Performing an auriculopalpebral block. **A,** The auriculopalpebral nerve *(yellow line)* is palpated by running a finger up and down over the zygomatic process of the facial bone *(white arrows).* **B,** Approximately 2 mL of lidocaine is then injected over the nerve.

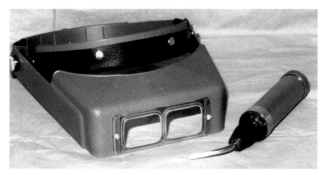

Figure 5-8. Finoff transilluminator and Optivisor magnifying loupe.

both eyes as a test of CN V and CN VII function. These tests are more thoroughly described later. Finally, globe movements and position are examined. As the head is elevated, depressed, and moved laterally, the eye should return to or remain in the center of the palpebral fissure, producing a physiologic nystagmus. Both globes should retropulse normally and symmetrically.

Examination in dim ambient light is then commenced with a magnifying loupe and a focal light source (Figure 5-8). A Finoff transilluminator, which fits to the direct ophthalmoscope or otoscope handset, produces a brighter and more focused beam of light than a penlight and is therefore preferred. A source of magnification is absolutely essential to conduct a complete ocular examination. The most useful instrument for general practice is a simple magnifying loupe with a power of 2 to 4× and a focal length of 15 to 25 cm (6 to 10 inches). Using this combination of a focal light source and magnification, the clinician should examine the eye from many angles while the light is directed from many contrasting angles. Particular attention should be paid to the Sanson-Purkinje images, which result from reflections from ocular structures. When a focal light beam is examined from an oblique angle as it passes through the eye, three reflections can usually be seen: the cornea, the anterior lens capsule, and, sometimes, the posterior lens capsule (Figure 5-9). The combination of variable viewing and illumination angles permits the examiner to gain intra-ocular depth perception by virtue of parallax, shadows, perspective, and reflected light (Figure 5-10).

The slit-lamp biomicroscope (Figure 5-11) is a more sophisticated optical instrument that combines up to 40× magnification and illumination and can be used to examine many different microscopic and optical features of the patient's

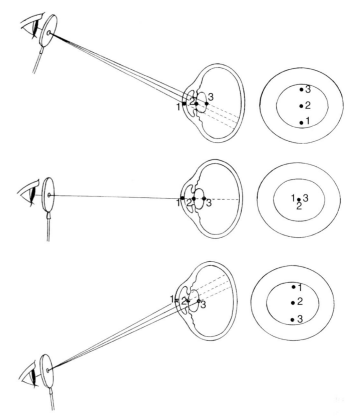

Figure 5-10. The use of parallax to localize intraocular opacities. *1,* Corneal opacity; *2,* cataract on anterior lens capsule; *3,* cataract on posterior lens capsule. The pupil is dilated for this examination. (From Komar G, Szutter L [1968]: Tierarztliche Augenheilkunde. Paul Parey, Berlin.)

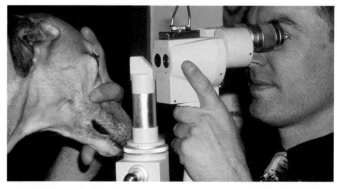

Figure 5-11. A slit-lamp biomicroscope in use. Slit-lamp biomicroscopes provide binocular magnification (with stereopsis) and a focal light source whose angle, shape, and intensity can all be altered. These greatly facilitate ophthalmic examinations in all animals.

eye such as individual layers of the cornea that normally are invisible to the naked eye of the examiner. As such, it allows pathologic processes to be described more accurately so as to better guide diagnosis, prognosis, and treatment. Because of the requirement for training and skill in their use, slit-lamp biomicroscopes are usually found only in specialty practices and teaching institutions.

Using a source of focal light and magnification, the clinician examines ocular structures sequentially according to a mental checklist (see Figure 5-2). A logical order appears to be to work simultaneously from peripheral to axial and from anterior to

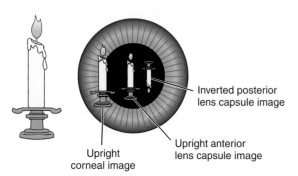

Inverted posterior lens capsule image

Upright anterior lens capsule image

Upright corneal image

Figure 5-9. The Sanson-Purkinje reflections off the cornea and anterior and posterior lens capsules provide perspective during the examination and should be used to judge the depth of lesions within the eye.

posterior, as follows. More detail can be found in the specific chapters relating to diseases of these individual tissues.

Eyelids

The eyelids should be examined with particular attention to the periocular skin, eyelid margin, and meibomian gland orifices. Look in particular for the following:

- Periocular discharge: serous ("epiphora"), mucoid, purulent, sanguineous, or a combination of these
- Periocular dermatitis/blepharitis: alopecia, scaling, hyperemia, crusting, swelling, ulceration, maceration, etc.
- Palpebral fissure size: narrowed or macropalpebral fissure
- Eyelid position and motion: entropion, ectropion, ptosis, blepharospasm
- Disorders of the cilia or periocular hair: ectopic cilia, distichia, trichiasis

Third Eyelid

The position of the third eyelid should be examined at rest, and then its anterior face further examined through gentle digital retropulsion of the globe through the upper lid. This later step should be omitted if a deep or penetrating corneal or scleral lesion renders the globe unstable. The posterior or bulbar face of the third eyelid may be examined by means of protrusion and eversion of the third eyelid with a pair of fixation forceps or mosquito hemostats after application of topical anesthetic (Figure 5-12). Look in particular for the following:

- Increased prominence at rest: orbital mass, enophthalmos, phthisis, microphthalmos, Horner's syndrome, Haw's syndrome
- Scrolled third eyelid cartilage
- Masses: prolapse of the gland of the third eyelid ("cherry eye"), neoplasia
- Irregularities of the margin or surfaces: chronic conjunctivitis ("pannus" or conjunctivitis), trauma
- Foreign bodies
- Changed color: melanosis, hyperemia, anemia
- Surface moistness and discharge: dacryocystitis, keratoconjunctivitis sicca

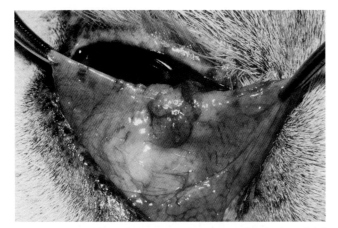

Figure 5-12. Use of two hemostats to exteriorize the third eyelid for examination following application of a topical anesthetic. This horse has a squamous cell carcinoma on the leading edge of the third eyelid.

Conjunctiva

In addition to the conjunctiva that lines both surfaces of the third eyelid, the remaining conjunctiva lining the eyelids (palpebral conjunctiva) and the anterior globe (bulbar conjunctiva) must also be examined. This requires opening and eversion of the upper and lower eyelids and examination with the globe in many positions of gaze. Look in particular for the following:

- Change in color: hyperemia, anemia, icterus, melanosis
- Chemosis: conjunctival edema
- Surface irregularities, thickening, or masses
- Inadequate or excessive surface moistness or discharge
- Subconjunctival hemorrhage or emphysema

Nasolacrimal Apparatus

The only components of the nasolacrimal apparatus visible during the external eye examination are the ventral and dorsal puncta in the palpebral conjunctiva near the medial canthus. However, pathology in any part of the nasolacrimal drainage apparatus can produce ocular and periocular signs. Look in particular for the following:

- Ocular discharge (epiphora, mucoid, purulent, sanguineous, or a combination of these)
- Tear staining at the medial canthus
- Negative fluorescein passage (Jones) test result (see later section on vital dyes)
- Occlusion or absence of one or both puncta: atresia, fibrosis/ cicatrization, canalicular foreign body (typically a grass awn)
- Abscess, swelling, or purulent dermatitis near the medial canthus (dacryocystitis)

Cornea

The normal cornea is transparent owing to a number of anatomic and physiologic features. As a result, pathology within the cornea manifests as opacity, often of a color and pattern highly suggestive of the pathologic process (see Chapter 10). Look in particular for the following:

- Loss of transparency: fibrosis, edema, melanosis, vascularization, cellular infiltrate, lipid or mineral accumulation, keratic precipitates
- Changes in contour: keratoconus, keratoglobus, globe rupture, corneal ulcer
- Surface irregularities or dullness: corneal mass/plaque, corneal ulcer/facet, keratoconjunctivitis sicca, iris prolapse/staphyloma
- Change in corneal diameter: buphthalmos, microphthalmos, phthisis

Sclera

Only the anterior portion of the scleral coat may be seen on direct external examination of the eye. Even then, it is seen through the almost transparent bulbar conjunctiva. The posterior sclera also is usually not directly visualized except in dogs with a subalbinotic fundus. In these patients, the inner aspect of the posterior sclera (the lamina fusca) is visible between and through choroidal tissue. This tends to have a more tan appearance than the external anterior sclera and is discussed more fully later as part of the ocular fundus. Pathology of the posterior aspects of the sclera can sometimes create notable changes in the adjacent choroid or retina, which can be seen during the fundic exam or using ultrasound. However, scleral changes can go unnoticed unless special care is taken to include this tissue on the mental checklist for the eye examination. When examining the anterior portion of the sclera, one should in particular look for the following:

- Changes in thickness: thinning with or without staphyloma or diffuse thickening with scleritis
- Surface irregularities: nodular granulomatous episcleritis, neoplasia, staphyloma, globe rupture
- Alteration in scleral "show": increased due to exophthalmos, phthisis, microphthalmos, tetanus, macropalpebral fissure; decreased due to symblepharon, ptosis, blepharospasm
- Change in contour: due to globe rupture (often at or near the limbus)
- Change in color: episcleral injection, hemorrhage, icterus, melanosis, melanocytic tumor

Anterior Chamber

The anterior chamber is the aqueous humor–filled space between the iris and posterior cornea. As such, it can be difficult to examine. The following three techniques assist with this problem:

1. Assess the globe from the lateral side, looking "across" the anterior chamber (Figure 5-13).
2. Assess the clarity of the view of the rest of the intraocular structures, especially the iris face. If this is decreased, then corneal disease and/or anterior chamber debris is likely.
3. Give attention to the Sanson-Purkinje images as described previously.

When assessing the anterior chamber, one should look in particular for the following:

- Alterations in depth: increased with posterior lens dislocation, microphakia, buphthalmos, hypermature cataract or after surgical lens removal. Decreased with anterior lens dislocation, iris or ciliary body tumors/cysts,

iris bombé, many acute glaucomas, intumescent cataracts, and aqueous misdirection in cats.
- Abnormal contents: anterior lens luxation, foreign body, hyphema, fibrin, hypopyon, aqueous flare, iris cysts, tumors, persistent pupillary membranes, vitreous, and anterior synechia

Iris and Pupil

The iris and pupil are assessed together because alterations in one often produce changes in the other. Both should be examined before and after pupil dilation. Obviously the iris face is best examined before dilation, but abnormalities of the posterior iris (and ciliary body) are sometimes not visible until full pupil dilation is achieved. Horses and ruminants normally have cystic excrescences of posterior iris epithelium that emerge to varying degrees through the pupil, especially dorsally and ventrally, as the corpora nigra or granula iridica. This is very highly developed in the camelids, in which it forms a series of interdigitating pleats. Look in particular for the following:

- Altered pupil shape (dyscoria) or position (corectopia): synechia, iris atrophy, iris hypoplasia, iris coloboma
- More than one aperture in the iris: iris coloboma, persistent pupillary membranes, iris atrophy, iris hypoplasia
- Iridal masses: iris cysts, neoplasia, abscess/granuloma
- Altered iris color: heterochromia iridis, rubeosis iridis, edema, melanosis, melanocytic neoplasia, iris granuloma/abscess, chronic or acute uveitis
- Altered pupil size: uveitis, glaucoma, Horner's syndrome, iris atrophy, retinal or optic nerve disease, central nervous system (CNS) disease, CN III paralysis, drug administration, lens dislocation
- Iridodonesis (fluttering of the iris): surgical aphakia or lens dislocation
- Altered pupil color: cataract, nuclear sclerosis, vitreous hemorrhage, retinal detachment, asteroid hyalosis

Lens

Examination of the lens, like that of other clear ocular structures, can be confusing. Here, too, the Sanson-Purkinje images are useful (see earlier). The examiner can use parallax (see Figure 5-10) or the slit beam of the direct ophthalmoscope and a source of manification to determine position of opacities within the lens. Lens pathology is relatively limited, with altered clarity (nuclear sclerosis or cataract) and dislocation (luxation or subluxation) predominating. Look in particular for the following:

- Altered size: microphakia, hypermature cataract, intumescent cataract
- Altered shape: spherophakia, lenticonus, lentiglobus, hypermature cataract, intumescent cataract, lens capsule rupture
- Altered position: luxation, subluxation, aphakic crescent
- Lens opacity: cataract, nuclear sclerosis, anterior lens capsule melanosis, intralenticular hemorrhage, persistent hyaloid artery, persistent hyperplastic primary vitreous, persistent tunica vasculosa lentis

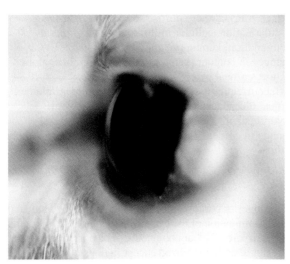

Figure 5-13. Transverse view of the left eye of a cat. The view from this angle is very useful for examination of the anterior chamber in animals. Magnification and a focal light source are also essential.

Examination of the lens completes examination of the anterior segment, which will identify the vast majority of ocular lesions encountered in general practice. However, a complete examination also necessitates examination of those structures in the posterior segment: the vitreous and various structures of the ocular fundus. This requires some equipment and techniques additional to those used for examination of the anterior segment, which are described in the following sections.

OPHTHALMOSCOPY

The clinician can examine the fundus of larger eyes (notably those of the horse, cow, and many raptors) directly through a widely dilated pupil by aligning the light beam with his/her visual axis and standing a short distance from the patient, as for retroillumination (see Figure 5-5). However, this maneuver is not possible for dogs and cats, and even for horses and cows, accurate assessment requires examination using one of three methods of ophthalmoscopy:

- The direct ophthalmoscope
- The indirect lens
- The monocular indirect ophthalmoscope

Although various writers describe one or others of these ophthalmoscopes as easier to use, the old adage that practice makes perfect applies, and persistence and practice are essential to master any ophthalmoscopic technique. Therefore rather than concentrating on the technique that is alleged to be easier to learn, budding ophthalmoscopists should perhaps focus on the technique most likely to be useful to them throughout their careers with the aim being to become competent at that technique. Most ophthalmologists prefer to scan the whole fundus with an indirect lens and then to examine more closely any regions of interest using the direct ophthalmoscope. This approach takes advantage of the greater field of view associated with indirect ophthalmoscopy and the higher magnification permitted by direct ophthalmoscopy. Regardless of the ophthalmoscope used, thorough examination of the fundus requires complete pupil dilation, which is achieved approximately 15 to 20 minutes after application of 1 drop of tropicamide. The extent and speed of dilation can be enhanced in some patients by application of a second drop about 5 minutes after the first.

Direct Ophthalmoscopy

The direct ophthalmoscope directs a beam of light into the patient's eye and places the observer's eye in the correct position to view the reflected beam and details of the interior of the eye (Figure 5-14). It is called a *direct* ophthalmoscope because it provides a direct and upright image of the fundus rather than a virtual and inverted image as provided by the indirect ophthalmoscope. The direct ophthalmoscope (Figure 5-15) has a rheostat to control the light intensity, colored filters, a slit beam for viewing elevations and depressions within the fundus, an illuminated grid to project onto the fundus to measure lesions, and a series of lenses on a rotating wheel that adjusts the depth of focus within the eye. These lenses may be used to examine structures other than the fundus or to measure the height of lesions by changing the focus from the tip of the lesion to the surrounding retina and determining the dioptric difference. However, many of these features are of limited use in noncompliant veterinary patients.

To avoid interference between the examiner's and patient's noses, the observer should use the left eye to examine the patient's left eye and the right eye to examine the patient's right

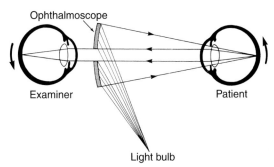

Figure 5-14. Direct ophthalmoscopy. Arrows show orientation of images in examiner's and patient's eyes. (Modified from Vaughan D, Asbury T [1983]: General Ophthalmology, 10th ed. Lange Medical, Los Altos, CA.)

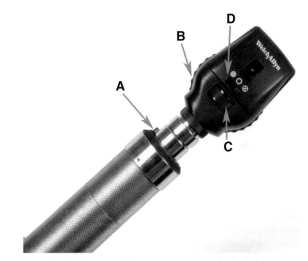

Figure 5-15. The direct ophthalmoscope. Controls for light intensity **(A)**, focusing lenses **(B)**, light aperture size and shape **(C)**, and filters **(D)**.

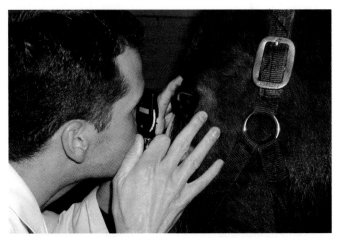

Figure 5-16. The direct ophthalmoscope being used to examine a horse's fundus.

eye. This is less important with laterally placed eyes such as in horses (Figure 5-16). Ideally, the examiner's opposite eye is left open. With the ophthalmoscope set on 0 D and so that the largest circle of light is emitted, the ophthalmoscope is rested firmly against the examiner's brow and the patient's eye is viewed in a darkened room from approximately 25 cm away. The tapetal reflection is located, and then the observer moves in to within 2 to 3 cm of the patient's eye. If necessary, adjustment may be made to the lens settings to bring the fundus into focus. The fundus is then searched in quadrants, with the optic nerve head used as a reference point. The direct ophthalmoscope is analogous to the high-power lens of a microscope and provides an upright image magnified 15 to 17×, varying somewhat with the size of the patient's eye. Therefore thorough examination of the fundus by direct ophthalmoscopy is at best time-consuming and often impossible because the field examined is so small and the patient's eye is constantly moving.

Indirect Ophthalmoscopy

With indirect ophthalmoscopy, a convex lens (typically 20 to 30 D) is placed between the observer's eye and the patient's eye and an inverted virtual image is formed between the lens and observer (Figure 5-17). The magnification and field of view depend on the dioptric power of the lens and on the size of the patient's eye. However, with the lenses typically used in veterinary medicine, the magnification is always less and the field of view greater than that achieved with use of a direct ophthalmoscope. Therefore indirect ophthalmoscopy allows examination of a greater percentage of the fundus with each field and is faster and more thorough than direct ophthalmoscopy. The ability to compare all regions of the fundus present in one field of view is another important advantage. With the binocular indirect ophthalmoscope (Figure 5-18), a head-mounted light source between the examiner's eyes permits both eyes to be used for the examination and creates depth perception to better interpret raised and depressed lesions within the fundus. This technique also leaves both hands of the examiner free; one hand can then be used to position the patient's head and eyelids at arm's length from the examiner, and the other to position the lens and further control the patient's eyelids (Figure 5-19).

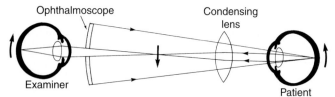

Figure 5-17. Indirect ophthalmoscopy. (Modified from Vaughan D, Asbury T [1983]: General Ophthalmology, 10th ed. Lange Medical Publications, Los Altos, CA.)

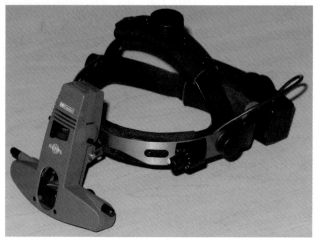

Figure 5-18. A portable binocular indirect ophthalmoscope.

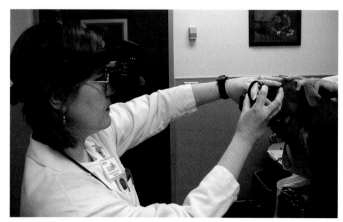

Figure 5-19. The binocular indirect ophthalmoscope and a 2.2 panretinal lens are ideal for funduscopic examination of most domestic veterinary patients.

Monocular Indirect Ophthalmoscopy

A number of new monocular indirect ophthalmoscopes that fit onto the standard battery handset used for the direct ophthalmoscope have become available (Figure 5-20). Monocular indirect ophthalmoscopy has features intermediate between those of direct ophthalmoscopy and the indirect lens. It produces an upright image of moderate magnification and moderate field of view. The instrument can be used with one hand and is relatively easy for the beginner and infrequent user to master. However, because the observer uses only one eye, there is little depth perception. Views of a canine fundus that would be obtained using the three methods of ophthalmoscopy are shown in Figure 5-21.

NORMAL FUNDUS

The fundus of each domestic species has a characteristic but highly variable appearance, which must be learned through regular practice with a reliable ophthalmoscope. The interpretation of fundic lesions is probably one of the most difficult components of the ocular examination and is a common and justifiable reason for referral to a veterinary ophthalmologist. The following structures are found in the fundus of domestic species (Figure 5-22):

- *Tapetum:* A highly reflective structure in the dorsal portion of the fundus. The pig, bird, and camelids have no tapetum, and absence of tapetum in other species usually having one

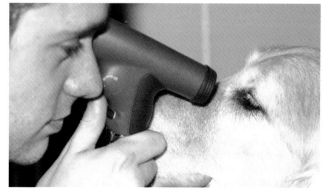

Figure 5-20. The monocular indirect ophthalmoscope (Panoptic) in use.

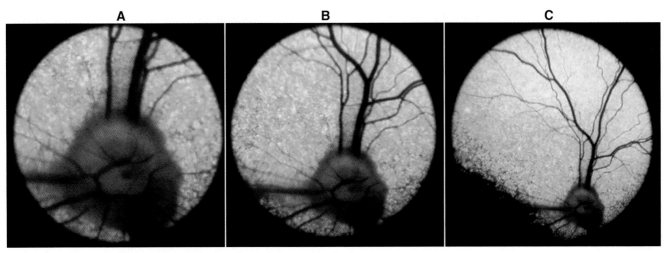

Figure 5-21. View of a canine fundus as seen through the direct ophthalmoscope **(A)**, the monocular indirect (Panoptic) ophthalmoscope **(B)**, and a 20-D indirect lens **(C)**. Note that as magnification increases, field of view decreases. (Courtesy Dr. David Ramsey.)

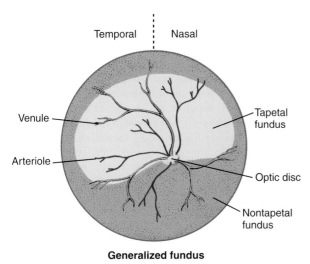

Generalized fundus

Figure 5-22. Structures in the normal fundus. For this diagram, species differences have been ignored. For individual and species differences, see Figures 5-23 through 5-29.

is considered a normal variation. When present the tapetum typically occupies the dorsal half or less of the fundus. The nonreflective ventral portion, termed the *nontapetal area,* may be variably melanotic with choroidal vessels evident if melanin is sufficiently lacking. Tapetal development continues postnatally. In young dogs and cats the fundus is grayish soon after the eyes open (7 to 10 days). With tapetal development the dorsal fundus progresses through lilac and successively lighter blues to the adult color and reflectivity by approximately 4 months of age.

- *Optic disc, optic nerve head, or optic papilla:* The region of the optic nerve where axons that form the nerve fiber layer of the inner retina turn through about 90 degrees to exit the eye and orbit as the optic nerve. It is ventrolateral to the posterior pole of the globe. The degree of myelination varies among species and even individuals of the same species (but minimally between eyes of the same individual). As for the tapetum, postnatal development of the optic papilla occurs and myelination can continue in dogs until approximately 4 months of age. When

present, myelin produces some irregularities in the border (and therefore the shape) of the optic disc. Also, a small depression of variable size is seen in the middle of the optic disc in myelinated nerves and is known as the physiologic cup.

- *Retina:* The funduscopically important parts of the retina are the retinal vessels, the retinal pigment epithelium (RPE), and the neurosensory retina. The retinal vascular pattern varies among species. When present, retinal arterioles and venules can be seen emanating from the optic disc. The RPE is perhaps poorly named because it is not always pigmented (melanotic). When the tapetum (which it overlies) is present, the RPE is typically nonpigmented to permit light to pass through it and reach the tapetum. In nontapetal animals and in those nontapetal regions of tapetal fundi, the RPE may be more melanotic and may obscure the view of the choroid behind it. In some subalbinotic animals the melanin content of the RPE is limited and a clear view of the choroid is possible (Figure 5-23). The neurosensory retina itself is translucent (rather like wax paper) and, as

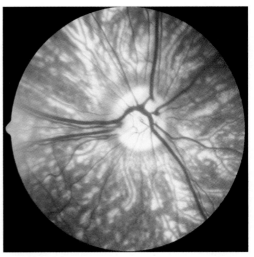

Figure 5-23. Subalbinotic fundus of a dog. The choroidal vessels can be seen easily because of sparse melanin within the choroid and retinal pigment epithelium.

such, is not seen directly. Rather, its major effect on funduscopic appearance is that it reduces the tapetal reflection dorsally and makes the ventral nontapetal area seem slightly more gray than black. This effect is usually not appreciated until retinal thickness is reduced in various forms of retinal degeneration. The effect consists of tapetal hyperreflectivity, a more mosaic pattern to the nontapetal fundus, and retinal vascular attenuation.

- *Choroid:* The choroid is a highly vascular, variably melanotic structure. Unlike the retinal vessels, which are relatively fine, dark red, branching vessels, choroidal vessels appear as broad, orange to pink, spokelike vessels emanating from the optic disc. The choroid is seen when there is no overlying tapetum and when the overlying RPE is not highly melanotic. This most commonly occurs in the ventral fundus of subalbinotic animals (see Figure 5-23).

Dog

Typically, tapetal and nontapetal areas are present in the canine fundus (Figure 5-24), although the tapetum can be normally absent in dogs. Tapetal color is usually gold, bluish green, or orange-brown. The tapetum has a fine beaded or granular appearance. The junction between tapetal and nontapetal areas is often irregular. The nontapetal fundus is deep brown to black and relatively homogeneous to slightly mottled. The choroid is normally visible in the nontapetal fundus of subalbinotic, lightly colored, or merle animals (see Figure 5-23).

The optic disc usually lies near the tapetal-nontapetal junction (depending on the size of the tapetum). When it lies in the tapetal region, a small hyperreflective ring immediately adjacent to the margin of the disc is normal and is called peripapillary conus. The disc surface tends to be white to pink, owing to admixing of myelin and numerous small capillaries. The physiologic cup is a small gray depression in the center of the optic disc. The retinal vascular pattern is holangiotic, meaning that vessels should extend from the optic nerve head to the periphery of the retina. The major retinal venules typically anastomose on the surface of the disc. The anastomoses may appear complete or incomplete, depending on the degree of myelination covering the vessels. These venules penetrate the lamina cribrosa with the nerve fibers but soon leave the nerve to enter the orbit. Retinal arterioles (about 20) emerge from the outer portions and margin of the disc and are considerably smaller than the venules. There typically are three major retinal venules—superior, ventromedial, and ventrolateral—although additional veins and variation in orientation are common. Over the nontapetal fundus, the retinal vessels may normally exhibit a grayish silver sheen or "reflex" in the center of the vessel, which is not seen over the tapetum.

Cat

The feline fundus tends to be more uniform in appearance than the canine fundus (Figure 5-25). A large, highly reflective, relatively uniform tapetal region of gold or green is usually present. The nontapetal region tends to be highly melanotic but can be amelanotic in subalbinotic animals, especially oriental breeds. The optic disc is smaller and more circular and does not have an obvious physiologic cup because of the lack of myelin. The optic nerve head is usually present in the tapetal area. Like the dog, the cat has a holangiotic retinal vascular pattern. However, the retinal vessels emanate from the edge of the optic disc, and there is no venous circle on the optic nerve head. As with the dog, there are generally three arterioles—superior, ventromedial, and ventrolateral—which are ciliary in origin. The area centralis is a region of high cone density for enhanced visual acuity. It is superior and temporal to the optic disc, within the tapetal fundus, and is usually visible as an oval to elliptical area devoid of large blood vessels and with a slightly granular appearance.

Horse

The equine fundus retina (Figure 5-26) differs greatly in appearance from the canine or feline fundus. Most horses have a tapetum with the junction between tapetal and nontapetal areas being relatively uniform. The tapetum varies in color from bluish purple to green and yellow. As with other

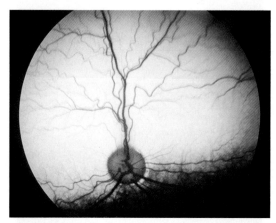

Figure 5-24. Typical canine fundus. Note tapetum, holangiotic retinal vascular pattern, with anastomotic ring on the optic nerve head, melanotic retinal pigment epithelium and choroid, and myelinated optic nerve head.

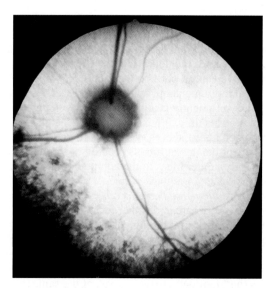

Figure 5-25. Typical feline fundus. Note tapetum, holangiotic retinal vascular pattern, with vessels extending only to the periphery of the optic nerve head, melanotic retinal pigment epithelium and choroid, and nonmyelinated optic nerve head.

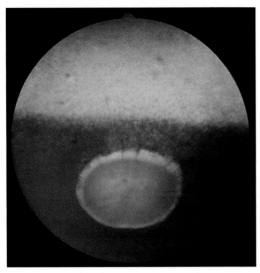

Figure 5-26. Typical equine fundus. Note tapetum, paurangiotic retinal vascular pattern, melanotic retinal pigment epithelium and choroid, and oval, salmon pink, nonmyelinated, optic nerve head. This horse has the diffuse color dilute region seen dorsal to the optic nerve head in a number of normal horses.

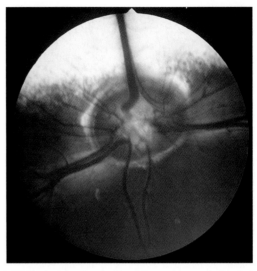

Figure 5-27. Typical bovine fundus. Note tapetum, holangiotic retinal vascular pattern, with large retinal vessels, melanotic retinal pigment epithelium and choroid, and horizontally ovoid optic nerve head.

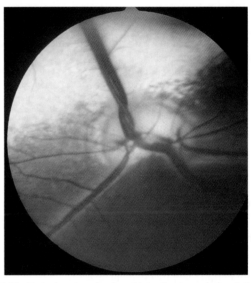

Figure 5-28. Typical ovine fundus. Note tapetum, holangiotic retinal vascular pattern, with large, intertwined retinal vessels, melanotic retinal pigment epithelium and choroid, and kidney bean–shaped optic nerve head.

herbivores, the horse's tapetum tends to be less reflective than that of the carnivores with the stars of Winslow being far more readily appreciated. These are small, uniformly scattered red or dark pink dots and lines representing end-on views of capillaries of the choriocapillaris traversing the tapetum to supply the outer retina. The nontapetal area is typically brown and relatively homogeneous. Absence of the tapetum or amelanotic nontapetal area allows the choroidal circulation to be seen but occurs relatively infrequently in horses compared with dogs and cats. However, a common normal variant is a relative reduction in tapetal coloration dorsal to the disc with variable exposure of the choroidal circulation (see Figure 5-26). The optic disc lies in the nontapetal fundus, is a horizontal oval, and has 30 to 60 short vessels supplying the surrounding retina. This is a paurangiotic vascular pattern with the arterioles and venules indistinguishable from each other. The lamina cribrosa is often visible within the optic nerve head.

Sheep, Goats, and Cattle

The fundi of sheep, goats, and cattle are similar. They are typically tapetal with a heavily myelinated optic nerve head. The optic nerve head varies in shape among these three domesticated ruminant species. In cattle it tends to be horizontally ovoid (Figure 5-27), in sheep it is kidney shaped (Figure 5-28), and in goats it forms an irregular circle (Figure 5-29). The nontapetal area is homogeneous brown/black except in albinotic and subalbinotic animals, in which it may lack melanin, revealing the subjacent choroidal vasculature. The retinal vascular pattern is holangiotic with three or four major venules and arterioles radiating from the optic disc. The retinal vessels are of large diameter and bulge (with the inner retina) into the vitreous. The dorsal retinal venule and arteriole often intertwine, and tributaries of the dorsal vessels often appear like the hanging branches of a tree. Remnants of the hyaloid vascular system may persist centrally on the optic nerve head as Bergmeister's papilla.

EXAMINATION OF THE POSTERIOR SEGMENT

Vitreous

The anterior vitreous can be partially examined along with the anterior segment after pupil dilation and if a bright light source is used. However, examination of the vitreous is completed with ophthalmoscopy. As for the aqueous humor, the vitreous should be transparent and should effectively go unnoticed during the examination if it is normal. Therefore look in particular for the following:

- Opacities within the vitreous: persistent hyaloid artery or its remnants (perfused or nonperfused), asteroid hyalosis, synchysis scintillans, inflammatory exudates, vitreous hemorrhage, traction bands, obvious vitreous plicae

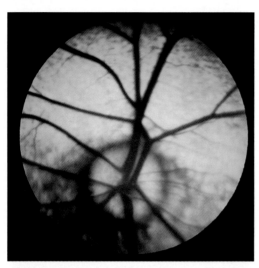

Figure 5-29. Typical caprine fundus. Note tapetum, holangiotic retinal vascular pattern, melanotic retinal pigment epithelium and choroid, and roughly circular optic nerve head. (Courtesy University of California, Davis, Veterinary Ophthalmology Service Collection.)

- Swirling of the vitreous with globe movement: liquefaction of the vitreous (syneresis)
- Retinal detachment/dialysis/tears

Retina

Retinal disease is usually best observed as changes in the appearance of the underlying tapetum, choroid, or RPE. Look in particular for the following:

- Changes in color: inflammatory cells, edema, melanin, hemorrhage, fibrosis (gliosis), retinal folds, neoplasia, and lipid accumulation, all of which obscure the view of the tapetum
- Changes in tapetal reflectivity: hyporeflectivity (typically active and acute processes) or hyperreflectivity (indicative of more chronic and inactive changes)
- Difficulty focusing on all of the retina at once: vitreous debris, retinal edema, retinal detachment, scleral coloboma/ectasia
- Changes in the vascular appearance: retinal vessels may appear attenuated (retinal degeneration, anemia) or enlarged/tortuous (systemic hypertension, chorioretinitis, vasculitis, collie eye anomaly)

Optic Nerve

Interpretation of optic nerve head changes requires an appreciation of the normal species-related variations as well as some individual variations. Look in particular for the following:

- Increased size or prominence: optic neuritis, papilledema, excessive myelination
- Decreased size or prominence: coloboma, optic nerve hypoplasia, micropapilla, optic nerve atrophy, glaucomatous cupping
- Vascular changes: hemorrhages, anemia, engorgement, Bergmeister's papilla

ADDITIONAL DIAGNOSTIC TESTING

Following a through examination of the anterior and posterior segments, additional testing should be chosen on the basis of presenting complaint, history, signalment, examination findings, and disease suspicion. Discussion of such tests forms the remainder of this chapter.

Aqueous Flare

Aqueous flare (sometimes just called "flare") is a pathognomonic sign of anterior uveitis due to breakdown of the blood-ocular barrier with subsequent leakage of plasma proteins (often along with cells) into the aqueous humor within the anterior chamber. Aqueous flare is best detected with the use of magnification and a very focal, intense light source in a totally darkened room after pupil dilation. The path taken by the beam of light is viewed from an angle. In the normal eye, a focal reflection is seen where the light strikes the cornea. The beam is then invisible as it traverses the almost protein- and cell-free aqueous humor in the anterior chamber. The light beam becomes visible again as a focal reflection on the anterior lens capsule and then as a diffuse beam through the body of the normal lens because of the presence of lens proteins (Figure 5-30, *A*). If uveitis has allowed leakage of serum proteins from the iris or ciliary body into the aqueous humor, the light will scatter as it passes through the anterior chamber. Aqueous flare is therefore detected when a beam of light is visible traversing the anterior chamber and joining the focal reflections on the corneal surface and the anterior lens capsule (Figure 5-30, *B*).

A slit-lamp biomicroscope provides ideal conditions for detecting flare (Figure 5-31); however, the beam produced by the smallest circular aperture on the direct ophthalmoscope held as closely as possible to the cornea in a completely darkened room and viewed transversely with some source of magnification also has excellent results (Figure 5-32). The smallest circle of light is preferred over the slit beam on the direct ophthalmoscope because the slit beam is not as intense and does not provide as many "edges" of light where flare can be

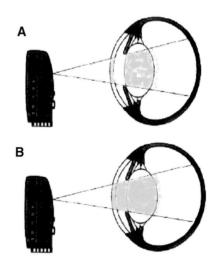

Figure 5-30. Detection of aqueous flare. **A,** In the normal eye a focal light beam is visible only where it traverses the cornea and lens but not within the anterior chamber. **B,** With leakage of serum proteins from the iris or ciliary body into the aqueous humor (anterior uveitis), the beam of light is also visible traversing the anterior chamber.

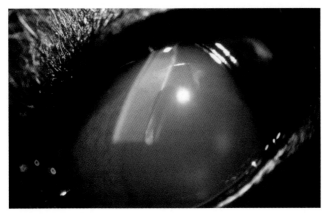

Figure 5-31. Photograph of a dog with aqueous flare. Note that the beam of light is visible within the anterior chamber behind the cornea.

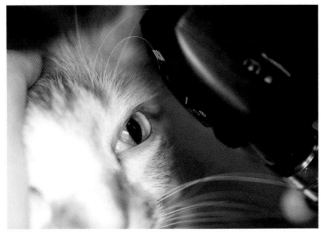

Figure 5-32. The direct ophthalmoscope can be used to assess aqueous flare. It is turned to the small circle of light, held very close to the patient's cornea, and the light beam is viewed at a transverse angle in a darkened room using a source of magnification.

appreciated more easily. Assessment of flare may be easier after complete pupil dilation because the dark space created by the pupil provides an excellent "backdrop" against which the light beam can be seen traversing the anterior chamber. If flare is seen, then anterior uveitis can be diagnosed with certainty. However, it is important to note that not all eyes with uveitis have flare. The absence of this sign should not be used to eliminate the diagnosis of uveitis, and other signs of uveitis (low intraocular pressure, miosis, rubeosis iridis, keratic precipitates, etc.) should be searched for.

All red, inflamed, or painful eyes should undergo assessment for aqueous flare to facilitate the diagnosis of uveitis.

Tonometry

Tonometry is the measure of intraocular pressure (IOP) and is perhaps one of the most important but underused diagnostic tests in veterinary medicine. For too long, tonometry has been taught as simply a method of diagnosing glaucoma (in which IOP is raised). However, it is far more than this. It is also a method of diagnosing anterior uveitis (where IOP is typically reduced) and of confirming the diagnosis of all other causes of

reddened eye, such as keratitis, conjunctivitis, scleritis, and orbital cellulitis (in which IOP should be unaffected). Following confirmation of uveitis or glaucoma, tonometry should be an essential and perhaps the most important method of monitoring response to therapy and judging the tapering or augmentation of therapy. The ready availability of the Tono-Pen—a reasonably priced, user-friendly, applanation tonometer—has made tonometry an achievable goal in all private practices and is the basis of this section. However, other methods of tonometry are also described.

Cannulation measures IOP directly; it is used experimentally but not clinically. Other methods employ measurements of corneoscleral tension to estimate IOP. Digital palpation of the globe through closed lids provides an extremely unreliable, nonreproducible measure of IOP and will fail to identify animals in which IOP is within a range for which treatment is likely to be successful. Dependence on this method leads to inaccurate diagnosis and inappropriate ocular therapy, with unacceptable consequences such as blindness or ongoing ocular pain. Therefore a method of IOP measurement is an essential part of a thorough ophthalmic evaluation.

Indentation Tonometry

The Schiøtz tonometer relies upon indentation tonometry. In this method, a standard force is applied with a metal rod to the anesthetized cornea. The distance the rod indents the cornea is measured and is inversely related to the IOP (i.e., the greater the tonometer scale reading, the lower the patient's IOP). This method is easily understood if one regards the eye as analogous to a water-filled balloon. If the blunt end of a pencil is applied to the balloon with a given force (e.g., the weight of the pencil placed vertically), the pencil indents the surface of the balloon by a certain distance. If the pressure in the balloon is decreased (some of the water is let out), the tension in the rubber wall decreases, and the same pencil resting on the balloon indents it farther. Conversely, if the pressure in the balloon is increased, the same pencil indents it less. The Schiøtz tonometer (Figure 5-33) consists of three parts: the plunger (analogous to the pencil), the footplate assembly (a device to measure indentation), and the handle. A further refinement is added: The weight applied to the eye through the rod may be varied by adding or subtracting weights (5.5 g, 7.5 g, 10.0 g, or 15.0 g). The greater

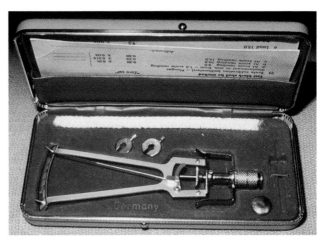

Figure 5-33. The Schiøtz tonometer.

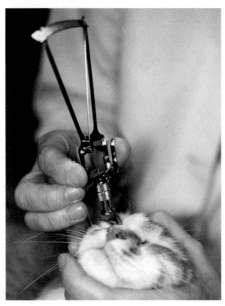

Figure 5-34. The Schiøtz tonometer in use on a cat. Note that the tonometer must be held vertically, making its use awkward or impossible in many veterinary patients.

the weight applied to the eye at a given IOP, the greater the penetration of the rod.

Before use of the Schiøtz tonometer, a drop of local anesthetic is placed on the surface of the eye. The patient is then restrained and the lids are carefully retracted without placing pressure on the globe. Since the indentation tonometer relies on gravity for an accurate reading, it must be placed vertically upon the cornea (Figure 5-34). This requires that the head be elevated so that the corneal surface is horizontal. The tonometer is placed on the eye, either with no weight in place (the plunger weighs 5.5 g) or with the 7.5-g weight in place. The scale reading is recorded. The calibration table supplied with the instrument is then used to convert the scale reading to the IOP via the appropriate column, selected according to the weight used. Human calibration tables supplied with the instrument are more accurate than veterinary versions. The data are recorded as scale reading/weight/pressure (e.g., 5.0 units/5.5 g/21 mm Hg).

Because of difficulties in head positioning and patient cooperation, Schiøtz tonometry is difficult in many small animals and impossible for large domestic animals. Also, if, under the influence of the Schiøtz plunger, the sclera and cornea stretch because of the slight increase in IOP caused by the indentation, a higher scale reading and a lower IOP are measured, because the ocular rigidity has changed. This ocular rigidity varies considerably in dogs. A quick check to determine the influence of ocular rigidity on the accuracy of the readings may be performed by measuring the pressure with two different tonometer weights (using the lighter weight first). If the pressures obtained are similar, the influence of ocular rigidity is small. If the pressure obtained with the heavier weight is considerably less, the ocular rigidity is low and the walls of the globe are stretching. The plunger assembly of the Schiøtz tonometer must be kept clean because mucus and salts from tears can dry on the plunger rod surfaces, prevent free movement of the plunger, and cause inaccurate results. The instrument may be sterilized with ethylene oxide to prevent transfer of pathogenic microorganisms between patients.

Owing to ease of use, the Tono-Pen has largely replaced the Schiøtz tonometer in progressive practices.

Applanation Tonometry

Unlike indentation tonometry, applanation tonometry using the Tono-Pen is suitable for large animals, is unaffected by variations in ocular rigidity, requires no conversion tables, and needs no sterilization. The principle of applanation tonometry is that the force required to flatten a given area of a sphere is equal to the pressure within the sphere (the Imbert-Fick law). Therefore if the area is known (the size of the footplate) and the force is measured, the pressure can be calculated. Although there are numerous types of applanation tonometers, the most commonly used in general and specialty veterinary practice is the Tono-Pen. This instrument has changed design somewhat over the years but the basic utility of the instrument is unchanged (Figure 5-35).

The advantages of the Tono-Pen include the following:

- It is accurate and easy to use.
- The animal's head does not need to be held vertically, although the probe must applanate the corneal surface at right angles.
- Errors induced by different sizes and curvatures of corneas in different species are less important.
- Because of the small instrument head, irregular or diseased corneal areas may be avoided, and accurate readings obtained from even small corneas of exotic species.
- The probe tip is covered with a disposable latex cap, which is changed between uses and prevents transfer of infections.
- Minimal restraint is required.
- The pressure is displayed in mm Hg without need for conversion via tables.

Before use, a drop of topical anesthetic is applied to the cornea. The patient is minimally restrained by an assistant so as not to artificially raise IOP via direct pressure on the jugular veins, and the operator carefully retracts the eyelids using the nondominant hand. Care must be taken not to place pressure on the globe. The dominant hand holding the Tono-Pen should then be stabilized against the hand holding the eyelids, and the central cornea gently touched with the instrument's tip using multiple, very light "blotting" movements. Particular attention

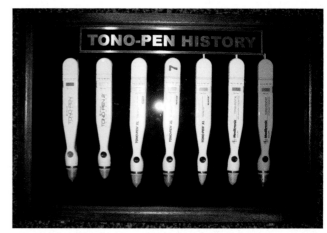

Figure 5-35. A series of Tono-Pens showing the evolution of the instrument through the years. Despite these changes, the utility of this instrument is unchanged.

should be paid to the "approach angle" of the tip to the cornea so that the tip's flat surface is parallel to the corneal surface (i.e., so that the Tono-Pen itself is perpendicular to the corneal surface). This is best achieved by viewing the interface between the cornea and the tip from the side. The cornea is "blotted" sufficient times to elicit an average reading. The digital display is in mm Hg. The reliability (coefficient of variance) of the result should be 5%, or tonometry should be repeated.

Rebound Tonometry

Rebound (or impact or dynamic) tonometry is a third mechanism by which IOP may be measured and which uses a different mechanical principle. Rebound tonometers eject a small probe (such as a metal pin with a rounded end) at a fixed distance from the cornea and assess the motion of the probe as it strikes the cornea and is returned (rebounds) to the instrument. Eyes with higher IOP cause a more rapid deceleration of the probe and shorter return time to the instrument. This technique is affected by ocular surface tension and so should be performed before application of any topical medications, including topical anesthetic. This feature raises some questions as to how readings by such tonometers might be affected by keratoconjunctivitis sicca (in which surface tension would be altered) and by the presence of corneal pathology as is frequently encountered in animals with glaucoma or uveitis. Additionally, the probe distance from the eye is likely to exert some influence on readings, and ensuring the proper distance can be difficult in uncooperative animals. The technique was developed more than 50 years ago and only recently has undergone a resurgence in popularity owing to the release of a new rebound tonometer, manufactured as TonoVet or iCare (Figure 5-36). This instrument has so far been calibrated for dogs, cats, and horses only, and one must select the correct software for each species before beginning IOP measurements. In a study using normotensive dog eyes, the TonoVet consistently reported lower IOP than the Tono-Pen did; however, the difference was only about 1 to 2 mm Hg. The reliability of the rebound tonometer in patients with diseased corneas or when measured through a contact lens has not yet been assessed.

The IOP should be measured in all red, inflamed, or painful eyes to diagnose or eliminate from consideration both glaucoma and uveitis.

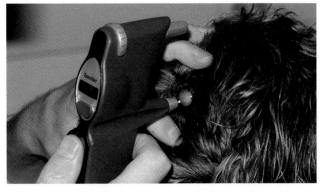

Figure 5-36. The TonoVet rebound tonometer in use.

Normal Intraocular Pressure

Across large populations, normal canine and feline IOP is reported as approximately 10 to 20 mm Hg. However, significant variation is noted among individuals as well as among techniques and the time of day at which IOP is measured. Therefore comparison of IOP between right and left eyes of the same animal is critical to interpretation of results. A good rule of thumb is that IOP should not vary between right and left eyes of the same patient by more than 20%. As with all other measured biologic values, one should not treat a low or high IOP but should use it as an indicator of uveitis or glaucoma, respectively, and should assess the patient for other signs consistent with those diagnoses. Additionally, IOP can vary with some exogenous and endogenous factors. Sedatives, tranquilizers, and anesthetic drugs can cause lowered IOP readings because of reduced extraocular and adnexal muscle tone. By the same mechanism, ketamine may cause a slightly elevated reading. Patient cooperation is an important factor, and care should be taken to minimize pressure applied around the neck or orbital area, or in retracting the eyelids.

Tonography

Tonography is the study of aqueous outflow facility in response to pressure applied to the eye. It is based on the observation that applied pressure softens an eye because fluid is forced out through the iridocorneal (or "drainage") angle. This softening occurs to a lesser extent in a glaucomatous eye because aqueous is less able to pass out of the anterior chamber (i.e., outflow facility is decreased). In tonography, a Schiøtz-type weight and plunger are placed on the cornea of a still patient and the gradual reduction in IOP over 4 minutes is measured graphically on a strip chart recorder. The outflow facility coefficient (C) can be calculated from this graph. This technique is used predominantly in research settings.

Gonioscopy

Gonioscopy describes examination of the iridocorneal or "drainage" angle (the junction between the iris and cornea). In the normal eye of most species light rays that are reflected from the drainage angle strike the posterior cornea and undergo total internal reflection as in a prism (Figure 5-37, *A*). This occurs because of the difference in refractive index between the cornea and the surrounding air, and the high angle of incidence of the light rays from the drainage angle. By replacing the air surrounding the cornea with a goniolens that has an index of refraction close to that of the cornea, total internal reflection is avoided and light rays from the drainage angle can be viewed directly through the goniolens. Additional modifications may be made to the goniolens to provide magnification. Magnifying instruments such as the biomicroscope, gonioscope, head loupe, and fundus camera may also be used. Direct goniolenses (e.g., Koeppe; Figure 5-37, *B*), through which the angle is viewed directly and indirect goniolenses (e.g., Goldmann; Figure 5-37, *C*), in which the image is viewed in a mirror, are both available. Low-vacuum goniolenses are very useful for veterinary use, as they are held in place by low-pressure vacuum applied by a 2-mL syringe and a column of saline held below the level of the eye. All goniolenses are bonded to the cornea with a liquid medium such as saline (for low-vacuum goniolenses) or methylcellulose solutions (for nonvacuum goniolenses).

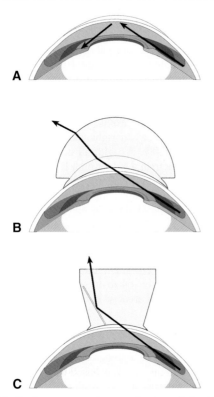

Figure 5-37. Gonioscopy permits examination of the iridocorneal or "drainage" angle. **A,** Normally, light rays from the drainage angle undergo total internal reflection at the posterior cornea. **B,** A direct goniolens refracts light so that the drainage angle may be viewed directly. **C,** An indirect goniolens refracts light so that the image is viewed in a mirror.

Gonioscopic examination is a frequent part of the examination of patients in which suspected glaucoma or ocular hypertension is suspected and complements tonometry and tonography. In cooperative patients topical anesthesia is usually sufficient (Figure 5-38); however, tranquilization may be necessary in refractory animals. The normal structures of the canine drainage angle are shown in Figure 5-39. Gonioscopy is used primarily to determine whether the angle is open, narrow, closed, or obstructed by mesodermal remnants, and to check for the presence of foreign bodies, tumors, and inflammatory

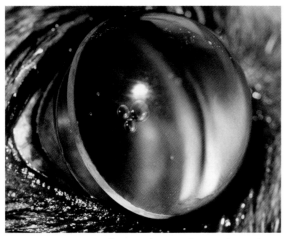

Figure 5-38. A gonioscopic lens in place on the anesthetized cornea of an unsedated dog.

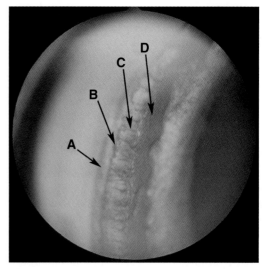

Figure 5-39. Gonioscopic view of a normal canine iridocorneal (drainage) angle. **A,** Outer pigment band; **B,** inner pigment band; **C,** pectinate ligaments; **D,** iris root.

exudates. The technique is applicable to all domestic species but is most commonly used in dogs. In cats and horses the anterior chamber is deeper than in dogs and parts of the drainage angle can be examined without a goniolens.

Vital Dyes

Vital dyes stain living tissues. Fluorescein and rose bengal are most commonly used in veterinary ophthalmology.

Fluorescein

Fluorescein is a water-soluble dye that is retained by all hydrophilic but not hydrophobic structures. The classic example of its use is in the identification of a corneal ulcer, in which the fluorescein is retained by the hydrophilic stroma wherever it is exposed by loss of the hydrophobic epithelium. Fluorescein should always be applied from an impregnated paper strip. Prepared solutions should not be used because they can become contaminated by bacteria. The strip is removed from the packet, moistened with a drop of sterile saline or eye rinse, and touched very briefly to the conjunctival and not the corneal surface. Direct application of the strip to the cornea can cause artifactual stain retention. Excess dye should always be rinsed with sterile saline, and the eye examined with magnification and a blue light from a cobalt filter attached to a Finoff transilluminator or from the direct ophthalmoscope. A Wood's light also may be used.

Defects in the corneal epithelium appear as bright green areas. However, various ulcer types demonstrate different and characteristic staining patterns. Recognizing these patterns will greatly assist in differentiating simple (superficial) ulcers from complicated (deep, infected, or indolent) ulcers. In superficial ulcers the stain adheres only to the ulcer floor and has distinct margins (Figure 5-40). In deeper stromal ulcers both the walls and floor of the ulcer will stain and there may be some diffusion of fluorescein into the neighboring stroma, producing less distinct margins (Figure 5-41). With descemetoceles the center of the ulcer will fail to take up stain and will appear black because Descemet's membrane, which does not stain

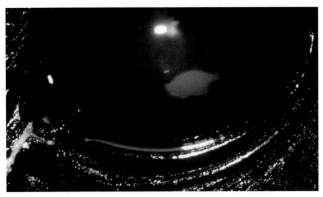

Figure 5-40. Characteristic staining pattern of a superficial ulcer. Note that the fluorescein stain adheres only to the floor of the ulcer and has distinct margins.

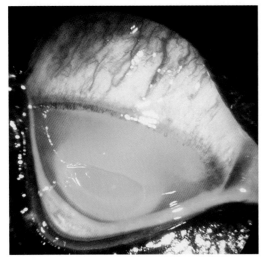

Figure 5-41. Characteristic staining pattern of a deeper stromal ulcer. Note that the fluorescein stain adheres to the walls and floor of the ulcer and that there is some diffusion of fluorescein into the neighboring stroma, producing less distinct margins.

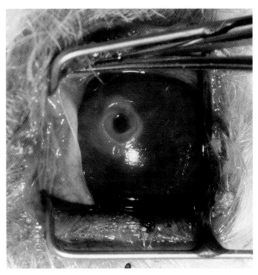

Figure 5-42. Characteristic staining pattern of a descemetocele. Note that the fluorescein stain adheres only to the walls of the ulcer; the center ("floor") of the ulcer fails to take up stain and appears black because the exposed regions of Descemet's membrane do not retain fluorescein stain.

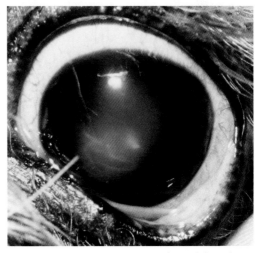

Figure 5-43. Characteristic staining pattern of an indolent ulcer. Note that fluorescein stains the floor of the ulcer but that this area does not have distinct margins. Rather, it is surrounded by a halo of less distinct stain seen through the nonadherent epithelial lip.

with fluorescein, is exposed (Figure 5-42). Indolent ulcers (see Chapter 10) have a characteristic fluorescein staining pattern because they are superficial and therefore have a stained floor (like other superficial ulcers) surrounded by a halo of less distinct stain seen through their nonadherent epithelial lip (Figure 5-43). A penetrating corneal wound will also produce a characteristic stain pattern. In addition to all areas of exposed corneal stroma retaining fluorescein dye, the egress of aqueous resulting from the globe rupture will produce tiny rivulets in the fluorescein dye as they dilute it at the corneal surface. Evaluating for this feature is called a *Seidel test*. This test is performed by applying a concentrated solution of fluorescein and not rinsing it off but rather allowing the aqueous humor to do so, while viewing with a blue light source and a source of magnification.

Nonulcerative lesions sometimes stain and can cause confusion unless they are recognized. For example, the surface of a vascularized or roughened corneal lesion may show diffuse, faint fluorescein staining because of pooling of stain due to surface tension. Fibrovascular ("granulation") tissue will also retain stain owing to its hydrophilic nature. Finally, an epithelialized stromal defect (a *facet*) pools stain and must be differentiated from a corneal ulcer. One can make this distinction by examining the

eye with a blue light and magnification while an assistant rinses the cornea. Fluorescein stain cannot be rinsed from an ulcer, whereas stain pooling in a facet can easily be rinsed.

All red, inflamed, or painful eyes should be stained with fluorescein to diagnose or eliminate from consideration corneal ulcers.

Fluorescein dye may also be used for other ocular diagnostic tests. Topical ophthalmic application of fluorescein dye and observation for its appearance at the nares confirms patency of the nasolacrimal duct on that side and is referred to as the Jones or fluorescein passage test (Figure 5-44). The interval required for fluorescein to appear is variable (up to 5 to 10 minutes in some normal dogs). In some dogs and cats, especially brachycephalic breeds, drainage from the nasolacrimal duct may occur into the posterior nasal cavity, resulting in false-

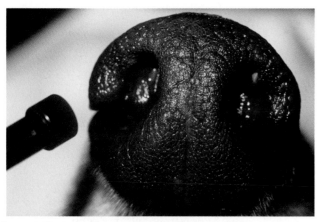

Figure 5-44. A positive Jones or fluorescein passage test result, as evidenced by the appearance of fluorescein stain at the nostril following its application to the ipsilateral corneal surface.

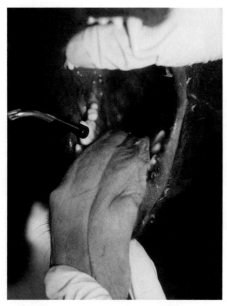

Figure 5-45. In some dogs the nasolacrimal duct opens caudally within the nasopharynx, and fluorescein stain is found in the mouth rather than the nostril after application of the stain to either corneal surface.

negative result of the Jones test unless the mouth is also examined (Figure 5-45).

The tear film break-up time (TFBUT) is an assessment of the stability of the precorneal tear film. The clinician applies a drop of fluorescein stain to the cornea and immediately closes the lids until a pre-prepared source of magnification and a blue light are moved into the viewing position. The lids are then opened, and the dorsolateral quadrant of the precorneal tear film is observed closely while the lids are held apart. The time is recorded from lid opening until the tear film "breaks up" as evidenced by dark spots appearing in the dorsolateral quadrant of the otherwise green fluorescein stain. In the presence of a normal lipid layer of the tear film the TFBUT is a quantitative measure of mucin quantity and quality. Decreased mucin quantity or quality causes tear film instability and a shortening of the TFBUT. Average TFBUT in dogs is approximately 20 seconds, and in cats is about 17 seconds. In cats with tear film disturbances TFBUTs as short as 1 second have been recorded.

Rose Bengal

Rose bengal stains dead and devitalized cells and therefore is retained by corneas in which the epithelium is eroded to less than its full thickness. Therefore there is no exposure of corneal stroma, and fluorescein stain would not be retained. It is even retained by surface squamous cells that have altered surface characteristics or altered mucin coating. As such, it is very useful for the diagnosis of keratoconjunctivitis sicca, qualitative tear film deficiencies, or early dendritic corneal ulcers associated with the herpesviruses, in which there is necrosis and desquamation of corneal and conjunctival epithelium but not exposure of the underlying stroma.

Tests of Lacrimal Patency

Blockage of the nasolacrimal ducts causes overflow of tears (epiphora) at the lid margin near the medial canthus, with staining of the surrounding hair. For more detailed discussion of the lacrimal system, see Chapter 9. Blockage of the nasolacrimal ducts may be evaluated by:

- The fluorescein passage (or "Jones") test as described previously
- Flushing the upper and lower puncta in dogs or cats or the lower (nasal) punctum in horses
- Dacryocystorhinography with radiographs or computed tomography (see later)

Neuroophthalmic Testing

Many cranial nerves are involved to varying degrees with ocular function (see also Chapter 16), as follows:

- CN II: vision and PLRs
- CN III: globe movement via the medial, ventral, and dorsal rectus and inferior oblique muscles; eyelid opening; pupil constriction (via parasympathetic fibers carried with CN III)
- CN IV: globe movement via the superior oblique (extraocular) muscle
- CN V: facial and ocular sensation; lacrimation (via parasympathetic innervation of the lacrimal gland); pupil dilation (via sympathetic innervation of the dilator muscle)
- CN VI: globe movement via the retractor bulbi and lateral rectus muscles
- CN VII: eyelid closure

Basic neuroophthalmic tests therefore form a critical part of the complete ophthalmic examination. In most cases they are extremely simply performed. Commonly employed neuroophthalmic tests include the following:

- PLRs (described previously)
- Swinging flashlight test
- Dazzle reflex
- Palpebral reflex
- Menace response
- Behavioral testing of vision

Swinging Flashlight Test

The swinging flashlight test is a modification of PLR testing. Owing to incomplete decussation in most mammals, the pupil under direct illumination usually constricts slightly more than the contralateral pupil. Therefore when a light source is directed rapidly from one eye to the other (as would be done to test and verify the consensual PLR), the newly illuminated pupil should constrict a little farther than it had already constricted due to the consensual PLR. In patients with a unilateral prechiasmal lesion (i.e., a lesion of the optic nerve between the chiasm and the retina, or of the retina itself), the pupil on the affected side will constrict when stimulated via the contralateral, normal retina (i.e., will have a normal consensual PLR) but will dilate as the light is swung from the normal eye to the affected eye. This is a called a positive swinging flashlight test result or a Marcus Gunn pupil and is pathognomonic for a prechiasmal lesion on the side on which the pupil dilates when illuminated.

Dazzle Reflex

The dazzle reflex is manifested as partial or complete eyelid closure on the illuminated side (and sometimes on both sides) when a bright light is directed at the eye. The reflex follows the same afferent pathway as the PLR but synapses with fibers of the facial nerve in the nucleus of CN VII in the midbrain (presumptively at the rostral colliculus). Therefore it can be used in association with the PLR to further localize some lesions. The reflex is absent in the presence of severe retinal, optic nerve, optic tract, or facial nerve lesions.

Palpebral Reflex

The palpebral reflex consists of a partial or complete closure of the eyelids in response to touching the eyelid skin. Interpretation of the palpebral reflex requires an understanding of the neurologic reflex as well as other potential confounding factors. The afferent arm of the neural arc being tested includes the sensory fibers of the trigeminal nerve; the efferent pathway uses the motor fibers of the facial nerve and the muscles of eyelid closure (principally the orbicularis oculi). In addition to pathology at any point along this neurologic pathway, lagophthalmos due to a physical obstruction of eyelid closure, such as severe buphthalmos or exophthalmos, can cause decrease or absence of the palpebral reflex. The reflex can be overridden in very fearful animals, especially birds and exotic species. The palpebral reflex should be tested through stimulation of the skin at both the medial canthus and lateral canthus. Most animals respond with complete eyelid closure to stimulation at the medial canthus. Fearful animals and animals with breed-related lagophthalmos may not completely close the eyelids in response to stimulation at the lateral canthus.

Menace Response

A normal menace response is evident as eyelid closure when the examiner stimulates the eye in a visually "threatening" way, usually by waving a hand in front of it. However, this response has a number of limitations that must be understood, as follows:

- The stimulus must be visual only. No direct contact with the patient's periocular tissues or creation of air currents, odors, or noise can be associated with the gesture. Achieving this goal is very difficult in any animal in which these senses are heightened, especially in cats and in most visually impaired animals. To prevent air currents, the threatening motion can be performed behind a transparent sheet of Plexiglas.
- Each eye must be tested individually (with the nontested eye closed) because unilaterally blind animals are adept at protecting both eyes when the sighted eye is stimulated.
- Placid or fearful animals may show little response, preferring to watch the menacing gesture.
- The eye should be menaced from the nasal (medial) and temporal (lateral) directions.
- The menace response is a learned response that is absent for the first 10 to 14 weeks of life in puppies and kittens and the first 10 to 14 days in foals.

Even when the test is performed correctly, however, the menace response is a particularly coarse assessment of vision. To put it in perspective, the equivalent test in humans—the ability to simply see hand motions—is considered one grade better than "light perception," after which total blindness is diagnosed. The afferent arm of the menace response includes all components of the eye necessary for vision, especially the retina and optic nerve; and the efferent pathway requires normal facial nerve (CN VII) and eyelid function. However, the arc also passes through the cerebellum, so absence of the menace response is also associated with degenerative lesions of the cerebellar cortex. Whenever the menace response is absent, the palpebral reflex (see earlier) should be tested as a second method of evaluating the efferent pathway shared by the two reflexes.

Behavioral Testing of Vision

Evaluation of vision in veterinary patients remains one of the most challenging parts of the ophthalmic examination (see Chapter 1). Because vision is a cortical function and many neuroophthalmic tests are actually tests of the visual pathways (or segments of them) but not truly tests of vision, vision is best assessed with various behavioral tests. However, results of these tests are affected by some subjectivity and must be very critically analyzed. Each test must be interpreted by the clinician, with consideration given to the animal's personality, emotional state, state of consciousness, and cognitive function. Given the subjective nature of visual testing, visual deficits can be described at best as mild, moderate, severe, or total.

Much can be gained from an accurate history. In particular, information should be sought about the extent and rapidity of vision loss, whether both night vision and day vision are affected, and whether the owner believes the visual impairment is unilateral or bilateral. When judging apparent unilateral visual loss, one must recall the physiologic effects of optic nerve fiber decussation at the optic chiasm. Objects approaching from the left of the patient are perceived by the medial (or nasal) half of the left retina and the lateral (temporal) half of the right retina. The inverse is true for the right visual field. Therefore patients blind in only one eye may still retain vision in the visual field on the side of the affected eye; from the lateral retina of the opposite, functioning eye (see Figure 1-15 in Chapter 1).

During any behavioral tests of vision, individual eyes should ideally be tested independently by "patching" of the remaining eye if the animal will tolerate it.

Various visual "tracking" tests form the basis of vision testing in small animals. A small cotton ball is dropped 20 to 30 cm in front and to each side (i.e., in each visual field) of the patient. Most dogs and cats follow the object to the floor, especially on the first one or two attempts. Alternatively, some animals "track" a silent toy or a laser pointer or other light source directed onto the wall or floor in front of them. A maze test is an excellent method of assessing vision in dogs and horses but is of little value in most cats. In this test, a variety of test obstacles of different sizes and shapes (e.g., chairs, buckets) are placed around a room or pen. With a small animal, the owner is placed on one side of the obstacles and calls the animal from the clinician, once only. Both the client and clinician remain still and quiet during the test. With horses, the patient is led through the maze on a long (3 to 4 m) lead rope. Horses, cattle, and sheep that are unused to being led can be released in a pen or barn that they are not used to, and their movements watched. If the result of such a passive test is negative, large animal patients may be driven through the obstacles.

Regardless of style used, maze testing should be performed in the dark (to test scotopic vision) and in lighted conditions (to test photopic vision). Scotopic maze tests assess rod dysfunction (e.g., early retinal degeneration in dogs or cats, vitamin A deficiency in cattle) and should be performed before photopic testing or the obstacles should be changed between scotopic and photopic testing because animals with decreased visual function often become very adept at memorizing their way through tight spaces.

Electroretinography and Visual Evoked Potentials

Electroretinography (ERG) is the study of electrical potentials produced by the retina when light strikes it. Light of varying intensity, wavelength, and flash duration is directed onto the retina and the resulting potential differences are detected by electrodes placed around the eye (Figure 5-46). These are then amplified and form a characteristically shaped wave that can be recorded on paper or stored electronically and assessed for amplitudes and implicit times (Figure 5-47). For accurate results the ERG is performed with the animal under general anesthesia or deep sedation to minimize periocular muscle

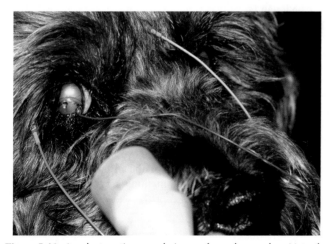

Figure 5-46. An electroretinogram being performed on a dog. Note the ground and reference (subcutaneous) electrodes as well as the corneal contact lens electrode.

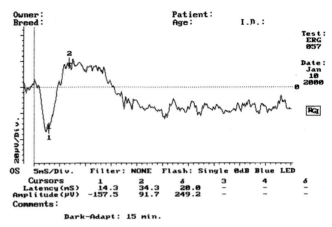

Figure 5-47. A normal electroretinogram.

movements. It is useful in all species. Electroretinography is a test of retinal but not optic nerve or visual function. It is usually available only at specialty ophthalmology practices. The ERG may be used for the following purposes:

- Preoperative evaluation of retinal function before cataract extraction when fundic examination is not possible
- Diagnosis and differentiation of inherited retinal disorders (e.g., rod-cone dysplasias, progressive retinal degeneration, hemeralopia)
- Investigation of unexplained visual loss (amaurosis) in which retinal lesions are not visible ophthalmoscopically (e.g., sudden acquired retinal degeneration [SARD], optic neuritis, CNS disease)

These diagnoses are discussed more fully in Chapter 15.

Following placement of additional electrodes in the skin over the visual cortex and with some alterations in the stimulatory and analytical protocols, electrical potentials at points in the visual pathways central to the retina can be recorded in response to a flash of light into each eye. These responses, called *visual evoked potentials* (VEPs), are rarely used clinically.

Retinoscopy

Retinoscopy is a technique for objective evaluation of the refractive state of the eye and allows determination of refractive errors such as hyperopia ("farsightedness"), myopia ("nearsightedness"), and astigmatism. It is used to evaluate refractive errors after cataract extraction and for evaluation of the visual state of animals with apparent visual problems but in which no abnormalities are found on ophthalmoscopy or electroretinography.

Imaging Techniques

Radiography

Dorsoventral, lateral, anterior-posterior, and oblique plain film radiographs of the orbit and surrounding skull may reveal disease processes in and around the orbit, maxillary dental arcade, and paranasal sinuses. Sometimes a radiopaque ring of stainless steel wire is placed around the limbus to serve as an anatomic reference point. Occasionally contrast techniques are also used, although these are now used less commonly because cross-sectional imaging techniques such as magnetic resonance imaging (MRI) and computed tomography (CT) have become more widely

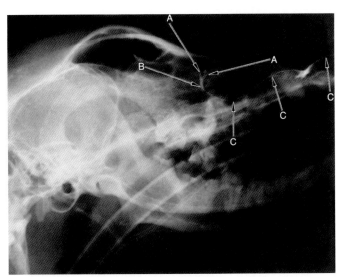

Figure 5-48. A lateral dacryocystorhinogram in a dog. *A,* Lacrimal canaliculus; *B,* lacrimal sac; *C,* nasolacrimal duct. (Courtesy Dr. R. Wyburn.)

available and provide more information with less risk to the patient. Plain films are always assessed before contrast techniques are commenced. All radiographic techniques for ocular disease require general anesthesia for maximal diagnostic yield and radiologic safety, except perhaps a simple lateral or DV radiograph to assess for a radioopaque foreign body. Contrast techniques still in reasonably common use include the following:

• Dacryocystorhinography: injection of contrast medium into the lacrimal canaliculi, lacrimal sac, and nasolacrimal duct for assessment of nasolacrimal obstruction/dysfunction

(Figure 5-48). Lateral and dorsoventral views are both useful. The technique is equally applicable to large and small animals. CT dacryocystorhinography combines the opportunity for two-dimensional cross-sectional images with the contrast-assisted outlining of the nasolacrimal apparatus and is particularly useful.

• Contrast zygomatic sialogram: injection of contrast medium into the zygomatic salivary gland duct within the mouth to outline the gland in the ventral orbit

Orbital venography (injection of contrast medium into the angularis oculi vein) and contrast orbitography (injection of air or radiopaque contrast agents into the orbit) have now been replaced by CT and MRI.

Ultrasonography

In ultrasonography, high-frequency sound waves above the audible range are directed posteriorly through the eye from the cornea, and the echoes are detected, amplified, and displayed on an oscilloscope screen. In B-scan ultrasonography a two-dimensional cross section of the eye and orbit is obtained (Figure 5-49). A-scan ultrasonography is less commonly used. In this technique the echoes are viewed as a series of peaks (Figure 5-50) and permit measurements of various anterior-posterior distances within the eye (biometry). Ultrasonography is used to examine the contents of eyes in which opacity of one of the usually clear ocular media (cornea, aqueous humor, lens, or vitreous) prevents visualization of the structures caudal to it. It is also useful to assess orbital structures and to guide fine-needle aspiration of intraocular and orbital structures.

Ultrasonography is easy to perform, and gives immediate results with excellent definition. However, differentiation

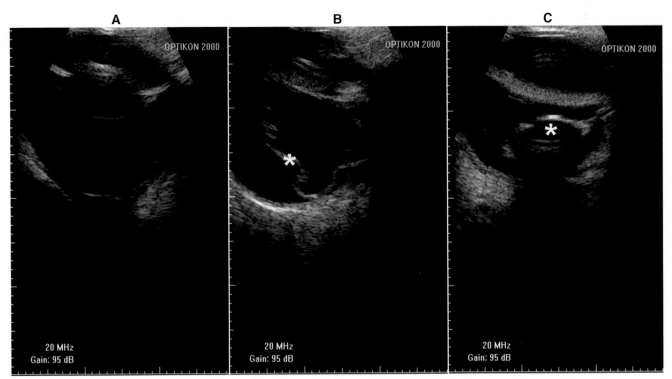

Figure 5-49. B-mode ultrasound images of **A,** a normal globe; **B,** a detached retina *(*);* **C,** a posteriorly luxated lens (*).

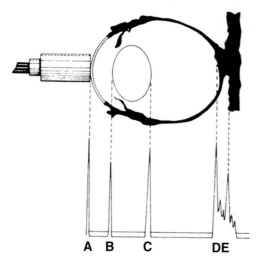

Figure 5-50. Schematic of A-mode ultrasonography of a normal eye, showing the transmitter pulse **(A)**, anterior lens capsule echo **(B)**, posterior lens capsule echo **(C)**, posterior globe wall echo **(D)**, and retrobulbar tissue echoes **(E)**. (From Rubin LF, Koch SA [1968]: Ocular diagnostic ultrasonography. J Am Vet Med Assoc 153:1706.)

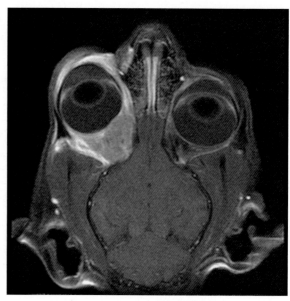

Figure 5-51. T1-weighted, post–contrast injection, frontal magnetic resonance image of a cat with a space-occupying mass behind the right eye. Cytology and culture testing performed on material aspirated from this mass permitted diagnosis of a bacterial retrobulbar abscess/cellulitis that responded well to antibiotic therapy. (Courtesy Dr. Winnie Lo.)

between neoplasia and inflammation is not reliable. The patient is best examined without general anesthesia or sedation, which causes enophthalmos and reduces the clarity of the image obtained. A drop of topical anesthetic is applied to the ocular surface, and the ultrasound probe with sterile coupling gel is applied directly to the cornea or eyelids as the patient permits. Direct corneal contact yields slightly superior images. A transcutaneous temporal technique also has been described and is useful for visualization of retrobulbar structures.

Ultrasonography is particularly useful for the following:

- Detection of retinal detachment (see Figure 5-49, *B*)
- Detection of lens dislocation or rupture (see Figure 5-49, *C*)
- Detection of vitreous degeneration
- Detection of intraocular tumors or foreign bodies
- Characterization of retrobulbar disease
- Guidance of fine-needle aspirates of orbital and ocular lesions

Computed Tomography and Magnetic Resonance Imaging

CT and MRI provide superb detail for localization of orbital lesions (Figure 5-51) and, with increasing availability, have largely replaced skull radiography. Contrast sialography and dacryocystorhinography are as applicable to CT as they are to radiography and provide superior detail. The normal CT and MRI appearances of canine, feline, and equine orbital, ocular, and periocular structures have now been well described, and case reports and case series are expanding knowledge of the CT and MRI appearances of various pathologic conditions. The superior detail shown by these cross-sectional imaging techniques not only greatly assists surgical planning but also may be used to help differentiate individual tumor types on the basis of differing invasion patterns. In cats, for example, indentation of the globe is more frequently seen with lymphomas, whereas squamous cell carcinomas are more likely to produce lysis of orbital bones. In dogs adenocarcinomas were associated with diffuse bony lysis. However, there are exceptions to these trends, and histopathologic or cytologic confirmation of retrobulbar

mass type remains essential. Therefore one or sometimes both of these imaging techniques are now performed almost routinely before biopsy or surgical excision of orbital masses in animals.

Fluorescein Angiography

Fluorescein angiography is used to investigate retinal and choroidal vascular patency, vessel-wall permeability, and pigmentary abnormalities of the fundus. For this technique the patient is sedated or anesthetized, fluorescein is injected intravenously, and the fundus is illuminated with a light of a specific wavelength that stimulates fluorescence. The emitted light is photographed in a series of approximately 30 photographs taken in the first 30 seconds, followed by single photographs 20 and 30 minutes later (Figure 5-52). Circulation of the fluorescein proceeds through the following phases:

- Choroidal phase: Choroidal vasculature has filled.
- Arteriolar phase: Retinal arterioles have filled.
- Arteriovenous phase: Retinal arterioles and venules have filled.
- Venous phase: Retinal arterioles have emptied and veins have begun to fill.
- Late phase: Certain tissues (e.g., optic nerve head) stain with fluorescein.

In the normal eye fluorescein does not penetrate the endothelium of retinal or choroidal vessels but does pass the choriocapillaris. In disease states these relationships are altered. For example, with neovascularization, hypertension, vasculitis, or chorioretinitis, retinal and/or choroidal blood vessels may show increased permeability to the dye. Fluorescence of the tapetum in domestic animals and the lower frequency of retinal vascular disease in domestic animals than in humans decrease the utility of the technique in veterinary medicine.

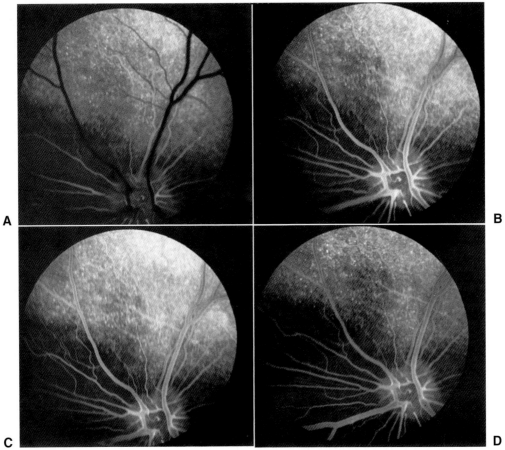

Figure 5-52. Normal canine fluorescein angiogram. **A,** Choroidal phase; **B,** arteriovenous phase; **C,** venous phase; **D,** late phase. (Courtesy Dr. R.W. Bellhorn.)

BIBLIOGRAPHY

Abrams K, et al. (1990): Evaluation of the Schirmer tear test in clinically normal rabbits. Am J Vet Res 51:1912.

Acland GM (1988): Diagnosis and differentiation of retinal disease in small animals by electroretinography. Semin Vet Med Surg 3:15.

Bauer GA, et al. (1996): Exfoliative cytology of conjunctiva and cornea in domestic animals: a comparison of four collecting techniques. Vet Comp Ophthalmol 6:181.

Bedford PGC (1973): A practical method of gonioscopy and goniophotography in the dog and cat. J Small Anim Pract 14:601.

Bellhorn RW (1973): Fluorescein fundus photography in veterinary ophthalmology. J Anim Hosp Assoc 9:227.

Calia CM, et al. (1994): The use of computed tomography scan for the evaluation of orbital disease in cats and dogs. Vet Comp Ophthalmol 4:24.

Carastro SM (2004): Equine ocular anatomy and ophthalmic examination. Vet Clin North Am Equine Pract 20:285.

Cottrill NB, et al. (1989): Ultrasonographic and biometric evaluation of the eye and orbit of dogs. Am J Vet Res 50:898.

Dziezyc J, et al. (1987): Two dimensional real-time ocular sonography in the diagnosis of ocular lesions in dogs. J Am Anim Hosp Assoc 23:501.

Fike JR, et al. (1984): Anatomy of the canine orbital region. Vet Radiol 25:32.

Gelatt KN, et al. (1976): Fluorescein angiography of the normal and diseased ocular fundi of the laboratory dog. J Am Vet Med Assoc 169:980.

Gelatt KN, et al. (1975): Evaluation of tear formation in the dog, using a modification of the Schirmer tear test. J Am Vet Med Assoc 166:368.

Gelatt KN, et al. (1970): Radiographic contrast techniques for detecting orbital and nasolacrimal tumors in dogs. J Am Vet Med Assoc 156:741.

Görig C, et al. (2006): Comparison of the use of new handheld tonometers and established applanation tonometers in dogs. Am J Vet Res 67:134.

Hager DA, et al. (1987): Two-dimensional real-time ocular ultrasonography in the dog—technique and normal anatomy. Vet Radiol 28:60.

Hamor RE (2001): Techniques for collection and interpretation of tissue samples in ocular disease. Clin Tech Small Anim Pract 16:17.

Karpinski LG (2004): The prepurchase examination. Vet Clin North Am Equine Pract 20:459.

Knollinger AM, et al. (2005): Evaluation of a rebound tonometer for measuring intraocular pressure in dogs and horses. J Am Vet Med Assoc 227:244.

Komaromy AM, et al. (2006): Effect of head position on intraocular pressure in horses. Am J Vet Res 67:1232.

Lavach JD, et al. (1977): Cytology of normal and inflamed conjunctivas in dogs and cats. J Am Vet Med Assoc 170:722.

LeCouteur RA, et al. (1982): Computed tomography of orbital tumors in the dog. J Am Vet Med Assoc 180:910.

Leiva M, et al. (2006): Comparison of the rebound tonometer (ICare) to the applanation tonometer (Tonopen XL) in normotensive dogs. Vet Ophthalmol 9:17.

Lim CL, Cullen CL (2005): Schirmer tear test values and tear film break-up times in cats with conjunctivitis. Vet Ophthalmol 8:305.

Manning JP, St. Clair LE (1976): Palpebral, frontal, and zygomatic nerve blocks for examination of the equine eye. Vet Med Small Anim Clin 71:187.

Martin CL (1969): Gonioscopy and anatomical correlations of the drainage angle of the dog. J Sm Anim Pract 10:171.

Martin CL (1969): Slit lamp examination of the normal canine anterior ocular segment part I: introduction and technique. J Small Anim Pract 10:143.

Martin CL (1969): Slit lamp examination of the normal canine anterior ocular segment part II: description. J Small Anim Pract 10:151.

Martin CL (1969): Slit lamp examination of the normal canine anterior ocular segment part III: discussion and summary. J Small Anim Pract 10:163.

Massa KL, et al. (1999): Usefulness of aerobic microbial culture and cytologic evaluation of corneal specimens in the diagnosis of infectious ulcerative keratitis in animals. J Am Vet Med Assoc 215:1671.

Miller PE, Pickett JP (1992): Comparison of the human and canine Schiøtz tonometry conversion tables in clinically normal cats. J Am Vet Med Assoc 201:1017.

Miller PE, Pickett JP (1992): Comparison of the human and canine Schiøtz tonometry conversion tables in clinically normal dogs. J Am Vet Med Assoc 201:102.

Miller WM, Cartee RE (1985): B-scan ultrasonography for the detection of space-occupying masses. J Am Vet Med Assoc 187:66.

Moore PA (2001): Examination techniques and interpretation of ophthalmic findings. Clin Tech Small Anim Pract 16:1.

Penninck D, et al. (2001): Cross-sectional imaging techniques in veterinary ophthalmology. Clin Tech Sm Anim Pract 16:22.

Rubin LF (1974): Atlas of Veterinary Ophthalmoscopy. Lea & Febiger, Philadelphia.

Rubin LF (1967): Clinical electroretinography in animals. J Am Vet Med Assoc 151:1456.

Rubin LF, Koch SA (1968): Ocular diagnostic ultrasonography. J Am Vet Med Assoc 153:1706.

Schiffer SP, et al. (1982): Biometric study of the canine eye, using A-mode ultrasonography. Am J Vet Res 43:826.

Slatter DH (1973): Differential staining of canine cornea and conjunctiva with rose bengal and alcian blue. J Small Anim Pract 14:291.

Stuhr CM, Scagliotti RH (1996): Retrobulbar ultrasound in the mesaticephalic and dolichocephalic dog using a temporal approach. Vet Comp Ophthalmol 6:91.

van der Woerdt A, et al. (1995): Effect of auriculopalpebral nerve block and intravenous administration of xylazine on intraocular pressure and corneal thickness in horses. Am J Vet Res 56:155.

Veith L, et al. (1970): The Schirmer tear test in cats. Mod Vet Pract 51:48.

Villagrasa M, Cascales MJ (2000): Arterial hypertension: angiographic aspects of the ocular fundus in dogs. A study of 24 cases. Eur J Comp Anim Pract 10:177.

Willis M, et al. (1997): Conjunctival brush cytology: Evaluation of a new cytological collection technique in dogs and cats with a comparison to conjunctival scraping. Vet Comp Ophthalmol 7:74.

Willis MA, Wilkie DA (1999): Avian ophthalmology part 1: anatomy, examination, and diagnostic techniques. J Av Med Surg 13:160.

Yakely WL, Alexander JE (1973): Dacryocystorhinography in the dog. J Am Vet Med Assoc 159:1417.

Zook BC, et al. (1981): Anatomy of the beagle in cross section: head and neck. Am J Vet Res 42:844.

EYELIDS

David J. Maggs

ANATOMY, FUNCTION, AND
 PATHOLOGIC RESPONSES
DELAYED OR PREMATURE OPENING OF
 THE EYELIDS IN NEONATES
EYELID AGENESIS (COLOBOMA)

PROMINENT NASAL FOLDS
DISORDERS OF THE CILIA
ENTROPION
ECTROPION
EYELID INJURIES

CHALAZION
HORDEOLUM AND MEIBOMIAN ADENITIS
NEOPLASIA
SKIN DISEASES AFFECTING THE EYELIDS

ANATOMY, FUNCTION, AND PATHOLOGIC RESPONSES

Anatomy and Function

The eyelids consist of a fibrous tarsal plate and muscle, bounded by skin on the outer surface and conjunctiva on the inner surface (Figure 6-1). In addition, there are a number of adnexal specializations, such as cilia (eyelashes) and glands. These components vary by species; however, some general comments are possible. The skin on the outer surface of the eyelid is thinner, more mobile, and more pliable than skin elsewhere on the body. Cilia are present on the outer surface of the upper eyelid margin in dogs, horses, cattle, pigs, and sheep. A few cilia also are present on the lower eyelids of horses, cattle, and sheep. Cats have no cilia but do have a line of modified hairs that are essentially identical. Modified sweat glands—the glands of Moll—open onto the eyelid margin near the base of the cilia. The glands of Zeis are rudimentary sebaceous glands that open into the follicles that produce the cilia. The tarsal or meibomian glands (Figures 6-1 and 6-2) are modified sebaceous glands that are embedded in the tarsal plate, a layer of fibrous tissue that gives some structural rigidity to the eyelid. The meibomian glands open right at the eyelid margin posterior to the cilia. Their orifices are visible grossly, and a grayish white secretion rich in phospholipids can be expressed from them. This secretion has two functions: It coats the eyelid margins to minimize overflow of tears and it forms the superficial lipid layer of the precorneal tear film. This lipid layer has high surface tension and thereby adds stability to and reduces evaporation of the aqueous layer of the tear film.

Tear film components drain from the ocular surface through the lacrimal puncta, which lie on the inner surfaces of the upper and lower eyelids 3 to 4 mm lateral to the medial canthus, approximately opposite the last of the meibomian gland openings. The lacrimal canaliculi drain into the lacrimal sac, which lies in a fossa of the lacrimal bone. Blinking creates a negative pressure within the sac, thereby drawing tears into it. During the relaxation phase of blinking, pressure is placed on the sac, thereby forcing tears down the nasolacrimal duct. This forms the so-called lacrimal pump. Blinking occurs with contraction of the orbicularis oculi muscle, which encircles and closes the palpebral fissure (Figures 6-3 and 6-4). It is innervated by the palpebral nerve, a branch of the facial nerve (cranial nerve [CN] VII) (Figure 6-5). Localization of this nerve is important for injection of local anesthetic and induction of akinesia of the upper eyelid in large animals.

The general pattern and innervation of muscles surrounding the eyelids is similar in all species, although the names and relative development differ somewhat among species. The orbicularis oculi muscle is the major muscle responsible for eyelid closure. It is anchored medially to the wall of the orbit by the medial palpebral ligament (see Figure 6-5) and laterally by the retractor anguli oculi lateralis (see Figures 6-3 and 6-4). In cattle and sheep this latter structure is fibrous in nature and is known as the lateral palpebral ligament (see Figure 6-5). In horses it is visible as a fibrous raphe within the orbicularis muscle. The medial and lateral attachments of the orbicularis oculi preserve the elliptical shape of the palpebral fissure and prevent it from becoming circular during contraction of the orbicularis. Excessive muscle tone in the orbicularis oculi muscle, called blepharospasm, may result in spastic entropion.

Opening of the eyelids requires not only relaxation of the orbicularis oculi muscle but also elevation of the upper eyelid and depression of the lower eyelid. The upper eyelid is more mobile than the lower eyelid in mammals, although the opposite is true in birds and reptiles. The major elevators of the upper eyelid are the levator palpebrae superioris, which originates near the optic foramen, inserts into the tarsal plate, and is innervated by the oculomotor nerve (CN III), and Müller's muscle, which lies posterior to the levator and is sympathetically innervated (see Figure 6-1). The levator and superior rectus muscles have common innervation (CN III), so that elevation of the globe by the superior rectus muscle is coordinated with elevation of the upper eyelid. If it were not, the animal would see the inner surface of the upper eyelid on elevation of the globe. The levator anguli oculi medialis and frontalis muscles are minor elevators of the upper eyelid and are both innervated by the palpebral nerve (see Figures 6-3 and 6-4).

The lower eyelid is depressed by the malaris muscle, which is innervated by the dorsal buccal branch of the facial nerve. Note that different branches of the facial nerve supply the orbicularis, which narrows the palpebral fissure, and the malaris, which widens it. Actions of the muscles of the eyelids are summarized in Figure 6-6. Sensory innervation for the dog, horse, and ox is shown in Figures 6-7 to 6-9. Interference with sensory or motor innervation of the eyelids may result in severe desiccation of the cornea and conjunctiva.

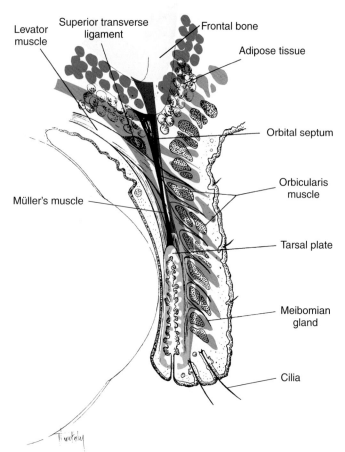

Figure 6-1. Anatomy of the normal eyelid. (From Remington LA [2005]: Clinical Anatomy of the Visual System, 2nd ed. Butterworth-Heinemann, St. Louis.)

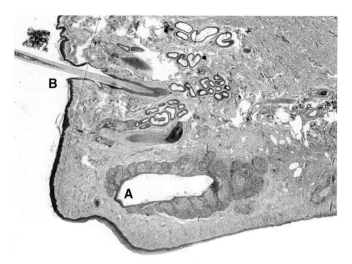

Figure 6-2. Photomicrograph of the normal eyelid stained with trichrome (Masson) showing tarsal (meibomian) gland **(A)** and cilium **(B)**. (Courtesy Dr. Richard Dubielzig.)

The eyelids protect the eye in the following ways:

- Sensory and protective effects of the cilia and sensory vibrissae surrounding the eye
- Secretions of the meibomian glands and conjunctival goblet cells, which contribute to the outer lipid and inner

mucopolysaccharide layers of the precorneal tear film, respectively
- Physical protection against trauma
- Reduction of evaporation of tears
- Distribution of the precorneal tear film by eyelid movements
- "Pumping" of tears down the nasolacrimal duct, preventing epiphora and promoting a precorneal tear film of uniform thickness and optical properties

Pathologic Responses

The eyelids show pathologic reactions and diseases characteristic of skin. However, these may be modified by the extremely vascular nature of eyelids and by the numerous associated specialized structures (glands, cilia, etc.). In addition, malfunction and poor conformation of the eyelids are very common causes of ocular disease in animals, especially dogs, and frequently result in painful and potentially blinding secondary ocular disease, especially of the conjunctiva and cornea.

DELAYED OR PREMATURE OPENING OF THE EYELIDS IN NEONATES

In the newborn foal or calf the eyelids are open at birth; whereas in the kitten and puppy they open at about 10 to 14 days of age. Premature opening occurs infrequently in dogs and cats but when it does, it results in corneal desiccation, keratitis, corneal ulceration, and conjunctivitis because tear production takes several weeks to reach adequate levels. If these consequences are left untreated, corneal perforation and endophthalmitis may occur. Treatment consists of frequent application of a topical lubricating ophthalmic ointment. Rarely, a temporary tarsorrhaphy may be necessary to further limit evaporation of tears and aid in corneal healing (see Chapter 10). A small gap should be left at the medial canthus to permit administration of bactericidal antibiotic or bland lubricating ointment. Sutures are removed after 7 to 10 days, but topical treatment may be necessary for a few days longer.

More commonly, delayed opening of the eyelids (ankyloblepharon) occurs in dogs or cats. This is often associated with accumulation of mucus and sometimes with infection (ophthalmia neonatorum). Typical infectious agents vary somewhat by species: *Chlamydophila felis* or feline herpesvirus is common in cats, and *Staphylococcus* spp. may infect dogs or cats. Ankyloblepharon can be treated conservatively with warm compresses for a short period in the expectation that the eyelids will open. However, if they do not open within a day or so, the eyelids should be gently pried open with firm digital pressure or by inserting the nose of a closed pair of small mosquito hemostats at the medial canthus, where there is often a small gap between the eyelids. The hemostats can then be gently opened in this position but should not be reclosed while inserted between the eyelids, so as to avoid damage to surface ocular structures. A sharp instrument should never be used for this purpose, and the fused eyelid margins should never be incised to separate them, because either action would cause irreversible damage to the eyelid margins themselves and/or the meibomian glands with subsequent lifelong keratitis. After the eyelids are pried apart, the ocular surface should be liberally irrigated with saline or dilute (1:50) povidone-iodine *solution* (not povidone-iodine *scrub*) and the cornea checked with fluorescein stain for evidence of ulceration. A topical antibiotic ointment with a

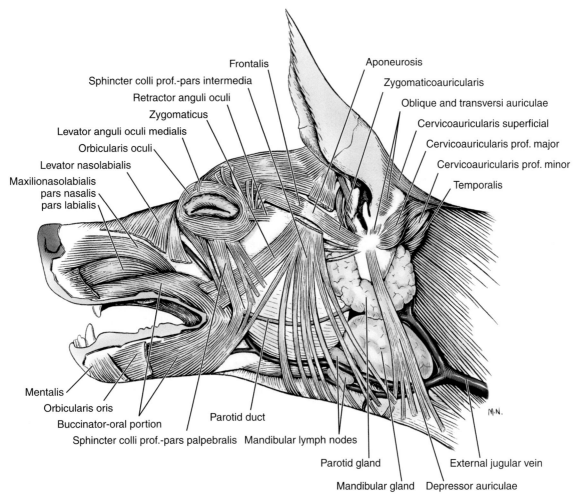

Frontalis
Sphincter colli prof.-pars intermedia
Retractor anguli oculi
Zygomaticus
Levator anguli oculi medialis
Orbicularis oculi
Levator nasolabialis
Maxilionasolabialis
pars nasalis
pars labialis

Aponeurosis
Zygomaticoauricularis
Oblique and transversi auriculae
Cervicoauricularis superficial
Cervicoauricularis prof. major
Cervicoauricularis prof. minor
Temporalis

Mentalis
Orbicularis oris
Buccinator-oral portion
Sphincter colli prof.-pars palpebralis
Mandibular lymph nodes
Parotid duct

Parotid gland
Mandibular gland
Depressor auriculae
External jugular vein

Figure 6-3. Lateral view of the superficial muscles of the canine head (platysma and sphincter colli muscles removed). (Modified from Evans HE [1993]: Miller's Anatomy of the Dog, 3rd ed. Saunders, Philadelphia.)

spectrum appropriate for the suspected organisms should be applied a few times daily for approximately 1 week.

EYELID AGENESIS (COLOBOMA)

Eyelid coloboma refers to congenital absence of a portion of an eyelid. It can occur in all species but it is most common in cats, in which it usually affects the lateral portion of the upper eyelid (Figure 6-10). In piebald and Karakul sheep it has been described as affecting the middle of the upper eyelid. Coloboma is believed to be a hereditary condition. Dermoids may be seen in association with coloboma (see Chapter 10). Eyelid colobomas are associated with excessive evaporation and inadequate dispersion of the precorneal tear film, and sometimes with trichiasis. Together, these lead to secondary keratoconjunctivitis, pain, and sometimes corneal ulceration. If the lower eyelid is affected, epiphora may occur owing to escape of tears through the defect. With time, corneal scarring, pigmentation, and vascularization are common.

Eyelid colobomas are repaired with a variety of blepharoplastic procedures; the choice depends on the size and position of the defect. Larger defects require more extensive reconstructive procedures and are best referred to a veterinary ophthalmologist. However, simple defects affecting less than one third of the eyelid margin can be restored by removal of the edges of

the defect so as to create a wedge defect (Figure 6-11). This is then closed in two layers with special care to accurately appose the sides of eyelid margin without leaving sutures that may abrade the cornea (Figure 6-12). Sutures are removed 10 days later. Postoperatively, an Elizabethan collar is used. The two-layer eyelid closure also should be used for reapposition of any incisions or lacerations involving the eyelid margin, including traumatic injuries, medial canthoplasty, tumor resection, and treatment of some cases of entropion or ectropion.

PROMINENT NASAL FOLDS

In Pekingese, pugs, English bulldogs, Boston terriers, and similar brachycephalic breeds the nasal folds may be unusually prominent. When this feature is combined with a shallow orbit and prominent globe, the hair on these skin folds may contact the cornea with resultant epiphora, corneal melanosis, vascularization, and, in some cases, ulceration. A careful inspection should be made for other causes of irritation (e.g., distichiasis, medial entropion) that also are common in these same breeds. When this syndrome is seen in young puppies of breeds at risk but before the development of keratitis, the owner should be advised to observe the eyes carefully for signs of ocular disease as the animals mature.

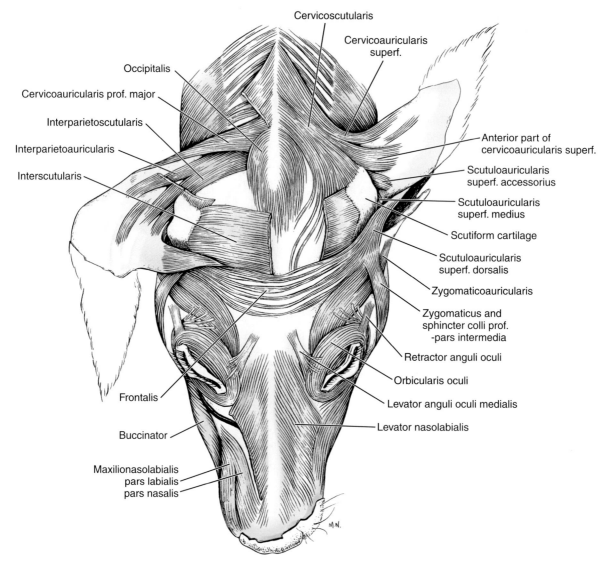

Figure 6-4. Dorsal view of the deep muscles of the canine head. (Modified from Evans HE [1993]: Miller's Anatomy of the Dog, 3rd ed. Saunders, Philadelphia.)

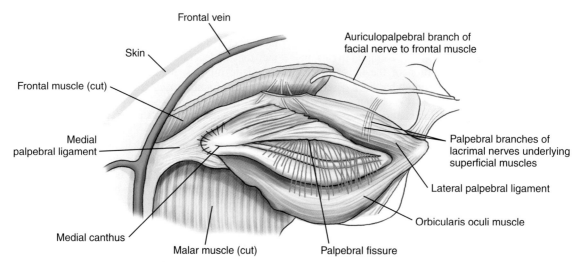

Figure 6-5. Frontal view of the normal bovine orbit and adnexa, also showing the terminations of the lacrimal and facial nerves. Note the position of the auriculopalpebral branch of the facial nerve for injection of local anesthetic for akinesia of the upper lid. (Modified from Getty R [1975]: Sisson and Grossman's The Anatomy of the Domestic Animals, 5th ed, Vol 1. Saunders, Philadelphia.)

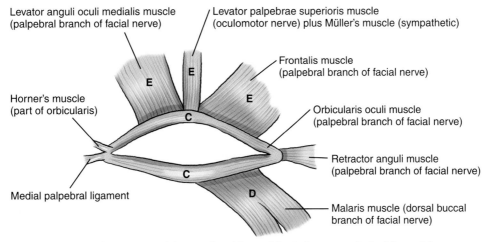

Figure 6-6. Action and innervation of the muscles of the eyelids. *C*, Contracts palpebral fissure (closes upper and lower lids); *D*, depresses lower lid; *E*, elevates upper eyelid.

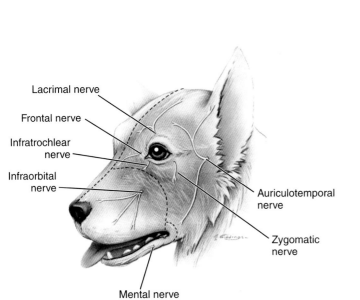

Figure 6-7. Sensory innervation of the canine periocular area. (Modified from Westhues M, Fritsch R [1964]: Animal Anaesthesia, Vol 1: Local Anaesthesia. Oliver & Boyd, London.)

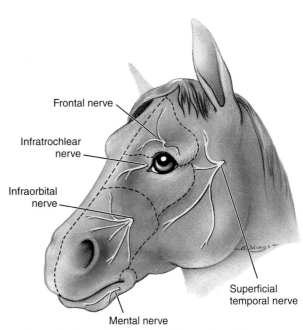

Figure 6-8. Sensory innervation of the equine periocular area.

If nasal folds are causing keratitis, they should be removed either partially (Figure 6-13) or totally (Figure 6-14). In partial removal, only the medial portion of the fold is removed, where it touches the cornea, resulting in less alteration from the breed "norm" desired by some owners. The wound is closed with simple interrupted sutures of 4/0 silk placed 2 mm apart. In both methods the suture ends should be short enough to prevent corneal irritation. Sutures are removed 10 days later. Postoperatively, an Elizabethan collar is used. Nasal fold removal should be performed in conjunction with reconstructive medial canthoplasty when there is associated corneal drying, corneal exposure, and keratitis due to macropalpebral fissure and lagophthalmos or lower medial entropion (see later discussion of brachycephalic ocular syndrome).

DISORDERS OF THE CILIA

Normally positioned cilia emerge from the dermal side of the eyelid margin (Figure 6-15, *A*). The three common disorders in which aberrant cilia or hair cause corneoconjunctival irritation are as follows:

- *Distichiasis* (Figure 6-15, *B*): Cilia emerge from the openings of the meibomian glands. A few soft distichia can be seen in many dogs, especially poodles and cocker spaniels. Without clinical evidence of irritation, they are considered insignificant. The typical clinical appearance of distichiasis is shown in Figure 6-16.
- *Ectopic cilia* (Figure 6-15, *C*): Cilia arise from the meibomian glands and emerge through the palpebral conjunctiva where

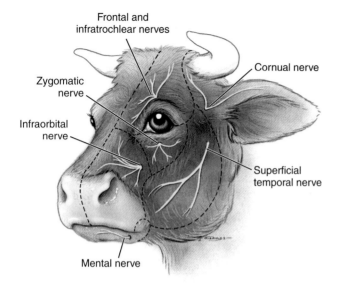

Figure 6-9. Sensory innervation of the bovine periocular area.

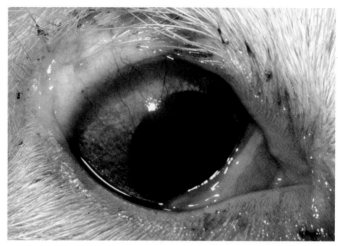

Figure 6-10. Eyelid agenesis of the right eye in a cat. Note the congenital absence of upper eyelid margin laterally and the subsequent chronic keratitis evident as superficial corneal vascularization due to trichiasis. (Courtesy University of California, Davis, Veterinary Ophthalmology Service Collection.)

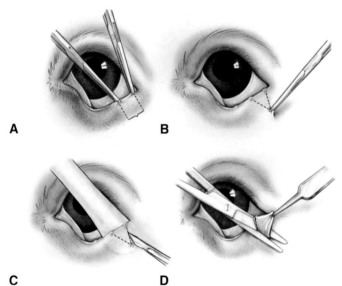

Figure 6-11. Eyelid wedge resection. This general technique may be used for correction of some cases of entropion or ectropion and smaller eyelid colobomas, freshening and closure of eyelid lacerations, and removal of eyelid tumors. **A,** The extent of eyelid margin to be resected may be identified by gently crimping the eyelids with hemostats or with a dermatologic marker pen. **B,** The apex of the triangle or "wedge" to be resected is then marked in a similar manner. Usually the height of this triangle is approximately twice its base. **C,** The skin incision is made with a No. 15 Bard-Parker scalpel while the eyelid is supported by a Jaeger lid plate. **D,** The subcutis and conjunctiva are cut with straight Mayo or Stevens tenotomy scissors, so that the tissue wedge is completely resected. The method of closure is described in Figure 6-12.

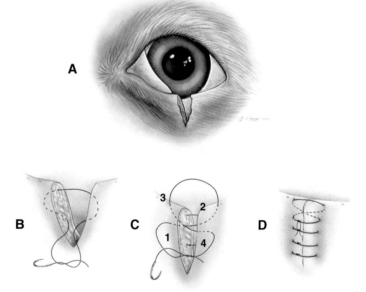

Figure 6-12. Standard two-layer closure technique. **A,** This technique is used for all eyelid wounds or incisions that involve the eyelid margin. **B,** A buried 3/0 to 5/0 absorbable horizontal mattress suture is placed without penetrating the skin, the margin itself, or the conjunctiva. The suture is placed so that the appositional forces are at the margin, but the knot is distal from it so as to avoid corneal contact. This buried suture may be continued if necessary in a continuous or interrupted pattern from the eyelid margin to the apex of the incision so as to close the subcutis. **C,** The skin is closed using a figure-of-eight suture of 3/0 or 4/0 silk or braided nylon. Numbers identify order of needle passage through the tissue so that appositional forces are again at the margin but the knot is distal from it. Both suture ends are left long at this stage. **D,** The rest of the skin incision is closed with a series of closely spaced simple interrupted sutures. The ends of the figure-of-eight suture are incorporated into the knot of the first simple interrupted suture so that they are directed away from the eye.

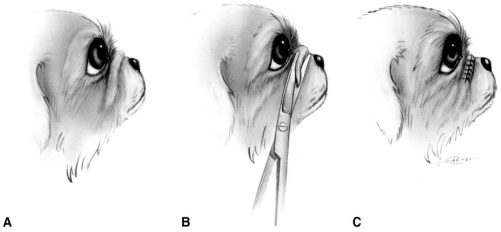

A   **B**   **C**

Figure 6-13. Partial removal of the nasal fold. **A,** Lateral view of nasal fold. **B,** Removal of nasal portion with curved scissors. Note that the nasal portion of the fold is removed. **C,** The sutured wound with a small fold remaining that is more prominent laterally. The knots are placed on the anterior side of the incision in order to limit corneal contact. (Redrawn from Severin GA [2000]: Severin's Veterinary Ophthalmology Notes, 3rd ed. Severin, Ft. Collins, CO.)

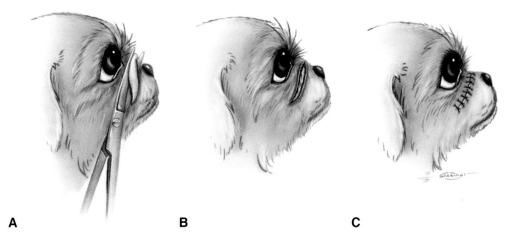

A   **B**   **C**

Figure 6-14. Total removal of the nasal fold. **A,** Removal of the fold, starting laterally. **B,** The fold removed. **C,** The fold sutured. The knots are placed on the anterior side of the incision in order to reduce the chance of corneal contact. (Redrawn from Severin GA [2000]: Severin's Veterinary Ophthalmology Notes, 3rd ed. Severin, Ft. Collins, CO.)

they cause marked corneal irritation and usually ulceration. Cilia may be white or pigmented, and considerable diligence may be needed to find them. On occasions, they are visible only with the illumination and magnification provided by a slit-lamp or operating microscope.
- *Trichiasis* (Figure 6-15, *D*): Cilia or adjacent skin hairs arising from a normal location are misdirected so that they touch the cornea. This may be a primary condition but is also a consequence of nasal folds, eyelid coloboma, eyelid agenesis, and entropion.

Cilia disorders can be bilateral or unilateral and can affect upper or lower eyelids. However, ectopic cilia are more common on the upper eyelid. Although not necessarily congenital, disorders of the cilia usually are seen early in life and rarely make their first appearance after full maturity. Disorders of cilia are most common in dogs, in which they are breed-related and familial. Horses are sometimes affected with ectopic cilia; however trichiasis acquired following eyelid trauma is the most frequent cilia disorder in horses. Cats are uncommonly affected by cilia disorders.

Clinical Signs of Cilia Disorders

All cilia disorders produce similar signs, as follows:

- *Epiphora:* Excess tearing and staining of facial hairs is usually present despite patency of the nasolacrimal apparatus. Purulent discharge is unusual except with corneal ulceration.
- *Blepharospasm:* Pain associated with constant irritation and sometimes corneal ulceration is evident as blepharospasm and occasionally rubbing. In some dogs pain and epiphora are intermittent.
- *Chronic conjunctival hyperemia:* The surface vessels of the conjunctiva are engorged, and a reddish pink capillary flush is present. It is unusual for clinically significant disorders of cilia to be present without this sign.
- *Corneal ulceration:* Disorders of the cilia, particularly ectopic cilia, can cause corneal ulceration. Ulcers caused by cilia are usually shallow and are frequently eccentrically placed on the cornea, corresponding to the position of the cilia. As with ulcers due to any other cause, secondary

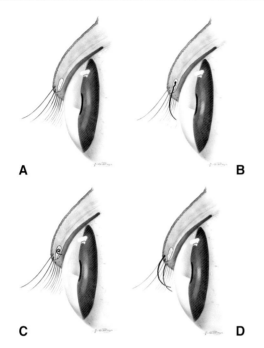

Figure 6-15. A, Normal eyelid. Note the position of cilia in relation to the orifice of the meibomian gland. **B,** Distichiasis. Cilia emerge from the meibomian gland orifice. **C,** Ectopic cilium. The cilium arises from the meibomian gland but emerges through the palpebral conjunctiva. **D,** Trichiasis. Normal cilia or hairs arising from a normal location reach the cornea due to altered facial or eyelid conformation.

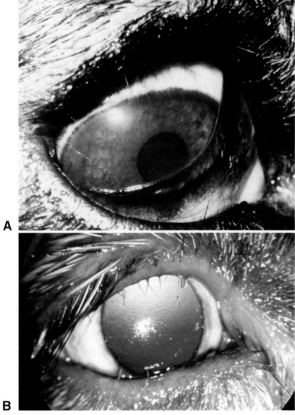

Figure 6-16. Distichiasis in two dogs. **A,** This dog has distichia on both upper and lower eyelids, which are best seen when viewed against the third eyelid or sclera. **B,** Retroillumination also provides an excellent method of detecting more subtle distichia. (Courtesy University of Missouri, Columbia, Veterinary Ophthalmology Service Collection.)

infection may cause corneal malacia or stromal loss (see Chapter 10). In all cases of corneal ulceration a thorough search for cilia should be undertaken, with magnification and use of general anesthesia if necessary.

Adequate magnification is essential for detecting abnormal cilia.

Treatment of Distichiasis

Numerous methods have been advocated for the correction of canine distichiasis. "Eyelid-splitting" and partial tarsal plate excision techniques have been abandoned because of post-operative cicatricial entropion, scarring of the eyelid margin, and destruction of the meibomian glands. Cryoepilation or electroepilation is used most commonly now. Electroepilation is useful for treating a small number of follicles but tends to be less reliable and convenient than cryoepilation, especially when large numbers of follicles are to be treated. Simple epilation by forceps without adjunctive cryotherapy or application of an electric current is a temporary measure because the cilia regrow within 3 to 4 weeks. However, it can be useful to determine the clinical significance of the epilated cilia.

Cryoepilation

Cryoepilation takes advantage of the selective susceptibility of hair follicles to cold. A nitrous oxide or liquid nitrogen cryo-probe is applied to the conjunctiva overlying the meibomian glands that contain the offending cilia (Figure 6-17). The ice ball is observed as it advances over the line of gland openings on the eyelid margin. Two rapid freeze–slow thaw cycles are used. Following thawing of the second freeze, all visible cilia

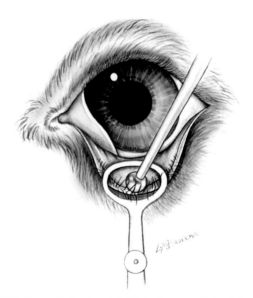

Figure 6-17. Cryoepilation for distichiasis. The tarsal glands from which the distichia originate are isolated with a chalazion clamp. The clamp assists with exposure and slows thawing to enhance follicular cell death. The lid is everted and the cryoprobe is applied over the tarsal gland from the conjunctival surface. The ice ball is allowed to advance to the eyelid margin. A double freeze-thaw cycle is performed. Care must be taken to avoid corneal contact. After thawing of the second freeze, all visible cilia are manually epilated.

are manually epilated. Postoperatively, the eyelid swells and the meibomian glands undergo cryonecrosis. However, eyelid tissues other than the follicle are relatively spared. By 4 weeks, the treated meibomian glands have regenerated without cilia; however, new cilia may appear from untreated areas.

Postoperative swelling can be reduced by perioperative use of a systemically administered corticosteroid or nonsteroidal antiinflammatory drug (NSAID). An oral NSAID may be continued postoperatively for analgesia. An antibiotic-steroid ophthalmic ointment may also help diminish conjunctival swelling. Some depigmentation of the eyelid margin may occur, but most of this pigment returns within 6 months.

Failures with cryoepilation may be attributed to the following:

- Use of a "counting" or timed technique to determine the size of the ice ball rather than actual, precise observation of the frozen area through the operating microscope
- Failure to appreciate the spherical nature of an ice ball, and the potential for inadequate freezing at depth when adjacent areas are frozen. Overlapping of frozen areas avoids this problem.
- Departure from the principles of controlled cryonecrosis. The ideal is a double cycle of rapid freeze–slow thaw. A Desmarres chalazion clamp with screw lock (see Figure 6-17) helps speed the freeze and slow the thaw by reducing blood supply to the area being treated.
- Failure to identify all aberrant cilia

Electroepilation

The ideal electroepilator supplies direct current (1 to 5 mA) to the offending meibomian gland, destroying it by electrolysis. A fine needle (25 or 26 gauge) can be used as the applying electrode. It is passed alongside the cilium and into the follicle with use of adequate magnification. Current is applied for 20 to 30 seconds. Easy removal of the cilium, which often adheres to the epilation needle, indicates follicle destruction. Low currents, supplied by a small battery, prevent contraction of the orbicularis oculi, excessive damage to surrounding structures, as well as postoperative scarring. High-frequency alternating current supplied by electrosurgical units must not be used for epilation, because it may cause severe necrosis and scarring.

Treatment of Ectopic Cilia

Ectopic cilia are treated with resection of the affected cilium and meibomian gland under magnification. An elliptical Desmarres chalazion clamp with screw lock is placed around the cilium for hemostasis, and the eyelid is everted. A block of tissue containing the offending follicle and meibomian gland is removed with a small (No. 65 Beaver) scalpel blade (Figure 6-18), leaving the eyelid margin intact. No sutures are placed. Digital pressure for several minutes is sufficient to control hemorrhage. A topical broad-spectrum antibiotic ointment is applied three times daily for 5 to 7 days postoperatively. If correctly performed, this technique is highly effective and is rarely associated with recurrence, although follicles may arise in the future from different sites.

Focal tarsoconjunctival resection is the method of choice for removal of ectopic cilia.

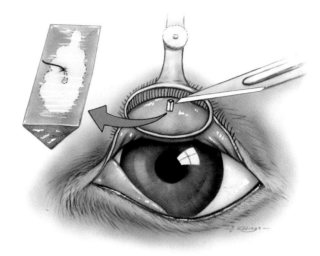

Figure 6-18. Resection of an ectopic cilium. The eyelid surrounding the cilium is clamped with a chalazion clamp for hemostasis, and the eyelid is everted. A wedge of palpebral conjunctiva including the ectopic cilium and its follicle is resected en bloc.

Treatment of Trichiasis

Depending on location of the offending hairs, trichiasis is treated with any of the following:

- Regular trimming of the periocular hairs by the owner. This is often neglected by inexperienced owners and is important in breeds such as the poodle, shih tzu, and Lhasa apso.
- Cryoepilation of the offending hairs (Figure 6-19). This method is especially useful at the medial canthus when there are a large number of hairs on the inner surface of the canthus and on the medial caruncle. As with cryotherapy elsewhere on the eyelids the owner must be warned that the frozen area may be depigmented for up to 6 months.
- Surgical correction of the deformity causing the trichiasis (e.g., entropion, nasal folds, eyelid coloboma).

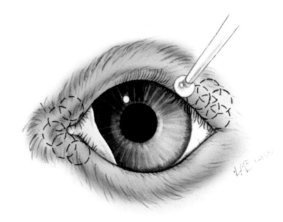

Figure 6-19. Cryoepilation for trichiasis. The offending hairs are identified and the cryoprobe is applied over the dermal surface. A lid plate is necessary to protect the cornea. The ice ball is allowed to advance to the eyelid margin. A double freeze-thaw cycle is performed. After thawing of the second freeze, offending hairs are manually epilated.

ENTROPION

Entropion, or inward rolling of the eyelid margin, is common in many species. It may be conformational, spastic, or cicatricial or may occur subsequent to alteration in globe position (enophthalmos) or size (phthisis/microphthalmos). Conformational entropion occurs most frequently in dogs and sheep but is uncommon in cats, horses, and cattle. Conformational entropion usually affects both eyes, although occasionally only one eye is affected or there is marked asymmetry in severity of the entropion. The upper eyelid is less commonly affected than the lower. The whole length of the eyelid may be affected in severe cases, but the affected area is usually restricted to one portion of the margin. In brachycephalic animals entropion is more notable medially, whereas in large, broad-skulled dogs conformational entropion frequently affects the lateral part of the lower eyelid and the lateral canthus. Conformational entropion is believed to be inherited in a large number of dog breeds, including the chow chow, English bulldog, Irish setter, Labrador and golden retrievers, Saint Bernard, shar-pei, Rottweiler, Great Dane, and Chesapeake Bay retriever. Although conformational entropion may be manifest soon after eye opening, it often does not become clinically evident in many affected breeds until later in life as the skull and associated facial skin gain their adult conformation. Occasionally maturation is associated with reduction or sometimes even resolution of entropion. For these reasons, surgery is always delayed until facial maturity is achieved.

Spastic entropion occurs with spasm of the orbicularis oculi muscle (blepharospasm) due to painful ocular conditions such as ulcerative or nonulcerative keratitis, conjunctivitis, or uveitis. It is relatively common in cats, possibly owing to the frequency with which feline herpesvirus causes corneal disease and associated pain in this species. However, because clinically significant entropion—regardless of cause—is always associated with some degree of trichiasis, spastic entropion is a component of all cases of entropion. It is important to eliminate this spastic component before permanent surgical correction of entropion; otherwise postoperative ectropion may occur. Therefore thorough assessment of entropion includes determination of the cause and relative contribution of blepharospasm through the use of the following steps:

1. Examination of the patient before and after the application of a topical anesthetic.
2. Assessment of the tear film with the Schirmer tear test.
3. Fluorescein staining. (Ulcers may be the cause or result of entropion. Regardless, they will exacerbate the spastic component.)
4. Examination with magnification for coexistent cilia disorders.
5. Assessment of aqueous flare and intraocular pressure.

Although treatment of the underlying condition sometimes relieves the spasm, surgical correction, as for conformational entropion, may be necessary.

Clinical Signs of Entropion

- Rolling in of the eyelid (Figure 6-20). This can be very subtle in some mild cases, especially if the dog is excitable in the examination room.
- Blepharospasm with further rolling in of the eyelid ("spastic entropion")

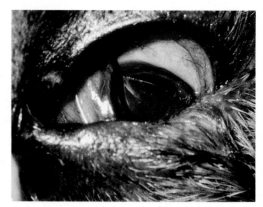

Figure 6-20. Entropion of the lower eyelid of a dog with consequent epiphora and conjunctival hyperemia.

- Excoriation and maceration of the eyelid surface from constant contact with tears
- Rubbing of the affected area
- Corneal ulceration
- Corneal melanosis and vascularization in chronic cases
- Conjunctival hyperemia
- Epiphora or mucoid discharge

Treatment of Entropion

The various methods of treating entropion are summarized here. The choice of procedure depends on the level of facial maturity, species, severity and position of eyelid abnormality, and (in lambs) economic factors. Although there are surgical techniques specific to each procedure, the following general principles apply to all:

1. Always eliminate other causes of spastic entropion before deciding on the extent of surgical resection.
2. Accurately assess extent of skin resection before sedation, premedication, or induction of anesthesia. Consider use of a dermatologic marker pen. If bilateral surgery is planned, make careful preoperative note of whether the extent of resection required is symmetric.
3. Undercorrection, with the need for a second operation, is preferable to overcorrection, which causes cicatricial ectropion.
4. Minimize surgical tissue trauma.
5. It is not necessary to remove orbicularis oculi muscle; doing so increases hemorrhage, operating time, postoperative edema, and risk of infection.
6. Use fine suture material (4/0 or smaller in dogs and cats).
7. Use fine, swaged-on, cutting suture needles.
8. Place multiple, closely spaced sutures of small "bites."
9. Use an Elizabethan collar until 2 to 3 days *after* suture removal.
10. Provide adequate postoperative analgesia for the first 7 to 10 days.
11. For the first few days after surgery, while the tissues are swollen, the eyelid may appear overcorrected, but as swelling subsides (over 5 to 7 days) the correction can be better evaluated. Delay any decision regarding a second operation for at least 4 to 6 weeks, when wound contraction is complete.

Temporary "Tacking" Techniques

Because entropion progresses or improves with maturity in some animals, permanent surgical correction of entropion is best delayed until facial maturity is reached. Likewise, surgery should not be performed in patients with a temporary cause of entropion, such as transient enophthalmos due to lack of orbital fat, as seen in young animals, especially foals. However, all these patients will benefit from some form of temporary relief of the entropion until surgery is performed. This has traditionally been achieved with a series of temporary tacking sutures placed so as to evert the eyelid (Figure 6-21). More recently, surgical staples have been used in place of sutures because they are quicker, less traumatic, and less irritating, persist in the tissue longer than sutures, and can be applied without general anesthesia (Figure 6-22). An Elizabethan collar is necessary when sutures are placed but can often be removed a few days after staples are placed because the latter are less irritating. A topical antibiotic ointment is used initially but is often not necessary once surgical inflammation and corneoconjunctival irritation from the entropion have resolved. The staples or sutures are left in place for as long as necessary. In some animals tacking may have to be repeated several times until facial maturity is reached and permanent corrective surgery can be performed.

Injection Technique in Lambs

For economic reasons entropion in lambs has been treated with subcutaneous injection of a liquid to physically alter lid alignment. However, manual eversion of the eyelid alone may be successful if performed within 48 hours of birth, and stapling as described previously is preferable to injection techniques. Various fluids have been injected to evert the lower eyelid. A subcutaneous injection of sterile air along the affected area of

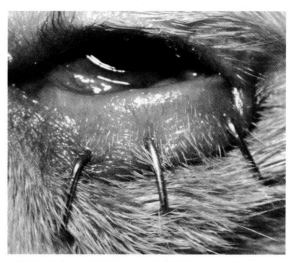

Figure 6-22. Lower eyelid entropion in a Labrador retriever puppy that has been temporarily everted with surgical staples. These can be placed without sedation and often do not require use of an Elizabethan collar.

lid is often effective. However, if air from sheep yards is used, injection of airborne spores of *Clostridium tetani* may occur. Injection of procaine penicillin or long-acting tetracycline has also been described. The use of paraffin for this technique is often associated with severe lipogranuloma formation and should be avoided. As entropion is often hereditary in lambs, breeding stock should be examined for evidence of entropion, and the affected animals culled.

Wedge Resection

When entropion is due to euryblepharon (elongated eyelids), the lower eyelid can be shortened by resection of a full-thickness wedge from its lateral end as described previously for correction of eyelid coloboma (see Figure 6-11). If the entropion is associated with a "notch" deformity, the wedge can be repositioned to remove the deformed tissue. However, the medial canthal area and nasolacrimal apparatus must be avoided. As with all incisions that involve the eyelid margin, accurate apposition with a two-layer closure is essential (see Figure 6-12).

Hotz-Celsus Procedure

The majority of cases of simple, breed-related or conformational entropion can be addressed using a Hotz-Celsus procedure (Figure 6-23). The initial incision parallel to the eyelid margin should be made at the haired-nonhaired border. A common error is to place this incision too far from the eyelid margin. This placement causes a significant loss of "mechanical advantage" and achieves less eversion for the same amount of tissue resection. The length of this first incision is dictated by the length (extent) of inverted eyelid. Gentle pressure with the thumb on the lower lid at the point of entropion until the eyelid margin (meibomian gland orifices) can be seen along the whole length will assist with outlining the full lateral and medial extent of entropion. Other clues are provided by the pale discoloration, blepharedema, and alopecia that occur secondary to maceration of eyelid skin from constant exposure to the tear film. The tendency is to make this incision too short. In fact, given that the amount of resected tissue will taper sharply at each end of the incision, very little eversion is

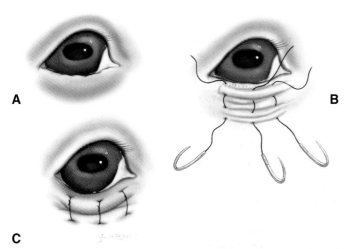

Figure 6-21. Temporary "tacking" sutures used to correct entropion in immature animals or animals with a transient cause for entropion. **A,** Lower eyelid entropion. **B,** Placement of a series of vertical mattress sutures. The first bite is taken very close to the eyelid margin, and the second bite is taken a few millimeters distant to the first. It is important to not penetrate through the conjunctival surface because doing so would irritate the cornea. The suture is directed exactly perpendicular to the eyelid margin. A 2/0 or 3/0 nylon suture is recommended. **C,** As the suture is tightened a small furrow between the two bites is created and causes the eversion of the eyelid. The sutures are tied with the knots as distant from the eye as possible.

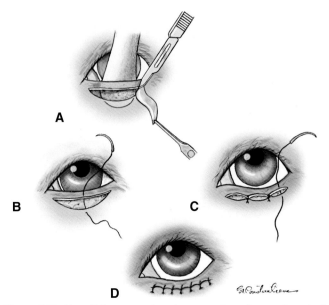

Figure 6-23. Hotz-Celsus procedure for correction of entropion. **A,** A Jaeger lid plate is inserted into the conjunctival fornix to provide support for the incisions. The initial incision is made parallel to the eyelid margin at the haired-nonhaired border. A second incision is made that arcs between the ends of the first incision. The width of the skin to be removed determines the extent of eversion this procedure will create. **B,** The defect is closed with a series of simple interrupted skin sutures. The first suture placed should be at the widest point of the resected tissue. **C,** Each of the following sutures is then placed so as to bisect the space remaining. **D,** Final appearance. (Modified from Moore CP, Constantinescu GM [1997]: Surgery of the adnexa. Vet Clin North Am Small Anim Pract 27:1011.)

caused at the lateral and medial extremes of the incision, and the surgeon should err on the side of a longer rather than a shorter incision. The real "art" of entropion surgery is in deciding on the amount of tissue to be resected at the widest point. The same clues used for the decision regarding incision length can be used to determine the amount of tissue that needs to be resected. The most important point is to ensure that the widest tissue resection is planned for the most inverted section of the eyelid, even if this creates an asymmetric area of resected tissue. In general, it is better to err on the side of under-treatment as a subsequent entropion operation can always be performed. Use of calipers or some other simple method of measurement may assist in resection of a symmetric portion of the contralateral eyelid if that is required.

The skin incisions are best made with a No. 15 Bard-Parker or No. 64 Beaver scalpel blade. The eyelid tissue is then best resected with a small pair of tenotomy scissors such that it has a V-shaped or boat keel–shaped profile. This shape ensures maximal eversion and excellent wound apposition. The wound is then closed with multiple, small, closely spaced, simple interrupted sutures of 3/0 or 4/0 braided nylon or silk. Despite being an absorbable suture, polyglactin is sometimes used to close the skin because of its other desirable features. Sutures should be placed perpendicular to the eyelid margin with use of the "rule of bisection." This technique both permits apposition of two wound margins of unequal length while minimizing tissue redundancy at the far end of the wound and ensures that the widest point of resection is not displaced laterally or medially as would occur if the wound were sutured from one end to the other. It is easily performed by placement of the first suture centrally (at the widest point of resection) and placement of each subsequent suture such that it bisects the distance still to be sutured. Standard postoperative

management consists of topical antibiotic ointment, an Elizabethan collar, and a systemically administered NSAID for analgesia. Systemic antibiotics are not necessary. Sutures can be removed approximately 10 days postoperatively.

The Hotz-Celsus procedure is a very effective method of surgically correcting many simple forms of entropion in all species.

Arrowhead Procedure for Lateral Entropion

For a number of years it was recognized that dogs with broad skulls, such as Rottweilers, retrievers, and Great Danes, had a peculiarly lateral entropion that could be quite subtle and seemed less responsive to Hotz-Celsus procedures than other, simpler forms of entropion. Subsequently, an anatomic study revealed that the lateral canthal ligament in these breeds was directed in such a way that it caused an inversion of the lateral canthus. The arrow-head procedure with lateral canthal tenotomy was developed to correct these anatomic variations. It has greatly improved management of these cases with a single procedure.

The lateral canthal tenotomy should be performed first. An eyelid speculum is placed, and the eyelid margins are firmly grasped at the lateral canthus with tissue forceps. The canthus is elevated away from the orbit in a lateral and rostral direction. This tightens the lateral canthal tendon, which is really simply a condensation of subconjunctival fibrous tissue extending from the lateral canthus to the orbital rim. Blunt-tipped tenotomy scissors can then be used in a closed position to identify the tendon by gently "strumming" across this conjunctival surface. A small conjunctival incision is then made over this tendon using scissors. The tendon is further localized with the same strumming motion and then cut blindly. A gradual "relaxation" of the tension with which the lateral canthus is attached to the lateral orbit can be appreciated. Although some authors recommend removal of a small section of the ligament, it is usually not necessary. The conjunctival incision is not sutured.

The second part of the procedure follows basic principles almost identical to those described earlier for the Hotz-Celsus procedure. The initial skin incision is placed along the haired-nonhaired border as for the Hotz-Celsus procedure, except that it includes parts of the upper and lower eyelids and lateral canthus (Figure 6-24). Sufficient tissue to evert the entropic regions of the upper and lower eyelids is then resected as for the Hotz-Celsus procedure. The outer curvilinear incisions are joined at a point sufficiently lateral to the lateral canthus to laterally evert the inverted canthus. Some authors recommend augmenting this everting force by placement of a buried everting mattress suture at the lateral canthus to further ensure correction of any entropion of the lateral canthus. However, this step is usually not necessary and tends to cause additional conjunctiva to show lateral to the globe. The incisions are closed with use of the rule of bisection, beginning with a suture placed at the lateral canthus. All sutures must be placed perpendicular to the eyelid margin if maximal eversion is to be achieved. Postoperative management is as for the Hotz-Celsus procedure.

Medial Canthoplasty for Lower Medial Entropion and Brachycephalic Ocular Syndrome

A syndrome of eyelid, conjunctival, and corneal lesions is seen commonly in brachycephalic dogs and, to a lesser extent, cats.

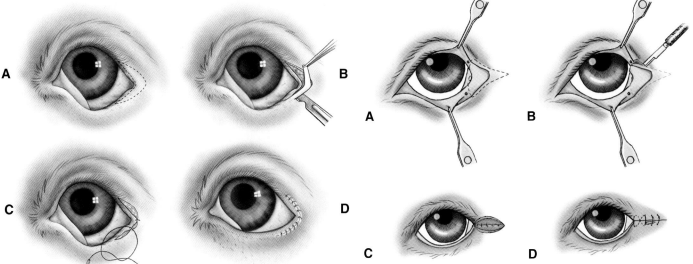

Figure 6-24. Lateral arrowhead procedure for entropion of the lateral aspects of the upper and lower eyelids and the lateral canthus. This is usually performed after a lateral canthal tenotomy. **A,** An arrowhead-shaped section of tissue to be removed is outlined surrounding the lateral canthus. Its dimensions are dictated by the severity and extent of the entropion and may be asymmetric. **B,** The tissue is resected with a scalpel blade and tenotomy scissors. **C,** The incisions are closed using the rule of bisection, beginning with a suture placed at the lateral canthus. **D,** All sutures must be placed perpendicular to the eyelid margin if maximal eversion is to be achieved.

Figure 6-25. Medial canthoplasty. **A,** The area to be resected is outlined and should include approximately the medial one fourth of the upper and lower eyelid margins, the medial caruncle, and a section medial to the medial canthus. Care is taken to not resect the nasolacrimal puncta. **B,** The outlined tissue is resected using a No. 64 Beaver blade. The incisions should be perpendicular to the upper and lower eyelid margins where they cross them. **C,** A buried mattress suture is used to appose the fresh edges of the canthus, as described in Figure 6-12. This may be continued as a series of mattress sutures if required. **D,** The skin is closed with a figure-of-eight suture at the new canthus and a series of simple interrupted sutures medial to that (as described in Figure 6-12). (Modified from Moore CP, Constantinescu GM [1997]: Surgery of the adnexa. Vet Clin North Am Small Anim Pract 27:1011.)

This so-called brachycephalic ocular syndrome consists of any combination of the following features:

- Lower medial entropion
- Breed-related exophthalmos (shallow orbits)
- Macropalpebral fissure (evident as excessive limbal or scleral exposure)
- Lagophthalmos (and/or sleeping with the eyelids incompletely closed)
- Medial caruncular trichiasis
- Nasal fold trichiasis
- Pigmentary keratitis
- Epiphora due to "kinking" of the nasolacrimal canaliculi and obscuring of the puncta

Brachycephalic ocular syndrome is sometimes exacerbated by distichiasis and decreased tear production or quality.

The medial canthoplasty provides a way to neatly correct many of the contributing features of this syndrome, by shortening the lower and upper eyelids, removing the medial caruncle, and everting the lower medial entropion, thereby reducing corneal exposure, frictional irritation, and functional nasolacrimal apparatus obstruction. It is recommended for dogs with progressive corneal lesions. It is also suitable for patients with postproptosis exophthalmos that does not resolve and causes lagophthalmos and secondary corneal lesions. In very severe cases, medial and lateral canthoplasties may be required. The technique is illustrated in Figure 6-25 but is best performed by those with some experience at eyelid surgery and with use of magnification. The animal may be placed in dorsal recumbency with the neck ventroflexed or may be placed in sternal recumbency with the head elevated so that the symmetry of the surgical technique may be accurately assessed during the procedure. Important features of the procedure are avoidance of the lacrimal puncta, meticulous removal of all hair

follicles from the medial caruncle and conjunctiva, careful incision of the eyelids, perfect realignment of the eyelid margin, and appropriate postoperative management as for other eyelid procedures.

ECTROPION

Ectropion, or eversion of the eyelid, invariably affects the lower eyelid only. Clinically significant ectropion is much less common than entropion. The most common type is conformational or breed-related ectropion, which is seen in dogs with loose facial skin, such as retrievers, Saint Bernards, bloodhounds, and cocker spaniels (Figure 6-26). Ectropion is so common in these breeds that a degree of clinically insignificant ectropion is sometimes considered "normal." Cicatricial ectropion is an alternate form of ectropion due to contraction of scar tissue from previous injuries or surgical procedures such as overcorrection of entropion. Cicatricial ectropion is most common in horses and dogs. Regardless of cause, ectropion may result in severe secondary corneoconjunctival lesions if severe enough and left untreated.

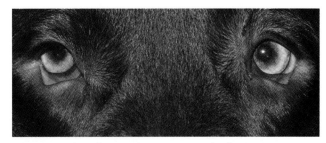

Figure 6-26. Bilateral ectropion in a young Labrador retriever. (Courtesy University of California, Davis, Veterinary Ophthalmology Service Collection.)

Treatment of Ectropion

Ectropion requires surgical correction when it causes conjunctivitis, keratitis, or exfoliative blepharitis due to epiphora or when it exacerbates keratoconjunctivitis sicca. However, many animals tolerate slight ectropion with no ill effects and correction is required much less frequently than for entropion. A variety of techniques has been described for the correction of ectropion. Only commonly used methods suitable for the majority of simpler cases are described here. Patients with more complex ectropion and combined entropion-ectropion should be referred to an ophthalmologist.

Wedge Resection

When there is marked conformational ectropion, the lower eyelid can be shortened by resection of a full-thickness wedge from the lateral end of the lower eyelid as is done for eyelid coloboma (see Figure 6-11). A standard two-layer closure (see Figure 6-12) is then used to perfectly appose the sides of the eyelid margin. For ectropion due to either focal cicatricial contraction or a "notch" deformity in the lower eyelid, the wedge should be repositioned to remove the deformed or scarred tissue. However, the medial canthal area and nasolacrimal apparatus must be avoided.

"V-to-Y" Blepharoplasty

The V-to-Y (Wharton-Jones) blepharoplasty procedure is used for cicatricial ectropion and in cases in which a small wedge resection is insufficient (Figure 6-27). It is particularly well suited

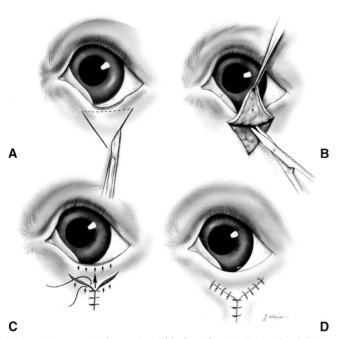

Figure 6-27. V-to-Y (Wharton-Jones) blepharoplasty. **A,** A triangle of skin is outlined. The base is determined by the extent (width) of the lid margin affected by ectropion. The height of the triangle is determined by the extent of eversion to be corrected. A scalpel is used to incise the skin along the two sides but not the base of the triangle. **B,** The skin flap created is elevated and undermined, along with any scar tissue. **C,** The two sides of the triangle are sutured together to form the vertical portion of the Y. The length of the vertical portion of the wound is determined by the extent of eyelid eversion. Arrows show the tissue forces created. **D,** The incisions are closed so as to form the two arms of the Y.

to correction of ectropion due to a broad, contracted scar. The V-to-Y blepharoplasty is begun with outlining of a triangular piece of skin with the base parallel and equal in length to the affected eyelid margin. A skin incision is made along the two lower sides of the triangle, and the skin between them is undermined to elevate a V-shaped flap. Scar tissue beneath the flap is excised. The ventral ends of the incisions then are sutured together with simple interrupted sutures of 3/0 to 5/0 braided nylon or silk to form a vertical line perpendicular to the eyelid margin. This vertical portion forces the triangle and eyelid margin superiorly. The length of the vertical portion depends on how much elevation/inversion of the eyelid margin is required to return it to its normal position. To allow for subsequent wound contraction, it should be about 2 to 3 mm longer than required. Finally, the remaining parts of the two incisions are sutured to the free edges of the flap so that the sutured skin forms a Y.

EYELID INJURIES

The eyelids have an excellent blood supply, and injuries to them heal rapidly when repaired correctly. The following considerations are important to ensure an optimal outcome:

1. Because of this rich blood supply, the eyelids are susceptible to severe edema and distortion after even relatively minor injury (or surgery).
2. Although it is preferable to treat eyelid injuries as soon as possible, the patient's general condition must be stabilized before eyelid injuries are repaired.
3. When an eyelid injury is noted, a thorough search must be made for concurrent injuries to the cornea, sclera, and nasolacrimal apparatus in particular, and to the globe as a whole.
4. In all cases, the nasolacrimal puncta should be identified and cannulated, and the nasolacrimal apparatus flushed to ensure patency.
5. Sutures in the eyelids must be kept away from the globe and should be soft and pliable to prevent injury to the cornea.
6. The margin should always be accurately reapposed with a standard two-layer closure (see Figure 6-12).
7. Bacterial flora in the conjunctival sac and surrounding area may readily invade this area, but severe postoperative septic blepharitis is uncommon if a course of systemic antibiotics with good spectrum of activity against gram-positive organisms (such as amoxicillin-clavulanic acid or a cephalosporin) is instituted.
8. Severe pruritus and self-trauma may occur during wound healing, especially if inflammation is present as a result of infection, tissue trauma, or large or tight sutures. Control of these primary factors as well as provision of an Elizabethan collar and postoperative use of warm packs and analgesics will minimize this problem and are essential.

Treatment of Eyelid Injuries

Provided that one third or less of the eyelid margin is missing, direct closure of the wound via the same technique used to close a wedge resection (see Figure 6-12) may then be used (Figure 6-28). If the defect is more extensive, an advancement flap or other reconstructive procedure may be necessary.

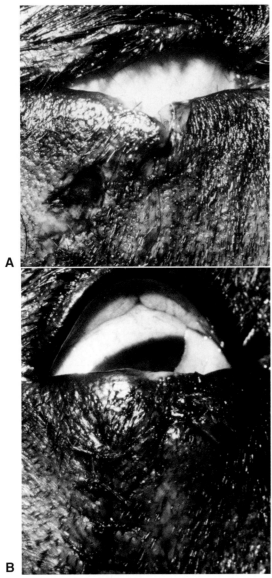

Figure 6-28. A, Lower eyelid laceration in a dog. Note that the eyelid margin is involved and must be apposed accurately to avoid trichiasis. **B,** Immediate postoperative appearance. A standard two-layer closure as described in Figure 6-12 was used.

Surgical preparation and clipping should be gentle to prevent further edema. Tissue débridement must be minimal so as not to further shorten the eyelid; this minimal approach is possible because the extensive blood supply of the eyelid limits secondary infection at this site, especially if antibiotics are provided. An excellent technique to "freshen" wound margins on the eyelid while resecting the minimum tissue necessary involves gentle scraping (not incising) of tissue edges with a scalpel blade until they are cleaned of obvious debris and exudates and bleeding is noted. This also permits identification of viable tissue. A standard two-layer closure with soft, braided suture can then be used to close the eyelid laceration as for all other incisions involving the eyelid margin (see Figure 6-12). Systemic and topical antibiotics should be used perioperatively. Postoperatively, an ophthalmic ointment is preferred as it provides lubrication and protects the cornea during wound healing. Topical corticosteroids are usually unnecessary and should be avoided if there is coincident corneal ulceration.

Systemically administered NSAIDs and application of warm packs may minimize pain and swelling, and an Elizabethan collar is essential to prevent self-trauma.

Lacerations and injuries involving the nasolacrimal apparatus will cicatrize, leading to impaired drainage of tears and epiphora. Although many animals with dysfunction of one punctum or canaliculus (especially if it is the dorsal punctum) show no epiphora, this is not constant or reliable. Therefore every effort should be made to repair damage to the nasolacrimal apparatus as soon as possible after injury. Because this repair requires magnification and experience, referral to a veterinary ophthalmologist is frequently indicated. If primary repair of the nasolacrimal apparatus is unsuccessful, drainage of tears into the nasal cavity can be effected with conjunctivorhinostomy (see Chapter 9).

CHALAZION

A chalazion is a nonneoplastic enlargement of the meibomian gland caused by blockage of its duct and inspissation of its secretory products. It is generally a painless swelling that appears yellowish-white when viewed through the palpebral conjunctiva or skin (Figure 6-29). However, if the gland ruptures, lipid-laden sebaceous material escapes into the eyelid stroma and causes a lipogranuloma that may become quite inflamed. Meibomian gland duct obstruction (and therefore a chalazion) is commonly seen with meibomian gland neoplasms. Treatment of a chalazion (with or without meibomian gland neoplasia) involves surgical incision and drainage. Manual expression is contraindicated because it might spread infection and/or glandular secretions into surrounding tissues. With general anesthesia, the affected area is clamped with Desmarres chalazion forceps and a small incision is made into the mass through the palpebral conjunctiva. The contents are removed with a chalazion curette (Figure 6-30). Conjunctival sutures are not placed because they would abrade the cornea and are not required because the conjunctiva heals rapidly. Some ophthalmologists follow up with two cycles of rapid freeze–slow thaw cryotherapy if there is concern about an associated meibomian gland neoplasm. Postoperative application of a topical corticosteroid-antibiotic ointment is advisable. As with all other forms of blepharitis,

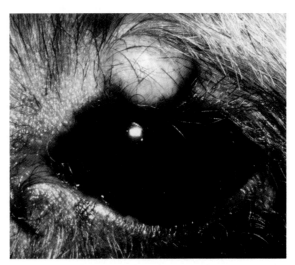

Figure 6-29. Chalazion in a dog.

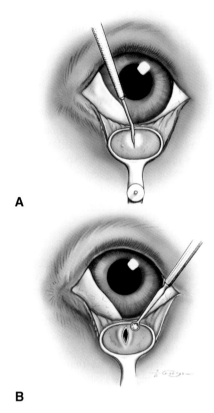

A

B

Figure 6-30. Treatment of chalazion. **A,** A chalazion clamp is applied to the affected region of the eyelid, and the chalazion is incised through the palpebral conjunctiva with a small scalpel blade. **B,** Granulomatous material and glandular secretions are removed with a chalazion curette. Two freeze-thaw cycles of cryotherapy may be applied as for distichiasis (see Figure 6-17).

warm compresses are useful in cooperative patients and reduce postoperative edema, swelling, and pain. A similar disease, lipogranulomatous conjunctivitis, is seen in cats, although it involves multiple meibomian glands (see Chapter 7).

HORDEOLUM AND MEIBOMIAN ADENITIS

An external hordeolum (or stye) or internal hordeolum is a purulent bacterial infection of a gland of Zeis or meibomian gland, respectively. The infecting bacterium is often *Staphylococcus aureus* and therefore these lesions tend to be more painful and inflamed than chalazia. Involvement of multiple glands is common, especially in dogs, and is then termed meibomitis, meibomian or tarsal adenitis, or marginal blepharitis. Clinical signs include variable erythema and swelling of the eyelid margins, pruritus, pain, chemosis, and purulent conjunctivitis (Figure 6-31). Because the meibomian glands secrete the lipid layer of the tear film, which is critical to tear function, meibomian adenitis is often associated with corneal and conjunctival disease and may precipitate keratoconjunctivitis sicca. Therapy should be scaled to match disease severity and chronicity (Table 6-1). Systemic antibiotic therapy and topical antibiotic-corticosteroid administration are required. Without culture and sensitivity data or while waiting for these results, administration of amoxicillin-clavulanic acid, doxycycline, or a cephalosporin is advisable. Protracted therapy is often necessary as with deep pyoderma elsewhere. If there is significant lipogranulomatous inflammation or hyper-

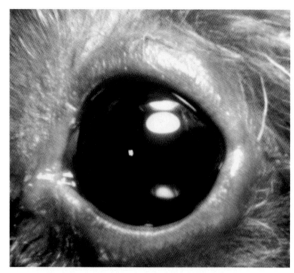

Figure 6-31. Meibomitis or marginal blepharitis in a dog.

Table 6-1 | Therapy for Canine Meibomitis or Marginal Blepharitis

DISEASE SEVERITY	MEANS OF DIAGNOSIS	THERAPY
Early/mild	Clinical signs ± Culture and sensitivity testing	Topical antibiotic-corticosteroid preparations Systemic antibiotics (e.g., doxycycline, cephalosporin, clavulanic acid–amoxicillin, or as dictated by culture and sensitivity results) Continue therapy for at least 3-4 wks
Moderate	Clinical signs Culture and sensitivity testing Conjunctival and skin scrapings for cytologic assessment	Initially as for early/mild disease Revise according to diagnostic test results Continue therapy for at least 6-8 wks If no fungal or parasitic agents found, systemic prednisolone (0.5 mg/kg PO q24h for 7 days) during the third wk of antibiotic therapy
Severe, chronic, or recurrent	As for moderate disease Biopsy	As for moderate disease but may need longer or indefinite course of appropriate antibiotics and corticosteroids Consult veterinary dermatologist Consider bacterin injections

sensitivity to staphylococcal antigens is suspected, systemic administration of a corticosteroid is required. Systemic antibiotics should be initiated before, during, and after corticosteroid use.

Chronic, severe, or recurrent meibomitis requires patience and protracted treatment for control (and usually not cure). Some authors claim success with administration of appropriately prepared staphylococcal bacterin of animal origin. Therapy can gradually be tapered according to clinical improvement. In unresponsive cases, confirmation of microbial involvement through careful collection of meibomian secretions for cytologic examination, fungal culture, or bacterial culture and sensitivity testing may be necessary. Purulent blepharitis may also be caused by dermatologic fungi (e.g., *Microsporum canis, Microsporum gypseum, Trichophyton mentagrophytes, Aspergillus niger*). Involvement of Demodex mites should also be investigated through microscopic examination of secretions from the meibomian glands as well as skin scrapings or hair plucked from adjacent eyelid skin. Immune-mediated dermatopathies that target mucocutaneous borders should also be considered and require biopsy for definitive diagnosis.

NEOPLASIA

Eyelid tumors are relatively common in all domestic species. However, the most common eyelid neoplasms vary by species, as follows:

- Dog: meibomian adenoma, papilloma, histiocytoma, melanoma (Table 6-2)
- Cat: squamous cell carcinoma
- Horse: squamous cell carcinoma, equine sarcoid, melanoma
- Cattle: squamous cell carcinoma

Although each of these tumors has some characteristic or suggestive clinical features, only histologic examination of an incisional or excisional biopsy specimen or cytologic examination of an aspirate, impression smear, or scraping is definitively diagnostic, and resected tumors should always be submitted for histologic examination. Therapy should be tailored to the individual tumor type and the patient after systemic assessment and in accordance with owner concerns. In particular, variations in therapy may be chosen according to malignancy, rate of growth, position, presence of metastases, local invasiveness, degree of corneoconjunctival irritation, and response to previous and current therapy. Eyelid tumors are typically treated surgically, often with adjunctive therapy such as cryotherapy, radiation therapy, chemotherapy, or immunotherapy (see Chapter 3). Cryotherapy is particularly useful for eyelid lesions, as most eyelid tissues (including the nasolacrimal apparatus) are relatively resistant to the effects of cryotherapy and the lid retains function after cryonecrosis sufficient to produce tumor cell death. Cryotherapy is particularly useful for small or early tumors, especially in elderly or debilitated patients.

Surgical Excision

As much of the neoplasm as possible should be removed, including the regional lymph node if affected, and margins of the excised tissue should be examined histologically. For smaller tumors involving one third or less of the eyelid margin, a simple, full-thickness wedge resection with two-layer closure similar to that used to correct coloboma, entropion, or ectropion is indicated (Figure 6-32). As much of the eyelid margin as possible is retained. When more than one third of the eyelid length must be removed, total excision is usually not possible without some sort of blepharoplastic procedure, and referral may be indicated. One of the more straightforward blepharoplastic procedures is the H-plasty or full-thickness advancement flap (Figure 6-33). For more extensive lesions, a variety of advancement, rotation, axial pattern skin flaps, and myocutaneous free grafts can be used, depending on the size and location of the tissue to be replaced. These procedures should be performed by a surgeon experienced in reconstructive surgery and microsurgical vascular anastomoses.

Specific Tumor Types

Squamous Cell Carcinoma

Squamous cell carcinoma may involve the eyelids of all species but is especially common in poorly pigmented areas of the eyelids in horses, cattle, and cats (Figure 6-34). The tumor is associated with exposure to ultraviolet light. The pathogenesis

Table 6-2 | **Frequency of Canine Eyelid Tumors**

TUMOR TYPE	TOTAL NO.	PERCENTAGE
Meibomian (tarsal) adenoma	58	28.7
Squamous papilloma	35	17.3
Meibomian (tarsal) adenocarcinoma	31	15.3
Benign melanoma	26	12.9
Malignant melanoma	16	7.9
Histiocytoma	7	3.5
Mastocytoma	5	2.5
Basal cell carcinoma	5	2.5
Squamous cell carcinoma	5	2.5
Fibroma	4	2.1
Fibropapilloma	2	1.0
Lipoma	2	1.0
Adnexal carcinoma	1	0.5
Hemangiopericytoma	1	0.5
Malignant lymphoma	1	0.5
Neurofibroma	1	0.5
Neurofibrosarcoma	1	0.5
Atypical epithelioma	1	0.5
Undetermined	1	0.5
Total benign	**148**	**73.3**
Total malignant	**54**	**26.7**

From Krehbiel JD, Langham RF (1975): Eyelid neoplasms of dogs. Am J Vet Res 36:115.

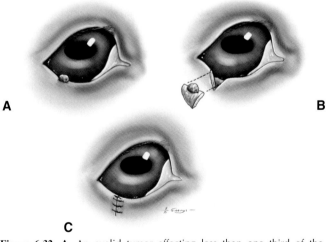

Figure 6-32. A, An eyelid tumor affecting less than one third of the margin. **B,** The tumor and a surrounding area of normal tissue are removed by full-thickness wedge excision (see Figure 6-11 for more detail). **C,** The defect is closed with a standard two-layered closure as described in Figure 6-12.

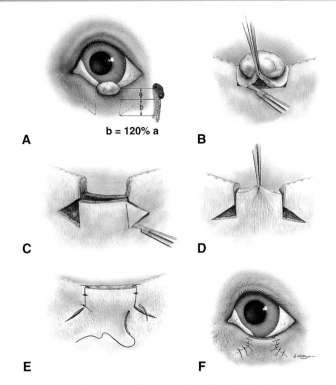

b = 120% a

A

B

C

D

E

F

Figure 6-33. Advancement flap or H-plasty for eyelid lesions greater than one third of the eyelid length. **A,** The tumor before excision. Incisions are outlined by dotted lines. Vertical sides of the triangles (b) are 20% longer than the vertical incisions adjacent to the tumor (a), to allow for wound contraction. **B,** The tumor (with adequate margins) is outlined with a square or rectangular incision. The tumor and associated eyelid are then completely resected and submitted for histopathologic examination. **C,** A full-thickness marginal deficit remains. Two triangular areas are excised as originally outlined. **D,** A sliding half-thickness "flap" of lower eyelid is created by blunt and sharp dissection and is elevated into the marginal deficit. **E,** Figure-of-eight sutures of 5/0 or 6/0 nylon or silk are placed at the two marginal wounds, as for simple eyelid closures (see Figure 6-12, C). The apices of the triangles are then sutured with simple interrupted sutures using the same suture material. **F,** Remaining sutures are placed approximately 2 mm apart. If the palpebral conjunctiva is mobile, it is elevated and sutured to the outer aspect of the skin edge with a simple continuous suture of 6/0 or 7/0 Vicryl to minimize trichiasis. If trichiasis occurs subsequently, cryotherapy may be required (see Figure 6-19).

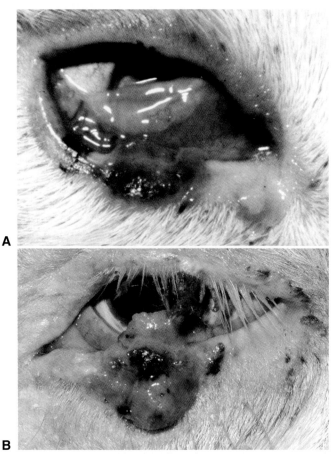

A

B

Figure 6-34. Erosive lower eyelid squamous cell carcinoma in a cat **(A)** and a more proliferative but ulcerated lower eyelid squamous cell carcinoma in a horse **(B).** (Courtesy University of California, Davis, Veterinary Ophthalmology Service Collection.)

of eyelid squamous cell carcinoma is shown in Figure 6-35. Although squamous cell carcinomas may metastasize to regional lymph nodes and eventually to the lungs, these tumors are typically characterized by local invasiveness. The invading neoplasm results in local inflammation with blepharitis and conjunctivitis. Clinical signs include chronic purulent ocular discharge, which may be temporarily or partially responsive to antibiotics. Periocular excoriation, chronic conjunctivitis, and encrusted or hemorrhagic lesions of the eyelids are common. Squamous cell carcinoma must be distinguished from other causes of chronic blepharitis, for which it is frequently mistaken. Diagnosis is confirmed with cytologic assessment of scrapings or by biopsy.

In horses, squamous cell carcinoma of the eyelid is common, although less so than that of other ocular sites. In a survey of 49 equine cases, single lesions involved the eyelids in 14% of patients, the third eyelid in 26%, and the limbus in 25%. Multiple lesions in one eye were present in 8% of patients, and 16% of patients had bilateral lesions. The mean age of affected horses was approximately 10 years. In cattle, squamous cell carcinoma occurs more commonly on the conjunctiva and third

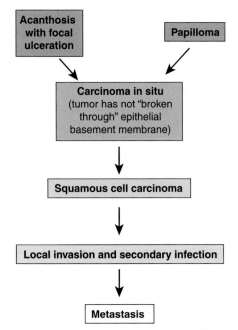

Acanthosis with focal ulceration

Papilloma

Carcinoma in situ (tumor has not "broken through" epithelial basement membrane)

Squamous cell carcinoma

Local invasion and secondary infection

Metastasis

Figure 6-35. Pathogenesis of eyelid squamous cell carcinoma.

eyelid (75%) than on the eyelids (25%). However, the rate of metastasis is greater from lesions on the eyelids and third eyelid than from the cornea or conjunctiva. More detailed discussion of ocular squamous cell carcinoma in cattle is found in Chapter 7. Squamous cell carcinoma of the eyelid is frequent in white cats and often occurs along with lesions involving the nasal planum and pinnae. Ocular squamous cell carcinoma is uncommon in dogs. In one study, squamous cell carcinoma represented only 2.5% of 202 canine eyelid neoplasms (see Table 6-2).

Squamous cell carcinomas should undergo complete surgical resection whenever possible. For larger lesions, this requires a blepharoplastic procedure to ensure retention of proper eyelid function. If excision is not likely to be complete, debulking followed by cryotherapy or radiation therapy may be necessary. In cattle, large (>50 mm in diameter) squamous cell carcinomas of the eyelid respond poorly to cryotherapy, hyperthermia, and immunotherapy. For such tumors surgical excision followed by interstitial brachytherapy and/or immunotherapy is recommended if available. For advanced recurrent or infiltrative lesions, enucleation or exenteration may be necessary. In horses interstitial brachytherapy with iridium-192 or intralesional cisplatin injection has also been recommended.

Meibomian Adenoma

Meibomian adenoma is the most common eyelid tumor in dogs, occurring most frequently after middle age. It is uncommon in other species. The tumors originate in the meibomian glands, and although many grow rapidly and sometimes appear histologically malignant, they are usually clinically benign. Typically they appear as proliferative masses appearing from the meibomian gland orifice (Figure 6-36). Enlargement of the gland itself is often visible, especially when viewed from the conjunctival surface. These tumors also may be associated with glandular enlargement due to retained secretions and associated lipogranuloma formation (chalazion). The tumor may cause frictional keratoconjunctivitis and should be removed as soon as the diagnosis is made.

Simple removal of the section of the mass protruding from the eyelid margin is inadequate, because the tumor arises from the meibomian gland and will recur if not totally removed.

However, smaller lesions may be debulked in this manner and via curettage through a conjunctival incision as for treatment of chalazion (see Figure 6-30). This must be followed by two freeze-thaw cycles of cryotherapy as described for distichiasis (see Figure 6-17) to reduce recurrence. Debulking and cryotherapy can be done with sedation and regional anesthesia, making it preferable in older dogs. Full-thickness wedge excision (see Figure 6-11) followed by two-layer closure (see Figure 6-12) reduces recurrences further but requires general anesthesia and more postoperative care. A 15% recurrence rate and mean recurrence time of 7.4 months have been shown after cryosurgery, compared to an 11% recurrence rate and mean recurrence time of 28.3 months after surgical excision.

Equine Sarcoid

Equine sarcoid or fibrosarcoma is the second most common tumor of the equine eyelid. Lesions may be present elsewhere on the face and body, but the tumor is often restricted to the eyelids (Figure 6-37). Sarcoids are nodular masses usually beneath intact skin and firmly adherent to the overlying dermis and subcutaneous tissues. Occasionally they can be ulcerated and must be distinguished from the eyelid lesions of habronemiasis in endemic areas. In a survey of 10 cases of sarcoid, the mean age of the affected animals was 4.4 years and there was no sex predilection. Because of the infiltrative nature, poor definition, and often advanced state at clinical presentation, complete surgical excision of sarcoids is difficult and recurrence is likely. If surgical excision is used, a wide surrounding margin of normal

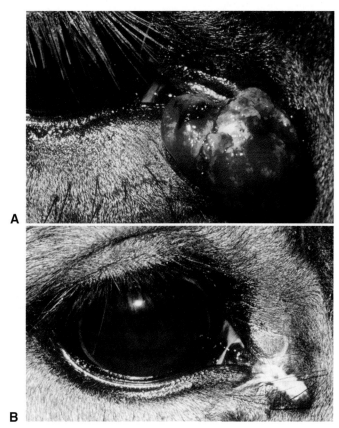

Figure 6-37. A, Equine sarcoid at the medial canthus of the right eye. **B,** Same tumor 2 months later after surgical debulking and three treatments with radiofrequency hyperthermia given at 2-week intervals.

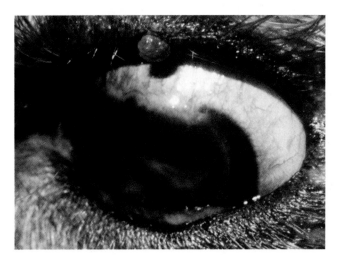

Figure 6-36. Upper eyelid meibomian adenoma in a dog. Note that a section of the tumor protrudes from a meibomian gland orifice on the eyelid margin.

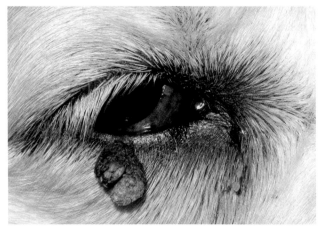

Figure 6-38. Lower eyelid papilloma in a dog. Note the lack of marginal involvement in this case compared with the meibomian adenoma in Figure 6-36.

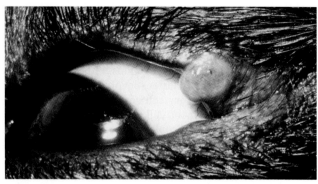

Figure 6-39. Solitary histiocytoma of the upper eyelid of a young dog.

tissue should be removed with reconstruction via a preplanned method. Because of these difficulties, treatment with immunotherapy (usually bacille Calmette-Guérin [BCG]), cryotherapy, or radiation therapy is often preferred. Radiofrequency hyperthermia has also given good therapeutic results. The following 12-month nonrecurrence rates have been reported:

- Iridium-192 brachytherapy: 86.6% (74.0% at 5 years)
- Radon-222 brachytherapy: 92%
- Cobalt-60 radiotherapy: 58%
- Gold-198 brachytherapy: 83%
- Orthovoltage therapy: 33%
- BCG injection: 100%

Viral Papillomatosis

Viral papillomas of the eyelids and conjunctiva occur in young dogs and cattle as part of oral or generalized papillomatosis. They can also occur as solitary eyelid lesions in older dogs (Figure 6-38). When continually moistened by tears, the tumors are grayish white and soft. The disease is often self limiting, especially in younger animals, and excision or cryotherapy is required only if the tumors are causing secondary mechanical damage to the eye.

Histiocytoma

Histiocytic masses involving the eyelids occur occasionally in dogs. They may occur as single or multiple eyelid lesions in an otherwise well dog, as part of a broader cutaneous histiocytosis complex, or as part of the systemic histiocytosis syndrome. Bernese mountain dogs, Irish wolfhounds, Rottweillers, retrievers, and basset hounds seem to be predisposed to this

group of diseases. The tumors vary from benign lesions that regress spontaneously to tumors that are metastatic from or to the eyelids and therefore may involve regional lymph nodes or other organ systems. All affected dogs therefore warrant a thorough dermatologic and general physical examination as well as histologic assessment of the mass, often with immunophenotyping by a pathologist with some expertise in this group of diseases. Histiocytomas involving the eyelid typically appear as tan to pink, somewhat alopecic masses that may grow relatively quickly and may ulcerate quickly (Figure 6-39).

Treatment should be chosen after thorough assessment of the extent of disease and the effect of the mass upon ocular function (lid closure, corneoconjunctival irritation, etc.). Solitary masses in young dogs may spontaneously regress, usually within the first few weeks to months. If not, surgical resection of solitary eyelid masses is possible as for other eyelid tumors (see Figures 6-32 and 6-33). Dogs with systemic or widespread cutaneous involvement carry a more guarded prognosis and may require systemic immunotherapy.

SKIN DISEASES AFFECTING THE EYELIDS

The preceding sections of this chapter describe blepharitis when it occurs as a distinct entity. However, the lids are frequently inflamed as part of more widespread dermatitis. In some patients, blepharitis may be more overt than dermatitis in other regions because the eyelids are so vascular and prone to exaggerated inflammatory responses. Alternatively, they may simply be a site where dermatitis is more likely to be noticed owing to anthropomorphic attention to the eyes or because the eyelid margin is one of the more clearly visible mucocutaneous junctions affected in a wide variety of skin diseases. As such, all patients with blepharitis should undergo a complete dermatologic examination. Table 6-3 provides a comprehensive list of common skin disorders that may affect the eyelids, their clinical signs, important diagnostic steps, and suggested treatment.

Table 6-3 | **Skin Diseases Affecting the Eyelids**
Drs. C.A. Outerbridge and P.J. Ihrke

DISORDER AND AFFECTED ANIMALS	CLINICAL SIGNS	DIAGNOSIS	TREATMENT
PARASITIC Sarcoptic acariasis (scabies) *Sarcoptes scabiei* Dogs, horses, pigs, cattle, sheep	Eyelids alone unlikely. Head and ears often initial sites; also hocks and elbows are preferential sites in dogs. Intense pruritus and papular eruptions are important features. Alopecia, erythema, crusting, scaling, and ulceration secondary to self-trauma are common.	Clinical signs (intense pruritus) and appropriate history (abrupt onset). Skin scrapings to identify the mite (can be difficult to find). Occasionally skin biopsy. Response to therapy.	All in-contact animals must be treated. *Dogs:* Numerous topical parasiticides: Lime sulfur is safest topical for all ages and species. Systemic ivermectin (SC or PO) or milbemycin (PO), 4-6 sequential weekly treatments. *Do not use* in ivermectin-sensitive breeds. Cheek swab sample can be submitted for MDR-1 gene analysis to determine whether dog is an ivermectin-sensitive individual. Selamectin applied topically every 2 wks for 4 sequential treatments. *Cattle:* Topicals applied at 10-day intervals for 6 treatments: lindane, coumaphos, diazinon, malathion, toxaphene, and lime sulfur. Ivermectin SC; repeat in 2 wks. *Horses:* Rare disease worldwide eradicated in United States so diagnosed cases should be reported to the USDA
Demodicosis* *Demodex* spp. Dogs, goats, cattle, pigs, cats, sheep, horses	Facial lesions and periorbital distribution common; patchy alopecia and mild erythema with scaling and follicular plugging. Chronic secondary lesions of lichenification, hyperpigmentation, and scale common, especially in goats. Ruminants can have nodular lesions involving face, neck, and shoulders.	Appropriate history and physical exam findings. Skin scrapings of affected areas to identify the mite. Skin biopsy rarely necessary except in the shar-pei and in cases of pododemodicosis.	Treatment may not be required in all cases because lesions may regress spontaneously. *Dogs:* 1. Localized: therapy not required 2. Generalized: topical therapy: Amitraz dips: Clip long coats and shampoo with benzoyl peroxide as follicular flushing agent before dipping. Systemic therapy: ivermectin or milbemycin daily until two consecutive negative scrapings 4-6 wks apart. *Do not use* in ivermectin-sensitive breed unless MDR-1 gene analysis confirms individual is not sensitive. *Horses: Do not use* Amitraz. Disease usually regresses without treatment. Daily ivermectin may have efficacy. *Ruminants:* Surgical excision or topical iodide
Notoedric acariasis *Notoedres cati* Cats	Eyelids are not the only affected site. Lesions, typically bilaterally symmetrical, start at medial edge of pinna and spread to involve face, eyelids, and neck. Skin is thickened, partially alopecic, with adherent yellowish to gray crusts. Intense pruritus.	Distribution of lesions and intense pruritus should heighten suspicion. Skin scrapings to identify the mite.	Many topical therapies can be toxic to cats. Lime sulfur 2% to 3% is safe for use in cats. Clipping of hair and soaking of crusts may be required. Systemic therapy: ivermectin SC or PO 3-4 sequential weekly treatments; all in-contact cats must be treated Selamectin applied topically every 2 wks for 2-3 treatments should be effective.

MDR-1, Multiple-drug resistance–1; *USDA,* U.S. Department of Agriculture.
*Diseases that might manifest only as lesions on the eyelid in some species.

Continued

Table 6-3 | **Skin Diseases Affecting the Eyelids—cont'd**

DISORDER AND AFFECTED ANIMALS	CLINICAL SIGNS	DIAGNOSIS	TREATMENT
Psoroptic acariasis *Psoroptes equi* *Psoroptes hippotis* *Psoroptes bovis* *Psoroptes ovis* *Psoroptes capri* *Psoroptes cuniculi* Horses, pigs, cattle, sheep, goats, rabbits; not in horses or sheep in the United States	Eyelids rarely affected alone. Pruritus is often intense with crusted papules and secondary excoriations and serocellular crusts. Weight loss, anemia, and secondary infections can be associated.	Skin scrapings to identify the mite. Appropriate clinical signs.	Topical therapies: Lindane, coumaphos, diazinon, toxaphene, chlordane, malathion, or lime sulfur should be applied to all affected and contact animals weekly for at least 2 wks. Ivermectin 0.2 mg/kg SC is approved for use in cattle.
Echidnophaga gallinacea "Sticktight flea"* Dogs, cats, rabbits, horses	Adherent flea found often on pinnal margins, eyelids, and muzzle.	Identifying flea. Possible exposure to poultry.	Avoid reexposure. Topical flea adulticides.
Cutaneous onchocerciasis *Onchocerca cervicalis* Horses	Preferential sites for microfilaria: ventral midline, lower eyelid, and lateral limbus of the eye. Hypersensitivity reaction results in patchy alopecia, erythema, and scaling. Focal depigmentation can occur.	History, clinical signs, skin biopsy, onchocerca microfilarial saline preparation Disease now rare in those regions where ivermectin is routinely used as anthelmintic	Ivermectin PO

Ticks*
Small animals: *Dermacentor* spp.
  Rhipicephalus sanguineus
  Ixodes
  Amblyomma
Large animals: *Boophilus* (cows)
  Haemaphysalis spp.
  Ixodes spp.
  Amblyomma
	Preferentially attach to mucocutaneous junctions such as eyelids and to poorly haired regions. Cause focal swollen, erythematous lesion at site of attachment. Can transmit rickettsial and protozoal diseases.	Find and identify the tick.	Remove the tick. Acaricides.

Cutaneous habronemiasis (summer sores) *Habronema* spp. *Draschia megastoma* Spread by *Musca* spp. and *Stomoxys* spp. Horses	Cutaneous lesions occur when larvae are deposited on damaged skin or moist areas: medial canthus of eye, urethral process, and lower limbs. Ulcerative, nodular masses may have necrotic, yellow mineralized foci.	History and clinical findings. Skin biopsy.	Surgical débridement if possible. Corticosteroids: systemic, intralesional, topical. Systemic insecticidal therapy to eradicate adults and prevent reinfestation. Control vectors.
Flies Flesh-eating: larvae of *Lucilia* *Protophormia* *Phormia* *Calliphora* *Sacrophaga* spp. Sheep, cattle, dogs, horses, cats	Fly strike is uncommon around the eyes, found typically in wet, contaminated areas of the body. Poll strike in sheep may affect eyelids.	Clinical signs, presence of larvae	Remove larvae, clip affected areas of hair, clean and débride.

Biting:
  Musca
  Tabanidae
  Hydrotaea
  Stomoxys
  Haematobia
Horses, cattle, dogs
	Ear margins, periorbital, preferential sites on face to find bleeding or scabbed bites. Often very painful bites with some species (*Stomoxys, Tabanidae*) and may cause livestock to become very agitated.	Clinical signs, presence of flies	Avoid exposure. Fly control.

ARTHROPOD HYPERSENSITIVITY			
Eosinophilic folliculitis and furunculosis Dogs	Acute onset (hours) of well-demarcated, alopecic, erythematous papules and nodules that often coalesce, involve dorsal muzzle, and can be periorbital. Fistulous tracts may also be present. Lesions are often bilaterally symmetrical with ulcerative and hemorrhagic surface. Pruritus and pain can be intense.	History and clinical signs: distinctive lesions with possible exposure to wasps, bees, hornets, spiders, or ants Seasonality linked to arthropod exposure. Cytologic demonstration of eosinophils on impression smears of lesions. Skin biopsy.	Avoid exposure to causative arthropods. Corticosteroid therapy for 2-3 wks.

Table 6-3 | **Skin Diseases Affecting the Eyelids—cont'd**

DISORDER AND AFFECTED ANIMALS	CLINICAL SIGNS	DIAGNOSIS	TREATMENT
Mosquito-bite hypersensitivity Cats	Bilaterally symmetrical lesions include papules, nodules on the pinnae, erythema, erosive, hemorrhagic crusting of dorsal muzzle, self-trauma. Affects dorsal muzzle, preauricular area, periorbital area, and pinnae.	Distinctive lesions, distribution with possible exposure. Seasonality. Skin biopsy.	Avoid exposure. Corticosteroids.
FUNGAL Dermatophytosis* *Microsporum canis, Microsporum equinum,* and *Microsporum gypseum* *Trichophyton mentagrophytes, Trichophyton equinum,* and *Trichophyton verrucosum* Dogs, cats, horses, cattle; rare in sheep and goats	Young animals most susceptible. Pleomorphic and often multifocal lesions of alopecia, scaling, and crusting. Periorbita commonly affected in dogs, cats, and cattle. Cattle have marked lichenification. Kerion dermatophytosis: well-demarcated nodule with erythema and ulceration. Pruritus is typically minimal.	Microscopic evaluation of hairs. Fungal culture. Skin biopsy.	*Large animals:* Dermatophytosis may spontaneously resolve. Topical therapies: chlorhexidine, lime sulfur, miconazole, captan, povidone-iodine. *Small animals:* Clip hair. Topical therapies: lime sulfur, enilconazole Systemic therapies: griseofulvin, ketoconazole, itraconazole Environmental decontamination
Deep systemic mycosis Histoplasmosis (cats) Blastomycosis (dogs) Cryptococcosis (cats)	Cutaneous lesions include dermal or subcutaneous nodules that may ulcerate and form fistulous tracts. Lesions may be found anywhere cutaneously but can involve the face, including eyelids.	Skin biopsy of lesions and identification of fungal agent. Other organ systems may be affected. Serology.	Appropriate systemic antifungal therapy
BACTERIAL Focal folliculitis and furunculosis* Small animals: *Staphylococcus* spp. Large animals: variable bacteria: *Staphylococcus* spp. *Corynebacterium* spp. Dogs, cats, horses, goats, cattle	Hair projects from surface of the papule or pustule. Crusts, alopecia.	Cytologic evaluation and Gram stain of pustular contents Culture of a pustule	Appropriate antibiotic therapy. Evaluate for underlying predisposing causes.
Dermatophilosis *Dermatophilus congolensis* Cattle, horses, sheep, goats	Proliferative crusts with matted hair, exudation, and crust formation. Crusted papules. Removal of crusts reveals a granulation bed. Lesions often involve muzzle, neck, dorsum, and distal extremities. Periorbital involvement is uncommon. Painful, not pruritic. Nonpigmented skin is more susceptible.	Cytologic examination of crusts for characteristic actinomycete. Culture. Skin biopsy.	Removal of crusts. Topical therapy with povidone-iodine shampoo or chlorhexidine daily for 7 days, then twice weekly. Systemic therapy for severe cases: penicillin or oxytetracycline (ruminants).
Feline leprosy *Mycobacterium lepraemurium* Cats and possibly ferrets	Single or multiple cutaneous nodules: often fistulous or ulcerated. Affects face, including eyelids and distal extremities. May be associated with underlying immunosuppression, although most cats are not systemically unwell.	Finding of acid-fast organisms on cytologic or histologic samples. Diffuse granulomatous inflammatory response is seen histologically. Appropriate test for FeLV/FIV. Culture is difficult.	Surgical excision, enrofloxacin, clarithromycin, clofazimine

FeLV/FIV, Feline leukemia virus/feline immunodeficiency virus.

Continued

Table 6-3 | **Skin Diseases Affecting the Eyelids—cont'd**

DISORDER AND AFFECTED ANIMALS	CLINICAL SIGNS	DIAGNOSIS	TREATMENT
PROTOZOAL			
Leishmaniasis *Leishmania* spp. Dogs; rare in cats	Exfoliative dermatitis with silvery adherent scales on face; can be generalized. Periocular alopecia. Ulcerative dermatitis: lips, eyelids. Sterile pustular dermatitis, nasal depigmentation, or nodules may also be seen. Concomitant systemic signs.	Exposure to *endemic area* and compatible clinical signs. Identification of amastigotes in lymph node aspirates or bone marrow specimens. Skin biopsy reveals organisms in 50% of cases. Immunohistochemistry can be helpful in identifying organisms in tissue. Serologic assay can cross-react with *Babesia* spp. and *Trypanosoma cruzi*.	Meglumine antimonate, allopurinol
VIRAL			
Feline pox virus Cats Rare and regional	Ulcerated crusted papules or nodules that progress to scar. Often introduced through bite wound on head or forelimb.	Skin biopsy may demonstrate viral inclusions. Virus isolation or PCR from skin biopsy.	None
Feline herpesvirus 1 (FHV-1) Cats	Ulcerative and sometimes proliferative crusting skin lesions most commonly involve the dorsal muzzle and nasal planum but may progress to involve medial canthi.	Skin biopsy may reveal intranuclear viral inclusions. PCR of skin biopsy may reveal FHV-1 DNA.	SC interferon, PO lysine, PO famciclovir
ALLERGIC			
Atopic dermatitis (environmental allergy to pollens and molds) Dogs, cats, horses, goats	Bilaterally symmetrical periorbital erythema; alopecia and crusting due to self-trauma. Pruritus often present elsewhere, in particular feet, ears, groin, and axillae in dogs. Horses may be presented with urticarial reactions.	Seasonal history of pruritus is helpful (seasonality varies with geography and chronicity). Diagnosis of exclusion; all other causes of pruritus must be eliminated. All secondary opportunistic infections must be identified and treated.	Antihistamines and essential fatty acid supplements. Judicious use of low-dose corticosteroids. Allergen-specific immunotherapy (hyposensitization therapy) based on results of intradermal skin testing of ELISA for antigen-specific IgE. Systemic cyclosporine.
Food allergy (cutaneous adverse food reaction) Dogs, cats, horses	Bilaterally symmetrical periorbital erythema; alopecia and crusting due to self-trauma Distribution of pruritus involves feet, face, ears, axillae, inguinal regions. In cats, head, periorbita, and neck involved. Horses may be presented with urticarial reactions.	Nonseasonal history of pruritus. Resolution of pruritus with feeding of a single novel protein-source diet. Diagnosis confirmed by rechallenge with previous diet for return of pruritic signs. All secondary opportunistic infections must be identified and treated.	Strict diet using a single novel protein source. Treat all secondary infections.
Contact dermatitis (irritant or allergic) Dogs, cats, horses, ruminants	Erythema, papules, exudation and crusting, alopecia. Lesions are seen in sparsely haired regions or areas with known contact with substance (consider topical therapies, i.e., eye medications).	Distribution of lesions Provocative exposure or patch testing	Avoid exposure. Remove offending substance with bathing. Corticosteroids.
Drug hypersensitivity/drug eruption/fixed drug eruption Dogs, cats, horses, cattle	Pleomorphic cutaneous or mucocutaneous reactions. Can look like other skin diseases. Often bilaterally symmetrical.	Accurate past drug history. Skin biopsy.	Remove offending drug.

ELISA, Enzyme-linked immunosorbent assay; *IgE*, immunoglobulin E; *PCR*, polymerase chain reaction.

Table 6-3 | **Skin Diseases Affecting the Eyelids—cont'd**

DISORDER AND AFFECTED ANIMALS	CLINICAL SIGNS	DIAGNOSIS	TREATMENT
AUTOIMMUNE			
Pemphigus foliaceus Dogs, cats, horses, goats Breed predilections: chow chow, Akita, bearded collie, Newfoundland, schipperke, Doberman dogs; appaloosa horses	Exfoliative crusting, pustular dermatitis Individual pustules may be large. Often begins on the face (dorsal muzzle, periorbital) with bilaterally symmetrical generalize, often involving footpads. Often involves coronary bands in horses ± concurrent pitting edema. Can be predominantly facial.	Skin biopsy: broad subcorneal pustules often spanning several follicles. Neutrophilic or eosinophilic infiltrate with rafts of acantholytic cells.	Immunosuppressive doses of corticosteroids (all species). Can also consider gold salts (chrysotherapy; all species), chlorambucil (dogs and cats), or azathioprine (not in cats).
Pemphigus vulgaris Dogs, cats Rare	Vesicobullous eruptions lead rapidly to ulcerative lesions with irregular margins. Oral cavity (90%) and mucocutaneous junctions are affected. Nikolsky's sign may be present.	Skin biopsy: suprabasilar clefting with acantholysis leading to bulla formation	Immunosuppressive therapy with corticosteroids, azathioprine, chlorambucil. Poor prognosis.
Pemphigus erythematosus Dogs, cats Breed predilections: collie, German shepherd Rare	Erythematous, pustular dermatitis of face and ears with crusts, exudation, alopecia, and erosions. Typically, lesions are bilaterally symmetrical. Depigmentation of nasal planum may be seen. Restricted to head and neck.	Skin biopsy ± DIF, positive ANA result *Histology:* Subcorneal pustule formation with acantholysis. There may be some lichenoid interface inflammation at the epidermal-dermal junction. Ideally, DIF-positive at intercellular and possibly basement membrane zones.	Topical corticosteroids, tetracycline, niacinamide, systemic corticosteroids, azathioprine in dogs
Discoid lupus erythematosus Dogs Breed predilections: collie, Shetland sheepdog, German shepherd, Siberian husky Common autoimmune skin disease in dogs	Lesions restricted to face: depigmentation, erythema, scaling, ulceration of the nasal planum causing loss of cobblestone appearance; can involve dorsal muzzle, periorbital, lip margins. Typically, lesions are bilaterally symmetrical. Scarring and fibrosis cause flaring of alar folds.	Skin biopsy ± DIF, negative ANA result *Histology:* Patchy vacuolar degeneration of the basal cell layer. Lichenoid or interface dermatitis. Heavily lymphoplasmacytic infiltrate. Apoptotic cells may be evident. Pigmentary incontinence.	Avoid sun exposure; use topical sunscreens and corticosteroids, topical tacrolimus. Systemic tetracycline and niacinamide.
Systemic lupus erythematosus Dogs, cats Breed predilections: collie, Shetland sheepdog, spitz, poodle, German shepherd dogs; Siamese cats at increased risk	Multisystemic disease. Cutaneous signs are seen in <20% of cases. Pleomorphic lesions: erythema, alopecia, scaling, crusting, depigmentation often partially bilaterally symmetrical Ulcerations of footpads, mucocutaneous junctions, and oral cavity can occur.	Skin biopsy ± DIF, positive ANA result, systemic evaluation for immune-mediated disease in other organ systems: polyarthritis, anemia, uveitis, myositis, thrombocytopenia, neutropenia, glomerulonephritis. *Histology:* Lichenoid interface dermatitis with vacuolar degeneration of the basal cell layer. Presence of apoptotic cells. Ideally, DIF-positive at basement membrane; often in a clumped pattern.	Immunosuppressive therapy with corticosteroids ± azathioprine or other immunosuppressive drugs. Appropriate supportive therapy: fluids, transfusion.
Bullous dermatosis affecting basement membrane zone: bullous pemphigoid, epidermolysis bullosa acquisita Dogs, horses	Vesiculobullous; intact lesions and multifocal ulcerative lesions may be seen; affects oral cavity, mucocutaneous junctions, and intertriginous areas of groin and axillae	Skin biopsy ± DIF *Histology:* Subepidermal cleft formation. Acantholysis is not seen. Ideally, DIF-positive at basement membrane; zone in bullous pemphigoid.	Immunosuppressive therapy: corticosteroids, azathioprine, chlorambucil

ANA, Antinuclear antibody; *DIF,* direct immunofluorescence.

Continued

Table 6-3 | **Skin Diseases Affecting the Eyelids—cont'd**

DISORDER AND AFFECTED ANIMALS	CLINICAL SIGNS	DIAGNOSIS	TREATMENT
Vogt-Koyanagi-Harada (VKH)–like (or uveodermatologic) syndrome Dogs Breed predilection: Akita	Symmetric depigmentation of nasal planum, muzzle, periorbital. Erythema and crusting may be noted in affected areas. Concurrent uveitis.	Skin biopsy. Clinical signs (concurrent uveitis) and breed affected. *Histology:* Decreased or absent epidermal melanin. Early lesions have dermal inflammation with large macrophages containing melanin pigment.	Systemic corticosteroids and azathioprine as well as topical (ophthalmic) prednisolone. Level of therapy usually dictated by severity of ophthalmic lesions. Cutaneous lesions are generally milder and are markers for the ophthalmic disease.
Alopecia areata Dogs, cats, horses Breed predilection: dachshund	Focal or multifocal patches of alopecia with no associated inflammation. Pinnal and symmetrical periorbital alopecia may be present.	Skin biopsy *Histology:* Epidermis is normal. Hair follicles are atrophic and sometimes distorted. Inflammatory cells around the distal portion of the follicle.	None. Can recover spontaneously.
Nodular panniculitis Dogs	Focal or multifocal dermal nodules that rupture with greasy exudate and crust formation. Smaller nodules may be present on eyelid margins. Animals often appear systemically unwell.	Skin biopsy, negative fungal and bacterial cultures from macerated tissue. Systemic workup; rule out pancreatitis and infectious causes. *Histology:* Multiple dermal granulomas or pyogranulomas composed of large macrophages and neutrophils may extend to involve panniculus.	Immunosuppressive therapy with corticosteroids, azathioprine
ISCHEMIC/VASCULAR DISEASES			
Canine familial dermatomyositis Dogs Breed predilections: collie, sheltie, fox terrier, corgi	Alopecia, crusting, erosions, and scarring. Often facial, particularly over bony prominences, distal extremities, tip of tail. Signs of muscle involvement may be present: weakness, megaesophagus.	Skin biopsy ± EMG and muscle biopsy	Pentoxifylline, vitamin E, corticosteroids, niacinamide, and tetracycline. Treat secondary infections.
Vaccine-induced ischemic dermatopathy Dogs	Alopecia, erythema, scaling. Ulceration. Often tail tip, ear margins, periocular.	Skin biopsy. May be associated with recent vaccinations, particularly rabies vaccine.	Pentoxifylline, vitamin E, corticosteroids, niacinamide, and tetracycline. Treat secondary infections.
NUTRITIONAL/METABOLIC DISEASES			
Zinc-responsive dermatitis Dogs Breed predilections: arctic breeds (husky, malamute)	Adherent fine scale, crusting, erosions, and ulcers. Often perioral and periorbital distribution.	Compatible signalment and clinical signs. Skin biopsy.	Zinc supplementation
Generic dog food–associated Dogs	Well-demarcated lesions of severe adherent scale, crusting, erosions and ulceration; perioral and periocular in distribution. Animals appear systemically unwell.	Skin biopsy and history of inappropriate diet	Good-quality diet
Superficial necrolytic dermatitis (hepatocutaneous syndrome) Dogs	Ulceration, severe crusting, alopecia. Perioral, periorbital, pinnae, perianal, scrotal. Almost always involves foot pads with severe hyperkeratosis and fissuring.	Skin biopsy. Systemic workup is indicated. Associated with hepatic or pancreatic disease. Characteristic hepatic changes on ultrasonography and characteristic hepatic histopathology. Minority of dogs may have pancreatic glucagonoma. Plasma amino acids, if measured, are markedly depleted.	Palliative therapy with protein supplementation, fatty acids, and zinc may improve the cutaneous manifestations. Parenteral therapy with intravenous amino acids may be beneficial for some dogs. Long-term prognosis is poor.

EMG, Electromyography.

Table 6-3 | **Skin Diseases Affecting the Eyelids—cont'd**

DISORDER AND AFFECTED ANIMALS	CLINICAL SIGNS	DIAGNOSIS	TREATMENT
NEOPLASTIC			
Squamous cell carcinoma* Dogs, cats, horses, cattle	Erosions, ulceration, particularly of nonpigmented skin	Biopsy	Surgical resection, cryosurgery, radiation therapy, strontium therapy, photodynamic therapy
Sarcoid Horses	Verrucous or proliferative plaques or nodules	Biopsy	Cryosurgery, BCG, intralesional chemotherapy
Melanoma* Dogs, horses, cats Breed predilection: gray-coated horses	Firm, raised, alopecic lesions. Epithelium is usually intact but may be ulcerated, and tumor is typically pigmented. May be epidermal or dermal.	Cytology of fine-needle aspirate. Biopsy.	Wide surgical excision, radiation, photodynamic therapy *Horses:* surgical excision, cryosurgery, cimetidine
Histiocytoma* Dogs	Rapidly growing, alopecic, erythematous, raised nodules in young dogs. May have ulcerated surface.	Cytology of fine-needle aspirate. Biopsy.	Spontaneous regression typical over weeks to months
Reactive histiocytosis (two forms: cutaneous and systemic) Dogs Breed predilections: Bernese mountain dog, golden retriever	Skin lesions include multiple papules, nodules, and plaques anywhere on the body. Lesions may ulcerate. Frequently on muzzle, eyelids, nasal planum. Lesions of cutaneous histiocytosis are limited to the skin; if lymph nodes, conjunctiva, sclera, nasal cavity, lungs, spleen, or bone marrow is involved, dog has systemic histiocytosis.	Skin biopsy. Systemic workup: radiography and ultrasonography to evaluate for hepatic and splenic involvement.	Therapies to consider include systemic corticosteroids, cyclosporine, and leflunomide.
Mastocytoma/mast cell tumor* Dogs, cats, horses	Single cutaneous nodule; surface may be alopecic, haired, or ulcerated; may be associated with erythema.	Cytology of fine-needle aspirate. Biopsy. Often benign in horses	Wide surgical excision, radiation therapy, intralesional therapy, various chemotherapy protocols
Epitheliotrophic cutaneous T-cell lymphoma (*Mycoses fungoides*) Dogs, cats, horses	Pleomorphic, exfoliative lesions with erythema Depigmentation of nasal philtrum	Biopsy	Corticosteroids, retinoids, lomustine, other chemotherapeutics associated with variable, often poor, results, resection for solitary lesions, radiation therapy
PIGMENTARY DISORDERS			
Vitiligo* Dogs, horses, cats, cattle Breed predilection: Rottweiler	Focal loss of pigment in skin and hair. Often macular depigmentation that involves muzzle, nasal planum, eyelid margins, and eyelashes. Can also affect foot pads.	Clinical signs. Skin biopsy.	Consider tetracycline and niacinamide; dietary supplements in large animals. Therapy may not restore pigment in all cases.
Lentigo simplex* Orange cats	Macular pigmentation of nasal planum, gingival margins, eyelid margins.	Clinical signs	None
MISCELLANEOUS			
Juvenile cellulitis Dogs	Pustules, nodules, fistulous tracts, exudative. Pronounced lymphadenopathy. Affects ears, muzzle, periorbital area, and eyelids. Animals often appear systemically unwell: concurrent fever, lameness.	Distinctive lesions in young puppy. Skin biopsy. Cytology of fine-needle aspirate of lymph nodes. Negative cultures.	Corticosteroids ± antibiotics?

BCG, Bacille Calmette-Guérin.

BIBLIOGRAPHY

Bonney CH, et al. (1980): Papillomatosis of the conjunctiva and adnexa in dogs. J Am Vet Med Assoc 176:48.

Bowman DD (2003): Georgi's Parasitology for Veterinarians, 8th ed. Saunders, St. Louis.

Bussieres M, et al. (2005): The use of carbon dioxide laser for the ablation of meibomian gland adenomas in dogs. J Am Anim Hosp Assoc 41:227.

Cantaloube B, et al. (2004): Multiple eyelid apocrine hidrocystomas in two Persian cats. Vet Ophthalmol 7:121.

Chambers ED, Severin GA (1984): Staphylococcal bacterin for treatment of chronic staphylococcal blepharitis in the dog. J Am Vet Med Assoc 185:422.

Chambers ED, Slatter DH (1984): Cryotherapy of canine distichiasis and trichiasis. An experimental and clinical report. J Small Anim Pract 25:647.

Collins BK, et al. (1992): Idiopathic granulomatous disease with ocular adnexal and cutaneous involvement in a dog. J Am Vet Med Assoc 201:313.

Degner DA, Walshaw R (1997): Medial saphenous fasciocutaneous and myocutaneous free flap transfer in eight dogs. Vet Surg 26:20.

Donaldson D, et al. (2005): Surgical management of cicatricial ectropion following scarring dermatopathies in two dogs. Vet Ophthalmol 8:361.

Dziezyc J, Millichamp NJ (1989): Surgical correction of eyelid agenesis in a cat. J Am Anim Hosp Assoc 25:515.

Greene CE (2006): Infectious Diseases of the Dog and Cat, 3rd ed. Saunders, St. Louis.

Gross TL, et al. (2005): Skin Diseases of the Dog and Cat: Clinical and Histopathologic Diagnosis, 2nd ed. Blackwell Science, Oxford, England.

Hamilton HL, et al. (2000): Diagnosis and blepharoplastic repair of conformational eyelid defects. Compend Cont Ed Pract Vet 22:588.

Helper LC, Magrane WG (1970): Ectopic cilia of the canine eyelid. J Small Anim Pract 11:185.

Hoffman A, et al. (2005): Feline periocular peripheral nerve sheath tumor: a case series. Vet Ophthalmol 8:153.

Hurn S, et al. (2005): Ectopic cilium in seven horses. Vet Ophthalmol 8:199.

Johnson BW, Campbell KL (1989): Dermatoses of the canine eyelid. Comp Cont Ed 11:385.

Krehbiel JD, Langham RF (1975): Eyelid neoplasms of dogs. Am J Vet Res 36:115.

Lackner PA (2001): Techniques for surgical correction of adnexal disease. Clin Tech Small Anim Pract 16:40.

Lavach JD, Severin GA (1977): Neoplasia of the equine eye, adnexa and orbit—a review of 68 cases. J Am Vet Med Assoc 170:202.

Lewin G (2003): Eyelid reconstruction in seven dogs using a split eyelid flap. J Small Anim Pract 44:346.

Martin CM, et al. (1996): Ocular adnexal cryptococcosis in a cat. Vet Comp Ophthalmol 6:225.

Mosunic CB, et al. (2004): Effects of treatment with and without adjuvant radiation therapy on recurrence of ocular and adnexal squamous cell carcinoma in horses: 157 cases (1985-2002). J Am Vet Med Assoc 225:1733.

Newton SA (2000): Periocular sarcoids in the horse: three cases of successful treatment. Equine Vet Ed 12:137.

Owen RA, Jagger DW (1987): Clinical observations on the use of BCG cell wall fraction for treatment of periocular and other equine sarcoids. Vet Rec 120:548.

Pellicane CP (1994): Eyelid reconstruction in five dogs by the semicircular flap technique. Vet Comp Ophthalmol 4:93.

Poli A, et al. (2002): Feline leishmaniosis due to Leishmania infantum in Italy. Vet Parasitol 106:181.

Roberts SM, et al. (1986): Prevalence and treatment of palpebral neoplasms in the dog—200 cases (1975-1983). J Am Vet Med Assoc 189:1355.

Scherlie PH (1992): Ocular manifestation of systemic histiocytosis in a dog. J Am Vet Med Assoc 201:1229.

Scott DW, et al. (2001): Muller & Kirk's Small Animal Dermatology, 6th ed. Saunders, Philadelphia.

Scott DW, Miller WH (2003): Equine Dermatology. Saunders, St. Louis.

Smith BP (2002): Large Animal Internal Medicine, 3rd ed. Mosby, St. Louis.

Stiles J, et al. (2003): Use of a caudal auricular axial pattern flap in three cats and one dog following orbital exenteration. Vet Ophthalmol 6:121.

Theon A, et al. (1993): Intratumoral chemotherapy with cisplatin in oily emulsion in horses. J Vet Med Assoc 202:261.

Theon AP, Pascoe JR (1995): Iridium-192 interstitial brachytherapy for equine periocular tumors: treatment results and prognostic factors in 115 horses. Equine Vet J 27:117.

van der Woerdt A (2004): Adnexal surgery in dogs and cats. Vet Ophthalmol 7:284.

Withrow SJ, Vail DM (2007): Withrow & MacEwen's Small Animal Clinical Oncology, 4th ed. Saunders, St. Louis.

Wolfer JC (2002): Correction of eyelid coloboma in four cats using subdermal collagen and a modified Stades technique. Vet Ophthalmol 5:269.

CONJUNCTIVA

David J. Maggs

ANATOMY AND PHYSIOLOGY

CLINICAL SIGNS OF CONJUNCTIVAL
DISEASE

CONJUNCTIVITIS
OTHER CONJUNCTIVAL DISORDERS

ANATOMY AND PHYSIOLOGY

The conjunctiva is a mobile mucous membrane covering the inner surface of the lids, the inner and outer surfaces of the third eyelid, and the anterior portion of the globe adjacent to the limbus (Figure 7-1). The space lined by the conjunctiva is called the conjunctival sac. The palpebral conjunctiva is tightly bound to the inner surface of the lids. In the dorsal fornix the conjunctiva is supported by an anterior extension of the muscle sheath of the levator palpebrae and dorsal rectus muscles. This band moves the loose conjunctiva of the fornix with the globe and prevents it from falling down over the cornea. The bulbar conjunctiva is loosely attached to the episclera over the globe and is anchored more firmly near the limbus.

The conjunctiva consists of a nonkeratinized columnar epithelium with goblet cells, subtended by the substantia propria and overlaid by the tear film (Figure 7-2). The tear film that coats and nourishes the cornea is also an essential protective and nutritional layer for the conjunctiva. Alterations in tear film quantity or quality, as seen with keratoconjunctivitis sicca, cause marked deterioration in conjunctival as well as corneal health. Additionally, the conjunctival goblet cells contribute the mucin layer of the tear film, which gathers in the conjunctival fornices as a mucous thread. The mucous thread migrates medially, gathering dust particles and cells for eventual disposal down the nasolacrimal duct or onto the surface of the skin at the medial canthus. In animals with a deep inferior fornix (e.g., Irish setters, Dobermans, collies), the normal mucous thread may be particularly prominent, accumulating as a grayish gelatinous mass at the medial canthus (so-called medial canthal pocket syndrome).

The conjunctiva is the most exposed mucous membrane in the body. To respond rapidly to noxious stimuli, it has well-developed defense mechanisms and has been compared with an everted lymph node (Figure 7-3). The subepithelial substantia propria comprises loose fibrous connective tissue but also contains numerous lymphocytes that, when stimulated by antigens, form active follicles. These follicles are present throughout the conjunctiva but are particularly numerous on the bulbar surface of the third eyelid. Two layers of lymphatic drainage are present—one adjacent to the superficial conjunctival blood vessels and one in the deeper fibrous layer.

The arterial supply of the conjunctiva is prolific, coming from the peripheral and marginal arcades of the eyelids and the anterior ciliary arteries. The superficial conjunctival vessels overlie the deeper, straighter episcleral vessels, although the two systems communicate. The superficial conjunctival vessels form loops or arcades at the limbus. It is from these loops that "endothelial budding" occurs in response to superficial corneal disease, resulting in superficial corneal vascularization. Deep corneal vascularization originates from the deeper episcleral and scleral blood vessels.

Conjunctival Wound Healing

Simple, uncomplicated wounds of the conjunctiva heal rapidly, usually within 24 to 48 hours. Denuded areas of sclera are also rapidly reepithelialized in this manner. Within a few hours, conjunctiva attaches to the episclera, and healing occurs by epithelial sliding and mitosis.

Cellular Responses in Conjunctival Disease

Identification of predominant cell type(s) in the conjunctiva may be useful in differentiating possible causes and chronicity of conjunctivitis (Table 7-1). Neutrophils are typically seen in acute conjunctivitis, especially of bacterial or viral origin. Lymphocytes and plasma cells are more typical of chronic and often immune-mediated conjunctivitis and sometimes organize into follicles visible both histologically and clinically (Figure 7-4). Lymphoid follicles indicate chronic antigenic stimulation and do not signify a specific disease. Eosinophils are seen in allergic or immune-mediated conjunctivitis, especially in cats and horses. As conjunctivitis becomes more chronic, goblet cells can increase in number, and the epithelium proliferates and is thrown into folds (papillary hypertrophy), which give it a "velvety" appearance. Metaplasia of the conjunctiva may occur with chronic vitamin A deficiency, especially in chickens and turtles/tortoises. Inflammatory membranes may also form as conjunctivitis becomes chronic. True membranes consist of cellular debris and fibrin, are firmly attached to the underlying epithelium, and when removed leave a raw, bleeding surface. Pseudomembranes consist of similar material that is nonadherent and easily removed.

CLINICAL SIGNS OF CONJUNCTIVAL DISEASE

The accurate observation and interpretation of conjunctival signs are essential in the differential diagnosis of "the red eye." Too frequently, serious intraocular diseases such as uveitis and

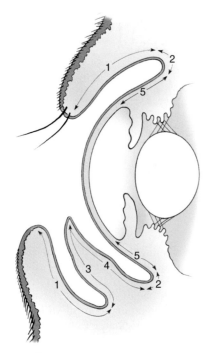

Figure 7-1. Areas of conjunctiva: *1,* palpebral; *2,* fornix; *3,* anterior third eyelid; *4,* posterior third eyelid; *5,* bulbar.

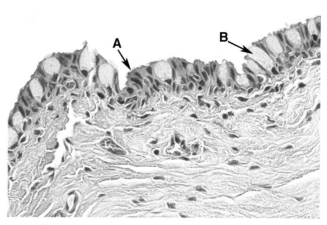

Figure 7-2. Normal conjunctival histology. **A,** Columnar epithelial cells; **B,** goblet cells. Substantia propria lies beneath the epithelium and contains numerous spaces and blood vessels of significance in the formation of chemosis.

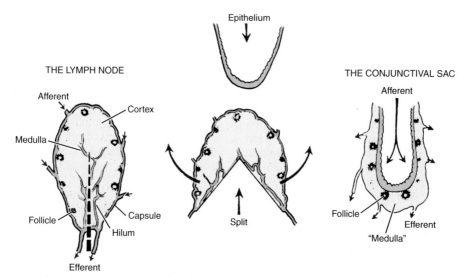

Figure 7-3. The relationship between a lymph node and the conjunctival sac. (Modified from Duke-Elder S [1965]: System of Ophthalmology, Vol 8, Part II. Henry Kimpton, London.)

glaucoma, which also produce redness, are misdiagnosed as conjunctivitis, and the underlying disorder continues, destroying vision or the eye and leading to chronic discomfort or occasionally death of the animal from systemic disease.

Conjunctival inflammation is typically characterized by conjunctival hyperemia, ocular discharge, and chemosis (conjunctival edema). Other changes seen in conjunctival disease are summarized in Box 7-1.

Conjunctival Hyperemia

Conjunctival hyperemia generally occurs as a result of local release of inflammatory mediators (conjunctivitis). Occasion-

ally, conjunctival hyperemia can occur as a result of reduced venous drainage due to increased central venous pressure (e.g., ventricular septal defect) or, more commonly, obstruction of local venous drainage by cervical or orbital neoplasms. It is essential to distinguish hyperemia (or injection) of episcleral vessels from hyperemia of conjunctival vessels, because this distinction permits the critical differentiation of deep and potentially vision-threatening diseases, such as uveitis, glaucoma, and deep (stromal) keratitis, from more superficial surface ocular diseases, such as conjunctivitis and superficial keratitis (Table 7-2).

Episcleral and conjunctival injection can coexist. Therefore it is essential to realize that although more serious deep corneal

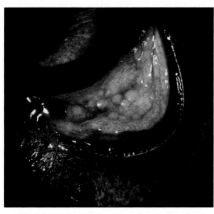

Figure 7-4. Follicular conjunctivitis in a dog. Note the follicle formation in the ventral conjunctival fornix and on the anterior face of the third eyelid.

Table 7-1 | **Cellular Responses Associated with Specific Conjunctivitides**

DISEASE	CELLULAR RESPONSE
Acute bacterial conjunctivitis	Predominantly neutrophils; few mononuclear cells; many bacteria; degenerating epithelial cells
Chronic bacterial conjunctivitis	Predominantly neutrophils; many mononuclear cells; degenerate or keratinized epithelial cells; goblet cells; bacteria may or may not be seen; mucus; fibrin
Feline herpesvirus conjunctivitis	Pseudomembrane formation; giant cells; fibrin; erythrocyte, neutrophil, and mononuclear cell numbers depend on stage of infection
Feline mycoplasmal conjunctivitis	Predominantly neutrophils; fewer mononuclear cells; basophilic coccoid or pleomorphic organisms on cell membrane
Feline chlamydial conjunctivitis	Predominantly neutrophils; in subacute cases mononuclear cells increased in number; plasma cells; giant cells; basophilic cytoplasmic inclusions early in the disease
Keratoconjunctivitis sicca	Keratinized epithelial cells; goblet cells; mucus; neutrophilic response marked if there is much infection; bacteria
Canine distemper	Varies with stage of disease: early—giant cells and mononuclear cells; later—neutrophils, goblet cells, and mucus; infrequent intracellular inclusions
Allergic conjunctivitis	Eosinophils; neutrophils may be marked; basophils possible

From Lavach JD, et al. (1977): Cytology of normal and inflamed conjunctivas in dogs and cats. J Am Vet Med Assoc 170:772.

Box 7-1 | **Clinical signs of conjunctival pathology**

Ocular discharge (typically mucoid)
Chemosis
Conjunctival hyperemia
Abnormal swellings
Emphysema
Follicle formation
Pruritus
Hemorrhage

Table 7-2 | **Differentiation of Episcleral and Conjunctival Injection**

CONJUNCTIVAL VESSELS	EPISCLERAL VESSELS
Finer	Larger
Branch frequently	Branch occasionally
Form arcades or loops at limbus	Dive through sclera just before limbus
Pink/red	Dark red
Mobile	Fixed
Bulbar, palpebral, forniceal, and third eyelid all involved	Seen only overlying sclera
Tortuous route	Relatively straight
Blanch rapidly with topical application of dilute epinephrine (1:100,000) or phenylephrine (0.25%)	Blanch slowly if at all with topical application of dilute epinephrine (1:100,000) or phenylephrine (0.25%)
Individual vessels tend to be indistinct	Individual vessels tend to be distinct
Ocular discharge often mucoid or mucopurulent	Ocular discharge often serous
Pupil size usually normal	Miosis or mydriasis possible
Intraocular pressure (IOP) usually normal	IOP usually high or low
Chemosis often present	Chemosis sometimes present
Diffuse corneal edema usually not present	Diffuse corneal edema often present
Presence indicates conjunctival or superficial corneal disease	Presence indicates scleral or deep corneal disease, glaucoma, or uveitis

or intraocular disease can cause "innocent bystander" inflammation of the conjunctival vessels, the reverse is not true.

Ocular Discharge

Mucopurulent discharge is a common sign of conjunctival disease, especially keratoconjunctivitis sicca. Epiphora alone is rarely a sign of primary conjunctival pathology unless accompanied by other signs, such as increased production of mucus, follicle formation, hyperemia, or blepharospasm. With severe ocular discharge the eyelid margins may stick together, especially upon waking. Change in color of the mucous thread from transparent or gray to yellow is due to accumulation of inflammatory cells and cellular debris within it. Sanguineous discharge is seen in ulcerative or traumatic conjunctivitis.

Chemosis (Conjunctival Edema)

Chemosis may be caused by any stimulus that results in acute inflammation. It is especially common in acute allergic conjunctivitis, toxic injuries, and trauma. It is usually but not always seen with concurrent hyperemia and can be dramatic enough to prevent full eyelid closure and to predispose to conjunctival desiccation.

Conjunctival and Subconjunctival Hemorrhage

Subconjunctival extravasations and ecchymoses are seen relatively frequently with severe, acute, systemic inflammation (septicemia), vasculitis, and coagulopathies as well as after trauma. Large subconjunctival hemorrhages are usually traumatic in origin. The hemorrhage is resorbed over 7 to 10 days and changes successively from bright red to dark red, yellow, and white.

Subconjunctival Emphysema

Subconjunctival emphysema manifests as a subconjunctival swelling with crepitus. It is caused by the entry of air into the periorbita from surrounding paranasal sinuses, usually after traumatic damage to the sinus walls. Subconjunctival emphysema is an indication for thorough imaging of the sinuses and a complete ocular examination. Depending on the severity of the initial trauma, subconjunctival hemorrhages and intraocular damage may also be present. In the absence of more severe lesions the air is usually absorbed in 7 to 14 days. A systemic antibiotic should be administered to prevent orbital infection by normal flora from the damaged sinus.

Follicle Formation

Lymphoid follicles frequently occur after chronic antigenic stimulation (see Figure 7-4). Slight epiphora and follicle formation are often the only signs of mild allergic conjunctivitis. Follicles are normally present on the bulbar surface of the third eyelid but, after stimulation, may appear in other parts of the conjunctiva.

Pruritus

Conjunctivitis is commonly associated with pruritus, although the history provided by the owner, plus secondary lesions (e.g., periocular alopecia and erythema, stained or matted hair on the medial aspect of the metacarpus) may be the only indication. Deep ocular pain, as in glaucoma or uveitis, is more likely to cause blepharospasm or changes in behavior or appetite suggestive of pain. Superficial pruritus usually causes rubbing motions with the paws.

Swellings or Conjunctival Masses

Swellings and infiltrates are examined for color, rate of growth, position, and attachment to conjunctiva, sclera, or adjacent structures. Although not all swellings and infiltrates are tumors, the diagnostic approach and some potential causes are discussed in the section on conjunctival neoplasia.

CONJUNCTIVITIS

Classification

Conjunctivitis has been classified on the basis of duration, nature of discharge, appearance, and etiology (Boxes 7-2 and 7-3). Of these, etiology is the most important, and an etiologic diagnosis should always be sought as a basis for rational therapy. Classification according to duration or appearance is useful only as a step toward an etiologic diagnosis. Numerous systemic diseases—canine distemper, feline herpesvirus, *Chlamydophila* spp., and infectious bovine rhinotracheitis—may also cause conjunctivitis and must be considered.

Differential Diagnosis

The general and common clinical signs of conjunctivitis (hyperemia, discharge, chemosis, and follicle formation) do not assist with an etiologic diagnosis or with the differentiation of primary from secondary conjunctivitis. In fact, conjunctiva is often secondarily inflamed with almost all other ocular and periocular diseases, including primary keratitis, orbital disease,

---

Box 7-2 | Means of classifying conjunctivitis

Etiology	Duration	Appearance
Bacterial	Acute	Mucoid ("catarrhal")
Viral	Subacute	Purulent
Fungal	Chronic	Mucopurulent
Parasitic	Recurrent	Hemorrhagic
Immune-mediated		Follicular
Toxic or chemical		Membranous
Tear film abnormalities		Pseudomembranous
Frictional (see Box 7-3):		Ligneous
Endogenous		
Exogenous		

Box 7-3 | Frictional irritants causing conjunctivitis

Exogenous	Endogenous
Foreign body	Qualitative tear film deficiencies
Dust	Quantitative tear film deficiencies
Sand	Entropion
Smoke	Distichiasis
Smog/pollution	Nasal fold trichiasis
Low humidity	Ectopic cilia
Allergens	Ectropion
Wind	Lagophthalmos
Contaminated water	
Toxins	

---

blepharitis, keratoconjunctivitis sicca, dacryocystitis, uveitis, and glaucoma. Therefore conjunctivitis should be seen as a potential sign of numerous, diverse, and often blinding ocular diseases and occasionally as a sign of systemic and potentially life-threatening disease. As a result every eye in which conjunctival inflammation is identified should undergo thorough diagnostic testing including at the very least comparison of pupil size between eyes, Schirmer tear testing, assessment of aqueous flare and intraocular pressure, globe retropulsion, and application of fluorescein stain. An algorithm showing the diagnostic approach to a patient with conjunctival inflammation is shown in Figure 7-5.

Once it has been verified that the patient has primary conjunctivitis and not conjunctival inflammation as a sign of more serious ocular and/or systemic disease, a specific etiologic diagnosis should be sought (see Box 7-2, Box 7-3, and Figure 7-5). The major causes of conjunctivitis vary by species. For example, feline conjunctivitis is largely infectious (*Chlamydophila felis* or feline herpesvirus), whereas canine conjunctivitis is almost exclusively noninfectious (e.g., pannus, keratoconjunctivitis sicca, entropion, foreign bodies, etc.). By contrast, horses are rarely affected with primary infectious conjunctivitis and are more likely to have conjunctival inflammation as a sign of keratitis or uveitis, and ruminants are more prone to infectious conjunctivitides. These guidelines should be used to aid in prioritizing differential diagnoses in each species.

Diagnostic Methods

Bacterial Culturing

Bacterial culturing is not the first diagnostic procedure in determining the cause of conjunctivitis. Very few primary bacteria cause conjunctivitis, especially in small animals, and most (*Chlamydophila, Mycoplasma,* etc.) require special collection

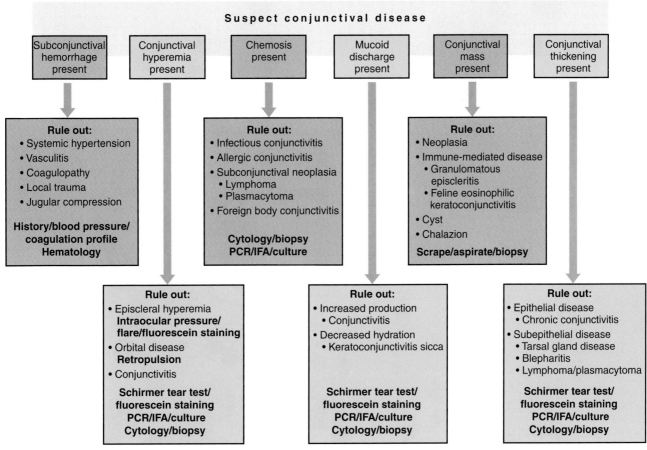

Figure 7-5. Diagnostic algorithm for common pathological responses in patients with conjunctival disease. *IFA,* Immunofluorescent antibody; *PCR,* polymerase chain reaction. (Modified from Slatter D [2003]: Textbook of Small Animal Surgery, 3rd ed. Saunders, Philadelphia.)

and/or culture conditions. Therefore cultures are performed rarely and usually after initial antibiotic therapy has been unsuccessful. In fact, cultures usually show either an organism present in the normal flora or a common pathogen. Failure of conjunctivitis to respond to antibiotics is more commonly the result of incorrect diagnosis and failure to determine the etiology rather than incorrect choice of antibiotic. Many causes of conjunctivitis result in increased numbers of bacteria from the normal flora or growth of common pathogens, and, therefore the cause of the conjunctivitis typically should not be ascribed to the bacteria isolated.

When culture specimens are taken, swabs should be moistened (with saline solution), and the sample plated onto blood agar or into nutrient and thioglycollate broth as soon as possible. See Tables 3-1, 3-3, 3-4, and 3-6 to 3-9 in Chapter 3 for normal ocular surface flora of common domestic species.

Conjunctival Scrapings

Unlike culture, scrapings and biopsies are frequently extremely useful for better defining cause and chronicity of conjunctivitis and for guiding therapy. Scrapings are particularly useful to determine the potential malignancy of cells associated with conjunctival masses, such as squamous cell carcinoma. For method of collection, see Chapter 5. Scrapings are examined for cellular alterations (Giemsa stain) and bacteria (Gram stain) as well as inclusion bodies. Intracytoplasmic melanin granules should be differentiated from other inclusions (e.g., chlamydial

elementary bodies, and *Mycoplasma* spp. in cats and sheep). The types of cells commonly encountered are described in Figure 7-6 and Table 7-1.

Conjunctival Biopsy

A small "snip biopsy" of conjunctiva can be obtained with use of only topical anesthesia. After topical application of two drops of anesthetic 5 minutes apart, a cotton-tipped applicator soaked in proparacaine (or other topical ophthalmic anesthetic) should be applied gently to the surface. A small area of the conjunctiva to be sampled is then delicately "tented" with fine tissue forceps and resected with small tenotomy scissors (Figure 7-7). The sample should be minimally handled to avoid artifactual changes, spread onto a flat surface, and fixed for histologic processing. Before fixation, equine conjunctival samples also may be sliced and incubated in saline at 37° C, and the supernatant centrifuged and examined for *Onchocerca* microfilaria.

General Treatment Considerations for Conjunctivitis

After determination of the etiology and treatment of non-conjunctival factors (e.g., correction of lid defects, removal of foreign bodies, replacement of deficient tear film, protection from exogenous factors), the following therapeutic agents can be employed:

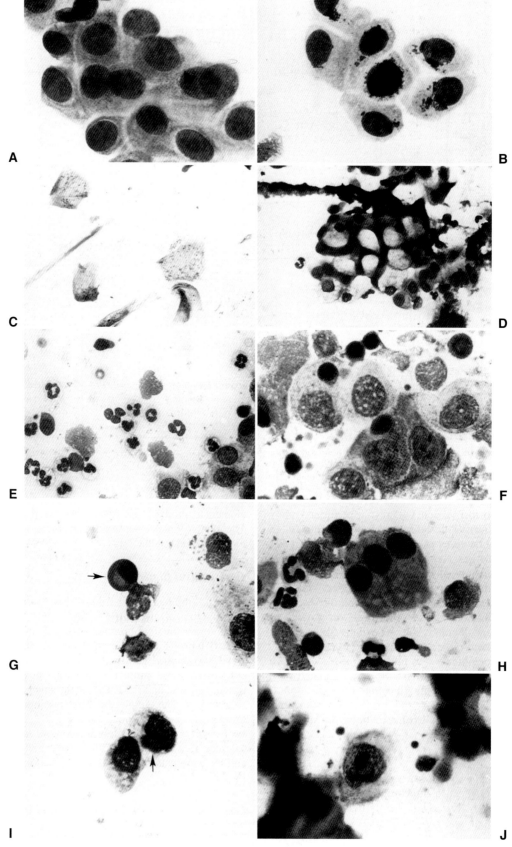

Figure 7-6. *For legend, see opposite page*

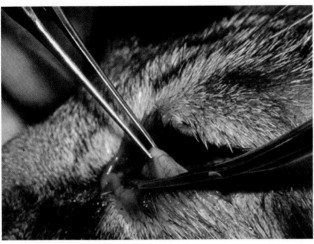

Figure 7-7. A conjunctival "snip" biopsy specimen being taken from the ventral conjunctival fornix of a cat with chronic conjunctivitis.

Antibiotics

Topical antibiotics are frequently prescribed for patients with conjunctivitis. This approach is appropriate, however, only for treating a primary bacterial conjunctivitis (which is relatively rare) or if the goal is simply to limit overgrowth of the normal conjunctival flora while the primary cause of conjunctivitis is simultaneously addressed by another therapy. The reflex use of an antibiotic whenever conjunctival inflammation is seen and without further testing or thought as to the primary cause of conjunctival inflammation must be avoided. Apparent (but temporary) response to antibiotic therapy can entrench such prescribing patterns. For example, conjunctivitis due to aqueous tear film dysfunction (keratoconjunctivitis sicca) will improve *while* but not *because* the patient is treated with an antibiotic. The improvement is due to both reduction of overgrowth of flora (which occurred because of tear film disturbance) and the lubricating property of the vehicle in which the antibiotic is delivered. Meanwhile, though, nothing has been done to limit the ongoing destruction of the lacrimal gland, thus reducing prognosis for response to cyclosporine at a later date. Giving consideration to the primary cause of conjunctivitis before prescribing an antibiotic (alone) is always warranted. See Chapter 3 for rational choices of antibiotics for specific conjunctival pathogens and overgrowth of flora.

Corticosteroids

Corticosteroids are commonly used to treat conjunctivitis, often in conjunction with antibiotics. However, as with anti-biotics, use of corticosteroids is not always rational. As a rule, they should be used in noninfectious disorders after correction of nonconjunctival factors. Their major role is in those conjunctivitides, such as pannus and allergic conjunctivitis, in which an immune-mediated cause is suspected. By contrast, corticosteroids are contraindicated in most feline conjunctivitides because the vast majority are infectious in nature (feline herpesvirus and *C. felis*). Corticosteroids should not be a routine part of conjunctivitis therapy or be used in the absence of a specific diagnosis.

Cleansing Agents

Removal of accumulated ocular discharge is important to prevent maceration, blepharitis, periocular dermatitis, and eyelid or conjunctival adhesions, and to improve patient comfort and penetration of ophthalmic medications. Therefore cleaning, flushing, and warm-packing of the eyelids is a useful adjunct in the early therapy of many conjunctival disorders, particularly when done in conjunction with more specific therapy. However, removal of one sign of conjunctivitis (discharge) is no substitute for specific treatment and resolution of the primary cause. Many commercial solutions are available. Cleansing may be followed by application of a bland protective ointment.

Topical Mast Cell Stabilizers and Antihistamines

Sodium cromoglycate, olopatadine, lodoxamide, and other mast cell–stabilizing agents have been used topically to treat allergic and eosinophilic conjunctivitis. However, anecdotal reports of the efficacy of these products vary, and controlled studies on their safety or efficacy in veterinary patients are lacking.

Vasoactive Agents

Sympathetic agents in low concentration are available and are used for their vasoactive effects. Their empirical use to reduce hyperemia and chemosis in acute conjunctivitis or allergy may be effective, but topical corticosteroids are more potent and better address the cause.

Bacterial Conjunctivitis

Primary bacterial conjunctivitis is common in cattle and sheep, in which *Moraxella bovis,* often in association with other agents, causes infectious keratoconjunctivitis (see Chapter 10). *Moraxella* spp. have also been isolated from horses with conjunctivitis in North America and Australia. In dogs, *Staphylococcus aureus, Staphylococcus epidermidis,* and *Streptococcus* spp. can be isolated from animals with external

Figure 7-6. Cell types found in different types of conjunctivitis. **A,** Epithelial conjunctival cells from a normal dog. The cells are found in sheets and are round to oval, with large nuclei. **B,** Conjunctival epithelial cells containing melanin granules. Melanin occurs in varying amounts and may be identified as dark green to black granules after Giemsa staining. **C,** Keratinized epithelial cells. These cells are abnormal in large numbers. **D,** Conjunctival goblet cells. Goblet cells contain a large amount of mucus, which displaces the nucleus to the periphery. **E,** Scraping from a dog with acute bacterial conjunctivitis. Large numbers of neutrophils and degenerating epithelial cells are present. **F,** Scraping from a kitten with herpesvirus infection. Mononuclear cells predominate. Viral inclusions are not visible. **G,** Plasma cell *(arrow).* This finding is abnormal and suggests inflammatory disease but is not associated with any specific disease. **H,** Multinucleated cell in a scraping from a dog with distemper. Neutrophils, mononuclear cells, and degenerating epithelial cells are also present. **I,** Chlamydial inclusion *(arrow)* in the cytoplasm of an epithelial cell from a cat with acute conjunctivitis. **J,** Neoplastic epithelial cell from a cat with squamous cell carcinoma of the lid margin. The cell is unusually large and vacuolated. (From Lavach JD, et al. [1977]: Cytology of normal and inflamed conjunctivas in dogs and cats. J Am Vet Med Assoc 170:722.)

ocular disease (see Table 3-2 in Chapter 3), but these organisms are frequently found in normal eyes and likely represent overgrowth of normal flora in an eye debilitated from another cause. Acute bacterial conjunctivitis can occur, however, especially in outdoor dogs that swim in contaminated water. Such cases should respond rapidly and completely to a short (7-day) course of a topical broad spectrum antibiotic and should not recur.

Conjunctivitis that does not respond or responds only temporarily to topical antibiotic therapy is unlikely to be bacterial in origin. Examination of the lids, lid margins, and nasolacrimal system, measurement of tear production and intraocular pressure, and fluorescein staining should form a routine part of examination in such eyes. Chronic bacterial conjunctivitis is frequently associated with lid abnormalities or with infections in the ear and skin; as such, it forms part of a spectrum of surface inflammatory conditions, including generalized seborrhea, pyoderma, and severe periodontal disease. These are sometimes exacerbated by endocrinopathies, and a complete diagnostic approach is recommended. Typically the conjunctival signs improve as these other disorders are controlled. Successful treatment depends on improvement of the patient's general condition and treatment of associated infections.

Treatment

1. Correction of the primary cause.
2. Topical broad-spectrum antibiotics (see Chapter 3 for choice of antibiotic).
3. Removal of crusts and exudates by soaking with saline-moistened cotton or commercial eye cleaning solutions.
4. Systemic antibiotic therapy if conjunctivitis is associated with blepharitis, generalized dermatitis, or otitis.
5. Prevention of self-trauma with an Elizabethan collar.
6. Topical therapy with a combined antibiotic-steroid is sometimes necessary in chronic conjunctivitis but should not be used routinely.

Chlamydial Conjunctivitis

Members of the family Chlamydiaceae have undergone reclassification and renaming as a result of better characterization using new molecular biology techniques. However, the range of diseases these organisms cause remains largely unchanged by this reclassification. Table 7-3 shows the previous and current names for the major organisms of veterinary importance. Chlamydial spp. cause notable conjunctivitis in cats, birds, and small ruminants. The potential for zoonosis

Table 7-3 | **Nomenclature for Chlamydial Organisms of Veterinary and Human Importance**

PREVIOUS NAME	CURRENT NAME(S)	SPECIES AFFECTED
Chlamydia psittaci	Chlamydophila felis	Cats
	Chlamydophila caviae	Guinea pigs
	Chlamydophila abortus	Humans, horses, ruminants, and pigs
	Chlamydophila psittaci	Humans and birds
Chlamydia pneumoniae	Chlamydophila pneumoniae	Koalas, frogs, and horses
Chlamydia pecorum	Chlamydophila pecorum	Pigs, cattle

exists, especially from birds, but appears to be minor in other species.

In cats, chlamydial conjunctivitis initially may be unilateral but typically spreads to the other eye within 7 days of primary infection. Mild rhinitis, fever, and submandibular lymphadenopathy are typically seen coincident with ocular signs in primary exposure but often resolve more promptly and completely than the conjunctival signs, which can be very persistent. Chemosis is a predominant feature. With chronicity, membranous or follicular conjunctivitis can be notable. If untreated the disease may last for months, and a protracted carrier state can occur. Chlamydial conjunctivitis is diagnosed from its clinical signs, a history of exposure, occasional demonstration of characteristic intracytoplasmic elementary bodies in scrapings of epithelial cells (see Figure 7-6, I), or polymerase chain reaction (PCR) testing. The major differential diagnosis is herpetic conjunctivitis due to feline herpesvirus type 1 (FHV-1). Table 7-4 provides some guidelines for differentiating these two diseases.

Chlamydial conjunctivitis also occurs in sheep, often in association with lameness due to polyarthritis. This condition is distinguishable from infectious ovine keratoconjunctivitis by the presence of lameness and lack of corneal lesions. Chlamydial conjunctivitis also occurs in birds and in the Australian koala, in which a high proportion of the population may be affected with chronic keratoconjunctivitis and infertility. Different strains of *Chlamydia* are responsible for infection of the conjunctiva and genitalia. Stress is believed to play a major role in the pathogenesis in koalas. Many koalas harbor the organism but lack clinical signs.

Treatment

Recent information shows that cats may "sequester" *Chlamydophila* in nonocular sites. This finding, along with controlled studies comparing topical and systemic therapy, has led to the recommendation that systemic antibiotics (typically doxycycline) be used in addition to or instead of topical ophthalmic ointments. The same information, although not confirmed as applying to all other host or chlamydial species, could be used to justify systemic treatment (usually in conjunction with topical therapy) in most individuals in which chlamydial infection is diagnosed. Azithromycin initially reduces clinical signs and shedding of *C. felis* in experimentally infected cats but does so only temporarily and less effectively than doxycycline.

Mycoplasmal Conjunctivitis

Mycoplasma spp. have formerly been described as a cause of conjunctivitis in cats. However, approximately 90% of normal cats harbor the organisms, and their clinical significance as a cause of feline conjunctivitis is debatable. Likewise, the importance of *Mycoplasma* spp. in infectious ovine and bovine keratoconjunctivitis and in many infectious conjunctivitides in other animals is questionable or undetermined. It is possible that culture of *Mycoplasma* spp. from debilitated eyes represents only an overgrowth of flora.

Mycoplasma spp. have been isolated from numerous outbreaks of conjunctivitis in house and wild finches in the United States. Clinical signs consisted of severe unilateral or bilateral chemosis with serous to mucopurulent drainage and nasal

Table 7-4 | **Characteristic Features of Infectious Feline Keratoconjunctivitis**

CLINICAL SIGNS	FELINE HERPESVIRUS 1	FELINE CALICIVIRUS	CHLAMYDIA
Malaise/anorexia	+ + +	+ +	±
Sneezing	+ + +	+	+ +
Nasal discharge	+ + +	+ +	+ +
Oral ulceration	–	+ + +	–
Ptyalism	+	+ + +	±
Ocular discharge	+ + +	+	+ +
Conjunctivitis	+ + +	–	+ + +
	(Hyperemic)		(Chemotic)
Keratitis	+ + +	–	–

From August JR (2001): Consultations in Feline Internal Medicine, 4th ed. Saunders, Philadelphia. Modified from Gaskell RM, Dawson S (1994): Viral-induced upper respiratory tract disease, in Chandler EA, Gaskell CJ, Gaskell RM (eds): Feline Medicine and Therapeutics, 2nd ed. Blackwell Scientific, Boston.
+, Mild; ++, moderate; +++, severe; –, absent; ±, variably present.

exudate. Transfer of infection at shared feeders was incriminated in the epidemiology of many of the outbreaks.

Treatment

Mycoplasma and *Chlamydia* have similar susceptibility patterns. Topically and systemically administered tetracyclines are an excellent choice of therapy for mycoplasmal conjunctivitis.

Viral Conjunctivitis

Conjunctivitis is caused by a variety of viruses in all species. The following general considerations are important:

- Although the conjunctiva is frequently an important portal of entry of systemic viral diseases, it is not always the site of severe pathology or predominant clinical signs.
- Conjunctivitis is present in both mild and severe forms in numerous systemic diseases (e.g., infectious bovine rhinotracheitis, canine distemper, feline herpesvirus infection).
- Severe viral conjunctivitis is commonly the most obvious clinical signs, although other systems may be involved (e.g., herpetic conjunctivitis in cats).
- Not all viruses isolated from the conjunctiva are pathogenic, nor is their significance completely understood. For example, adenoviruses have been found in cattle with infectious bovine keratoconjunctivitis.

Feline Viral Conjunctivitis

FHV-1 is considered the most common cause of conjunctivitis (and keratitis) in cats. In fact, FHV-1 and *C. felis* probably account for the vast majority of all feline conjunctivitides. Differentiation of these two organisms is guided largely by clinical signs (see Table 7-4) because diagnostic test results can be falsely positive or negative for these organisms.

Critical to the interpretation of diagnostic test results for FHV-1 and the management of cats infected with this organism is knowledge that FHV-1 establishes a permanent latent or carrier state in most cats infected. Additionally, FHV-1 is a ubiquitous and highly conserved virus worldwide. Serologic studies suggest that at least 95% of cats have been exposed to the virus via either vaccination or transfer of wild-type virus between cats by macrodroplets or fomites (including hands of owners). Although long-lived within the ganglia of cats, FHV-1 is extremely labile in the environment and susceptible to commonly used disinfectants.

Lifelong latency within the trigeminal ganglia of carrier cats occurs in at least 80% of cats and should be considered the norm. At least half of these cats assume epidemiologic importance owing to later reactivation and shedding of virus. Such episodes of reactivation may be stimulated by stress such as rehousing, intercurrent illness, or changes in the human or pet population within a household. The administration of corticosteroids is a very reliable method of reactivating latent virus under experimental conditions, and this possibility should be considered whenever one is tempted to administer a topical or systemic corticosteroid to a cat.

FHV-1 causes disease via a number of theorized mechanisms, each of which requires a different therapeutic approach. After primary inoculation of oral, nasal, or conjunctival mucosa there is an initial period of rapid replication within and associated cytolysis of epithelial cells at these sites. This can sometimes be observed directly in the cornea as the pathognomonic dendritic ulcers. This phase of cell destruction also causes rhinitis and conjunctivitis. If cytolysis is severe enough to cause ulceration of mucosal surfaces, serosanguineous ocular or nasal discharge can be seen. Exposure of conjunctival substantia propria and corneal stroma permits formation of symblepharon, or adhesions between these tissues (Figure 7-8). If viral infection occurs before the eyelids open, large amounts of inflammatory debris may accumulate in the conjunctival sac (conjunctivitis neonatorum).

Primary disease is usually self-limiting within 10 to 20 days. However, during this period, viral latency is established in the majority of cats (Figure 7-9). Intermittent, and usually recurrent, episodes of viral reactivation from the latent state may be followed by centrifugal spread of virus back along the sensory axons to peripheral epithelial sites in a minority of animals. Association of these episodes of reactivation with clinically evident disease at peripheral sites is termed *recrudescence*. Recrudescent disease may be ulcerative or nonulcerative and may involve the same tissues (cornea, conjunctiva, nose) as in primary disease; however, it may be unilateral, unassociated with systemic or nonocular signs, and is usually milder although often more chronic and/or recurrent than primary bouts of disease.

During recrudescent or primary disease, FHV-1 induces tissue damage via two classic mechanisms—as a direct result of viral replication (cytolysis) and indirectly through immunopathologic processes mediated by inflammatory cells. The most striking example of immunopathologic herpetic disease in cats is stromal keratitis (see Chapter 10), but chronic immunologic conjunctivitis also occurs.

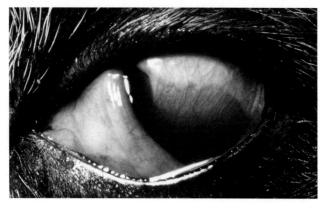

Figure 7-8. Symblepharon (conjunctival and corneal adhesion) in a cat after recovery from feline herpesvirus 1 infection. Forniceal conjunctiva has adhered to the cornea. (From August J [2001]: Consultations in Feline Internal Medicine, 4th ed. Saunders, Philadelphia.)

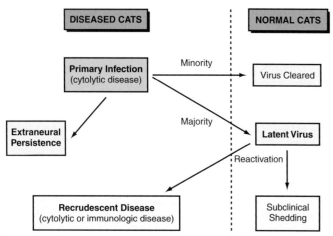

Figure 7-9. Pathogenesis of feline herpesvirus 1 (FHV-1). Traditionally, three phases of viral activity have been described for FHV-1: primary infection, neural latency, and recrudescent infection. Recent evidence suggests that extraneural persistence of virus may also occur. (Modified from August J [2001]: Consultations in Feline Internal Medicine, 4th ed. Saunders, Philadelphia.)

The basic epidemiologic factors that must always be considered in the diagnosis and management of cats infected with FHV-1 are summarized in Box 7-4.

There are two broad categories of testing methods for FHV-1:

- Viral detection using virus isolation (VI), immunofluorescent antibody (IFA) testing, or PCR testing
- Detection of antibodies (usually in serum) using serum neutralization (SN) or enzyme-linked immunosorbent assay (ELISA)

As always, understanding the limitations of these tests is critical (Table 7-5). It is important to note that no test differentiates vaccine virus from wild-type virus.

Because of the widespread exposure of cats to wild-type or vaccine virus, serologic test results are predictably positive in a majority of cats and are therefore not useful for diagnosing FHV-1 in individual cats. When it comes to viral detection, a major paradox exists with respect to the diagnosis of FHV-1. Cats experiencing primary FHV-1 infection shed virus in sufficient quantities that viral detection is relatively easy. However, clinical signs during this phase of infection tend to be charac-

---

Box 7-4 | Epidemiologic factors to consider in the management of cats with feline herpesvirus (FHV-1)

- Feline populations (not the environment) are the reservoir of infection.
- FHV-1 infection (but not necessarily disease) is common.
- FHV-1 establishes lifelong latency in most cats.
- FHV-1 commonly reactivates from latency with or without obvious cause and with or without clinical evidence of reactivation.
- FHV-1 reactivation is associated with recrudescent disease in only a small percentage of cats.
- FHV-1 induces disease via two distinct mechanisms with important therapeutic implications:
  - Cytolysis due to viral replication: An antiviral agent may be needed; immunomodulation is contraindicated.
  - Immunopathology: Antiinflammatory therapy may be indicated, usually along with antiviral agents.

---

teristic and self-limiting, making definitive diagnosis less necessary. By contrast, during the more chronic FHV-1–associated syndromes, the diversity and ambiguity of clinical signs make viral identification more desirable, especially if specific antiviral therapy is being considered. However, the elusive nature of the virus in these chronic syndromes and subclinical shedding in some animals make this issue difficult. Indeed, the diagnosis of FHV-1 in individual cats represents one of the greatest challenges in the management of chronic FHV-1-related diseases.

Canine Viral Conjunctivitis

The major viral cause of conjunctivitis in dogs is canine distemper virus. Canine adenovirus and canine herpesvirus have also historically been blamed for mild conjunctivitis. With distemper virus, conjunctivitis is frequently present in the early stages, appearing as severe hyperemia and serous discharge combined with tonsillitis, pharyngitis, pyrexia, anorexia, and lymphopenia, especially in young pups. Cytoplasmic inclusion bodies in epithelial cells are difficult to find in conjunctival scrapings, but viral antigen may be detected by IFA, or viral DNA detected by PCR. In advanced stages of distemper, chronic bilateral conjunctivitis and a dull and sometimes scarred cornea result from low Schirmer tear test readings due to keratoconjunctivitis sicca. Bilateral mucopurulent rhinitis is often also present. Secondary bacteria (e.g., *S. aureus*) are common.

Canine adenovirus I (infectious canine hepatitis) and adenovirus II (infectious tracheobronchitis) can cause conjunctivitis in dogs, although the former is a rare cause. Marked bilateral hyperemia and serous or seromucous exudate are present. Age, vaccination history, recent contacts and environment, and systemic signs help to differentiate dogs infected with one of the adenoviruses from those infected with canine distemper, except in severe complicated tracheobronchitis. Other ocular lesions of infectious canine hepatitis are discussed in Chapter 10.

Equine Viral Conjunctivitis

Viral conjunctivitis in horses is frequently associated with (but usually forms a relatively minor component of) upper

Table 7-5 | **Attributes of Commonly Used Diagnostic Tests for Feline Herpesvirus (FHV-1)**

ATTRIBUTES	VIRUS ISOLATION	POLYMERASE CHAIN REACTION TEST	IMMUNOFLUORESCENT ANTIBODY TEST	SEROLOGY
Detects	Virus	Virus	Virus	Host response
Viable virus necessary	Yes	No	No	No
Prior use of vital stains affects test result	Yes	Maybe	Yes	No
Collection and transport techniques	Detailed	Simple	Simple	Simple
Differentiates vaccine from wild type virus	No	No	No	No

respiratory tract infections. The most common diseases are those due to equine herpesvirus (EHV), parainfluenza, and influenza. Conjunctivitis usually resolves simultaneously with or before the more major systemic signs, and specific conjunctival treatment is not necessary.

Bovine Viral Conjunctivitis

Infectious bovine rhinotracheitis (IBR) and malignant catarrhal fever (MCF) are the only common viral diseases resulting in conjunctivitis in cows. Infectious bovine keratoconjunctivitis (IBK or "pink eye") also causes a severe conjunctivitis but largely as a result of and in association with the more significant and serious keratitis (see Chapter 10). Numerous diseases exotic to many parts of the world (e.g., Rift Valley fever, foot-and-mouth disease) cause conjunctivitis in ruminants, in addition to the more important systemic signs. Table 7-6 lists some clinical features useful for differentiating IBR, MCF, and IBK.

Treatment of Viral Conjunctivitis

No antiviral agents have been developed for treatment of viruses of veterinary ophthalmic importance. However, various antiviral agents developed for human use have been tried in animals. Unless these have been tested for efficacy against the virus of interest or for safety in the host species, such therapeutic extrapolations may not necessarily be safe or effective. Safety is rarely of importance for a topically applied medication but is often important for a systemically administered antiviral drug. Efficacy concerns exist regardless of route of administration. The major studies in veterinary medicine have involved the safety of these drugs in the cat and their efficacy against FHV-1.

Antiviral agents should be considered when signs are severe, persistent, or recurrent, especially when there is corneal involvement (with or without ulceration). Some important general concepts about antiviral agents assist with selection and expectations of this class of drugs. Because viruses reside intracellularly and utilize host cellular "machinery," antiviral agents tend to exhibit greater host toxicity compared with antibacterial drugs. This tendency rarely limits topical application of these drugs but may severely limit their systemic use. Antiviral agents in common use are virostatic; therefore they require frequent dosing or topical application. In some cases hourly application of ophthalmic preparations is recommended for at least the first 24 hours of therapy in humans. Given owner and veterinary limitations as to therapeutic frequency, antiviral agents should be applied at least 5 times daily, especially in the early stages of disease. Therapy with any of these drugs should be continued for at least 1 week beyond resolution of ocular lesions, which typically occurs within 2 to 3 weeks.

The in vitro efficacy against FHV-1 of many drugs developed for the human herpesviruses has been studied and their relative potencies reported as follows:

Trifluridine >> idoxuridine ≅ ganciclovir > vidarabine ≅ cidofovir ≅ penciclovir >> acyclovir >> foscarnet

The in vitro efficacy of these antiviral drugs against EHV-1 is somewhat different (ganciclovir > acyclovir > adefovir ≅ cidofovir > foscarnet).

Only four antiviral drugs have received relatively widespread clinical use in cats over a number of years and are discussed here. The others require clinical testing before they can be recommended in cats or other species.

The superior in vitro potency and corneal penetration of trifluridine suggest that it should be the first choice for topical

Table 7-6 | **Characteristic Features of Infectious Bovine Keratoconjunctivitis**

CLINICAL SIGNS	INFECTIOUS BOVINE RHINOTRACHEITIS	MALIGNANT CATARRHAL FEVER	INFECTIOUS BOVINE KERATOCONJUNCTIVITIS
Conjunctivitis	+++ Acute hyperemia	+++ Acute hyperemia Chemosis	+++ Acute hyperemia Blepharospasm
Systemic signs	Respiratory	Mucosal necrosis Lymphadenopathy	Few/None
Keratitis	+ (Limbal)	+++ (Limbal)	++++
Corneal ulceration	–	–	+
Other ocular disease	None	Anterior uveitis Panophthalmitis Blepharitis	Severe keratitis
Cause	Bovine herpesvirus 1	Alcelaphine herpesvirus 1	Moraxella bovis

+, Mild; ++, moderate; +++, severe; –, absent.

therapy. Unfortunately, however, cats often show marked aversion to application of this drug, suggesting that it is irritating. It is available as a 1% solution. Idoxuridine may be a more practical choice in veterinary patients owing to its high clinical efficacy, lower cost, and reduced irritancy. In many countries, idoxuridine is no longer available as a commercial ophthalmic solution; however, compounding pharmacists can formulate a 0.1% ophthalmic solution or a 0.5% ointment. Vidarabine as a 3% ointment appears to be well tolerated by a majority of cats. Treatment is recommended at least 4 times daily. With all topically administered agents, use of an ointment may be particularly helpful when keratoconjunctivitis sicca is apparent.

Acyclovir and its prodrug, valacyclovir, are the only systemic antiherpetic drugs that have received adequate clinical and research attention in feline medicine. Acyclovir must be activated by multiple phosphorylation steps. The initial phosphorylation is catalyzed by viral thymidine kinase. It is this feature that accounts for the drug's relative safety in humans as a systemic antiviral agent. The capacity of FHV-1 thymidine kinase to perform this phosphorylation step is believed to be limited and may explain the poor efficacy of acyclovir against FHV-1. Poor bioavailability further limits use of this drug in cats. Doses as high as 100 mg/kg in cats failed to attain plasma acyclovir concentrations that approximate the effective dose to kill FHV-1, and some cats showed toxic effects at these doses. The principal toxic effects seen in cats are leukopenia and anemia, although normalization of the complete blood count usually accompanies withdrawal of acyclovir therapy and appropriate supportive care. Valacyclovir is an acyclovir prodrug that has superior bioavailability but unfortunately causes severe renal and hepatic toxicity in cats. Valacyclovir must *not* be used in cats. Neither orally nor intravenously administered acyclovir achieved therapeutic concentrations in horses.

In addition to specific antiviral therapy, the following supportive/adjunctive care should be considered:

- *Supportive therapy* remains the mainstay of therapy for viral conjunctivitis. It consists of frequent cleaning of eyelid margins followed by application of a suitable lubricant ointment, as well as maintenance of adequate nutrition and hydration in systemically affected animals. Corticosteroids (by any route) are generally contraindicated.

- *Antibacterial therapy:* No antiviral agents are reported to have antibacterial activity and so antibacterial drug administration may be wise, especially if there is concurrent corneal ulceration or severe systemic debilitation. Given the frequent involvement of *Chlamydia* or *Mycoplasma* spp. in the eyes of species often affected by viral agents of ocular importance, systemically and locally administered tetracyclines may be a good choice.
- *Lysine:* Lysine reduces in vitro replication of FHV-1, and its oral administration decreases shedding of feline herpesvirus from latently infected cats and severity of conjunctivitis in cats undergoing primary infection with the virus. Oral administration of 500 mg of lysine twice daily appears safe and can be given long term to cats with recurrent infections.
- *Interferon:* Neither topical nor systemic therapy with interferons has been conclusively shown by controlled studies to be effective for the treatment of viral conjunctivitis.

Mycotic Conjunctivitis

Mycotic conjunctivitis is uncommon in all species and tends to be chronic. Exudates can be relatively tenacious and form crusts around the eyelid margins. Organisms involved are *Candida* spp., *Aspergillus* spp., and yeasts. The history is usually one of chronic conjunctivitis with little or no response to previous antibiotic or antibiotic-steroid therapy. Diagnosis is made via culture and cytology. Causes of local or systemic immunodeficiency should be considered. Mycotic keratitis in horses usually lacks conjunctival involvement. The same topical preparations used for mycotic keratitis are recommended for mycotic conjunctivitis (see Chapters 3 and 10).

Parasitic Conjunctivitis

Parasites that may cause conjunctivitis in various species are shown in Table 7-7. Additionally, a chronic blepharoconjunctivitis associated with constant irritation from flies *(Musca domestica)* is sometimes seen in horses during summer. Mucopurulent discharge, epiphora, and moist eyelid margins are the usual signs. Control of flies using repellents and fly veils/masks is essential. Treatment consists of local antibiotic preparations and application of corticosteroids to conjunctiva and eyelid margins in severe cases. In very severe cases, insect-proof stables are sometimes

Table 7-7 | **Parasitic Conjunctivitis**

PARASITE	SPECIES AFFECTED	TREATMENT AND PREVENTION
Thelazia spp.	Dog, cat, cattle, horse, pig, sheep, deer, human	Removal under local anesthesia Topical demecarium bromide Topical echothiophate iodide Systemic ivermectin
Onchocerca cervicalis	Horse	Systemic ivermectin Topical corticosteroids
Draschia megastoma	Horse	Fly control/repellents Systemic ivermectin
Oestrus ovis	Sheep	Mechanical removal Systemic ivermectin
Oxyspirura mansoni	Poultry (especially turkeys)	Removal of parasites Control of intermediate host (cockroach)
Habronema spp.	Horses	Ivermectin Intralesional corticosteroids

necessary. In some areas this "summer conjunctivitis" is due to release of *Habronema* larvae by feeding flies.

Immune-Mediated Conjunctivitis

Because of the conjunctiva's exposed position and resident lymphoid tissue, immunopathology may occasionally initiate and often exacerbates conjunctivitis. In this chapter, the terms "immune-mediated" and "autoimmune" are not used interchangeably as is sometimes the case. Rather, disease caused by an autoimmune response form a subgroup of the broader immune-mediated group of diseases—that is, they are immune-mediated disease in which the antigen is identified and is an autoantigen. Four reasonably common examples of conjunctival immunopathology are seen in small animal and equine practice: nodular granulomatous episclerokeratoconjunctivitis, allergic conjunctivitis, eosinophilic keratoconjunctivitis, and pannus (or chronic superficial keratoconjunctivitis). Because all except allergic conjunctivitis typically produce more overt signs of keratitis than of conjunctivitis, they are described in Chapter 10. Allergic conjunctivitis is discussed here.

Allergic Conjunctivitis

Allergic conjunctivitis can occur after exposure of the conjunctiva to antigens as a result of direct contact (airborne or topically applied agents), inhalation, or ingestion and may be seen with signs of more widespread atopy or allergic responses. The response is elicited by many different kinds of antigens and can occur in all species. The clinical signs are as follows:

- Periocular erythema and conjunctival hyperemia (Figure 7-10)
- Serous to mucoid discharge
- Chemosis
- Concurrent inflammation of the skin, paws, nasal cavity, ears, or pharynx

As with all other forms of conjunctivitis, achieving an etiologic diagnosis is essential. Trials whereby potential antigens are removed from and then reintroduced to the animal's environment are useful. However, it is most important to eliminate other, more common causes of conjunctivitis. Therefore a Schirmer tear test should always be performed to eliminate keratoconjunctivitis sicca. Conjunctival cytology is important in the accurate diagnosis of allergic conjunctivitis. Eosinophils are not always present, but lymphocytes and

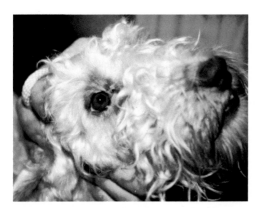

Figure 7-10. Allergic dermatitis (blepharitis) and conjunctivitis. (From Muller GH, Kirk RW [1989]: Small Animal Dermatology, 4th ed. Saunders, Philadelphia.)

plasma cells are frequently seen. Secondary bacterial conjunctivitis may occur after inflammation has been initiated by an antigen. Toxins produced by bacteria (e.g., *S. aureus*) present in the conjunctival sac or meibomian glands may also initiate allergic conjunctivitis, but the clinical appearance differs from that of spontaneous or atopic conjunctivitis. Food allergy also results in allergic conjunctivitis in calves. Hypersensitivity to medications such as neomycin and other aminoglycosides may occur.

Treatment of Immune-Mediated Conjunctivitis

1. Topical corticosteroid therapy at a frequency and concentration as low as possible to control (but usually not cure) the condition is the mainstay of therapy. In mild cases, a low-potency corticosteroid such as hydrocortisone may be used intermittently. More commonly, especially early in the disease course, topical application of a more potent, penetrating corticosteroid such as dexamethasone or prednisolone is required.
2. Topical application of cyclosporine has been used for some time to treat immune-mediated conjunctivitis in dogs and is now under investigation for vernal conjunctivitis in humans.
3. Mast cell–stabilizing agents and antihistamines have been used topically to treat allergic and eosinophilic conjunctivitis. However, anecdotal reports of the efficacy of these products vary, and controlled studies on their safety or efficacy in veterinary patients are lacking.
4. Local antibiotic preparations may help in the short term if secondary bacterial conjunctivitis is present. However, many antibiotics (such as neomycin) can *cause* allergic conjunctivitis. Although this drawback is insufficient to prevent their routine use, it should be considered if the conjunctivitis worsens when a new drug is begun.
5. Systemic therapy with corticosteroids, more potent immunosuppressive agents, antihistamines, antibiotics, and hyposensitization therapy may be required in severe cases with skin (including eyelid) involvement.

OTHER CONJUNCTIVAL DISORDERS

Drug Plaques

Certain repository medications (e.g., methylprednisolone) leave unsightly, creamy-white subconjunctival plaques months after injection in some animals (Figure 7-11). The material in these plaques may also incite a local granulomatous conjunctivitis around the material. In such cases surgical excision is required.

Conjunctival Lacerations

Traumatic lacerations of the conjunctiva heal very rapidly, and small lacerations usually require only short-term topical antibiotic therapy. More severe lacerations are flushed with saline to remove foreign material, sutured with 6/0 or 7/0 polyglactin 910 (Vicryl) or polydioxanone (PDS) suture, and treated with topical antibiotics.

Ligneous Conjunctivitis

Ligneous conjunctivitis is a chronic, membranous conjunctivitis with gross thickening of palpebral and third eyelid con-

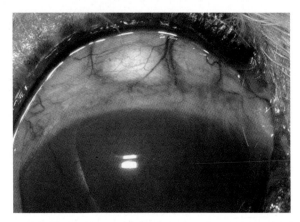

Figure 7-11. Plaque formation following subconjunctival injection in the dorsal bulbar conjunctiva of a dog.

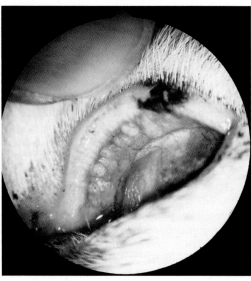

Figure 7-13. Lipogranulomatous conjunctivitis of the upper eyelid of a 16-year-old domestic cat. (From Read RA, Lucas J [2001]: Lipogranulomatous conjunctivitis: clinical findings from 21 eyes in 13 cats. Vet Ophthalmol 4:93.)

junctivae bilaterally (Figure 7-12). There is some evidence that younger, female Doberman pinschers may be predisposed. A conjunctival biopsy should be performed to confirm the diagnosis. Histology demonstrates a characteristic amorphous, eosinophilic hyaline material throughout the subconjunctiva. In some animals, other mucous membranes may also be involved and most dogs have evidence of nonocular disease, especially involving the upper respiratory or urinary tract. A vascular basis for the disease is proposed. Topically administered cyclosporine is often effective at controlling the disease, although systemic administration of immunomodulatory agents may be necessary, and recurrence is relatively common.

Lipogranulomatous Conjunctivitis

Lipogranulomatous conjunctivitis has been described in cats. It is an inflammatory condition that arises from the meibomian glands and therefore manifests superficially as blepharitis and on the inner eyelid surface as a nodular conjunctivitis (Figure 7-13). Involvement of multiple tarsal glands across one or more eyelids, producing a multifocal nodular white thickening of involved lids, is common. The upper eyelid is involved more commonly than the lower lid. Actinic radiation may be important in the pathogenesis of these lesions because they have been reported more commonly in white-skinned cats and sometimes

in association with squamous cell carcinoma (SCC). If meibomian glands rupture, secretions leak into the surrounding tissue and cause a marked lipogranulomatous reaction. Histologic appearance is similar to that of chalazia in dogs (see Chapter 6).

Surgical extirpation of glandular material and associated granulomatous infiltrate has been recommended for this condition. A conjunctival approach is preferred because of the rapidity with which conjunctiva heals and to avoid surgical disruption of the eyelid margin. Surgical treatment involves resection of lipogranulomas and overlying conjunctiva as a single strip of tissue outlined by two incisions parallel to the eyelid margin. The defect is allowed to heal without suturing.

Conjunctival Neoplasia

Neoplasia of the conjunctiva may occur in any species and may represent primary or metastatic disease. Of the conjunctival neoplasms, SCC is the most common. Others commonly recorded are hemangioma and hemangiosarcoma, melanoma, papilloma, and mastocytoma. As with masses elsewhere, cytologic assessment of scrapings or aspirates, or histologic assessment of biopsy specimens is essential for accurate diagnosis because neoplastic and nonneoplastic masses may appear similar on clinical examination alone. Involvement of neighboring eyelids, cornea, or sclera is common, and the reader is referred also to chapters dealing with these tissues for additional information.

Conjunctival Dermoid

Dermoids are examples of a choristoma or congenital circumscribed overgrowth of microscopically normal tissue in an abnormal place. Conjunctival dermoids represent histologically normal skin arising in the conjunctiva, usually laterally, and frequently involving the limbus (Figure 7-14). Dermoids occasionally involve the eyelids and may coexist with an eyelid coloboma. Dermoids containing hair follicles have hair growing from the surface, which causes conjunctival and corneal irritation

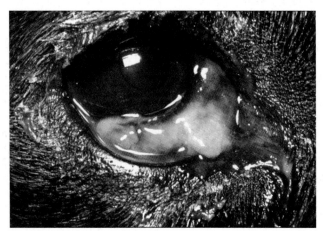

Figure 7-12. Ligneous conjunctivitis in a dog. (Courtesy Dr. David Ramsey.)

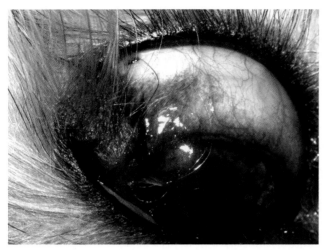

Figure 7-14. A conjunctival dermoid with obvious tufts of irritating hairs in a 6-month-old shih tzu.

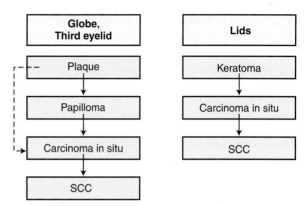

Figure 7-15. Pathogenesis of bovine squamous cell carcinoma *(SCC)* at various ocular sites.

and leads to epiphora and keratitis. Dermoids usually grow slowly, if at all. In Hereford cattle they are inherited, with recessive and polygenic genetic characteristics being reported.

Treatment for dermoid is careful surgical excision via conjunctivectomy and dissection down to bare sclera. If the lesion extends onto the cornea, referral to an ophthalmologist for combined conjunctivectomy and keratectomy is recommended.

Ocular Squamous Cell Carcinoma

SCC is probably the most common conjunctival neoplasm in veterinary medicine. It is regularly seen in horses, cattle, small ruminants, and cats but occurs very infrequently in dogs. Some general comments regarding clinical signs, progression, malignancy, diagnosis, and therapy are possible. Some specific comments regarding this tumor in cattle are found in the next section.

ETIOLOGY. The exact etiology is unknown. However, incidence of SCC is much higher in animals with hypopigmentation and in areas of high sunlight or altitude, in which exposure to ultraviolet radiation is greater. About 75% of cases in cattle occur in animals lacking pigment in the eyelids, third eyelid, or conjunctiva. Therefore selection for lid pigmentation has been used as a control measure in cattle. Lid pigmentation is highly heritable and is present at birth, whereas conjunctival pigmentation has a lower heritability and develops throughout life. Although viral particles have been demonstrated in SCC lesions, an etiologic relationship has not been established.

CLINICAL SIGNS AND PATHOGENESIS. For the globe (conjunctiva, cornea, and limbus) and third eyelid, plaque is the initial precursor lesion of SCC (Figure 7-15). Plaques are grayish-white areas of thickened epithelium occurring most frequently at the nasal and temporal limbus. On the lids, the precursor lesion is the keratoma, a brown, crusty, and sometimes hornlike structure, that occurs at mucocutaneous junctions (Figure 7-16). Papilloma is the next stage and has a similar distribution, but the surface is roughened and the mass is frequently pedunculated or moveable. The base often merges with an underlying plaque. Carcinoma in situ may arise from any of these lesions. This term is used for the stage before the neoplastic cells have penetrated the basement membrane of the epithelium and entered the subepithelial connective tissue to become true

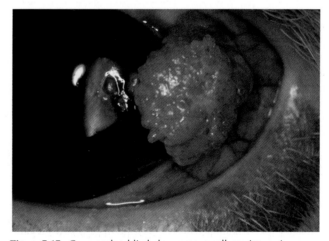

Figure 7-16. Eyelid keratoma on the lower eyelid of a cow. This is a precursor lesion for squamous cell carcinoma. (Courtesy Dr. David Ramsey.)

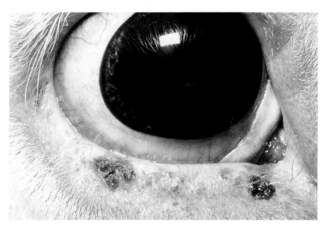

Figure 7-17. Corneoscleral limbal squamous cell carcinoma in a cow.

SCC. The surface of carcinomas may be roughened or papillary, hemorrhagic, or ulcerated. (Figure 7-17).

The tumor is often aggressively invasive locally and may involve eyelids, intraorbital space and tissues, and even bone and paranasal sinuses. Metastasis is less common and typically involves local lymph nodes. The rate of progression of SCC is variable, with lesions ranging from slow-growing to highly malignant. Both cell-mediated and humoral immunity to tumor antigens has been demonstrated.

DIFFERENTIAL DIAGNOSIS. SCC must be distinguished from the following conditions:

- Other neoplastic lesions of the conjunctiva, including but not limited to melanoma (which can be poorly pigmented), lymphangiosarcoma, hemangioma, hemangiosarcoma, dermoid (which are not always haired), and lymphoma
- Granulation tissue, as seen with any chronic inflammatory process but especially pannus of dogs, eosinophilic keratoconjunctivitis of horses and cats, and chronic ulceration of any species but especially infectious bovine keratoconjunctivitis in ruminants. Differentiation of granulation tissue from SCC is particularly challenging when it occurs after resection of SCC when it may be mistaken for early tumor recurrence.

Biopsy or cytologic scraping (see Figure 7-6, *J*) of suspicious lesions is indicated and usually diagnostic, with up to 90% accuracy having been reported.

TREATMENT. Treatment depends on species, tumor location, value of the animal, and stage of the disease. Treatment options include surgical excision or debulking, cryotherapy, hyperthermia, immunotherapy, radiation therapy (numerous types), intralesional chemotherapy, and photodynamic therapy (see Chapter 3). Cryotherapy has the advantages of simplicity and rapidity, economy, analgesia, minimal preoperative and postoperative treatment, repeatability, and minimal side effects. Economic and radiologic health considerations may limit the use of radiotherapy.

Bovine Ocular Squamous Cell Carcinoma

INCIDENCE. SCC of the eye and adnexa is one of the most common and most important ocular conditions affecting cattle. It is uncommon in breeds with pigmented conjunctiva and lids but may occur in any breed. Herefords are affected most frequently (incidence may reach 10%), but SCC also occurs in shorthorn and Friesian cattle. Both the precursors to SCC and the disease itself are usually unilateral (10% are bilateral). Ocular lesions outnumber lid lesions by a ratio of 3:1, whereas lesions of the third eyelid account for less than 5% of the total lesions. Precursor lesions are not uncommon in animals younger than 4 years, whereas SCC is more common at 7 to 9 years and is rare before 5 years. Fifty percent of precursor lesions manifesting at the end of one summer may disappear by the next summer.

TREATMENT. In a large study of cryotherapy using a double freeze-thaw cycle to −25° C, an overall cure rate of 97% was achieved, and even quite large lesions responded well. Treatment with bacille Calmette-Guérin (BCG) cell wall vaccine injected into the tumor caused regression in 71% of affected animals. Intratumoral injection of 200,000 units of interleukin (IL-2) resulted in a 67% complete regression at 20 months after injection.

CONTROL. Incidence of ocular SCC within a herd may be reduced by selective breeding for lid, limbal, and conjunctival pigmentation, which are genetically related and heritable. Use of breeding animals whose progeny have not demonstrated SCC is also recommended because genetic factors other than periocular pigmentation are believed to be involved.

Canine Conjunctival Papillomatosis

Papillomas usually occur on the eyelids or mucocutaneous junctions and may be multiple, especially in young animals. For those arising from the conjunctiva, the most important differential diagnosis is SCC. The relationship to oral and cutaneous papillomatosis is not established. Surgical removal or cryotherapy is the treatment of choice, especially if the lesion is causing pain from friction. Recurrence has been observed. Spontaneous regression of ocular papillomas occurs, especially in young animals.

Equine Conjunctival Angiosarcoma

Conjunctival angiosarcomas occur in aged horses, grow slowly, and metastasize despite excision and radiation therapy. They must be differentiated from SCC by biopsy. Enucleation may be necessary because these tumors are often very aggressive.

BIBLIOGRAPHY

Barkyoumb SD, Leipold HW (1984): Nature and cause of bilateral ocular dermoids in Hereford cattle. Vet Pathol 21:316.

Bentz BG, et al. (2006): Pharmacokinetics of acyclovir after single intravenous and oral administration to adult horses. J Vet Intern Med 20:589.

Bonney CH, et al. (1980): Papillomatosis of conjunctiva and adnexa in dogs. J Am Vet Med Assoc 176:48.

Browning GF (2004): Is *Chlamydophila felis* a significant zoonotic pathogen? Aust Vet J 82:695.

Collins BK, et al. (1993): Biologic behavior and histologic characteristics of canine conjunctival melanoma. Prog Vet Comp Ophthalmol 3:135.

Garre B, et al. (2007): In vitro susceptibility of six isolates of equine herpesvirus 1 to acyclovir, ganciclovir, cidofovir, adefovir, PMEDAP and foscarnet. Vet Microbiol (in press).

Hacker DV, et al. (1986): Ocular angiosarcoma in four horses. J Am Vet Med Assoc 189:200.

Johnson BW, et al. (1988): Conjunctival mast cell tumors in two dogs. J Am Anim Hosp Assoc 24:439.

Haesebrouck F, at al. (1991): Incidence and significance of isolation of *Mycoplasma felis* from conjunctival swabs of cats. Vet Microbiol 26:95.

Lavach JD, et al. (1977): Cytology of normal and inflamed conjunctivas in dogs and cats. J Am Vet Med Assoc 170:722.

Longbottom D, Coulter LJ (2003): Animal chlamydioses and zoonotic implications. J Comp Pathol 128:217.

Maggs DJ (2005): Update on pathogenesis, diagnosis, and treatment of feline herpesvirus type 1. Clin Tech Small Anim Pract 20:94.

Maggs DJ, et al. (2003): Efficacy of oral supplementation with L-lysine in cats latently infected with feline herpesvirus. Am J Vet Res 64:37.

Maggs DJ, Clarke HE (2004): In vitro efficacy of ganciclovir, cidofovir, penciclovir, foscarnet, idoxuridine, and acyclovir against feline herpesvirus type-1. Am J Vet Res 65:399.

Mosunic CB, et al. (2004): Effects of treatment with and without adjuvant radiation therapy on recurrence of ocular and adnexal squamous cell carcinoma in horses: 157 cases (1985-2002). J Am Vet Med Assoc 225:1733.

Mughannam AJ, et al. (1997): Conjunctival vascular tumors in six dogs. Vet Comp Ophthalmol 7:56.

Nasisse MP, et al. (1997): Effects of valacyclovir in cats infected with feline herpesvirus 1. Am J Vet Res 58:1141.

Nasisse MP, et al. (1993): Clinical and laboratory findings in chronic conjunctivitis in cats: 91 cases (1983-1991). J Am Vet Med Assoc 203:834.

Owens JG, et al. (1996) Pharmacokinetics of acyclovir in the cat. J Vet Pharmacol Ther 19:488.

Pentlarge VW (1991): Eosinophilic conjunctivitis in five cats. J Am Anim Hosp Assoc 27:21.

Pusterla N, et al. (2003): Cutaneous and ocular habronemiasis in horses: 63 cases (1988-2002). J Am Vet Med Assoc 222:978.

Ramsey DT, et al. (1996): Ligneous conjunctivitis in four Doberman pinschers. J Am Anim Hosp Assoc 32:439.

Read RA, Lucas J (2001): Lipogranulomatous conjunctivitis: clinical findings from 21 eyes in 13 cats. Vet Ophthalmol 4:93.

Sparkes AH, et al. (1999): The clinical efficacy of topical and systemic therapy for the treatment of feline ocular chlamydiosis. J Feline Med Surg 1:31.

Stewart RJ, et al. (2005): Local interleukin-2 and interleukin-12 therapy of bovine ocular squamous cell carcinomas. Vet Immunol Immunopathol 106:277.

Stiles J, et al. (2002): Effect of oral administration of L-lysine on conjunctivitis caused by feline herpesvirus in cats. Am J Vet Res 63:99.

Sykes JE (2005): Feline chlamydiosis. Clin Tech Small Anim Pract 20:129.

von Bomhard W, et al. (2003): Detection of novel chlamydiae in cats with ocular disease. Am J Vet Res 64:1421.

THIRD EYELID

Chapter 8

David J. Maggs

ANATOMY AND PHYSIOLOGY
EXAMINATION
DISEASES OF THE THIRD EYELID

NEOPLASMS AFFECTING THE THIRD
EYELID
TRAUMA TO THE THIRD EYELID

INFLAMMATORY DISORDERS OF THE
THIRD EYELID

ANATOMY AND PHYSIOLOGY

The third eyelid (or nictitating membrane) is a mobile, protective, and glandular structure lying between the cornea and the lower eyelid in the medial portion of the inferior conjunctival sac (Figure 8-1).

The third eyelid (Figure 8-2) consists of the following:

- A T-shaped cartilaginous "skeleton"
- The gland of the third eyelid
- Conjunctiva covering the bulbar and palpebral surfaces
- Numerous superficial lymphoid follicles under the bulbar surface

The T cartilage provides essential rigidity to the third eyelid. Its "horizontal" arm lies parallel to and about 1.5 mm from the leading edge of the third eyelid. The "vertical" arm runs perpendicular to the free edge and at its base is encircled by the gland of the third eyelid (see Figure 8-2). The gland of the third eyelid is seromucoid and produces up to 50% of the normal tear film in dogs. In the dog, this gland has both adrenergic and cholinergic innervation, with cholinergic being the denser. In the pig and many rodents a portion of the gland of the third eyelid or a separate gland (the Harderian gland) is found deeper within the orbit. The cartilage and gland are covered on both bulbar and palpebral surfaces by conjunctiva that is tightly adherent at the free margin of the third eyelid but looser over the base and gland. The free margin and a portion of the anterior face of the third eyelid are often but not always pigmented. Lymphoid follicles, which are pinkish red, are normally present beneath the conjunctiva on the bulbar surface of the third eyelid (Figure 8-3).

A poorly defined fascial retinaculum secures the base of the gland and the cartilage to the periorbita surrounding the ventral oblique and rectus muscles. The musculature controlling the third eyelid is largely vestigial in domestic species, and the membrane moves passively across the eye when the globe is retracted by the retractor bulbi muscles innervated by the abducens nerve. Movement is in a dorsolateral direction, toward the orbital ligament. The position of the third eyelid is also partially determined by sympathetic tone of the orbital smooth muscles. Interruption of this sympathetic supply, as in Horner's syndrome, results in enophthalmos (posterior displacement of the globe within the orbit) and prominence of the third eyelid.

In birds the third eyelid is almost transparent and is under voluntary control (Figure 8-4). It sweeps over the globe in a ventromedial direction from the dorsolateral quadrant, although there is some species variation in direction of move-

ment. The third eyelid in birds does not have a gland associated with it.

The third eyelid has the following important functions:

- Distribution of the precorneal tear film
- Protection of the cornea
- Production of aqueous and immunoglobulin for the tear film (in domestic mammals)

Therefore removal of the third eyelid or its gland predisposes to the following problems:

- Increased corneal exposure, drying of the cornea, corneal trauma, and chronic keratitis
- A chronic conjunctivitis that is often purulent and frequently resistant to treatment
- Decreased tear production, which contributes to the first two problems

The third eyelid is a useful and important structure. The only indications for its removal are severe, irreparable trauma and histologically confirmed malignant neoplasia.

EXAMINATION

The clinician can easily examine the palpebral surface of the third eyelid by digitally retropulsing the globe through the upper lid. The bulbar surface is examined after application of topical anesthesia and the use of forceps or mosquito hemostats to grasp the leading edge of the third eyelid just outside the horizontal arm of the cartilage. The membrane can then be reflected to examine the bulbar surface and the space between the third eyelid and the globe (see Figure 8-3). This is a common site for foreign bodies to become lodged. The bulbar surface is normally follicular and may become more so with so-called follicular conjunctivitis (see Chapter 7).

Perhaps the most common abnormality of the third eyelid noted during an ocular examination is unusual prominence. This sign is seen with a number of third eyelid diseases discussed in this chapter. However, prominence of the third eyelid can also indicate other orbital, neurologic, or ocular diseases, which are discussed elsewhere; they include the following:

- Horner's syndrome (sympathetic denervation)
- Third eyelid protrusion (or "haws") syndrome
- Space-occupying orbital lesions that push the membrane across the eye from its base

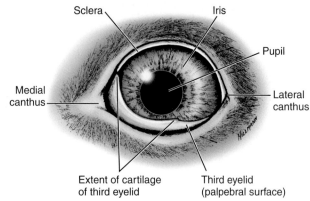

Figure 8-1. Diagram of the eye showing normal position of the third eyelid. (Modified from Evans HE [1993]: Miller's Anatomy of the Dog, 3rd ed. Saunders, Philadelphia.)

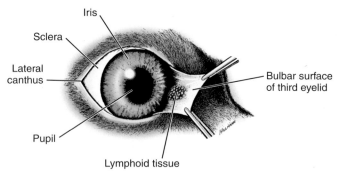

Figure 8-3. Diagram of the third eyelid manually everted to show normal lymphoid follicles on the bulbar surface. (Modified from Evans HE [1993]: Miller's Anatomy of the Dog, 3rd ed. Saunders, Philadelphia.)

- With a small globe due to microphthalmos or phthisis bulbi
- With enophthalmos due to active retraction of the globe in painful ocular conditions or due to loss of orbital contents as in dehydration, atrophy, or fibrosis
- With tetanus, especially in large animals
- Tranquilization (e.g., with acetylpromazine)

DISEASES OF THE THIRD EYELID

Because the third eyelid has two surfaces of conjunctiva and is intimately associated and confluent with the rest of the conjunctiva, it is predictably involved in many conjunctival disorders. These are discussed more fully in Chapter 7. This chapter emphasizes conditions peculiar to the third eyelid.

Amelanotic Leading Edge of the Third Eyelid

Congenital absence of melanin on the free or leading edge of the third eyelid in some individuals reveals normal, well-vascularized conjunctiva, which is frequently mistaken by owners or breeders for third eyelid protrusion or inflammation. This appearance is not abnormal, however, and does not require surgical correction.

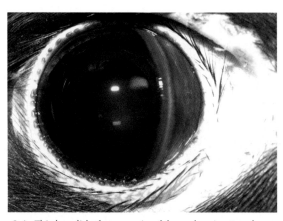

Figure 8-4. Third eyelid of a peregrine falcon showing translucency and voluntary dorsal-to-ventral movement typical of the avian third eyelid.

When such eyes become inflamed for other reasons, the amelanotic third eyelid may appear more visible because the conjunctival vasculature is not obscured by pigment. Also, such eyelids are presumed to be at higher risk for solar-induced neoplasms, such as hemangioma, hemangiosarcoma, and squamous cell carcinoma.

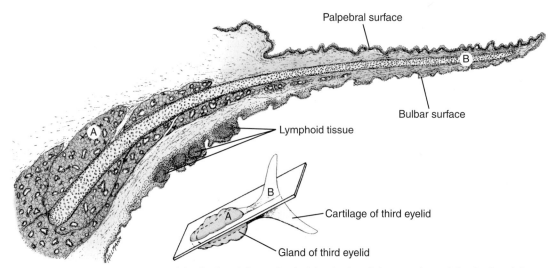

Figure 8-2. Transverse section of the third eyelid. A, Gland of the third eyelid; B, cartilage of the third eyelid. (Modified from Evans HE [1993]: Miller's Anatomy of the Dog, 3rd ed. Saunders, Philadelphia.)

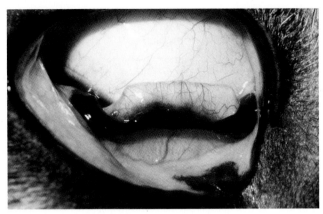

Figure 8-5. Everted or "scrolled" cartilage of the third eyelid in a dog.

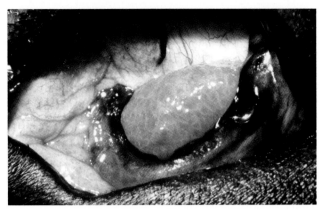

Figure 8-7. Protrusion of the gland of the third eyelid ("cherry eye") in a dog.

Eversion or Scrolling of the Third Eyelid

Eversion of the third eyelid or "scrolled third eyelid" refers to rolling out of the margin of the membrane due to abnormal curvature of the vertical portion of the T-shaped cartilage (Figure 8-5). This condition may be unilateral or bilateral, and although most commonly seen in young dogs, it occasionally develops in middle-aged dogs. It is common in Weimaraners, Saint Bernards, Newfoundlands, Great Danes, German short-haired pointers, and Irish setters, and a hereditary basis has been suggested. Injuries and improper suturing of the third eyelid may also result in eversion.

Treatment

Eversion of the third eyelid is corrected surgically because of its undesirable cosmetic appearance and the resultant second-ary conjunctivitis and keratitis in some animals. The deformed or buckled section of excessive cartilage is removed via a surgical approach from the bulbar surface (Figure 8-6). The

defective, scrolled portion of cartilage is usually found in the vertical arm of the cartilage, near its junction with the horizontal arm of the T. A topical antibiotic ointment should be used for approximately 1 week after surgery.

Protrusion of the Gland of the Third Eyelid

Protrusion of the gland of the third eyelid (or "cherry eye") occurs most commonly in dogs and occasionally in cats. The appearance is characteristic, with the gland of the third eyelid protruding as a reddish follicular mass from behind a usually "floppy" margin of the third eyelid (Figure 8-7). It likely results from lymphoid hyperplasia (in young animals exposed to environmental antigens for the first time) and laxity of the retinaculum that should attach the third eyelid to the periorbita (in genetically predisposed, especially brachycephalic, animals). This combination of events allows the gland to evert while remaining attached to the cartilage of the third eyelid.

The gland should be surgically replaced to retain essential lacrimal function and to prevent the exposed gland and over-lying conjunctiva from becoming dry, inflamed, secondarily infected, and cosmetically unappealing. Prolapsed glands of the third eyelid should never be removed because the gland of the third eyelid is a significant contributor to precorneal tear film production. Studies confirm clinical experience that kerato-conjunctivitis sicca is commonly seen, often years later, in animals, especially those of susceptible breeds in which the third eyelid or its gland was removed. Also, complications have been reported in prolapsed glands left in the prolapsed position.

Treatment

Occasionally in the early stages, a prolapsed gland can be manipulated into its normal position. However, recurrence is almost inevitable. For these reasons surgical replacement is practiced. If the gland is severely inflamed or the conjunctival surface secondarily infected, preoperative treatment for a few days with a topical antibiotic-steroid ointment is advisable; however, this treatment will not result in resolution of protrusion.

Corrective surgical procedures may be broadly categorized as "anchoring" or "pocket" techniques. The original anchoring method involved suturing the gland to the ventral aspect of the globe. This had a relatively high rate of recurrence owing to difficulty accessing and suturing to the sclera, and too frequently resulted in globe penetration during suturing. Therefore it is no

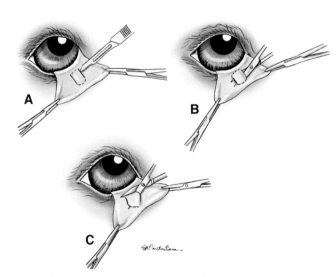

Figure 8-6. Surgical correction of third eyelid cartilage eversion. **A,** On the bulbar side of the third eyelid, the conjunctiva is incised overlying each side of the scrolled vertical part of the third eyelid cartilage. **B,** The scrolled cartilage and overlying conjunctiva are undermined with tenotomy scissors. **C,** The undermined section of scrolled cartilage and overlying conjunctiva is resected. No sutures are required.

longer recommended. Numerous variations of the anchoring techniques have been proposed, with one of the methods in which the gland is sutured to the periosteum of the ventral orbital margin now being preferred (Figure 8-8). This procedure is associated with some reduction in third eyelid mobility. As a result, pocket techniques may be more physiologic. Of the pocket techniques, the technique of Morgan is very useful (Figure 8-9). Medical treatment after any replacement technique includes topical antibiotic-steroid ointment or solution and use of an Elizabethan collar. Oral administration of a nonsteroidal antiinflammatory agent may be indicated for postoperative analgesia. Recurrence is possible, even with a correctly performed pocket or anchoring technique, especially in the very large breed dogs such as mastiffs and Newfoundlands.

Prolapsed glands of the third eyelid are treated by replacement, *not* by excision.

Protrusion of the harderian gland occurs in dwarf lop rabbits with clinical signs and sequelae similar to those of third eyelid gland protrusion in dogs and cats. Replacement of the gland by anchoring to the orbital rim is recommended.

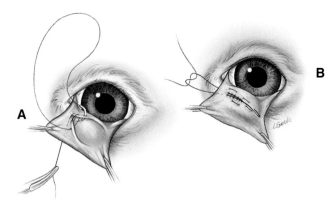

Figure 8-9. Surgical replacement of a prolapsed gland of the third eyelid ("cherry eye") via a modification of the conjunctival pocket technique of Morgan. **A,** Two semielliptical incisions are made through the bulbar conjunctiva around the periphery of the prolapsed gland. The outer (free) edges of conjunctiva created by these incision are then apposed over the prolapsed gland using 4/0 to 6/0 absorbable suture, such as polyglactin 910 (Vicryl) in a simple continuous pattern. The initial and final anchoring knots are placed on the anterior face of the third eyelid to avoid frictional irritation of the cornea. **B,** The second (Cushing) layer of a continuous Connell-Cushing pattern is then placed with bites parallel to the conjunctival incisions, and, again, knots are placed on the anterior face of the third eyelid.

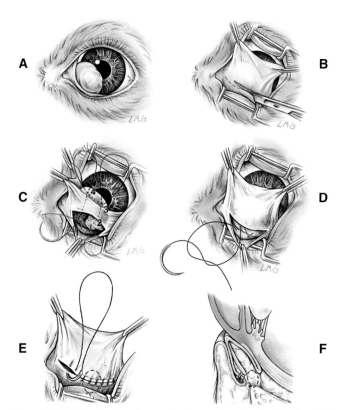

Figure 8-8. A, Surgical replacement of a prolapsed gland of the third eyelid ("cherry eye") via anchoring to the ventral orbital rim. **B,** A small incision is made in the ventral conjunctival fornix to allow access to the orbital rim. **C,** A 2/0 nylon suture is anchored to the orbital fascia immediately adjacent to the orbital rim *(1)* passed up through the lateral side of the exposed gland *(2),* across the dorsal aspect of the gland *(3),* and down through the medial side of the gland *(4)* to re-emerge opposite the initial bite *(1).* **D,** The suture is tied in a surgeon's throw and with sufficient tension to reduce the prolapsed gland. **E,** The conjunctival incision is closed with 6/0 polyglactin 910 (Vicryl) in a simple continuous pattern. **F,** Cross-sectional view showing position of both sutures and the reduced gland.

NEOPLASMS AFFECTING THE THIRD EYELID

Squamous cell carcinoma commonly involves the third eyelid in cattle and horses (Figure 8-10). Amelanotic or poorly pigmented third eyelids appear more susceptible. Third eyelid squamous cell carcinoma is sometimes also seen in small animals, but lymphoma (Figure 8-11), hemangioma or hemangiosarcoma (Figure 8-12), and adenocarcinoma (Figure 8-13) of the third eyelid also are common. Wilcock and Peiffer (1988), who described seven cases of adenocarcinoma of the canine third eyelid in dogs between 10 and 16 years of age, observed frequent local recurrence (57%) and suspected metastasis after excision.

Identification of a third eyelid neoplasm should stimulate a thorough assessment of the orbit, regional lymph nodes, and distant sites for metastases or extension. Surgical excision is recommended for all malignant tumors other than lymphoma, which can be treated via systemic chemotherapy. For focal masses near the third eyelid free margin resection of the mass and surrounding normal tissue may be possible (Figure 8-14).

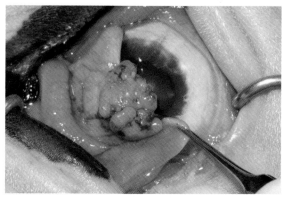

Figure 8-10. Squamous cell carcinoma of the third eyelid in a lightly melanotic horse.

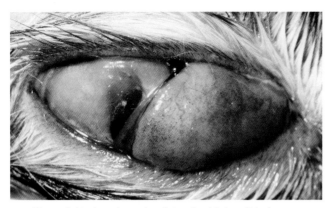

Figure 8-11. Lymphoma involving the third eyelid of a cat.

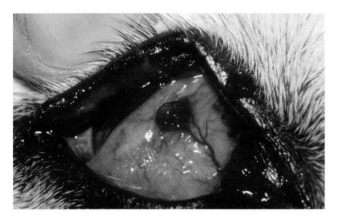

Figure 8-12. Hemangiosarcoma of the third eyelid of a dog.

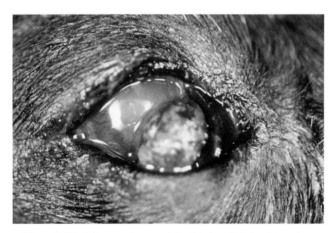

Figure 8-13. Adenocarcinoma of the third eyelid gland in a dog.

Larger tumors necessitate complete excision of the third eyelid and surrounding conjunctiva (Figure 8-15).

TRAUMA TO THE THIRD EYELID

Injuries to the third eyelid occur as a result of fights, motor vehicle accidents, and foreign body penetration. Usually, tears involving the conjunctiva only do not require suturing. Small

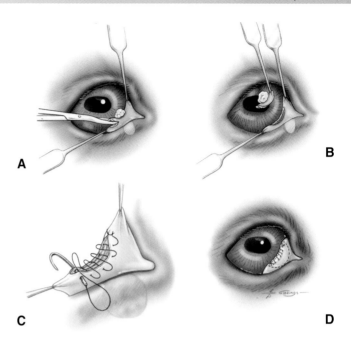

Figure 8-14. Surgical removal of a small neoplasm on the free margin of the third eyelid. **A** and **B,** The third eyelid is grasped with forceps or mosquito hemostats, and the mass plus adequate margin are removed with tenotomy scissors. **C** and **D,** The bulbar and anterior conjunctival surfaces are sutured over the edge of any exposed cartilage using 6/0 absorbable suture in a simple continuous pattern. Adjunctive radiation or cryotherapy may be necessary in the region outlined by a dotted line.

flaps off the leading edge can be safely removed. Larger lacerations, especially those involving the free margin and creating larger loose flaps, may benefit from careful appositional suturing with knots placed on the anterior surface so as to avoid frictional irritation of the cornea (Figure 8-16). Although some retraction takes place during healing, a functional third eyelid can often be retained. In some circumstances grafting of oral mucous membrane may be useful for replacing large defects.

INFLAMMATORY DISORDERS OF THE THIRD EYELID

The third eyelid is predictably involved in most conjunctival disorders. These are discussed more fully in Chapter 7. The third eyelid can be involved more obviously than or, rarely, to the exclusion of other conjunctival surfaces in so-called atypical pannus (see Chapter 10), eosinophilic keratoconjunctivitis of cats and horses (see Chapter 10), ligneous conjunctivitis of dogs (see Chapter 7), habronemiasis of horses (see Chapter 7), and nodular granulomatous episclerokeratoconjunctivitis of dogs (see Chapter 10). Although these disorders may represent clinically unusual distribution of the lesions, diagnosis and therapy are the same as for the more "typical" forms, and prognosis may be better than for those forms that also or only involve cornea.

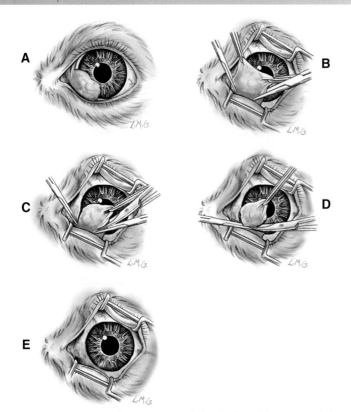

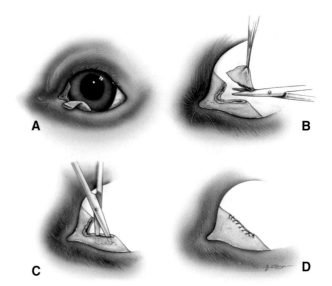

Figure 8-16. Repair of a more major third eyelid laceration (minor lacerations do not need surgical correction). **A,** Torn third eyelid with a loose necrotic flap. **B,** Any loose or necrotic tissue should be resected. **C,** The bulbar and palpebral conjunctiva is mobilized from the underlying cartilage with tenotomy scissors. **D,** The mobilized conjunctiva is sutured with a continuous suture of 6/0 or 7/0 polyglactin 910 (Vicryl), with the knots tied on the anterior (palpebral) surface.

Figure 8-15. A, Complete resection of the third eyelid is required for larger tumors of the third eyelid. **B,** An eyelid speculum and mosquito hemostats are used to ensure adequate exposure of the third eyelid. Hemostats are then placed along the dorsomedial and ventrolateral borders of the third eyelid. **C,** Scissors are used to cut on the third eyelid side of each hemostat, and the anterior and posterior (bulbar) surfaces of sectioned conjunctiva are oversewn in a simple continuous pattern using 6/0 or 7/0 polyglactin 910 (Vicryl). **D,** The base of the third eyelid is clamped deep enough within the orbit that the gland and cartilage are completely resected, and the conjunctival edges are oversewn in the same manner as described in **C. E,** Final appearance showing the three lines of simple continuous suture, which ensure against orbital fat prolapse.

BIBLIOGRAPHY

Constantinescu GM, McClure RC (1990): Anatomy of the orbital fasciae and the third eyelid in dogs. Am J Vet Res 51:260.

Dugan S, et al. (1992): Clinical and histologic evaluation of the prolapsed third eyelid gland in dogs. J Am Vet Med Assoc 201:1861.

Keil SM, et al. (1997): Bilateral nodular eosinophilic granulomatous inflammation of the nictitating membrane of a cat. Vet Comp Ophthalmol 7:258.

Komaromy AM, et al. (1997): Primary adenocarcinoma of the gland of the nictitating membrane in a cat. J Am Vet Med Assoc 33:333.

Kuhns EL (1977): Oral mucosal grafts for membrana nictitans replacement. Mod Vet Pract 58:768.

Larocca RD (2000): Eosinophilic conjunctivitis, herpes virus and mast cell tumor of the third eyelid in a cat. Vet Ophthalmol 3:221.

Martin CL (1970): Everted membrane nictitans in German shorthaired pointers. J Am Med Assoc 157:1229.

Moore C, et al. (1992): Distribution and course of secretory ducts of the canine third eyelid gland. Vet. Pathol 29:480.

Morgan RV, et al. (1993): Prolapse of the gland of the third eyelid in dogs: a retrospective study of 89 cases (1980-1990). J Am Anim Hosp Assoc 29:56.

Powell CC, Martin CL (1989): Distribution of cholinergic and adrenergic nerve fibers in the lacrimal in dogs. Am J Vet Res 50:2084.

Rebhun WC, Del Piero F (1998): Ocular lesions in horses with lymphosarcoma: 21 cases (1977-1997). J Am Vet Med Assoc 212:852.

Stanley RG, Kaswan RL (1994): Modification of the orbital rim anchorage method for surgical replacement of the gland of the third eyelid. Am J Vet Res 205:1412.

Stuhr CM, et al. (1999): Surgical repair of third eyelid lacerations in three birds. J Adv Med Surg 13:201.

Wilcock BL, Peiffer RL (1988): Adenocarcinoma of the third eyelid in seven dogs. J Am Vet Med Assoc 15:193.

LACRIMAL SYSTEM

Paul E. Miller

ANATOMY AND PHYSIOLOGY

The lacrimal system consists of the following structures:

- Lacrimal and third eyelid glands
- Accessory lacrimal glands
- Precorneal tear film
- Lacrimal puncta and canaliculi (Figure 9-1)
- Lacrimal sac
- Nasolacrimal duct
- Nasal puncta

Lacrimal and Third Eyelid Glands

The *gland of the third eyelid,* which lies within the stroma of the third eyelid, is partially visible on the inner surface of the third eyelid (see Chapter 8 and Figure 9-2). The tubulo-alveolar lacrimal gland is flattened and lies over the superior-temporal part of the globe. In the dog it lies beneath the *orbital ligament* and supraorbital process of the frontal bone and is related to the medial surface of the zygomatic bone (Figure 9-3). The position is similar in species with a fully enclosed bony orbit.

Lacrimal secretions enter the superior conjunctival fornix from the canine lacrimal gland via three to five microscopic ducts, and from the gland of the third eyelid via multiple ducts opening on the bulbar surface of the third eyelid between the normal lymphoid follicles. The *precorneal tear film* is distributed over the ocular surface by gravity, blinking, and movement of the third eyelid.

Accessory Lacrimal Glands

The accessory lacrimal glands (Figure 9-4), which are near the lid margins and contribute to the precorneal tear film, are composed of the following:

- The meibomian (tarsal) glands. In the dog, 20 to 40 of these glands open onto the lid margin. They produce the superficial layer of the precorneal tear film.
- The glands of Moll (modified sweat glands)
- The glands of Zeis (modified sebaceous glands associated with the cilia)

The functional significance of the glands of Moll and Zeis in animals is unknown, although infections of the glands of Zeis occur clinically and are called *external hordeolum* (stye).

Precorneal Tear Film

The precorneal tear film covers the cornea and conjunctiva (Figure 9-5). It consists of three layers, differing in composition, and is about 8 to 9 μm thick.

The *outer superficial (lipid) layer* (0.1 μm thick) is composed of oily materials and phospholipids from the tarsal glands and the glands of Zeis along the lid margin. Its two functions are as follows:

- To limit evaporation of the aqueous layer
- To bind the precorneal tear film to the cornea at the lid margins and prevent overflow by its high surface tension

Drugs containing preservatives with detergent properties and commercial shampoos remove this layer and can lead to corneal drying and possibly corneal ulceration. The layer is difficult to appreciate clinically but may be observed as an oil-like film over the ocular surface if the eye is examined with oblique illumination and at high magnification. Alternatively, the layer has been evaluated experimentally with polarized light biomicroscopy.

The *middle,* or *aqueous, layer,* consisting predominantly of water derived from the lacrimal gland and the gland of the third eyelid is the thickest layer (approximately 7 μm) and serves the following functions:

- To flush foreign material and bacteria from the conjunctival sac
- To lubricate the lids and third eyelid as they move over the cornea
- To supply the cornea with nutrients, including oxygen, amino acids, vitamin A, growth factors, and antibodies (immunoglobulin [Ig] A), and to remove metabolic waste products. White blood cells also reach the ocular surface via the tear film.
- To give a smooth surface to the cornea for optimal optical efficiency. The inner mucin layer also performs this function by filling in irregularities in the corneal surface.
- To act as a source of antibacterial substances, such as immunoglobulins, lactoferrin, and lysozyme. Tears also contain protease inhibitors that protect the cornea from degradative enzymes released by bacteria, inflammatory cells, and keratocytes.

The *inner mucoid layer* (1.0 to 2.0 μm thick) consists of hydrated glycoproteins derived from the conjunctival goblet cells. This layer is critical in binding the lipophobic aqueous layer to the lipophilic corneal surface and in preventing the tear

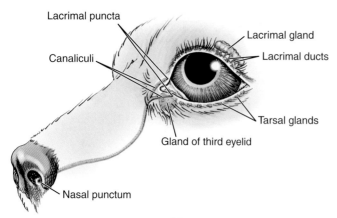

Figure 9-1. Components of the nasolacrimal system.

Lacrimal puncta

Canaliculi

Lacrimal gland

Lacrimal ducts

Tarsal glands

Gland of third eyelid

Nasal punctum

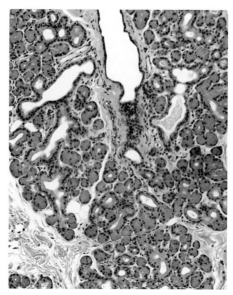

Figure 9-2. Tubuloalveolar structure of the canine gland of the third eyelid. (Courtesy Dr. Richard R. Dubielzig.)

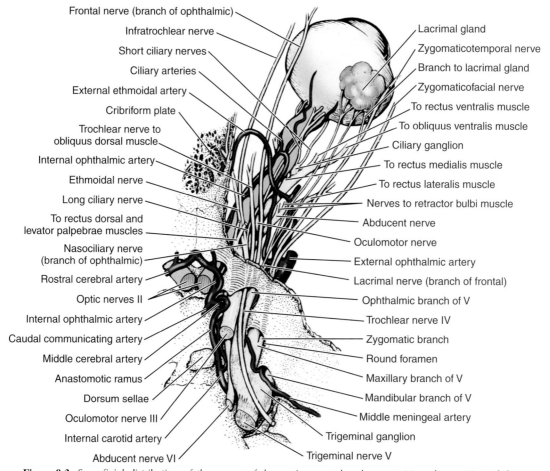

Frontal nerve (branch of ophthalmic)

Infratrochlear nerve

Short ciliary nerves

Ciliary arteries

External ethmoidal artery

Cribriform plate

Trochlear nerve to obliquus dorsal muscle

Internal ophthalmic artery

Ethmoidal nerve

Long ciliary nerve

To rectus dorsal and levator palpebrae muscles

Nasociliary nerve (branch of ophthalmic)

Rostral cerebral artery

Optic nerves II

Internal ophthalmic artery

Caudal communicating artery

Middle cerebral artery

Anastomotic ramus

Dorsum sellae

Oculomotor nerve III

Internal carotid artery

Abducent nerve VI

Lacrimal gland

Zygomaticotemporal nerve

Branch to lacrimal gland

Zygomaticofacial nerve

To rectus ventralis muscle

To obliquus ventralis muscle

Ciliary ganglion

To rectus medialis muscle

To rectus lateralis muscle

Nerves to retractor bulbi muscle

Abducent nerve

Oculomotor nerve

External ophthalmic artery

Lacrimal nerve (branch of frontal)

Ophthalmic branch of V

Trochlear nerve IV

Zygomatic branch

Round foramen

Maxillary branch of V

Mandibular branch of V

Middle meningeal artery

Trigeminal ganglion

Trigeminal nerve V

Figure 9-3. Superficial distribution of the nerves of the canine eye, dorsal aspect. Note the position of the lacrimal gland beneath the orbital ligament. (Modified from Evans HE [1993]: Miller's Anatomy of the Dog, 3rd ed. Saunders, Philadelphia.)

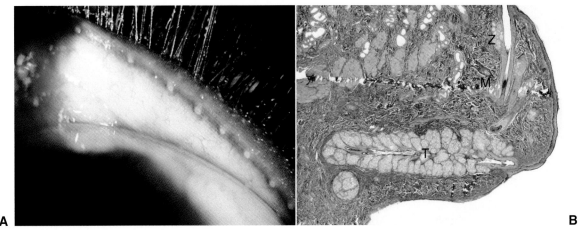

A   **B**

Figure 9-4. A, The openings of the meibomian (tarsal) gland ductules are apparent as multiple, circular, lightly pigmented foci at the eyelid margin in this goat. The sebaceous secretions of these glands contribute to the lipid layer of the tear film. **B,** Cross-sectional view of the normal canine eyelid. The accessory lacrimal glands of the eyelid margin include the tarsal (meibomian) glands *(T)*, glands of Moll *(M)*, and glands of Zeiss *(Z)*. (**B** courtesy Dr. Richard R. Dubielzig.)

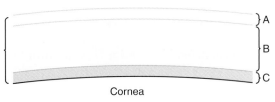

Cornea

Figure 9-5. Precorneal tear film. *A,* Superficial lipid layer; *B,* aqueous layer; *C,* inner mucoid layer.

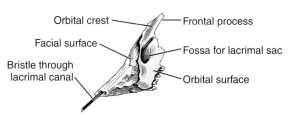

Figure 9-6. Left canine lacrimal bone, lateral aspect, showing the lacrimal fossa. (Modified from Evans HE 1993]: Miller's Anatomy of the Dog, 3rd ed. Saunders, Philadelphia.)

film from "beading up" on the corneal surface much like water does on the surface of a freshly waxed car. The mucoprotein molecules are thought to be bipolar, with one end lipophilic (associated with the corneal epithelium) and one end hydrophilic (associated with the aqueous layer). This layer is also difficult to appreciate clinically but may be indirectly evaluated by determination of the tear film break-up time (TFBUT).

Mucous Threads

Fine mucous threads lie in the superior and inferior conjunctival fornices in the normal animal. These strands are accumulations of mucus derived from the conjunctival goblet cells and exfoliated epithelial cells. The threads migrate nasally in a predictable fashion, collecting debris from the conjunctival sac. Vacuoles within the threads contain debris and exhibit enzymatic activity. Dehydrated remnants of these threads are frequently found on the skin at the nasal canthus in the morning ("sleep" or "sleepy seeds"). These accumulations are normally grayish and translucent and may be quite large in animals with deep conjunctival fornices (e.g., Irish setters, Doberman pinschers). In cats it is not uncommon for the threads to be deep red to black because they are stained with tear porphyrins. In an animal without signs of conjunctival inflammation or epiphora, larger accumulations are normal if they are grayish or translucent (possibly reddish black in cats). Increased quantities are often a sensitive indicator of ocular surface inflammation. A change in color of the mucous thread to green or yellow is a reliable indicator of the presence of inflammatory cells and mandates a careful clinical examination.

Accumulations of normal mucus are frequently mistaken by owners for signs of ocular disease. Yellowish or green mucus, however, is a sign of inflammatory cells in the mucus.

Lacrimal Puncta, Canaliculi, and Nasolacrimal Duct

In most domestic mammals the *inferior* and *superior puncta* lie on the inner conjunctival surface of the eyelids, near the nasal limit of the tarsal glands (see Figure 9-1). Rabbits possess only one large inferior puncta that is a few millimeters from the eyelid margin.

The *lacrimal canaliculi* (*superior* and *inferior*) lead to a variable dilation in the common nasolacrimal duct—the *lacrimal sac.* The lacrimal sac varies in size, in some animals consisting only of a slight dilation in the duct. The sac lies within a depression in the lacrimal bone called the *lacrimal fossa* (Figure 9-6).

From the lacrimal sac, the *nasolacrimal duct* passes via a canal on the medial surface of the maxilla to open in the nasal cavity (Figure 9-7). In dogs the opening is ventrolateral near the attached margin of the alar fold; in horses it is ventral on the mucocutaneous junction; and in cattle it is more lateral. In cattle and horses the nasal opening is readily visible and can be cannulated, but in dogs it can be seen only after exposure with a speculum or other suitable instrument with the animals under general anesthesia. In dogs the nasolacrimal duct commonly has an opening into the nasal cavity between the lacrimal sac

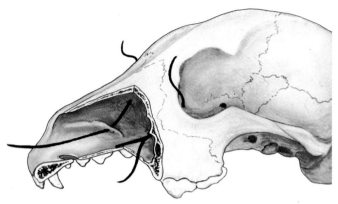

Figure 9-7. Cutaway drawing of the canine skull, showing the lacrimal fossa, lacrimal foramen, and relative position of the nasolacrimal duct. (Modified from Severin GA [2000]: Severin's Veterinary Ophthalmology Notes, 3rd ed. Severin, Ft. Collins, CO.)

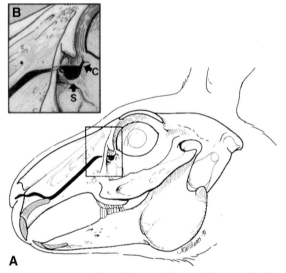

Figure 9-8. Diagram of the rabbit nasolacrimal duct. **A,** The duct bends and narrows at two points, proximally as it passes through the maxillary bone and distally as it bends near the incisor tooth root. This anatomy makes the rabbit prone to dacryocystitis and nasolacrimal duct obstruction. **B,** Higher magnification of the area outlined in the box in **A,** showing the single canaliculus and the location of the lacrimal sac. (From Burling K, et al. [1991]: Anatomy of the rabbit nasolacrimal duct and its clinical implications. Prog Vet Comp Ophthalmol 1:33.)

and the nasal opening, although the remainder of the duct is intact. In rabbits the nasolacrimal duct has multiple sharp bends and constricted areas, which may be associated with the frequency of duct obstruction and dacryocystitis in this species. Cannulation is also difficult in most rabbits (Figure 9-8).

Approximately 25% of the precorneal tear film is lost by evaporation. The remainder passes into the puncta and via the canaliculi, sac, and duct to the nasal cavity. A large proportion of the precorneal tear film accumulates in the inferior fornix as the *lacrimal lake*. Most of this fluid enters the inferior punctum through capillary attraction and movements of the lids. During contraction of the orbicularis oculi, the wall of the sac is tensed, creating lower pressure within the lumen and causing tears to enter; this mechanism is called the *lacrimal pump*.

Innervation

Innervation of the lacrimal gland and control of secretion are complex, and the exact details are undetermined in domestic animals. Fibers from the ophthalmic division of the trigeminal nerve, facial nerve, pterygopalatine ganglion, and sympathetic fibers from the carotid plexus have been traced to the lacrimal gland.

DISTURBANCES OF LACRIMAL FUNCTION

The two categories of lacrimal dysfunction are as follows:

- Inability of the drainage system to remove the tears produced. This may be caused either by *obstruction* of the drainage system or *overproduction* of tears. The clinical signs depend on the relative amounts of tears produced and drained away.
- Failure to produce a normal precorneal tear film (or one of its components), usually resulting in secondary conjunctivitis and keratitis. Abnormalities are *quantitative* (insufficient aqueous component) or *qualitative* (abnormalities in components or function of the superficial lipid layer, or the inner mucoid layer).

Effects of Precorneal Tear Film Dysfunction

Abnormalities in the quantity or quality of the tear film may compromise function. Deficiency of the tear film may cause the following:

- Hypertonicity of the remaining tear film
- Dehydration of the conjunctival and corneal epithelium
- Hypoxia of the corneal epithelium and subepithelial stroma
- Lack of lubrication with frictional irritation of the ocular surface by the eyelids and third eyelid
- Increase in numbers of microorganisms and mucus on the ocular surface and on the eyelids
- Secondary inflammation of the conjunctiva and cornea with stromal vascularization and later pigmentation
- Corneal erosions or ulcers

Examination

The techniques for examination of lacrimal disorders have been discussed in Chapter 5. The reader is referred to that chapter for descriptions of the following specific tests:

- Schirmer tear test (STT) (p. 81) for quantitative abnormalities
- TFBUT for qualitative disorders
- Fluorescein stain for corneal ulceration
- Rose bengal stain (p. 100) to detect epithelial abnormalities caused by quantitative and qualitative disorders
- Fluorescein passage or Jones test (p. 99) for drainage disorders
- Nasolacrimal cannulation and flushing (p. 95) for drainage disorders
- Dacryocystorhinography (p. 103) for drainage disorders

The fluorescein passage test (Jones test) is reliable only when its result is positive. Because of communications between the nasolacrimal duct and the nasal cavity, false-negative results occur even though the duct is patent. If epiphora is due to over-production of tears, the eye is usually red and the STT values are higher than normal.

Disorders Characterized by Epiphora

The conjunctiva is usually quiet in patients with epiphora due to passive or simple mechanical obstruction of the nasolacrimal system, whereas it is reddened in patients with epiphora due to chronic irritation/inflammation of the cornea, conjunctiva, or lacrimal sac.

Dacryocystitis

Dacryocystitis is inflammation within the lacrimal sac and nasolacrimal duct. It occurs most frequently in dogs and cats and less frequently in horses. Although foreign bodies (e.g., grass awns, sand, dirt, and concretions of mucopurulent material) can be expressed in some patients, the primary cause is often undetermined. Cystic dilations of the nasolacrimal duct causing chronic dacryocystitis in dogs have been described. They are treated by creation of a drainage stoma into the nasal cavity (Figure 9-9). The infected focus within the proximal portion of the duct may reinfect the conjunctival sac, resulting in chronic, unilateral conjunctivitis of apparent unexplained cause. Often the amount of ocular discharge in dacryocystitis is far in excess of what would be expected in view of the severity of conjunctivitis present.

Chronic dacryocystitis may cause recurrent unilateral conjunctivitis with no other apparent clinical signs.

CLINICAL SIGNS. The clinical signs of dacryocystitis are as follows:

- Ocular discharge ranging from clear tears to more commonly thick mucopurulent exudate at the medial canthus; the exudate may have layers of purulent and clear material or gas bubbles within it
- Mild conjunctivitis—especially medially
- Expression or flushing of mucopurulent material from the nasal or lacrimal puncta; this area often is painful to the touch but sometimes is totally painless
- Painful, erythematous dermatitis at the medial canthus in some cases
- Abscessation of the sac in severe cases; in chronic cases, this abscessation may cause a large cavity to form
- History of recurrent unilateral conjunctivitis with temporary responses to topical antibiotics and attempted flushing

DIAGNOSIS. Diagnosis is based on clinical signs, especially expression of purulent material from the puncta. The exact site of the obstruction may be determined by cannulation, dacryocystorhinography, or magnetic resonance imaging.

TREATMENT

Nasolacrimal Catheterization. Because of its tendency to recur, definitive surgical catheterization (Figure 9-10) is

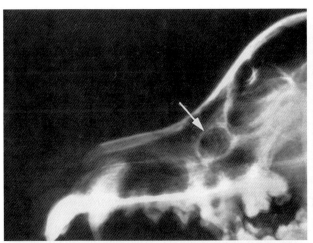

A

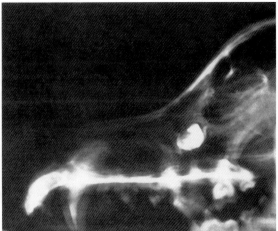

B

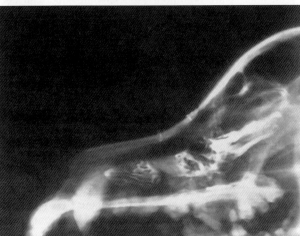

C

Figure 9-9. A, Lateral radiographic view of the skull of a 4-year-old golden retriever with recurrent intermittent episodes of purulent discharge from the right eye. A radiolucent area with sclerotic margins *(arrow)* is evident dorsal and rostral to the maxillary process of the maxillary bone (dorsal to the upper right fourth premolar). **B** and **C,** Dacryocystorhinogram of the right nasolacrimal duct of the same dog before surgery **(B)** and 9 months after surgery **(C).** Before surgery, contrast material accumulated in the cyst indicated in **A,** and the nasolacrimal duct was visible proximal to the radiolucency. After surgery, contrast material was evident in the nasal passage but did not accumulate in the cyst. (From van der Woerdt A, et al. [1997]: Surgical treatment of dacryocystitis caused by cystic dilatation of the nasolacrimal system in three dogs. J Am Vet Med Assoc 211:445.)

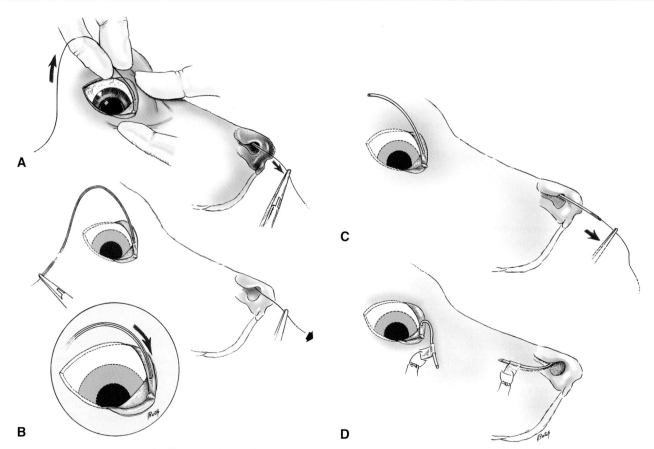

Figure 9-10. Indwelling nasolacrimal duct catheterization for correction of recurring obstruction. **A,** A monofilament nylon thread (2/0 with a smooth melted end) is passed via the superior punctum to emerge from the nose. If an obstruction is present in the sac, the duct is threaded from the nasal end, and the thread is manipulated to emerge from the superior punctum. **B,** Fine polyethylene (PE90), polyvinyl, or silicone tubing with a beveled end is passed over the thread. Halsted forceps are clamped behind the tubing, which is pulled from the nasal end by forceps on the thread. In horses, larger tubing is used. **C,** Care is taken as the tubing enters the punctum. *Note:* The inferior punctum may also be used if threading via this punctum was used. The tubing is pulled down the nasolacrimal duct, past any obstructions. **D,** The tube is sutured in place for 2 to 3 weeks. An Elizabethan collar should be considered to prevent the tubing from being dislodged. (Modified from Bistner SI, et al. [1977]: Atlas of Veterinary Ophthalmic Surgery. Saunders, Philadelphia.)

indicated for dacryocystitis. Although daily flushing and topical medication are effective in some cases, they are less reliable than catheterization and there is a greater chance of recurrence. The tube is left in place for 2 to 3 weeks. The inserted tubes rarely cause discomfort unless they become loose. For the first few days the uncannulated punctum may be flushed daily with a topical ophthalmic antibiotic solution, and topical antibiotic/corticosteroid solution is also applied to the ocular surface. If abscessation of the sac or severe dermatitis is present, systemic antibiotics are added.

Dacryocystotomy. For patients in which obstruction prevents the passage of a catheter, the lacrimal sac may be exposed ab externo, through an incision parallel to the lower lid, followed by removal of the outer surface of the lacrimal bone with a Hall Surgitome bur over the sac, flushing of the sac, and placement of the catheter (Figure 9-11). In some chronically affected animals a cavity may develop in the region of the sac. If the catheter is left in place and antibiotic therapy is continued, the space usually fills with fibrous tissue and a patent duct remains. This may take several months.

Congenital Atresia, Ectopia, and Imperforate Puncta

In dogs, imperforate puncta (usually of the inferior puncta) and punctal aplasia are common, especially in American cocker spaniels, Bedlington terriers, golden retrievers, miniature and toy poodles, and Samoyeds. The condition is congenital and is often characterized by epiphora, although some animals are relatively asymptomatic and epiphora may not become apparent until several weeks of age, when tear production increases. Diagnosis is made by examination of the normal location of the puncta with magnification and from the inability to cannulate or probe the puncta with a small polytetrafluoroethylene (Teflon) IV catheter (minus needle), a lacrimal cannula, or fine nylon thread. In most cases the obstruction consists of a layer of conjunctiva over the lumen, but occasionally obstructions are present in other parts of the nasolacrimal duct. The overlying conjunctiva may be removed with fine scissors after it is elevated with liquid under pressure (Figure 9-12) or through retrograde probing with fine nylon thread (2/0) from the nasal opening (Figure 9-13). Some patients require short-term (1 to

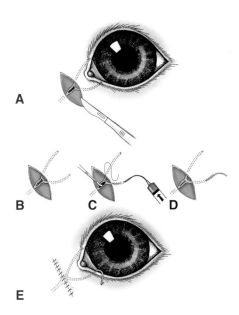

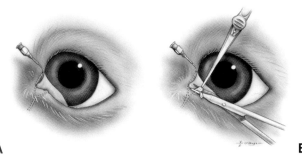

Figure 9-11. Dacryocystostomy in the dog. **A,** An incision is completed ventral to the medial canthus into the lacrimal sac. **B** and **C,** The foreign material is removed and submitted for laboratory evaluation. The nasolacrimal duct system is cannulated with a Silastic tube **(D),** and the incision is closed routinely **(E).** (Modified from Grahn B [1999]: Disorders and surgery of the canine nasolacrimal system, in Gelatt KN (editor): Veterinary Ophthalmology, 3rd ed. Lippincott Williams & Wilkins, Philadelphia.)

Figure 9-12. Repair of imperforate punctum through the use of pressurized fluid. **A,** The opposing punctum is cannulated, and pressure is applied via a saline-filled syringe to elevate the obstructing conjunctiva over the other punctum. The use of methylene blue solution aids in the location of the bleb. Some loss of saline occurs down the nasolacrimal duct. **B,** The tissue is grasped with fine forceps and incised with strabismus scissors or other fine scissors. Antibiotic-corticosteroid preparations are applied for 7 to 10 days to prevent scarring and obstruction. Daily dilation and flushing may be needed for a few days to prevent closure. If the membrane is thick or bleeds when incised the nasolacrimal system may need to be cannulated for 1 to 3 weeks to prevent fibrosis of the newly created stoma.

3 weeks) placement of an indwelling catheter to prevent fibrosis of the newly created stoma, especially if the wound bleeds after excision.

In foals (and crias) the obstruction is usually at the nasal puncta instead of the inferior puncta. The nasal puncta may be covered with mucosa, and a variable portion of the nasolacrimal duct may be missing. Additional or abnormally positioned openings may also be present. For treatment, the lumen of the duct is distended with saline via the lacrimal puncta, or with

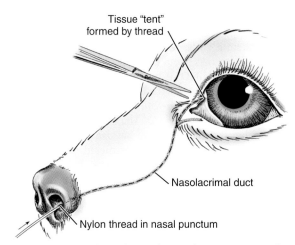

Figure 9-13. Retrograde probing of imperforate punctum. The nasal meatus of the nasolacrimal duct is probed using a nylon (2/0) thread. The probe is passed up to elevate the obstructing conjunctiva, which is excised. This procedure is most useful for the superior punctum, because it is more difficult to pass a probe into the inferior punctum from the nasal end.

polyethylene tubing, and the nasal mucosa is incised until the lumen is entered. The stoma is cannulated with the tubing, which is sutured in place for 7 to 21 days. Daily application of a topical antibiotic-corticosteroid preparation for 3 to 4 days after removal of the tube is advisable to reduce the chance of postoperative stricture formation. A variety of diverse congenital anomalies of the nasolacrimal duct occur in all species, but all are rare.

In young cats, the most common cause of apparent congenital lacrimal obstruction is cicatrization of the puncta due to feline herpesvirus type 1 conjunctivitis.

Cystic Disorders

Cystic disorders of the lacrimal system and tissues are uncommon but may affect the lacrimal gland, canaliculi, nasolacrimal duct, gland of the third eyelid, zygomatic salivary gland, conjunctival goblet cells, lacrimal sac, and parotid duct after transplantation. Clinical signs are usually restricted to localized swelling, and treatment consists of careful surgical excision and, sometimes, cannulation (see also section on dacryocystitis). Periorbital epidermoid cysts have also been described at the medial canthus in dogs.

Cicatricial Nasolacrimal Obstructions

In cats, especially kittens, scarring and blockage of the puncta or nasolacrimal ducts are common sequela of presumed herpetic keratoconjunctivitis and upper respiratory tract infections. Similar changes due to variety of causes may be seen in any species and frequently accompanies symblepharon. If the puncta and ducts cannot be cannulated, conjunctivorhinostomy or drainage procedures to the oral cavity (conjunctivobuccostomy) are the only remedy. Conjunctivorhinostomy and conjunctivobuccostomy are usually performed by a veterinary ophthalmologist in animals without evidence of active conjunctivitis or chronic respiratory disease. Active, or recurrent, disease increases the chance the newly created opening will scar closed and usually means that surgery will fail to correct the problem. If recurrent respiratory disease is present in cats, a careful examination for evidence of herpetic keratitis is performed and serologic tests for feline leukemia virus, feline immunodeficiency virus, and possibly cryptococcosis should be considered.

CONJUNCTIVORHINOSTOMY. In conjunctivorhinostomy a communication is made from the medial conjunctival sac to the nasal cavity and is kept open with a stent of plastic or silicone tubing until healed (Figure 9-14). The method is most suitable for dogs lacking lacrimal drainage but can be used in cats. In cats the opening tends to become obstructed with scar tissue, and the stent is left in longer (8 to 12 weeks) before initial removal. During the postoperative period the topical antibiotic therapy is continued and the stent is cleaned frequently. Also, the eye is checked weekly to ensure that the stent is not causing ocular irritation (e.g., by pressing on the cornea through the third eyelid).

CONJUNCTIVOBUCCOSTOMY. Conjunctivobuccostomy is an alternative method of providing lacrimal drainage (Figure 9-15).

Tear-Staining Syndrome in Dogs

The miniature and toy poodle and the Maltese terrier are most commonly affected by tear-staining syndrome (Figure 9-16), a primarily cosmetic defect in which the hair around the medial canthus is stained reddish brown from constant epiphora. The condition is usually present from a young age and is rarely accompanied by other significant ocular disorders. Some animals may also have a localized dermatitis in the medial canthal region. Although it is most obvious in animals with a lightly

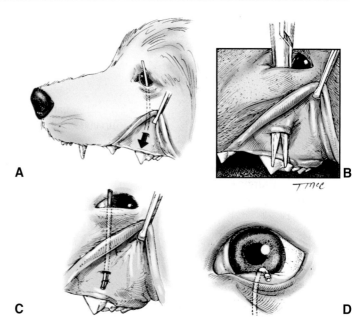

Figure 9-15. Conjunctivobuccostomy. **A,** Direction of the final drainage canal. **B,** A canal is made from the inferior conjunctival fornix to the oral cavity with straight hemostats. **C,** A tube is passed and sutured to the oral mucosa. **D,** The upper end of the tube is sutured to the skin in the region of the nasal canthus so as not to rub on the cornea. The tube is left in place for a minimum of 2 months. (Modified from Lavach JD [1985]: Lacrimal system, in Slatter DH [editor]: Textbook of Small Animal Surgery, Saunders, Philadelphia.)

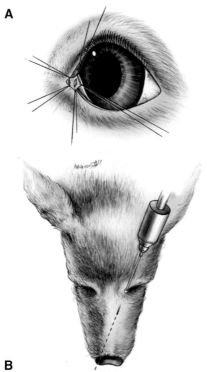

Figure 9-14. Conjunctivorhinostomy. **A,** The conjunctiva is removed from the inferior nasal area overlying the lacrimal bone. **B,** A communication is made from the conjunctival sac to the nasal cavity with a Steinmann orthopaedic pin. The pin is directed toward the contralateral external nares but is advanced only until it enters the nasal cavity. A stent of plastic tubing is sutured in place.

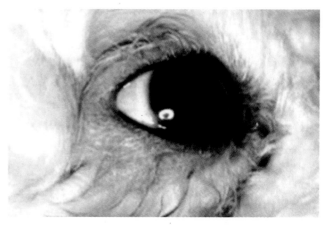

Figure 9-16. Chronic tear-staining syndrome in a miniature poodle.

colored hair coat, it occurs in animals with dark hair coats as well. The staining is believed to be due to lactoferrin-like pigments in the tears, which overflow because of a functional or partial obstruction of the drainage system.

Various causes of tear-staining syndrome have been proposed, including caruncular hairs, which wick tears onto the face; medioventral entropion or trichiasis; kinking of an otherwise patent inferior puncta; small lacrimal lake; tight medial canthal ligaments; folds of conjunctiva, which prevent entry of tears into the puncta; and abnormal lid closure resulting in failure of the lacrimal pump. In some animals multiple factors may be involved, and in others an obvious cause is not apparent. Epiphora also occurs commonly in brachycephalic Persian cats owing to obstruction of the nasolacrimal duct.

TREATMENT. Treatment for tear-staining syndrome in dogs consists of the following approaches:

- If a specific cause can be identified, treatment of that condition may alleviate the epiphora. Often, if a specific cause cannot be identified, the owner simply needs to be reassured that the problem is primarily cosmetic in nature and that the pet's vision or comfort is not threatened.
- If medial lower lid entropion or trichiasis is present, temporary eversion of the inferior-medial lower eyelid with a single suture in the medial canthus or eversion with one or two small surgical staples (Precise DS-15 surgical staple or similar) may be used diagnostically (Figure 9-17). If after 1 to 2 weeks the owner reports that eversion of the inferior eyelid has reduced the wetness (staining may not improve until the hair grows out), a permanent medial entropion correction may resolve the problem.
- Oral tetracycline 5 mg/kg once daily provides definite short-term improvement. Similar results may be achieved with oral metronidazole. Staining normally reappears 2 to 3 weeks after cessation of therapy. How these antibiotics reduce staining is unknown, but because tear production remains normal and the face still remains wet (if less stained), it is possible that they act by interfering with bacteria that create the compounds staining the hair.
- Treatment of concurrent allergies with topical and antibiotic steroid drops, mast cell stabilizers, and systemic low-dose steroids is helpful if these agents are used judiciously in patients with allergic disease.
- Affected animals should not be bred. Since the 1960s the incidence of very severely affected individuals appears to have decreased markedly.
- Although controversial and not the procedure of choice, partial removal of the gland of the third eyelid may result in improvement (Figure 9-18) in patients with severe disease that cannot otherwise be controlled. Because this procedure permanently removes a portion of the tear production mechanism, it is performed only if STT values exceed

15 mm/min. This procedure is not used indiscriminately or as a substitute for full ophthalmic investigation of the epiphora. It is essential to obtain fully informed consent on the part of the owner before performing this procedure as keratoconjunctivitis sicca (KCS) may occur postoperatively.

Other Causes of Epiphora

Other causes of epiphora, discussed in Chapters 6 and 7, are as follows:

- Prominent nasal folds
- Entropion
- Disorders of cilia
- Allergic inhalant dermatitis and conjunctivitis

Deficiency of the Precorneal Tear Film

Mucin Deficiency

Decreased numbers of conjunctival goblet cells, caused by chronic inflammation, metaplasia, hypoplasia, or fibrosis, can cause mucin deficiency—especially in dogs and probably cats. Affected animals may have many of the signs of the milder forms of KCS except that the STT values may be normal to slightly subnormal. Because mucin helps bind the aqueous portion of the tear film to the ocular surface, moisture does not uniformly wet the surface of the eye but instead "beads up" on the ocular surface effectively leaving some areas of the cornea dry. Decreases in TFBUT and numbers of goblet cells on histologic evaluation can confirm the diagnosis (Moore et al., 1987). Unless these tests are performed, it is often hard to make the diagnosis of mucin deficiency because of the difficulty in identifying this layer clinically. Treatment is best accomplished with cyclosporine, which may improve ocular mucins, and the use of tear replacement solutions, preferably by one of the polyvinylpyrrolidone or methylcellulose derivatives, which more closely simulate natural mucins.

Lipid Deficiency

Deficiencies of the precorneal tear film are typically due to inflammation of the eyelid margin and meibomian glands. Common causes are staphylococcal and *Malassezia*-associated blepharitis, generalized seborrhea, atopy, and demodicosis. Aberrant lipids may be directly toxic to epithelial cells, and loss of this layer may allow premature dispersion of the aqueous layer of the tear film, resulting in corneal drying. Clinical signs include sometimes subtle blepharitis manifested as swollen, rounded eyelid margins, swelling of the openings of the meibomian glands, hyperemia of the mucocutaneous junction, dry crusty lid margins, chalazia, and a yellow-white appearance to individual meibomian glands when viewed from the conjunctival surface. Gentle expression of the meibomian glands does not yield the normal clear, viscous oil but instead often yields a thick, opaque, cream-cheese–looking substance. Chronic keratitis, usually much less severe than in patients with deficiency of the aqueous layer, may also be present. The conjunctiva is often hyperemic, there is a mucoid to mucopurulent discharge, and the corneal epithelial surface may have faint localized areas of edema, multifocal areas of epithelial roughening, and, possibly, overt corneal erosion. Surface disease in these animals is

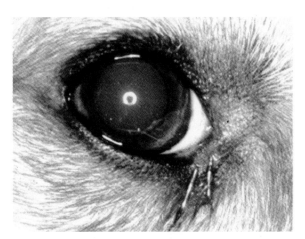

Figure 9-17. Diagnostic stapling for epiphora. A fine surgical staple (3M's Precise DS-15 or similar) or temporary everting suture is placed so as to evert the medial canthus. If this procedure alleviates the epiphora over a period of several days, a permanent procedure that everts the medial canthal area would be expected also to alleviate the epiphora. If this temporary procedure does not resolve the epiphora, eversion surgery is also unlikely to be of benefit, and additional possible causes of the epiphora should be explored.

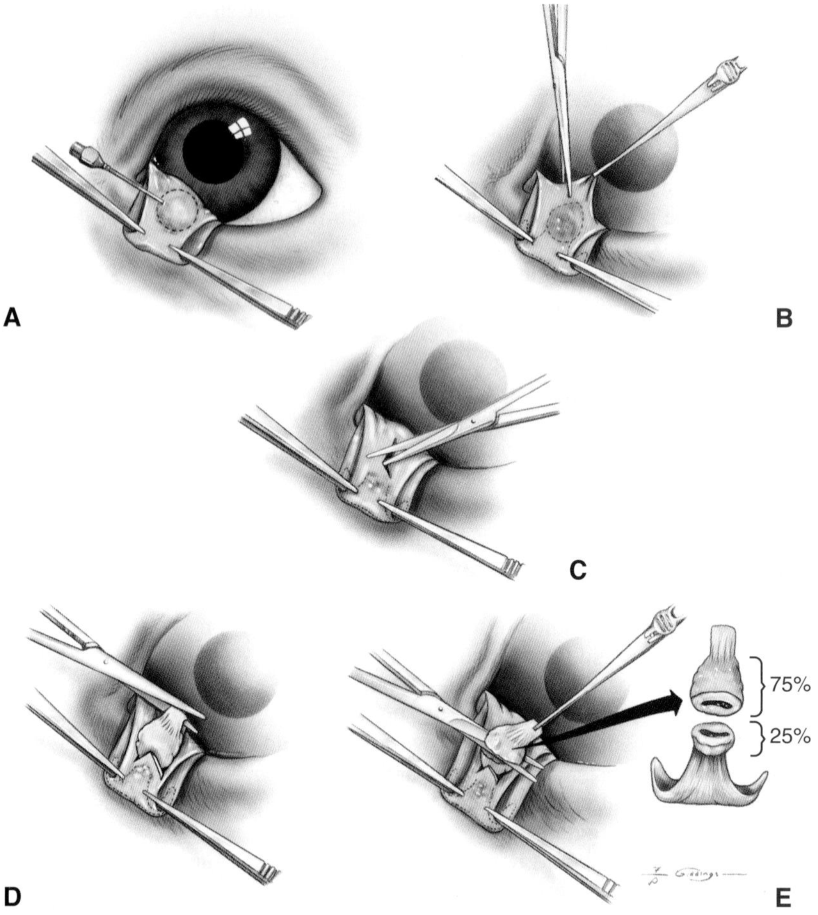

Figure 9-18. Partial removal of the gland of the third eyelid. **A,** Fixation forceps are applied to the edges of the cartilaginous T portion of the third eyelid. **B,** The gland is exposed by traction, and 0.25 mL of 1:100,000 epinephrine solution is injected subconjunctivally for hemostasis *(avoid use of epinephrine with halothane anesthesia).* **C,** With strabismus scissors, the conjunctiva is incised at the base of the gland. **D,** The gland is exposed by blunt subconjunctival dissection. **E,** Twenty-five to seventy-five percent of the gland is removed.

believed to be the result of poor surfacing of the tear film, frictional irritation from swollen lid margins, and perhaps toxic effects of abnormal lipids or inflammatory products.

This condition is treated with warm, moist compresses for several minutes two to three times per day and topical and systemic antibiotics, choice of which is ideally based on results of culture and sensitivity testing of secretions expressed from the eyelid margin. In select cases systemic or topical corticosteroids may also be helpful, especially if granulomas have developed in the eyelid as a result of the escape of meibomian lipids into the surrounding tissue. Topical therapy with a lipid substitute, such as petrolatum, mineral oil, or lanolin, may also be beneficial. Often the disease is chronic, and some form of long-term maintenance therapy is required.

Deficiency of the Aqueous Phase

Deficiency of the aqueous phase of the precorneal tear film is a common disorder in dogs (less so in cats and horses) that leads to xerosis (abnormal dryness) and KCS. Drying resulting from decreased secretion by the lacrimal glands is distinguished from drying attributable to increased evaporation of the aqueous layer in animals with congenitally open eyelids, facial paralysis, and exophthalmos.

Keratoconjunctivitis Sicca

The incidence of KCS in canine patients has been estimated at 1% (Moore, 1999).

ETIOLOGY. The etiology of KCS can be classified as follows:

Drug-Induced. KCS in dogs has been associated with the nonsteroidal antiinflammatory drug (NSAID) etodolac as well as with many sulfa derivatives, including trimethoprim-sulfamethoxazole, sulfadiazine, and sulfasalazine. Sulfa-derivative KCS is associated with a direct toxic effect on the lacrimal acinar cells by the nitrogen-containing pyridine and pyrimidine rings of these drugs. Up to 50% of dogs in which KCS develops after they receive a sulfa derivative do so within 30 days of starting the drug, and KCS has been reported to occur as soon as within the first week. Animals weighing less than 12 kg may be at increased risk. Sulfasalazine and its derivatives (used to treat chronic colitis in dogs) also cause KCS in dogs, but not all drugs of the group do so. 5-Amino salicylic acid (5-ASA), a derivative of sulfasalazine that is the active constituent in the treatment of colitis, also causes KCS in dogs. KCS has also been associated with phenazopyridine, a rarely used urinary analgesic, which also contains a nitrogen ring. It causes KCS after 7 to 10 days of use in most dogs, but not in cats. Temporary reduction in tear production may also be caused by general anesthesia and topical or systemic atropine.

Surgically Induced. KCS commonly occurs after removal of a prolapsed gland of the third eyelid, but the median time for this occurrence is 4.5 years after the operation. It may also been seen in patients in which the facial nerve is disrupted (e.g., ear canal ablation).

Immune-Mediated. KCS in dogs is most often immune-mediated. The lacrimal acinar epithelial cells may be an immune-privileged site and may be protected by a blood-tear barrier. Disruption of this barrier may allow immune-mediated destruction of these tissues, resulting in KCS. Indeed, in some dogs with KCS circulating autoantibodies to the lacrimal glands, salivary glands, and gland of the third eyelid are present. As in humans, animals with KCS may also be affected with a variety of autoimmune or immune-mediated disorders, including Sjögren's syndrome (dry mouth as well as eyes), systemic lupus erythematosus, pemphigus foliaceus, rheumatoid arthritis, hypothyroidism, diabetes mellitus, polymyositis and polyarthritis, atopy, glomerulonephritis, and ulcerative colitis.

Idiopathic. The majority of cases of idiopathic KCS may actually be immune-mediated, both in dogs and in the less commonly affected cat.

Orbital and Supraorbital Trauma. Trauma that either affects the glands directly or damages the nerves that innervate them may cause KCS. The disorder frequently accompanies traumatic proptosis. In horses KCS is rare, but the most common cause is regarded as trauma to the facial nerve.

Infectious. Canine distemper virus affects the lacrimal glands and glands of the third eyelid and may result in temporary or permanent dysfunction. KCS has also been associated with Leishmania infection and with chronic viral or bacterial conjunctivitis with fibrosis of the glands or their ducts. Feline herpesvirus may induce KCS through fibrosis of the lacrimal gland ductules.

Locoweed Poisoning. In cattle, sheep, and horses, locoweed poisoning can cause KCS.

Other Causes. Debilitated or dehydrated animals frequently have decreased tear production. Vitamin A deficiency rarely causes KCS in dogs, although it may do so somewhat more frequently in other species. Eosinophilic granulomatous dacryoadenitis, perhaps secondary to parasitic invasion into the lacrimal glands, has been reported as a cause in horses.

Congenital. Congenital acinar hypoplasia occurs in miniature breeds such as the pug, Chihuahua, and Yorkshire terrier. Cats with eyelid agenesis may also exhibit KCS due to absence of the glands or their ductules.

Senile Atrophy. Dogs 10 years or older are at increased risk for KCS due to senile atrophy of the lacrimal glands.

Radiation. The lacrimal gland and gland of the third eyelid, if in the field, may be damaged by radiation therapy.

Neurogenic. KCS may be seen in conjunction with loss of parasympathetic innervation of the lacrimal glands (cranial nerve [CN] VII) and in certain other neurogenic disorders, especially those involving the trigeminal nerve (CN V) and dysautonomia. Often, neurogenic KCS is unilateral and the nares on the affected side is also dry if the parasympathetic innervation is damaged proximal to the pterygopalatine ganglion.

KCS is a *common and important ocular disease* in dogs. It should be suspected whenever chronic conjunctivitis, keratitis, or ocular discharge is present.

Excision of the gland of the third eyelid is a common cause of KCS in dogs.

PATHOLOGIC CHANGES. A reduction in the aqueous portion of the tear film may result in compensatory conjunctival cell hyperplasia and increased mucin production. Additionally, at least in the acute phase, the tear film becomes more hypertonic, leading to dehydration of the ocular surface epithelium (corneal and conjunctival), in turn resulting in edema, vacuolar degeneration, and generalized thinning of the corneal/conjunctival epithelium. Corneal epithelial cells are more readily exfoliated by the greater friction associated with blinking and a roughened, keratinized conjunctival epithelium. Overt epithelial erosion or corneal ulceration may then occur, leading to substantial ocular pain as the trigeminal nerve endings in the cornea are exposed. Over time the conjunctiva becomes hyperemic and chemotic, and the epithelium undergoes squamous metaplasia and hyperkeratinization. The corneal epithelium also thickens and keratinizes. The resulting irregular epithelial surface may reduce the adhesion of the remaining tear film to the ocular surface, further worsening the condition. Inflammatory cells and blood vessels infiltrate the anterior corneal stroma, and pigment, lipid, and calcium may be secondarily deposited. When this occurs the cornea is typically less susceptible to ulceration, and if an ulcer develops it may be less painful because of loss of the superficial corneal sensation. Loss of antimicrobial substances normally suspended in the aqueous portion of the tear film (IgA, lysozyme) predisposes the dry eye to secondary bacterial and sometimes fungal infections. Not only may the bacteria lead to corneal malacia and perforation but the increased protease and inflammatory debris present within the remaining tear film may also raise the risk of corneal melting and perforation. A dry eye should be regarded not only as an immunocompromised eye but also as a nutritionally deficient one because the precorneal tear film supplies the anterior cornea with a significant portion of its metabolic needs.

BREED PREDISPOSITION. KCS occurs more commonly in the American cocker spaniel, bloodhound, Boston terrier, Cavalier King Charles spaniel, English bulldog, English springer spaniel, Lhasa apso, miniature schnauzer, Pekingese, poodle, pug, Samoyed, shih tzu, West Highland white terrier, and Yorkshire terrier.

CLINICAL SIGNS. The signs of KCS depend on whether the condition is bilateral or unilateral, acute or chronic, and temporary or permanent (Figures 9-19 to 9-21).

Mucoid and Mucopurulent Discharge. A thick, often ropy ocular discharge that clings to the ocular surface is the most consistent clinical sign of KCS. The discharge may be the result of increased mucin production by the conjunctival goblet cells and/or a reduction in the rinsing function of the tear film. The purulent component of the discharge may be sterile and the

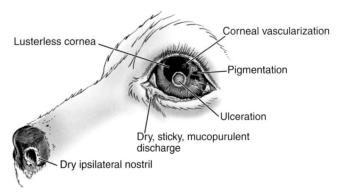

Figure 9-19. Clinical signs of keratoconjunctivitis sicca.

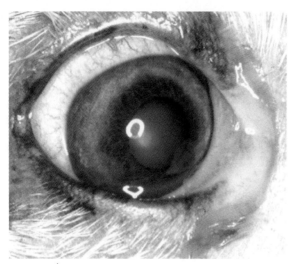

Figure 9-20. Mild keratoconjunctivitis sicca in a dog with a history of intermittent conjunctival hyperemia and discharge. At this stage tear production may wax and wane, and it is easy to misdiagnose the condition as intermittent conjunctivitis presumably of bacterial or allergic origin.

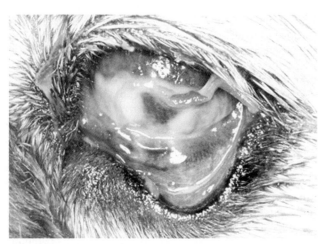

Figure 9-21. Severe keratoconjunctivitis sicca in an American cocker spaniel. Note the thick mucopurulent discharge that clings to the cornea, the hyperemia conjunctiva, and corneal roughening and pigmentation.

result of inflammatory cell infiltrate into the conjunctiva or cornea, or it may be septic if secondary bacterial infection has occurred. Dried discharge is often present on the eyelids. The conjunctiva is usually hyperemic, thickened, and chemotic.

Blepharospasm. Variable severity of blepharospasm and protrusion of the third eyelid (presumably from frictional irritation as the lids move over a dryer ocular surface) are common. The level of pain depends on the amount of ocular surface sensitivity remaining.

Corneal Ulceration. In severe or acute cases the corneal epithelium is lost, especially centrally. Mucopurulent material or malacic corneal stroma may adhere to the ulcer bed. Corneal perforation and endophthalmitis may occur.

Corneal Vascularization and Pigmentation. Superficial and deep corneal vascularization and pigmentation often occur in chronic KCS. These changes are common causes of vision loss in this disorder.

Dry, Lusterless Cornea. The dry appearance of the cornea due to lack of the precorneal tear film is characteristic of KCS but occurs in only 25% of dogs with the disorder.

Dry Ipsilateral Nostril. The nares and nostril may also be dry on the affected side, especially in neurogenic KCS. This sign is thought to be due to impaired innervation of the lateral nasal gland in addition to the lacrimal glands.

Chronic Staphylococcal Blepharitis. Chronic infection of the eyelids and the tarsal glands, sometimes with hypersensitivity, may occur. Deficiency of the lipid layer of the tear film may accompany deficiencies of the aqueous and mucin layers.

Intermittent KCS is a common clinical entity and often can be diagnosed only with repeated performance of the STT. Unilateral cases of KCS may be more likely to be intermittent in nature than bilateral cases. Many patients show fluctuations in STT values above and below the normal lower limit of 10 mm/min, with clinical signs being more common either in the winter when humidity in the home is low or at hot, dry times of the year when evaporation of the tear film is the greatest. In brachycephalic breeds intermittent instances of KCS may result in ulceration. KCS should be suspected as a cause of the ulcer if the cornea is ulcerated and the STT value is less than 10 to perhaps 15 mm/min, because the normal response of the eye to ulceration should be to increase tear production above normal.

DIAGNOSIS. The diagnosis of KCS is suggested by the history (drug administration, "cherry eye" excision, repeated bouts of conjunctivitis that recur when topical medication is discontinued), clinical signs, and STT values. STT values less than 10 mm/min are suspicious for KCS, especially in brachycephalic breeds of dogs or in patients that should have epiphora (corneal erosion, conjunctivitis, etc.). Rose bengal staining may also be of value. Rose bengal stains conjunctival cells and mucus a bright rose red when devitalized by drying. The clinician should consider a complete hematologic and serum chemistry profile and other diagnostic tests to rule out other concurrent disorders or immune-related diseases that have been associated with KCS, including diabetes mellitus, hypothyroidism, polyarthritis and polymyositis, rheumatoid arthritis, and immune-mediated skin disorders.

NATURAL COURSE OF THE DISEASE. KCS caused by drugs, systemic diseases, and orbital and supraorbital trauma may resolve spontaneously in 45 to 60 days, but many patients do not recover. The majority of cases of idiopathic KCS do not improve without treatment. Patients with untreated, or under-treated, KCS are at substantial risk for vision loss.

Failure by owners to apply treatment adequately and consistently is a common cause of poor therapeutic results in KCS. The importance, aims, cost, and alternatives for therapy must be discussed with the owner at the start and reinforced throughout therapy.

TREATMENT. Initial therapy is medical, and in the majority of patients consistent medical therapy adequately controls the disease. In select cases surgery may be of benefit. In general, when multiple medications are being given to the same eye, it is best to space the applications out as evenly as possible. If such spacing is difficult, or impossible, solutions and suspensions should be given no closer than 5 minutes apart and ointments should be given no closer than 30 minutes apart. Given the current range of treatment options, poor owner compliance or low patient acceptance of therapy is the primary cause of visual impairment in KCS.

Medical Therapy. All medications should be applied to an eye that is as free of discharge and as clean as possible to ensure adequate contact of the preparation with the target tissue. Application of any medication to a dry eye filled with debris and caked with discharge is almost invariably ineffective. Cleaning of the eyes and periocular tissue is usually best accomplished with a sterile eye wash and gentle wiping of the eyes with soft gauze or tissue. The aims of medical therapy are as follows.

Stimulate Natural Tear Production. Topical cyclosporine forms the cornerstone of KCS therapy. Available preparations include 0.2% ointment, which is approved by the U.S. Food and Drug Administration (FDA) for use in dogs, and 1% or 2% compounded formulations in an olive oil or corn oil base. All three formulations are clinically effective, although some patients may be more responsive to the 1% or 2% compounded formulations than to the commercially available ointment preparation. The compounded formulations, however, may be more irritating than the ointment in a small proportion (5% to 10%) of animals, and 2% cyclosporine may suppress systemic lymphocytes. There have been no reports of systemic adverse effects with topical cyclosporine.

The exact mechanism by which cyclosporine increases tear production is somewhat uncertain but involves immunomodulation by inhibition of helper T cells and by direct stimulation of tear production by binding to the cyclophilin receptor and thereby inhibiting prolactin, which in turn limits tear production. Additional effects of cyclosporine that are independent of its tear stimulatory effects are a reduction in corneal pigmentation and an improvement in conjunctival goblet cell mucin secretion.

A common regimen is to begin with topical cyclosporine ophthalmic ointment every 12 hours for a month and recheck tear production several hours after the medication has been administered. Topical cyclosporine therapy often requires a month or more before an effect may be seen (perhaps because of the time required to immunomodulate helper T cells and to allow the gland to regenerate), but once tear production does increase, the response to the drug is more immediate (minutes to hours after application). The latter response may be a function of a neurohormonal mechanism of action of the drug. If STT values are not substantially increased (> 10 mm/min), the same regimen may be continued for 2 more months or 1% or 2% compounded cyclosporine every 12 hours may be used for several months. During this time an STT, performed a few hours after cyclosporine has been applied to the eye, is performed monthly. If tear production still has not increased, 1% cyclosporine every 8 hours or topical tacrolimus every 12 hours may be tried. If tear production (STT value) consistently exceeds 20 mm/min (uncommon), tear stimulant therapy may be reduced to once a day and all the other medications may be discontinued.

Tacrolimus (formerly FK506) is a potent immunomodulator with a mechanism of action believed to be similar to cyclosporine A but with a reported 10- to 100-fold higher potency. In one study, compounded 0.02% tacrolimus suspension applied every 12 hours was highly effective at improving tear production. All dogs that were controlled with cyclosporine A also could be controlled with tacrolimus, and in about one quarter of those dogs, tear production rose an additional 5 mm/min or more. Additionally, a significant number of dogs who did not experience increased tear production with cyclosporine did so with tacrolimus. In addition to increasing tear production, tacrolimus also reduced many of the other symptoms of KCS. Despite these promising results the potential toxic side effects of the drug and the potential carcinogenicity of the compound do indicate that further studies are required before the drug can be

determined to be safe for the animal as well as for the human who applies the medication. A related compound, pimecrolimus, also experimentally improved tear production in dogs treated with a 1% corn oil–based formulation three times a day, but its long-term safety is also unknown.

Pilocarpine, administered either topically or systemically, may be used in selected cases in an effort to stimulate tear production. In view of its mechanism of action, it would be expected to be most effective in patients with neurogenic KCS secondary to parasympathetic denervation, in which peripheral cholinergic receptors have undergone upregulation and are more sensitive to the effects of cholinergic stimulation than other cholinergically innervated tissues. Pilocarpine may be used topically in a dilute form in artificial tears (0.125% or 0.25%) given every 6 to 8 hours or orally by being mixed with the animal's food. In the latter instance the initial dose applied to the food is 1 drop of 2% topical pilocarpine per 10 kg of body weight twice daily. The dose is increased in 1-drop increments every 2 to 3 days until signs of systemic toxicity develop (inappetence, hypersalivation, vomiting, diarrhea, bradycardia). Because the efficacy of this approach depends on a differential sensitivity of the lacrimal glands than other tissues (gastrointestinal, cardiac), the therapeutic window is quite narrow, and one needs to see subtle signs of toxicity in other tissues before concluding that the drug is ineffective. In my experience the drug is seldom effective in treating KCS, and its side effects (local ocular irritation, inappetence, vomiting/ diarrhea) may preclude its long-term use.

Other promising tear stimulants in dogs in the experimental setting are the use of 100 μL of nerve growth factor ointment every 12 hours and oral administration of low-dose interferon-α. The long-term safety and efficacy of these compounds remain to be elucidated.

Replacement of the Precorneal Tear Film. Wetting agents are second best to drugs, which increase natural tears. They do, however, play an important role in improving the ocular health of animals in which tear stimulant therapy does not raise tear production to adequate levels or while waiting for tear stimulant therapy to begin to work. There are many types of artificial tears, and in addition to a wetting agent, they contain varying amounts and types of preservatives. A preparation is initially selected on the basis of the tear function that needs replacement and the individual needs of the patient. If a particular brand of tear replacement therapy is effective but irritating, a related compound with a different or no preservative should be tried. Often a variety of agents are tried before the optimal formulation is identified for an individual patient.

Preparations with polyvinyl alcohol (common in many over-the-counter formulations) are relatively watery in consistency, resulting in a relatively short contact time and the need for frequent application. They are best selected when the goal is to keep the eye free of debris, and by themselves they are typically inadequate to treat a substantially dry eye. The addition of dextrans (e.g., Hypotears) results in a slightly more viscous material that better mimics natural mucins and should be considered if the goal is to replace the mucin layer. The addition of methylcellulose (e.g., Isopto Tears, Tears Naturale, GenTeal lubricating eyedrops, GenTeal gel, Refresh Celluvisc Tears) makes the solution more viscous, slows its evaporation rate, increases the corneal contact time, and also is beneficial if the goal is to replace the mucin layer. The greater viscosity of these agents also makes them good choices when the goal is to lubricate the eye, although they may result in more debris around the eyelids. The addition of viscoelastic agents such as chondroitin sulfate and sodium hyaluronate (Hylashield) result in one of the longest contact times, but these compounds may not be readily available in the United States.

Ointments containing petrolatum, mineral oil, or lanolin (e.g., Duratears, Lacri-Lube, Puralube, Lubri-Tears) are very thick and have the longest contact time but are the least like natural tears. They are best used in animals with exposure keratitis expected to go long periods without treatment, just before bedtime, or in patients with lipid layer deficiencies. Although the long contact time makes it appealing to use these compounds in severely dry eyes, their viscous nature usually results in a thick "gummy" material that may be uncomfortable. Severely dry eyes typically respond better to less viscous compounds than the ointments.

Reduce Ocular Surface Inflammation. Topical cyclosporine or tacrolimus may have some efficacy at reducing ocular surface inflammation—even if they do not increase tear production. If these agents are inadequate, a short course (1 to 4 weeks) of topical 0.1% dexamethasone or 1% prednisolone acetate applied every 6 to 8 hours may be used to reduce corneal vascularization, pigmentation, and inflammation. Topical corticosteroids may also be useful in patients in which conjunctival swelling around the lacrimal ductules precludes tear secretion stimulated by cyclosporine or tacrolimus. Topical corticosteroids are usually not used long term, and it is mandatory to perform fluorescein staining of the cornea before their use to ensure absence of even minor corneal erosions or abrasions. In general these compounds should be used with extreme caution in acute KCS because of the risk of corneal ulceration or perforation. Alternatively a topical NSAID such as flurbiprofen could be used.

Control Secondary Infection. Because white blood cells may be present within the cornea/conjunctiva and on the ocular surface simply as a result of inflammation associated with drying, the presence of a purulent discharge does not necessarily indicate a secondary bacterial infection. Conjunctival cytology can be a useful guide in determining whether the discharge is sterile or septic and whether topical antibiotics are required. If bacterial overgrowth or secondary infection has occurred, topical antibiotics such as neomycin/bacitracin/polymyxin B may be used every 6 to 8 hours. If corneal ulceration has occurred, topical antibiotics should be applied more frequently and corneal cytology and culture/sensitivity testing should be considered (see Chapter 10 for details). Additionally, the response to therapy should be closely followed because ulcerative keratitis in patients with KCS often becomes malacic and corneal perforation is not uncommon. In general topical antibiotics are not typically required on a long-term basis, and their continual application typically results only in ocular irritation or resistant organisms.

Removal of Excess Mucus. Rinsing the eyes with sterile eye wash is often sufficient to remove excess mucus. Mucolytics may be used in selected patients with copious discharge that clings tenaciously to the ocular surface and eyelids. Although 5% acetylcysteine may be used as a mucolytic, its low pH may result in irritation, it has a shelf-life of only a few days once opened, and it is expensive. Nevertheless it may be useful, at least in the short term, in patients with unusually thick and tenacious discharge.

Owner noncompliance with frequent medication regimens is an important cause of treatment failure, especially when response to cyclosporine is poor.

Follow-up. Initial therapy typically consists of cleaning the eyes at least once daily with sterile eye wash, topical application of cyclosporine ophthalmic ointment every 12 hours, use of an artificial tear (selected on the basis of the most pressing need for replacement—cleaning, lubrication, or addressing exposure) every 2 to 4 hours, and topical application of antibiotics if bacterial overgrowth has occurred. If the conjunctiva is quite chemotic and the cornea is negative to fluorescein stain, topical corticosteroids or an NSAID may be considered. In select cases with copious discharge a mucolytic may also be used. A lubricating ointment is usually given at bedtime. The patient is examined at 1 month (ideally a few hours after receiving cyclosporine), and tear stimulant therapy is adjusted as described previously. Unless advised otherwise, many owners do not treat the pet on the day of the visit, thereby making it difficult for the clinician to assess the efficacy of cyclosporine therapy. If a corneal ulcer or erosion was present at the initial examination, the timing of the recheck appointment is dictated by the corneal defect and not by the KCS.

In many animals cyclosporine or tacrolimus may increase tear production to the extent that other medications may be reduced or eliminated. Even if tear production does not increase, therapy with cyclosporine and the other compounds often results in substantial clinical improvement and retention of vision. A higher proportion of dogs with an initial STT value above 2 mm/min show a beneficial response to cyclosporine than those with a reading below 2 mm/min. If the STT value is 0 at commencement of treatment, the chance of response to cyclosporine is less, although overall clinical response to the regimen may be good. Corneal pigmentation may be reduced in about 80% of affected dogs. In rare cases or in patients with intermittent KCS, cyclosporine may be discontinued and tear production remains at normal levels. Topical cyclosporine is ineffective in KCS secondary to distemper, trauma, or advanced glandular fibrosis and in many drug-induced forms of the disorder.

If severe ulceration is present, the above topical therapy, including cyclosporine, is used in addition to aggressive antibiotic therapy, and the eye is treated as described in Chapter 10. Some patients need immediate surgical therapy if corneal rupture is imminent, and such high-risk patients should be referred to an ophthalmologist.

A minimum of 3 to 6 months of medical therapy is desirable before surgical therapy for KCS is considered, because some dogs regain tear production during this time. If surgical treatment is performed too early, epiphora may result when tear production returns, requiring surgical reversal. By the end of 3 to 6 months, the owner has often decided in favor of either medical or surgical treatment. For long-term medical treatment, antibiotics, corticosteroids, and acetylcysteine may be reduced or deleted from the regimen. For cases that fail to respond with increased tear production or in animals that demonstrate sensitivity to cyclosporine or tacrolimus or for whose owners topical treatment is inconvenient, surgical therapy is a viable alternative.

Complications of KCS with medical therapy include vascularization, scarring, and pigmentation of the cornea to varying degrees. Surgical attempts to remove this opaque tissue by keratectomy have a low success rate, with postoperative return of the tissue in a high proportion of patients. Complications of such keratectomy include reduced tear flow, thought to be due to section of the corneal nerve and reduced reflex lacrimation, bacterial keratitis, predominantly with gram-positive organisms, and delayed reepithelialization of the cornea. The best candidates for this procedure are patients with an excellent response to cyclosporine, STT values above 15 mm/min, absence of recent or current bacterial conjunctivitis, and minimal limbal or conjunctival pigment.

Surgical Therapy

Parotid Duct Transposition. The parotid duct conducts saliva from the parotid gland to an oral papilla near the carnassial tooth. In the transposition procedure the duct and papilla are mobilized and transferred to the conjunctival sac to provide substitute lubrication. The technique is technically demanding and requires precision and practice. Even if successful, it rarely eliminates the need to treat the eye topically.

Because of potential complications (occurring in 9% to 37% of cases, as reported by various authorities), parotid duct transposition should be undertaken only by a competent surgeon experienced in the technique and after medical treatment has been evaluated for at least 3 to 6 months.

Before this technique is performed, the teeth are cleaned, and if periodontal disease is present, systemic antibiotics are given for 14 days. Before surgical intervention, the clinician confirms function of the parotid gland and patency of the duct and eliminates the possibility of xerostomia by placing one or more drops of 1% atropine onto the oral mucosa and observing the papilla for secretion. In this circumstance, 1% atropine is used not for its parasympatholytic effects (which would reduce saliva production) but because it is very bitter tasting and acutely induces profuse salivation when administered via this route.

Under general anesthesia the oral cavity is cleaned and packed with gauze soaked in povidone-iodine solution. The lateral surface of the face is prepared for surgery, and the parotid papilla is cannulated with 2/0 nylon (colored) with a smooth blunt end (Figure 9-22). This cannula facilitates later identification and manipulation of the duct. Because of a right-angle bend in the duct as it enters the papilla, perseverance may be necessary to effect cannulation. Grasping the papilla and moving it rostrally reduces the bend and makes passage of the nylon easier.

Subcutaneous approaches ("closed procedures") in which no facial skin incision is made have also been described. In this version the papilla and duct are dissected free via the oral cavity to the point near where the duct attaches to the gland. From there a subcutaneous tunnel is made by blunt dissection to the inferior-lateral conjunctival cul-de-sac, where the papilla is sutured in place. Extreme care must be taken not to twist or rotate the duct as it is being transposed.

Both the "open" and "closed" procedures are effective, and the decision as to which one to use is largely personal preference because both procedures have their proponents and detractors.

Postoperative Treatment. Until a regular supply of parotid secretions is established, cyclosporine, artificial tears, and topical antibiotics are used several times a day. Small, regular amounts of food (e.g., a dry dog biscuit every hour or so at the owner's convenience) and soft food are used to establish a continuous supply of secretion until skin sutures are removed at 10 days.

Operative and Postoperative Complications. Postoperative subcutaneous edema is common for the first few days and can be limited by careful suturing of the oral mucosal incision to prevent saliva from entering the wound.

The most severe intraoperative complication is severing the duct from the papilla, which results in scar formation and constriction around the junction with the conjunctiva. If the end of the duct is opened with an incision along both sides for 2 to 2.5 mm, a wider opening with less chance of constriction can be obtained. Careless or traumatic handling of the duct with instruments leads to cicatricial constriction and obstruction. Microsurgical resection and anastomosis of obstructions is possible but cannot be relied on to repair the results of poor surgical technique.

The most common postoperative complication is accumulations of whitish crystalline mineralized material from salivary secretions on the ocular surface and lid margins. These accumulations cannot be prevented and, if substantial, result in blepharoconjunctivitis and blepharospasm. They can be reduced by frequent applications of 1% to 2% ethylene-diaminetetraacetic acid (EDTA) in artificial tears. Continued use of cyclosporine may be helpful because of its lubricant and antiinflammatory properties. Facial irritation from over-production of saliva may occur, but ligation of the parotid duct is rarely necessary. After parotid duct transposition, the numbers of bacteria on the surface of the eye increase, with many uncommon organisms isolated. Usually these organisms are nonproblematic although they may contribute to blepharo-conjunctivitis in some patients. If glandular function returns after transposition, epiphora can result. It may be prevented in the majority of patients by adequate medical evaluation before surgery is attempted. If epiphora should occur, ligation of the duct or re-transposition to the mouth is curative. Salivary flow can also be reduced by surgical reduction of the diameter of the parotid duct.

NEOPLASIA

Neoplasms of the lacrimal gland are rare in dogs and manifest as space-occupying lesions that can be removed by suitable orbital approaches (see Chapter 17). Lacrimal adenocarcinoma has a good prognosis if removed early, while still localized. Conjunctival neoplasms may invade the nasolacrimal duct and spread to the nasal cavity; likewise, neoplasms in the nasal cavity may invade the nasolacrimal duct. Space-occupying nasal lesions may obstruct the nasolacrimal duct, causing epiphora. Cryotherapy may be used near the lacrimal puncta and canaliculi without causing permanent obstruction.

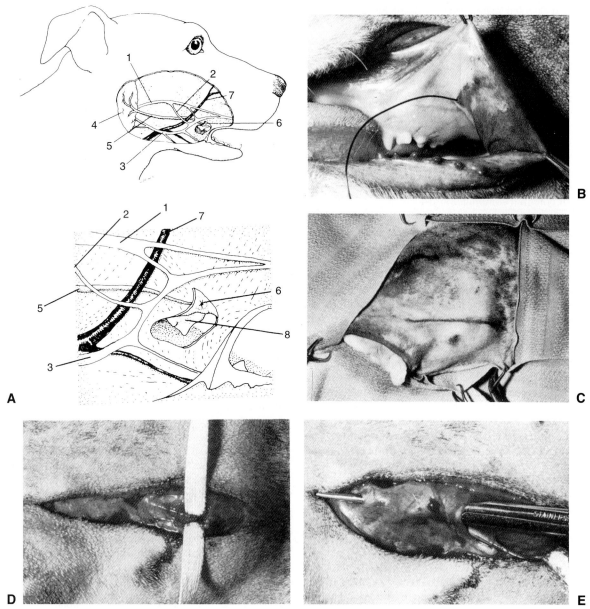

Figure 9-22. Parotid duct transposition. **A,** Diagram of the face *(top)* and enlargement of the area where the duct enters mouth *(bottom)*. *1,* Dorsal buccal nerve; *2,* anastomosis of dorsal buccal and ventral buccal nerves; *3,* ventral buccal nerve; *4,* parotid salivary gland; *5,* parotid duct; *6,* papilla of parotid duct; *7,* facial vein; *8,* upper carnassial tooth. **B,** Monofilament nylon suture marker in place of the parotid duct. **C,** Cotton soaked with 1:750 aqueous benzalkonium chloride placed over the parotid duct papilla. The course of the duct is marked on the skin. **D,** Umbilical tape passed beneath parotid duct so that the duct can be manipulated without being damaged by forceps. **E,** Completed dissection beneath the facial vein and branches of buccal nerve with blunt scissors. (From Severin GA [1973]: Keratoconjunctivitis sicca. Vet Clin North Am 3:407.)

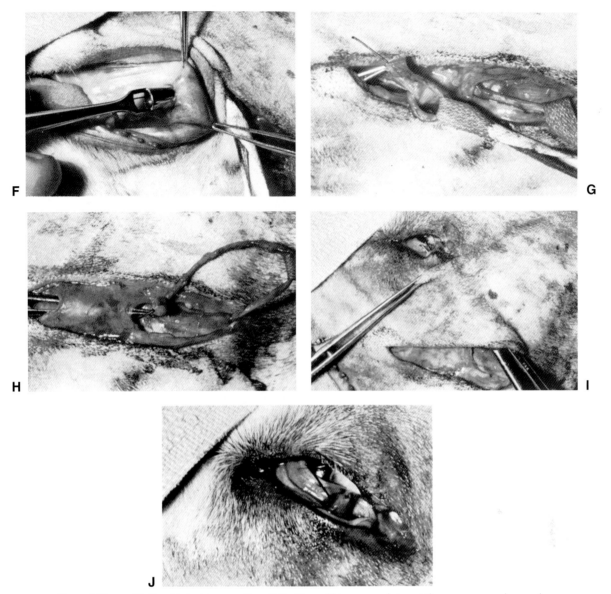

Figure 9-22, cont'd. Parotid duct transposition. **F,** Position of biopsy punch to cut the mucous membrane plug containing the parotid papilla and duct. **G,** Pulling the parotid duct and papilla into the facial wound. **H,** Parotid duct dissected free to the angle of the mandible. **I,** Tunneling to the lower lateral fornix with blunt delicate scissors. **J,** Oral mucous membrane plug with parotid duct papilla positioned for suturing to the conjunctiva. (From Severin GA [1973]: Keratoconjunctivitis sicca. Vet Clin North Am 3:407.)

BIBLIOGRAPHY

Barnett KC, et al. (1995): Treatment of keratoconjunctivitis sicca in dogs with cyclosporine ophthalmic ointment: a European clinical field trial. Vet Rec 137:504.

Berdoulay A, et al. (2005): Effect of topical 0.02% tacrolimus aqueous suspension on tear production in dogs with keratoconjunctivitis sicca. Vet Ophthalmol 8:225.

Berger S, et al. (1995): A quantitative study of the effects of Tribrissen on canine tear production. J Am Anim Hosp Assoc 31:236.

Burling K, et al. (1991): Anatomy of the rabbit nasolacrimal duct and its clinical implications. Prog Vet Comp Ophthalmol 1:33.

Carter R, Colitz CMH (2002): The causes, diagnosis, and treatment of canine keratoconjunctivitis sicca. Vet Med 97:683.

Carrington SD, et al. (1987): Polarized light biomicroscopic observations on the precorneal tear film. 2: keratoconjunctivitis sicca in the dog. J Small Anim Pract 28:671.

Coassin M, et al. (2005): Efficacy of topical nerve growth factor treatment in dogs affected by dry eye. Graefes Arch Clin Exp Ophthalmol 243:151.

Collins BK, et al. (1994): Immune-mediated keratoconjunctivitis sicca in a horse. Vet Comp Ophthalmol 4:61.

Collins BK, et al. (1986): Sulfonamide-associated keratoconjunctivitis sicca and corneal ulceration in a dysuric dog. J Am Vet Med Assoc 189:924.

Covitz D, et al. (1977): Conjunctivorhinostomy: a surgical method for the control of epiphora in the dog and cat. J Am Vet Med Assoc 171:251.

Cullen CL, et al. (2005): Tear film breakup times in young healthy cats before and after anesthesia. Vet Ophthalmol 8:159.

Gao J, et al. (1998): The role of apoptosis in the pathogenesis of canine keratoconjunctivitis sicca: the effect of topical cyclosporin A therapy. Cornea 17:654.

Gilger BC, et al. (1999): Low-dose oral administration of interferon-alpha for the treatment of immune-mediated keratoconjunctivitis sicca in dogs. J Interferon Cytokine Res 19:901.

Gilger BC, et al. (1995): Cellular immunity in dogs with keratoconjunctivitis sicca before and after treatment with 2% cyclosporine. Vet Immunol Immunopathol 49:199.

Glen JB, Lawson DD (1971): A modified technique of parotid duct transposition for the treatment of keratoconjunctivitis sicca in the dog. Vet Rec 88:210.

Grahn BH, Mason RA (1995): Epiphora associated with dacryops in a dog. J Am Anim Hosp Assoc 31:15.

Hartley C, et al. (2006): Effect of age, gender, weight and time of day on tear production in normal dogs. Vet Ophthalmol 9:53.

Harvey CE, Koch SA (1971): Surgical complications of parotid duct transposition in the dog. J Am Anim Hosp Assoc 7:122.

Headrick JF, et al. (2004): Canine lobular orbital adenoma: a report of 15 cases with distinctive features. Vet Ophthalmol 7:47.

Hicks SJ, et al. (1998): Biochemical analysis of ocular surface mucin abnormalities in dry eye: the canine model. Exp Eye Res 67:709.

Izci C, et al. (2002): Histologic characteristics and local cellular immunity of the gland of the third eyelid after topical ophthalmic administration of 2% cyclosporine for treatment of dogs with keratoconjunctivitis sicca. Am J Vet Res 63:688.

Kaswan RL, et al. (1995): Diagnosis and management of keratoconjunctivitis sicca. Vet Med 90:539.

Kaswan RL, et al. (1985): Keratoconjunctivitis sicca: immunological evaluation. Am J Vet Res 46:376.

Laing EJ, et al. (1988): Dacryocystotomy: a treatment for chronic dacryocystitis in the dog. J Am Anim Hosp Assoc 24:223.

Latimer CA, Wyman M (1984): Atresia of the nasolacrimal duct in three horses. J Am Vet Med Assoc 184:989.

Lavach JD, et al. (1984): Dacryocystitis in dogs: a review of 22 cases. J Am Anim Hosp Assoc 20:463.

Lim CC, Cullen CL (2005): Schirmer tear test values and tear film break-up times in cats with conjunctivitis. Vet Ophthalmol 8:305.

Martin CL, et al. (1987): Cystic lesions of the periorbital region. Comp Cont Ed 9:1022.

Moore CL (1999): Diseases and surgery of the lacrimal secretory system, in Gelatt KN (editor): Veterinary Ophthalmology, 3rd ed. Lippincott Williams & Wilkins, Philadelphia.

Moore CP, et al. (1987): Density and distribution of canine conjunctival goblet cells. Invest Ophthalmol Vis Sci 28:1925.

Naranjo C, et al. (2005). Characterization of lacrimal gland lesions and possible pathogenic mechanisms of keratoconjunctivitis sicca in dogs with leishmaniosis. Vet Parasitol 133:37.

Nell B, et al. (2005): The effect of topical pimecrolimus on keratoconjunctivitis sicca and chronic superficial keratitis in dogs: results from an exploratory study. Vet Ophthalmol 8:39.

Nykamp SG, et al. (2004): Computed tomography dacryocystography evaluation of the nasolacrimal apparatus. Vet Radiol Ultrasound 45:23.

Olivero DK, et al. (1991): Clinical evaluation of 1% cyclosporine for topical treatment of keratoconjunctivitis sicca in dogs. J Am Vet Med Assoc 199:1039.

Petersen-Jones SM (1997): Quantification of conjunctival sac bacteria in normal dogs and those suffering from keratoconjunctivitis sicca. Vet Comp Ophthalmol 7:29.

Petersen-Jones SM, Carrington SD (1988): Pasteurella dacryocystitis in rabbits. Vet Rec 122:514.

Playter RF, et al. (1997): Lacrimal cyst (dacryops) in 2 dogs. J Am Vet Med Assoc 171:736.

Reilly L, Beech J (1994): Bilateral keratoconjunctivitis sicca in a horse. Equine Vet J 26:171.

Salisbury MR, et al. (1995): Microorganisms isolated from the corneal surface before and during topical cyclosporine treatment in dogs with keratoconjunctivitis sicca. Am J Vet Res 56:880.

Sansom J, et al. (1985): Keratoconjunctivitis sicca in the dog associated with the administration of salicylazosulphapyridine (sulphasalazine). Vet Rec 116:391.

Schlegel T, et al. (2003): IgA and secretory component (SC) in the third eyelid of domestic animals: a comparative study. Vet Ophthalmol 6:157.

Schmidt G, et al. (1970): Parotid duct transposition: a follow-up study of sixty eyes. J Am Anim Hosp Assoc 6:235.

Slatter D, Davis WJ (1974): Toxicity of phenazopyridine: electron microscopical studies on canine lacrimal and nictitans glands. Arch Ophthalmol 91:484.

Speiss BM, et al. (1989): Eosinophilic granulomatous dacryoadenitis causing bilateral keratoconjunctivitis sicca in a horse. Equine Vet J 21:226.

Stiles J, et al. (1995): Keratectomy for corneal pigmentation in dogs with cyclosporine responsive chronic keratoconjunctivitis sicca. Vet Comp Ophthalmol 5:25.

Termote S (2003): Parotid salivary duct mucocele and sialolithiasis following parotid duct transposition. J Small Anim Pract 44:21.

van der Woerdt A, et al. (1997): Surgical treatment of dacryocystitis caused by cystic dilatation of the nasolacrimal system in three dogs. J Am Vet Med Assoc 211:445.

Wilkie DA, Rings MD (1990): Repair of anomalous nasolacrimal duct in a bull by use of conjunctivorhinostomy. J Am Vet Med Assoc 196:1647.

CORNEA AND SCLERA

David J. Maggs

ANATOMY, PHYSIOLOGY, AND WOUND
  HEALING
PATHOLOGIC RESPONSES

CORNEAL DISEASES BELIEVED TO BE
  INHERITED
ACQUIRED CORNEAL DISEASES

SCLERAL DISORDERS BELIEVED TO BE
  INHERITED
ACQUIRED SCLERAL DISORDERS

ANATOMY, PHYSIOLOGY, AND WOUND HEALING

Cornea

The outer, fibrous coat of the eye consists of the posterior, opaque sclera and the anterior, transparent cornea. The anterior-most sclera is covered by the translucent bulbar conjunctiva. The point at which the cornea, sclera, and bulbar conjunctiva merge is called the limbus. In domestic species the horizontal diameter of the cornea is greater than the vertical diameter. This difference is especially notable in the large herbivores. The corneal thickness varies among species and across regions of the cornea but is usually between 0.5 and 0.8 mm.

The cornea has the following four layers (Figure 10-1):

- Stratified epithelium and its basement membrane
- Collagenous stroma
- Descemet's membrane (basement membrane of the endothelium)
- Endothelium

The corneal epithelium is stratified, squamous, and non-keratinized. From deep to superficial it comprises the basement membrane, basal epithelial cells, wing cells, and squamous surface cells (Figure 10-2). Basal cells are attached to the basement membrane by hemidesmosomes. As basal cells divide, daughter cells are forced toward the surface, become flattened as wing cells, and gradually lose many of their organelles. Basal cells are replaced by stem cells at the limbus that are constantly undergoing mitosis and migrating centripetally. Surface squamous cells possess microvillous projections that anchor the deep mucin layer of the precorneal tear film. The corneal stroma, composed of keratocytes, collagen, and ground substance, constitutes 90% of the corneal thickness and lends rigidity to the globe. The parallel collagen fibrils form lamellae of interlacing sheets (Figure 10-3), with occasional interspersed keratocytes (which are modified fibroblasts), lymphocytes, macrophages, and neutrophils. The regular spacing of stromal collagen fibrils maintains corneal transparency and distinguishes corneal stroma from the collagen in scar tissue and sclera.

Descemet's membrane is the basement membrane of the endothelium, lying between the posterior stroma and the endothelium (see Figures 10-1 and 10-4). Because it is continuously secreted by endothelial cells throughout life, this membrane thickens with age. It is very elastic but can break from globe stretching (buphthalmos), as seen with advanced glaucoma, or with penetrating injuries or ruptured ulcers. Descemet's membrane becomes exposed in ulcers in which there is complete stromal loss (descemetoceles). It does not stain with fluorescein and therefore appears as a dark, transparent, sometimes outwardly bulging structure in the center of a deep corneal ulcer or wound.

The endothelium is one cell layer thick and lies posterior to Descemet's membrane, lining the anterior chamber. Its role is to pump ions from the stroma into the aqueous. The movement of water that follows these ions ensures that the corneal stroma remains relatively dehydrated. This function is a major contributor to corneal transparency. Endothelial cells in the adult animal are postmitotic and have a limited capacity to replicate in most species. With advancing age, endothelial cells are lost and the corneal stroma becomes thicker owing to subtle edema. The normal canine endothelial cell density in young dogs is approximately 2800 cells/mm². Corneal decompensation and inability to remove water from the stroma occur when endothelial cell density falls below 500 to 800 cells/mm². The endothelium may be prematurely lost or damaged because of genetic predisposition (endothelial dystrophy), trauma (exogenous and due to anterior lens luxation), intraocular or corneal surgery, intraocular inflammation (uveitis), or glaucoma. Such loss of corneal endothelium, beyond the ability of surrounding cells to compensate, usually causes permanent corneal edema and opacity.

The cornea is the most powerful optical refracting surface in the eye. This ability relies mainly on appropriate corneal curvature and transparency. Corneal transparency is maintained by numerous specialized anatomic and physiologic features. The following features keep the cornea transparent:

- Lack of blood vessels
- Relatively low cell density
- Lack of melanin (or other pigments)
- Maintenance of a relatively dehydrated state
- A smooth optical surface (provided by the precorneal tear film)
- A highly regular arrangement of stromal collagen fibrils
- Lack of keratinization

Factors that alter the collagen lattice or spacing of collagen fibrils, the optical surface, or the type of collagen all reduce corneal transparency (see Figure 10-3). Common examples are corneal edema, corneal scarring, loss of epithelium, alterations in the precorneal tear film, elevated intraocular pressure (IOP), damage to endothelium, formation of scar tissue, altered glycosaminoglycan content, melanosis, corneal vascularization, and infiltration of the stroma with white blood cells.

Because the cornea is avascular, oxygen and nutrients must be obtained and metabolites disposed of through alternate

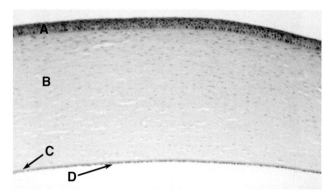

Figure 10-1. Photomicrograph of the feline cornea. **A,** Epithelium; **B,** stroma; **C,** Descemet's membrane; **D,** endothelium.

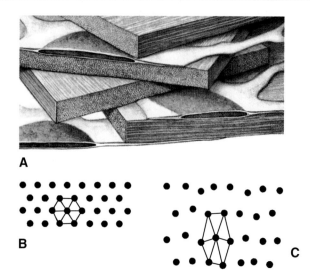

Figure 10-3. The corneal stroma. **A,** Collagen lamellae. Parallel collagen fibrils lie within a lamella and run the full length of the cornea. Successive lamellae run across the cornea at angles to one another. Fibroblasts are shown between the lamellae. **B,** Cross-sectional orientation of normal stromal collagen fibrils. Each of the fibrils is separated from its fellows by equal distances because of mucoproteins, glycoproteins, and other components of the ground substance. Maurice has explained the transparency of the cornea on the basis of this very exact equidistant separation, which results in the elimination of scattered light by destructive interference. **C,** Cross-sectional view of disoriented collagen fibrils, which scatter light and result in reduction of corneal transparency. The orderly position of the fibrils can be disturbed by edema, alterations in the ground substance, scar formation, or infiltration of the interlamellar spaces by cells or substances such as mineral and lipid. (Modified from Hogan MJ, et al. [1971]: Histology of the Human Eye. Saunders, Philadelphia.)

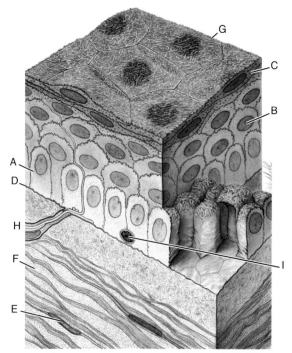

Figure 10-2. Drawing of the corneal epithelium comprising columnar basal cells *(A)*, polyhedral wing cells *(B)*, and nonkeratinized surface squamous epithelial cells *(C)*. The basal cells are subtended by the epithelial basement membrane *(D)*, stromal keratocytes *(E)*, and collagenous stroma *(F)*. Note also the extensive arrays of microplicae and microvilli at the corneal surface *(G)*, which help retain the tear film. A sensory (trigeminal) nerve fiber *(H)* is shown penetrating the epithelium at its base, and a lymphocyte *(I)* can be seen migrating through the basal epithelium. (Modified from Hogan MJ, et al. [1971]: Histology of the Human Eye. Saunders, Philadelphia.)

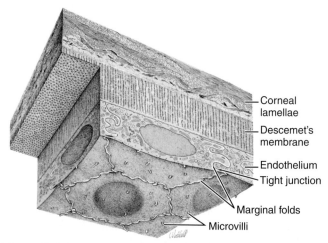

Figure 10-4. Inner cornea showing the deepest corneal lamellae, Descemet's membrane, and the endothelium. The deeper stromal lamellae split, and some branches curve posteriorly to merge with Descemet's membrane. Descemet's membrane is seen in meridional and tangential planes. The endothelial cells are polygonal. Microvilli on the apical surface of the endothelial cells and marginal folds at the intercellular junctions protrude into the anterior chamber. Intercellular spaces near the anterior chamber are closed by a tight junction. (Modified from Hogan MJ, et al. [1971]: Histology of the Human Eye. Saunders, Philadelphia.)

routes (Figure 10-5). Such routes include the aqueous humor, the precorneal tear film and the atmosphere, and adjacent capillary beds in the sclera and bulbar and palpebral conjunctiva. The endothelium and posterior stroma receive most of their nutrients from the aqueous humor, but the tear film and atmospheric oxygen are the major sources for the anterior cornea.

Normal Corneal Healing

Each component of the cornea heals to a different degree, at a different rate, and via completely different mechanisms.

An understanding of these differences will help the clinician better assess whether healing is progressing abnormally, take appropriate steps to halt delayed healing or clinical deterioration, and offer more accurate prognoses after ocular injury or disease.

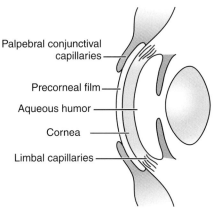

Figure 10-5. Sources of oxygen available to the cornea. (Modified from Scheie HG, Albert DM [1977]: Textbook of Ophthalmology, 9th ed. Saunders, Philadelphia.)

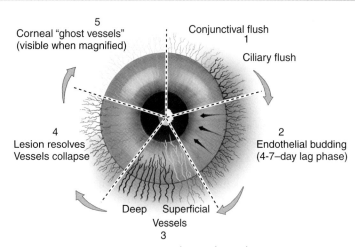

Figure 10-6. Sequence of corneal vascularization.

Epithelium

The corneal epithelium has great regenerative capacity. Within minutes after an injury, epithelial cells surrounding the margin of the lesion begin to slide and cover the affected area. During sliding, melanocytes from the limbus may be carried into formerly transparent areas and may be grossly visible as corneal melanosis. The entire cornea can reepithelialize within 4 to 7 days although it takes longer for the epithelium to regain full thickness and maturity. Once epithelial cells have slid to cover the defect, mitosis occurs and the multilayered epithelial surface is reconstituted. Finally, firm attachment to the basement membrane via the hemidesmosomes is reestablished.

Stroma

Stromal collagen is replaced slowly by fibrovascular ingrowth from the adjacent limbus (vascular healing), activation of keratocytes into active fibroblasts (avascular healing), or a combination of the two mechanisms. Uncomplicated stromal wounds tend to undergo avascular healing, but infected or destructive lesions usually stimulate, and require, vascularized healing, as in other sites in the body. After injury, stromal keratocytes are capable of synthesizing collagen, glycosaminoglycans, and mucoprotein of the ground substance and of transforming to fibroblasts that produce nontransparent collagen. However, stromal collagen replacement rate and repair vary with species and may extend to years. Because epithelium heals more rapidly than stroma, stromal defects are often covered by new epithelium before they are filled with new collagen, resulting in a facet. Stromal regeneration then occurs beneath the new epithelial surface.

Avascular healing of corneal stroma occurs as follows:

1. Due to chemotactic influences, neutrophils infiltrate and surround the lesion. These cells reach the lesion from the tear film, from the aqueous humor, and by migration through the corneal stroma after release from limbal vessels.
2. Keratocytes in the immediate area die. Surrounding keratocytes transform to fibroblasts and migrate to the damaged area, where they synthesize collagen and ground substance. The collagen fibrils laid down during stromal regeneration are irregular and decrease corneal transparency.
3. About 48 hours after injury, macrophages invade the lesion and remove cellular debris.
4. Within the ensuing weeks to months, the density of the scar decreases but it does not disappear. Scar resolution varies somewhat with the species and age of the affected individual.

In vascularized healing of destructive lesions, cellular infiltration is more extensive, and the area is invaded by blood vessels originating from the limbus (Figure 10-6). Granulation tissue is laid down and forms a denser scar than in avascular healing. Eventually the blood vessels cease to be perfused, but they remain as "ghost vessels" and are visible on slit-lamp examination. If inflammation recurs at a later date, these ghost vessels may rapidly become perfused, creating the clinical appearance of more severe or chronic inflammation than is actually present. Corneal nerves damaged by the lesion gradually regenerate, and sensation returns slowly to the affected area.

Endothelium and Descemet's Membrane

Because of its elasticity, Descemet's membrane retracts when damaged, forming tight curls and exposing the subjacent posterior stroma. Neighboring endothelial cells slide in to cover the area, and a new Descemet's membrane is eventually laid down. In extensive lesions, however, endothelium may not cover the area, and an area of swollen and edematous stroma persists. Endothelial regenerative capability varies with species and age but is generally minimal in mature animals of common domestic species.

Effects of Corticosteroids on Corneal Healing

Topical corticosteroids limit corneal opacification by inhibiting fibroplasia, decreasing vascularization, and reducing melanosis. They also control the potentially blinding consequences of anterior uveitis that frequently accompanies corneal wounds. However, corticosteroids also inhibit epithelial regeneration, corneal infiltration with inflammatory cells, fibroblastic activity, and endothelial regeneration. The strength of the resulting wound is lessened, collagenases are potentiated up to 15 times, and the risk of infection is greatly enhanced when corticosteroids are used. These potential negative and positive effects on wound outcome and healing must be considered carefully. Typically there is good justification for the use of topical corticosteroids provided that:

- Infection has been controlled
- An epithelial covering, as demonstrated by lack of fluorescein retention, has been established
- The structural integrity of the cornea is not compromised
- The corneal disease was not caused by feline herpesvirus or another primary infections agent

Using these guidelines, clinicians tend to use topical corticosteroids for control of inflammation associated with surgically induced corneal wounds when close monitoring is possible and usually in combination with topical antibiotics.

Sclera

The sclera forms a larger portion of the fibrous coat of the eye than the cornea. The sclera is composed of three layers. From outside to inside they are the episclera, the sclera proper or scleral stroma, and the lamina fusca. The episclera is composed of a dense, highly vascular, fibrous layer that binds Tenon's capsule to the sclera. Collagenous fibers within the episclera blend into the superficial scleral stroma. Anteriorly, the episclera thickens and blends with Tenon's capsule and subconjunctival connective tissue near the limbus. The scleral stroma, like the corneal stroma, is composed of collagen fibers and fibroblasts. However, scleral collagen fibers differ in diameter and shape, run in different directions in different parts of the globe, and are not regularly spaced, thus making the sclera nontransparent. The lamina fusca is the zone of transition between the sclera and the outer layers of the choroid and ciliary body.

Numerous channels exist in the sclera through which vessels and nerves pass. These channels also provide routes by which disease processes such as infections and neoplasia may enter or leave the eye. The optic nerve leaves the eye through a sievelike perforation of the sclera at the posterior pole called the lamina cribrosa. Alterations in tension on the lamina cribrosa during glaucoma reduce the size of the spaces through which nerve axons pass and interfere with axoplasmic flow within the optic nerve, thereby contributing to optic nerve degeneration in this disease. The short posterior ciliary arteries and nerves pierce the sclera around the optic nerve and enter the choroid. The long posterior ciliary arteries and nerves pierce the sclera near the optic nerve and pass anteriorly around the eye to the ciliary body. Anterior ciliary arteries and vortex veins enter and leave the sclera in the area overlying the ciliary body. The intrascleral venous plexus lies anteriorly in the outer portion of the scleral stroma. It receives aqueous humor from the area of the iridocorneal angle via the angular aqueous plexus and aqueous veins and then passes the aqueous humor to the choroidal venous system (see Chapter 12).

In fish, lizards, birds, and some amphibians, cartilaginous and/or bony ossicles may form part of the sclera. These structures are thought to enhance ocular rigidity and aid in accommodation. Surgical techniques for removal of the eye (enucleation) must allow for these ossicles (see Chapter 20).

PATHOLOGIC RESPONSES

Because of its avascularity and compact construction, pathologic reactions in the cornea tend to vary greatly in their speed of onset and recovery, and can become intractable. Also, changes that would be mild or even unnoticed in other tissues, such as edema, slight scar formation, lipid accumulation, or change in tissue tension, may greatly alter transparency and therefore are more significant in the cornea.

Corneal disorders are of three general categories with respect to origin, as follows:

- Exogenous
- Extension from other ocular tissues
- Endogenous

Exogenous insults must first pass through or damage the corneal epithelium, which—despite its special properties and precarious position—is an extremely effective barrier to most microbial organisms. With the exception of *Moraxella bovis* and the herpesviruses, microorganisms cannot *initiate* primary keratitis in animals. However, once the epithelium has been breached, most microorganisms can readily establish themselves and spread within the avascular stroma. The efficiency of the epithelial barrier is indicated by the frequency with which pathogenic bacteria are found in the normal conjunctival sac of domestic animals but the relative rarity of primary disease arising from their presence (see Chapter 3).

Extension of disease processes from adjacent ocular tissues is a common cause of corneal disorders. Examples are the entry of infectious canine hepatitis virus into the cornea from the aqueous, the effects of uveitis, anterior lens luxation, or glaucoma on the cornea, and the infiltration of corneal stroma by inflammatory cells and blood vessels in some systemic diseases, most notably neoplasias such as lymphoma.

Endogenous disorders of the cornea include the corneal dystrophies, which are familial and likely inherited.

Corneal Reactions to Disease

The majority of clinically important keratopathies manifest as one or more of the following major pathologic reactions:

- Corneal edema
- Corneal vascularization
- Corneal fibrosis (scar formation)
- Corneal melanosis
- Stromal infiltration with white blood cells
- Accumulation of an abnormal substance within the cornea (usually lipid or mineral)
- Stromal malacia (or "melting")

Corneal Edema

Control of entry of water into the cornea and maintenance of a state of relative dehydration is critical to corneal transparency. Corneal edema results when excess fluid accumulates within the stroma and forces the collagen lamellae apart, leading to loss of transparency (Figure 10-7). The endothelium makes the major contribution to control corneal stromal fluid balance by moving solutes (and therefore water) from the stroma to the aqueous against the IOP gradient that forces water into the cornea. The epithelium plays a lesser but critical role by preventing tears from entering the stroma. Dysfunction of either of these cell layers leads to stromal edema and loss of transparency. For example, if the corneal epithelium becomes ulcerated, water enters the stroma from the precorneal film, and gross swelling

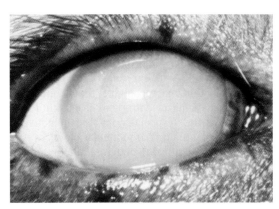

Figure 10-7. Corneal edema produces a diffuse blue corneal opacification. (Courtesy University of California, Davis, Veterinary Ophthalmology Service Collection.)

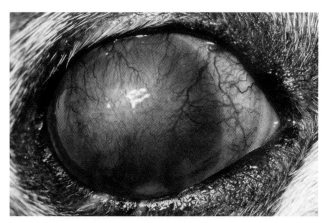

Figure 10-8. Superficial corneal vascularization in a dog with keratoconjunctivitis sicca.

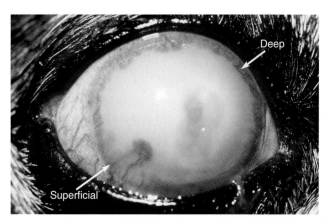

Figure 10-9. Deep corneal blood vessels in a dog with a deep corneal ulcer. Note also the superficial vessels and diffuse corneal edema.

and discoloration occur until a new layer of epithelium has covered the area and fluid balance is restored. Endothelial cell loss tends to cause more marked and more diffuse corneal edema. Because endothelial cells are postmitotic and do not regenerate, some degree of endothelial cell loss and dysfunction occur as part of the normal aging process in all domestic species. This physiologic loss of endothelium does not cause appreciable edema. Hastened cell loss may also occur as a result of primary corneal or intraocular disease processes such as corneal endothelial dystrophy, glaucoma, uveitis, and anterior lens luxation. Regardless of cause, corneal edema appears hazy blue and may be localized or diffuse. Corneal edema is reversible if the underlying cause is removed, sufficient endothelial cell function remains, and fluid balance is reestablished. Severe corneal edema may result in epithelial bullae formation (bullous keratopathy) and sometimes corneal vascularization (see later).

Corneal Vascularization

The normal cornea contains no blood vessels; however, vessels invade the corneal stroma in response to various pathologic processes and especially during vascularized stromal healing. Corneal vascularization may be superficial, deep, or both. Superficial vessels occur in the anterior third of the stroma and appear "treelike"; that is, they usually begin at the limbus as a single vessel and branch extensively within the cornea (Figure 10-8). Very superficial vessels may be seen crossing the limbus because they are continuous with the conjunctival circulation. Deep intrastromal vessels appear more "hedgelike"; that is, they are shorter and straighter, branch less, and look like paintbrush strokes (Figure 10-9). They appear to arise from under the limbus because they are continuous with the ciliary circulation. The depth of the invading vessels is usually a very accurate indication of the depth of the initiating lesion—deep vessels suggest corneal stromal or intraocular disease, whereas superficial vessels are induced by surface (usually corneal epithelial) disease. The sequence of vascularization is shown in Figure 10-6. In complicated and persistent corneal lesions, aggressive vascularization with granulation tissue formation occurs.

Corneal vascularization is generally beneficial, especially in stromal repair. Clinical evidence of this tendency is seen in repair of corneal stromal abscesses, especially in horses. In such cases, as corneal blood vessels advance from the limbus toward and through a lesion, resolution of other corneal disease and corneal clearing occur in the vascularized zone between the vessel extremities and the limbus. Therefore, although corneal blood vessels may result in ingrowth of melanin, influx of inflammatory cells, and facilitate stromal fibrosis, control of vascularization with the use of topical corticosteroids during the repair process may not always be indicated.

Corneal vascularization may be either deep or superficial. Depth of the invading vessels indicates depth of the inciting lesion.

Corneal Fibrosis

Collagen fibrils produced during repair of a stromal lesion are not laid down in a regular lattice pattern and so interfere with light transmission. This produces a grey "wispy" or "feathery" opacity within the cornea under a normal epithelium that is not associated with other signs of inflammation except perhaps some residual corneal blood vessels (Figure 10-10). With time, scars may clear optically but often do not do so completely. The tendency to clear is greater in young animals and also in cattle, sheep, and cats. Melanosis of the scarred area often occurs in dogs. In dogs lipid deposition may also occur near the scar. The deeper the initial injury, the more dense and permanent the scar and the lesser the tendency for transparency to return. With increasing size, a corneal scar is termed a *nebula, macula,* and

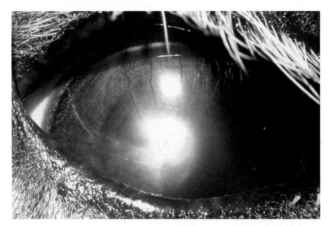

Figure 10-10. Corneal fibrosis and superficial vascularization in a horse.

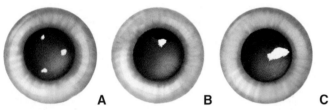

Figure 10-11. Types of corneal scars. **A,** Nebula; **B,** macula; **C,** leukoma.

leukoma (Figure 10-11). If the iris attaches to the posterior surface of the leukoma owing to anterior synechia, the lesion is called an *adherent leukoma*.

Corneal Melanosis

Corneal melanosis is frequently called *corneal pigmentation* or *pigmentary keratitis* (Figure 10-12). This term ignores the fact that pigments other than melanin (such as hemoglobin or the soluble pigment in corneal sequestra of cats) may cause opacification of the cornea; therefore *corneal melanosis* is the preferred term. Regardless of the term chosen, it is often used as if it were a clinical diagnosis; actually, corneal melanosis is merely a sign of chronic corneal irritation that may arise from any number of causes, each with a different treatment and prognosis. Melanin is deposited in the corneal epithelium and sometimes the anterior stroma and originates from proliferation

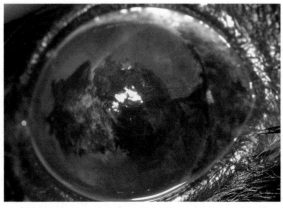

Figure 10-12. Corneal melanosis and vascularization due to brachycephalic ocular syndrome in a shih tzu. (Courtesy University of California, Davis, Veterinary Ophthalmology Service Collection.)

and migration of normal limbal melanocytes during corneal inflammation. The more heavily melanotic the limbus, the more likely and the denser the corneal melanosis.

Corneal melanosis is a nonspecific response to chronic corneal irritation as seen with exposure (due to lagophthalmos, facial nerve dysfunction, macropalpebral fissure, etc.), frictional irritation (due to distichiasis, entropion, nasal skin folds, etc.), tear film abnormalities (especially keratoconjunctivitis sicca [KCS]), or chronic immunologic stimulation such as pannus (chronic superficial keratoconjunctivitis). In these disorders, removal of the stimulus usually prevents or slows progression of the melanosis but may not cause it to recede. With severe and/or chronic irritation, melanosis is accompanied by changes in the corneal epithelium such as thickening, rete peg formation, metaplasia, vascularization, and keratinization. Species variation in the tendency for development of corneal melanosis exist, with birds being extremely resistant, horses and cats moderately resistant, and dogs extremely susceptible.

Corneal melanosis itself is not normally treated unless it is rapidly progressive in susceptible breeds (e.g., pug) or is interfering with vision. However, detection of corneal melanosis should always stimulate thorough diagnostic investigation for the underlying source of irritation. The underlying cause should be removed when possible (e.g., immunomodulation in pannus, removal of source of frictional irritation, reconstructive blepharoplasty, tear replacement therapy).

At the very least, animals with corneal melanosis should undergo the following evaluations:

* Schirmer tear test
* Assessment of palpebral reflex
* Application of fluorescein stain
* Examination for presence of trichiasis, distichiasis, ectopic cilia
* Assessment for entropion or ectropion
* Corneal cytology if there are masslike or plaquelike lesions as seen with pannus (chronic superficial keratoconjunctivitis)

Corneal melanosis ("pigmentary keratitis") is not a diagnosis but a nonspecific sign of chronic corneal irritation. It should stimulate a thorough diagnostic investigation of potential underlying causes.

Stromal Infiltration with White Blood Cells

Inflammatory cell infiltration of the corneal stroma appears as yellowish green discoloration (Figure 10-13). It usually occurs in response to an infection or in association with a corneal foreign body. However, nonseptic infiltration of the cornea can occur. This finding is most dramatic in the equine cornea, is commonly seen in dogs, and is relatively infrequently seen in cats. Inflammatory cells originate from the tear film, limbus, or uveal tract (via the aqueous humor) and can accumulate within the corneal stroma surprisingly quickly, indicating a potent chemotactic stimulus. Corneal cytology along with culture and sensitivity testing should be performed, and broad-spectrum antibiotic therapy initiated promptly. Frequent reexamination of the cornea is justified because liberation of lytic enzymes from inflammatory cells, microbes, and corneal cells can be associated with rapid collagenolysis (i.e., malacia or corneal "melting").

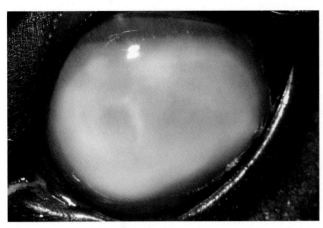

Figure 10-13. Corneal stromal infiltration with white blood cells (equine stromal abscess). Note also the deep corneal blood vessels. (Courtesy University of California, Davis, Veterinary Ophthalmology Service Collection.)

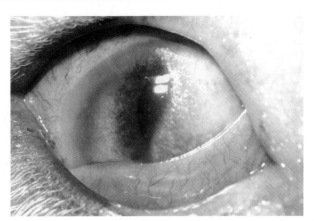

Figure 10-15. Corneal lipid degeneration and edema in a dog with episcleritis. (Courtesy University of California, Davis, Veterinary Ophthalmology Service Collection.)

Accumulation of Abnormal Substances (Lipid or Mineral) within the Cornea

Lipid and/or mineral accumulation appears as sparkly, crystalline, or shiny white areas in the cornea. These accumulations frequently contain cholesterol and/or calcium in varying combinations. All corneal layers may be involved, but lipid/mineral deposits are usually subepithelial, so the cornea does not retain fluorescein stain. Such accumulation occurs as a primary or inherited, but not necessarily congenital, condition in many canine breeds (corneal lipid dystrophy) but rarely in other species. It may also occur as an acquired, inflammatory condition (corneal lipid degeneration) in dogs and horses but rarely in cats. Lipid dystrophy is typically bilateral and nonpainful, has minimal effect on vision, and requires no therapy (Figure 10-14). Corneal lipid degeneration, by contrast, is usually unilateral and frequently associated with inflammation (keratitis, scleritis, or uveitis). Coincident corneal edema, vascularization, fibrosis, and melanosis are common (Figure 10-15). Occasionally there is a history of ocular trauma, often with ulceration that healed with lipid deposition. Corneal lipid accumulation may also occasionally be seen with long-term corticosteroid use.

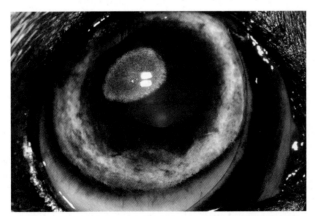

Figure 10-14. Corneal lipid/mineral dystrophy in a dog. (Courtesy University of California, Davis, Veterinary Ophthalmology Service Collection.)

In some animals, deposition of lipid in the cornea is due to elevated serum lipid concentrations. Investigation of common causes of systemic hyperlipidemia, such as hypothyroidism, diabetes mellitus, hyperadrenocorticism, and primary hyperlipidemia, is therefore warranted. Both serum cholesterol and triglyceride concentrations should be assessed. If serum lipid values are elevated, dietary management and treatment for the underlying cause are necessary. Surgical removal of lipid plaques is contraindicated until hyperlipidemia is corrected, because keratitis from the keratectomy increases lipid deposition during healing. A specific lipid keratopathy is noted in frogs (see Chapter 20).

Stromal Malacia (or "Melting")

Stromal malacia or "melting" occurs as a result of collagenolysis due to collagenase liberation from invading white blood cells, especially neutrophils within the corneal stroma, microorganisms, or corneal epithelial cells or keratocytes. The result is loss of rigidity and structure of the corneal collagen with subsequent "sagging" or "oozing" of the stroma over the ventral cornea or eyelid (Figure 10-16), followed by stromal loss with development of a deep ulcer or descemetocele. This change can occur very quickly and in relative isolation if the stimulus for collagenase production is marked and rapid but is more commonly seen in association with other corneal pathology, notably stromal white cell infiltration and edema.

CORNEAL DISEASES BELIEVED TO BE INHERITED

Microcornea

Microcornea can be diagnosed through measurement of the horizontal and vertical diameters of the cornea and comparison of the results with values from the other eye (Figure 10-17). The condition is usually unilateral and associated with microphthalmia (see Chapter 2).

Dermoid

Dermoids are examples of a choristoma or congenital circumscribed overgrowth of microscopically normal tissue in an

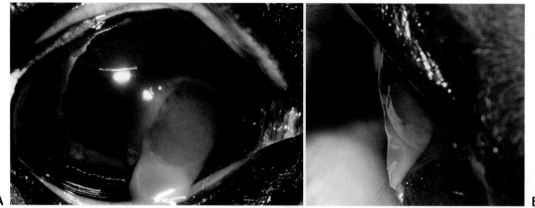

Figure 10-16. Corneal malacia ("melting") and stromal edema in a horse. **A,** Frontal view; **B,** profile. (Courtesy University of Missouri, Columbia, Veterinary Ophthalmology Service Collection.)

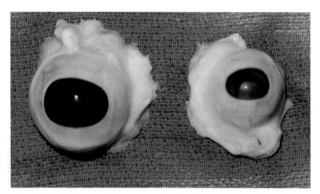

Figure 10-17. Right and left globes from a Limousin calf. Note the unilateral microphthalmia and microcornea. This calf also had arthrogryposis. (Courtesy University of California, Davis, Veterinary Ophthalmology Service Collection.)

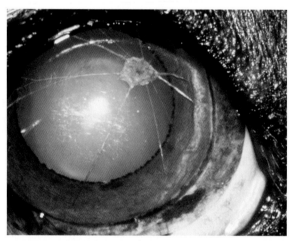

Figure 10-19. Iris-to-cornea persistent pupillary membranes. (Courtesy University of Missouri, Columbia, Veterinary Ophthalmology Service Collection.)

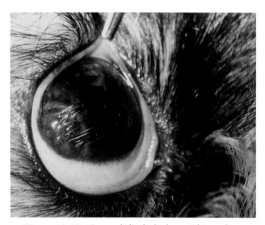

Figure 10-18. Corneal (limbal) dermoid in a dog.

abnormal place (Figure 10-18). They may involve conjunctiva, third eyelid, eyelid margin, limbus, or cornea in various combinations. In dermoids containing hair follicles, hair grows from the surface, which causes conjunctival and corneal irritation evident as corneal opacity, conjunctival hyperemia, and ocular discharge. Dermoids usually grow slowly, if at all. They are believed to be inherited in Hereford cattle, Birman and Burmese cats, Saint Bernard dogs, dachshunds, and Dalmatians. Treatment requires careful surgical excision with conjunctivectomy, combined with keratectomy if they cross the

limbus. Because the cornea underlying dermoids may be thinner than normal, referral to an ophthalmologist is recommended.

Persistent Pupillary Membranes

Persistent pupillary membranes (PPMs) are an inherited failure of the uveal tract to regress appropriately during embryologic and immediate postnatal development. They are more fully discussed in Chapter 11. However, they can cause corneal opacity if they arc from the iris collarette to the corneal endothelium (Figure 10-19), where they are associated with corneal edema, melanosis, and/or fibrosis. These are noninflammatory and vary in their effect on vision according to severity. No therapy is possible or necessary for PPMs; however, affected animals should not be bred.

Congenital Subepithelial Geographic Corneal Dystrophy

Congenital subepithelial geographic corneal dystrophy is transient and occurs in many dog breeds. It appears as hazy, grayish-white, geographic or mosaic areas of usually subtle superficial corneal opacity in the interpalpebral fissure of neonatal puppies. It is painless and often goes unnoticed. The condition usually resolves by 10 weeks of age. Treatment is not required.

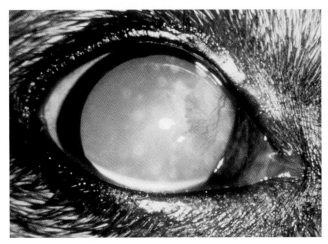

Figure 10-20. Superficial punctate keratitis in a dog. (Courtesy University of Missouri, Columbia, Veterinary Ophthalmology Service Collection.)

Superficial Punctate Keratitis

The term *superficial punctate keratitis* is applied to multiple, superficial, circular defects in the corneal epithelium that may or may not stain with fluorescein (Figure 10-20). The affected areas are scattered diffusely across the corneal surface, sometimes leaving the cornea looking like the skin of an orange. The condition is recognized as familial in shelties and dachshunds, may be due to a qualitative tear film deficiency (most likely mucin deficiency), and often responds to cyclosporine applied topically twice daily. Recurrences are frequent. Similar (nonrecurrent and noninherited) keratopathies may be induced by mild corneal insults, such as exposure during general anesthesia and use of topical anesthetics.

Corneal Lipid Dystrophy

Deposition of lipid or, occasionally, mineral in the anterior stroma (immediately subjacent to the epithelium) is relatively common in dogs and is seen rarely in cats and horses. Deposits are usually central or isolated from the limbus and are bilateral although they may be asymmetrical (see Figure 10-14). The condition appears to be familial and may be static or slowly progressive. The lipid may take a variety of forms, including circles, ovals, and arcs concentric with the limbus. This condition can be differentiated from corneal degeneration (see Figure 10-15) or diseases caused by circulating hyperlipidemia, because corneal lipid dystrophy is noninflammatory, lacks connection with the limbus, and is associated with normal fasting serum cholesterol and triglyceride concentrations.

Corneal Endothelial Dystrophy

Corneal endothelial dystrophy is relatively common in Boston terriers, boxers, dachshunds, poodles, and Chihuahuas. The condition is believed to be inherited and results in a premature and clinically relevant loss of corneal endothelial cells to the point at which corneal edema results. Unless the edema becomes severe enough to cause bullae formation and secondary ulceration, the disease is characteristically nonpainful. Symptomatic treatment with hyperosmotic 5% sodium chloride ointment may minimize epithelial edema and subsequent bullae formation. Unless the ointment is applied at least four times daily, this therapy usually does not appreciably reduce stromal edema or the blue discoloration of the cornea. Thermokeratoplasty may be beneficial in advanced cases. This technique involves making multiple, small, superficial stromal burns with a specialized ophthalmic cautery unit. Referral to an ophthalmologist for this procedure is recommended because the cornea can be perforated by the heat of the cautery unit. Corneal endothelial dystrophy is usually progressive and permanent.

ACQUIRED CORNEAL DISEASES

Acquired disorders of the cornea may be categorized as ulcerative or nonulcerative, infectious or noninfectious, or by cause, topography, species affected, or depth. However, regardless of the classification system used, some overlap occurs. For example, ulcerative disease may have numerous causes and stromal diseases may also be ulcerative. Therefore the following discussion of the common acquired keratopathies of the domestic species is made without regard to classification systems.

Corneal Ulcers

Broadly defined, a corneal ulcer is any keratopathy in which there is loss of epithelium. *Ulcerative keratitis* is an equivalent term because there is always some inflammation associated with corneal ulceration. Corneal ulcers occur commonly in veterinary practice, and although simple (uncomplicated) ulcers would likely heal without veterinary attention, a complicated ulcer requires optimal management if the affected eye is to be saved.

Optimal management of corneal ulcers requires knowledge of the following information:

- Common causes of ulceration
- Expected healing times for ulcers
- Classification of ulcers as simple or complicated
- Classification of complicated ulcers into three therapeutically relevant categories
- General medical therapy
- Indications for surgery

Common Causes of Corneal Ulceration

Corneal epithelium is constantly being physiologically abraded by normal blinking and desiccation and being replaced by normal cell turnover. Rate of regeneration and surface protective mechanisms are usually sufficient to ensure that ulceration does not occur. Therefore, from a purely mechanistic viewpoint, corneal ulcers may be thought of as arising when this situation becomes unbalanced owing to decreased corneal epithelial protection or increased corneal abrasion (Figure 10-21). Corneal protection is provided by the tear film along with the upper, lower, and third eyelids. Inadequate production, retention, or dispersion of the tear film is therefore frequently associated with corneal ulceration.

Excessive abrasion can be further divided into endogenous causes, such as abnormal lid position or anatomy and eyelash abnormalities, and exogenous causes, such as trauma and foreign body retention in the conjunctival fornix—all of which are common in dogs but less common in most cats because of breeding practices and the relatively more protected environment in which cats tend to live. Brachycephalic cats are more

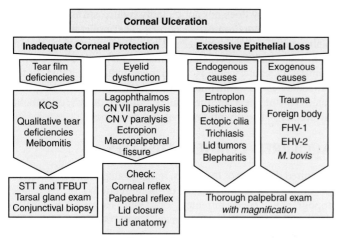

Figure 10-21. Diagnostic algorithm for patients with corneal ulcers. *CN,* Cranial nerve; *EHV-2,* equine herpesvirus type 2; *FHV-1,* feline herpesvirus type 1; *KCS,* keratoconjunctivitis sicca; *STT,* Schirmer tear test; *TFBUT,* tear film break-up time.

likely to have these eyelid/cilia abnormalities. Horses are susceptible to exogenous trauma but rarely suffer eyelid or tear film abnormalities. Infectious agents also qualify as exogenous causes of corneal ulceration, but it should be noted that other than *M. bovis* and the herpesviruses, primary infectious ulceration does not occur.

Ulceration due to exogenous trauma is a diagnosis by exclusion and can be reached only after all other potential causes are eliminated through consideration of limited infectious agents, thorough examination of lid function and anatomy, and measurement of tear production.

With consideration of the known causes of ulcers, the basic diagnostic approach to corneal ulceration should consist of the following evaluations:

- Schirmer tear test
- Assessment of corneal and palpebral reflex
- Thorough examination of lid and conjunctival anatomy and function, including the posterior face of the third eyelid
- Microbiologic assessment if the ulcer is believed to be infected
- Fluorescein staining

Simple versus Complicated Ulcers

Corneal wound healing was fully described earlier. An ulcer should heal (i.e., become reepithelialized and no longer retain fluorescein stain) within 7 days and without progression to involve the stroma. Failure of occurrence of *both* of these events is abnormal. Therefore at every examination all ulcers should be classified as "simple" or "complicated" on the basis of two defining features—duration and depth. Simple ulcers heal without stromal involvement *and* within 7 days. Complicated corneal ulcers involve the stroma (i.e., are deeper) *and/or* persist longer than 7 days. It is important to note that to be classified as simple, ulcers must be *both* acute and superficial; whereas to be classified as complicated, ulcers need only be deep *or* chronic, although of course they can be both.

At every examination all ulcers should be classified as "simple" or "complicated" on the basis of their duration and depth.

Nonhealing ulcers in all patients can be assigned to one of the following three categories:

- *The underlying cause went undiagnosed or untreated and is still present.* Reexamination of the eye, with special attention to trichiasis, distichia, ectopic cilia, tear film health, presence of herpesvirus or *M. bovis,* lagophthalmos, ectropion, entropion, neuroparalytic/neurotrophic keratitis, or a foreign body, is essential.
- *The ulcer has become infected by bacteria.* Such ulcers typically have stromal involvement or loss and frequently appear malacic or "gelatinous." The surrounding corneal stroma may be greenish yellow, suggesting inflammatory cell infiltration.
- *The ulcer has become indolent.* A canine-specific diagnosis, *indolent ulcer* describes a superficial ulcer with a lip of nonadherent corneal epithelium (see later). Recently a similar syndrome has been suggested in horses, but histologic confirmation is lacking so far. By contrast, nonhealing superficial ulcers with nonadherent lips in cats are presumed to be due to feline herpesvirus until proven otherwise. In horses, fungi and herpesvirus are often implicated in nonhealing ulcers. Therefore persistent superficial ulcers in cats and horses fit into one of the two preceding categories in this list—that is, the original cause (herpesvirus) is still present or they have become infected (with a fungus).

All complicated ulcers should be further characterized as indolent (in dogs), infected, or having a persistent (and perhaps unrecognized) cause.

General Medical Therapy for Corneal Ulcers

Regardless of cause, chronicity, severity, and whether the ulcer is complicated or simple, some general comments about medical therapy are possible. Most important is identification and removal or correction of the cause. Without this step, ulcers will not resolve and may progress. At the very best, they will heal only to recur shortly afterwards. Other important therapeutic considerations are the topical use of an antibiotic and a mydriatic agent along with prevention of self-trauma. Some patients may also benefit from analgesic or antiinflammatory medication, which are more fully described later.

ANTIBIOTICS. Topically applied antibiotics are indicated for all corneal ulcers. Although no bacteria are believed to be primary corneal epithelial pathogens and therefore initiate ulcers in small animals, disruption of epithelium does predispose the corneal stroma to infection. In ruminants, *M. bovis* and perhaps *Chlamydia* and *Mycoplasma* spp. may initiate keratitis; these plus other bacteria will certainly complicate ulcers and delay healing. A full discussion of each of the major antibiotics appears in Chapter 3. The following discussion is a brief summary of some useful antibiotics.

Triple antibiotic (neomycin and polymyxin B along with bacitracin or gramicidin) is an excellent first choice for prophylaxis because it is broad spectrum and polymyxin B is effective against many *Pseudomonas* spp. Gentamicin and tobramycin are widely used and inexpensive, but they have relatively poor efficacy against the majority of organisms constituting normal conjunctival flora and therefore are not ideal first choices for broad-spectrum prophylaxis. Frequency of antibiotic application is determined by severity of the condition. Ointments should be avoided when there is a risk of corneal perforation because the petrolatum vehicle causes a severe granulomatous uveitis if it enters the eye.

More aggressive therapy is needed if there are initial signs of infection (stromal loss, infiltration with white blood cells, or malacia), rapid progression of the ulcer, or poor response to standard therapy, or when cytology and/or culture results suggest that organisms are present. Fortified and compounded solutions can be formulated in such cases (Box 10-1). Alternatively, some of the newer topical fluoroquinolone preparations are particularly effective, especially for *Pseudomonas* spp. In all situations in which more resistant organisms are suspected, corneal culture and sensitivity testing should be performed, and antibiotics chosen wisely to minimize development of resistant organisms. Widespread use of any of these preparations for prophylaxis in noninfected ulcers is strongly discouraged. Subconjunctival injection of antibiotics may be beneficial in therapy of rapidly progressive ulcers but is not intended as a substitute for frequent topical therapy, and extreme care must be taken to avoid globe penetration at the time of injection. Topical ophthalmic preparations must *not* be used for injection; this route of therapy is discussed more fully in Chapter 3. Most systemically administered antibiotics are not expected to achieve therapeutic concentrations in the cornea because it is avascular. These agents may be indicated, however, if perforation has occurred or is impending, in heavily vascularized corneas, and after conjunctival graft placement.

MYDRIATIC THERAPY. Stimulation of corneal nerves can produce a significant "reflex" anterior uveitis. This exacerbates pain associated with ulceration and can cause animals to rub their eyes and worsen corneal ulceration. Topical application of a mydriatic agent is therefore justified in most cases of corneal ulceration. Atropine 1% ointment or ophthalmic solution should be used at a frequency sufficient to effect mydriasis—usually between one and three times daily initially with rapid tapering of dose frequency as adequate pupil dilation is achieved.

Box 10-1 | Compounding fortified and noncommercial topical antibiotic solutions

Amikacin

1. Remove 2 mL from a 15-mL squeeze bottle of artificial tear solution* and discard.
2. Add 2 mL of injectable amikacin (50 mg/mL).

Final concentration = 6.7 mg/mL (0.67% solution).
Shelf life[†] = 30 days.

Cefazolin

1. Remove 2 mL from a 15-mL squeeze bottle of artificial tear solution and discard.
2. Reconstitute a 500-mg vial of cefazolin with 2 mL of sterile water.
3. Add entire 500 mg of the reconstituted cefazolin (2.4 mL) to the bottle of artificial tear solution.

Final concentration = 33 mg/mL (3.3% solution).
Shelf life[‡] = 14 days.
Keep the solution refrigerated.

Cephalothin

1. Remove 6 mL from a 15-mL squeeze bottle of artificial tear solution and save.
2. Add the 6 mL of tear solution to a 1-g vial of cephalothin.
3. Add the entire 1 g of the reconstituted cephalothin (6.4 mL) to the bottle of artificial tear solution.

Final concentration = 65 mg/mL (6.5% solution).
Shelf life[§] = 14 days.
Keep the solution refrigerated.

Gentamicin (Fortified)

1. Add 2 mL of injectable gentamicin (50 mg/mL) to the 5-mL bottle of commercial ophthalmic gentamicin solution (0.3%).

Final concentration = 14 mg/mL (1.4% solution).
Shelf life[†] = 30 days.

Ticarcillin

1. Reconstitute a 1-g vial of ticarcillin with 9.4 mL of sterile water.
2. Add 1.0 mL (100 mg) of this solution to a 15-mL squeeze bottle of artificial tears.

Final concentration = 6.3 mg/mL (0.63% solution).
Shelf life[†] = 4 days.
Keep the solution refrigerated.

Tobramycin (Fortified)

1. Add 1.0 mL of injectable tobramycin (40 mg/mL) to a 5-mL bottle of commercial ophthalmic tobramycin solution (0.3%).

Final concentration = 9.2 mg/mL (0.92% solution).
Shelf life[†] = 30 days.

Vancomycin

1. Remove 9 mL from a 15-mL squeeze bottle of artificial tear solution and discard.
2. Reconstitute a 500-mg vial of vancomycin with 10 mL of sterile water.
3. Add the entire 500 mg of reconstituted vancomycin (10.2 mL) to the bottle of artificial tear solution.

Final concentration = 31 mg/mL (3.1% solution).
Shelf life[†] = 4 days.
Keep the solution refrigerated.

Adapted from Baum JL (1988): Antibiotic use in ophthalmology, in Tasmen W, Jaeger EA (editors): Duane's Clinical Ophthalmology, 4th vol. JB Lippincott, Philadelphia.
*Recommended artificial tear solutions are Isopto Alkaline (Alcon), which contains 1% hydroxypropylmethylcellulose; and Adapt (Alcon), which contains polyvinyl alcohol. These solutions are a little more viscous than others, which helps to increase the contact time.
[†]Data from Glasser DB, Hyndiuk RA (1987): Antibiotics, in Lamberts DW, Potter DE (editors): Clinical Ophthalmic Pharmacology. Little, Brown & Co, Boston.
[‡]Shelf life for cefazolin is a conservative estimate based on data from Bowe BE, et al. (1991): An in vitro study of the potency and stability of fortified ophthalmic antibiotic preparations. Am J Ophthalmol 111:686.
[§]Data from Osborne E, et al. (1976): The stability of ten antibiotics in artificial tear solutions. Am J Ophthalmol 82:775.

Atropine compromises tear production and should be used cautiously if at all in the treatment of ulcers associated with KCS. Monitoring of gastrointestinal function of horses receiving topically administered atropine is also important.

ANALGESIC/ANTIINFLAMMATORY AGENTS. Topical corticosteroids are totally contraindicated in the therapy of corneal ulcers because they predispose to infection, delay corneal healing, and potentiate enzymatic destruction of the cornea. The increasing array of topical nonsteroidal antiinflammatory drugs (NSAIDs) (see Chapter 3) also may delay corneal healing, and use of such agents has recently been associated with devastating ulcer progression and globe rupture in some humans with infected ulcers. Therefore these drugs are contraindicated in the presence of herpesvirus and for other infected ulcers. Systemic administration of NSAIDs may be indicated, and systemic corticosteroids can be used judiciously to treat severe concurrent uveitis, even if the corneal wound is infected. With long-term use, however, they may impede vascular ingrowth, which is required for healing of deep stromal ulcers.

PREVENTION OF SELF-TRAUMA. Prevention of self-trauma is an elementary but often overlooked part of ulcer management. Exacerbation of ulceration through self-trauma often goes unobserved but is common and especially important in treatment of indolent ulcers, in which poorly adherent corneal epithelium may be easily abraded if the patient rubs the eye.

All ulcers should be treated by removal or correction of the cause, application of a topical antibiotic, and prevention of self-trauma.

Treatment of Uncomplicated (Simple) Corneal Ulcers

The basic tenets for treatment of superficial ulcers are identification and treatment of the cause and institution of broad-spectrum antibiotic therapy. Prevention of self-trauma and induction of mydriasis are considered on an individual basis. A recheck examination should always be scheduled within 7 days. Uncomplicated, superficial ulcers treated in this manner should have healed at the recheck. If they have not, one of the most common errors in ulcer treatment is frequently made: It is assumed that the wrong antibiotic was chosen and a different one is tried. Rather, an ulcer that has not healed at the 1-week recheck should be recognized as a complicated ulcer and should be further categorized as complicated by the primary cause still being present, by secondary infection, or because it is indolent.

When a superficial ulcer does not heal in 7 days, change the diagnosis, not the antibiotic.

Treatment of Deep (Stromal) Corneal Ulcers or Descemetoceles

Ulcers that are rapidly progressive or that have areas of stromal melting (see Figure 10-16), stromal loss (Figure 10-22), or marked cellular infiltrate (see Figure 10-13) are considered complicated and assumed to be infected. A scraping should be collected and assessed cytologically, and a sample submitted for aerobic bacterial and sometimes fungal culture and sensitivity testing. If the stroma is entirely destroyed exposing

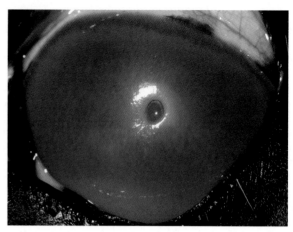

Figure 10-22. Deep stromal ulcer with diffuse corneal edema, deep corneal vascularization, and stromal white blood cell infiltration. There is also hypopyon ventrally. (Courtesy University of California, Davis, Veterinary Ophthalmology Service Collection.)

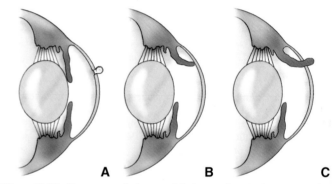

Figure 10-23. Deep corneal ulcers and their sequelae. **A,** Descemetocele; **B,** anterior synechia; **C,** iris prolapse.

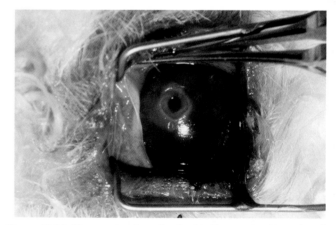

Figure 10-24. Descemetocele stained with fluorescein. Note that the ulcer's "walls" retain stain but the "floor" does not. This photograph was obtained while the patient was under general anesthesia before placement of a conjunctival graft. An eyelid speculum has been placed, and the globe is being rotated with a pair of forceps.

Descemet's membrane (which is sometimes forced outward by the IOP), the lesion is called a *descemetocele* (Figure 10-23, *A*). Descemet's membrane does not stain with fluorescein (Figure 10-24). If untreated, Descemet's membrane may rupture with escape of aqueous, which carries the iris forward into the hole.

If the iris is incorporated into the healing wound, an *anterior synechia* is formed (Figure 10-23, *B*). If the iris is carried out of the wound, *iris prolapse* results (Figure 10-23, *C*).

Medical treatment for stromal ulcers and descemetoceles is similar to (although usually more intensive than) that for simple ulcers: An initiating cause should be sought and removed or controlled if possible, broad-spectrum topical antibiotic and mydriatic therapy should be initiated, and an Elizabethan collar should be provided. Stromal ulcers should be topically medicated with antibiotics as often as hourly for the first 1 to 2 days. If the ulcer is deeper than half corneal thickness, it will also benefit from surgery because the corneal stroma has only a limited ability to regenerate, and healing is slow, often requiring fibrovascular infiltration. This process may take weeks if it occurs spontaneously from the limbus but can be rapidly provided by conjunctival grafting.

Conjunctival grafts provide the following advantages:

- Mechanical support for a thin or weakened cornea
- A continuous supply of serum, which contains anticollagenases and growth factors
- An immediate source of actively replicating fibroblasts for collagen regeneration in the stroma
- A route for systemic antibiotics to be delivered to the corneal ulcer

Conjunctival grafts are somewhat tedious and time-consuming to perform and require advanced training, excellent magnification, correct instrumentation, access to and familiarity with use of 7/0 or smaller suture material with a swaged-on, spatula-tipped needle, and knowledge of basic microsurgical principles. In most cases the patient needing a conjunctival graft should be referred to an ophthalmologist. Probably the most difficult skill to acquire is judgment of depth for placement of corneal sutures. Ideally, they should be placed approximately three-quarter corneal thickness and without penetrating the anterior chamber.

There are at least five broad types of conjunctival grafts:

- Island or free grafts (Figure 10-25, *A* and *B*)
- Complete or 360-degree grafts (Figure 10-25, *C* and *D*)
- Simple advancement or hood grafts (Figure 10-26, *A*)
- Rotational pedicle grafts (Figure 10-26, *B*)
- Bridge grafts (Figure 10-26, *C*)

Advancement-type (hood or 360-degree) grafts are probably easiest to harvest and place; however, rotational pedicle grafts more easily reach a defect in the central cornea. For rotational pedicle grafts, dissection is typically begun with tenotomy scissors at the temporal bulbar conjunctiva (Figure 10-27). A strip of conjunctiva of sufficient length and width to reach and cover the ulcer is freed from the underlying Tenon's capsule. The conjunctival graft should be thin and mobile. A useful rule of thumb is that if tenotomy scissors can be readily visualized through the conjunctiva, the graft is thin enough. Corneal epithelium should be gently débrided for approximately 1 mm around the ulcer before suturing the graft to ensure union between the subconjunctival tissue of the graft and the corneal stroma in the ulcer bed. Débrided material may be submitted for cytologic and microbiologic examination. The graft is sutured to viable cornea surrounding the ulcer with simple interrupted sutures. An alternative approach is to tack the graft with four to six simple interrupted sutures and then oversew the graft perimeter with a

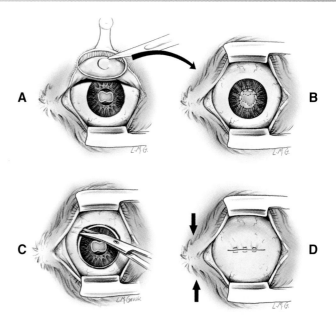

Figure 10-25. A, A conjunctival island graft is harvested from the palpebral conjunctiva with use of a chalazion clamp for tissue fixation. **B,** The island graft is sutured into the corneal defect around its whole perimeter. **C** and **D,** A 360-degree conjunctival graft is harvested by complete perilimbal incision and centripetal advancement of conjunctiva. This graft type should be reserved for large corneal defects and is usually a globe salvage technique because scarring is commonly extensive. This graft does not require corneal sutures, although they can aid in reducing the chance of dehiscence.

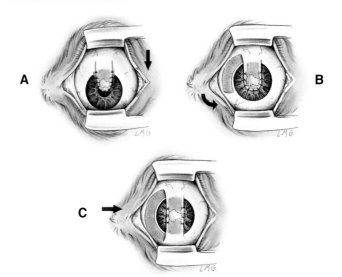

Figure 10-26. A, A conjunctival advancement graft is harvested from the bulbar conjunctiva adjacent to the corneal defect. This works best for paraxial corneal defects. **B,** A rotational pedicle graft in which a conjunctival pedicle is harvested from the lateral bulbar conjunctiva and rotated over the corneal defect. These grafts provide support and vascularity to axial defects. **C,** A conjunctival bridge graft is also harvested from bulbar conjunctiva but is left attached at both ends to enhance the vascular supply and equalize retraction forces that may cause dehiscence. In all three graft types, the conjunctiva is moved to cover the corneal defect in the direction of the arrow.

simple continuous pattern. Additional sutures at the limbus may help secure the graft. It is not essential to close the rent in the bulbar conjunctiva; however, doing so tends to reduce postoperative pain. The rent can be closed with a simple continuous pattern.

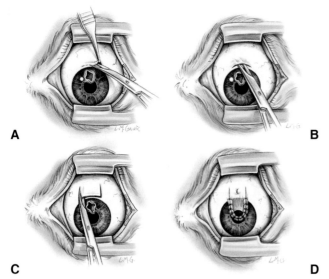

Figure 10-27. Fornix-based advancement flap for smaller lesions near the limbus. **A,** A small limbal incision is made adjacent to the lesion. **B,** The flap is undermined using blunt dissection. **C,** Parallel or slightly divergent conjunctival incisions are made toward the fornix, with the flap width sufficient to cover the corneal lesion. **D,** The conjunctival flap is advanced centrally to cover the corneal lesion and sutured in place with simple interrupted sutures of 7/0 to 9/0 polyglactin.

Medical therapy for ulcerative keratitis is continued, and the graft can be trimmed when the cornea is healed (Figure 10-28). Trimming is usually done at least 6 to 8 weeks after graft placement, although thin grafts may slowly integrate with the cornea and not require trimming. Use of topical corticosteroids to minimize scarring and reduce vascularization was traditionally recommended. More current information suggests that avascularity is the natural state for the cornea and will be regained spontaneously as the biologic need for blood vessels wanes. Cyclosporine (2% solution) does have some antiangiogenic properties and may be a safer alternative if anything is needed.

Other types of conjunctival grafts vary mostly in extent of dissection. Free or island grafts provide mechanical support to the cornea and may be sutured around their whole perimeter, thus ensuring a good "seal"; however, they lack the vascular advantages of other grafts. The 360-degree graft is unique in that it does not require corneal sutures; rather, the free con-

junctival edges are simply apposed to each other with horizontal mattress sutures of 6/0 or 7/0 polyglactin 910 (see Figure 10-25, *C* and *D*). Although this feature makes the graft technically easier to perform, early graft retraction is the major disadvantage. The 360-degree graft may be necessary, however, for very large central corneal ulcers.

TEMPORARY TARSORRHAPHY VERSUS THIRD EYELID FLAP. Third eyelid flaps have been used widely for treatment of ulcers. Although they do provide a "bandage" that reduces desiccation and frictional irritation of the cornea by the upper and lower eyelids, they are also associated with some unwanted and potentially deleterious effects. Penetration of medications through or around the third eyelid to the affected cornea is questionable at best; indeed the anterior face of the third eyelid provides a slick, and direct "chute" to the nasolacrimal puncta. Inability of the owner and clinician to monitor progress or, more important, worsening of the ulcer behind the third eyelid is another serious limitation of this technique. Some of the more serious, progressive ulcers presented to veterinary ophthalmologists have developed behind a third eyelid flap.

In comparison, a temporary lateral tarsorrhaphy is extremely easy to perform, provides adequate corneal protection, and allows medication and monitoring of the ulcer (Figure 10-29). A temporary tarsorrhaphy is performed using 3/0 or 4/0 silk or braided nylon on a $\frac{3}{4}$- or $\frac{1}{2}$-curved, cutting micropoint needle, with the aid of 3× to 5× magnification. The upper eyelid is grasped gently with fine tissue forceps, and the needle is passed

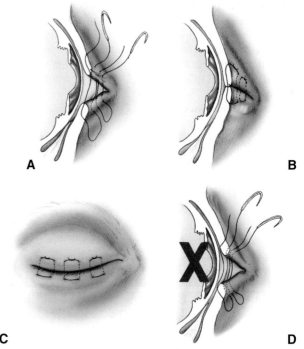

Figure 10-29. Temporary tarsorrhaphy. **A** to **C,** A series of intermarginal horizontal mattress sutures are placed with knots on the upper eyelid to minimize accumulation of secretions. Stents are not necessary unless the lids are under a great deal of pressure as with exophthalmos or replacement of traumatic proptosis. Correctly placed sutures enter at the hairednonhaired junction and emerge at the eyelid margin, just anterior to the meibomian gland orifices **(B)** so that they do not abrade the cornea even if the lids subsequently gap slightly. **D,** Sutures placed too deeply so as to emerge through the conjunctival surface result in corneal ulceration. (Modified from Severin GA [2000]: Severin's Veterinary Ophthalmology Notes, 3rd ed. Severin, Ft. Collins, CO.)

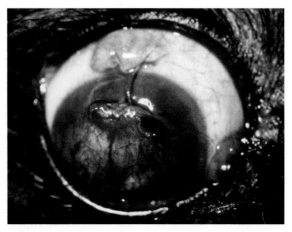

Figure 10-28. Conjunctival pedicle graft immediately after being trimmed.

through the skin, entering at the haired-nonhaired junction approximately 3 mm from the eyelid margin and emerging just anterior to the meibomian (tarsal) gland orifices, which appear as a gray line of small circles along the margin. Care is taken not to penetrate the conjunctiva, as doing so would cause suture to rub on the cornea. The suture is then continued through the lower lid, entering just anterior to the meibomian gland orifices and emerging at the haired-nonhaired junction. A mattress suture is completed by passing of the needle back through the lower and then upper lids in an identical manner approximately 5 to 7 mm medial to the point where the original "bites" were taken. The suture should be knotted firmly to further reduce the chance of corneal contact with the suture if "gapping" of the eyelids occurs. This completes a horizontal mattress-type pattern in which the knot is on the upper lid and less likely to be coated with ocular secretions. Usually one or two mattress sutures in this style beginning at the lateral canthus will close the lids to an extent that still permits monitoring and topical treatment medially but provides adequate corneal protection.

CYANOACRYLATE ADHESIVES (TISSUE GLUE). In some cases medical-grade ophthalmic cyanoacrylate adhesives may be used as an alternative to surgery. These provide structural support for deep stromal ulcers but none of the biologic advantages of conjunctival grafts. Cyanoacrylate has some inherent antimicrobial properties and helps stimulate vascular ingrowth but should be reserved for ulcers in which the health of the surrounding stroma is adequate and certainly not malacic. The technique is simple, but optimal position of the globe should be obtained to avoid inadvertently gluing adnexal structures. The patient is anesthetized and the eyelids are held open with a wire eyelid speculum. To facilitate adhesion, the corneal wound edges are gently débrided of epithelium, and the ulcer bed is cleaned and dried very gently with sterile cellulose sponges. A single drop of cyanoacrylate is applied through a 27- or 30-gauge needle or painted onto the ulcer with a tuberculin syringe lacking a needle. The smallest drop can be generated by turning rather than pushing the plunger. The goal is not to *fill* the entire defect but rather to apply a thin *coat* over the ulcer bed and adjacent normal cornea for approximately 1 mm. The glue is typically extruded within 7 to 14 days as corneal blood vessels and/or epithelium migrate underneath it. A soft contact lens and/or a partial temporary tarsorrhaphy may be placed for added protection and to reduce frictional irritation from the rough glue surface.

PROTEASE INHIBITORS. Corneal "melting" (or malacia) is one of the most devastating consequences of severe ulceration as well as a prerequisite for stromal involvement. Collagenases are enzymes produced by certain bacteria, especially gram-negative organisms such as *Pseudomonas* spp. They are also elaborated by degranulating neutrophils and damaged corneal stromal or epithelial cells. Therefore deep (stromal) ulcers are assumed to be infected until proven otherwise. For patients with deep ulcers and for which surgery is not an option, protease inhibitors may be applied topically. Anticollagenase products are used in hope of inhibiting corneal melting. Acetylcysteine was once widely advocated for this purpose. More recently, autologous serum has been promoted as a preferred product. In addition to serum's broad-spectrum anticollagenase properties, it also contains numerous growth factors assumed to be beneficial.

Serum is harvested from a venous blood sample collected aseptically and allowed to clot in a red-top tube. After centrifugation, serum is separated and stored in a sterile multidose vial or commercially available eyedrop container. Autologous serum can then be applied to the infected eye as needed (as frequently as every 30 to 60 minutes for a rapidly melting corneal ulcer). Serum should be stored in the refrigerator and replaced every few days.

Treatment of Indolent Corneal Ulcers in Dogs

Indolent ulcers (also known as refractory or "boxer" ulcers, spontaneous chronic corneal epithelial defects, and recurrent erosions) are a unique type of superficial ulcer in dogs that is frustrating for veterinarians and clients alike. This type of ulcer is due to a failed union between epithelial basement membrane and the anterior layers of the corneal stroma and, defined as such, has been proven to occur in dogs only thus far, although a clinically similar ulcer has been described in horses. These ulcers are typically chronic, superficial, noninfected, and minimally to moderately painful. They usually vascularize slowly if at all and are characterized by a nonadherent lip of corneal epithelium at the ulcer perimeter that is easily débrided with a cotton-tipped applicator (Figure 10-30). The epithelial lip often produces a characteristic "halo" fluorescein staining pattern because the stain runs under and is then seen through the lip (Figure 10-31). Indolent ulcers, which are seen regularly in

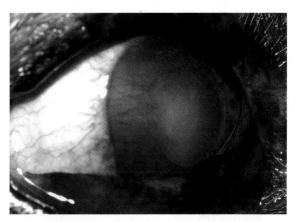

Figure 10-30. Indolent corneal ulcer in an elderly golden retriever. Note the indistinct ulcer margins and the mild corneal edema. There is also some superficial vascularization. (Courtesy University of California, Davis, Veterinary Ophthalmology Service Collection.)

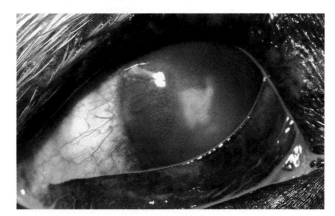

Figure 10-31. The same indolent corneal ulcer as in Figure 10-30, here shown after fluorescein staining. Note the indistinct manner in which the ulcer bed stains and that there is a "halo" of stain rather than a stained area with sharp borders. (Courtesy University of California, Davis, Veterinary Ophthalmology Service Collection.)

older dogs of any breed and boxer dogs of any age, are believed to represent a defect in either the epithelial basement membrane or, more likely, the anterior stromal surface that prevents adhesion between these two structures. Diagnosis relies on characteristic signalment, chronicity, clinical appearance, and staining pattern of the ulcer as well as the ease with which the epithelium is débrided.

Grid keratotomy is the treatment of choice for indolent ulcers (Figure 10-32). Indolent ulcers should probably be pretreated for a few days with a broad-spectrum ophthalmic antibiotic (such as a triple-antibiotic formulation) to sterilize the corneal surface before the grid keratotomy is performed. The first stage in this therapeutic procedure is conveniently the final step required for diagnosis—removal of any redundant, nonadherent epithelium via débridement with a dry cotton-tipped applicator after corneal application of topical anesthetic. The epithelial lip surrounding indolent ulcers is very easily débrided, which sometimes results in an extensive ulcer. Occasionally, epithelium can be débrided out to the limbus over part or all of the corneal surface. This is, however, a necessary first step, and inadequate débridement is one of the more common reasons for treatment failure. A simple (nonindolent) ulcer cannot be débrided in this fashion.

Grid keratotomy is performed after débridement. General anesthesia or sedation is recommended for fractious dogs and for a clinician learning this technique. With compliant animals and an experienced operator, topical anesthesia and good restraint or sedation may be sufficient. Grid keratotomy consists of making linear striations in the cornea in a "cross-hatch" or grid pattern using the tip of a 25-gauge needle. A tuberculin syringe seems to make the ideal "handle" for directing the needle. Striations must extend from normal adherent epithe-lium through the ulcer bed and must emerge in normal adherent epithelium on the other side of the ulcer. They must be multiple and deep enough to create obvious, visible score marks in the corneal stroma.

Medical therapy is continued afterward as for any superficial ulcer. A single postoperative dose of atropine is usually sufficient to control reflex uveitis. Hyperosmotic (5%) sodium chloride ointment is recommended if corneal edema is marked, because it might further decrease already impaired epithelial adhesion. Grid keratotomy may be combined with application of a soft contact lens and partial temporary tarsorrhaphy. This step provides greater protection for the healing cornea and contact lenses may increase surface tension via a gentle "suction-cup" effect, thereby enhancing epithelial adhesion. When a contact lens is in place, ophthalmic solutions rather than ointments should be used to ensure drug delivery to the corneal surface and to minimize chances of dislodging the contact lens. A success rate of approximately 80% can be expected with grid keratotomy alone. Treatment failures tend to arise when patients are "under-treated" by inadequate débridement or by making too few, too superficial, and/or too short score marks in the cornea. For indolent ulcers that have not healed 10 to 14 days after an initial grid keratotomy, the procedure should be repeated. Recurrent or unresolved cases should be referred for a superficial keratectomy.

Grid keratotomy is a potent treatment for indolent ulcers in dogs, but it is contraindicated in all other ulcer types in dogs and in ulcers in other species. The indolent ulcer diagnosis has not been proven to occur in cats or horses, and grid keratotomy is absolutely contraindicated in cats, in which it frequently induces a corneal sequestrum.

Grid keratotomy is the treatment of choice for indolent ulcers in dogs. It should *never* be used in cats.

Epithelial Inclusion Cysts

Epithelial inclusion cysts are an uncommon sequela to corneal ulceration or trauma. They occur when epithelial cells become disorganized during healing such that they form small, epithelium-lined cysts that, with progression, become fluid-filled, yellow corneal masses (Figure 10-33). They protrude from the corneal surface and indent the stroma itself but are not

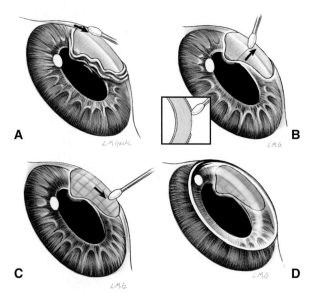

Figure 10-32. Corneal débridement and grid keratotomy. **A,** After application of a topical anesthetic, all loose corneal epithelium is débrided with a cotton-tipped applicator in radial sweeps toward the limbus. **B,** A 25-gauge needle is dragged on a shallow angle and with its bevel up across the ulcerated cornea until a series of approximately parallel score marks has been made in the corneal stroma to a depth not exceeding 25% of the stroma; inset shows greater detail. **C,** A second set of stromal grooves is made at about 90 degrees to the first set. **D,** A therapeutic soft contact lens or biodegradable collagen shield can be placed over the ulcerated cornea. *Note:* This technique is contraindicated in feline corneas.

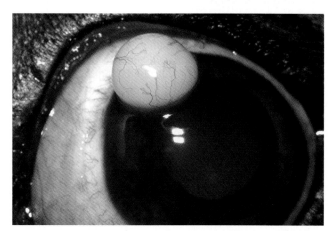

Figure 10-33. Corneal epithelial inclusion cyst. (Courtesy University of California, Davis, Veterinary Ophthalmology Service Collection.)

infected and cause little corneal reaction or pain. The cysts are removed with superficial keratectomy.

Mycotic Keratitis

Bacterial and viral infections of the cornea are much more commonly recognized than fungal infections in most parts of the world. However, particularly in tropical and subtropical areas, any corneal ulcer that does not respond to antibiotic therapy, especially one associated with stromal infiltration with white blood cells and especially in a horse, should be scraped. The exfoliated tissue should then be examined cytologically and cultured for possible mycotic involvement. Antifungal sensitivity testing can be done but is slow and expensive. There is also some controversy about the clinical applicability of in vitro sensitivity data. In a study of equine ulcerative keratomycosis in Florida, the frequency of fungal isolates was *Aspergillus*, 41%; *Fusarium*, 32%; *Penicillium*, 9%; *Cylindrocarpon*, 4%; *Scyalidium*, 4%; *Torulopsis*, 4%; and yeast, 4%. The in vitro susceptibility of the isolates to different antifungal agents was natamycin = miconazole > itraconazole > ketoconazole. The organisms were significantly less susceptible to fluconazole than to the other medications. In a separate series of 35 fungal isolates from equine eyes, the following susceptibilities were reported: natamycin, 97%; nystatin, 74%; miconazole, 69%; amphotericin, 51%; 5-fluoro-cytosine, 49%; and ketoconazole, 31%. Such reports must be interpreted with caution, however, because frequency of different organisms shows geographic variation.

The clinical appearance of mycotic keratitis can also vary greatly. Generally, fungal infections have a much slower onset and course than bacterial infections as well as a classic history of having been resistant to conventional antibiotic therapy. Horses with keratomycosis may be presented with ulcerative keratitis or corneal abscessation underneath an intact epithelium (see later). Regardless, one of the more characteristic features is focal, creamy yellow, somewhat "fluffy" corneal opacities at the advancing edge of the lesion—so-called satellite lesions (Figure 10-34). These are sometimes characteristically deep within the corneal stroma or at the inner endothelial surface. Other clinical signs are as expected for corneal lesions and include blepharospasm, conjunctival and episcleral

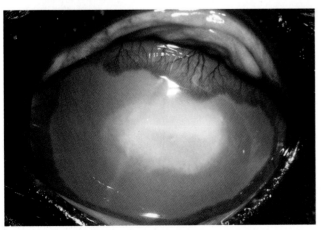

Figure 10-34. Equine stromal keratomycosis. Note the "fluffy" stromal infiltrate as well as the associated diffuse corneal edema and deep and superficial corneal blood vessels. (Courtesy University of California, Davis, Veterinary Ophthalmology Service Collection.)

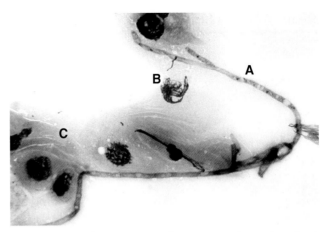

Figure 10-35. Cytologic specimen from a corneal scraping showing septate, branching fungal hyphae (**A**), a neutrophil (**B**), and some corneal epithelial cells (**C**). (Courtesy University of California, Davis, Veterinary Ophthalmology Service Collection.)

hyperemia, epiphora, and corneal edema and neovascularization. Patients with keratomycosis often appear to have more pain than would be expected for a similarly severe bacterial keratitis. Diagnosis requires observation of fungal elements within samples submitted for cytology (Figure 10-35), culture, or histopathology.

A subpalpebral lavage tube is essential in severe cases owing to the pain as well as the frequency and number of medications needed. Medical therapy should include topical or systemic treatment with an antifungal drug. Commonly used topical agents are shown in Table 10-1. Systemically administered agents are discussed in Chapter 3. Some authors recommend treatment as infrequently as once or twice daily at first, especially if reflex uveitis is poorly controlled because rapid fungal death is alleged to incite a potent immune reaction and worsening uveitis. Control of secondary uveitis with flunixin meglumine, and of ciliary spasm with 1% atropine ophthalmic drops or ointment, is essential. Because most antifungal agents do not have antibacterial properties, topical application of a broad-spectrum antibiotic is also required if ulceration is present. If the cornea is malacic, serum should be applied topically for its anticollagenase properties. In many horses an early decision to surgically debulk the lesion will hasten healing time, reduce pain, lessen the chance of globe rupture, and permit the harvesting of diagnostic samples from deep in the cornea. Keratectomy of the lesion and surrounding stromal opacities, followed usually by placement of a conjunctival graft to cover and vascularize the stromal defect, is also an excellent choice. Referral for penetrating or posterior lamellar keratoplasty may be required for very deep lesions.

Stromal Abscess

Corneal stromal abscesses are believed to occur when small corneal puncture wounds allow bacteria or fungi to gain entrance to the stroma. The epithelium then rapidly heals over these sites, leaving the infectious organisms sequestered in the avascular cornea, where they can replicate and elicit a marked inflammatory response known as a *corneal abscess*. Stromal abscesses are seen most commonly in horses. They appear as focal yellowish white corneal opacities, with evidence of usually marked uveitis (Figure 10-36, *A*). Corneal vascularization is variable and is the means by which these lesions

Table 10-1 | **Topical Treatment of Mycotic Keratitis**

DRUG	PREPARATION FOR TOPICAL OPHTHALMIC USE	COMMENTS
POLYENES		
Natamycin	5% ophthalmic suspension	Only commercial ophthalmic preparation
		Usually well tolerated
		Has broad spectrum and good efficacy against common fungal isolates from equine keratomycosis
		Expensive
Amphotericin B	0.10%-0.25% solution	Dilute with sterile water or 5% dextrose (not saline)
		Irritating when injected; do not use subconjunctivally
		Antagonizes miconazole
Nystatin	50,000-200,000 U/mL	Highly effective against yeasts
		Limited activity against filamentous fungi
IMIDAZOLES		
Miconazole	0.5%-1.0% solution	Dilute with saline or 5% dextrose (not artificial tears)
		Broad-spectrum activity similar to that of natamycin
		Some activity against gram-positive bacteria
		Antagonizes amphotericin B
		Subconjunctival use recommended by some authors
Fluconazole	0.2% solution	Some studies have suggested low susceptibility among equine corneal isolates
		Good corneal penetration
		Subconjunctival use recommended by some authors
Itraconazole	1%	Equivalent to 5% natamycin in one study
		Addition of 30% dimethyl sulfoxide improves corneal penetration
Voriconazole	1%	Experimental application to normal horses only
		Good corneal penetration
		No clinical reports available

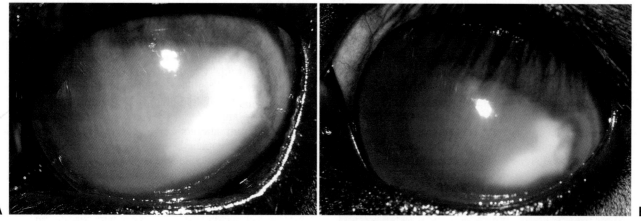

Figure 10-36. A, Equine stromal abscess. Note the marked inflammatory cell infiltrate within the cornea and intense vascular response. **B,** The same eye after 5 days of medical treatment. Note the decrease in stromal cellular infiltrate, especially peripheral to the advancing corneal blood vessels. (Courtesy University of California, Davis, Veterinary Ophthalmology Service Collection.).

ultimately heal if not surgically resected and treated with a corneal or conjunctival graft (Figure 10-36, *B*).

Etiologic diagnosis is challenging because the depth of these lesions within the cornea limits collection of samples to those obtained surgically during keratectomy. Likewise, penetration of antimicrobial agents is often limited by the intact epithelium overlying these abscesses. For these two reasons, referral for diagnosis and surgical treatment is recommended. Recently some success has been achieved with systemic administration of an antifungal agent such as fluconazole, which penetrates the blood-ocular barrier and achieves adequate concentrations in the aqueous humor (see Chapter 3).

Corneal Lacerations

Corneal lacerations occur commonly in all species. In dogs and cats they are frequently secondary to cat-scratch injuries. In horses sharp trauma from objects in the environment is most common. Blunt trauma also causes globe rupture; however, this tends to be along the limbus rather than dissecting across the central cornea. An attempt to differentiate blunt from sharp trauma is important because the former carries a greater risk of intraocular damage. Regardless of cause, three prognostic factors should be established in all corneal lacerations: depth of the laceration, involvement of the lens, and extension of the

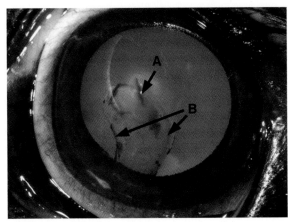

Figure 10-37. Corneal laceration (**A**) and associated anterior lens capsule rupture (**B**). Owing to the elasticity of the anterior lens capsule, a simple linear laceration usually "gaps" open to become elliptical, as seen here. Note also the intralenticular melanin and iris from the neighboring iris. This appearance is strongly suggestive of lens capsule rupture. (Courtesy University of California, Davis, Veterinary Ophthalmology Service Collection.)

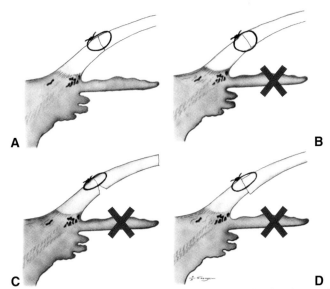

Figure 10-38. Repair of a corneal laceration. **A,** Correctly placed corneal suture. **B** to **D,** Incorrectly placed sutures: **B,** Suture made too deep penetrates the anterior chamber. **C,** Suture made too superficial results in poor endothelial closure and persistent edema. **D,** Uneven suture bites lead to poor apposition of wound edges. (Modified from Slatter D [editor] [2003]: Textbook of Small Animal Surgery, Vol II, 3rd ed. Saunders, Philadelphia.)

laceration beyond the limbus. Whenever possible, referral to an ophthalmologist is recommended.

Lacerations that penetrate the superficial corneal layers only, rather than the entire corneal thickness, usually have a good prognosis with appropriate care. They are treated in essentially the same way as ulcers. Perforating wounds with globe rupture have a poorer prognosis because of intraocular damage and greater tissue disruption at the wound edge. They heal by vascularization (either slowly and naturally from the limbus or prolapsed iris, or via a conjunctival graft). Regardless, there is more scar tissue and corneal opacification.

A careful examination is made to evaluate the extent of intraocular injuries. Great care must be taken to prevent pressure on the globe so as to avoid the risk of further intraocular damage. One of the most common causes of severe endophthalmitis and often secondary glaucoma leading to enucleation is unrecognized damage to the lens and its capsule from a perforating corneal injury (Figure 10-37). This damage causes phacoclastic uveitis that is usually unresponsive to medical treatment and may require emergency lensectomy (see Chapter 13). A careful assessment of the limbus for the full 360 degrees should be conducted. Lacerations that extend beyond the limbus carry a great risk of involvement of the underlying ciliary body and retina with marked uveitis, retinal detachment, and sometimes phthisis being likely. If a menace response cannot be elicited and the intraocular structures cannot be fully examined, a consensual pupillary light reflex from the affected to the normal eye should be evaluated. If major intraocular damage is evident, a consensual pupillary light reflex is present, and the limbus is intact, the patient should be referred for suturing of the corneal wound (Figure 10-38).

Removal of Corneal Foreign Bodies

Corneal foreign bodies are usually of two different types, those that adhere to the corneal surface by surface tension and may subsequently become even more firmly attached by creating an ulcerated region at their borders (Figure 10-39) and those that penetrate into the cornea and sometimes into the globe itself (Figure 10-40). They must be removed to limit

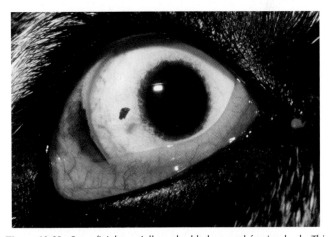

Figure 10-39. Superficial, partially embedded corneal foreign body. This was a piece of plant material that could be forcibly rinsed from the corneal surface.

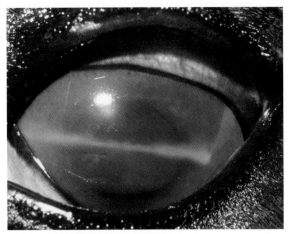

Figure 10-40. Penetrating plant material foreign body in a horse. This foreign body penetrated at the medial limbus and crossed the anterior chamber without penetrating or damaging the lens or iris. It required surgical removal.

pain, reduce the risk of infection, and prevent vascularization and scar formation. Small adhered foreign bodies are best removed with a fine stream of eye rinse or saline directed forcefully at the corneal surface after application of a topical anesthetic. This procedure is safe only if the cornea is not weakened, because a stream of fluid can rupture a descemetocele or other deep ulcer. Penetrating foreign bodies are more problematic and should be referred for surgical removal by means of an incision made in the cornea over the long axis of the foreign body under an operating microscope. After removal of either class of foreign body, a broad-spectrum topical antibiotic and atropine are administered to limit infection and the effects of secondary uveitis, respectively. If globe perforation has occurred, a systemically administered antibiotic should also be used. Corneal epithelial healing is normally rapid as long as secondary infection is controlled.

Keratoconjunctivitis Sicca

KCS is discussed in detail in Chapter 9.

Pigmentary Keratitis

Pigmentary keratitis is sometimes used as a clinical diagnosis when corneal melanosis is noted. In fact, corneal melanosis is simply a sign of chronic keratitis due to any number of causes, each with a different treatment and prognosis. Corneal melanosis (see Figure 10-12), its causes, and the diagnostic steps to follow when it is noted were previously described in the section on pathologic responses. The most common causes of corneal melanosis (and the chapters in which they are discussed) are as follows:

- Chronic exposure due to brachycephalic ocular syndrome (see Chapter 6)
- Cilia disorders (see Chapter 6)
- Tear film dysfunction (see Chapter 9)
- Any combination of the preceding conditions

Treatment is directed at halting progress of the melanosis through correction of the underlying cause. This usually stops further melanin deposition, but melanin already present may be slow to recede if it does so at all. For this reason, the importance of early detection of subtle melanosis and correction of causes before melanosis is advanced cannot be overstated.

"Pannus" or Chronic Immune-Mediated Superficial Keratoconjunctivitis

Pannus classically refers to nonspecific vascularization of avascular tissue (e.g., cartilage or cornea). However, it has been used so commonly to describe a characteristic immune-mediated disease of the cornea and conjunctiva of dogs that it is also used here by common convention. Other synonyms that have been used are Uberreiter's syndrome and chronic immune-mediated keratoconjunctivitis syndrome. Although a distinct breed predilection for this disorder is seen in German shepherds and greyhounds, it can affect any dog breed and should never be discounted as a diagnosis simply because the patient is not one of the commonly affected breeds.

The exact etiology is unknown. Cell-mediated immunity to corneal and uveal antigens has been demonstrated in affected corneas; however, this can also occur in many other chronic inflammatory corneal disorders. Epidemiologic evidence of increased severity and greater resistance to treatment in patients residing more than 4000 feet above sea level suggests that ultraviolet radiation is important in the pathogenesis. It has been proposed that ultraviolet radiation alters the antigenicity of tissue in susceptible corneas, resulting in cell-mediated "auto-immunity."

In the early stages, corneal epithelial cells proliferate and the superficial stroma is infiltrated by plasma cells and lymphocytes. As the disease progresses, melanocytes, histiocytes, and fibrocytes also enter the cornea, and edema and neovascularization occur. In the advanced stage, the corneal epithelium and anterior stroma become heavily melanotic and vascularized, and the epithelium may become keratinized (Figure 10-41). The epithelium remains intact in this disease, but frequently the mounds of fibrous granulation tissue retain fluorescein and the irregular corneal surface permit pooling of fluorescein. Both findings provide the illusion of ulceration. The syndrome tends to affect the temporal, nasal, inferior, and superior corneal quadrants, listed in descending order of occurrence and severity. Corneal vascularization and melanosis occur first at the temporal limbus and gradually move centrally. The other quadrants are gradually affected, and eventually the whole cornea may be involved. Edema and corneal degeneration often occur in the stroma 1 to 3 mm ahead of the advancing lesion. Depigmentation and thickening of the external surface of the third eyelid, usually near the margin, is common and can even occur without corneal lesions. This process contributes to the inflamed appearance of the eye. Mucoid ocular discharge is common.

The age of onset and breed of the affected animal are of prognostic significance. In animals affected when young (e.g., 1 to 2 years) the condition usually progresses to severe lesions, whereas animals first affected at a later age (e.g., 4 to 5 years) have less severe lesions. Severity of the disease also appears to vary with locality. Animals with higher sun exposure (because of latitude or elevation) show more severe lesions, which progress more rapidly to a more advanced state and respond to therapy less favorably, than do dogs with less ultraviolet exposure. Lesions must affect a large area of the cornea before vision is affected, and some cases may be quite advanced before first being noticed by the owner. Although the appearance of lesions is

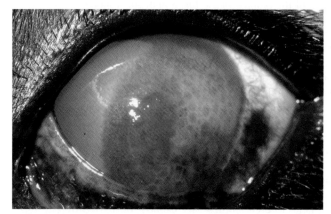

Figure 10-41. "Pannus" (chronic immune-mediated keratoconjunctivitis syndrome) in a dog. Note the cobblestone-like plaque of granulation tissue and melanin over the lateral cornea with a leading band of corneal edema. The third eyelid is similarly affected, as is common in this syndrome. (Courtesy University of California, Davis, Veterinary Ophthalmology Service Collection.)

often characteristic, especially if noted in a predisposed breed with appropriate sun exposure, diagnosis can be confirmed by cytologic assessment of a corneoconjunctival scraping, which is usually almost purely lymphocytic/plasmacytic. Pannus must be distinguished from corneal melanosis due to other chronic irritation, such as KCS, exposure, and frictional irritation, as well as from granulation tissue present in vascular healing of corneal stromal wounds.

Pannus is a chronic progressive corneal disorder that cannot be cured. The therapeutic goal should be control and sometimes regression of the lesions so that blindness can be avoided. The owner must understand that lifelong therapy is necessary at a level depending on the severity in each patient and the geographic locality. With the exception of susceptible patients living at high elevation, useful vision can usually be preserved with medical therapy alone. In patients living at low elevation or for mild lesions occurring in middle-aged dogs, treatment consists of topical application of a potent and penetrating corticosteroid eyedrop, such as 0.1% dexamethasone or 1% prednisolone two to four times daily and/or topical cyclosporine (1% to 2%) twice daily until an adequate response is seen. Therapy can then be tapered as dictated by severity of signs. Improvement usually takes a minimum of 3 to 4 weeks to become apparent. The goal should be the minimum number and frequency of medications needed to prevent progression or recurrence. If possible, the corticosteroid should be stopped and the animal maintained on cyclosporine alone, as the latter has fewer side effects with long-term use. In severe or resistant cases, subconjunctival corticosteroids (preferably short-acting repository preparations with 7 to 14 days' duration of action) may be necessary in addition to topical therapy.

Neurogenic Keratitis

Neurogenic keratitis is a collective term for neurotrophic keratitis due to loss of sensory innervation to the cornea (trigeminal nerve dysfunction) and neuroparalytic keratitis due to loss of motor innervation to the eyelids (facial nerve dysfunction). With neurotrophic keratitis, the corneal pathogenesis involves failure of the sensory stimulus to blink and protect the cornea as well as loss of the trophic factors supplied to the cornea via axoplasmic flow through the trigeminal nerve. There may also be associated masticatory muscle atrophy and enophthalmos. In neuroparalytic keratitis, interruption of motor innervation of the eyelids causes inadequate blink, lack of distribution of the precorneal tear film, and lack of protection of the corneal and conjunctival surfaces from friction and exposure. Instead of the normal blinking action of the upper and lower eyelids, the globe is often retracted, with subsequent passive movement of the third eyelid across the cornea.

Owing to anatomic position of the relevant nerves, neurotrophic keratitis tends to be associated with orbital disease, whereas neuroparalytic keratitis is seen most commonly in horses with guttural pouch disease and in other animals (especially dogs) with chronic otitis or after surgery for chronic otitis. In the early stages of both diseases, corneal epithelial degeneration and stromal edema occur. More advanced lesions include corneal desiccation and opacification due to vascularization and melanosis. Ulceration may occur with either form of neurogenic keratitis and may progress to perforation. Treatment involves temporary or permanent partial (usually lateral) tarsorrhaphy (see Figure 10-29) to prevent corneal trauma and desiccation. Supplementation of the tear film is essential, and topical antibiotic therapy is necessary if corneal ulceration is present. Prognosis totally depends on the cause and treatment options for the primary condition causing the neurologic deficit. If treatment is not possible, enucleation may be required.

Feline Herpetic Keratitis

Feline herpesvirus type 1 (FHV-1) is a very common pathogen of the cornea and conjunctiva of the cat. Although the virus preferentially infects and replicates within the conjunctiva, it does commonly cause corneal disease. Only the corneal syndromes are discussed here. The reader is referred to Chapter 7 for a full discussion of relevant virology, pathogenesis, and conjunctival signs, along with methods of diagnosis and treatment. Feline herpesvirus may affect the corneal epithelium or stroma and produce different clinical entities in each. Epithelial replication results in severe ulcerative keratitis, which is dendritic at first (Figure 10-42) but rapidly becomes geographic (i.e., maplike). Disease within the corneal stroma is believed to result from viral particles or antigens entering through ulcerated epithelium and may result more from immunopathology than from viral replication. Both forms can occur in young kittens after primary infection or in adult cats as a result of reactivation of virus quiescent in sensory ganglia after periods of stress or administration of corticosteroids.

Herpetic keratitis in cats, like herpetic conjunctivitis, is frequently resistant to treatment, and relapses are common. Therapy usually involves topical use of antiviral agents, topical antibiotics if ulceration is present, and, sometimes, oral administration of lysine. Occasionally, surgical removal of the affected tissue by superficial keratectomy is also useful. The use of corticosteroids and cyclosporine is controversial and usually contraindicated, and these agents certainly should never be used without concurrent antiviral therapy and close clinical monitoring.

Corticosteroids are contraindicated in feline herpetic keratitis and should be used with caution in any feline eye because of the frequency of herpesvirus infection.

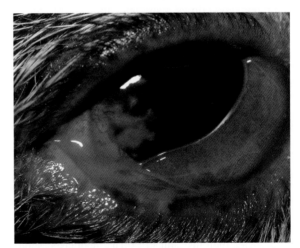

Figure 10-42. Dendritic corneal ulcers in a cat. These lesions are considered pathognomonic for feline herpesvirus infection. (Courtesy University of California, Davis, Veterinary Ophthalmology Service Collection.)

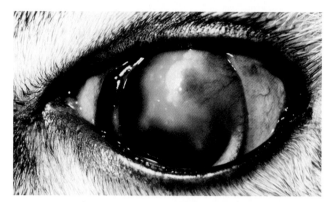

Figure 10-43. Feline eosinophilic keratoconjunctivitis. Note the raised chalky plaque in the dorsolateral cornea and the leading zone of corneal ulceration with dendritic margins. (From August JR [2001]: Consultations in Feline Internal Medicine, ed 4. Saunders, Philadelphia.)

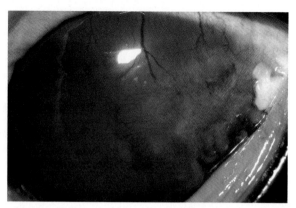

Figure 10-44. Equine eosinophilic keratoconjunctivitis. Note the similarities in clinical appearance to feline eosinophilic keratitis as shown in Figure 10-43.

Feline Eosinophilic Keratoconjunctivitis

Feline eosinophilic keratitis (FEK) is an enigmatic disease of cats. Clinically, it appears as single or multiple focal, raised, pink plaque(s) resembling granulation tissue. Sometimes the plaques have a chalky appearance (Figure 10-43). Most cases are unilateral, but bilateral involvement is possible. Typically the lateral cornea is initially involved, but in advanced cases the entire cornea may be affected. Areas of corneal ulceration are also possible, particularly on the leading edge of the lesion. Third eyelid and/or conjunctival involvement is seen relatively commonly along with keratitis and occasionally alone. Eyelids can also be involved. Diagnosis is suggested by clinical appearance and confirmed with cytologic demonstration of eosinophils and mast cells along with neutrophils and hyperplastic or dysplastic epithelial cells. The cause is undetermined, but the condition appears to be due to an aberrant immune response. In many cases the antigenic stimulus is unrecognized; however, a recent investigation suggests that FHV-1 DNA can be detected in corneal samples from approximately 75% of cats with FEK.

This disease has traditionally been treated with topical corticosteroids and/or systemic megestrol acetate. However, recurrences are common with this protocol. Potential involvement of FHV-1 presents clinicians with a dilemma, because use of immunomodulatory drugs, especially topical corticosteroids, for treatment of an eye that is potentially infected with FHV-1 warrants caution. Some cases improve with antiviral medications alone, and so it appears wise to begin therapy with a topical antiviral agent only and to recheck the patient in a week or so. If there is improvement and the owner is compliant, continuation of this regimen may be all that is necessary. At the very least, antiviral treatment should be continued for as long as there is evidence of active viral replication and certainly while ulceration is present. More commonly, a form of immunomodulatory therapy must be added to the regimen. Topical corticosteroids may be used if no ulcers are present, but even then, reactivation of FHV-1 and/or ulcer formation may occur once corticosteroid therapy is begun. This problem has led to the recommendation of oral megestrol acetate for FEK. However, potential complications of its use, such as mammary hyperplasia, diabetes mellitus, and mammary neoplasia, should be explained to the animal's owner. Early diagnosis and treatment as described of recurrences will limit the need for protracted therapy.

Equine Eosinophilic Keratoconjunctivitis

A disease similar in appearance and cytologic appearance to FEK is also recognized in horses (Figure 10-44). Like cats, horses affected with equine eosinophilic keratoconjunctivitis demonstrate blepharospasm, epiphora or sometimes more caseous mucoid discharge, chemosis, conjunctival hyperemia, and, often, a white corneoconjunctival plaque surrounded by a region of superficial corneal ulceration and vascularization. The lateral limbal area is most commonly affected, and patients may be unilaterally or, less commonly, bilaterally affected. As in cats, diagnosis is confirmed by demonstration of large numbers of eosinophils in corneal scrapings. Once infectious organisms, especially fungus, have been eliminated by cytologic examination and culture, treatment should be initiated with topical dexamethasone or prednisolone (usually with a broad-spectrum antibiotic such as neomycin–bacitracin–polymyxin B) applied three or four times daily. In resistant lesions, superficial keratectomy may enhance healing and shorten the course of the disease.

Corneal Sequestration

Corneal sequestration is a corneal disease unique to the cat. Synonyms include feline corneal necrosis, corneal mummification, and keratitis nigrum. Although any cat can be affected, Persian, Burmese, Himalayan, and maybe Siamese cats appear to be more susceptible. The cause of the disease is unknown, but it usually occurs after chronic ulceration. As such, feline herpesvirus is frequently incriminated and can be detected in at least 50% of biopsy specimens from cats with this disease. Occasionally corneal sequestration is seen in cats with no previous history of ulcerative corneal disease. The clinical signs are classic, with the appearance of a focal amber to black, usually central corneal plaque surrounded by a broader area of superficial ulceration (Figure 10-45). These lesions tend to be painful, and blepharospasm and epiphora are expected. Depending on chronicity, sequestra are often accompanied by corneal vascularization, edema, and stromal white blood cell infiltration due to a foreign body reaction stimulated by the necrotic tissue. The black material is pigmented and necrotic cornea, not melanin.

The necrotic plaque sometimes sloughs without the need for surgical intervention. In such cases ongoing medical manage-

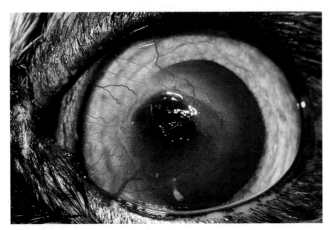

Figure 10-45. Corneal sequestrum in a cat. Note also the surrounding corneal edema and vascularization. (Courtesy University of California, Davis, Veterinary Ophthalmology Service Collection.)

ment of the ulcer and secondary uveitis with topical antibiotics and atropine, respectively, along with antiviral therapy if herpesvirus is believed to be the initiating cause should be provided until sloughing occurs. Corticosteroids should not be used for sequestra. However, most animals exhibit signs of marked ocular pain during this period, and removal of the plaque by keratectomy is preferred as it shortens this period of discomfort. Associated keratitis should be controlled before keratectomy is performed. Manual removal of sequestra should not be attempted, because some sequestra extend to Descemet's membrane and globe rupture is possible. After keratectomy, most ophthalmologists graft the corneal defect with conjunctiva or corneoconjunctival transposition. Recurrences after treatment may occur, but results are normally excellent.

Feline sequestra are painful and may take many months to slough. Keratectomy hastens healing and resolves discomfort.

Bullous Keratopathy

Bullous keratopathy is a nonspecific diagnosis that describes the formation of small vesicles in the epithelium and stroma of an edematous cornea (Figure 10-46). These vesicles ultimately coalesce to form larger bullae. The surrounding epithelium and stroma are edematous and often vascularized, either in response to the bullae or as a result of the underlying corneal disorder. Rupture of the bullae with subsequent ulceration is expected once they become severe.

Treatment relies on resolution of the underlying condition, although this is often not possible. Symptomatic therapy with hyperosmotic sodium chloride ointment may reduce the edema and limit rupture of bullae. Topical antibiotics should be applied if bullae rupture and fluorescein is retained by the exposed stroma. In intractable, progressive bullous keratopathy, thermokeratoplasty may be used. In this technique the cornea is treated carefully with focal application of heat. A scar forms in treated areas, and the associated tissue contraction "squeezes" out stromal fluid and limits further stromal distention. Alternatively, complete corneal coverage with a very thin, 360-degree conjunctival graft may reduce bullae formation. The patient is best referred to an ophthalmologist for these treatments. The prognosis for mild bullous keratopathy is good, especially if the

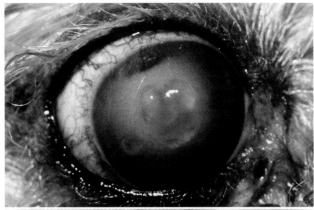

A

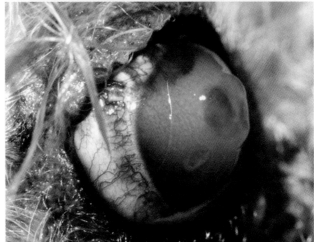

B

Figure 10-46. Bullous keratopathy. **A,** Frontal view; **B,** profile.

underlying cause can be cured. Extensive bullous keratopathy has a poor prognosis.

"Florida Keratopathy" or "Florida Spots"

Small, usually multifocal, white corneal stromal opacities unique to tropical and subtropical climates have been described in both dogs and cats. These opacities, called *Florida keratopathy* or *Florida spots,* are not associated with inflammation or pain, do not respond to any therapy, and are apparently self-limiting. Their cause is unknown.

Infectious Bovine Keratoconjunctivitis

Infectious bovine keratoconjunctivitis (IBK), one of the most common diseases of cattle, is of major economic importance in beef- and milk-producing areas throughout the world. Synonyms include "pink eye" and "New Forest eye." *M. bovis* is considered the causative agent as well as one of very few organisms considered to be a primary corneal pathogen—that is, one that can attach to and penetrate through intact corneal epithelium. In fact, *M. bovis* is the only bacterium of veterinary importance that can *initiate* corneal ulceration. Piliated *M. bovis* organisms adhere to the corneal epithelium and produce cytotoxins, epithelial detachment factor, and hemolysins, which, together with collagenases from host cells, cause necrosis of epithelium and stroma. Other organisms, including *Mycoplasma bovoculi,* infectious bovine rhinotracheitis virus (BHV-1),

Box 10-2 | **Microbial, host, and environmental or husbandry factors involved in the pathogenesis of infectious bovine keratoconjunctivitis**

Microbial Factors

- Pili
- Hemolysins
- Epithelial detachment factor
- Cytotoxins
- Presence of other infectious organisms:
  - Infectious bovine rhinotracheitis virus (BHV-1)
  - *Mycoplasma* spp.
  - *Ureaplasma* spp.
- Ability to use iron bound by lactoferrin

Host Factors

- Genetics (*Bos indicus* less susceptible)
- Age
- Periocular pigmentation?

Environmental or Husbandry Factors

- Ultraviolet radiation
- Herding animals together
- Infectious bovine rhinotracheitis vaccination
- Dust
- Fly vectors:
  - *Musca autumnalis*
  - *Musca domestica*
  - *Stomoxys calcitrans*
- Heavy snowfall
- Transport stress
- Dry tall weeds?

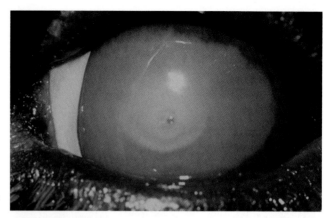

Figure 10-47. Infectious bovine keratoconjunctivitis. Note the central ulceration with stromal white blood cell infiltration along with diffuse edema and deep corneal vascularization.

Ureaplasma spp., and adenoviruses, have been isolated from field outbreaks of IBK and are likely also involved in the pathogenesis of some outbreaks. Other microorganisms and environmental and host factors are also critical in the pathogenesis of IBK; these cofactors are listed in Box 10-2.

In herds with no previous outbreaks, young and older animals are equally severely affected. After the initial occurrence, however, younger animals are more frequently and severely affected. Affected animals possess some immunity that becomes less effective after 1 or 2 years, frequently allowing reinfection. The effectiveness of this immunity depends directly on the severity of the initial disease. Unfortunately, attempts to produce either live or killed vaccines against *M. bovis* have been disappointing. Recent commercial vaccines using pili antigens require further field evaluation before their true value is known. Peak outbreaks usually occur in summer, especially when ultraviolet radiation, flies, and dusty conditions prevail.

The initial lesion is severe, ulcerative keratoconjunctivitis (Figure 10-47) associated with intense epiphora, blepharospasm, and marked corneal edema. There is a usually central corneal opacity due to stromal cell infiltration, which enlarges, ulcerates, and vascularizes. Secondary (so-called reflex) uveitis is marked. Ulceration may progress to involve the stroma, and descemetocele formation with perforation and subsequent panophthalmitis may occur. At the peak of disease, the animal is in considerable pain, may be totally blind, and may have difficulty walking and finding food and water. Such animals are often dangerous for farm staff to handle, and extensive weight losses and reduced

milk yields may occur. In less severe cases recovery takes 1 to 3 weeks, with vascularization and clearing from the limbus toward the center of the cornea. Some residual scar formation is expected. However, the bovine cornea possesses remarkable reparative properties, and many extensively scarred corneas are completely healed a year later, especially in young animals. Nevertheless, severe scarring does remain in a proportion of affected eyes.

If possible, affected animals should be segregated to limit spread of the disease and provided with shade. Attempts to reduce the vector fly population may be instituted. Individual animals may be treated with injections of procaine penicillin G beneath the *bulbar* conjunctiva. In a study in which penicillin was injected into the superior *palpebral* conjunctiva of naturally infected calves, the therapy did not shorten healing time, proving that site of injection is critical. A single systemic dose of repository oxytetracycline (20 mg/kg) followed by 10 days of oral oxytetracycline has been shown to be superior to 300,000 U procaine penicillin G injected subconjunctivally and to no treatment and may be used if withholding regulations are followed. Florfenicol, given once subcutaneously (40 mg/kg) or twice 2 days apart intramuscularly (20 mg/kg) to experimentally infected calves, also significantly reduced healing times compared with that in untreated calves. This finding was subsequently verified in a natural outbreak. Finally, a single dose of ceftiofur injected subcutaneously into the pinnae has also shown to be a useful therapy. Severe lesions can be protected by a temporary tarsorrhaphy (see Figure 10-29) or third eyelid flap.

Control measures include genetic selection, elimination of carrier animals, and good fly control. After an outbreak or in newly introduced animals, carrier status can be shortened by two systemic injections of long-acting tetracycline (20 mg/kg). The use of vaccines cannot be recommended to prevent IBK, although decreased prevalence and severity have been reported when vaccination is performed 6 weeks before the expected onset of the disease season. Calves are vaccinated at 21 to 30 days of age with a second vaccination 21 days later. Powders and sprays are contraindicated in the treatment of IBK because they provide suitable antibiotic concentrations only for short periods and are irritating.

Infectious Bovine Rhinotracheitis

Infectious bovine rhinotracheitis (IBR) is due to bovine herpesvirus. In affected animals, conjunctivitis is more prominent than keratitis (see Chapter 7). However, peripheral corneal edema, ulceration, and vascularization are occasionally present. Keratitis due to IBR virus must be distinguished from corneal lesions of malignant catarrhal fever (bovine malignant catarrh), IBK, and squamous cell carcinoma.

Malignant Catarrhal Fever

Malignant catarrhal fever (MCF) is discussed more fully in Chapter 18. The corneal signs only are emphasized here. Ocular lesions are typically seen in the "head and eye" form of the disease. Lesions begin in the central cornea and move toward the limbus. If the cornea remains clear, signs of uveitis, including aqueous flare, cells, fibrin, miosis, and iris swelling, may be observed. MCF is suspected when nasal, oral, and ocular lesions occur with persistent pyrexia, enlarged lymph nodes, and encephalitis. The presence of ocular lesions differentiates MCF from rinderpest, bovine viral diarrhea mucosal disease, infectious stomatitis, and calf diphtheria. IBR is distinguished by its infectious nature, respiratory signs, recovery rate, and predominance of conjunctivitis rather than endophthalmitis. Ocular signs arise from the necrotizing effect of the virus on vascular tissues and vary according to the form of the disease.

Infectious Canine Hepatitis

Infectious canine hepatitis due to infection with canine adenovirus type 1 causes hepatic and renal disease in dogs and is discussed in Chapter 18. The major ocular effect is corneal edema, leading to its lay name "blue-eye." The corneal edema is due, in part, to anterior uveitis, which can be extremely marked and can even lead to secondary glaucoma. However, corneal edema also arises from endothelial cell death or dysfunction as a direct result of viral replication as well as antigen-antibody complex deposition within corneal endothelial cells themselves (Figure 10-48). If endothelial damage is temporary, corneal edema usually resolves in 1 to 2 weeks, but some animals have permanent partial or total corneal opacity.

Treatment is directed at limiting permanent endothelial cell death or dysfunction, anterior uveitis, and secondary glaucoma. In the acute stages, topical corticosteroids, sometimes in combination with topical NSAIDs, should be used to control uveitis. Systemic administration of corticosteroids or NSAIDs may also be necessary. Frequent reexaminations with regular measurements of IOP are advisable. Topical atropine should be applied if IOP is not elevated. Topical hyperosmotic sodium chloride ointment may be used to limit edema or bullae formation, but its effect is mild and transitory. If response is not evident in 4 to 5 weeks, permanent corneal edema is likely. Once glaucoma has occurred, intraocular prosthesis or enucleation is necessary.

SCLERAL DISORDERS BELIEVED TO BE INHERITED
Colobomatous Defects

Colobomatous or notch defects in the sclera most commonly occur toward the equator or posterior pole of the globe. Their clinical appearance varies greatly according to location, but in both situations the areas of scleral absence (coloboma) or thinning (ectasia) are associated with protrusion of the underlying uveal tract through the affected sclera. At the equator the protrusion appears as a black or blue bulge often almost completely hidden by the eyelids in most normal positions of gaze (Figure 10-49). Unless they are large and cause significant weakening of the globe, such protrusions can be monitored. Repair involves a scleral or other tectonic grafting procedure and requires referral to a veterinary ophthalmologist. At the posterior pole, scleral thinning or absence typically involves the optic nerve as well as the choroid. If it is severe, the overlying retina may detach. This is a common feature of collie eye anomaly, which is discussed in the chapter on retinal disease (see Chapter 15).

ACQUIRED SCLERAL DISORDERS
Scleritis/Episcleritis

Anteriorly, the sclera is overlaid by a loose connective tissue called the *episclera,* which connects it to the bulbar conjunctiva. At the limbus, the sclera is confluent with the cornea. Posteriorly, the sclera overlies the choroid and retina and externally it is adjacent to the orbital tissues. Because all of these layers are so

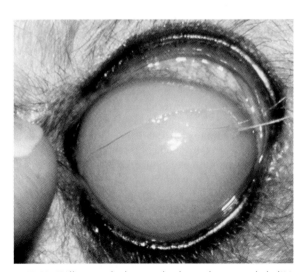

Figure 10-48. Diffuse marked corneal edema due to endotheliitis and anterior uveitis in association with infectious canine hepatitis virus. (Courtesy University of Missouri, Columbia, Veterinary Ophthalmology Service Collection.)

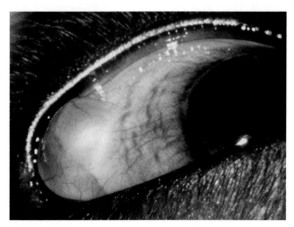

Figure 10-49. Equatorial scleral coloboma with associated staphyloma. (Courtesy University of Missouri, Columbia, Veterinary Ophthalmology Service Collection.)

intimately related anatomically and physiologically, inflammation of the sclera and episclera inevitably involves adjacent tissues and therefore can lead to chorioretinitis (and potentially retinal detachment), orbital cellulitis, keratitis, conjunctivitis, and blepharitis in any combination. Partly because of this variation in clinical involvement, the terms *scleritis, episcleritis, episclero-conjunctivitis, episclerokeratitis,* and *episclerokeratoconjunctivitis* have become somewhat jumbled in the literature. Here the term *episcleritis* is used with the acknowledgment that the neighboring tissues are almost inevitably involved to varying degrees.

Episcleritis has been broadly divided into necrotizing and nodular variants. In the necrotizing form, there is inflammation, necrosis, and thinning and loss of sclera and surrounding tissues. In the nodular form, there is granulomatous thickening of the sclera and/or episclera. The latter has commonly been called *nodular granulomatous episclerokeratoconjunctivitis* (NGE). Regardless of their histologic and clinical nature, this group of diseases is believed to be immune-mediated and is typically treated with immunomodulation. Some of the disorders are remarkably resistant to therapy, frequently recur, and often require prolonged treatment.

Typically, NGE appears as a single or sometimes multiple, raised, tan to red subconjunctival mass(es) at the limbus (Figure 10-50). Occasionally there is a more diffuse thickening of a broader region of episclera. The dorsolateral limbus is most commonly affected, but other limbal regions and even the third eyelid are occasionally affected. There is associated conjunctivitis and often the cornea becomes affected as the lesion advances into the corneal stroma. Crystalline opacities (presumably cholesterol or triglycerides) and corneal edema are the classic lesions. The syndrome occurs predominantly in collies, but many other breeds may be affected. Commonly used synonyms are *nodular fasciitis, fibrous histiocytoma, limbal granuloma,* and *collie granuloma.* The etiology is unknown. Lesions may be bilateral but are usually not symmetrical. Although clinical appearance is usually highly suggestive, histologic analysis is required to definitively confirm the diagnosis and differentiate this syndrome from neoplastic diseases such as squamous cell carcinoma and amelanotic limbal melanoma. The lesions consist of masses of histiocytes and fibrocytes.

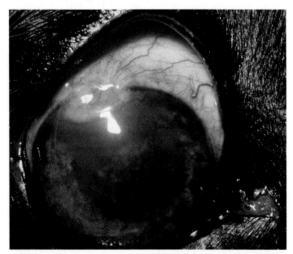

Figure 10-50. Nodular granulomatous episclerokeratoconjunctivitis in a dog. Note extension into the neighboring corneal stroma. (Courtesy University of California, Davis, Veterinary Ophthalmology Service Collection.)

Because of the alleged immune-mediated nature of the condition, long-term immunomodulatory treatment is usually necessary for its control, although some cases regress completely. Without treatment, the condition is usually slowly progressive. Immunomodulatory therapy must be provided at the maximum level tolerated by the animal and the minimum level that causes some regression of the lesion. Frequency of application as well as concentration or dose of medications should be tapered as rapidly as possible as the patient improves. Additionally, medication type and route can be altered so as to cause the minimum of side effects as the disease regresses.

Recommended therapies and routes of administration are as follows:

- Corticosteroids:
  - Systemic
  - Subconjunctival
  - Intralesional
  - Topical (dexamethasone or prednisolone only)
- Topical cyclosporine (1% or 2 %)
- Systemic tetracycline and niacinamide (not niacin):
  - For dogs weighing less than 10 kg: 250 mg of each drug q8h
  - For dogs weighing 10 kg or more: 500 mg of each drug q8h
- Systemic azathioprine
- Surgical removal/debulking
- Cryotherapy
- β-Irradiation

Scleral Trauma

Blunt or sharp trauma to the sclera may result in thinning or rupture of the sclera with subsequent protrusion of the underlying uveal tract—a *traumatic staphyloma*. As with corneal perforations, prognosis depends largely on the extent of damage to the intraocular structures. Hyphema, iris prolapse, vitreous hemorrhage, lens capsule rupture, lens luxation, and retinal detachment are all possible and obviously indicate a poor prognosis. For simple uncomplicated penetrating wounds, surgical closure along with control of postoperative uveitis with corticosteroids and prostaglandin inhibitors is often successful. Systemic antibiotics and antiinflammatory agents should also be administered. For more extensive injuries, referral to an ophthalmologist for more sophisticated procedures (e.g., lens removal, vitrectomy, scleral allografting) may be indicated.

Severe blunt or concussive injuries can also cause scleral rupture, usually with even more devastating intraocular consequences than those of sharp trauma. In such instances, the eye usually ruptures adjacent to and concentric with the limbus (Figure 10-51). This situation is particularly common in the horse, especially when kicked by another horse. These ruptures may vary in size from a few millimeters in length to involvement of almost the entire circumference, with prolapse of lens, vitreous, iris, and ciliary body. Less extensive ruptures should be referred for primary closure and control of uveitis. The prognosis for extensive ruptures depends on damage to intraocular structures but is always guarded to poor. Damage to the ciliary body frequently leads to phthisis bulbi, and enucleation is recommended.

Penetrating and concussive scleral injuries are often associated with phthisis, especially when hyphema is marked.

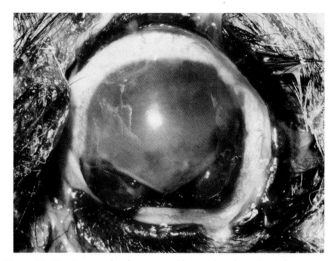

Figure 10-51. Corneoscleral rupture with uveal prolapse in a dog.

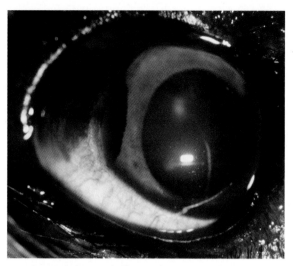

Figure 10-52. Limbal (or epibulbar) melanoma in a dog. Note extension into the neighboring corneal stroma. (Courtesy University of California, Davis, Veterinary Ophthalmology Service Collection.)

Limbal Neoplasia

Primary scleral and corneal tumors are rare. In fact, rather than being a site of neoplastic origin, the sclera and cornea are important barriers, typically preventing spread of intraocular neoplasms to other parts of the body and intraocular spread of adnexal or orbital tumors. However, intraocular neoplasms may leave the eye via the optic nerve, ciliary and vortex veins, and intrascleral nerve canals.

In contrast to the cornea and sclera proper, the corneoscleral limbus is a relatively common site of origin for neoplasms. Perhaps this is because it is a region of very high mitotic activity and, particularly dorsolaterally, experiences notable exposure to ultraviolet light. The most frequently observed tumors are hemangioma/hemangiosarcoma (particularly in dogs and horses), limbal melanoma (dogs), and squamous cell carcinoma (horses and cattle). Squamous cell carcinomas are discussed in Chapter 7, because they almost always extend caudally from the limbus to involve the conjunctiva in addition to or instead of the cornea.

Limbal (Epibulbar) Melanocytoma

Limbal melanocytomas are relatively common in dogs. They arise from melanocytes in the superficial tissues near the limbus but often invade the adjacent corneal stroma or, less frequently, extend posteriorly into the sclera (Figure 10-52). Outward growth such that the tumor protrudes from the ocular surface is common, but intraocular penetration of the sclera and invasion of the iris or ciliary body is uncommon. When it does occur, intraocular extension makes differentiation of a melanocytic tumor of limbal origin from one of anterior uveal origin challenging. Although they are sometimes referred to as "limbal melanomas," these tumors have a low metastatic potential and are often slow growing, especially in older dogs. Therefore they are best called *limbal melanocytomas* because of their biologic behavior. In younger dogs or when there is rapid growth, these tumors may be surgically debulked and treated with cryosurgery or with en bloc resection followed by a corneoscleral allograft. The prognosis for survival is excellent, and vision can also frequently be saved. Reduction in tumor size can also be achieved by laser photocoagulation; however, a 25% recurrence rate has been recorded for this approach.

BIBLIOGRAPHY

Andrew SE, et al. (2002): Density of corneal endothelial cells, corneal thickness, and corneal diameters in normal eyes of llamas and alpacas. Am J Vet Res 63:326.

Andrew SE, et al. (2001): Density of corneal endothelial cells and corneal thickness in eyes of euthanatized horses. Am J Vet Res 62:479.

Andrew SE, et al. (1998): Equine ulcerative keratomycosis: visual outcome and ocular survival in 39 cases (1987-1996). Equine Vet J 30:109.

Angelos JA, et al. (2000): Efficacy of florfenicol for treatment of naturally occurring infectious bovine keratoconjunctivitis. J Am Vet Med Assoc 216:62.

Ball MA, et al. (1997): Evaluation of itraconazole-dimethyl sulfoxide ointment for treatment of keratomycosis in nine horses. J Am Vet Med Assoc 211:199.

Befanis PJ, et al. (1981): Endothelial repair of the canine cornea. Am J Vet Res 21:113.

Bentley E (2005): Spontaneous chronic corneal epithelial defects in dogs: a review. J Am Anim Hosp Assoc 41:158.

Bentley E, Murphy CJ (2004): Thermal cautery of the cornea for treatment of spontaneous chronic corneal epithelial defects in dogs and horses. J Am Vet Med Assoc 224:250.

Bosscha MI (2004): The efficacy and safety of topical polymyxin B, neomycin and gramicidin for treatment of presumed bacterial corneal ulceration. Br J Ophthalmol 88:25.

Brooks DE, et al. (1998): Antifungal susceptibility patterns of fungi isolated from cases of ulcerative keratomycosis in Florida horses. Am J Vet Res 59:138.

Brown MH, et al. (1998): Infectious bovine keratoconjunctivitis: a review. J Vet Intern Med 12:259.

Chmielewski NT, et al. (1997): Visual outcome and ocular survival following iris prolapse in the horse: a review of 32 cases. Equine Vet J 29:31.

Clode AB, et al. (2006): Evaluation of concentration of voriconazole in aqueous humor after topical and oral administration in horses. Am J Vet Res 67:296.

Crispin S (2002): Ocular lipid deposition and hyperlipoproteinaemia. Prog Retin Eye Res 21:169.

Deykin AR, et al. (1997): A retrospective histopathologic study of primary episcleral and scleral inflammatory disease in dogs. Vet Comp Ophthalmol 7:245.

Dueger EL, et al. (2004): Efficacy of a long-acting formulation of ceftiofur crystalline-free acid for the treatment of naturally occurring infectious bovine keratoconjunctivitis. Am J Vet Res 65: 1185.

Eastman TG, et al. (1998): Combined parenteral and oral administration of oxytetracycline for control of infectious bovine keratoconjunctivitis. J Am Vet Med Assoc 212:560.

Featherstone HJ, Sansom J (2004): Feline corneal sequestra: a review of 64 cases (80 eyes) from 1993 to 2000. Vet Ophthalmol 7:213.

Gaarder JE, et al. (1998): Clinical appearances, healing patterns, risk factors, and outcomes of horses with fungal keratitis: 53 cases (1978-1996). J Am Vet Med Assoc 213:105.

Gionfriddo JR, et al. (2003): Idiopathic ocular and nasal granulomatous inflammatory disease in a dog. Vet Ophthalmol 6:163.

Gwin RL, et al. (1982): Decrease in canine corneal endothelial cell density and increase in corneal thickness as functions of age. Invest Ophthalmol Vis Sci 22:267.

Gwin RL, et al. (1982): Primary canine corneal endothelial cell dystrophy: specular microscopic evaluation, diagnosis and therapy. J Am Anim Hosp Assoc 18:471.

Hendrix DV, et al. (1995): Corneal stromal abscesses in the horse: a review of 24 cases. Equine Vet J 27:440.

Hurn S, et al. (2005): Ectopic cilium in seven horses. Vet Ophthalmol 8:199.

Marrion RM, Riley LK (2000): Detection of cell detachment activity induced by *Moraxella bovis*. Am J Vet Res 61:1145.

Martin CL (1981): Canine epibulbar melanomas and their management. J Am Anim Hosp Assoc 17:83.

Michau TM, et al. (2003): Superficial, nonhealing corneal ulcers in horses: 23 cases (1989-2003). Vet Ophthalmol 6:291.

Michau TM, et al. (2003): Use of thermokeratoplasty for treatment of ulcerative keratitis and bullous keratopathy secondary to corneal endothelial disease in dogs: 13 cases (1994-2001). J Am Vet Med Assoc 222:607.

Moore CW, et al. (1995): Antibacterial sensitivity patterns for microbial isolates associated with infectious keratitis in horses: 63 cases (1986-1994). J Am Vet Med Assoc 207:928.

Morgan RH, et al. (1996): Feline eosinophilic keratitis: a retrospective study of 54 cases (1989-1994). Vet Comp Ophthalmol 6:131.

Nasisse MP, et al. (1998): Detection of feline herpesvirus 1 DNA in corneas of cats with eosinophilic keratitis or corneal sequestrum. Am J Vet Res 59:856.

Ollivier FJ, et al. (2004): Profiles of matrix metalloproteinase activity in equine tear fluid during corneal healing in 10 horses with ulcerative keratitis. Vet Ophthalmol 7:397.

Paulsen ME, et al. (1987): Nodular granulomatous episclerokeratitis in dogs: 19 dogs (1973-1985). J Am Vet Med Assoc 190:1581.

Sauer P, et al. (2003): Changes in antibiotic resistance in equine bacterial ulcerative keratitis (1991-2000): 65 horses. Vet Ophthalmol 6:309.

Skorobohach BJ, Hendrix DVH (2003): Staphyloma in a cat. Vet Ophthalmol 6:93.

Smith PC, et al. (1990): Effectiveness of two commercial infectious bovine keratoconjunctivitis vaccines. Am J Vet Res 51:1147.

Sullivan TC, et al. (1996): Photocoagulation of limbal melanoma in dogs and cats: 15 cases (1989-1993). J Am Vet Med Assoc 208:891.

Sweeney CR, Irby NL (1996): Topical treatment of *Pseudomonas* sp-infected corneal ulcers in horses: 70 cases (1977-1994). J Am Vet Med Assoc 209:954.

Watte CM, et al. (2004): Clinical experience with butyl-2-cyanoacrylate adhesive in the management of canine and feline corneal disease. Vet Ophthalmol 7:319.

Williams DL (2005): Major histocompatibility class II expression in the normal canine cornea and in canine chronic superficial keratitis. Vet Ophthalmol 8:395.

Yamagata M, et al. (1996): Eosinophilic keratoconjunctivitis in seven horses. J Am Vet Med Assoc 209:1283.

UVEA

Paul E. Miller

ANATOMY AND PHYSIOLOGY
PATHOLOGIC REACTIONS
CONGENITAL UVEAL ABNORMALITIES

UVEITIS
TRAUMA
HYPHEMA

UVEAL CYSTS AND NEOPLASMS
MISCELLANEOUS DISORDERS
SURGICAL PROCEDURES

The uvea plays an important role in ocular physiology, and disorders of this tissue are common in veterinary practice. The iris controls the amount of light entering the eye, and the ciliary body alters the focal power of the lens, produces aqueous humor that supplies nutrition to ocular structures, and aids in regulating intraocular pressure (IOP). Together they also form a blood-aqueous barrier so as to maintain the clarity of the aqueous humor and vitreous. The choroid plays a major role in providing nutrition to the retina. Because of these diverse roles, uveal disorders are frequently associated with alterations in vision and IOP.

ANATOMY AND PHYSIOLOGY

The eye consists of the following basic layers (Figure 11-1):

- Fibrous (outer) layer—the sclera and cornea
- Vascular (middle) layer—the uvea, or uveal tract
- Neuroectodermal inner layer—the retina and optic nerve

The *uveal tract* has three parts: the *iris* and the *ciliary body,* which together form the *anterior uvea,* and the *choroid,* which is also known as the *posterior uvea.*

Iris

The *iris* controls the amount of light entering the eye by varying the size of the pupil. Reduction in the size of the pupil also increases the depth of field for near objects and reduces certain optical aberrations. To accomplish this goal, the iris has two sets of muscles:

- *Musculus constrictor pupillae:* A circular band of muscle fibers concentric with the pupil. These fibers have predominantly *parasympathetic* innervation (Figure 11-2).
- *Musculus dilator pupillae:* Radially oriented fibers passing from near the root of the iris toward the pupillary margin. These fibers have predominantly *sympathetic* innervation.

Viewed from the anterior surface, the iris has two zones, the *pupillary zone* (Figures 11-3 and 11-4) and the *ciliary zone.* A variable thickening of the iris at the junction of these two zones is called the *collarette.* The anterior surface of the iris is covered by a modified layer of stromal cells, the *anterior border layer* (Figure 11-5). The remaining parts of the iris are the *stroma* and *sphincter muscle,* the *anterior epithelium* and *dilator muscle,* and the *posterior pigmented epithelium* and

pigment ruff. The posterior pigmented epithelium is continuous with the nonpigmented epithelium covering the ciliary body and eventually with the retina.

The bulk of the iris is stroma, which consists of fibrous connective tissue with bundles of collagen, pigmented and non-pigmented cells, and blood vessels in a mucopolysaccharide matrix. Variations in iris color are due to variations in pigmentation of the stroma and posterior pigmented epithelium and in the arrangement of the anterior border layer (Figure 11-6).

The *temporal and nasal long ciliary arteries* enter the iris near its root (see Figure 11-3) and form the major arterial circle, which may be incomplete. The vascular supply of the iris of domestic animals greatly exceeds that of the human iris. Therefore surgical procedures near the iris root in animals often result in profuse hemorrhage if the major arterial circle is transected.

The dilator pupillae muscle extends as a continuous sheet in front of the anterior epithelium (see Figure 11-4) and is intimately related with it. The constrictor pupillae muscle is a flat ring of smooth muscle surrounding the pupil in the posterior iris stroma (see Figure 11-5).

In horses, cattle, sheep, and goats, which have a horizontally elliptical pupil, black masses suspended from the superior and occasionally the inferior rim of the pupil are termed *corpora nigra* (e.g., in horses) or *granula iridica* (e.g., in ruminants). These masses aid in further control of light entering the pupil and should not be mistaken for tumors or cysts.

Ciliary Body

The *ciliary body* lies immediately posterior to the iris. On its posterior surface the ciliary body has numerous folds known as the *ciliary processes* (Figures 11-7 and 11-8). This area of the ciliary body, termed the *pars plicata* (folded part), merges posteriorly into a flat area *(pars plana),* which joins the retina. The *zonular fibers,* which support the lens, originate from the pars plana and between the ciliary processes (Figures 11-9 and 11-10).

Viewed in section, the ciliary body is triangular, with one side joining the sclera, one side facing the vitreous body, and the base giving rise to the iris and *iridocorneal angle* (Figure 11-11). The ciliary body is covered with two layers of epithelium, the inner layer of which is nonpigmented and the outer layer of which is pigmented. It is continuous with similar epithelium on the posterior surface of the iris and the pigment epithelium of the retina (Figure 11-12). The smooth muscle fibers of the *ciliary muscle* (parasympathetic innervation) together with blood

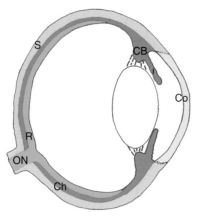

Figure 11-1. The three layers of the eye. *CB,* Ciliary body; *Ch,* choroid; *Co,* cornea; *ON,* optic nerve; *R,* retina; *S,* sclera. (Modified from Fine BS, Yanoff M [1972]: Ocular Histology. Harper & Row, New York.)

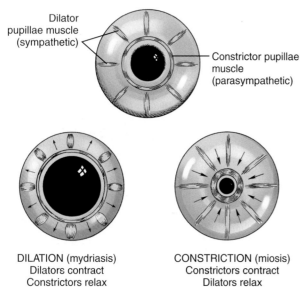

Figure 11-2. Control of pupil size. The arrangement of the constrictor fibers varies among domestic species, but the principles are similar.

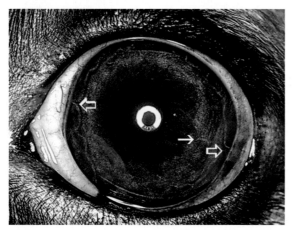

Figure 11-3. Clinical anatomy of the iris. The pupillary zone of the iris is typically darker than the surrounding, lighter-colored ciliary zone. The junction between the two zones is termed the iris collarette *(solid arrow).* Persistent pupillary membranes, if present, typically originate at the iris collarette region. The sinuous posterior ciliary artery enters the iris near the limbus at the 3 and 9 o'clock position *(open arrows).* From there it divides into superior and inferior branches to form the major vascular circle of the iris.

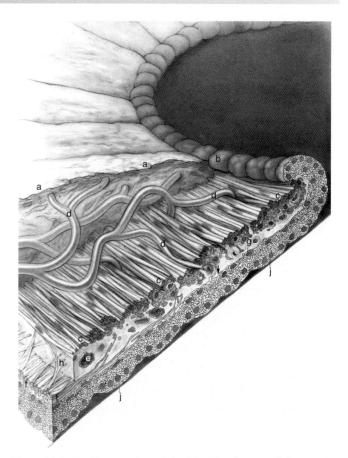

Figure 11-4. Pupillary portion of the iris. The dense, cellular anterior border layer *(a)* terminates at the pigment ruff *(b)* in the pupillary margin. The sphincter muscle is at *(C).* The arcades *(d)* from the minor circle extend toward the pupil and through the sphincter muscle. The sphincter muscle and the iris epithelium are close to each other at the pupillary margin. Capillaries, nerves, melanocytes, and clump cells *(e)* are found within and around the muscle. The three to five layers of dilator muscle *(f)* gradually diminish in number until they terminate behind the midportion of the sphincter muscle *(arrow),* leaving low, cuboidal epithelial cells *(g)* to form the anterior epithelium to the pupillary margin. Spurlike extensions from the dilator muscle form Michel's spur *(h)* and Fuchs's spur *(i)* (these spurs are not commonly described in domestic animals). The posterior epithelium *(j)* is formed by columnar cells with basal nuclei. Its apical surface is contiguous with the apical surface of the anterior epithelium. (From Hogan MJ, et al. [1971]: Histology of the Human Eye. Saunders, Philadelphia.)

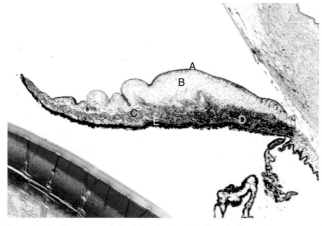

Figure 11-5. Structure of the iris. *A,* Anterior border layer; *B,* stroma; *C,* constrictor muscle; *D,* dilator muscle; *E,* posterior epithelium. (Courtesy Dr. Richard R. Dubielzig.)

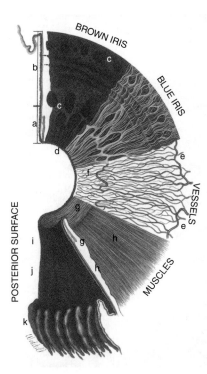

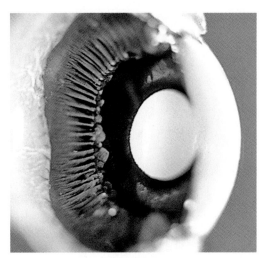

Figure 11-8. Posterior aspect of the canine iris and ciliary body (with the lens removed), showing the arrangement of the numerous bladelike ciliary processes. In this golden retriever multiple small ciliary cysts are also present at the tips of these processes. (Courtesy Dr. Richard R. Dubielzig.)

Figure 11-6. Surfaces and layers of the iris. Clockwise from the top the iris cross-section shows the pupillary *(a)* and ciliary *(b)* portions, and the surface view shows a brown iris with its dense, matted anterior border layer. The blue iris surface shows a less dense anterior border layer and more prominent trabeculae. Arrows indicate circular contraction furrows. *c,* Fuchs's crypts; *d,* pigment ruff; *e,* major arterial circle. Radial branches of arteries and veins extend toward the pupillary region. The arteries form the incomplete minor arterial circle *(f),* from which branches extend toward the pupil, forming capillary arcades. (*Note:* The incomplete minor arterial circle is variable or absent in many animals.) *g,* Circular arrangement of the sphincter muscle; *h,* radial processes of the dilator muscle; *i,* radial contraction furrows; *j,* structure folds of Schwalbe; *k,* pars plicata of the ciliary body. (Modified from Hogan MJ, et al. [1971]: Histology of the Human Eye. Saunders, Philadelphia.)

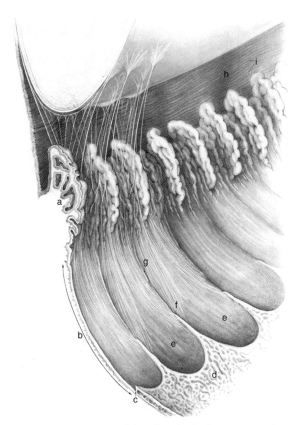

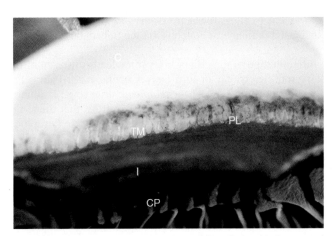

Figure 11-7. Dissecting microscope view of the relationship between the iris, ciliary body, and iridocorneal angle. *C,* Endothelial surface of the cornea; *CP,* ciliary processes; *I,* iris at pupil margin; *PL,* pectinate ligament; *TM,* trabecular meshwork. (Courtesy Dr. Mitzi Zarfoss.)

Figure 11-9. Posterior aspect of the ciliary body, showing pars plicata *(a)* and pars plana *(b).* The junction between ciliary body and retina is at *c,* and the retina at *d.* In primates this junction is scalloped with bays *(e),* dentate processes *(f),* and striae *(g)* (ora serrata), but in most domestic species it is a straight line (ora ciliaris retinae). (From Hogan MJ, et al. [1971]: Histology of the Human Eye. Saunders, Philadelphia.)

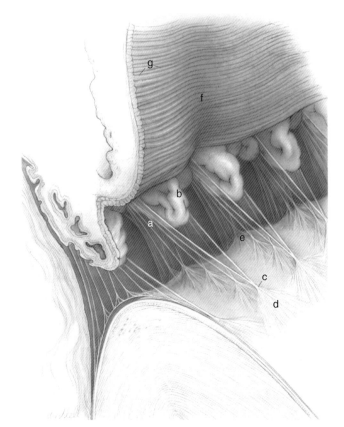

Figure 11-10. Anterior view of ciliary processes showing zonules attached to the lens: *a*, lens zonules; *b*, ciliary process; *c, d,* and *e,* attachment of zonules to lens capsule; *f,* radial folds in iris; *g,* circular folds in iris. The precise arrangement of the lens zonules with the lens capsule varies considerably among species. (From Hogan MJ, et al. [1971]: Histology of the Human Eye. Saunders, Philadelphia.)

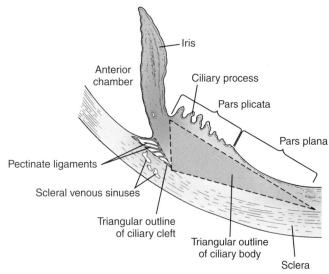

Figure 11-11. Parts of the ciliary body.

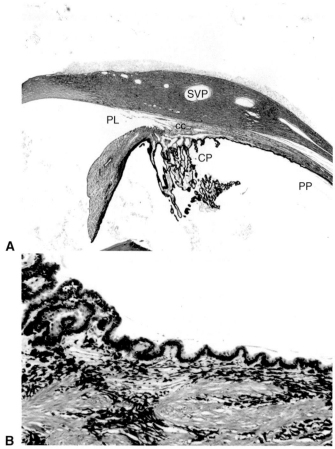

Figure 11-12. A, Normal ciliary body of a cat: *CC,* region of the ciliary cleft; *CP,* ciliary processes; *I,* iris; *PL,* pectinate ligament, *PP,* pars plana; *SVP,* scleral venous plexus. **B,** The ciliary body epithelium is bilayered, with the innermost layer being nonpigmented and the outer layer containing pigment. (Courtesy Dr. Richard R. Dubielzig.)

- Relaxation of lens zonules and change in shape or position of the lens to allow for near vision
- Increased drainage of aqueous via the trabecular meshwork

Inflammation of the ciliary body often leads to spasm of the ciliary muscle, which in turn causes ocular pain. Pain relief may be achieved by use of a *cycloplegic* drug (e.g., atropine), which relaxes the ciliary body. Although drugs that dilate the pupil (mydriatics) may also relax the ciliary muscle (atropine), not all do so (e.g., epinephrine).

Choroid

The *choroid* is a thin, variably pigmented, vascular tissue forming the posterior uvea. It joins the ciliary body anteriorly and lies between the retina and sclera posteriorly. The choroid is extremely vascular, with its capillaries arranged in a single layer on the inner surface to nourish the outer retinal layers (Figure 11-14). In species with limited retinal vasculature (e.g., horse, rabbit, guinea pig) the retina depends to a large extent on the choroidal blood supply. The choroidal stroma typically contains numerous melanocytes, which form a dark optical background to the retina. In most domestic mammals except the pig, a reflective layer—the *tapetum lucidum*—lies within the inner capillary layer. In large animals the tapetum is penetrated by

vessels, connective tissue, and nerves occupy a large portion of the ciliary body (Figure 11-13). The muscle fibers originate near the apex of the triangle and insert into the region of the ciliary cleft and trabecular spaces of the iridocorneal angle. *Contraction* of the ciliary muscle causes the following:

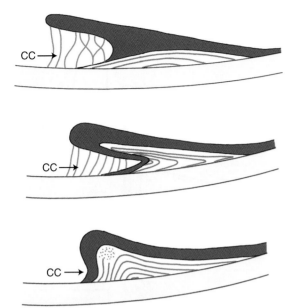

Figure 11-13. Degree of development of the ciliary body musculature among mammalian iridocorneal angles in the ungulate *(top)*, carnivore *(middle)*, and ape *(bottom)*. Development is most pronounced in primates (ape) and least pronounced in herbivorous species (ungulate), with carnivore development between. The size of the iridocorneal angle and its cilioscleral cleft or sinus *(CC)* is inversely large or most pronounced in the ungulate. (Modified from Samuelson DA [1999]: Ophthalmic anatomy, in Gelatt KN [editor]: Veterinary Ophthalmology, 3rd ed. Lippincott Williams & Wilkins, Philadelphia, p. 77; which was drawn after Duke-Elder S [1958]: System of Ophthalmology, Vol 1: The Eye in Evolution. Henry Kimpton, London.)

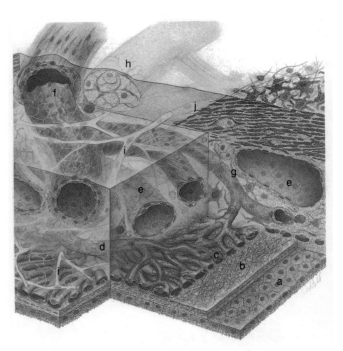

Figure 11-14. Choroidal blood supply and innervation, and Bruch's membrane. The retina is located at the bottom and the sclera at the top of the drawing. The retinal pigment epithelium *(a)* is in close contact with Bruch's membrane *(b)*. The choriocapillaris *(c)* forms an intricate network along the inner choroid. Bruch's membrane is very thin in some domestic species. In the superior fundus the tapetum lies between the branching vessels in the choroid and the single layer of the choriocapillaris under the retina. Venules *(d)* leave the choriocapillaris to join the vortex system *(e)*. The short ciliary artery is shown at *f*, before its branching *(g)* to form the choriocapillaris. A short ciliary nerve enters the choroid at *h* and branches into the choroidal stroma *(i)*. *j,* Suprachoroidea. (Modified from Hogan MJ, et al. [1971]: Histology of the Human Eye. Saunders, Philadelphia.)

numerous small capillaries, which appear as small focal dark spots (the *stars of Winslow*) when viewed end-on with the ophthalmoscope. The arteries and nerves to the anterior parts of the eye pass forward through the choroid. The choroid receives its main arterial supply from the following vessels:

- *Short posterior ciliary arteries,* which penetrate the sclera around the optic nerve
- *Long posterior ciliary arteries,* which enter near the optic nerve and branch near the ora ciliaris retinae and lead back into the choroid
- *Anterior ciliary arteries,* which send branches back into the choroid after penetrating the anterior sclera

Histologically the choroid consists of the following layers (see Figure 11-14):

- *Suprachoroidea*: avascular, pigmented connective tissue lying adjacent to the sclera
- Large-vessel layer: typically also contains numerous melanocytes
- Intermediate-vessel layer: also contains the tapetum in the superior fundus
- *Choriocapillaris*: a layer of capillaries adjacent to Bruch's membrane and the retina

In herbivores the tapetum is fibrous in nature *(tapetum fibrosum),* whereas in carnivores the tapetum is cellular and composed of reflective crystals *(tapetum cellulosum)* (Figure 11-15). The reflective properties of the tapetum, and not the presence of pigments, causes the distinctive color of the fundi of different animals and is the reason an animal's eyes "shine" in the dark. This color varies with thickness of the tapetum,

breed, age, and species. Reflecting light through the retina a second time improves the animal's ability to function in dim light.

Blood-Ocular Barrier

The uveal tract plays a key role in maintaining the blood-ocular barrier (Figure 11-16). Diseases involving the uveal tract frequently cause a breakdown of this barrier, which leads to exudation of excessive amounts of proteins or cells into the aqueous humor, vitreous, or subretinal space. The blood-ocular barrier is composed primarily of a blood-retinal barrier and a blood-aqueous barrier. The blood-retinal barrier is formed at the level of the retinal capillary vascular endothelium, which is nonfenestrated and has tight junctions, and the retinal pigment epithelium, which also has tight junctions and separates the relatively leaky choroidal blood vessels from the overlying retina. The blood-aqueous barrier is formed by tight junctions at the level of the nonfenestrated iridal vascular endothelium and between cells constituting the nonpigmented ciliary body epithelium. Most large molecules, especially proteins, are unable to pass through or between the cells in this barrier system. The exact anatomic location of the barrier is probably different for different substances (e.g., capillary endothelial cells, endothelial basement membrane, and intercellular junctions). By limiting the amount of

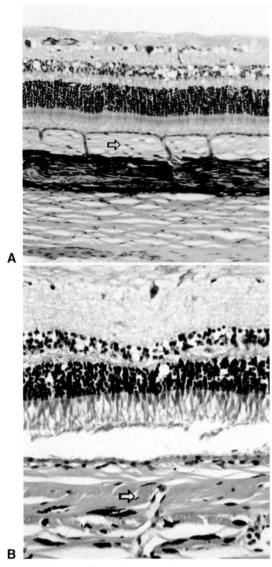

Figure 11-15. A, Normal canine tapetum cellulosum *(arrow).* It is located between the choroid and the photoreceptor layer and pierced by the choriocapillaris. **B,** Normal tapetum fibrosum of a bovine *(arrow).* (Courtesy Dr. Richard R. Dubielzig.)

protein and other large molecules that may scatter light in the aqueous and vitreous humor, these barriers serve to create a more optically perfect media. They are, however, frequently disrupted by inflammation or other disease processes.

PATHOLOGIC REACTIONS

Definitions

Although the uvea exhibits the same range of reactions as other tissues, inflammation is the most important. The following terms describe inflammation of the various parts of the uveal tract:

- *Uveitis:* inflammation of the uvea
- *Iritis:* inflammation of iris
- *Cyclitis:* inflammation of ciliary body
- *Iridocyclitis:* inflammation of iris and ciliary body
- *Choroiditis:* inflammation of choroid

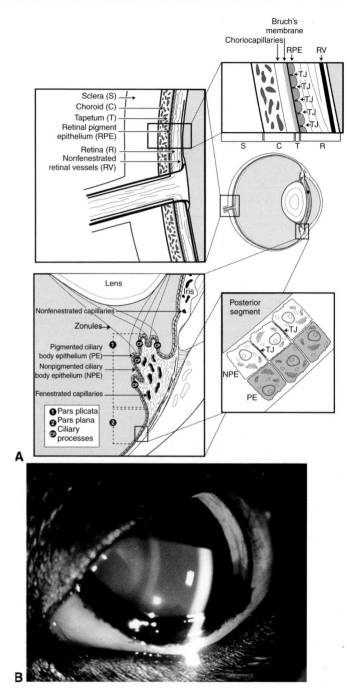

Figure 11-16. A, Blood-ocular barrier. The barrier normally prevents large molecules and cells from leaving the blood vessels and entering the eye, thereby maintaining clarity of the aqueous humor and vitreous. **B,** Aqueous flare in a cat with uveitis. This finding, which represents breakdown of the blood-aqueous barrier, is a hallmark of anterior uveitis. (**A** from Gilger B [2005]: Equine Ophthalmology. Saunders, St. Louis.)

Because of the continuity between the various parts of the uvea, aqueous humor, and vitreous, however, uveal inflammation often involves many ocular structures. The retina and choroid are adjacent, with no major barriers between, so they are frequently inflamed together. Consequently, the following terms are often preferable:

- *Anterior uveitis:* inflammation of iris and ciliary body
- *Posterior uveitis:* inflammation of choroid

- *Chorioretinitis:* inflammation of choroid and retina with primary focus in choroid
- *Retinochoroiditis:* inflammation of choroid and retina with primary focus in retina
- *Panuveitis:* inflammation of all uveal components

Immune Mechanisms

The uvea is an immunologically competent tissue that behaves as an accessory lymph node. Intraocular antigens may enter the systemic circulation and stimulate distant lymphoid organs. In 5 to 7 days sensitized B and T lymphocytes migrate toward the antigen within the eye, enter the uvea, and engage in antibody formation or cell-mediated immune reactions, which may create intraocular inflammation. Subsequent exposure to the same antigen results in a faster and greater (anamnestic) response.

The uvea is often secondarily inflamed when other parts of the eye are inflamed (e.g., secondary anterior uveitis frequently accompanies keratitis). Although such reactions are commonly beneficial in resolution of the primary disease (e.g., production of immunoglobulins and sensitized lymphocytes), excessive secondary uveitis may irreparably damage the eye.

Autoimmune phenomena also occur in the uvea. Preceding tissue damage (e.g., previous inflammation) releases tissue-specific retinal or uveal antigens that are normally intracellular or otherwise immunologically isolated. Hence one cause of uveal inflammation (e.g., trauma, infection by various organisms) may subsequently lead to a secondary, immune-mediated mechanism that results in persisting or recurring inflammation. Such a response may be involved in recurrent equine uveitis. Immune-mediated inflammation may also occur after exposure to lens proteins that have been immunologically isolated by the lens capsule before birth (e.g., lens-induced uveitis) or in response to antigens associated with uveal melanocytes (e.g., uveo-dermatologic syndrome).

Autoimmune diseases may originate with, or be perpetuated by, the following processes, which may also lead to recurrent episodes of uveitis:

- *Molecular mimicry:* Externally derived antigens (bacterial, viral, other) mimic host antigens, thereby directly stimulating T cells to attack sequestered host antigens.
- *Bystander damage:* An agent (viral or otherwise) damages tissue, releases sequestered antigens, and re-stimulates resting autoreactive T cells.
- *Epitope spreading:* The immune response spreads from one autoantigenic molecule to another (intermolecular) or from one site on the same molecule to another (intramolecular).

CONGENITAL UVEAL ABNORMALITIES

Abnormalities of the Pupil

Pupillary abnormalities are as follows:

- *Dyscoria:* abnormally shaped pupil
- *Corectopia:* eccentrically placed pupil
- *Polycoria:* more than one pupil
- *Aniridia:* lack of iris
- *Coloboma:* sector defect in iris (see later)

Corectopia (which is congenital) must be distinguished from a pupil pulled out of shape by synechia (which is acquired). In synechiation the pupil is distorted by adhesions between the lens and iris. Pupillary abnormalities are rarely significant by themselves, but they may be an important indication of other abnormalities.

Persistent Pupillary Membrane

During development the pupillary membrane (anterior portion of the tunica vasculosa lentis) spans the pupil from one portion of the iris collarette to another and supplies nutrients to the developing lens (see Chapter 2). In dogs this membrane is usually resorbed during later fetal development and the first 6 weeks of life, leaving a clear pupillary aperture. It is not uncommon, however, for remnants to remain for several months or longer. In general small remnants spanning from one portion of the iris to another (iris-to-iris persistent pupillary membranes [PPMs]) have no visual consequences, although visual impairment may occur if strands contact the cornea (iris-to-cornea PPMs) or lens (iris-to-lens PPMs) and create an opacity within the visual axis (Figure 11-17).

PPMs occur in a large number of dog breeds, most notably the basenji, in which they are recessively inherited (see Appendix I). A genetic basis is also likely in many other dog breeds, but the mode of inheritance is probably not simply mendelian. PPMs may span from one region of the iris to another (sometimes crossing the pupil) or they may extend to the cornea or lens, creating opacities in these structures. PPMs can usually be differentiated from inflammatory anterior or posterior synechia on the basis of their origin near the iris collarette region (versus an origin at the pupillary margin for synechia) and their presence at birth. It usually is possible to see the membrane extending from the iris collarette region to the cornea or lens, although occasionally the membrane may have broken free and the cornea or lens opacity (often pigmented) is all that remains. Therapy is not typically required or possible. The best method of preventing the disorder is to examine breeding stock and breed only animals that are free of PPMs. Slit-lamp biomicroscopy is essential for the examinations.

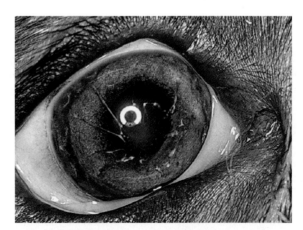

Figure 11-17. Persistent pupillary membranes (iris to cornea) in a young Saint Bernard dog. Unlike postinflammatory anterior synechia, these iridal strands originate near the iris collarette region. Anterior synechia would originate at the pupillary border or in the far periphery of the iris, near the iridocorneal angle. (Courtesy University of Wisconsin–Madison Veterinary Ophthalmology Service Collection.)

Coloboma

A *coloboma* is a defect in the eye resulting from incomplete closure of the embryonic fissure. Typical colobomas occur in the inferomedial portion of the iris or choroid or adjacent to the optic disc (Figure 11-18). Colobomas of the sclera also occur in the collie eye anomaly. Although the embryonic fissure is not involved, *coloboma* is also applied to lid defects and to sector defects in the iris and lens.

Anterior Segment Dysgenesis

Anterior segment dysgenesis is an autosomal recessive trait in the Doberman pinscher characterized by variable degrees of microphthalmia, corneal opacity, lack of anterior chamber, undifferentiated iris and ciliary body, hyaloid artery remnants, absence of or rudimentary lens, retinal dysplasia and separations, and congenital blindness. There is no treatment for this disorder.

Anterior segment dysgenesis syndrome occurs frequently in Rocky Mountain horses and has two distinct ocular phenotypes: (1) large cysts originating from the temporal ciliary body or peripheral retina (Figure 11-19) and (2) multiple anterior segment anomalies, including ciliary cysts, iris hypoplasia, iridocorneal adhesions and opacification, nuclear cataract, and megalocornea (Figure 11-20). This condition may be codominantly inherited, so

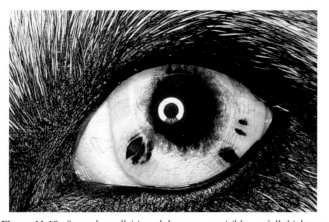

Figure 11-18. Several small iris colobomas are visible as full-thickness defects in the iris in this Australian shepherd dog.

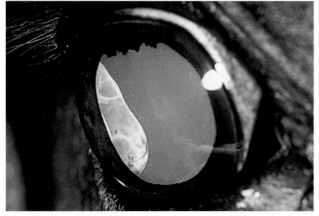

Figure 11-19. A temporally located cyst involving the posterior iris, ciliary body, and peripheral retina in a Rocky Mountain horse presumed to be heterozygous for the responsible gene.

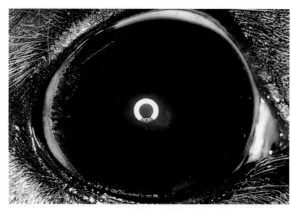

Figure 11-20. Anterior segment dysgenesis in a Rocky Mountain horse presumed to be homozygous for the responsible gene. The iris is smooth, dark, and histologically hypoplastic. The pupil resists dilation, presumably owing to defects in the iris musculature. This horse had other anterior segment anomalies, including ciliary cysts, iris hypoplasia, iridocorneal adhesions and opacification, nuclear cataract, and megalocornea.

that ciliary cysts are seen in heterozygous animals and multiple anterior segment anomalies are seen in homozygous animals.

Disorders of Pigmentation

Partial albinism (subalbinism) refers to reduction in ocular pigmentation. Part or all of the iris may lack pigment and appear blue. In a true albino the iris is pink.

Heterochromia

Heterochromia refers to variations in iris coloration. Both eyes, one eye only, or only part of an iris may be affected, and often there are concurrent variations in coat color (Table 11-1). *Heterochromia*

Table 11-1 | **Breeds Affected by Heterochromia Iridis**

SPECIES	BREED	CHARACTERISTICS
Cat	Siamese	Subalbinism
	Burmese	Variable iris hypopigmentation
	Abyssinian	Variable iris hypopigmentation
	Persian	Variable iris hypopigmentation
Dog	Australian cattle dog	Dappling
	Australian shepherd	Merling
	Boxer	White coat
	Collie	Merling (autosomal dominant)
	Great Dane	Harlequin coat (autosomal dominant)
	Long-haired dachshund	Harlequin coat (autosomal dominant)
	Dalmatian	Dappling (autosomal dominant)
	Malamute	Dappling
	Old English sheepdog	Heterochromia iridis
	Siberian husky	Dappling (autosomal dominant)
	Weimaraner	Iris hypopigmentation varies
Horse	Pinto, appaloosa, white and gray horses	Variable heterochromia
Cattle	Hereford, shorthorn	Albinism, subalbinism

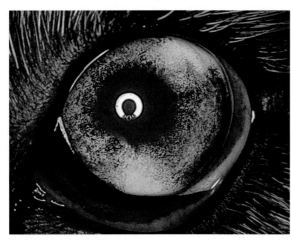

Figure 11-21. Heterochromia iridis (blue and brown iris) in an otherwise normal Australian shepherd dog.

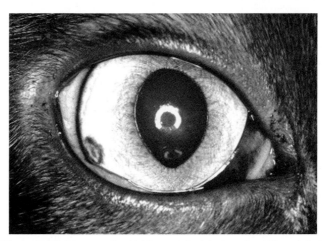

Figure 11-22. Iris nevus (freckle) in a cat. Such lesions should be regularly monitored for signs of progression.

iridis refers to variations in pigmentation of different regions of the iris in the same eye (Figure 11-21), and *heterochromia iridium* refers to variations in coloration between the two eyes of the same animal. Although heterochromia may be normal, blue iridal tissue has also been associated with iris hypoplasia, iris coloboma, and corectopia as well as with absence of or a small tapetum and lack of pigmentation of the nontapetal fundus. An association between congenital deafness and heterochromia has also been recognized in blue-eyed white cats and in the Dalmatian, Australian cattle dog, English setter, Australian shepherd, Boston terrier, Old English sheepdog, and English bulldog.

Lay terms for heterochromia are as follows:

- Wall eye: blue and white iris or part of an iris
- China eye: blue iris or part of an iris
- Watch eye: blue and yellow/brown iris or part of an iris

In dogs, heterochromia is due to incomplete maturation or absence of pigment granules in the iris stroma or anterior pigmented layer. Heterochromia iridis is proposed to be due to decreased availability of tyrosine hydrolase, necessary for the synthesis of melanin, as follows:

$$\text{L-tyrosine} \rightarrow \text{L-dihydroxyphenylalanine} \rightarrow \text{melanins}$$

$$\text{tyrosine}$$

$$\text{hydrolase}$$

In most species heterochromia is of no clinical significance. In cattle ocular albinism has been further subdivided (Table 11-2).

Table 11-2 | **Ocular Albinism in Cattle**

TYPE OF ALBINISM	FEATURES
Partial	Iris blue and white centrally, brown peripherally Hair color normal
Incomplete	Iris light blue, gray, and white Hair color white Some brown sectors in iris, and some colored hair patches Nontapetal fundus incompletely pigmented and choroidal vasculature visible
Complete	Iris very pale blue or white Hair pure white Variable fundus colobomas and tapetal hypoplasia

Iris Nevus

Iris nevi (Figure 11-22) are most commonly observed in cats and dogs. They may consist of focal spots of hyperpigmentation. They must be differentiated from neoplasms that require surgical treatment. Iris nevi do not protrude above the surface of the iris and do not enlarge. Nevi have a low malignant potential and show an increase in the number of cells or greater pigmentation of existing cells. They must be observed carefully for changes, especially in cats, in which they may transform into the early stages of diffuse malignant iris melanoma.

Waardenburg's Syndrome

Waardenburg's syndrome consists of deafness, heterochromia iridis, and white coat color. Although this hereditary syndrome occurs most commonly in blue-eyed white cats, it also occurs in dogs (especially the Australian cattle dog, Great Dane, and Dalmatian), mice, and humans. Not all blue-eyed white cats are affected. In the cat, the syndrome is inherited as a dominant trait with complete penetrance for the white coat and incomplete penetrance for deafness and blue irides.

UVEITIS

Clinical Signs

The detection of uveitis depends on familiarity with the clinical signs. In general the clinical signs of uveitis are similar regardless of cause. Signs of ocular discomfort are as follows:

- Photophobia and blepharospasm
- Pain (may manifest as anorexia or depression)
- Epiphora

Clinical signs more specific for uveitis are as follows:

- Aqueous flare
- Inflammatory cells free in the anterior chamber or adherent to the corneal endothelium (keratic precipitates)
- Hypopyon or hyphema
- Episcleral vascular injection or circumcorneal ciliary flush
- Corneal edema
- Miosis

- Resistance to mydriatics
- Lowered IOP
- Anterior or posterior synechiae
- Swollen or dull appearance of the iris
- Increased pigmentation of the iris
- Vitreous haze or opacity
- Retinal edema, exudate, or detachment
- Aqueous lipemia, which may be seen if circulating lipid levels are high

Aqueous flare is due to breakdown of the blood-aqueous barrier with increased permeability of vessels in the iris and ciliary body, resulting in release of protein into the aqueous. *Keratic precipitates* (KPs) are accumulations of inflammatory cells (neutrophils, lymphocytes, or macrophages) that adhere to the corneal endothelium. In large numbers these cells form a white layer in the anterior chamber called *hypopyon* (Figure 11-23). KPs may be small and scattered (in feline infectious peritonitis) or large and yellow ("mutton-fat" KPs) in granulomatous diseases. Miosis may be due to iridal edema or spasm of the iridal sphincter muscle. As the inflammation subsides, synechiae may form, causing an irregularly shaped pupil (Figure 11-24)

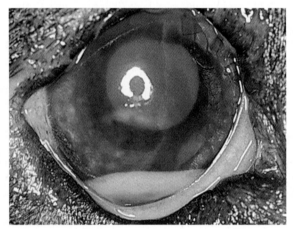

Figure 11-23. Hypopyon in the ventral anterior chamber in a dog that had suffered a penetrating ocular injury. Unless the cornea has been perforated, the anterior chamber is usually sterile in most patients with hypopyon.

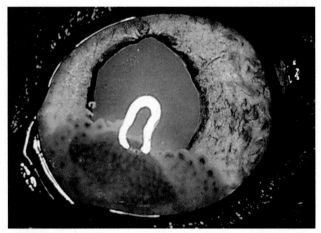

Figure 11-24. Dense "mutton fat" keratic precipitates with admixed blood in a cat with chronic anterior uveitis. The pupil is irregularly shaped (ectropion uveae) owing to small posterior synechia.

or a scalloped appearance on dilation, with pigment remnants on the anterior lens capsule. If posterior uveitis is present, the vitreous may become hazy, and retinal edema, exudates, or detachments may be seen.

Sequelae of Uveitis

Posterior Synechiae

Posterior synechiae occur when fibrinous adhesions form between the lens and iris, with fibrovascular organization occurring later (see Figure 11-24). Formation of synechiae is more likely when aqueous protein content is high. If synechiae form around the entire circumference of the pupil, *iris bombé* occurs, preventing aqueous flow to the anterior chamber, and secondary glaucoma almost invariably follows. An irregularly shaped pupil is frequently caused by synechiae. If blood or exudate organizes in the anterior chamber, a connective tissue membrane may occlude or obliterate the pupil.

Peripheral Anterior Synechiae

Adhesions may form between the iris and trabecular meshwork or between the iris and cornea. Swelling, iris bombé, and cellular infiltrates may reduce drainage of aqueous through the iridocorneal angle early in uveitis, but once peripheral anterior synechiae have formed, an alternative route for drainage must be provided, because the angle is held closed by the synechiae.

Cataract

Cataract (opacity of the lens) occurs frequently after uveitis. It is probably caused by altered composition of the aqueous that interferes with lens nutrition. When an animal with a cataract and signs of uveitis is examined, determination must be made as to whether the cataract caused the uveitis or the uveitis caused the cataract.

Glaucoma

IOP is usually *lowered* during uveitis because an inflamed ciliary body makes less aqueous humor and endogenous prostaglandins may increase uveoscleral outflow. If IOP is *normal* or *increased* in the presence of active inflammation, it is likely that aqueous humor outflow via the trabecular meshwork is impaired in one of the following ways:

- Blockage of the angle with inflammatory cells, debris, or neovascular membranes
- Peripheral anterior synechiae
- Occlusion of the pupil by posterior synechiae

Eyes with normal IOP and active uveitis may have impaired aqueous humor outflow and should be monitored carefully for glaucoma.

Intractable secondary glaucoma due to lens-induced uveitis is a common entity, especially in dogs. This condition may be seen after penetrating injuries to the lens, in patients with long-standing cataracts undergoing lens resorption, and sometimes after cataract extraction.

Retinal Detachment

Exudation and cellular infiltration from the choroid may cause retinal detachment.

Atrophy

The iris and ciliary body atrophy as the stroma is replaced by fibrous tissue. Defects may appear in the iris. Atrophy of areas of the choroid frequently results in atrophy of the overlying retina, which is visible ophthalmoscopically. Severe atrophy of the ciliary body causes *hypotony* (lowered IOP). In some animals the color of the iris becomes *darker* after uveitis. In severe cases the entire globe may shrink, a condition called *phthisis bulbi*.

Preiridal Fibrovascular Membranes

In some animals with chronic anterior uveitis new blood vessels and fibrous membranes form on the anterior surface of the iris. These may result in eversion of the pupillary margin, called *ectropion uveae*, or glaucoma as they cover the trabecular meshwork.

Cyclitic Membranes

A *cyclitic membrane* is a band of fibrovascular tissue extending from the ciliary body across either the pupil or the anterior face of the vitreous. It consists of fibrous tissue and blood vessels and may severely obstruct vision.

Sympathetic Ophthalmia

Sympathetic ophthalmia is a *rare* immune-mediated disorder in humans, and perhaps in animals, in which unilateral intraocular inflammation liberates previously immunologically isolated antigens. The resulting immune response to these ocular antigens leads to damage of the previously normal other eye.

Diagnosis of Uveitis

Anterior uveitis is distinguished from conjunctivitis, superficial keratitis, and glaucoma, the other causes of the red-eye syndrome (Table 11-3). The uvea is involved in numerous systemic dis-orders (Table 11-4). Such diseases usually affect other parts of the eye in addition to the uvea and are discussed in Chapter 18. Once uveitis is detected, every effort should be made to identify a specific cause of the inflammation so that the most effective therapy may be started. A thorough history and complete physical examination are essential for the proper diagnosis as to the cause of the inflammation in a given patient.

Numerous uveitis classification schemes have been proposed, including those based on the tissues affected (anterior uveitis, posterior uveitis, panuveitis), on the presumed histologic nature of the disorder (suppurative, nonsuppurative, granulomatous, nongranulomatous), on whether the cause starts inside the eye or from its surface (endogenous versus exogenous), and on a specific etiology (see Table 11-4). Although each of these schemes has its own advantages and disadvantages, classification into granulomatous or nongranulomatous and then by specific etiology is probably the most useful method in a clinical setting, because it also helps guide specific therapy (Table 11-5). This scheme, however, is plagued by the presence of a large percentage of patients having idiopathic uveitis in which the cause remains obscure and therapy can be only non-specific and directed at controlling inflammation and preventing further damage to the eye. Presumably, most of these cases are immune-mediated or involve microorganisms that are not yet recognized as pathogenic. It is hoped that over time the percentage of patients with idiopathic uveitis will decline as our understanding of the causes of this disorder improves.

Although classification as granulomatous or nongranulomatous uveitis is based on a histologic classification scheme, the criteria in Table 11-5 can also be used to make reasonable clinical inferences about the histologic nature of the inflammation and to allow for prioritization of the diagnostic tests to be performed. Most cases of granulomatous uveitis are associated with microorganism or foreign material stimulation of a chronic immune response, whereas nongranulomatous uveitis is often associated with phys-ical, toxic, or allergic causes. After determining whether a specific animal has granulomatous or nongranulomatous uveitis, the clinician should consider specific tests to try to determine the exact cause (e.g., serum titer measurement for *Toxoplasma*). In general the following specific categories of uveitis should be considered:

• Infectious associated—algal, bacterial, fungal, viral, protozoal, parasitic

Table 11-3 | **Differential Diagnosis of Ocular Inflammations**

PARAMETER	ANTERIOR UVEITIS	CONJUNCTIVITIS	SUPERFICIAL KERATITIS	GLAUCOMA
Conjunctiva	Variably thickened	Thick; folded	Variably thickened	Not thickened
Conjunctival vessels	Episcleral; not movable with conjunctiva, infrequently branch	Superficial, diffuse, extensive branching	Superficial, diffuse, extensive branching	Episcleral, not movable with conjunctiva, infrequently branch
Secretion or discharge	None to serous	Moderate to copious, serous to purulent	Moderate to copious, serous to purulent	None to serous
Pain	Moderate	None to slight	Moderate to severe	Moderate to severe
Photophobia	Moderate	None	Severe	Slight
Cornea	Clear to steamy	Clear	Clouded to opaque	Steamy
Pupil size	Small, sluggish, irregular, or fixed	Normal	Normal to small	Dilated, moderate to complete, and fixed
Pupillary light response	Variable	Normal	Normal	Absent
Intraocular pressure	Variable: may be normal, elevated, or diminished	Normal	Normal	Elevated

Modified from Lavignette AM (1973): Differential diagnosis and treatment of anterior uveitis. Vet Clin North Am 3:504.

Table 11-4 | **Causes of Uveitis**

CAUSE	MOST COMMONLY AFFECTED SPECIES	CAUSE	MOST COMMONLY AFFECTED SPECIES
NEOPLASTIC/PARANEOPLASTIC		**Viruses**	
Lymphosarcoma	Any	Canine adenovirus types 1 and 2 (immune-mediated)	Dog
Melanoma	Dog, cat	Canine distemper virus	Dog
Histiocytic proliferative disease	Dog	Coronavirus (feline infectious peritonitis)	Cat
Hyperviscosity syndrome	Dog	Feline leukemia virus	Cat
Granulomatous meningoencephalitis	Dog	Feline immunodeficiency virus	Cat
Miscellaneous primary intraocular tumors	Any	Herpesvirus (Marek's disease)	Chickens, turkeys
Miscellaneous metastatic tumors	Any	Herpesvirus	
METABOLIC		Feline herpesvirus 1	Cat
Diabetes mellitus (lens-induced uveitis)	Dog	Canine herpesvirus 1	Dog
Systemic hypertension	Cat, dog	Equine herpesvirus 1 and 2	Horse
Hyperlipidemia	Dog	Ovine herpes virus 2 (MCF)	Cattle
Coagulopathies	Any	Alcelaphine herpes virus 1 (MCF)	Cattle
IDIOPATHIC	Any	Rabies virus	Dog
		Equine influenza	Horse
IMMUNE-MEDIATED		Equine viral arteritis	Horse
Cataracts (lens-induced uveitis)	Any	Parainfluenza type 3	Horse
Lens trauma (phacoclastic uveitis)	Any	MCF	Cattle
Immune-mediated thrombocytopenia	Any		
Immune-mediated vasculitis	Any	**Parasitic**	
Uveodermatologic syndrome (Vogt-Koyanagi-Harada–like syndrome)	Dog	*Taenia multiceps*	Sheep, dog
		Echinococcus granulosis	Horse (rare)
INFECTIOUS		*Angiostrongylus vasorum*	Dog
Algae		*Dirofilaria immitis*	Dog
Geotricha spp.	Dog	*Setaria* spp.	Horse
Prototheca spp.	Dog	*Onchocerca cervicalis*	Horse (equine recurrent uveitis)
Bacteria			
Septicemia/endotoxemia due to any cause	Any	*Strongylus*	Horse
Leptospira spp.	Dog, horse	*Diptera* spp. (ophthalmomyiasis interna)	Various
Bartonella spp.	Dog, cat	*Toxocara* spp., *Baylisascaris* spp. (ocular larval migrans)	Dog, cat Sheep/Goats, cat
Borrelia burgdorferi	Dog, horse	*Trypanosoma* sp.	
Brucella spp.	Dog, horse	*Elaeophora schneideri*	Sheep/Goats
Escherichia coli	Cattle, horse		
Streptococcus spp.	Horse	**TOXIC**	
Rhodococcus equi	Horse	Drugs	
Listeria monocytogenes	Sheep, cattle	Pilocarpine, carbachol other parasympathomimetics	Any
Haemophilus spp.	Cattle		
Tuberculosis	Cattle, cat	Prostaglandin derivatives (latanoprost)	Any
		Sulfamethazine/trimethoprim (immune-mediated)	Dogs
Protozoa		Endotoxemia from any systemic source	Any
*Toxoplasma gondii**	Any	Infectious keratitis with bacterial toxin production	Any
Leishmania donovani	Dog	Radiation therapy	Any
Ehrlichia canis or *Ehrlichia platys*	Dog		
Rickettsia rickettsii	Dog	**TRAUMA**	
		Blunt or penetrating injuries	Any
Yeasts and Fungi		Corneal foreign bodies	Any
Aspergillus spp.	Chickens, turkeys, cat	**REFLEX UVEITIS**	
Blastomyces spp.	Dog, cat	Ulcerative keratitis of any cause	Any
Coccidioides immitis	Dog	Deep necrotizing or nonnecrotizing scleritis	Dog
Cryptococcus spp.	Dog, cat	Episcleritis	Dog
Histoplasma capsulatum	Dog, cat		
Pseudallescheria boydii	Dog		

MCF, Malignant catarrhal fever.

*Neosporum caninum has been found responsible for some cases of dogs previously diagnosed with *T. gondii* infection. The clinical significance is undetermined.

- Immune-mediated
- Neoplastic or paraneoplastic
- Metabolic
- Traumatic
- Toxic
- Reflex
- Idiopathic

Differential diagnosis of the cause of uveitis often requires specialist assistance, notably when potential zoonotic diseases may be involved or the cause remains unclear.

A few generalizations may be made. Uveitis associated with KPs is often associated with intraocular neoplasia, feline infectious

Table 11-5 | Classification Criteria for Anterior Uveitis

NONGRANULOMATOUS	GRANULOMATOUS
Acute onset	Gradual onset
Short course	Chronic or recurrent
No keratic precipitates	Keratic precipitates/greasy exudate on lens surface
No synechiae	Posterior synechiae
No iris nodules	Iris nodules may be present
Primarily anterior uveitis	Posterior uveitis may also be present

These criteria are useful but not absolute and are interpreted along with other clinical signs.

peritonitis, deep fungal agents, and intraocular foreign bodies. Severe uveitis that involves the anterior and posterior segments is often associated with a deep fungal agent, lymphosarcoma, or uveodermatologic syndrome. The last is also commonly associated with loss of pigment in the uveal tract, skin, or hair. Uveitis with hemorrhage is often associated with systemic hypertension, intraocular neoplasia, coagulopathy, or a tick-borne disorder.

General Therapeutic Principles

1: Make an Etiologic Diagnosis

The clinician must make a concerted attempt to find a cause for the uveitis. Although not all such attempts are successful, idiopathic uveitis is a diagnosis of exclusion. Often, if a specific cause is identified, more effective therapy may be instituted (e.g., removal of an abscessed tooth, treatment for deep mycosis, control corneal infection, chemotherapy for lymphosarcoma). Routine hematologic analysis and serum chemistry profiles are useful in indicating the presence of inflammatory disorders and concurrent systemic disease (see Table 11-4). In endemic areas appropriate serologic tests are indicated (e.g., for toxoplasmosis, coccidioidomycosis, blastomycosis, cryptococcosis). Blastomycosis is found most frequently in the central United States east of the Mississippi River, and coccidioidomycosis is found in Arizona, Nevada, and the central valley of California.

2: Control Inflammation

CORTICOSTEROIDS. Corticosteroids may be given via the topical, systemic, or, occasionally, subconjunctival route. These agents inhibit cell-mediated immune reactions, decrease antibody production, and stabilize lysosomal membranes, reducing release of intracellular proteolytic enzymes. If corticosteroids are administered via the topical or subconjunctival routes the cornea must not retain fluorescein stain. Additionally, immunosuppressive therapy should not be instituted if active infectious diseases, such as a deep fungal agent, have not been ruled out. In general the following approach is helpful:

- For mild uveitis (mild conjunctival hyperemia, no obvious or only minimal aqueous flare, hypotony, with/without miosis):
  1. Topical corticosteroids—0.1% dexamethasone or 1% prednisolone acetate q6-12h
- For moderate uveitis (moderate conjunctival hyperemia, readily detected aqueous flare, normal or decreased IOP, with/without miosis):
  1. Topical corticosteroids—0.1% dexamethasone or 1% prednisolone acetate q4-6h

  2. Systemic prednisone 0.25 mg/kg PO in dogs and cats; in horses a systemic nonsteroidal antiinflammatory drug (NSAID) should be used instead
- For severe uveitis (marked conjunctival hyperemia, marked aqueous flare/fibrin/hypopyon, with/without miosis):
  1. Topical corticosteroids—0.1% dexamethasone or 1% prednisolone acetate q1-4h
  2. Systemic prednisone 1.0 mg/kg PO in dogs and cats; in horses a systemic NSAID should be used instead
  3. Consider triamcinolone acetonide 1-2 mg per eye administered subconjunctivally.

NONSTEROIDAL ANTIINFLAMMATORY DRUGS. Significant protein leakage from uveal vessels during inflammation is mediated by prostaglandins. Inhibition of prostaglandin production decreases the amount of antibody present to engage in immunologic reactions and also decreases fibrin, which reduces synechia formation. Because endogenous prostaglandins also contribute to miosis by a mechanism that is not blocked by atropine, an NSAID may facilitate pupillary dilation with atropine. In general topical and systemic NSAIDs are not as potent as corticosteroids in the treatment of immune-mediated uveitis but may approximate or exceed the efficacy of corticosteroids in traumatic uveitis. Topical NSAIDS include flurbiprofen, suprofen, and diclofenac. These drugs are administered every 6 to 12 hours in most species. Systemic NSAIDS are typically dosed at levels recommended for the species being treated.

IMMUNOSUPPRESSIVE AGENTS. Topical 0.02% to 2.0% cyclosporine, oral cyclosporine, or oral azathioprine may be used in select cases of nonresponsive uveitis. Typically these agents require periodic laboratory evaluations for systemic side effects, especially those involving the bone marrow, liver, and kidney. Azathioprine has been suggested at 1 to 2 mg/kg/day for 3 to 7 days, followed by tapering to as low a dosage as possible.

3: Prevent Undesirable Sequelae

MYDRIATICS/CYCLOPLEGICS. Pupillary dilation (mydriasis) can help reduce synechiae formation and the likelihood of iris bombé with secondary glaucoma. Relaxation of the ciliary muscle (cycloplegia) can help lessen ocular pain. In general the dose required to dilate the pupil is somewhat lower than that necessary to induce cycloplegia and provide pain relief. One percent atropine ophthalmic ointment or solution is a parasympatholytic agent with potent mydriatic and cycloplegic activity, whereas 0.5% to 1.0% tropicamide solution is a shorter-acting parasympathomimetic with relatively potent mydriatic effects but milder cycloplegic effects. Sympathomimetics, such as 10% phenylephrine given every 8 to 12 hours, can boost the mydriatic effects of atropine and tropicamide, but these drugs afford no meaningful cycloplegia. On rare occasions mydriasis can compromise the drainage angle, leading to rises in IOP, or reduce tear production, especially in animals with keratoconjunctivitis sicca. In general atropine is used one to three times per day or to effect.

ANTIGLAUCOMA DRUGS. IOP is typically low in uveitis because an inflamed ciliary body makes less aqueous humor and endogenous prostaglandins increase uveoscleral outflow. If IOP is normal or elevated in the presence of inflammation, the drainage angle is probably compromised and the clinician must be concerned about impending glaucoma. It is essential that irreversible glaucomatous damage not be allowed to occur while antiinflammatory therapy works to clear the drainage angle. In general a topical or systemic carbonic anhydrase inhibitor (dorzolamide or methazolamide), a topical β-blocker (timolol), or an adrenergic agent (dipivefrin) is preferred to a parasympathomimetic (pilocarpine, demecarium bromide) or a prostaglandin derivative (latanoprost, travoprost), either of which may exacerbate intraocular inflammation.

4: Relieve Pain

The cycloplegic action of atropine relaxes the ciliary muscle and helps reduce ocular pain in uveitis. The patient may also be placed in a darkened room or stall to alleviate photophobia. Topical or systemic NSAIDs can provide pain relief as well as aid in controlling inflammation. For severe pain a systemic analgesic, such as butorphanol, morphine, or oxymorphone, may be used.

Specific Forms of Uveitis

Infectious Uveitis

The infectious causes of uveitis are summarized in Table 11-4. Many of these agents are located in specific geographic regions, a feature that helps narrow the list of possible causes in a given patient. Not all patients with infectious uveitis have living organisms within the eye. Uveitis may occur as a result of intraocular infection or in response to bacterial toxins generated within or outside the eye, or may stem from an immunologic response to the organism, which may be within the eye or elsewhere in the body. It is well recognized that uveitis may be associated with infection outside the eye, including prostatitis, endometritis, gingivitis and tooth root abscess, mastitis, metritis, navel ill, and pneumonia. In these cases uveitis may result from shedding of bacteria into the circulation, the uveitis being secondary to previously sensitized lymphocytes in the uvea, or may be due to bacterial toxins released from the primary site. Often the uveitis is recurrent in these cases, and hematologic examination or blood culture may be of value in arriving at a definitive diagnosis.

Blastomycosis, ehrlichiosis, histoplasmosis, and coccidioidomycosis are important causes of uveitis in dogs, as are cryptococcosis, toxoplasmosis, and feline infectious peritonitis in cats. If uveitis is present in association with lesions of lungs, bone, lymph nodes, skin, or testicles or if the animal is located in an area endemic for any of these organisms, appropriate serologic, radiographic, and cytologic tests are indicated.

Immune-Mediated Uveitis

Immune-mediated uveitis may be the result of a primary reaction to a foreign antigen, an autoimmune phenomenon directed against self-antigens, or a combination of the two. It is believed that the majority of idiopathic cases of uveitis are actually immune-mediated. Often the diagnosis is made through exclusion of all known causes of uveitis. In some cases specific clinical signs (depigmentation) or historical events (a complete cataract preceding the inflammation or cat-scratch injury involving the lens) support the diagnosis of immune-mediated uveitis, and a detailed evaluation is not required.

UVEODERMATOLOGIC SYNDROME. Synonym: Vogt-Koyanagi-Harada–like syndrome.

Uveodermatologic syndrome affects certain breeds more commonly than others—Akita, Old English sheepdog, golden retriever, Siberian husky, and Irish setter. It is a spontaneous autoimmune disease apparently directed against melanin that affects the anterior and posterior uvea, frequently resulting in blindness from retinal detachment or glaucoma. Antiretinal antibodies to previously sequestered retinal antigens may also be present. Presumably the antibodies develop after the initial insult has severely damaged the retina and may represent epitope spreading. Depigmentation of the mucocutaneous junctions, eyelids, and hair coat may precede or follow the ocular signs. Histologic examination of a biopsy specimen from the mucocutaneous junction (especially the lips), even if the tissue appears grossly normal, can be useful in the diagnosis of this disorder if results of a systemic evaluation are otherwise noncontributory and the animal has severe anterior and posterior uveitis. Neurologic signs are associated with the syndrome in humans but are rare in dogs. In some geographic regions the onset of the disease has a definite seasonal incidence (e.g., February to May in southern California).

Vigorous early antiinflammatory therapy with topical and systemic steroids, NSAIDs, and azathioprine is often necessary to save vision. Recurrences of the disease can be expected, with maintenance therapy using appropriate medications between recurrences. Given the severe and relentless nature of the uveitis, the *immediate* assistance of a veterinary ophthalmologist should be sought in the handling of dogs affected with uveodermatologic syndrome.

LENS-INDUCED UVEITIS. The embryology of the lens is such that the lens capsule essentially isolates the lens proteins immunologically from the immune system before birth. Therefore if the lens capsule ruptures or leaks, lens proteins may enter the aqueous and elicit an immune-mediated uveitis that may be acute or chronic. The most common causes of lens-induced uveitis are liquefaction of cataractous lens proteins that escape through an intact lens capsule, swelling of a cataractous lens with increased "porosity" of an otherwise intact lens capsule, small tears in the lens capsule from rapidly forming cataracts and lens swelling (diabetes mellitus), and traumatic disruption of the lens capsule (cat scratch, penetrating injuries).

Leakage through the Intact Lens Capsule. The most common form of lens-induced uveitis is caused by leakage through intact lens capsule, which is most frequently seen in conjunction with the advanced stages of cataract (complete on resorbing). It should be suspected in every animal in which a complete or resorbing cataract precedes the onset of a "red eye," or in animals with a "red eye" and a cataract. It may be differentiated from uveitis-induced cataract by the fact that in the latter, the "red eye" uveitis precedes the cataract. Lens-induced uveitis should be anticipated in all eyes with cataract, although it does not always occur. In this form of the disease the lens capsule becomes permeable, allowing liquefied cortex to leak into the aqueous and creating an immune-mediated uveitis and, possibly, secondary glaucoma. Without tonometry and biomicroscopy, this inflammation may not be evident, and many such eyes exhibit a dilated pupil—not a miotic pupil as would be expected in uveitis. Affected eyes, however, do typically exhibit at least some conjunctival hyperemia. Eyes with lens-induced uveitis before cataract surgery have a greater risk for many postoperative complications (glaucoma, retinal detachment) than eyes without it.

Therapy with topical corticosteroids or NSAIDs, often for relatively long periods, may be needed to control lens-induced uveitis. In particularly severe cases systemic antiinflammatory agents may be required. Corticosteroids, even those administered

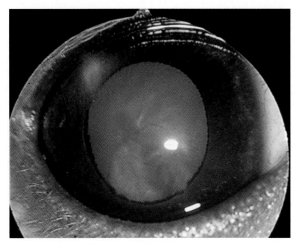

Figure 11-25. Chronic lens-induced uveitis in a basenji puppy after a cat claw injury. The lens capsule has been ruptured by the nail.

topically, should be used with caution in dogs with poorly regulated diabetes mellitus, cataract, and lens-induced uveitis so as to avoid worsening the glycemic control.

Lens-induced uveitis should be suspected in all red eyes in which cataract preceded the conjunctival hyperemia. Glaucoma should be ruled out in these cases.

Failure to recognize and treat lens-induced uveitis when cataracts are first diagnosed is a *very* common cause of lower success rates of cataract surgery in dogs. Medical therapy for lens-induced uveitis should be implemented as soon as the diagnosis is established.

Penetrating Lens Injuries. Penetrating injuries to the lens often quickly progress to endophthalmitis with secondary glaucoma (Figure 11-25). Bacteria are commonly inoculated during the injury, resulting in a mixed purulent inflammation with numerous neutrophils. Early lens extraction may offer the greatest chance for saving the eye, although large case studies to support this aggressive method of treatment are lacking. In many older dogs, medical treatment after lens capsule rupture cannot prevent loss of the eye through uncontrolled inflammation and secondary glaucoma. In young dogs (less than 12 months), much of the lens cortex may be resorbed, with less inflammation than in older animals, provided that infection is controlled. Nevertheless the long-term prognosis remains guarded in these animals.

Penetrating injury and lens capsule rupture are common causes of uveitis and endophthalmitis in dogs and cats.

UVEITIS ASSOCIATED WITH DENTAL DISEASE. Untreated gingivitis, periodontitis, and tooth root abscesses are very common causes of severe uveitis in dogs. Treatment of dental disorders is essential before any intraocular surgery is undertaken as well as for the patient's general health.

PIGMENTARY UVEITIS IN GOLDEN RETRIEVERS. In pigmentary uveitis in golden retrievers, pigment is dispersed in the anterior chamber, the iris becomes dark and thickened, and clumps of pigment may be seen on the lens capsule and corneal endothelium. Aqueous flare, posterior synechiae, cataract, and glaucoma may also occur. The cause of the disorder is undetermined, although some workers believe it to be immune-mediated and others have associated it with uveal cysts.

FELINE UVEITIS. Causes of uveitis in cats include feline infectious peritonitis, lymphosarcoma caused by feline leukemia virus, feline immunodeficiency virus, toxoplasmosis, cryptococcosis, histoplasmosis, blastomycosis, and coccidiomycosis. For details of the ocular manifestations of specific disorders, see Chapter 18. A specific type of nongranulomatous anterior uveitis described as *lymphocytic-plasmacytic uveitis* has been recognized as a common precursor to *glaucoma* if the uveitis is uncontrolled. It is also a common cause of glaucoma in cats. Idiopathic lymphocytic-plasmacytic uveitis occurs in both diffuse and nodular forms, with the nodular form being more commonly unilateral, and the diffuse form bilateral.

A minimum laboratory evaluation for cats with either unilateral or bilateral uveitis consists of the following procedures:

- Complete blood count
- Serum biochemical profile
- Urinalysis
- Thoracic radiography
- Serologic tests relevant to the geographic location: *Toxoplasma* (immunoglobulin [Ig] G and IgM), feline leukemia virus, feline immunodeficiency virus, *Cryptococcus, Blastomyces* spp., *Histoplasma* spp., and *Coccidioides* spp.

Uncontrolled or unobserved *idiopathic lymphocytic-plasmacytic uveitis* is a common cause of feline glaucoma.

In 93 cats with endogenous uveitis in Colorado in which a specific agent was identified, the following seroprevalence of infection was found: *Toxoplasma gondii*, 78.5%; feline immunodeficiency virus, 22.9%; feline leukemia virus, 4.95%; and feline coronavirus, 27%. The combination of topical corticosteroids and clindamycin hydrochloride (25 mg/kg, divided, twice daily) was beneficial in cats with uveitis associated with toxoplasmosis (Chavkin et al., 1992). It is highly probable that the various causes of feline uveitis vary greatly by geographic region.

EQUINE RECURRENT UVEITIS. Synonyms: "moon blindness," periodic ophthalmia.

As in other species, the horse may exhibit a single episode of uveitis due to any one of a multitude of causes. In addition to this form of uveitis, horses also frequently have apparently spontaneously recurring episodes of uveitis (equine recurrent uveitis [ERU]) that are presumably immune-mediated. ERU, however, is not a single disease as the name would imply but instead is a group of diseases united only by a clinical pattern of recurrent bouts of uveitis. With each subsequent uveitis attack, cumulative damage occurs to the ocular tissues, and blindness may result. The long-term prognosis is guarded, but with therapy, vision may be retained for a prolonged period in many animals.

History and Geographic Distribution. ERU has been recorded for millennia and is the most common cause of vision loss in the horse. As with many ancient disorders, the proposed causes and treatment have varied greatly over the years, and the disease has often been shrouded in folklore, ignorance, and misconceptions. For example, the term "moon blindness" has two origins: (1) the frequent recurrences were once thought coincident with the phases of the moon and (2) the cataract that often accompanies chronic ERU looked like a small moon in the eye.

The disease is worldwide in distribution, although distinct regional differences in frequency occur. It is more common in North America than in Australia, the United Kingdom, or

South Africa. An incidence of up to 12% has been recorded in eastern areas of the United States, and some investigators believe it is more prevalent in low-lying areas with high rainfall. There is no age or sex predilection. The Appaloosa breed appears to be at higher risk for development of recurrent uveitis, suggesting a genetic predisposition to ERU.

Etiology. There is no single cause of ERU (see Table 11-4). The most commonly held explanation is that the uveitis is an autoimmune phenomenon in which IgG antibodies and autoreactive T cells specific for retinal antigens are present. A cell-mediated immunity to uveal antigens has also been demonstrated in horses with ERU. The association between ERU and previous or current infection with *Leptospira* has been studied in greater detail than many of the other known etiologies of ERU. This organism appears to be capable of immunologically cross-reacting with the equine cornea and lens, and in horses with ERU, leptospiral antisera is also cross-reactive with the equine iris pigment epithelium and retina. In Europe leptospiral strains have been isolated from the ocular fluids of horses with chronic ERU, and it is postulated that persistent intraocular leptospiral infections by certain strains of the organism cause ERU. Many horses with ERU in the United States, however, do not appear to be infected with leptospiral organisms; also, potent immunosuppressive therapy with drugs such as intravitreal cyclosporine does not exacerbate the disease as would be expected with an active infectious process. Therefore the relative importance of the direct effects of the organism on the eye, locally produced antibodies against *Leptospira interrogans*, and autoantibodies against retinal autoantigens (retinal S-antigen and interphotoreceptor retinoid-binding protein) remain unclear in the pathogenesis of ERU. In any event, it is clear that ERU is a highly complex disorder with multifactorial causes related to the genetic constitution of the animal and that it is strongly immune-mediated. Common causes of ERU are *Leptospira*-associated uveitis and uveitis associated with migrating microfilariae of *Onchocerca cervicalis*.

Leptospira-Associated Uveitis. Although both experimental infections and natural outbreaks of leptospirosis have been associated with ERU, clinically apparent uveitis does not develop in most adult horses until 1 to 2 years after infection. Several reports have described isolation of *L. interrogans* from various ocular fluids, especially the vitreous, in horses with chronic ERU. The organism is difficult to culture, however, and results of polymerase chain reaction testing for leptospiral DNA are typically positive in many animals that are culture-negative, suggesting that the organism may be more prevalent than once thought. Serum antibody titers greater than 1:400 are suggestive of previous infection, although lower serologic titers may be found in many infected horses. In fact, negative serologic titers do not necessarily rule out leptospirosis as a possible cause, because the organism or its DNA is occasionally identified in the intraocular fluids of horses with negative serologic titer results. Interpretation of serologic test results may be further confounded by the occurrence of positive serologic titer results for *Leptospira* in horses without uveitis. Vitreal titers for *Leptospira* may also be elevated, although again the value of this test remains questionable.

Numerous serologic studies have shown widespread exposure (up to 30%) of the equine population to a variety of serotypes of *Leptospira* in North America, Britain, Europe, and Australia. Serotypes associated with the disease include *pomona, bratislava, autumnalis, grippotyphosa, canicola, icterohemorrhagiae, hardjo,* and *sejroe.*

There are at least two main theories as to the role of *Leptospira* in ERU. In the first theory, ERU after infection with *Leptospira* is primarily an immune-mediated disorder in which the organism is no longer present. In this scenario autoimmune inflammation tends to "burn out" as antiinflammatory regulatory cells get the upper hand in an active attack, leading to a clinically quiescent period. Recurrent active periods may be the result of the autoimmune response shifting from one site to another on the same autoantigen (intramolecular spreading) or to another entirely different autoantigen (intermolecular spreading). This theory is supported by the responsiveness of the disease to immunosuppressive therapy, which, if viable organism were to be present in the eye, would be expected to ultimately result in an exacerbation of the inflammation. Alternatively, it has been theorized that persistence of *L. interrogans* in the vitreous humor of horses with ERU can induce and maintain an autoimmune uveitis. During the periods between overt episodes, the number of leptospiral organisms may decline to such a level that overt inflammation is not clinically detectable, and antibody titers decline. When the antibody titer falls below a certain threshold, bacterial numbers may increase, resulting in a resurgence of antibodies that cross-react with host antigens, leading to greater inflammation, damage to adjacent tissues, and, perhaps, recognition of new antigenic epitopes. This theory is supported by the observation that infusion of antibiotics into the vitreal cavity in conjunction with a surgical vitrectomy may greatly reduce the frequency of recurrent episodes.

Clinical Signs. Clinical signs vary with the phase of the disease (Figure 11-26).

Active Phase. Clinical signs in the active phase are as follows:

- Marked blepharospasm
- Photophobia
- Lacrimation
- Pain
- Protrusion of the third eyelid
- Corneal edema
- Scleral injection
- Aqueous flare (with/without hypopyon)
- Miosis
- Thickened, infiltrated iris
- Anterior and posterior synechiae
- Fibrinous clots in anterior chamber
- Decreased IOP (occasionally increased)
- Depigmented butterfly lesions near optic disc (Figure 11-27)
- Any of the quiescent signs

In an animal with onchocerciasis, the following may be seen in addition to the typical ocular lesions of ERU:

- Focal dermatitis on the head, ventral thorax, and neck
- Vitiligo affecting the scrotum, lateral canthus, or lateral conjunctival limbus

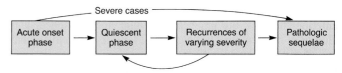

Figure 11-26. Clinical course of equine recurrent uveitis.

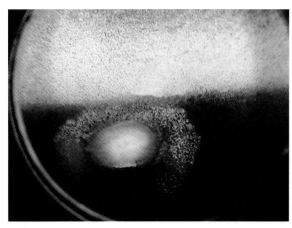

Figure 11-27. Wing-shaped hypopigmented lesions nasal and temporal to the optic disc ("butterfly lesions") are suggestive of previous uveitis. (Courtesy University of Wisconsin–Madison Veterinary Ophthalmology Service Collection.)

- Focal corneal opacities at the lateral limbus
- Hyperemia and chemosis of the perilimbal temporal conjunctiva

In the active phase, rapid intensive treatment is mandatory to prevent severe complications (e.g., synechiae, cataract, retinal detachment). Most active periods last several days to weeks.

Quiescent Phase. Typically an active period is followed by a quiescent phase of variable duration. Although inflammation may be clinically minimal or undetectable in the quiescent phase, histologic signs of inflammation and altered vascular permeability continue. During the quiescent phase immunologically active cells and cytokines also persist, and new antigenic epitopes or autoantigens may be recognized—prompting a resurgence of inflammation (Figures 11-28 and 11-29). It is not uncommon for horses in the quiescent phase to be offered for sale by unscrupulous individuals who represent the horse as "sound" or by those who are unaware of a horse's past history.

Clinical signs most likely to be seen during clinical examination of horses in the quiescent phase are as follows (Figures 11-30 and 11-31):

- Corneal opacity
- Pigment on anterior lens capsule
- Anterior and posterior synechiae
- Blunted and rounded corpora nigra
- Occluded pupil
- Iris atrophy
- Cataract (poor surgical candidates)
- Vitreous bands and opacities
- Butterfly lesions or retinal detachment
- Phthisis bulbi
- Partial or complete loss of vision

The presence of inflammatory sequelae in an equine eye indicates the possibility of ERU.

Treatment. In general the number of medications and frequency of the therapy are adjusted in accordance with the severity of the clinical signs. Mild disease may be treated with topical therapy alone, whereas more severe inflammation typically demands systemic therapy as well. Initial therapy usually includes the following measures:

1. Attempt to establish a definitive etiologic diagnosis, and specifically address the cause if possible.
2. Ensure good husbandry practices: Place the horse in a dark stall to relieve photophobia. Prevent ocular trauma by mowing pastures and removing sharp objects from the environment. Reduce contact with cattle and wildlife that may harbor leptospirosis, prevent access to ponds and swampy areas, and ensure good insect and rodent control. Minimize stress, ensure a good diet, and employ an optimal deworming schedule. Vaccinations should be optimized for each patient and based on the horse's use and specific needs. Multiple vaccinations should be spaced at least 1 week apart so as to avoid excessive antigenic stimulation and potential exacerbation of the disease.
3. Atropine ointment (1%) applied 1 to 4 times a day. This medication reduces pain by relaxing the ciliary muscle, aids in the prevention of synechia, and may help stabilize the blood-aqueous barrier. Atropine should be discontinued or reduced in frequency if the horse shows reduced gut motility and/or colic. Resistance to pupillary dilation is an indicator of the severity of the uveitis, the presence of synechia, or both. Once the uveitis is controlled, the pupil may remain dilated for days to weeks, especially if the drug was used frequently during an acute attack.
4. Systemic NSAIDs (listed here in order of potency—use only 1 at a time):
   - Flunixin meglumine 0.25 to 1.0 mg/kg q12h, IV, IM, or PO for 5 days; then, if required by the severity of the inflammation and if patient is appropriately monitored for gastric and renal side effects, 0.25 mg/kg PO q12-24h on a more long-term basis. If after 5 days systemic antiinflammatory therapy is still required, many ophthalmologists switch from flunixin meglumine to phenylbutazone. Flunixin meglumine may also facilitate pupillary dilation by atropine because endogenous prostaglandins can induce miosis by directly acting on the iris sphincter muscle; this action is blocked by NSAIDS but not by atropine.
   - Phenylbutazone 1 g per adult horse (or up to 4.4 mg/kg) q12-24h IV or PO. This drug typically is used after a 5-day course of flunixin meglumine if additional systemic antiinflammatory therapy is required. On occasion, with appropriate monitoring for gastric and renal toxicity, it is used as long-term therapy in an effort to reduce the frequency and severity of acute episodes, especially if aspirin is ineffective at such reductions.
   - Aspirin 25 mg/kg PO q12-24h (12.5 g/500 kg). Typically this agent is used in horses in which long-term topical antiinflammatory therapy cannot prevent recurrent outbreaks and long-term systemic NSAID therapy is required.
   - Consider ranitidine (6.6 mg/kg q8h) and sucralfate (20 mg/kg PO q8h) or omeprazole (4 mg/kg PO q24h) for gastric ulcer prophylaxis in foals.
5. Topical corticosteroids (e.g., 0.1% dexamethasone ointment, 1.0% prednisolone) applied every 1 to 6 hours, depending on severity. Long-term therapy is often required, and it is generally advisable to treat an acute episode for at least 2 weeks after the apparent resolution of all signs of

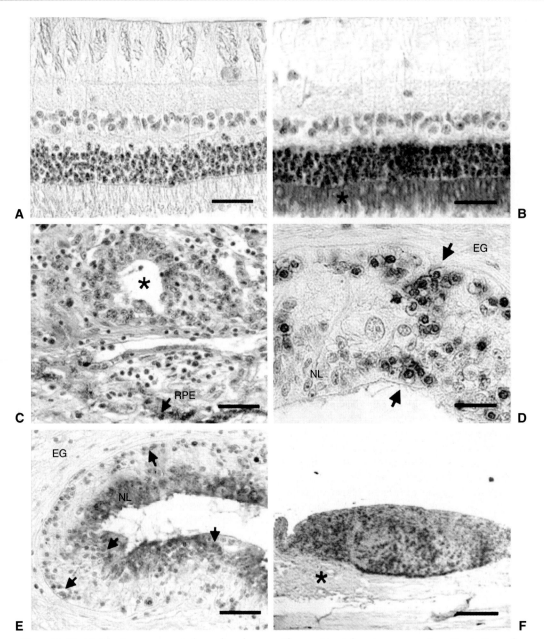

Figure 11-28. Histologic appearance of eyes from horses with experimental equine recurrent uveitis. **A,** Normal equine retina. *Bar,* 25 μm. **B,** Normal equine retina stained with antibodies to retinal S-antigen (S-Ag). Photoreceptor outer segments were clearly labeled *(red, *). Bar,* 20 μm. **C,** Affected horse with complete destruction of retinal architecture associated with immune-mediated disease directed against retinal S-Ag. CD3+ T cells *(brown)* are infiltrated around retinal neuronal cells. Leftover retinal pigment epithelial cells *(RPE)* and neovascularization were visible in the retina *(*). Bar,* 25 μm. **D,** Retinal infiltration by T cells (CD3+; *brown, arrows).* Destruction of photoreceptor outer segments with some remaining cells from the inner or outer nuclear layer and formation of epiretinal gliosis *(EG). NL,* Nuclear layer; *bar,* 15 μm. **E,** Severely destroyed retina in affected horse. Infiltration of CD3+ T cells *(brown, arrows)* in the nuclear layer *(NL)* of the remaining photoreceptor cells (visualized by red staining for S-Ag) and in the neuronal cell layer at the borderline to a severe epiretinal gliosis *(EG). Bar,* 40 μm. **F,** Subconjunctival lymphoid follicle (CD3+ cells stain red). **,* Sclera; *bar,* 120 μm. (From Deeg CA, et al. [2004]: The uveitogenic potential of retinal S-antigen in horses. Invest Ophthalmol Vis Sci 45:2286.)

active inflammation. In many patients long-term topical corticosteroid therapy is required to reduce the frequency and severity of subsequent attacks.

Additional approaches that can be used in unusually severe cases or cases refractory to the preceding approaches are as follows:

1. Topical NSAIDs (e.g., flurbiprofen 0.03%, 0.1% diclofenac, or another topical NSAID applied every 6 hours): These agents are not as potent as topical corticosteroids in ERU therapy, but in severe cases they may be used in addition to topical corticosteroids. Alternatively, they may be used long term, either alone or with topical corticosteroids in an effort to prevent recurrent

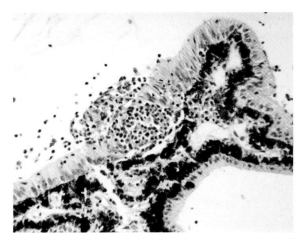

Figure 11-29. Lymphocytic inflammation of the ciliary body of a horse with chronic equine recurrent uveitis. (Courtesy Dr. Richard R Dubielzig.)

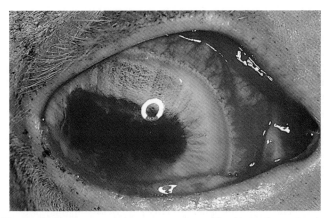

Figure 11-30. Acute equine recurrent uveitis. Note the extensive conjunctival hyperemia, miosis, and blue-green hue to the iris. The yellow serum of horses often makes a blue iris appear green.

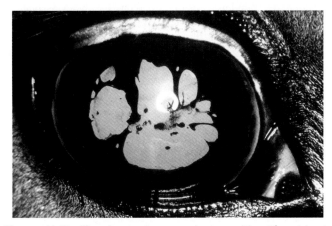

Figure 11-31. Chronic equine recurrent uveitis. The iris is hyperpigmented. Note also the numerous posterior synechiae and early cataract formation.

episodes. Topical NSAIDs can slow corneal epithelialization.

2. Cyclosporine A: Topical 0.2% cyclosporine ophthalmic ointment or 2% cyclosporine in oil applied every 6 to 12 hours has been suggested to be of value in the treatment of ERU. Because of the relatively limited intraocular penetration of this compound when applied topically, however, its efficacy appears to be somewhat less than that of topical corticosteroids. Experimentally, an intravitreal sustained-release insert containing cyclosporine has shown considerable promise in the treatment of ERU.

3. Subconjunctival corticosteroids (triamcinolone acetonide): Reported dosages for triamcinolone acetonide vary greatly from 1 to 2 mg per eye, to 20 mg per eye, to 40 mg per eye as often as every 1 to 3 weeks. Usual duration of action is 7 to 10 days. The major concern with this drug is that it creates a strong predisposition for bacterial and fungal keratitis and that, unlike topically applied corticosteroids, it cannot be withdrawn if the disease should occur. Therefore it is typically used as an adjunct to topical corticosteroids in the acute phase in especially severe cases or when the owner has difficulty medicating the horse as often as required. *Note:* The sustained-release vehicle in methylprednisolone acetate may result in an unsightly plaque and irritating granuloma.

4. Systemic corticosteroids (e.g., dexamethasone 5 to 10 mg/day PO or 2.5 to 5.0 mg daily IM or oral prednisolone 0.5 mg/kg q24h): In general, because of frequent adverse effects, systemic corticosteroids are used only as a last resort in the treatment of ERU. They can be considered in unusually severe cases or when the inflammation is refractory to systemic NSAIDS and topical corticosteroids. Side effects include laminitis and gastrointestinal upset.

5. Antibiotic therapy in horses with presumed leptospiral-associated uveitis: The efficacy of this therapy remains speculative, and side effects are not uncommon. Drugs that have been suggested include streptomycin (11 mg/kg IM q12h) and a 4-week course of oral doxycycline (10-20 mg/kg q12h). In one study by Gilmour et al., however, doxycycline at 10 mg/kg q12h orally did not result in appreciable drug concentrations in the aqueous humor or vitreous of normal eyes. Some researchers believe that the efficacy of vitrectomy for this disorder is due to the use of gentamicin in the irrigation fluid as much as the procedure itself. This theory has prompted some ophthalmologists to give a single intravitreal injection of 4 mg of **gentamicin** in an effort to prevent or eliminate recurrent episodes in severely affected eyes. Gentamicin injections, however, should be made with extreme caution because the drug may cause retinal degeneration, cataract formation, intraocular inflammation, endophthalmitis, and irreversible vision loss.

6. Surgical vitrectomy via a pars plana approach has been advocated by some workers to reduce the frequency and severity of attacks of ERU. The rationale for its use is based on the hypothesis that persistent organisms within the vitreal cavity (and perhaps the uveal tract) are capable of perpetuating an immune-mediated uveitis. Controlled clinical trials have yet to demonstrate the efficacy of this procedure, and cataracts are a common postoperative complication.

7. Vaccination is controversial. No approved vaccine is available for horses. The cross-reactivity of leptospiral antigens with normal constituents of the equine eye suggests that vaccination may actually cause the disease in some animals. Vaccination of seronegative horses with a multivalent bovine vaccine, with appropriate informed consent, may help suppress a herd outbreak. Vaccination as an adjunctive therapy in horses with ERU, however, failed

to slow the progression of the disease in one study (Rohrbach et al., 2005).

8. Enucleation is, on occasion, the only means of effectively treating a blind, painful globe.

Onchocerca Uveitis. *O. cervicalis* lives in the ligamentum nuchae of the horse. The microfilariae released by these adults migrate to the skin and ocular region and are transmitted by midges of the genus *Culicoides* and mosquitos. Ocular lesions are associated with the migration of the microfilariae from the ligamentum nuchae to the skin, some entering vessels of the bulbar and palpebral conjunctiva. The microfilariae are most readily found in the conjunctiva adjacent to the temporal limbus and in the corneal stroma adjacent to this area.

In 1971 Cello described the corneal lesions as "superficial subepithelial fluffy or feathery white opacities 0.5 to 1.0 mm in diameter, located 1 to 5 mm from the temporal limbus." The adjacent conjunctiva was hyperemic and chemotic, but biomicroscopic examination was required to demonstrate the corneal lesions.

The ocular lesions of onchocerciasis alone, including conjunctival vitiligo, are insufficient to indicate the presence of microfilariae. Unilateral ocular infestations with microfilariae may also occur.

ERU is said to be caused by the dead microfilariae or to be mediated by immunopathologic mechanisms involving IgE. Diethylcarbamazine stimulates IgE antibody responses. This feature, rather than a reaction by the host to killed microfilariae, may explain the inflammation seen after its administration.

Microfilariae are demonstrated by removing, under local anesthesia, (1) a small piece of conjunctiva from the affected area or (2) a piece of skin from the ventral thoracic midline. The tissue is minced with scissors and placed in 5 mL of saline at 37° C for 30 to 50 minutes (e.g., in a small vial in the clinician's pocket). The supernatant is centrifuged and examined for motile microfilariae. Alternatively, the tissue may be examined in saline on a slide immediately after collection. Interpretation of such slides must be made in association with other clinical findings, because many horses without ERU have microfilariae.

Microfilaricides must not be used during acute uveitis.

Treatment. The treatment is the same as that for *Leptospira*-associated uveitis. After the inflammation has subsided, ivermectin 0.2 mg/kg may be administered systemically. A single dose of ivermectin 0.2 mg/kg was found to be very effective in eliminating microfilariae from the skin of horses afflicted with dermatitis due to *O. cervicalis*. Alternatively, diethylcarbamazine 4 mg/kg daily is administered in the food for 21 days. At the first sign of recurrent inflammation during treatment, corticosteroid therapy is begun. In endemic areas prophylactic feeding of diethylcarbamazine and aspirin is recommended throughout the season when vectors are present. Aspirin may also be used continuously. The routine use of ivermectin and other highly effective anthelmintics appears to have substantially reduced the incidence of onchocercal uveitis in the United States.

UVEITIS DUE TO *Dirofilaria immitis*. Mature and immature adult dirofilaria are infrequently reported in the anterior chamber of dogs. Treatment is surgical removal. If adulticides are used while adult worms are present in the anterior chamber, severe uveitis and endophthalmitis may result. Severe

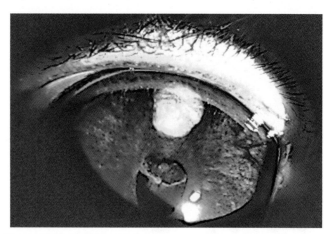

Figure 11-32. Uveitis and focal lens capsule rupture with cataract formation associated with the protozoan *Encephalitozoon cuniculi* in a rabbit.

endophthalmitis has also been observed when microfilariae are present in the eye and an adulticide is administered.

PHACOCLASTIC UVEITIS IN RABBITS. An unusual form of uveitis associated with apparent spontaneous lens capsule rupture, phacoclastic uveitis, occurs in the rabbit and frequently results in enucleation (Figure 11-32). Organisms believed to be *Encephalitozoon cuniculi* have been identified in affected lenses. Clinical signs of infection include a white or yellowish uveal or anterior chamber mass that progresses to severe uveitis and glaucoma that is usually refractory to treatment. Early lens removal has been suggested as a method of treatment to prevent development of uveitis.

TOXIC UVEITIS. The eye is exquisitely sensitive to bacterial endotoxins, and amounts as small as a few nanograms are capable of inducing substantial uveitis. Other toxic agents are pilocarpine and other topical parasympathomimetics as well as topical prostaglandins used in the treatment of glaucoma (e.g., latanoprost). Ethylene glycol poisoning has been associated with anterior uveitis in dogs. Sulfa-containing drugs and those associated with thrombocytopenia or coagulopathies have also been associated with uveitis (usually associated with hemorrhage).

TRAUMA

Traumatic Uveitis

Trauma is a common cause of uveitis in domestic animals.

Uveitis may result from either blunt or sharp trauma to the globe or may occur after intraocular surgical procedures. Therapy is the same as that for other forms of uveitis, although topical corticosteroids should be avoided if a corneal erosion or ulceration is present; in this case topical NSAIDS may be used, although they, too, may impair corneal epithelialization and there is some potential for topical NSAIDS to elicit a corneal melt. Topical and systemic NSAIDs are also typically avoided if significant intraocular hemorrhage is present. If the corneal epithelium is not intact, a topical antibiotic such as neomycin–polymyxin B–bacitracin combination product applied every 6 to 8 hours should be used prophylactically. If the globe has been penetrated, the wound may require suturing and systemic antibiotics in addition to topical therapy. Traumatic uveitis is aggressively treated in the horse because a traumatic breakdown of the blood-aqueous barrier may increase the risk of recurrent episodes of uveitis.

In severe ocular trauma, early and vigorous treatment is required to prevent permanent ocular damage and, perhaps, repeated episodes of uveitis.

In many cases the long-term prognosis of traumatic uveitis is determined more by the nature of the injury than by the therapy that was chosen.

Common uveal injuries are as follows:

* *Iris prolapse:* Protrusion of a portion of the iris through a corneal or scleral perforation
* *Hyphema:* Hemorrhage into the anterior chamber
* *Staphyloma:* A weakened or protruding lesion in the cornea or sclera into which a portion of the uvea protrudes from the inside; the uveal tissue usually adheres to the cornea or sclera
* *Concussion*
* *Iridodialysis:* Tearing of the iris from the ciliary body at its root. This condition is uncommon in domestic animals. Iris prolapse and hyphema are discussed in greater detail later.

Iris Prolapse

Iris prolapse is a common sequela to penetrating corneal wounds or ruptured corneal ulcers. The iris is carried forward into the corneal defect by escaping aqueous. Emergency treatment of such injuries is described in Chapter 19. When iris passes through such a corneal defect, its vascular supply is usually compromised, resulting in venous congestion and edema. This changes the appearance of the protruding mass so that it commonly looks like uvea-colored mucus adhering to the cornea.

Signs

Clinical signs of iris prolapse are as follows:

* The color of the prolapsed portion becomes lighter than the remaining iris.
* The protruding iris tissue forms a mound on the cornea.
* The tissue has a gelatinous mucoid appearance and frequently attracts adhering strands of conjunctival mucus.
* The pupil is eccentric as a result of traction of the protruding iris tissue.
* The corneal wound is often obscured by the edematous iris tissue. Protrusion of the ciliary body occurs most commonly in horses as a result of scleral rupture posterior to the limbus after blunt trauma.

Treatment

If the corneal wound is small, iris prolapse may be treated temporarily with a third-eyelid flap and topical and systemic antibiotic solutions until specialized assistance is available. In larger wounds requiring immediate repair, an attempt is made to replace the iris with an iris spatula before the cornea is sutured. If this is not possible, the protruding piece may be carefully excised with the use of an electrosurgical unit. The cornea is sutured, and the anterior chamber reconstituted with balanced salt solution or an air bubble. *Caution:* If the major arterial circle of the iris is transected, profuse intraocular hemorrhage can result. Enucleation or evisceration and intrascleral prosthesis are alternative therapies if the eye is blind.

Visual Outcome and Ocular Survival after Iris Prolapse in Horses

Iris prolapse is usually associated with a ruptured corneal ulcer or full-thickness corneal laceration. In a review of 32 cases, combined medical and surgical therapy (primary closure with or without a conjunctival graft) was successful in saving vision of 40% of eyes with perforating corneal disease (ulcers or stromal abscesses) and 33% of eyes with perforating lacerations (Chmielewski et al., 1997). Complications resulting in blindness included phthisis bulbi, extensive keratomalacia, and endophthalmitis. A favorable visual result was more likely in horses presented for specialist care with ulcers of less than 15 days' duration or corneal lacerations smaller than 15 mm.

HYPHEMA

The emergency treatment of hyphema is discussed in Chapter 19.

Etiology

Hyphema may be idiopathic or may result from many factors, such as the following:

* Traumatic disruption of a uveal blood vessel: sharp or blunt trauma, severe pressure around the neck as in choking or increased intrathoracic pressure in severe traumatic compression of the chest or dystocia
* Fragility of vessel walls, especially preiridal fibrovascular membranes that form in response to chronic disorders causing intraocular hypoxia (e.g., inflammation, glaucoma, retinal detachments, neoplasia, or after intraocular surgery)
* Clotting disorders, platelet disturbances, and blood dyscrasias
* Highly vascularized tumors
* Severe uveitis
* Retinal dysplasia with rupture of vessels
* Systemic disease (e.g., tropical canine pancytopenia, Rocky Mountain spotted fever)

Erythrocytes released into the anterior chamber undergo phagocytosis by the cells lining the trabecular meshwork. The surface of the iris provides fibrinolysin, which aids in resolving clots in the anterior chamber. The sequelae of hyphema often have a greater impact on the ultimate visual outcome than the hemorrhage itself (Figure 11-33).

Most hyphemas are small and are resorbed spontaneously in a few days.

Treatment

The treatment of hyphema is controversial because of conflicting experimental results with different drug regimens in different species. In the vast majority of patients surgical drainage of the hyphema is not useful because rebleeding is frequent. The

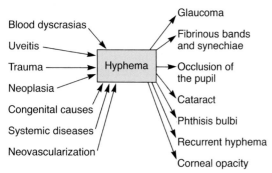

Figure 11-33. Causes and effects of hyphema. (Modified from Blogg JR [1980]: The Eye in Veterinary Practice. Saunders, Philadelphia.)

procedure may be considered, however, in patients with glaucoma secondary to blood in the anterior chamber in which the cause of the bleeding has been controlled. Although different methods are used, the aims are to:

- Identify the cause
- Prevent recurrent bleeding
- Control uveitis
- Limit the sequelae of uveitis

Surgical removal of clots from the anterior chamber is generally not an effective therapy.

The following treatment is recommended for hyphemia:

1. Prevent further trauma by immediate and enforced cage or stall rest.
2. Administer corticosteroid drops (dexamethasone 0.1%, prednisolone 1%) three times daily. NSAIDs are not used because of their effects on platelets and blood clotting.
3. Intracameral tissue plasminogen activator may be beneficial in select patients.

Additional Therapy for Mild Hyphemia

1. If the hyphema is not secondary to uveitis, administer 1% to 2% pilocarpine drops three times daily and attempt to dilate the pupil every second day with phenylephrine (10%) to prevent synechia formation.
2. If the hyphema is secondary to uveitis, dilate the pupil with 1% atropine every 8 to 12 hours.
3. Monitor IOP.

Additional Therapy for Severe Hyphemia

1. Instead of pilocarpine, use 1% atropine ophthalmic ointment or solution three times daily to relieve pain if present.
2. Administer systemic corticosteroids (e.g., prednisolone or dexamethasone) in appropriate systemic dosages.
3. Monitor IOP twice daily.
4. If glaucoma is incipient, use a topical or systemic carbonic anhydrase inhibitor or topical dipivefrin.

Recurrent Hyphema

If the hyphema is recurrent, a complete laboratory examination, including measurement of complete blood count, platelets, and clotting parameters, is indicated. In the absence of specific indi-

cations, use of vitamins C and K is not advised, nor are such agents as proteolytic enzymes or carbonic anhydrase inhibitors. Recurrent hyphema, especially with glaucoma, should prompt the clinician to rule out intraocular neoplasia as the cause of the bleeding.

UVEAL CYSTS AND NEOPLASMS

The uvea may be affected by cystic disorders that mimic neoplasia or by both primary and secondary neoplasms. Intraocular tumors frequently are also accompanied by glaucoma, intraocular hemorrhage, or chronic unresponsive uveitis.

Uveal Cysts

Uveal cysts are fluid-filled, ovoid to spherical structures that originate from the posterior pigmented epithelium of the iris or the ciliary body. Although they may represent a recessively inherited, congenital uveal defect (especially in Great Danes and golden retrievers), they are often not seen until adulthood. They also are commonly seen in Boston terriers and occasionally in cats and Rocky Mountain horses. A second type of cyst in horses may be seen within the iris stroma at its base in lightly pigmented irides. Uveal cysts may also occur secondary to inflammation. The cysts either remain attached or break free and float into the anterior chamber, either singly or in groups (Figure 11-34). In the anterior chamber they may float free or adhere to the iris or corneal endothelium, occasionally obstructing the visual axis and the pupil. Deflated cysts appear as patches of pigment adherent to the corneal endothelium. In rare circumstances large numbers of cysts may push the iris root forward, causing secondary closed-angle glaucoma. Uveal cysts may be differentiated from a pigmented neoplasm or iris nevus by the ability of the cyst to be transilluminated with a bright focal light, although this feature may be sometimes difficult to appreciate in horses or very heavily pigmented cysts. In such cases ultrasonography may be required to differentiate a cyst from neoplasia.

Removal of a uveal cyst is rarely indicated but should be considered in the following circumstances:

- The pupil is obstructed, impairing vision.
- Glaucoma is impending or present owing to anterior displacement of the iris by large numbers of cysts, or multiple cysts are present and the debris liberated by their collapse may obstruct the trabecular meshwork.

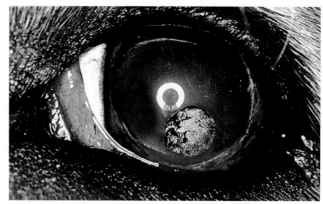

Figure 11-34. Causes and effects of hyphema. (Modified from Blogg JR [1980]: The Eye in Veterinary Practice. Saunders, Philadelphia.)

- The cyst is contacting the corneal endothelium, causing corneal edema.

Cysts may be removed by aspiration under microsurgical control or deflated by laser photocoagulation.

Cystic Corpora Nigra in Horses

Corpora nigra generally occupy the central portions of the upper and lower pupillary margins. Cystic corpora nigra appear as large, smooth structures at the pupillary margin. They may obstruct the pupil enough to cause visual impairment or blindness, manifested as decreased jumping performance or head shaking.

The differential diagnosis for such cysts is as follows:

- Cystic dilation of the iris stroma (blue or lightly pigmented irides)
- Free-floating iris cysts
- Pigmented neoplasms, such as melanoma
- Hypertrophic corpora nigra
- Inflammatory nodules

Cystic dilations of the iris stroma and free-floating iris cysts in horses rarely require treatment. Cystic corpora nigra must be distinguished from neoplasms, but they do not transilluminate readily. Cystic corpora nigra have a smooth appearance, whereas melanomas and hypertrophic corpora nigra have a roughened surface. Ultrasonography may be used to distinguish cystic corpora nigra from melanoma or hypertrophic corpora nigra. Cystic corpora nigra may be removed by aspiration under microsurgical control or with laser therapy.

Primary Tumors

Of the primary uveal tumor types listed in Box 11-1, adenoma, adenocarcinoma, and melanoma are the most common. Iris nevi were discussed earlier.

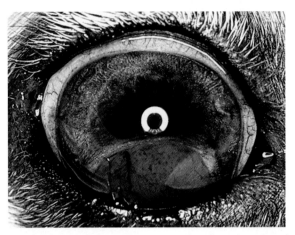

Figure 11-35. Ciliary body adenoma extending from the ciliary body through the iris and into the anterior chamber of a dog. (Courtesy University of Wisconsin–Madison Veterinary Ophthalmology Service Collection.)

Adenocarcinoma and Adenoma

Neoplasms of the ciliary epithelium are occasionally observed in dogs. Such a lesion usually appears as a single mass protruding from behind the iris into the pupil (Figure 11-35). The mass may be pigmented or unpigmented, depending on whether it arose from pigmented or unpigmented ciliary epithelium, and must be distinguished from melanocytoma or potentially malignant melanoma of the same site. The neoplasms infrequently infiltrate anteriorly into the drainage angle and iris, elevating IOP. The extent of the lesion may be outlined by transillumination and reflected light from the tapetum, and by ultrasonography. Treatment consists of removal of the tumor and adjacent ciliary body (iridocyclectomy), frequently including replacement of the defect with a scleral graft, laser cyclodestruction, or, if the tumor is extensive, enucleation. Provided that the tumor has remained within the globe, the prognosis for survival is good.

Melanocytoma and Melanoma

Although the vast majority of uveal melanomas are benign, malignant tumors arising from the iris, ciliary body, or, less commonly, the choroid do occur. They are most common in dogs and cats and less common in horses and cattle. Mitotic index is a more useful indicator of behavior and prognosis in dogs than the histologic criteria used for human ocular melanomas. The potential for metastasis is present, but different studies demonstrate wide variation in observed rates, making generalizations difficult. Intraocular and palpebral melanomas in cats have a greater tendency to metastasize and are more malignant than those in dogs, with higher rates of mortality and metastasis.

Melanoma in dogs and cats, unlike that in humans, occurs more frequently in the iris and ciliary body (Figure 11-36) than in the choroid and has a reasonable prognosis for survival if the eye is enucleated before the tumor has penetrated the sclera. Penetration may occur via ciliary arteries, veins, or nerves, by direct extension, or via the optic nerve. In a study of feline ocular melanomas by Patnaik and Mooney (1988) 10 of 16 uveal melanomas had metastases before enucleation. On the basis of tumor behavior in only three animals in the same study, feline palpebral melanomas may have a high rate of metastasis.

Box 11-1 | Classification of primary tumors

Melanocytes
Acquired

Iris nevus
Melanocytoma (benign)
Melanoma (potentially malignant)
Diffuse iris melanoma (feline)

Ciliary Epithelium
Congenital

Benign medulloepithelioma
Malignant medulloepithelioma
Benign teratoid medulloepithelioma
Malignant teratoid medulloepithelioma

Acquired

Nonpigmented:
   Adenoma
   Adenocarcinoma
Pigmented:
   Adenoma
   Adenocarcinoma

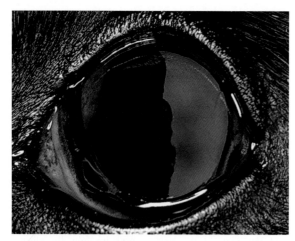

Figure 11-36. Ciliary body tumor (melanoma) in a dog. The mass is posterior to the iris but extends through the iris nasally. (Courtesy University of Wisconsin–Madison Veterinary Ophthalmology Service Collection.)

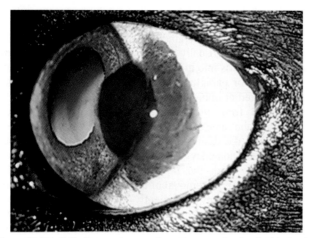

Figure 11-37. Epibulbar melanoma in a German shepherd. This benign tumor must be differentiated from an intraocular tumor that has broken through the sclera.

Epibulbar melanomas occur in dogs, cats, and horses (Figure 11-37). In dogs the average age of onset is 6 years, the most common site is the superior limbus, and the German shepherd has a higher incidence. These tumors grow slowly and are treated with local surgical excision, cryotherapy, or laser photoablation. The resulting defect may require structural support with a graft of autogenous or heterologous tissue or a synthetic material. Small, slow-growing tumors in older animals or animals with limited life span may simply be observed.

CLINICAL SIGNS. Melanomas usually cause the following clinical signs:

- Change in color or visible mass in the iris
- Uveitis or endophthalmitis due to necrosis of the tumor; cornea is often opaque
- Hyphema
- Secondary glaucoma

Melanomas often cause secondary glaucoma.

TREATMENT. Treatment of melanomas and melanocytomas consists of the following measures:

1. If the tumor is small or localized, local excision with *iridectomy* or *iridocyclectomy,* or alternatively with diode or neodymium:yttrium-aluminum-garnet (Nd:YAG) laser photocoagulation may be considered. By the time clinical signs are present, many tumors are too large for this treatment.
2. Enucleation of the globe is often mandated by the presence of intractable glaucoma, uveitis, or hyphema.

The prognosis for the animal's survival after enucleation is good; in one study, only 7 of 129 canine uveal melanomas had confirmed metastases. If there is any indication of scleral penetration, *orbital exenteration* is performed in an attempt to remove tumor cells. Frequent postoperative examinations (every 3 months for a year, then annually) are advisable, with special attention given to the submandibular, retropharyngeal, and bronchial lymph nodes. Adjunctive chemotherapy or radiation therapy may be used, although the efficacy of these treatments is unclear.

Primary Feline Ocular Sarcomas

Posttraumatic sarcomas of the feline eye have been reported to occasionally occur months to years after severe ocular trauma. Although the vast majority of cats with primary ocular sarcomas have a history of penetrating trauma that damaged the lens and/or other intraocular structures, a few cases have been described in which there is no history of trauma, infection, or ocular surgery. In addition to clinical signs consistent with the injury, signs of ocular sarcoma are chronic, relatively unresponsive uveitis, glaucoma with buphthalmos, and a previously phthisical eye that is now enlarging. Metastasis or local recurrence after enucleation is common. Because it lines the inner surface of the globe, the tumor commonly extends into the orbit via the optic nerve. Metaplastic bone has also been observed in ocular sarcomas. Although some researchers have suggested removal of all traumatized or phthisical feline eyes to prevent development of this rare tumor, the value of this approach remains to be determined.

Feline Diffuse Iris Melanoma

The diffuse iris melanoma seen in cats has specific features that differentiate it from other anterior uveal tumors. The tumor is often *very* slowly progressive, arising from pigmented areas on the anterior surface of the iris (see Figure 11-22) and perhaps eventually involve the iridocorneal angle, causing secondary glaucoma (Figure 11-38). In some cats, however, the tumor is rapidly progressive and quick to metastasize. Although the tumor is potentially malignant, the risk for metastasis in the majority of cats appears to be relatively low. Cats with this disorder should be regularly evaluated by a veterinary ophthalmologist to ascertain whether or when enucleation may be indicated. In single or multiple early iris melanomas that are progressing, tumor ablation with laser therapy may be useful. Because the disease is slowly progressive, the clinical conflict is whether to simply observe the patient or enucleate a functional eye if persistence of such an eye may present a risk to the animal's life through metastasis. Many affected cats, however, even those with metastatic disease, may live for long periods with few ill effects.

All pigmented iris tumors in cats should be referred to a veterinary ophthalmologist for evaluation and long-term therapy.

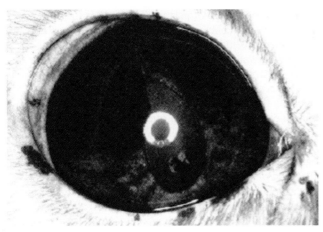

Figure 11-38. Diffuse iris melanoma in a cat. The iris is diffusely infiltrated, and the pupil is dyscoric. Enucleation is advised.

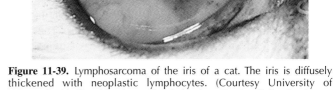

Figure 11-39. Lymphosarcoma of the iris of a cat. The iris is diffusely thickened with neoplastic lymphocytes. (Courtesy University of Wisconsin–Madison Veterinary Ophthalmology Service Collection.)

Criteria for considering enucleation of an eye with a progressively enlarging hyperpigmented iridal lesion are as follows:

- Noticeable thickening of the iris stroma with distortion of the pupil or its mobility
- Involvement of the ciliary body
- Extension into the sclera
- Secondary glaucoma
- Intractable uveitis

Secondary Tumors

With the exception of lymphosarcoma, tumors metastasizing to the uvea are uncommon. Although any metastatic tumor may potentially spread to the eye, the most common tumors to do so in dogs are mammary carcinoma, hemangiosarcoma, thyroid, pancreatic and renal carcinomas, malignant melanoma of the skin, seminoma, and rhabdomyosarcoma. Any metastatic tumor may spread to the eye, however.

Lymphosarcoma

Ocular manifestations of lymphosarcoma occur in the dog, cat, cow, and horse (see Chapter 18). In the dog ocular manifestations are clinically similar to those of uveitis and endophthalmitis; they include iridal swelling, hyphema, aqueous flare, retinopathy and retinal detachment, conjunctivitis, keratitis, noninflammatory chemosis, corneal edema with vascularization, KPs, intrastromal corneal hemorrhage, miosis, hypotony, ciliary injection, and secondary glaucoma. Approximately 40% of dogs with lymphosarcoma show some ocular signs. Histologically, the iris and ciliary body are more frequently affected than the choroid. Dogs with ocular signs may have a poorer prognosis for long-term remission and response to chemotherapy. Detailed consideration of chemotherapy for lymphosarcoma is beyond the scope of this book; however, animals blinded by lymphosarcoma *may* recover vision once chemotherapy with one of the standard regimens is begun. Adjunctive topical therapy with corticosteroids, atropine, and antiglaucoma drugs should be considered in animals with uveitis secondary to lymphosarcoma.

In cats similar but less common ocular lesions occur in lymphosarcoma, myeloproliferative disease, reticuloendotheliosis, feline immunodeficiency virus infection, and feline leukemia virus infection (Figure 11-39). Older male cats are more frequently affected with ocular lymphosarcoma; ocular signs were the initial presenting sign in more than 50% of affected cats in a retrospective pathologic study by Corcoran et al. (1995). In cattle ocular lesions in lymphosarcoma are restricted to infiltration of orbital tissues, often resulting in exophthalmos with exposure keratitis. Up to 10% of cattle with lymphosarcoma may have exophthalmos.

Lymphosarcoma should be considered in cattle with exophthalmos.

In poultry, infiltration of the iris and uveal tract with a change in color to bluish gray ("pearly eye") is seen in Marek's disease; it is called *epidemic blindness*.

MISCELLANEOUS DISORDERS

Iris Hypoplasia

In congenital iris hypoplasia in color-dilute, albinotic, and subalbinotic animals, the iridal holes may progress over time, leaving large spaces in the iris.

Iris Atrophy

Several types of iris atrophy occur, as discussed here.

Primary Iris Atrophy

A slowly progressive iris atrophy in previously normal adults occurs in dogs and cats. Spaces and holes develop in the iris, often leading to dyscoria, and are especially visible on retroillumination, in which light is reflected from the tapetum back toward the examiner. The condition is especially seen in Siamese cats, miniature schnauzers, poodles, and Chihuahuas but may occur in any breed. Although the disorder is not typically associated with obvious clinical signs, anisocoria may be present, and the pupillary light reflex may be diminished or, occasionally, absent.

Secondary Iris Atrophy

Atrophy of the iris may occur after the following conditions:

- Chronic glaucoma
- Chronic recurrent uveitis
- Severe ocular trauma

Senile Iris Atrophy

Senile iris atrophy occurs in older animals of all species and is characterized by irregular pupillary margins, spaces in the iris, and sluggishness or absence of pupillary reflexes. The condition must be distinguished from secondary iris atrophy. It is common in toy and miniature poodles, miniature schnauzers, and Chihuahuas and is significant in the evaluation of patients with cataract or visual impairment (Figure 11-40).

SURGICAL PROCEDURES

Surgical procedures for primary diseases of the iris are rarely performed, even in specialty practice. Examples are as follows:

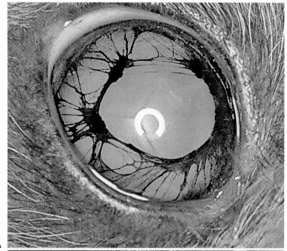

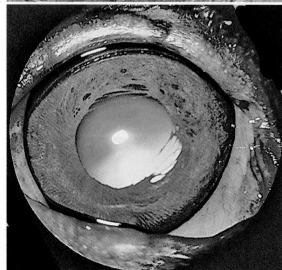

Figure 11-40. A, Marked iris atrophy in a miniature poodle. Full-thickness holes in the iris are readily visible. **B,** Milder form of iris atrophy. Note that the pupil is dyscoric and that the pupillary light reflex in such cases is often reduced.

- *Iridectomy* (removal of part of the iris): For focal circumscribed melanomas of the iris. Such lesions may also be treated by diode or Nd:YAG laser photocoagulation.
- *Iridocyclectomy* (removal of a portion of iris and ciliary body): For neoplasms of the ciliary body. Many neoplasms are too advanced at presentation for this procedure, but for those in the early stages the technique, although demanding, allows removal of affected tissue and salvage of the eye and vision. For larger neoplasms infiltrating the sclera, the scleral defect may be replaced with an autogenous graft.
- *Sphincterotomy* (incision of the sphincter): Performed occasionally during cataract surgery. The sphincter is cut in one or more places, if mydriasis is poor, to allow access to the lens and to reduce the chance of a small pupil postoperatively. Since the advent of NSAIDs the technique is rarely necessary. The use of iridectomy and iridencleisis for canine glaucoma has been superseded by cyclocryotherapy and laser cyclotherapy (see Chapter 12).

BIBLIOGRAPHY

Angles JM, et al. (2005): Uveodermatologic (VKH-like) syndrome in American Akita dogs is associated with an increased frequency of DQA1*00201. Tissue Antigens 66:656.

Bergsma DR, Brown KS (1971): White fur, blue eyes and deafness in the domestic cat. J Hered 62:171.

Bistner SI, et al. (1972): A review of persistent pupillary membrane in the basenji dog. J Am Anim Hosp Assoc 7:143.

Carter WJ, et al. (2005): An immunohistochemical study of uveodermatologic syndrome in two Japanese Akita dogs. Vet Ophthalmol 8:17.

Cello RM (1971): Ocular onchocerciasis in the horse. Equine Vet J 3:148.

Chavkin MJ, et al. (1992): Seroepidemiologic and clinical observations of 93 cases of uveitis in cats. Prog Vet Comp Ophthalmol 2:29.

Chmielewski NT, et al. (1997): Visual outcome and ocular survival following iris prolapse in the horse: a review of 32 cases. Equine Vet J 29:31.

Colitz CMH (2005): Feline uveitis: diagnosis and treatment. Clin Tech Small Anim Pract 20:117.

Collins BK, Moore CP (1999): Diseases and surgery of the canine uvea, in Gelatt KN: Veterinary Ophthalmology, 2nd ed. Lippincott Williams & Wilkins, Philadelphia.

Collinson PN, Peiffer RL (1994): Clinical presentation, morphology, and behavior of primary choroidal melanomas in eight dogs. Prog Vet Comp Ophthalmol 3:158.

Corcoran KA, et al. (1995): Histopathologic features of feline ocular lymphosarcoma: 49 cases (1978-1992). Vet Comp Ophthalmol 5:35.

Corcoran KA, Koch SA (1993): Uveal cysts in dogs: 28 cases (1989-1991). J Am Vet Med Assoc 203:545.

Davidson MG (2000): Toxoplasmosis. Vet Clin North Am Small Anim Pract 30:1051.

Davidson MG, et al. (1991): Feline anterior uveitis: a study of 53 cases. J Am Anim Hosp Assoc 27:77.

Davidson MG, et al. (1989): Ocular manifestations of Rocky Mountain spotted fever in dogs. J Am Vet Med Assoc 194:777.

Deeg CA, et al. (2006): Inter- and intramolecular epitope spreading in equine recurrent uveitis. Invest Ophthalmol Vis Sci 47:652.

Deeg CA, et al. (2004): Equine recurrent uveitis is strongly associated with the MHC class I haplotype ELA-A9. Equine Vet J 36:73.

Deeg CA, et al. (2004): The uveitogenic potential of retinal S-antigen in horses. Invest Ophthalmol Vis Sci 45:2286.

Deeg CA, et al. (2002): Immunopathology of recurrent uveitis in spontaneously diseased horses. Exp Eye Res 75:127.

Deeg CA, et al. (2002): Uveitis in horses induced by interphotoreceptor retinoid-binding protein is similar to the spontaneous disease. Eur J Immunol 32:2598.

Deeg CA, et al. (2001): Immune responses to retinal autoantigens and peptides in equine recurrent uveitis. Invest Ophthalmol Vis Sci 42:393.

Deehr AJ, Dubielzig R (1997): Glaucoma in golden retrievers, in Proceedings of the American College of Veterinary Ophthalmologists, 28th Annual Meeting, Santa Fe, NM, p. 105.

Denis HM, et al. (2003): Detection of anti-lens crystallin antibody in dogs with and without cataracts. Vet Ophthalmol 6:321.

Dubielzig RR (1995): Morphologic features of feline ocular sarcoma in 10 cats: light microscopy, ultrastructure and immunohistochemistry. Vet Comp Ophthalmol 4:7.

Duncan DE, Peiffer RL (1991): Morphology and prognostic indicators of anterior uveal melanomas in cats. Prog Vet Comp Ophthalmol 1:25.

Dwyer AE, et al. (1995): Association of leptospiral seroreactivity and breed with uveitis and blindness in horses: 372 cases (1986-1993). J Am Vet Med Assoc 207:1327.

Eule JC, et al. (2000): [Occurrence of various immunoglobulin isotopes in horses with equine recurrent uveitis (ERU)]. Berl Munch Tierarztl Wochenschr 113:253.

Ewart SL, et al. (2000): The horse homolog of congenital aniridia conforms to codominant inheritance. J Hered 91:93.

Faber NA, et al. (2000): Detection of *Leptospira* spp. in the aqueous humor of horses with naturally acquired recurrent uveitis. J Clin Microbiol 38:2731.

French DD, et al. (1988): Efficacy of ivermectin in paste and injectable formulations against microfilariae of *Onchocerca cervicalis* and resolution of associated dermatitis in horses. Am J Vet Res 49:1550.

Gelatt KN, et al. (1969): Ocular anomalies of incomplete albino cattle: ophthalmoscopic examination. Am J Vet Res 30:1313.

Gemensky-Metzler AJ, et al. (2004): The use of semiconductor diode laser for deflation and coagulation of anterior uveal cysts in dogs, cats and horses: a report of 20 cases. Vet Ophthalmol 7:360.

Gilger B, et al. (1997): Neodymium:yttrium-aluminum-garnet laser treatment of cystic granula iridica in horses: eight cases (1988-1996). J Vet Med Assoc 211:341.

Gilger BC, et al. (2001): Use of an intravitreal sustained-release cyclosporine delivery device for treatment of equine recurrent uveitis. Am J Vet Res 62:1892.

Gilger BC, et al. (2000): Effect of an intravitreal cyclosporine implant on experimental uveitis in horses. Vet Immunol Immunopathol 76:239.

Gilger BC, Michau TM (2004): Equine recurrent uveitis: new methods of management. Vet Clin North Am Equine Pract 20:417.

Gilmour MA, et al. (2005): Ocular penetration of oral doxycycline in the horse. Vet Ophthalmol 8:331.

Grahn BH, Cullen CL (2000): Equine phacoclastic uveitis: the clinical manifestations, light microscopic findings, and therapy of 7 cases. Can Vet J 41:376.

Halliwell RE, et al. (1985): Studies on equine recurrent uveitis II: the role of infection with *Leptospira interrogans* serovar *pomona*. Curr Eye Res 4:1033.

Halliwell RH, Hines MT (1985): Studies on equine recurrent uveitis I: levels of immunoglobulin and albumin in the aqueous humor of horses with and without intraocular disease. Curr Eye Res 4:1023.

Hartskeerl RA, et al. (2004): Classification of *Leptospira* from the eyes of horses suffering from recurrent uveitis. J Vet Med 51:110.

Herd RP, Donham JC (1983): Efficacy of ivermectin against *Onchocerca cervicalis* microfilarial dermatitis in horses. Am J Vet Res 44:1102.

Huston K, et al. (1968): Heterochromia iridis in dairy cattle. J Dairy Sci 51:1101.

Kalsow CM, Dwyer AE (1998): Retinal immunopathology in horses with uveitis. Ocular Immunol Inflamm 6:239.

Kern TJ, et al. (1985): Uveitis associated with poliosis and vitiligo in six dogs. J Am Vet Med Assoc 187:408.

Koutinas AF, et al. (1999): Clinical considerations on canine visceral leishmaniasis in Greece: a retrospective study of 158 cases (1989-1996). J Am Anim Hosp Assoc 35:376.

Krohne SG, et al. (1994): Prevalence of ocular involvement in dogs with multicentric lymphosarcoma: prospective evaluation of 94 cases. Vet Comp Ophthalmol 4:127.

Lappin MR (2000): Feline infectious uveitis. J Feline Med Surg 2:159.

Lappin MR, et al. (1995): Detection of *Toxoplasma gondii*-specific IgA in the aqueous humor of cats. Am J Vet Res 56:774.

Lappin MR, Black JC (1999): *Bartonella* spp infection as a possible cause of uveitis in a cat. J Am Vet Med Assoc 214:1205.

Leiva M, et al. (2005): Ocular signs of canine monocytic ehrlichiosis: a retrospective study in dogs from Barcelona, Spain. Vet Ophthalmol 8:387.

Loesenbeck G, et al. (1996): Immunohistochemical findings in eyes of cats serologically positive for feline immunodeficiency virus (FIV). Zentralbl Veterinaermed B 43:305.

Lucchesi PM, Parma AE (1999): A DNA fragment of *Leptospira interrogans* encodes a protein which shares epitopes with equine cornea. Vet Immunol Immunopathol 71:173.

Lucchesi PMA, et al. (2002): Serovar distribution of a DNA sequence involved in the antigenic relationship between *Leptospira* and equine cornea. BMC Microbiol 2:3.

Maggs DJ, et al. (1999): Detection of feline herpesvirus-specific antibodies and DNA in aqueous humor from cats with or without uveitis. Am J Vet Res 60:932.

Massa KL, et al. (2002): Causes of uveitis in dogs: 102 cases (1989-2000). Vet Ophthalmol 5:93.

Michau TM, et al. (2003): *Bartonella vinsonii* subspecies *berkhoffi* as a possible cause of anterior uveitis and choroiditis in a dog. Vet Ophthalmol 6:299.

Murphy CJ, et al. (1991): Anti-retinal antibodies associated with Vogt-Koyanagi-Harada-like syndrome in a dog. J Am Anim Hosp Assoc 27:399-402.

Patnaik AK, Mooney S (1988): Feline melanoma: a comparative study of ocular, oral and dermal neoplasms. Vet Pathol 25:105.

Peiffer RL, Wilcock BP (1991): Histopathologic study of uveitis in cats: 139 cases (1978-1988). J Vet Med Assoc 198:135.

Roberts SR (1963): Fundic lesions in equine periodic ophthalmia. Am J Ophthalmol 55:1049.

Rohrbach BW, et al. (2005): Effect of vaccination against leptospirosis on the frequency, days to recurrence and progression of disease in horses with equine recurrent uveitis. Vet Ophthalmol 8:171.

Romeike A, et al. (1998): Immunohistochemical studies in equine recurrent uveitis (ERU). Vet Pathol 35:515.

Ryan AM, Diters RW (1984): Clinical and pathologic features of canine ocular melanomas. J Am Vet Med Assoc 184:60.

Schaffer EM, Funke K (1985): Primary intraocular melanomas in dogs and cats. Tierarztl Prax 13:343.

Schmidt GM, et al. (1982): Equine ocular onchocerciasis: histopathologic study. Am J Vet Res 43:1371.

Spiess BM, et al. (1996): [Eye injuries in the dog caused by cat claws]. Schweiz Archiv Tierheilkd 138:429.

Sullivan TC, et al. (1996): Photocoagulation of limbal melanomas in dogs and cats: 13 cases. J Am Vet Med Assoc 208:891.

Trepanier LA (2004): Idiosyncratic toxicity associated with potentiated sulfonamides in the dog. J Vet Pharmacol Ther 27:129.

Trepanier LA, et al. (2003): Clinical findings in 40 dogs with hypersensitivity associated with administration of potentiated sulfonamides. J Vet Intern Med 17:647.

Trucksa RC, et al. (1985): Intraocular canine melanocytic neoplasms. J Am Anim Hosp Assoc 21:85.

van der Woerdt A (2001): Management of intraocular inflammatory disease. Clin Tech Small Anim Pract 16:58.

van der Woerdt A (1992): Lens induced uveitis in dogs: 151 cases (1985-1990). J Am Vet Med Assoc 201:921.

Verma A, et al. (2005): LruA and LruB, novel lipoproteins of pathogenic *Leptospira interrogans* associated with equine recurrent uveitis. Infect Immun 73:7259.

Vinayak A, et al. (2004): Clinical resolution of *Brucella canis*-induced ocular inflammation in a dog. J Am Vet Med Assoc 224:1804.

Wanke MM (2004): Canine brucellosis. Anim Reprod Sci 82-83:195.

Wilcock BP, et al. (1990): The cause of glaucoma in cats. Vet Pathol 27:35.

Wilcock BP, Peiffer RL (1987): The pathology of lens-induced uveitis in dogs. Vet Pathol 24:549.

Wilcock BP, Peiffer RL (1986): Morphology and behavior of primary ocular melanomas in 91 dogs. Vet Pathol 23:418.

Wilkie DA, Wolf D (1991): Treatment of epibulbar melanocytoma in a dog, using full-thickness eyewall resection and synthetic graft. J Am Vet Med Assoc 198:1019.

Wolfer J, et al. (1993): Phacoclastic uveitis in the rabbit. Prog Vet Comp Ophthalmol 3:92.

Wollanke B, et al. (2001): Serum and vitreous humor antibody titers in and isolation of *Leptospira interrogans* from horses with recurrent uveitis. J Am Vet Med Assoc 219:795.

THE GLAUCOMAS

Paul E. Miller

AQUEOUS PRODUCTION AND
  DRAINAGE
DIAGNOSTIC METHODS

CLINICAL SIGNS
CLASSIFICATION
PATHOGENESIS

TREATMENT
FELINE GLAUCOMA
EQUINE GLAUCOMA

The glaucomas are a diverse group of diseases united only by the fact that intraocular pressure (IOP) is too high to permit the optic nerve and, in some species, the retina to function normally. Characteristic changes of glaucoma include disrupted axoplasmic flow in the optic nerve head, death of retinal ganglion cells and their axons, cupping of the optic disc, and visual impairment or blindness.

AQUEOUS PRODUCTION AND DRAINAGE

The production and drainage of aqueous humor are influenced not only by the anatomy of the anterior segment but also by a large number of endogenous compounds, including neurotransmitters, hormones, prostaglandins, proteins, lipids, and proteoglycans. Indeed, so many factors influence the production and drainage of aqueous humor that it is difficult to identify a single pathway or drug that is capable of dramatically lowering IOP in every patient.

Aqueous humor is produced in the ciliary body by both active (selective transport of larger or charged molecules against a concentration gradient) and passive processes (diffusion and ultrafiltration). In *diffusion,* lipid-soluble substances enter the aqueous humor by passing through the ciliary epithelial cell membrane in proportion to their concentration gradient across the membrane. *Ultrafiltration* is the passage of water and water-soluble substances (which are generally limited by their size or charge) through theoretical micropores in the cell membrane in response to an osmotic gradient or hydrostatic pressure.

Many substances in the blood pass by ultrafiltration from the ciliary capillaries into the stroma of the ciliary processes before accumulating behind the tight junctions of the nonpigmented ciliary epithelium (the site of the blood-aqueous barrier). Some substances, such as sodium and chloride ions, are then actively pumped across the membrane into the posterior chamber, thereby drawing water passively along this concentration gradient. This process may account for the majority of actively formed aqueous.

Aqueous humor is also produced via the enzyme *carbonic anhydrase,* which catalyzes the formation of carbonic acid from carbon dioxide and water as follows:

$$CO_2 + H_2O \rightleftharpoons H_2CO_3 \rightleftharpoons HCO_3^- + H^+$$

Carbonic acid then dissociates, allowing negatively charged bicarbonate ions to pass to the aqueous. Although exactly how this leads to aqueous humor production is unclear, it appears that positively charged sodium ions, and eventually water, follow negatively charged bicarbonate ions into the posterior chamber. Drugs that inhibit carbonic anhydrase therefore decrease aqueous production and reduce IOP.

Aqueous exits the eye via several routes. In the *conventional* or *traditional outflow route* aqueous humor passes from the posterior chamber, through the pupil, and into the anterior chamber. Because of temperature differences between the iris and cornea, thermal convection currents occur in the anterior chamber, with aqueous near the iris rising and aqueous near the cornea falling. This is one reason cells and particulate matter in the anterior chamber may settle on the inferior corneal endothelial surface. Aqueous humor then leaves the anterior chamber by passing between the pectinate ligaments to enter the *ciliary cleft,* which contains the *trabecular meshwork* (Figure 12-1). After filtering between the beams of the sponge-like meshwork, aqueous crosses through the endothelial cell membranes of the meshwork to enter a series of radially oriented, blood-free collecting vessels collectively called the *angular aqueous plexus.* From there it enters an interconnected set of blood/aqueous-filled vessels (the *scleral venous plexus*) before draining either anteriorly via the episcleral and conjunctival veins or posteriorly into the vortex venous system and into the systemic venous circulation (Figure 12-2). Contraction of smooth muscle fibers of the ciliary muscle that insert into the trabecular meshwork are probably capable of increasing drainage of aqueous from the eye by enlarging the spaces in the trabecular meshwork. In most species the majority of aqueous humor (about 50% in horses, 85% in dogs, and 97% in cats) leaves the eye via the traditional outflow route.

The remainder of the aqueous humor leaves the eye via the *uveoscleral pathway* (see Figure 12-1). In this route aqueous humor passes through the root of the iris and interstitial spaces of the ciliary muscle to reach the *supraciliary space* (between the ciliary body and the sclera) or the *suprachoroidal space* (between the choroid and the sclera). From these locations aqueous humor may pass through the sclera into the orbit either via pores in the sclera where blood vessels and nerves enter the eye or between the scleral collagen fibers themselves. Outflow via this route may substantially increase in certain disease states and in response to certain antiglaucoma drugs, such as the prostaglandin derivatives.

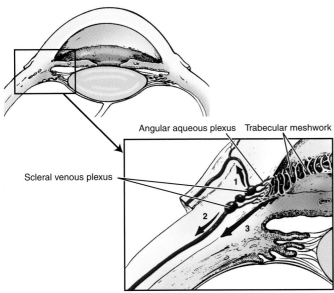

Figure 12-1. The routes of aqueous drainage from the canine iridocorneal angle. Aqueous humor passes between the beamlike pectinate ligament, then through the trabecular meshwork to enter the angular aqueous plexus and eventually the scleral venous plexus. From there, aqueous humor may drain *(1)* anteriorly to the episcleral and conjunctival veins, *(2)* posteriorly into the scleral venous plexus and vortex venous system, or *(3)* through the ciliary muscle interstitium to the suprachoroid and diffuse through the sclera (uveoscleral flow). (Modified from Martin CL [1993]: Glaucoma, in Slatter D [editor]: Textbook of Small Animal Surgery, 2nd ed. Saunders, Philadelphia.)

Balancing Aqueous Production and Outflow

IOP is the result of a delicate balance between production and outflow of aqueous humor (Figure 12-3). In glaucoma both production and outflow are altered. Usually a large percentage of the outflow pathway (perhaps as much as 80% to 90%) needs to be impaired before IOP starts to rise. If the outflow system is impaired to the point that IOP begins to increase, the eye usually attempts to compensate by reducing the passive production of aqueous humor. Active secretion, however, typically continues at a relatively normal rate, perhaps because if it did not, the avascular tissues of the eye that rely on aqueous humor for their nutrition would starve. Because the glaucomatous eye is functioning on a greatly diminished percentage of its normal levels of aqueous humor outflow and production, and because it has exhausted its usual compensatory pathways, pathologic processes or drugs that alter production or outflow only a small amount can have dramatic effects on IOP. This characteristic is one reason that glaucomatous eyes are typically more responsive to antiglaucoma drugs than normotensive eyes, but it also explains why IOP can rapidly rise to very high levels in a matter of 1 to 2 hours in some patients.

Often it is difficult to empirically predict the effect a given drug or its antagonist will have on IOP because many compounds affect both aqueous humor production and outflow—sometimes in complex and contradictory ways. For example, stimulation of β-adrenergic receptors in the ciliary processes increases intracellular cyclic adenosine monophosphate (cAMP), resulting in greater aqueous humor production. β-Adrenergic blocking drugs (e.g., timolol, betaxolol) decrease cAMP, thereby lowering aqueous humor production and ultimately reducing IOP. β-Blockers reduce IOP, however, only if the patient is

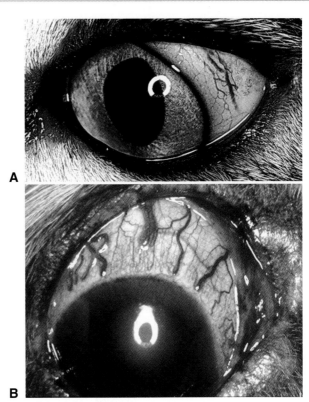

Figure 12-2. A, The scleral venous plexus is often visible in normal animals as a series of interwoven blood vessels several millimeters posterior to the limbus. **B,** Prominent episcleral and, to a lesser extent, conjunctival venous injection in a dog with glaucoma. Increased intraocular pressure compresses the intrascleral blood vessels, which drain posteriorly. This forces more blood through the episcleral and conjunctival veins—one reason the eye appears injected in glaucoma.

awake and adrenergic tone is present. This means that although a drug such as timolol can reduce IOP in a cat when it is awake, the agent may not control IOP for the more than 20 hours a day the cat is sleeping.

As expected, β-adrenergic drugs such as epinephrine and its derivative dipivefrin may transiently increase IOP, presumably by increasing aqueous humor production via stimulation of cAMP. A few minutes after application of these drugs, however, IOP begins to decrease, and it stays reduced for several hours. This is because epinephrine also increases aqueous outflow via β_2 receptors in the trabecular meshwork, and does so to a greater degree than it increases aqueous humor production. Epinephrine may also lower IOP by (1) reducing blood flow to the ciliary body (thereby lowering aqueous production) and (2) increasing uveoscleral outflow by relaxing the ciliary muscle and recruiting prostaglandins. The latter means, which can be blocked by topical nonsteroidal antiinflammatory drugs, may result in further increases in uveoscleral outflow and additional decreases in aqueous humor production. Complex interactions such as this are but one reason why both β-adrenergic agonists and β-blockers lower IOP in many species. When one considers species and individual differences in the density, distribution, and type of receptors as well as differences in the cause of the glaucoma, it is easy to see why it can be difficult to precisely predict what effect a given drug will have on IOP in a particular patient.

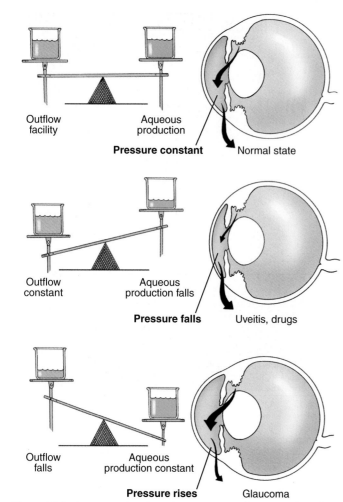

Figure 12-3. Common alterations in aqueous production and outflow facility and their effects on intraocular pressure.

Causes of Variations in Intraocular Pressure

Diurnal Variation

IOP varies slightly with time of day in many species, being the greatest in the morning and gradually declining over the course of the day in dogs and humans. The opposite phenomenon has been suggested to occur in cats, rabbits, and nonhuman primates.

Age

Both production and outflow of aqueous humor tend to decline with age, but production declines at a little faster rate than outflow in most individuals. In humans, aqueous production and IOP tend to decline after 60 years of age, although this tendency varies considerably with ethnic background and the presence of other diseases, such as systemic hypertension and obesity. Similarly, IOP in cats has been shown to decline approximately 1 mm Hg per year after 7 years of age. In a small percentage of humans, and perhaps animals, however, aqueous humor outflow is reduced to a greater degree than aqueous humor production, resulting in increased IOP with age.

Blood Flow

Disorders associated with substantially lower blood flow to the eye (e.g., dehydration, hypovolemic shock, cardiogenic shock) tend to result in lower IOP. A dog collar can significantly increase IOP if the dog is pulling against a leash or if the collar is too tight. Dogs with glaucoma probably should be exercised with a harness rather than a collar.

Drugs

In addition to the numerous antiglaucoma drugs that alter IOP, other drugs also may affect IOP. Most general anesthetics and tranquilizers cause IOP to fall. Ketamine may temporarily increase IOP, presumably owing to extraocular muscle spasm.

Ocular Inflammation

Both spontaneous and surgically induced inflammation lower aqueous production and IOP. A profound reduction in IOP is an important diagnostic clue to the presence of intraocular inflammation, especially uveitis.

DIAGNOSTIC METHODS

Tonometry

Measurement of and normal values for IOP are discussed in Chapter 5. It is suggested that the reader refer to that discussion before proceeding with this chapter. Despite its disadvantages, the most *economical* instrument in general veterinary practice is the Schiøtz tonometer with the *human* conversion tables. Surprisingly, dog-specific conversion tables for the Schiøtz tonometer do not agree as well with the more accurate applanation and rebound tonometers, and dog specific tables should *not* be used to convert Schiøtz scale readings to IOP estimates in dogs or cats. Two handheld tonometers that are more accurate and easier to use than the Schiøtz instrument are the Tono-Pen applanation tonometer and the TonoVet rebound tonometer. The ability to perform tonometry is essential to every veterinarian engaged in small animal practice. Tonometry minimizes the chances of making an important or even catastrophic error in diagnosis.

IOP should be determined in every red eye with an intact cornea and sclera.

Ophthalmoscopy

Direct and indirect ophthalmoscopy may be used to examine the optic nerve head for cupping of the optic disc, which is the hallmark of glaucoma. The red-free filter (green light) on many of these instruments facilitates examination of the optic nerve and retinal nerve fiber layer.

Gonioscopy

Gonioscopy is a very useful technique for examining the iridocorneal (filtration) angle and managing glaucoma. It is discussed in detail in Chapter 5. Gonioscopy allows the clinician to differentiate between *open-angle* and *closed-angle* glaucoma, to estimate the severity of the obstruction of the

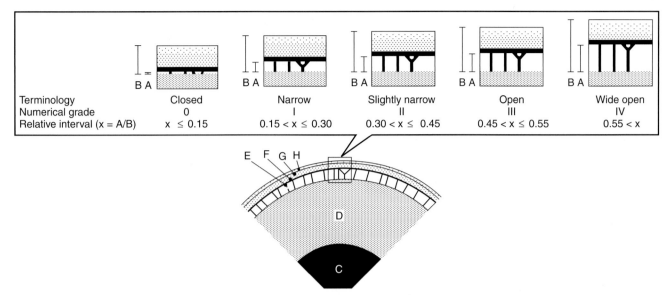

Terminology	Closed	Narrow	Slightly narrow	Open	Wide open
Numerical grade	0	I	II	III	IV
Relative interval (x = A/B)	x ≤ 0.15	0.15 < x ≤ 0.30	0.30 < x ≤ 0.45	0.45 < x ≤ 0.55	0.55 < x

Figure 12-4. Schematic drawing of a grading system for the width of the iridocorneal angle. The ratio of the width of the anterior opening of the ciliary cleft *(A)* and the distance from the origin of the pectinate ligaments to the anterior surface of the cornea *(B)* is estimated. *C,* Pupil; *D,* iris; *E,* pectinate ligament; *F,* deep pigmented zone; *G,* superficial pigmented zone; *H,* cornea. (From Ekesten, B, Narfström K [1991]: Correlation of morphologic features of the iridocorneal angle to intraocular pressure in Samoyeds. Am J Vet Res 52:1875.)

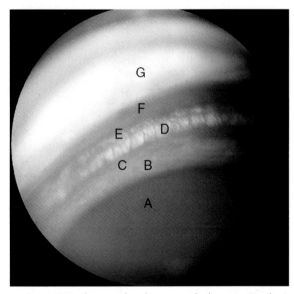

Figure 12-5. Goniophotograph of a normal dog. *A,* Pupil; *B,* iris; *C,* pectinate ligament strands *(thin brown lines); D,* bluish-white zone of the uveal trabeculae (trabecular meshwork); *E,* deep pigmented zone; *F,* superficial pigmented zone; *G,* cornea.

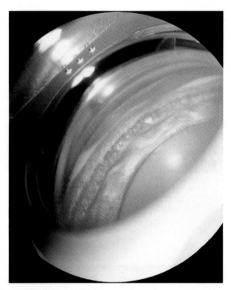

Figure 12-6. Normal canine iridocorneal angle as seen with a goniolens.

iridocorneal angle, and to evaluate the response to therapy (Figure 12-4). It does, however, require considerable practice to recognize the many normal variations and hence gonioscopy tends to be performed almost exclusively by veterinary ophthalmologists. Examples of gonioscopic findings are shown in Figures 12-5 to 12-11.

CLINICAL SIGNS

The effects of increased IOP on ocular tissues are similar regardless of the cause of the elevation. It is essential to con-

sider whether the lesions and clinical signs observed *are associated with* or *result from* the cause of the increased pressure.

Glaucoma is one of the most commonly misdiagnosed eye conditions. Failure of owners to recognize the disease early in its course may prevent effective treatment of the first eye. Failure of clinicians to recognize onset in the second eye may prevent retention of sight.

The clinical signs of glaucoma in the dog are summarized in Figure 12-12. The signs present in a particular animal depend on the duration, intensity, and cause of the pressure elevation. In general the most obvious signs are associated with end-stage

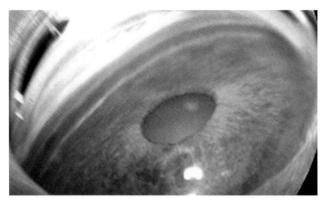

Figure 12-7. Gonioscopic view of the iridocorneal angle of a dog in which the angle is filled with liberated pigment. The physical width of the angle is normal, but the pigment occludes the trabecular meshwork and prevents readily identifying the pectinate ligament.

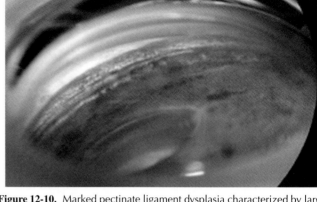

Figure 12-10. Marked pectinate ligament dysplasia characterized by large sheets of mesodermal tissue in a 7-year-old Bouvier dog. Although intraocular pressure is still within normal limits, aqueous humor can exit the eye only via a few small "flow holes" in the mesodermal sheets.

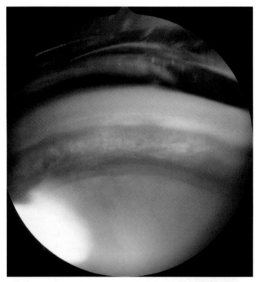

Figure 12-8. Gonioscopic view of a closed angle in a dog with secondary glaucoma. The retina was massively detached, resulting in forward shifting of the lens and, ultimately, of the iris into the iridocorneal angle. Note that the pectinate ligament cannot be seen.

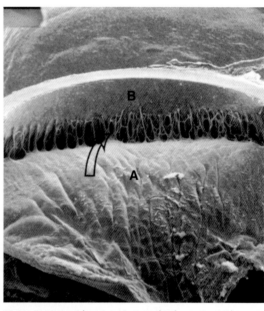

Figure 12-11. Scanning electron micrograph of a canine iridocorneal angle. *A*, Iris; *B*, cornea; *arrow*, pectinate ligament. (From Martin CL, Wyman M [1978]: Primary glaucoma in the dog. Vet Clin North Am 8:257.)

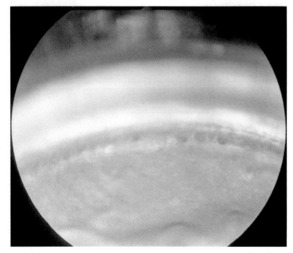

Figure 12-9. Mild pectinate ligament dysplasia characterized by broad-based pectinate ligament strands and a small region of "sheeting."

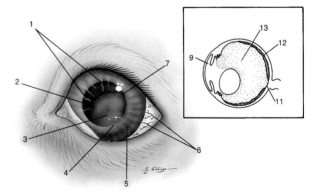

Figure 12-12. Clinical signs of canine glaucoma: *1*, Descemet's streaks (advanced cases); *2*, aphakic crescent; *3*, luxated lens (some cases); *4*, corneal edema; *5*, iris atrophy; *6*, enlarged episcleral vessels; *7*, fixed, dilated pupil; *9*, shallow anterior chamber; *11*, cupping of the optic disc; *12*, retinal atrophy and vascular attenuation; *13*, buphthalmos. Not shown: *8*, increased intraocular pressure; *10*, partial or complete loss of vision; *14*, ocular pain; *15*, loss of corneal sensitivity.

disease in which there is no hope of preserving vision. In the very early stages of glaucoma, in which there is a chance of preserving vision, the eye may appear normal and IOP may or may not be elevated. In some patients there is only a history of intermittent episcleral injection (especially in the evening) that spontaneously resolves, and IOP is normal on examination in the office. Glaucoma may be detected in these animals only by performing tonometry when the eye is red or, occasionally, by repeatedly measuring IOP over 24 hours. In other patients the eye may appear to be essentially normal and the only finding is increased IOP on tonometry. In these patients it is essential to differentiate glaucoma from increased IOP measurements associated with an uncooperative patient, technical problems with measuring IOP (excessive tension on the eyelids, a collar that is too tight, compression of the jugular veins during restraint, etc.), and malfunction of the instrument. Specialist assistance may be required to make the diagnosis of glaucoma in its early stages.

Increased Intraocular Pressure

IOP values exceeding 25 mm Hg in dogs and 27 mm Hg in cats in conjunction with compatible clinical signs are sufficient for a presumptive diagnosis of glaucoma. IOP values greater than 20 mm Hg are suspicious for glaucoma if other clinical signs, especially anterior uveitis, are present or if the patient is being treated for glaucoma. Often IOP exceeds 40 mm Hg by the time the owner notices changes in the eye. Frequent measurement of IOP is an integral part of diagnosis and treatment of the patient with glaucoma.

Pain, Blepharospasm, and Altered Behavior

An acute increase in IOP to 50 to 60 mm Hg or more is typically described by a human as "the worst headache of my life." It is likely that animals experience a comparable degree of pain with pressures in this range. If the IOP rise is acute, the dog may be blepharospastic, depressed, less active, timid, or, in rare cases, more aggressive. Some sleep more, eat less, vomit, and are less interested in play. On occasion they rub at the eye, but this behavior is an unreliable sign of glaucoma. Application of pressure to the affected eye through the upper lid or to the surrounding area may cause severe pain. If the condition is not treated, severe pain and blepharospasm are replaced by signs of chronic pain that many owners may not properly recognize as being attributable to glaucoma. Frequently the owner believes that the pet is simply "getting old" and this is why it is less active, sleeps more, and is less playful. A surgical procedure that alleviates the increased pressure (and accompanying pain) almost invariably results in a comment from the owner that the pet "acts like a new dog."

Elevated IOP should be considered to be painful even if the disease is chronic and the animal outwardly appears normal.

Engorged Episcleral Vessels

Engorgement of episcleral veins (see Figure 12-2, *B*) is one of the more common signs of increased IOP. Episcleral engorgement arises because the increased IOP reduces flow through the ciliary body to the vortex veins, and increased flow passes forward via anastomosing episcleral veins at the limbus (see Figure 12-1). Conjunctival capillaries may also be engorged, but usually to a lesser degree. Episcleral vascular engorgement is a sign of intraocular disease (anterior uveitis or glaucoma) and may be differentiated from superficial conjunctival vessel engorgement (which indicates ocular surface disease) by the following features:

* Episcleral vessels are larger, darker red, and more visible, and pass over a conjunctiva that is usually white or slightly pink. Superficial conjunctival vessels are brighter pink to red and cover a larger portion of the sclera.
* Episcleral vessels do not typically branch the closer they get to the limbus, whereas superficial conjunctival vessels do.
* Episcleral vessels blanch slowly or not at all after the application of topical 1% epinephrine, whereas superficial conjunctival vessels typically blanch within 1 to 2 minutes.

Corneal/Scleral Changes

Edema

Increased IOP impairs the function of the corneal endothelium, resulting in corneal edema. Typically the entire cornea is diffusely edematous in glaucoma, and the edema can be quite dramatic in acute glaucoma when IOP is very high (Figure 12-13). In advanced cases subepithelial bullae may form, which can lead to corneal ulceration if they rupture. In chronic glaucoma both superficial and deep vascularization, scarring, and pigmentation are common.

Buphthalmos and Descemet's Streaks

Chronic increases in IOP results in stretching of the cornea and sclera and enlargement of the globe (*buphthalmos;* Figure 12-14). Buphthalmos may be especially pronounced in young animals and in shar-peis, who have a more easily distended cornea and sclera than most adult dogs. Buphthalmic eyes are almost invariably blind, although limited vision may be retained for a while in some puppies and shar-peis. Buphthalmos is *irreversible* even if the pressure is later reduced, although a variety of surgical procedures are available to restore a cosmetically acceptable appearance.

By the time severe stretching has occurred, atrophy of the ciliary body may have reduced the IOP to normal and pain may be lessened. As the cornea stretches, linear ruptures in Descemet's

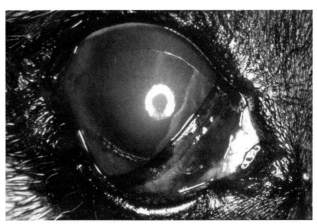

Figure 12-13. Diffuse corneal edema in a dog with glaucoma.

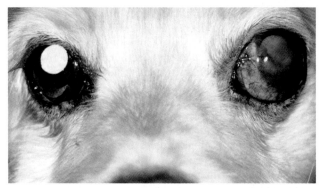

Figure 12-14. Buphthalmos in an American cocker spaniel with chronic primary angle-closure glaucoma. Exposure keratitis is also present.

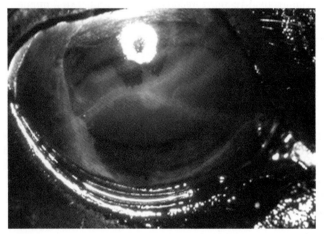

Figure 12-15. Curvilinear breaks in Descemet's membrane (Haab's striae) in the cornea of a horse with chronic glaucoma (intraocular pressure greater than 50 mm Hg).

membrane, called *Descemet's streaks (Haab's striae)*, may occur (Figure 12-15).

Changes in Anterior Chamber Depth

Depth of the anterior chamber (distance between cornea and iris) is evaluated with an oblique focal source of light or, better yet, by biomicroscopy. Decreased depth of the anterior chamber is often associated with impediments to outflow through the pupil (because the lens and iris are in greater contact) and the iridocorneal angle (because the anterior chamber is more crowded). A shallow anterior chamber is an especially prominent sign in cats in which aqueous humor is misdirected into the vitreal cavity (resulting in a forward displacement of the lens and iris) and in any animal in which the lens is anteriorly luxated or subluxated. Therefore a shallow anterior chamber should alert the clinician to the possibility of glaucoma. Glaucoma may also be associated with an abnormally deep anterior chamber in animals with posterior lens luxation or in buphthalmic eyes.

Fixed Dilated Pupil

As IOP rises, the pupillary constrictor muscle becomes ischemic and the pupil dilates to midrange or larger (Figure 12-16). A dilated pupil, along with episcleral injection and pain, may be among the first signs noticed by the owner. Mydriasis is not an

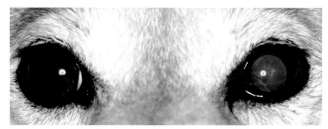

Figure 12-16. Mydriasis (and anisocoria) in a Shiba Inu dog with primary angle-closure glaucoma. A dilated pupil may be the result of ischemia of the iris sphincter muscle or interference with the function of the optic or ciliary nerves.

invariable sign of glaucoma— the pupil may be normal in mild IOP elevations, and miosis may be present in uveitis-induced glaucoma. In these latter cases, a careful examination is necessary to distinguish glaucoma from uveitis, and it is possible for both to be present in the same eye. In chronic glaucoma, or when IOP is acutely markedly elevated, the direct and consensual pupillary light reflexes are usually greatly impaired or absent. The longer glaucoma remains unresolved, the greater the chance that peripheral anterior synechiae will form and permanently block the drainage angle by fixing the peripheral iris in position.

Although a dilated, unresponsive pupil is consistent with glaucoma, it may be due to other diseases (e.g., progressive retinal degeneration, sudden acquired retinal degeneration syndrome, optic neuritis) and is not by itself diagnostic for glaucoma.

Lens Changes

Lens luxation in glaucoma may be either primary or secondary. A glaucomatous eye with a luxated, cataractous lens may have reached this state by one of several ways:

- Cataract (variety of etiologies) → lens-induced uveitis → glaucoma → buphthalmos → tearing of zonules → lens luxation
- Zonular malformation → lens luxation (or subluxation) → glaucoma → cataract
- Glaucoma (variety of etiologies) → buphthalmos → tearing of zonules → lens luxation → cataract

Lens luxation or subluxation may be recognized from the following signs:

- Presence of the lens *in front of* the iris (anterior luxation)
- Presence of an *aphakic crescent* in the pupil (most frequent in subluxation)
- Movement of the iris *(iridodonesis)* or lens *(phacodonesis)*
- Abnormally *shallow or deep anterior chamber*
- *Vitreous strands* in the pupil

If a luxated lens enters the anterior chamber and touches the corneal endothelium, a focal area of corneal edema may result. This opacity is frequently permanent, even if the lens is later removed. The continuous presence of a luxated lens in the anterior chamber damages the endothelium over a wider area and lowers the probability of successful surgical removal of the lens.

The recognition of how the final state was reached is important in determining which combination of therapeutic

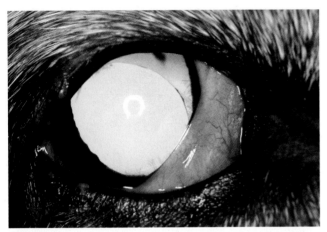

Figure 12-17. Chronic glaucoma in a basset hound resulting in buphthalmos and secondary tearing of lens zonules. The equator of the lens is visible superonasally that creates an aphakic crescent in this region.

Box 12-1 | **Inherited and breed predisposition to lens luxation in dogs**

Breeds in Which Lens Luxation Is Inherited

Border collie
Cairn terrier
Jack Russell terrier
Lakeland terrier
Manchester terrier
Miniature bull terrier
Norfolk terrier
Norwich terrier
Scottish terrier
Sealyham terrier
Skye terrier
Smooth haired fox terrier
West Highland white terrier
Tibetan terrier
Wirehaired fox terrier

Breeds with Predisposition to Lens Luxation

Australian shepherd
Basset hound
Beagle
Chihuahua
German shepherd
Greyhound
Miniature poodle
Miniature schnauzer
Norwegian elkhound
Pembroke Welsh corgi
Spaniel breeds
Welsh terrier
Toy poodle
Toy terrier

Modified from Gelatt KN, Brooks DE (1999): The canine glaucomas, in Gelatt KN (editor): Veterinary Ophthalmology, 3rd ed. Lippincott Williams & Wilkins, Philadelphia.

methods is required. History and signalment are critical factors in differentiating between these various possibilities. In all three pathways the lens may be displaced anteriorly or posteriorly or may be in the plane of the iris (either superiorly or inferiorly). An *aphakic crescent* is formed when the lens zonules have broken for a portion of the circumference of the lens, and it is possible to visualize the tapetal reflex through a crescent-shaped space between the lens equator and the pupillary border (Figure 12-17). After luxation the lens frequently, but not invariably, becomes cataractous.

Primary lens luxation, as occurs in terriers and certain other breeds (Box 12-1), may result in pupillary block with acute elevations in IOP. The presence of *vitreous strands* in the anterior chamber in the absence of buphthalmos suggests primary lens luxation. In these animals the lens may be completely luxated or only partially luxated (subluxation), and usually the lens is not cataractous until it becomes luxated (Figures 12-18 and 12-19).

Primary glaucoma tends to occur in middle-aged to somewhat older dogs of certain breeds (Box 12-2), and the lens

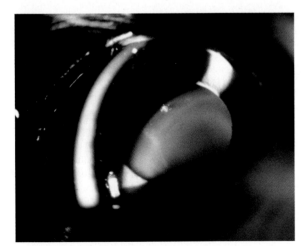

Figure 12-18. Lens subluxation in an 8-year-old wirehaired fox terrier. Notice that the anterior chamber is deeper superiorly than inferiorly, indicating that the lens has shifted position. The iris and lens also "trembled" when the eye moved (iridodonesis and phacodonesis).

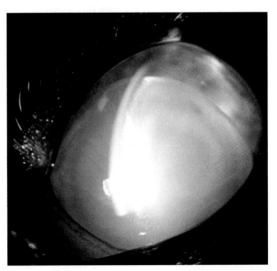

Figure 12-19. Complete anterior lens luxation associated with chronic uveitis in a cat. Secondary glaucoma was also present.

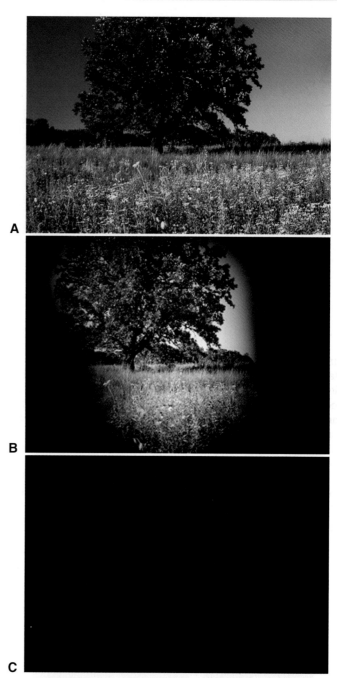

| Box 12-2 | Breeds of dog most commonly affected with different types of glaucoma |

Primary Open-Angle Glaucoma

Mixed breeds
American cocker spaniel
Basset hound
Boston terrier
Miniature schnauzer
Beagle
Chow chow
Siberian husky
Standard poodle

Closed-Angle Glaucoma

American cocker spaniel
Mixed breeds
Basset hound
Samoyed
Beagle
Siberian husky
Labrador retriever
Toy poodle

Secondary Glaucoma

Mixed breeds
American cocker spaniel
Wirehaired fox terrier
Toy poodle
Boston terrier
Miniature poodle
Labrador retriever
Siberian husky
Basset hound
Beagle

From Miller PE (1995): Glaucoma, in Bonagura JD (editor): Kirk's Current Veterinary Therapy XII: Small Animal Practice. Saunders, Philadelphia. Breeds are listed in descending order of frequency as recorded by the Veterinary Medical Data Base over a 20-year period.

Figure 12-20. Simulated changes in vision due to glaucoma. **A,** Normal visual field. **B,** Moderate vision loss in glaucoma; the peripheral visual field is reduced but central vision may persist. **C,** End-stage glaucoma; vision is completely lost.

subluxation or luxation does not occur until the globe has become buphthalmic and the lens zonules are stretched beyond the breaking point (secondary luxation). Similarly, primary cataract formation in a wide variety of breeds is frequently followed by lens luxation and glaucoma. Lens-induced uveitis from a secondarily luxated lens that has become cataractous from elevated IOP, and decreased IOP from the uveitis further complicate diagnosis and treatment. Thus the combination of glaucoma, cataract, and lens luxation in any particular eye may occur through several mechanisms and may be associated with a variety of IOP values at any given moment.

Lens luxation in a glaucomatous eye does not necessarily mean that luxation was the inciting cause of the glaucoma. The luxation may have *resulted from* the glaucoma.

Fundus Changes

Impaired Vision

Loss of some or all vision is a common sequela of glaucoma. In the early stages peripheral vision may be lost (Figure 12-20),

and it is difficult, if not impossible, to detect these changes in most animals. Complete vision loss can occur in a very short period (hours to a day) if the increase in IOP is very high, or over a period of weeks to months if the pressure increase is more insidious. Preservation of vision depends on control of IOP.

Optic Disc Cupping

Cupping, or posterior bowing of the optic disc through the lamina cribrosa, is the hallmark of glaucoma. Retinal nerve fibers run parallel to the surface of the retina and then turn

90 degrees to enter the multilayered, fenestrated meshwork of the lamina cribrosa before exiting the eye. Glial cells, blood vessels, and collagen beams form variably sized pores through which the optic nerve fibers pass. When IOP rises the scleral lamina cribrosa bows posteriorly, distorting the alignment of the pores and compressing the optic nerve fibers. Although this change may initially be so subtle as to not be detected ophthalmoscopically, it is sufficient to mechanically interfere with axonal axoplasmic flow and also probably with blood supply to the optic nerve head. Very large increases in IOP may also interfere with blood flow to the choroid and produce vision loss through ischemic damage to the photoreceptors and outer retinal layers. In acute glaucoma the optic disc may appear swollen in response to ischemia. Within a day or two the increased pressure may cause the disc to appear pale and compressed. As ganglion cell axons die, optic nerve head tissue is lost and pressure forces the lamina cribrosa outward (Figures 12-21 to 12-23). This change indicates irreversible damage to the optic nerve. Wallerian degeneration of the optic nerve follows (Figure 12-24).

Retinal Degeneration

In advanced glaucoma, profound retinal atrophy with increased tapetal reflectivity occurs together with attenuation or complete loss of retinal vessels, atrophy of the pigment epithelium in the nontapetal fundus, and optic atrophy (grayish-white appearance; Figure 12-25). These findings are also present in advanced progressive retinal degeneration (progressive retinal atrophy).

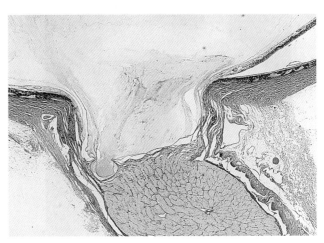

Figure 12-21. Cupping of the optic disc with loss of tissue anterior to the lamina cribrosa, which is bowing posteriorly. (From Slatter D [2003]: Textbook of Small Animal Surgery, 3rd ed. Saunders, Philadelphia.)

In progressive retinal degeneration the other signs of glaucoma are lacking, the disease is usually bilateral, the optic disc is not cupped, and differential diagnosis may be determined by the breed of dog and lack of other clinical signs of glaucoma. Ophthalmoscopically visible retinal and optic nerve lesions of glaucoma are irreversible.

Elevation of IOP decreases blood flow in the choroid, resulting in ischemia. This ischemia can be demonstrated func-

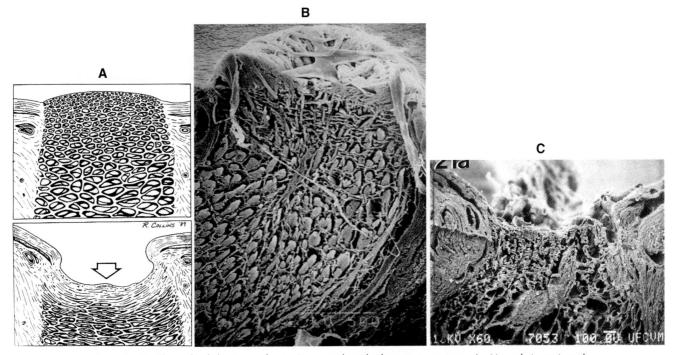

Figure 12-22. The scleral lamina cribrosa in normal and glaucomatous eyes. **A,** Normal (upper) and glaucomatous (lower) eye pore arrangement. From the normal pores in the normal eye, glaucoma causes pore misalignment and posterior movement or cupping of the lamina cribrosa. **B,** Trypsin digestion and scanning electron microscopy of a normal dog optic nerve head demonstrates the three-dimensional architecture of the scleral lamina cribrosa (original magnification, ×60). **C,** Trypsin digestion and scanning electron microscopy of a primary open-angle glaucomatous optic nerve head shows posterior displacement and loss of pore arrangement, which may impair axoplasmic and local capillary blood flow (original magnification, ×60). (From Brooks DE, et al. [1989]: Morphologic changes in the lamina cribrosa of beagles with primary open-angle glaucoma. Am J Vet Res 50:936.)

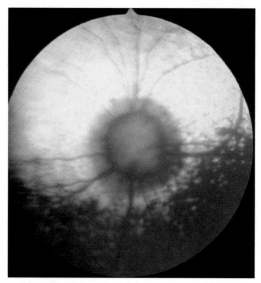

Figure 12-23. Optic disc cupping. Most retinal vessels disappear at the disc edge. The center of the disc is in focus below the level of the retinal surface and is grayish. There also is a peripapillary ring of altered retinal reflectivity. (Courtesy Dr. Christopher J. Murphy.)

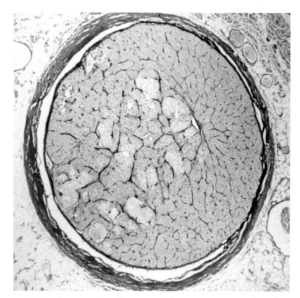

Figure 12-24. Cross-sectional view of the optic nerve of a dog with glaucoma. The paler blue areas represent degenerated nerve fiber axons. (Courtesy Dr. Richard R. Dubielzig.)

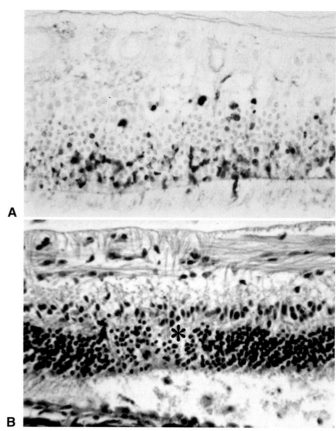

Figure 12-25. Retinal changes in acute primary angle-closure glaucoma. **A,** The retinal cells, which stain brown in this immunohistochemically stained section, are undergoing apoptosis. **B,** Histologic section of a retina showing segmental loss of nuclei in the photoreceptor layer *(*)*. (Courtesy Dr. Richard R. Dubielzig.)

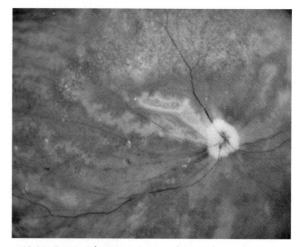

Figure 12-26. Postenucleation specimen from a dog with acute primary angle-closure glaucoma. Light-colored, roughly wedge-shaped regions of retinal necrosis, presumably secondary to impaired choroidal circulation, are apparent. (Courtesy Dr. Richard R. Dubielzig.)

tionally by depressed electroretinograms, and in some patients it is possible to visualize wedge-shaped defects in the retina that correspond to pressure-induced infarction of the choroidal blood supply (Figure 12-26). Early in glaucoma, if the pressure elevation is acute and very large, the photoreceptors in the retina undergo necrosis. In the next few days they begin to die by apoptosis as well. Ophthalmoscopically the cell death is seen as increased tapetal reflectivity. As in any other severe retinal atrophy, the condition is irreversible.

It has now been recognized that increased IOP may initiate a chain of events that can continue to impair vision despite return of IOP to within normal limits (Figure 12-27). In human primary open-angle glaucoma (POAG), in which the rise in IOP is more insidious and of usually smaller magnitude than in acute canine primary angle-closure glaucoma (PACG), vision loss is usually attributed mainly to retinal ganglion cell degeneration. Pressure-associated alterations in microcirculation and/or axoplasmic flow at the level of the lamina cribrosa may play a role in the death of ganglion cells in this form of glaucoma. Dying

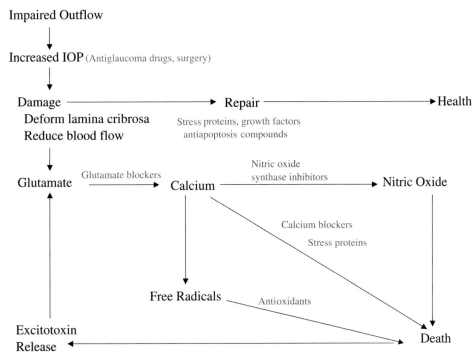

Impaired Outflow

↓

Increased IOP (Antiglaucoma drugs, surgery)

↓

Damage ————————————→ Repair ————————————→ Health
Deform lamina cribrosa   Stress proteins, growth factors
Reduce blood flow   antiapoptosis compounds

↓

Glutamate —— Glutamate blockers ——→ Calcium ——— Nitric oxide synthase inhibitors ——→ Nitric Oxide

                                              Calcium blockers
                                              Stress proteins

Free Radicals —— Antioxidants ——   Death

Excitotoxin
Release ←————————————————————————————

Figure 12-27. Cell death in glaucoma. Potential therapeutic interventions are in red. Once cell death begins, a self-perpetuating circle can occur that is not susceptible to intervention by current intraocular pressure–lowering medications or surgery.

ganglion cells may then release glutamate and other excitatory compounds that initiate a self-perpetuating circle of apoptotic cell death in previously unaffected neighboring ganglion cells. In dogs with acute PACG and more rapid/marked increases in IOP, one study found retinal damage to extend well beyond the ganglion cell layer. Within the first few days of an attack of acute PACG ganglion cell necrosis and segmental full-thickness areas of retinal attenuation consistent with infarction were apparent. As ganglion cell and retinal necrosis decreased over the ensuing days retinal cell death by apoptosis markedly increased. This finding suggests that in acute PACG, the marked increase in IOP not only interferes with axoplasmic flow through the lamina cribrosa but also causes ischemic necrosis of the retina. Again, as these cells die they initiate a vicious circle of progressive cell death due to apoptosis that continues despite normalization of IOP. This hypothesis would explain the clinical observation that even though IOP is controlled in some dogs with PACG, progressive vision loss still occurs.

Although this sequence of events is discouraging, it does offer the possibility for the development of additional therapeutic avenues for the treatment of glaucoma, including neuroprotective agents that prevent cell suicide via apoptosis, drugs that help maintain retinal/optic nerve blood flow and minimize ischemia, and modalities that interrupt reperfusion injuries when IOP is reduced from very high levels to normal. These differences in the histologic appearance among the various forms of glaucoma also reinforce the concept that glaucoma is not a single entity and that there are likely to be important differences in the cellular events leading to vision loss in patients with glaucoma.

CLASSIFICATION

Glaucoma almost invariably is the result of impaired aqueous humor outflow. In fact, in most patients with glaucoma aqueous humor production is less than normal (but still excessively high in view of the outflow capacity of the eye). The mechanism of this impairment may be etiologically classified as primary or secondary. *Primary glaucomas* have no consistent, obvious association with another ocular or systemic disorder, are typically bilateral, have a strong breed predisposition, and hence are believed to have a genetic basis (see Box 12-2). Primary glaucoma is subdivided into two main forms, *primary open-angle glaucoma,* in which the drainage angle appears gonioscopically normal (presumably because the impediment to aqueous outflow is deep to the pectinate ligaments) and *primary angle-closure glaucoma,* in which the drainage angle appears gonioscopically narrowed or closed (Figures 12-28 through 12-33). In the dog, PACG is at least eight times more common than POAG. Acute PACG also is two times more common in female dogs than in male dogs. A similar sex predisposition has been found in humans with PACG and has been attributed to a generally shallower anterior chamber in women than in men.

Secondary glaucomas are at least twice as common as primary glaucomas in dogs (and even more common in cats) and are associated with other ocular or systemic disorders that alter aqueous humor dynamics. Secondary glaucoma may be unilateral or bilateral and may or may not be inherited; the physical width of the gonioscopically visible drainage angle may also be classified as open or closed. Often the exact mechanism by which outflow is impaired in secondary glaucoma is unclear.

Because glaucoma is almost always due to the impaired flow of aqueous humor, it can be very useful to classify glaucoma according to the location(s) of those impediments (Box 12-3). Impediments to the normal flow of aqueous humor commonly occur at the level of the ciliary body, pupil, trabecular meshwork, angular aqueous plexus, scleral venous system, or episcleral veins. Frequently the obstruction to outflow starts at one place

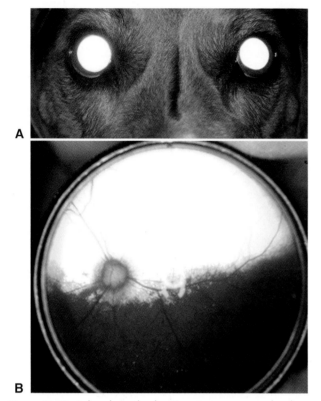

Figure 12-28. A beagle with chronic primary open-angle glaucoma. **A,** Both pupils are dilated and intraocular pressure is increased in both eyes (approximately 50 mm Hg). **B,** Fundus photograph of the same dog. The optic nerve is depressed from the surface of the fundus (cupped), has little myelin, and is darker than normal. The area surrounding the optic disc also has altered reflectivity.

(for example, the lens-pupil interface), but as the disease progresses, impediments to outflow also develop in more anterior structures (for example, at the iridocorneal angle; Figure 12-34), further worsening the problem. Therefore the longer the increased IOP persists, the more difficult it will be to successfully treat the patient.

The keys to successful therapy for glaucoma are early recognition of the problem, correct identification of the location of the impediment to outflow, and circumvention of that obstruction before additional impediments to outflow develop.

PATHOGENESIS

Primary Open-Angle Glaucoma

POAG is a bilateral disorder in which IOP tends to increase in a slow, insidious fashion simultaneously in both eyes in young to middle-aged dogs of certain breeds, most notably the beagle and the Norwegian elkhound (see Figures 12-28 and 12-29). Initially the gonioscopically visible angle is open. Over time the angle closes, the globe becomes buphthalmic, and the lens may subluxate. The precise mechanism of POAG in dogs is unclear, but it most likely results from subtle biochemical alterations in the trabecular meshwork that ultimately lead to greater resistance to aqueous outflow and increased IOP. In beagles, the defect appears to be inherited in an autosomal recessive fashion and may involve the glycosaminoglycan accumulation in the trabecular meshwork.

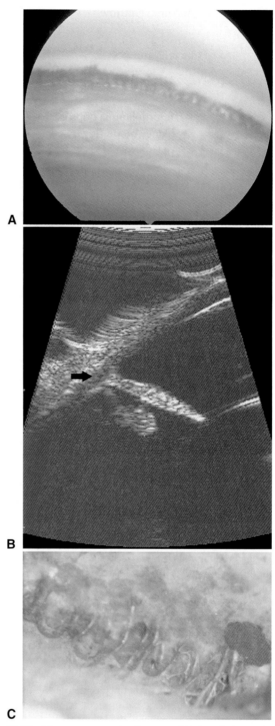

Figure 12-29. Primary open-angle glaucoma in a beagle (same dog as in Figure 12-28). **A,** The iridocorneal angle is gonioscopically relatively open. **B,** High-resolution ultrasound image of the anterior segment. Note that the iris does not have the same conformation as in dogs with primary angle-closure glaucoma (see Figure 12-31) and that the ciliary cleft is still open *(arrow)*. **C,** Dissecting microscope photo of a normal iridocorneal angle of a dog that has been stained to highlight the normal glycosaminoglycans (GAGs) in the trabecular meshwork (deep blue between the pigmented pectinate ligaments). Abnormal GAGs are believed to play a role in the genesis of primary open-angle glaucoma.

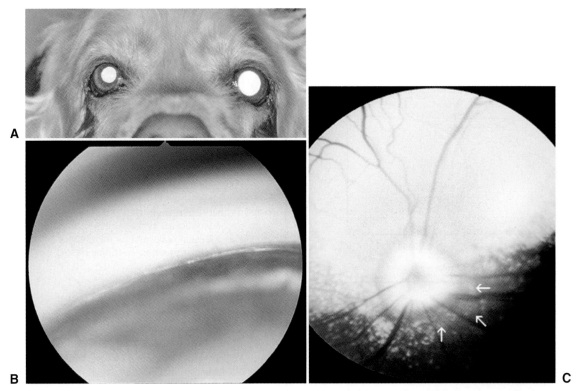

Figure 12-30. Acute angle-closure glaucoma in an American cocker spaniel. **A,** This disorder usually first manifests as a unilateral disease, but both eyes are ultimately affected. **B,** Gonioscopy shows that the iridocorneal angle is closed. **C,** In the acute stages the optic nerve is pale and there is subtle peripapillary swelling *(arrows)*.

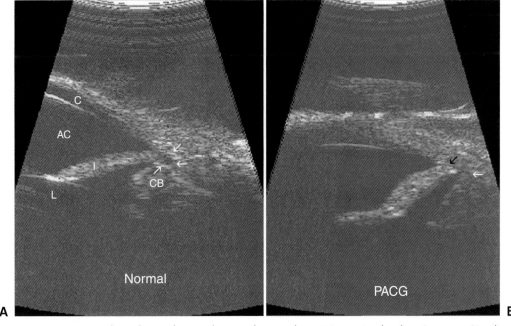

Figure 12-31. A, High-resolution ultrasound image of a normal eye. *AC,* anterior chamber; *C,* cornea; *CB,* ciliary body; *I,* iris; *L,* lens. White arrows outline the ciliary cleft. **B,** An eye with acute primary angle-closure glaucoma *(PACG).* Note the sigmoidal shape of the iris, increased contact of the peripheral iris with the cornea *(black arrow),* and collapse of the ciliary cleft *(white arrow).*

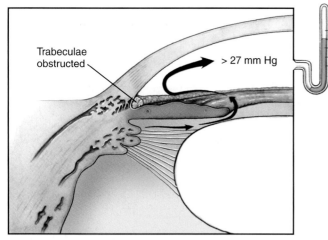

Figure 12-32. Open-angle glaucoma due to trabecular obstruction. The angle itself is normal gonioscopically.

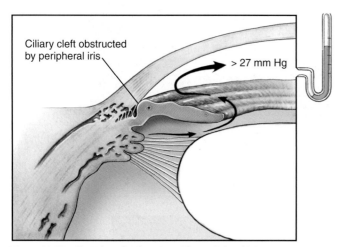

Figure 12-33. Closed-angle glaucoma. The peripheral iris prevents access by the aqueous to the ciliary cleft and drainage network. Obstruction at the pupil is also common in the closed-angle glaucomas.

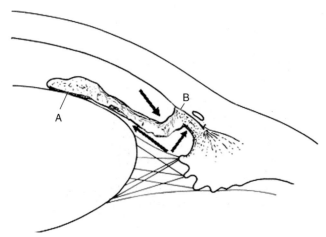

Figure 12-34. Proposed reverse pupillary block theory of the mechanism of primary angle-closure glaucoma in dogs. See text for complete description. Pectinate ligament dysplasia holds the peripheral iris in close contact with the inner surface of the cornea. Stress or excitement increases the choroidal pulse, forcing small aliquots of aqueous humor into the anterior chamber, which result in a slightly higher pressure in the anterior chamber than in the posterior chamber. This difference forces the iris against the lens near the pupil border, creating pupil block *(A)*. Prolonged increases in intraocular pressure lead to peripheral anterior synechia *(B)* and further impediment to aqueous humor outflow.

Box 12-3 | Glaucoma classification by location (posterior to anterior)

1. Ciliary body–vitreous–lens (malignant glaucoma):
   a. Block at ciliary body, vitreous, and lens with posterior pushing of lens-iris diaphragm
2. Pupil:
   a. Relative block due to iris to lens apposition
   b. Vitreous within pupil aperture
   c. Lens within pupil aperture:
      (1) Luxated lens
      (2) Intumescent lens
   d. Posterior synechia/iris bombé
3. Trabecular meshwork:
   a. Primary open-angle glaucoma
   b. Secondary obstructions:
      (1) Preiridal fibrovascular membranes
      (2) Cellular/proteinaceous material:
          (a) Vitreous
          (b) Plasma proteins
          (c) Neoplastic cells
          (d) Red blood cells
          (e) Pigment
          (f) Epithelial downgrowth through corneal perforation
   c. Primary angle-closure glaucoma:
      (1) Appositional closure
      (2) Synechial closure
   d. Secondary angle-closure glaucoma:
      (1) Peripheral anterior synechia
      (2) Ciliary body swelling/inflammation/cysts
      (3) Neoplasia
      (4) Anterior shifts of lens-iris diaphragm
4. Posttrabecular forms:
   a. Angular aqueous plexus
   b. Scleral outlet channels
   c. Episcleral vein obstructions
5. Developmental anomalies of the outflow system
6. Idiopathic mechanisms
7. Combined-mechanism glaucoma: more than one of the preceding mechanisms

Adapted from Slatter D (2003): Textbook of Small Animal Surgery, 3rd ed. Saunders, Philadelphia.

Primary Angle-Closure Glaucoma

PACG is also a bilateral disorder but it tends to manifest as an initially unilateral, rapid, marked increase in IOP in middle-aged to older dogs of certain breeds (see Figures 12-30 and 12-31, Box 12-2, and Table 12-1). An overt attack of glaucoma usually occurs in the initially normotensive fellow eye a median of 8 months after disease in the first eye becomes apparent. Again, the precise mechanism by which PACG occurs is uncertain, but there is a clear association with congenital pectinate ligament dysplasia (PLD or goniodysgenesis; see later). It is also associated with a female sex predisposition (approximately 2:1 female-to-male ratio), periods of stress or excitement, and dim light. Women also have a similarly higher risk of PACG than men, which has been attributed to a smaller, somewhat more "crowded" anterior chamber in women. Whether a similar phenomenon explains the female sex predisposition to PACG in dogs is unclear. Some dogs also experience transient, self-limiting episodes in which IOP spikes upwards but spontaneously returns to normal.

Table 12-1 | **Features of Canine Breed-Specific Glaucomas**

BREED	TYPE	USUAL PRESENTATION	ASSOCIATION WITH PECTINATE LIGAMENT DYSPLASIA	FEATURES
American cocker spaniel	Narrow to closed angle	Acute and chronic presentations	Infrequent	Most common primary glaucoma in United States. A series of self-limiting attacks may precede a final overt attack.
Chow chow	Narrow to closed angle	Acute and chronic presentations	Infrequent	Vision often retained with high pressures
Welsh springer spaniel	Narrow to closed angle	Acute and chronic presentations	No	Possible dominant inheritance
Bassett hound	Narrow to closed angle	Acute and chronic presentations	Common	Uveitis often also present but not clear if cause or effect
Flat-coated retriever	Narrow to closed angle	Acute and chronic presentations	Common	More common in England than in United States
Great Dane	Narrow to closed angle	Acute presentation	Common	More common in England than in United States
Samoyed	Narrow to closed angle	Acute and chronic presentations	Common	Lens is positioned anteriorly; pupil block may be involved
Bouvier des Flandres	Narrow to closed angle	Acute and chronic presentations	Common	May affect young dogs (1-3 yrs of age) as well as older (6-9 yrs of age)
Beagle	Open angle	Clinical cases rare; chronic syndrome	No	Autosomal recessive, angle closes late in disease. Clinical signs slow and insidious. Typically 2–5-yr-old dogs.
Norwegian elkhound	Open angle	Clinical cases rare; chronic syndrome	No	Vision often retained with high pressures Narrow to closed angle glaucoma with pectinate ligament dysplasia may also occur in breed

PLD is a condition in which the normally fine pectinate ligaments are replaced by tissues that range from a few broad-based, thick pectinate ligaments to large sheets of dysplastic tissue that cover varying amounts of the trabecular meshwork and deeper structures of the iridocorneal angle (see Figures 12-9, 12-10, 12-35, and 12-36). Large sheets of tissue may be punctuated by variably sized perforations ("flow holes") that permit aqueous humor to enter the trabecular meshwork. The deeper tissues of the iridocorneal angle may or may not be normal. Because the spaces within the trabecular meshwork tend to segmentally interconnect beneath the sheets of dysplastic pectinate ligaments, IOP tends to be normal even if only a few flow holes are present. Although virtually any breed of dog can be affected by PLD, the disorder is especially common in the basset hound, Bouvier des Flandres, American and English cocker spaniels, Norwegian elkhound, Siberian husky, dachshund, miniature poodle, Welsh terrier, wirehaired fox terrier, and Chihuahua.

PLD, however, is only one risk factor for PACG and in and of itself is insufficient to cause glaucoma in all but the most extreme and rare case in which the dog is born with glaucoma (congenital glaucoma). Evidence for this view comes from the observation that even though PLD is present at birth, glaucoma

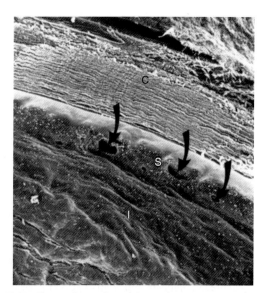

Figure 12-35. Sheets of mesodermal tissue obstructing access by aqueous to the ciliary cleft. Compare with the normal angle in Figure 12-11. Note the flow holes *(arrows)*. *C,* Cornea; *I,* iris; *S,* sclera. (From Martin CL, Wyman M [1978]: Primary glaucoma in the dog. Vet Clin North Am 8:257.)

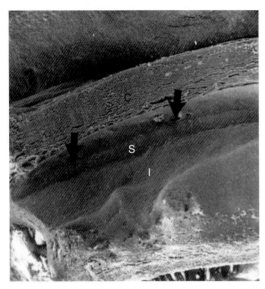

Figure 12-36. Lesion similar to the one shown in Figure 12-35, but with more extensive obstruction. *C,* Cut cornea; *I,* iris; *S,* sclera. Arrows delineate sheet with pores. (From Martin CL, Wyman M [1978]: Primary glaucoma in the dog. Vet Clin North Am 8:257.)

does not develop until the dog is typically middle-aged to old. Additionally, although virtually every dog in which PACG develops has PLD, only about 1% of dogs with PLD have glaucoma at some point in their lifetimes. This means that the vast majority of dogs with PLD never have glaucoma. Even if one limits the population to include only the dogs with the most extreme form of PLD (360-degree sheets with few flow holes), the risk of glaucoma increases to only about 15%. Finally, PLD alone does not explain the association of PACG with other risk factors, such as female sex predisposition, stress, and dim light. In the aggregate, these observations suggest that PLD is only the first step in a multistep process leading to PACG.

Recent imaging of the anterior segment in dogs experiencing an acute episode of PACG has led to a mechanistic theory, which holds that the event that initiates an attack may be impaired outflow at the level of the pupil (see Figures 12-30, 12-31, and 12-34). According to this theory, stress or excitement may raise heart rate and increase the difference between the systolic and diastolic blood pressures in the choroidal blood vessels. The increases in heart rate and pulse pressure result in a faster and larger forward "push" by the choroidal blood vessels on the posterior vitreous during systole. This force ultimately is transferred through the vitreous to the aqueous humor in the posterior chamber, causing an additional small bolus of aqueous humor to be forced through the pupil into the anterior chamber during systole. In the normal eye (or if the pulse pressure is normal) this fluid would simply flow back into the posterior chamber during diastole or, if trapped in the anterior chamber, it would force the iris more posteriorly, thereby opening the iridocorneal angle and allowing the additional fluid to exit via an expanded trabecular meshwork. In the eye at risk for PACG, however, exit of this small bolus of additional aqueous humor is impeded by abnormal pectinate ligaments, which may also prevent the angle from "popping open" in response to increased pressure in the anterior chamber. Alternatively, or perhaps in combination with PLD, age-associated declines in trabecular meshwork facility may also prevent the additional aqueous humor from escaping

the anterior chamber. This results in a transient pressure differential in which pressure is slightly greater in the anterior chamber than in the posterior chamber. If the pupil is midrange in size the iris can be pressed more firmly against the lens, resulting in a "ball-valve" effect and a so-called reverse pupillary block (see Figure 12-34). A midrange to somewhat dilated pupil (as occurs in dimmer light or during excitement) is more floppy and readily pressed against the lens than a very large or very small pupil. Very large pupils tend to cause the iris to "slide" off the more highly curved equatorial region of the lens, and very small pupils tend to have an iris that is taut and more resistant to compression against the lens. The next systole results in the forcing of a little more aqueous humor from the posterior chamber into the anterior chamber, further increasing IOP. This process continues until IOP reaches a physiologic maximum (typically 60 to 80 mm Hg) that is related to systemic blood pressure and the resistance of the intraocular tissues. Intermittent, spontaneously resolving attacks may occur if reverse pupil block develops but the pupil dilates to the point at which it can "slide" off the more highly curved equatorial region of the lens and break the block at the pupil; this block would then allow the excess aqueous humor to flow back through the pupil into the posterior chamber. If the block is not broken at the pupil, the iridocorneal angle and ciliary cleft may further collapse, thereby worsening the attack and making effective therapy much more difficult even though the whole process is of relatively short duration.

PACG may also be classified as having the following potentially overlapping phases:

- *Latent:* The fellow, normotensive eye has all the risk factors that the overtly affected eye exhibits, except that IOP has not increased. This eye should receive prophylactic therapy, because in 50% cases the fellow eye will experience overt PACG in 8 months if untreated.
- *Intermittent:* Characterized by transient (minutes to hours) increases in IOP that spontaneously resolve.
- *Acute congestive:* Characterized by very rapid, marked (50 to 80 mm Hg) increases in IOP with overt clinical signs.
- *Postcongestive:* Refers to an eye that has been successfully treated for acute congestive glaucoma and now has a normal or subnormal IOP.
- *Chronic:* IOP is chronically elevated. This state may follow an acute congestive episode that does not respond to therapy. Less commonly, multiple episodes of intermittent angle closure may slowly close the angle and create a clinical course that is characterized by multiple transient spikes in IOP and a gradually rising IOP between the spikes.
- *Absolute:* End-stage disease. Vision is lost, the eye is usually buphthalmic, and many secondary changes are typically present (lens luxation, corneal ulceration, etc.).

Secondary Glaucomas

Obstruction of the Iridocorneal Angle

The iridocorneal angle may be of normal width and simply filled with cells or substances that impair outflow (so-called secondary open-angle glaucoma) or the angle may very gradually narrow until closed by peripheral anterior synechia, fibrovascular membranes, and so on (so-called secondary closed-angle glaucoma). In general, secondary open-angle glaucomas carry a somewhat

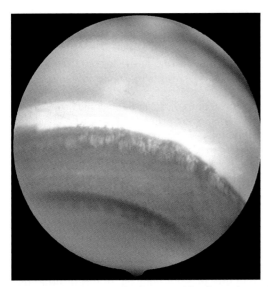

Figure 12-37. Goniophotograph showing blood in the trabecular meshwork. Intraocular pressure was elevated, but obvious hyphema was not clinically apparent.

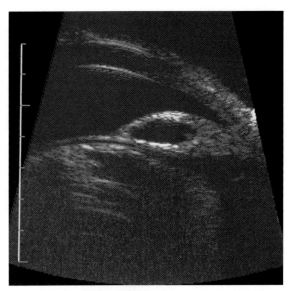

Figure 12-38. High-resolution ultrasound image in a dog with glaucoma secondary to iris bombé. The pupillary border is adherent to the anterior lens capsule and the remaining iris bows anteriorly. Additionally the ciliary cleft is collapsed, indicating that there are at least two obstructions to outflow in this patient. (Courtesy Dr. Ellison Bentley.)

better prognosis than secondary closed-angle glaucomas because the anatomy is less severely deranged. Examples of materials that may obstruct the trabecular meshwork are uveal cysts, neoplastic cells (especially melanocytes), inflammatory cells and debris, scar tissue (following chronic uveitis or intraocular surgery), red blood cells, macrophages filled with lens debris after capsule rupture (phacolytic glaucoma), vitreous, new blood vessels (preiridal fibrovascular membranes), air, viscoelastic materials used during intraocular surgeries, and epithelial cells originating from the cornea or conjunctiva. In many patients blocks may also exist at other locations in the eye (Figure 12-37).

Pupillary Block

In traditional pupillary block the flow of aqueous humor from the posterior chamber to the anterior chamber is impaired. This may result from direct physical adhesions between the iris and lens (*iris bombé*; Figure 12-38) due to chronic anterior uveitis or may simply reflect a condition in which the iris and lens are in tight apposition to each other but not physically fused (physiologic iris bombé). Pupillary block in the absence of physical adhesions commonly occurs in eyes in which the lens is very large (intumescent) or luxated into the pupillary aperture or when a portion of the lens zonules is disrupted and vitreous is able to move forward and occlude the pupil. In all forms of pupillary block glaucoma, however, aqueous accumulates in the posterior chamber, thereby increasing IOP. Very often, secondary angle-closure glaucoma complicates the latter stages of the process as the root of the iris is pushed forward into the angle. These apposed but not fused tissues (appositional closure) quickly lead to permanent adhesions and peripheral anterior synechia (synechial closure). Chronic low-grade uveitis due to lens movement also often leads to secondary angle closure.

Ciliary Body–Vitreous–Lens Block

Sometimes called "aqueous humor misdirection" or "malignant glaucoma," ciliary body–vitreous–lens block glaucoma develops when aqueous humor flows posteriorly into the vitreous cavity or

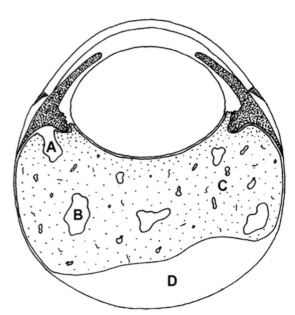

Figure 12-39. Proposed concept of ciliovitreolenticular block demonstrating the potential locations misdirected aqueous humor may collect in the vitreal cavity, including in the anterior peripheral vitreous (A), as lacunae in the central vitreous (B), diffusely throughout the vitreous (C), and between the posterior vitreous and retina (D). Increased fluid in the vitreal cavity displaces and condenses the anterior vitreal face, leading to anterior shifting of the lens-iris diaphragm. Eventually glaucoma occurs as more and more fluid is trapped within the vitreal cavity by a barrier created by the anterior ciliary body, displaced vitreous, and lens. Additionally, glaucoma may result from a cascade of obstruction to flow through the pupil and then at the iridocorneal angle/ciliary cleft. (From Czederpiltz JMC, et al. [2005]: Putative aqueous humor misdirection syndrome as a cause of glaucoma in cats: 32 cases. J Am Vet Med Assoc 227:1476.)

between the vitreous and the retina (Figures 12-39 and 12-40). The remaining vitreous is forced anteriorly, compressing its proteins and forcing them between the ciliary body and the lens. This tends to impair the forward flow of aqueous humor

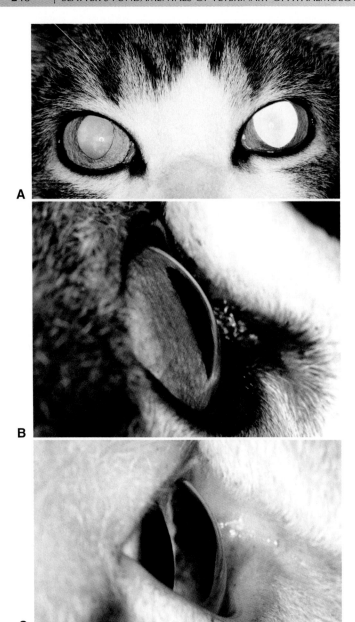

Figure 12-40. Feline aqueous humor misdirection syndrome. **A,** Frontal view; mild anisocoria is present. **B,** Affected cat eye viewed from the side. The anterior chamber is uniformly very shallow. **C,** Normal cat eye for comparison purposes. (From Czederpiltz JMC, et al. [2005]: Putative aqueous humor misdirection syndrome as a cause of glaucoma in cats: 32 cases. J Am Vet Med Assoc 227:1476.)

at the level of the ciliary body and to displace the entire lens–iris diaphragm anteriorly, shallowing the anterior chamber. Pupillary block is common, and in the later stages of the process secondary angle closure develops as well. A syndrome of aqueous humor misdirection, shallow anterior chamber, pupil dilation, and glaucoma is common in older cats. It can be differentiated from a luxated/subluxated lens by the absence of iridodonesis and phacodonesis.

Combined-Mechanism Glaucoma

Glaucoma also can occur via a combination of mechanisms, and in some patients it is not yet possible to definitively ascertain the mechanism by which IOP increases.

TREATMENT

The higher the IOP and the longer it remains increased, the less the chance that vision can be restored; 24 to 72 hours of very high IOP usually results in irreversible vision loss.

The specific actions of the antiglaucoma drugs are discussed in Chapter 3. Ideally the primary cause of the glaucoma should be treated directly. In some outflow obstructions, however, direct treatment may not be possible, and the surgeon is forced to treat the problem indirectly by reducing the production of aqueous humor. Regardless of cause, urgent therapy is required if vision is to be preserved. Often a combination of medical and surgical therapy is required, and the specific drugs and procedures chosen depend on the cause and stage of glaucoma and, to a significant extent, on the clinician's personal experiences.

Effective client education is essential in the therapy of glaucoma. Many owners' sole experience with glaucoma has been with POAG in older humans. In this disorder there is no pain, the rise in IOP is very slow and generally mild, and vision can often be maintained for the remainder of the person's life with medical therapy alone. The clinician should be careful to explain to the owner of an animal with glaucoma that there are many types of glaucoma and that treatment strategies used for POAG in older people are not appropriate for the vast majority of cases of glaucoma in animals (or other forms of glaucoma in humans, for that matter). Because many forms of glaucoma initially manifest with only one eye affected but are bilateral disorders, it is also imperative to inform the client about the clinical signs that should prompt him or her to seek medical attention in the event of an attack in the animal's fellow eye.

Primary glaucoma is a bilateral disease in dogs. Once a diagnosis of glaucoma has been made in one eye, the remaining eye should receive prophylactic medication and regular pressure checks.

The first step in the treatment of the animal with newly diagnosed glaucoma is to determine whether (1) the disorder is acute and the eye still has the potential for vision or (2) the problem is chronic and the eye is irreversibly blind (Figure 12-41). Regardless of the cause of the glaucoma, aggressive, potentially toxic, and expensive medical therapy is generally of limited to no value in patients with end-stage disease and an irrevocably blind eye. The clinician can more effectively treat such patients by identifying the cause of the glaucoma (neoplasia, lens luxation, primary angle closure, hyphema, etc.) and then performing the appropriate surgical procedure (cyclodestruction, enucleation, evisceration with intrascleral prosthesis, etc.) in conjunction with evaluating the risk of glaucoma in the remaining eye. If the affected eye has the potential for sight, however, aggressive attempts to lower IOP should be instituted. In these cases the next step is to determine the inciting cause of the glaucoma and directly address that cause, if possible.

Emergency Treatment of Acute Glaucoma

Glaucoma is usually treated by a veterinary ophthalmologist after the family veterinarian has made the initial diagnosis and provided emergency therapy.

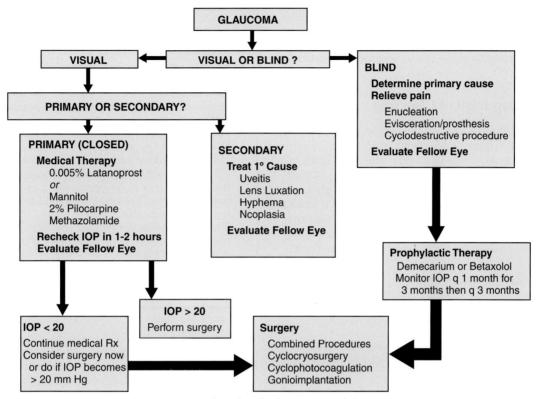

Figure 12-41. Flow chart for the treatment of glaucoma.

Box 12-4 | **Emergency therapy for primary angle-closure glaucoma in an eye with the potential for vision**

1. Latanoprost 0.005%: 1 to 2 drops topically and recheck intraocular pressure in 1 to 2 hours

If latanoprost is unavailable or ineffective:

1. Mannitol (1.0 to 1.5 g/kg IV): 5.0 to 7.5 mL/kg of 20% solution over 15 to 20 minutes
2. Methazolamide or dichlorphenamide: 2.2 to 4.4 mg/kg orally every 8 to 12 hours for dogs
3. Pilocarpine (2.0% drops): 1 drop every 10 minutes for 30 minutes, then every 6 hours

Water should be withheld for several hours after administration of mannitol.

Systemic dexamethasone (0.1 mg/kg IV) or topical 0.1% dexamethasone (every 6 to 8 hours) may be useful as well if pressure-induced ischemia has resulted in significant intraocular inflammation.

If the other eye is still normotensive, prophylactic therapy consisting of demecarium bromide (0.25% every 24 hours at bedtime with a topical corticosteroid) or betaxolol 0.5% every 12 hours should be instituted.

Early identification of the cause of the glaucoma and rapid reduction of IOP are essential to prevent permanent damage; Box 12-4 summarizes emergency treatment for PACG in an eye that still has the potential for vision. Although the initial response to medical therapy may be dramatic, *definitive treatment, usually surgical, must follow* medical therapy in order to control IOP in the long term in most patients. Except in very specific circum-

stances, medical therapy alone is generally not effective in the long-term control of most forms of glaucoma in animals and humans.

Reduction in pressure with this regimen is usually rapid (1 to 2 hours) but temporary (12 to 36 hours). If the eye responds to latanoprost, this medication should be continued every 12 hours until the patient can be evaluated by a specialist. Mannitol is very potent but it also can be quite toxic, so its use is limited to eyes with the potential for vision. If IOP remains elevated after a single injection of mannitol the 1.0 g/kg dose may be repeated in 4 hours if necessary, but long-term use should be avoided. Because mannitol solution is at or near the saturation point it may need to be heated or put through a 5-μm filter to avoid intravenous injection of crystals and potentially fatal consequences. Mannitol lowers IOP by dehydrating the vitreous along with the rest of the animal. Side effects include headache, osmotic diuresis, and worsening of dehydration, renal failure, or cardiovascular disease. Deaths due to pulmonary edema also have been reported if mannitol is given to animals anesthetized with methoxyflurane. A hyperosmotic agent should be used with caution if the blood-ocular barrier is not intact (uveitis, hyphema), because a leaky barrier may allow mannitol to enter the vitreous, thereby pulling water into the vitreal cavity and increasing IOP.

Oral glycerin at 1 to 2 mL/kg orally is an alternative to mannitol, although it is a less reliable ocular hypotensive drug and frequently induces vomiting. The probability of vomiting may be reduced by dividing the dose into thirds and giving it chilled or mixed with food. Glycerin is contraindicated in diabetic patients. On rare occasions glycerin may be used every 8 hours for up to 5 days if toxicity is not significant. Glycerin is occasionally dispensed for the owner to administer to treat a sudden attack of glaucoma immediately before seeking professional assistance.

Boxes 12-5 through 12-7 summarize emergency treatment for glaucoma associated with, or due to, specific circumstances or diseases.

Long-Term Management of Glaucoma

In most cases, definitive therapy for glaucoma is surgery (cyclocryotherapy, laser cyclophotocoagulation, gonioimplantation, evisceration with intraocular prosthesis insertion, or enucleation). If required, antiglaucoma drugs may supplement surgery and fine-tune IOP control. Certain types of glaucoma (e.g., uveitis-induced or hyphema-associated) may be treated medically first; if medical therapies fail, surgical methods may then be used. Glaucoma following primary lens luxation may be controlled medically if the lens remains posterior to the iris.

Surgical Therapy for Glaucoma

Particular attention should also be paid to the patient's general physical health before surgery, because alterations in hydration,

---

| Box 12-5 | **Emergency therapy for uveitis-induced glaucoma** |

1. Identify underlying cause and directly address it if possible.
2. Systemic dexamethasone (0.1mg/kg IV) or flunixin meglumine (0.1 mg/kg IV)
3. Topical dexamethasone (0.1% every 2 to 4 hours) or prednisolone acetate (1.0% every 2 to 4 hours)
4. Carbonic anhydrase inhibitors either topically (dorzolamide 2% alone or in combination with timolol, or brinzolamide 1%, both every 8 hours) or systemically (methazolamide or dichlorphenamide: 2.2 to 4.4 mg/kg orally every 8 to 12 hours for dogs and 1 to 2 mg/kg every 8 to 12 hours for cats)
5. If additional intraocular pressure lowering required, consider adding in topical timolol 0.5% every 8 to 12 hours, epinephrine 1% every 6 to 8 hours, or dipivefrin 0.1% every 6 to 8 hours.
6. Usually, pilocarpine, latanoprost, and systemic hyperosmotics should be avoided.

| Box 12-6 | **Emergency therapy for hyphema-associated glaucoma** |

1. Identify underlying cause and directly address it if possible.
2. Topical dexamethasone (0.1% every 2 to 4 hours) or prednisolone acetate (1.0% every 2 to 4 hours)
3. Carbonic anhydrase inhibitors either topically (dorzolamide 2% alone or in combination with timolol or brinzolamide 1%, both every 8 hours) or systemically (methazolamide or dichlorphenamide: 2.2 to 4.4 mg/kg orally every 8 to 12 hours for dogs and 1 to 2 mg/kg every 8 to 12 hours for cats) or together
4. If additional intraocular pressure lowering is required, consider adding in topical timolol 0.5% every 8 to 12 hours, epinephrine 1% every 6 to 8 hours, or dipivefrin 0.1% every 6 to 8 hours.
5. Usually, systemic hyperosmotics should be avoided.
6. The use of topical pilocarpine or atropine is controversial.

| Box 12-7 | **Emergency therapy for lens luxation–associated glaucoma** |

1. If lens in anterior chamber, dilate pupil with atropine 1% or tropicamide 1.0%.
2. Topical dexamethasone (0.1% every 2 to 4 hours) or prednisolone acetate (1.0% every 6 to 8 hours)

If ineffective:

1. Mannitol (1.0 to 1.5 g/kg IV): 5.0 to 7.5 mL/kg of 20% solution over 15 to 20 minutes
2. Carbonic anhydrase inhibitors either topically (dorzolamide 2% or brinzolamide 1%, both every 8 hours) or systemically (methazolamide or dichlorphenamide: 2.2 to 4.4 mg/kg orally every 8 to 12 hours for dogs and 1 to 2 mg/kg every 8 to 12 hours for cats)
3. If additional intraocular pressure lowering required, consider adding topical epinephrine 1% every 6 to 8 hours or dipivefrin 0.1% every 6 to 8 hours.
4. If the lens is in the anterior chamber, pilocarpine, timolol, and latanoprost should be avoided.

Referral to a specialist for further evaluation is advisable.

---

electrolyte, and acid-base status are common in animals that have malaise, inappetence, and so on from the pain associated with high IOP or that have received antiglaucoma drugs. Blood gas and acid-base status along with serum potassium levels may also need to be assessed before induction of anesthesia, especially if a systemic carbonic anhydrase inhibitor (CAI) has been administered recently. Preoperative rehydration may be necessary in animals that have received mannitol.

Glaucoma procedures used to treat eyes with the potential for vision are classified according to whether they increase aqueous humor outflow (e.g., gonioimplantation, filtering procedures) or decrease aqueous humor production (cyclophotocoagulation, cyclocryosurgery). A combination of outflow-enhancing and inflow-reducing procedures may be more effective than either one alone at controlling IOP and preserving vision. In current clinical practice gonioimplantation, cyclophotocoagulation, and cyclocryosurgery are by far the dominant surgical procedures used to treat an eye with the potential for retaining vision. If the eye is irreversibly blind, enucleation, evisceration with intrascleral prosthesis, and perhaps a cyclodestructive procedure are more appropriate.

Surgery to Increase Aqueous Humor Outflow

Historically a number of procedures to increase outflow (iridencleisis, corneoscleral trephination, cyclodialysis, and sclerectomy) have been used alone or in combination in an effort to address glaucoma due to impaired outflow of aqueous humor. These procedures would theoretically address the root cause of the glaucoma and allow for more normal nutritional support for the cornea and lens, because they would enable aqueous humor production to continue at more normal levels. Full- or partial-thickness holes in the sclera, however, have been plagued by fibrosis over the filtering site and long-term failure to control IOP in most patients. Artificial aqueous humor shunts (gonioimplants) with or without pressure-sensitive valves (to prevent IOP from getting too low) have also been used to try to create a pathway for aqueous to drain from the eye, but these also have the problem of development of a scar tissue–lined,

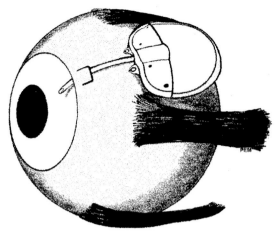

Figure 12-42. Positioning of an Ahmed gonioimplant. The conjunctiva has been removed for clarity. The implant is sutured to the sclera between the extraocular muscles so that the leading edge is 8 to 10 mm posterior to the limbus. A small tunnel incision is made in the sclera for the tubing to enter the anterior chamber. The implant has a one-way valve that opens when pressure exceeds approximately 8 mm Hg. (From Slatter D [2003]: Textbook of Small Animal Surgery 3rd ed. Saunders, Philadelphia.)

cystlike space that again becomes relatively resistant to the flow of aqueous humor (Figure 12-42). In an effort to avoid fibrosis around the drainage device, some surgeons have placed the distal end of the tubing into the frontal sinus, parotid salivary duct, nasolacrimal duct, or the orbit. None of these approaches, however, has been demonstrated to be more effective than subconjunctival drainage, and endophthalmitis is always a risk if the tube is placed in structures that communicate with the outside environment. Use of an antimetabolite such as mitomycin C or 5-fluorouracil may limit fibrosis over the body of the implant and improve its long-term filtering capacity. Adjunctive medical antiglaucoma therapy, or a limited cyclo-destructive procedure, may also be used to fine-tune IOP control once control is achieved grossly with the implant.

Surgery to Reduce Aqueous Humor Production

Although these procedures do not address the underlying reason for the glaucoma (impaired outflow), they can be quite effective at lowering IOP. Techniques for destroying the portion of the ciliary body that make aqueous humor include cyclo-cryotherapy with either liquid nitrogen or nitrous oxide, cyclophotocoagulation (cyclophotoablation) with either a diode or neodymium:yttrium-aluminum-garnet (Nd:YAG) laser, cyclodiathermy, focused ultrasound, and chemical ablation. In practical terms, however, only cyclocryosurgery and cyclo-photocoagulation are reliable and used with any regularity today. These are relatively crude procedures because they require the surgeon to estimate both the degree of outflow impairment and the amount of cyclodestruction necessary to match that impairment. Often the outflow facility is so severely compromised that the eye is highly sensitive to even minor alterations in aqueous production, resulting in a relatively narrow margin for error in these estimates. Too little destruction can result in persistence of the glaucoma, and too much can lead to phthisis bulbi. It is also not uncommon for outflow to be so severely impaired that aqueous humor production must be reduced to levels that cannot maintain normal ocular health, resulting in cataract formation or corneal endothelial decompensation and

vision loss even though IOP is controlled. Failure to control IOP in the long term with these procedures is the result of inadequate destruction of the ciliary body, regeneration of the ciliary epithelium, and progressive angle closure with loss of additional outflow capacity. Despite these limitations, however, a cyclo-destructive procedure is more appealing as a single procedure than a gonioimplant or filtering procedure because it is faster, technically easier, less expensive to perform, and repeatable.

Cyclodestruction is indicated in cases of medically uncontrollable primary glaucoma in an eye that still has the potential for vision and for the relief of chronic ocular pain in an irreversibly blind eye in an animal whose owner wishes to preserve the globe. The success rate is much lower in eyes with glaucoma secondary to chronic anterior uveitis, preiridal fibrovascular membrane formation, or retinal detachments. Relative contra-indications include intraocular neoplasia, hyphema, and anterior lens luxations.

Cyclocryotherapy

Controlled application of intense cold to the sclera overlying the ciliary body causes necrosis of the ciliary body and reduced aqueous production. Both liquid nitrogen and nitrous oxide are acceptable cryogens, but some surgeons believe liquid nitrogen to be a more reliable agent, perhaps because it achieves a colder temperature than nitrous oxide.

Preoperatively dexamethasone (0.1 mg/kg IV) and flunixin meglumine (0.1 mg/kg IV) are administered in anticipation of the severe uveitis than may follow cyclocryosurgery. Precise application of the cryoprobe over the ciliary processes and avoiding the 3 and 9 o'clock positions is essential. If the globe is approximately normal size, a 3-mm (diameter) nitrous oxide glaucoma cryoprobe is centered 5 mm posterior to the limbus (Figure 12-43). If the globe is enlarged, the cryoprobe is centered 5.5 to 6.0 mm posterior to the limbus. Gentle pressure on the globe, slightly indenting it, enlarges the extent of the ciliary destruction by shortening the distance between the cryoprobe and target tissue and by reducing blood flow to the area. Usually six to eight spots are frozen for 2 minutes when nitrous oxide instrumentation is used. Timing begins when the probe achieves a temperature of –70° to –80° C, a range that correlates with a temperature in the ciliary body of at least –10° C, which is

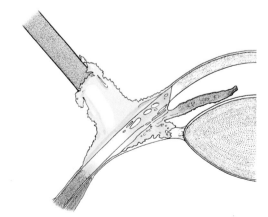

Figure 12-43. Cryoprobe cooled by liquid nitrogen, positioned 5 mm posterior to the limbus and adjacent to the ciliary body. (Modified from Roberts SM, et al. [1984]: Cyclocryotherapy. Part I: evaluation of a liquid nitrogen system. J Am Anim Hosp Assoc 20:823.)

necessary to cause cyclodestruction. If liquid nitrogen is used, the probe is placed in the same location, but the cryogen is circulated through the probe until the ice ball extends 1 mm past the limbus into clear cornea, after which the freeze is terminated. The larger size of the tip (2.5 × 6.5 mm) and the more profound freeze usually allows fewer sites to be frozen (perhaps as few as two to four).

At the conclusion of the procedure a subconjunctival injection of 0.5 to 1.0 mg of dexamethasone or other suitable corticosteroid may be given. Systemic analgesics may be necessary in some animals because freezing can induce significant ocular pain. The marked chemosis that follows freezing can result in exposure conjunctivitis and/or keratitis, so a partial temporary tarsorrhaphy may also be performed at the conclusion of the procedure.

Marked conjunctivitis, chemosis, and uveitis should be expected. Topical 0.1% dexamethasone/triple antibiotic ophthalmic ointment is administered every 4 to 6 hours, depending on the degree of inflammation. Antiglaucoma drugs are continued as before surgery, and if the eye has the potential for vision, the IOP is carefully followed for several days, and then at 1 and 2 weeks. If the eye is irreversibly blind, antiglaucoma drugs are continued for 10 to 14 days, after which the patient is reevaluated. Marked postoperative IOP spikes can persist for days after surgery, and occasionally aqueocentesis may be necessary to control IOP in the immediate postoperative period. Tapping the anterior chamber, however, can be detrimental because doing so exacerbates the uveitis, risks introducing bacteria or damaging the lens, and probably increases the chance of reperfusion injury to the retina and optic nerve. If IOP is well controlled 2 weeks postoperatively, the antiglaucoma medication dosage may be gradually tapered. The timing of further follow-up examinations varies according to response to therapy and whether the eye has the potential for vision.

Complications include the aforementioned IOP spike, uveitis, exposure keratoconjunctivitis, neurotrophic keratitis if the long posterior ciliary nerves are damaged, hyphema, retinal detachment, recurrence of glaucoma, and phthisis bulbi with a cosmetically unacceptable globe. The relatively high frequency of these complications indicates that cyclocryosurgery should not be performed as a prophylactic measure in the normotensive fellow eye of an animal with glaucoma.

Success rates vary with the duration of follow-up, whether IOP control or preservation of vision was the goal, and whether the owner permits more than one freezing episode. If IOP control, not vision, is the goal and the owner will allow multiple procedures to be performed, cyclocryosurgery can have a success rate as high as 90%. If the eye has the potential for vision at the outset, the rates of vision preservation may be as high as 60% at 6 months postoperatively. Unfortunately, as for all glaucoma procedures, the success declines with the length of follow-up. If IOP begins to rise again additional medical and or surgical therapy is required. In general cats seem to have a lower success rate than dogs. Certain breeds (cocker spaniel, Siberian husky, Norwegian elkhound, chow chow, and shar-pei) may require more aggressive ciliary body destruction to ensure long-term IOP control.

Laser Cyclophotocoagulation

An alternative method of destroying the ciliary body processes is transscleral irradiation of the ciliary body with a diode or Nd:YAG laser. Laser therapy has the advantages of being more controllable and potentially causing less reaction than cyclocryotherapy. It can also be repeated with less risk of hypotony. It suffers from the disadvantage of frequently requiring more than one treatment and of having a higher failure rate than cyclocryotherapy. Laser cyclophotocoagulation is exclusively performed by ophthalmic surgeons trained and experienced in its use.

Combined Procedures

The combination of a limited cyclodestructive procedure and a gonioimplant (with or without adjunctive medical therapy) offers some attractive theoretical advantages in treating glaucomatous eyes with the potential for vision. They include (1) blunting of the postoperative IOP spike that often accompanies a cyclodestructive procedure and can destroy the last vestiges of vision the patient has, (2) allowing for a greater level of aqueous humor production postoperatively so as to improve intraocular nutrition and reduce the chance a blinding cataract will occur, and (3) allowing for a finer control of IOP in the postoperative period. In one retrospective study a combination of the two procedures appeared to be more effective than a single procedure and allowed more than 50% of patients to retain vision for at least 1 year after an overt attack of angle-closure glaucoma. Combining procedures also allowed for a greater percentage of patients to maintain IOP within the normal range, even though vision was ultimately lost either because of progressive retinal and optic nerve degeneration secondary to an apoptotic cascade or because of cataract. The frequent follow-up visits, additional expense, and potentially greater complications of a combined procedure, however, do not allow for it to be advocated for the treatment of irrevocably blind eyes, for which the goal of therapy is simply pain relief.

Lens Luxation

The clinician should be aware that primary lens luxation is bilateral and usually hereditary, although very commonly the patient initially presents with an overt luxation in only one eye. An acute episode of glaucoma associated with lens luxation is managed as previously described in this chapter. If the eye is irreversibly blind the clinician should consider enucleation, evisceration with intrascleral prosthesis, or perhaps a cyclodestructive procedure. Lens extraction is seldom indicated in blind eyes because it is more costly than other procedures and because other impediments to outflow (e.g., at the angle) are usually present and cause glaucoma to persist postoperatively.

Longer-term therapy for an eye with the potential for vision and glaucoma attributable to a subluxated or luxated lens depends on the position of the lens and whether or not other impediments to outflow are present. If lens luxation is acute and the lens has luxated posteriorly, the eye may be treated with miotics to ensure that the lens does not enter the anterior chamber. Many animals tolerate a lens in the vitreous for long periods without recurrences of glaucoma, provided that medications are continued. If the lens is opaque and interferes with vision in the vitreous or has very recently become luxated, or if the pupil will not effectively constrict, intracapsular lens extraction may be performed, although the prognosis is guarded even when the procedure is performed by experienced surgeons.

If the lens has luxated into the plane of the pupil or anterior chamber, most surgeons prefer to remove it by either intracapsular lens extraction or phacoemulsification. Alternatively, the pupil may be dilated and an attempt made to get the lens to fall back into the vitreous. If the lens does fall into the vitreous, miotics may then be used in an effort to ensure that it remains there. If it does not, it should be surgically removed. The long-term success of any of these treatment strategies hinges on whether the patient has either POAG or peripheral anterior synechia and secondary angle-closure glaucoma in addition to the lens luxation. Unfortunately, both of these conditions commonly occur in patients with primary lens luxations thereby greatly reducing the probability of maintaining a comfortable and sighted eye over the long term.

Glaucoma Secondary to Uveitis

Gonioscopy is performed once emergency therapy has been implemented and the inflammation has been reduced. If the angle is open, medical therapy may be slowly reduced in accordance with control of the uveitis. The ability of topical dexamethasone 0.1% to increase IOP in normal dogs and dogs with POAG is of uncertain importance in the treatment of dogs with uveitis-induced glaucoma. In a clinical setting the relatively small rise in IOP attributable to topical corticosteroids is masked by the much more dramatic changes in IOP induced by inflammation of the ciliary body and the compromise of the drainage angle (both of which may be returned to more normal values by the use of topical corticosteroids). Therefore it seems reasonable to use topical corticosteroids for the treatment of uveitis-induced glaucoma, although these agents should not be employed indiscriminately.

If peripheral anterior and posterior synechiae are present, and pressure does not fall with emergency therapy, the prognosis for retaining vision is very poor. If the eye still has vision and an open iridocorneal angle, laser iridotomy may be attempted to create a new hole in the iris to allow aqueous to bypass the occluded pupil; however, the iris holes usually seal closed with time. Laser iridotomy is much less effective in eyes that also have peripheral anterior synechia and angle closure because it does not resolve this additional impediment to outflow at the level of the angle. Gonioimplantation may also be attempted, but frequently this procedure fails because the tube rapidly occludes with inflammatory debris and the subconjunctival filtering bleb rapidly scars. A cyclodestructive procedure may also be attempted although it frequently exacerbates the uveitis, possibly leading to even more synechia and outflow impairment. If the eye is irreversibly blind the clinician should consider enucleation (with histopathology to determine the cause of the uveitis), evisceration with an intrascleral prosthesis (again with histopathology; it should not be performed if neoplastic or infectious causes of the uveitis are suspected), or, in carefully selected cases, a cyclodestructive procedure.

Glaucoma Secondary to Intraocular Neoplasia

Melanoma of the iris or ciliary body is a relatively common cause of secondary glaucoma in dogs and a less common one in other species. In most cases, enucleation, with or without an orbital prosthesis, is the treatment of choice. In very select cases iridocyclectomy (removal of a portion of the iris and ciliary body), cyclocryotherapy, or laser photocoagulation is successful in treating circumscribed tumors. By the time glaucoma is present the tumor is usually too advanced for this type of therapy. Glaucoma secondary to lymphosarcoma may respond to medical antiglaucoma therapy and definitive systemic chemotherapy. In general evisceration with placement of an intrascleral prosthesis is to be avoided in patients with presumed intraocular neoplasia.

Absolute Glaucoma

Absolute glaucoma is the end stage of chronic, increased IOP with buphthalmos, severe degenerative changes in most ocular tissue, blindness, and, almost invariably, *pain*. Although the patient with absolute glaucoma frequently shows no pain on palpation of the eye, and the owner may not believe the animal has pain, enucleation of the affected eye almost invariably results in increased playfulness and improvements in the patient's demeanor. This observation leaves little doubt that chronic glaucoma is a painful condition in the vast majority of animals.

The goal of therapy for absolute glaucoma is to provide pain relief and address any cosmetic concerns the owner may have. Eyes with end-stage glaucoma are best treated by enucleation (with or without an intraorbital prosthesis), evisceration with intrascleral prosthesis, or a cyclodestructive procedure.

Evisceration with Intrascleral Prosthesis

Evisceration with intrascleral prosthesis is indicated if the owner desires to maintain a more cosmetically pleasing eye. After a careful assessment of the eye (Box 12-8), the globe is eviscerated via removal of the internal contents through a limbal incision, leaving a scleral and corneal shell. After hemorrhage is controlled a silicone prosthesis is inserted (Figure 12-44). The enlarged globe shrinks to the size of the prosthesis over the next 3 to 4 weeks. During this time the cornea may vascularize and appear red. This appearance eventually resolves, and the cornea assumes its final gray or black color. The extent of pigmentation is impossible to predict, and owners are so advised before surgery. Prostheses may also be used after severe injury, when phthisis bulbi is beginning, to preserve a

---

Box 12-8 | Indications and contraindications for intraocular prosthesis insertion

Indications

Chronic glaucoma ± buphthalmos
Prevention of phthisis bulbi
Blinding ocular trauma (may be used even after penetrating corneal wounds)
Chronic, noninfectious uveitis

Contraindications

Intraocular neoplasia
Panophthalmitis
Ulcerative keratitis
Senile degenerative keratopathy
Degenerative corneal disorders
Foci of bacterial infection (e.g., severe untreated dental disorders, discospondylitis, otitis externa)

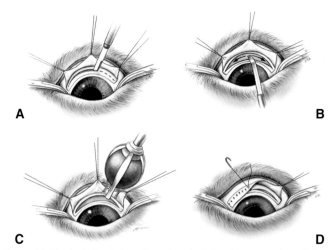

Figure 12-44. A, A fornix-based conjunctival flap is prepared, and the sclera is incised parallel to the limbus. **B,** Ocular contents are removed by dissection between the choroid and the inner scleral layers, leaving only the corneoscleral shell. **C,** A silicone prosthesis 1 mm larger than the limbal diameter of the other, normal eye is inserted with a prosthesis inserter. **D,** The sclera and conjunctiva are closed with interrupted or simple continuous absorbable sutures.

cosmetically acceptable eye. Prostheses have been successfully inserted into equine eyes with glaucoma previously unresponsive to medications and cyclocryotherapy. Although this procedure is generally quite successful, complications include ocular pain in the immediate postoperative period, ulcerative keratitis (potentially with exposure or extrusion of the prosthesis), keratoconjunctivitis sicca, infection, and recurrence of an unsuspected tumor. Because of the last possibility, all excised tissue should be histologically examined.

Enucleation

Once an eye has been thoroughly evaluated and a diagnosis of absolute glaucoma with pain has been made, the owner may decide to have the eye removed. An intraorbital prosthesis may or may not be placed, depending on the owner's wishes. See Chapter 17 for the technique.

All enucleated eyes should be examined by an experienced veterinary ophthalmic pathologist.

FELINE GLAUCOMA

The general principles of glaucoma therapy also apply to feline glaucoma. In general, normal feline IOP tends to be greater than that of the dog and to decline with age. One study found normal IOP for young cats with the Tono-Pen to be 20.2 ± 5.5 mm Hg with a range of 9 to 31 mm Hg, whereas the Tono-Pen yielded readings of 12.3 ± 4.0 mm Hg (range 4 to 21 mm Hg) in cats 7 years or older. The exact incidence of glaucoma in cats is unclear, although data from the Veterinary Medical Data Base suggested that 1 in 367 cats presenting to a University Teaching Hospital had glaucoma. In contrast, a prospective evaluation in a feline exclusive private practice found that 0.9% of cats 7 years or older had abnormally high IOP on tonometric screening.

Secondary glaucoma, most frequently due to chronic uveitis or intraocular neoplasia, is approximately 19 times more common than primary glaucoma in cats. Inherited congenital POAG has been described in Siamese cats, but acute PACG as seen in dogs is rare to nonexistent in cats. The rise in IOP in the vast majority of cats tends to be slow and insidious, and the condition is usually unilateral. Many cats with glaucoma initially present for another ocular disorder (chronic uveitis, iris color change, intraocular mass). Another common presentation, especially for those with aqueous humor misdirection syndrome (see earlier description in this chapter), is anisocoria with slowly progressing buphthalmos. The buphthalmos can be quite extreme in some animals. Ocular pain also tends to not be as obvious as in dogs, perhaps because the rise in IOP is typically not as abrupt or as high as in dogs, but there is no reason to believe that the condition is not painful in cats like it is in other species. Often the inciting cause is difficult to identify by the time the patient is first seen.

Common causes of glaucoma in cats include feline aqueous humor misdirection syndrome, chronic low-level lymphocytic plasmacytic uveitis with the formation of preiridal fibrovascular membranes, and neoplasia such as diffuse iris melanoma and uveal lymphoma. In one study *Toxoplasma* was implicated in 79%, feline corona virus in 27%, feline immunodeficiency virus in 23%, and feline leukemia virus in 6%. The most common clinical signs are dilated pupil, lens luxation, buphthalmos, exposure keratitis, and retinal degeneration. Cats with uveitis and prominent lymphoid nodules in the iris and iris erythema are considered to be at high risk for eventual development of glaucoma. Cats with positive *Toxoplasma* titers are more effectively treated with a combination of clindamycin and topical corticosteroid than with either drug alone.

Medical therapy for glaucoma in cats is similar to that in the dog, although cats tolerate some glaucoma medications poorly and may respond differently to antiglaucoma drugs. For example, latanoprost and the other commercially available prostaglandins do not lower IOP in cats, although they can induce profound miosis. The topical CAI brinzolamide did not lower IOP in normal cats when administered every 12 hours but may do so when given every 8 hours to cats with glaucoma. A related topical CAI, dorzolamide given every 8 hours, is effective in lowering IOP in glaucomatous cats. As in dogs, topical application of dexamethasone or 1% prednisolone acetate has increased IOP in cats, but the clinical significance of this finding is unclear. Additionally, unilateral topical administration of 0.5% tropicamide can raise IOP an average of approximately 3.5 mm Hg in both the treated and untreated eyes, and in some cats this increase may be as much as 17 to 18 mm Hg in the treated and untreated eyes. These observations reinforce the concept that cats are anatomically and physiologically distinct from dogs and that some therapies appropriate for the dog may not be transferable to the cat.

Although surgical therapy for feline glaucoma is similar to that for dogs, cyclocryotherapy must be quite aggressive if used, and liquid nitrogen is recommended as the cryogen to limit treatment failures. Cyclodestructive procedures are often unsuccessful in the long term in cats, perhaps because of the nature of their glaucoma. Evisceration with insertion of an intrascleral prosthesis may be performed, although the cosmetic results with a black silicone ball are less satisfactory than that achieved with dogs because of the normally brightly colored feline iris and vertically oriented slit pupil. Varying the color of the sphere and tattooing a slit pupil onto the cornea can improve the postoperative appearance of the globe. Enucleation, with or without the placement of an intraorbital prosthesis, is a reasonable procedure in cats. There are some suggestions, however, that cats may reject an intraorbital sphere more frequently than dogs.

EQUINE GLAUCOMA

Normal equine IOP is higher than a cat's or dog's, averaging approximately 23 mm Hg and ranging up to the low to mid 30s. Glaucoma is less commonly recognized in horses than in dogs or cats, perhaps because the uveoscleral pathway constitutes a greater percentage of the equine outflow pathway. Although primary glaucoma appears to occur in horses, the most common form is glaucoma secondary to chronic anterior uveitis or intraocular neoplasia. Appaloosas, horses with concurrent equine recurrent uveitis, and horses older than 15 years are at greater risk of glaucoma. Clinical signs of equine glaucoma include corneal striae (caused by rupture of Descemet's membrane), buphthalmos, decreased vision, lens luxation, loss of the pupillary light reflex, mild anterior uveitis, optic nerve atrophy, optic disc cupping, and elevated IOP. Because many horses with glaucoma also have anterior uveitis, the pupil is often miotic or normal in size and is not dilated as is common in other species. A feature that complicates both the diagnosis and therapy of equine glaucoma is that the IOP fluctuates markedly, and frequent measurements may be necessary to demonstrate the presence of glaucoma and the effects of treatment. The reason for this fluctuation is unclear but it may involve compression of the globe by the orbicularis oculi or extraocular muscles. Auriculopalpebral nerve block may be required to obtain accurate applanation tonometry in fractious horses, and sedatives may significantly decrease IOP.

The principles of medical and surgical therapy for glaucoma in other species apply to horses with glaucoma, although the response to antiglaucoma medications in horses may be different from that in dogs and cats. Studies of antiglaucoma drugs in horses often yield conflicting results, suggesting that there may be considerable interindividual variations in the responsiveness of this species to many antiglaucoma drugs. For example, topical pilocarpine given alone can increase IOP in many, but not all, horses. The mechanism for this finding is unclear but may involve exacerbation of preexisting uveitis, pupillary block, or a reduction in the uveoscleral outflow pathway. Atropine, which stabilizes the blood aqueous barrier and may increase uveoscleral outflow, can reduce IOP in many normal horses and in horses with glaucoma secondary to chronic uveitis. Atropine can, however, also raise IOP in some horses. The prostaglandin derivative latanoprost does not lower IOP in normal horses (or does so only by 1 to 2 mm Hg) and can be quite irritating. Other studies have indicated that topical prostaglandins exacerbate elevated IOP in horses with glaucoma. Only timolol or the topical CAIs seem to consistently lower IOP in horses. Systemic CAIs may be prohibitively expensive in horses, and their efficacy and safety has not been determined. Antiglaucoma therapy in the horse often involves a combination of antiglaucoma and antiinflammatory drugs. Unfortunately, the therapy of primary equine glaucoma is largely empirical owing to our lack of understanding of the pathogenesis of the condition.

A cyclodestructive procedure (cyclocryotherapy, laser cyclophotocoagulation) may be used in equine eyes that have the potential for vision and in an attempt to maintain a comfortable, but blind eye. One study suggested that an effective Nd:YAG laser protocol in horses with glaucoma is a power setting of 11 W, duration of 0.4 second, applied 5 mm posterior to the limbus at 60 sites, resulting in a total energy dose of 264 J. Additionally, equine glaucoma has been effectively treated with an intrascleral prosthesis and enucleation (with or without an intraorbital prosthesis). Despite the best efforts of the clinician, however, the long-term prognosis for retaining vision in a glaucomatous equine eye is poor.

BIBLIOGRAPHY

Abrams KL (2001): Medical and surgical management of the glaucoma patient. Clin Tech Small Anim Pract 16:71.
Bentley E, et al. (2003): Use of high-resolution ultrasound as a diagnostic tool in veterinary ophthalmology. J Am Vet Med Assoc 223:1617.
Bentley E, et al. (1999): Combined cycloablation and gonioimplantation for treatment of glaucoma in dogs: 18 cases (1992-1998). J Am Vet Med Assoc 215:1469.
Bentley E, et al. (1996): Implantation of filtering devices in dogs with glaucoma: preliminary results in 13 eyes. Vet Comp Ophthalmol 6:243.
Biros DJ, et al. (2000): Development of glaucoma after cataract surgery in dogs: 220 cases (1987-1998). J Am Vet Med Assoc 216:1780.
Bjerkas E, et al. (2002): Pectinate ligament dysplasia and narrowing of the iridocorneal angle associated with glaucoma in the English springer spaniel. Vet Ophthalmol 5:49.
Blocker T, van der Woerdt A (2001): The feline glaucomas: 82 cases (1995-1999). Vet Ophthalmol 4:81.
Brinkmann MC, et al. (1992): Neodymium:YAG laser treatment of iris bombé and pupillary block glaucoma. Proc Vet Comp Ophthalmol 2:13.
Brooks DE (1999): Equine ophthalmology, in Gelatt KN (editor): Veterinary Ophthalmology, 3rd ed. Lippincott Williams & Wilkins, Philadelphia.
Brooks DE, et al. (1997): Vitreous body glutamate concentration in dogs with glaucoma. Am J Vet Res 58:864.
Brooks DE, et al. (1995): Histomorphometry of optic nerves of normal dogs and dogs with hereditary glaucoma. Exp Eye Res 60:71.
Chavkin MJ, et al. (1992): Seroepidemiologic and clinical observations of 93 cases of uveitis in cats. Prog Vet Comp Ophthalmol 2:29.
Cook C, et al. (1997): Diode laser transscleral cyclophotocoagulation for the treatment of glaucoma in dogs: results of six and twelve months' follow-ups. Vet Comp Ophthalmol 7:148.
Cullen CL (2004): Cullen frontal sinus valved glaucoma shunt: preliminary findings in dogs with primary glaucoma. Vet Ophthalmol 7:311.
Cullen CL, Grahn BH (2000): Equine glaucoma: a retrospective study of 13 cases presented at the Western College of Veterinary Medicine from 1992-1999. Can Vet J 41:470.
Czederpiltz JM, et al. (2005): Putative aqueous humor misdirection syndrome as a cause of glaucoma in cats: 32 cases (1997-2003). J Am Vet Assoc 227:1434.
Davidson HJ, et al. (2002): Effect of topical ophthalmic latanoprost on intraocular pressure in normal horses. Vet Ther 3:72.
Davidson MG, et al. (1991): Phacoemulsification and intraocular lens implantation: a study of surgical results in 182 dogs. Vet Comp Ophthalmol 1:233.
Deehr AJ, Dubielzig RR (1998): A histopathological study of iridociliary cysts and glaucoma in golden retrievers. Vet Ophthalmol 1:153.
Ekesten B, Narstrom K (1991): Correlation of morphologic features of the iridocorneal angle to intraocular pressure in Samoyeds. Am J Vet Res 52:1875.
Ekesten B, Torrang I (1995): Age-related changes in ocular distances in normal eyes of Samoyeds. Am J Vet Res 56:127.
Ekesten B, Torrang I (1995): Heritability of the depth of the opening of the ciliary cleft in Samoyeds. Am J Vet Res 56:1138.
Gelatt KN, Brooks DE (1999): The canine glaucomas, in Gelatt KN (editor): Veterinary Ophthalmology, 3rd ed. Lippincott Williams & Wilkins, Philadelphia.
Gelatt KN, Mackay EO (2004): Prevalence of the breed-related glaucomas in pure-bred dogs in North America. Vet Ophthalmol 7:97.
Gelatt KN, Mackay EO (2004): Secondary glaucomas in the dog in North America. Vet Ophthalmol 7:245.
Gelatt KN, Mackay EO (2001): Changes in intraocular pressure associated with topical dorzolamide and oral methazolamide in glaucomatous dogs. Vet Ophthalmol 4:61.

Gelatt KN, Mackay EO (2001): Effects of different dose schedules of latanoprost on intraocular pressure and pupil size in glaucomatous beagles. Vet Ophthalmol 4:283.

Gelatt KN, Mackay EO (1998): The ocular hypertensive effects of topical 0.1% dexamethasone in beagles with inherited glaucoma. J Ocul Pharmacol Ther 14:57.

Gelatt-Nicholson KJ, et al. (1999): Comparative Doppler imaging of the ophthalmic vasculature in normal beagles and beagles with inherited glaucoma. Vet Ophthalmol 2:97.

Glover TL, et al. (1995): The intracapsular extraction of displaced lenses in dogs: a retrospective study of 57 cases (1984-1990). J Am Anim Hosp Assoc 31:77.

Gorig C, et al. (2006): Comparison of the use of new handheld tonometers and established applanation tonometers in dogs. Am J Vet Res 67:134.

Gum GG, et al. (1993): Effect of topically applied demecarium bromide and echothiophate iodide on intraocular pressure and pupil size in beagles with normotensive eyes and beagles with glaucoma. Am J Vet Res 54:287.

Gum GG, et al. (1992): Effect of hyaluronidase on aqueous outflow resistance in normotensive and glaucomatous eyes of dogs. Am J Vet Res 53:767.

Gwin RM, et al. (1978): Effects of topical L-epinephrine and dipivalyl epinephrine on intraocular pressure and pupil size in the normotensive and glaucomatous beagle. Am J Vet Res 39:83.

Gwin RM, et al. (1977): The effect of topical pilocarpine on intraocular pressure on pupil size in normotensive and glaucomatous beagles. Invest Ophthalmol Vis Sci 16:1143.

Hamor RE, et al. (1994): Intraocular silicone prostheses in dogs: a review of the literature and 50 new cases. J Am Anim Hosp Assoc 30:66.

Hampson EC, et al. (2002): Primary glaucoma in Burmese cats. Aust Vet J 80:672.

Herring IP, et al. (2000): Effect of topical 1% atropine sulfate on intraocular pressure in normal horses. Vet Ophthalmol 3:139.

Kato K, et al. (2006): Possible association of glaucoma with pectinate ligament dysplasia and narrowing of the iridocorneal angle in Shiba Inu dogs in Japan. Vet Ophthalmol 9:71.

Knollinger AM, et al. (2005): An evaluation of a rebound tonometer for measuring intraocular pressure in dogs and horses. J Am Vet Med Assoc 227:244.

Kroll MM, et al. (2001): Intraocular pressure measurements obtained as part of a comprehensive geriatric health examination from cats seven years of age or older. J Am Vet Med Assoc 219:1406.

Lannek EB, Miller PE (2001): Development of glaucoma after phacoemulsification for removal of cataracts in dogs: 22 cases (1987-1997). J Am Vet Med Assoc 218:70.

Martin CL (1975): Scanning electron microscopic examination of selected canine iridocorneal angle anomalies. J Am Anim Hosp Assoc 11:300.

Martin CL (1969): Gonioscopy and anatomical correlations of the drainage angle of the dog. J Small Anim Pract 10:171.

Martin CL, Wyman M (1978): Primary glaucoma in the dog. Vet Clin North Am 8:257.

Martin CL, Wyman M (1968): Glaucoma in the basset hound. Am J Vet Res 29:379.

McIlnay TR, et al. (2004): Evaluation of glutamate loss from damaged retinal cells in dogs with primary glaucoma. Am J Vet Res 65:776.

McLaughlin SA, et al. (1995): Intraocular silicone prosthesis implantation in eyes of dogs and a cat with intraocular neoplasia: 9 cases. J Vet Med Assoc 207:1441.

Meek LA (1988): Intraocular silicone prosthesis in a horse. J Am Vet Med Assoc 193:343.

Miller PE, et al. (2000): The efficacy of topical prophylactic antiglaucoma therapy in primary closed angle glaucoma in dogs: a multicenter clinical trial. J Am Anim Hosp 36:431.

Miller PE, et al. (1997): Mechanisms of acute intraocular pressure increases phacoemulsification lens extraction in dogs. Am J Vet Res 58:1159.

Miller PE, et al. (1990): Evaluation of two applanation tonometers in horses. Am J Vet Res 51:935.

Miller PE, Picket JP (1992): Comparison of the human and canine Schiøtz tonometry conversion tables in clinically normal cats. J Am Vet Med Assoc 201:1017.

Miller PE, Pickett JP (1992): Comparison of the human and canine Schiøtz tonometry conversion tables in clinically normal dogs. J Am Vet Med Assoc 201:1021.

Miller TL, et al. (2001): Description of ciliary body anatomy and identification of sites for transscleral cyclophotocoagulation in the equine eye. Vet Ophthalmol 4:183.

Miller TR, et al. (1995): Equine glaucoma: clinical findings and response to treatment in 14 horses. Vet Comp Ophthalmol 5:170.

Morris RA, Dubielzig RR (2005): Light-microscopy evaluation of zonular fiber morphology in dogs with glaucoma secondary to lens displacement. Vet Ophthalmol 8:81.

Mughannam AJ, et al. (1999): Effect of topical atropine on intraocular pressure and pupil diameter in the normal horse eye. Vet Ophthalmol 2:213.

Nasisse MP, et al. (1990): Treatment of glaucoma by use of transscleral neodymium:yttrium aluminum garnet laser cyclocoagulation in dogs. J Am Vet Med Assoc 197:350.

Nasisse MP, Glover TL (1997): Surgery for lens instability. Vet Clin North Am Small Anim Pract 27:1175.

O'Reilly A, et al. (2003): The use of transscleral cyclophotocoagulation with a diode laser for the treatment of glaucoma occurring post intracapsular extraction of displaced lenses: a retrospective study of 15 dogs (1995-2000). Vet Ophthalmol 6:113.

Pauli AM, et al. (2006): Effects of the application of neck pressure by a collar or harness on intraocular pressure in dogs. J Am Anim Hosp 42:207.

Pickett JP, et al. (1993): Equine glaucoma: a retrospective study of 11 cases. Vet Med 88:756.

Plummer CE, et al. (2006): Comparison of the effects of topical administration of a fixed combination of dorzolamide-timolol to monotherapy with timolol or dorzolamide on IOP, pupil size, and heart rate in glaucomatous dogs. Vet Ophthalmol 9:245.

Read RA, et al. (1998): Pectinate ligament dysplasia (PLD) and glaucoma in flat coated retrievers. I: objectives, technique and results of a PLD survey. Vet Ophthalmol 1:85.

Reilly CM, et al. (2005): Canine goniodysgenesis-related glaucoma: a morphologic review of 100 cases looking at inflammation and pigment dispersion. Vet Ophthalmol 8:253.

Ridgway MD, Brightman AH (1989): Feline glaucoma: a retrospective study of 29 clinical cases. J Am Anim Hosp Assoc 25:485.

Riggs C, Whitely RD (1990): Two cases of intraocular silicone prostheses in eyes with traumatic corneal lacerations. J Vet Med Assoc 196:617.

Roberts SM, et al. (1984): Cyclocryotherapy. Part I: evaluation of a liquid nitrogen system. J Am Anim Hosp Assoc 20:823.

Roberts SM, et al. (1984): Cyclocryotherapy. Part II: clinical comparison of liquid nitrogen and nitrous oxide cryotherapy on glaucomatous eyes. J Am Anim Hosp Assoc 20:828.

Rosenberg LF, et al. (1996): Cyclocryotherapy and noncontact Nd:YAG laser cyclophotocoagulation in cats. Invest Ophthalmol Vis Sci 37:2029.

Samuelson D, et al. (1989): Morphologic features of the aqueous humor drainage pathways in horses. Am J Vet Res 50:720.

Samuelson DA, et al. (1983): Orthograde rapid axoplasmic transport and ultrastructural changes of the optic nerve part II: beagles with primary open angle glaucoma. Glaucoma 5:174.

Sapienza JS, et al. (2000): Golden retriever uveitis: 75 cases (1994-1999). Vet Ophthalmol 3:241.

Sapienza JS, van der Woerdt A (2005): Combined transscleral diode laser cyclophotocoagulation and Ahmed gonioimplantation in dogs with primary glaucoma: 51 cases (1996-2004). Vet Ophthalmol 8:121.

Slater MR, Erb HN (1986): Effects of risk factors and prophylactic treatment on primary glaucoma in the dog. J Am Vet Med Assoc 188:1028.

Smith PJ, et al. (1996): Ocular hypertension following cataract surgery in dogs: 139 cases (1992-1993). J Am Vet Med Assoc 209:105.

Smith PJ, et al. (1986): Unconventional aqueous humor outflow of microspheres perfused into the equine eye. Am J Vet Res 47:2445.

Studer ME, et al. (2000): Effects of 0.005% latanoprost solution on intraocular pressure in healthy dogs and cats. Am J Vet Res 61:1220.

Stuhr CM, et al. (1998): The effects of intracameral carbachol on postoperative intraocular pressure rises after cataract surgery in dogs. J Am Vet Med Assoc 212:1885.

Takiyama N, et al. (2006): The effects of a timolol maleate gel-forming solution on normotensive beagle dogs. J Vet Med Sci 68:631.

Tinsley DM, Betts DM (1992): Clinical experience with a glaucoma drainage device in dogs. Vet Comp Ophthalmol 4:77.

van de Sandt RR, et al. (2003): Abnormal ocular pigment deposition and glaucoma in the dog. Vet Ophthalmol 6:273.

van der Linde-Sipman JS (1987): Dysplasia of the pectinate ligament and primary glaucoma in the Bouvier des Flandres dog. Vet Pathol 24:201.

van der Woerdt A, et al. (1998): Normal variation in, and effect of 2% pilocarpine on, intraocular pressure and pupil size in female horses. Am J Vet Res 59:1459.

Whigham HM, et al. (1999): Treatment of equine glaucoma by transscleral neodymium:yttrium aluminum garnet laser cyclophotocoagulation: a retrospective study of 23 eyes of 16 horses. Vet Ophthalmol 2:243.

Whitely D, et al. (1985): Implantation of intraocular prostheses in dogs. Comp Cont Ed Pract Vet 7:802.

Whiteman AL, et al. (2002): Morphologic features of degeneration and cell death in the neurosensory retina in dogs with primary angle-closure glaucoma. Am J Vet Res 63:257.

Wilcock BP, et al. (1991): Glaucoma in horses. Vet Pathol 28:74.

Wilkie DA, Gilger BC (2004): Equine glaucoma. Vet Clin North Am Equine Pract 20:381.

Willis AM, et al. (2002): Advances in topical glaucoma therapy. Vet Ophthalmol 5:9.

Willis AM, et al. (2001): Effects of topical administration of 0.005% latanoprost solution on eyes of clinically normal horses. Am J Vet Res 62:1945.

Wood JL, et al. (1998): Pectinate ligament dysplasia and glaucoma in flat coated retrievers. II: assessment of prevalence and heritability. Vet Ophthalmol 1:91.

ANATOMY AND PHYSIOLOGY   CATARACT   LENS LUXATION
CONGENITAL ANOMALIES

ANATOMY AND PHYSIOLOGY

Development of the lens is described in Chapter 2. The lens is a transparent, avascular, biconvex body with an anterior surface that is flatter or less curved than the posterior surface (Figure 13-1). The centers of the surfaces are called the *anterior* and *posterior poles.* The rounded circumference is the *equator,* which has numerous irregularities where zonular fibers attach. Its anterior aspect is in contact with the posterior surface of the iris and fills the pupil. Its posterior aspect is in contact with the vitreous or, more specifically, a depression in the vitreous called the *hyaloid* (patellar) *fossa.*

The lens consists of the *capsule, anterior epithelium,* and *lens fibers.* It is divided into two general regions, the *cortex* (outer areas near the capsule) and the *nucleus* (central area) (Figure 13-2). As the lens grows throughout life, layers of fibers are produced in the equatorial area and are laid down on top of the former layers, forcing older fibers toward the lens center in a process resembling the formation of rings in tree trunks. These successive layers are visible clinically with biomicroscopy. They are called the *adult, fetal,* and *embryonal nuclei,* respectively (Figure 13-3).

The lens is supported at the equator by the *lens zonules,* or suspensory ligaments—collagenous fibers that attach to the processes of the ciliary body and suspend the lens in the middle of the pupil (Figure 13-4). Alterations of tension in these fibers alter the refractive (optical) power of the lens. To view nearby objects, the animal *accommodates* through contraction of the ciliary body muscles, mediated by parasympathetic stimulation. In primates and birds, this contraction leads to an increase in the curvature of the lens (i.e., it becomes more spheroid), thus increasing its refractive power (Figure 13-5). In carnivores, the contraction of the ciliary muscle results in forward movement of the lens in the eye, allowing the animal to accommodate for nearby objects. To view distant objects, sympathetic stimulation causes the animal to *disaccommodate* by relaxing its ciliary muscle. In primates and birds the relaxation results in a flatter lens with reduced refractive power. In carnivores it results in posterior movement of the lens in the eye. In general, the accommodative ability of birds and primates is superior to that of carnivores; most herbivores, reptiles, and rodents possess virtually no accommodative capabilities. However, it is worth remembering in this context that the cornea is the most important refracting surface in the eye, accounting for the majority of the optical power (because light undergoes significant refraction as it passes from air into the cornea). The lens accounts only for 30% to 35% of the eye's refractive power and is used for fine adjustment for objects at different distances.

Lens Components

Capsule

The capsule is a transparent, elastic envelope surrounding the lens (Figure 13-6). It provides insertion for zonular fibers that suspend the lens in the eye. In primates, the capsule regulates lens shape through its elasticity. The capsule is impermeable to large molecules (e.g., albumin, globulin) but allows water and electrolytes to pass. The anterior lens capsule, which is associated with the underlying epithelium, is much thicker than the posterior lens capsule, which lost its underlying epithelium during embryonic development (see also Figure 13-2).

Lens Epithelium

Cuboidal epithelial cells lie beneath the anterior capsule (see Figure 13-6). Toward the equator, the cells proliferate (through mitosis), become more columnar, and elongate into new lens fibers (see Figure 13-2). Because of mitotic activity in this area, these cells are susceptible to toxic and pathologic influences, which may become apparent as equatorial opacities. The lens epithelium is important in transport of cations through the lens capsule. The posterior lens epithelium, which transforms into lens fibers of the embryonic lens nucleus, is not seen in newborns and adults.

Lens Fibers

Lens fibers make up the substance of the lens and are arranged in interdigitating layers (Figure 13-7). These fibers stretch from the equatorial region toward the anterior and posterior poles of the lens. However, they do not quite reach the poles but instead meet fibers from the opposite equator and form a Y-shaped suture pattern with them (Figure 13-8). The suture pattern may become visible as a prominent upright (anterior) or inverted (posterior) Y if the lens becomes cataractous (see Figures 13-1 and 13-3). Because new lens fibers are formed throughout life, the older fibers in the (central) lens nucleus are denser and less transparent than the younger fibers laid down around them in the cortex. This difference between nucleus and cortex becomes more pronounced as the animal ages and may result in the formation of *nuclear sclerosis* (see later).

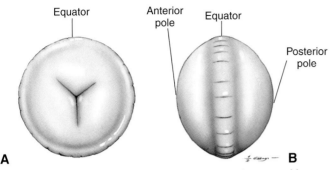

Figure 13-1. Canine lens. **A,** Anterior view of the upright anterior Y suture and equatorial margin. **B,** Lateral view of the poles and equator. Note the greater curvature of the posterior surface.

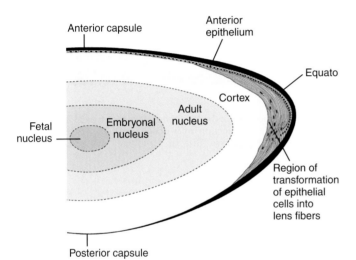

Figure 13-2. The adult lens, showing the nuclear zones, cortex, anterior epithelium, and capsule. Epithelial cells can be seen undergoing transformation into lens fibers at the equatorial region. The varying thickness of the lens capsule in various zones is also shown. (Modified from Hogan MJ, et al. [1971]: Histology of the Human Eye. Saunders, Philadelphia.)

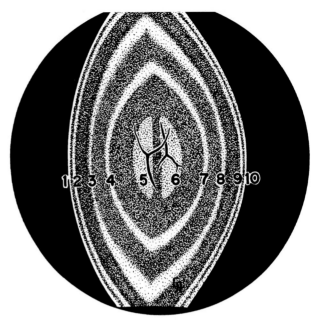

Figure 13-3. Optical section of normal adult lens. *1,* Anterior capsule; *2,* anterior line of disjunction (anterior epithelium); *3,* anterior surface of adult nucleus; *4,* anterior surface of fetal nucleus; *5,* anterior (upright) Y suture; *6,* inner layer of posterior half of fetal nucleus, containing posterior (inverted) Y suture; *7,* posterior surface of fetal nucleus; *8,* posterior surface of adult nucleus; *9,* posterior line of disjunction; *10,* posterior capsule. (From Remington LA [2005]: Clinical Anatomy of the Visual System, 2nd ed. Butterworth-Heinemann, St. Louis.)

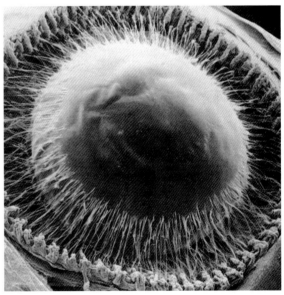

Figure 13-4. Scanning electron micrograph of anterior zonular insertion after removal of cornea and iris. (From Streeton BW [1982], in Jakobiec FA [editor]: Ocular Anatomy, Embryology, and Teratology. Harper & Row, Philadelphia.)

Metabolism and Composition

Because the lens is avascular, its metabolic needs are met by the aqueous humor. Therefore lens metabolism is precarious and depends on constant composition of the aqueous. Disturbances in aqueous composition (resulting from anterior uveitis) affect lens metabolism and transparency.

Metabolism of glucose provides most of the energy requirements of the lens. Glucose enters from the aqueous by both diffusion and assisted transport. Most of the glucose is broken down anaerobically to lactic acid via the hexokinase (pentose phosphate) pathway, although some aerobic glycolysis occurs via the citric acid cycle. Elevation in glucose levels (in diabetic patients) inhibits the hexokinase enzyme, and the glucose is diverted into the sorbitol shunt, where it is converted by aldose reductase into sorbitol (Figure 13-9).

The lens is high in protein (35%) and water (65%) and low in minerals. The proteins are divided into soluble proteins, or crystallins, and insoluble, or albuminoid, proteins. The former constitute approximately 85% of the lens protein content, but their proportion varies with species, location within the lens, age, and, most significantly, disease. The proportion of soluble proteins drops with age, and a similar process occurs when the lens becomes cataractous, as the proportion of insoluble proteins rises. During cataract formation, the lens proteins break into polypeptides and amino acids that diffuse through the lens capsule into the anterior and posterior chambers. Because these molecules are usually not recognized by the eye's immune system, the

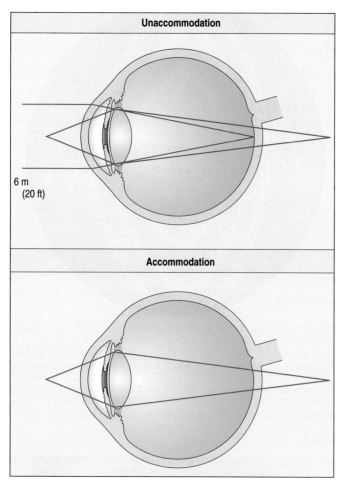

Figure 13-5. The accommodative power of the lens. At rest the unaccomodated eye focuses on distant objects but needs to accommodate to focus on near objects. (From Yanoff M, Duker JS [2004]: Ophthalmology, 2nd ed. Mosby, St. Louis.)

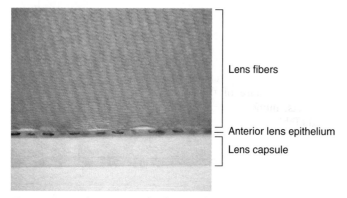

Figure 13-6. Light micrograph showing lens capsule, anterior lens epithelium, and lens fibers of the cortex. (From Remington LA [2005]: Clinical Anatomy of the Visual System, 2nd ed. Butterworth-Heinemann, St. Louis.)

breakdown and diffusion of cataractous lens protein usually trigger an inflammatory reaction known as *lens-induced uveitis* (LIU).

Nuclear Sclerosis

Throughout life, new lens cells are produced at the equator, forcing older cells toward the nucleus (see Figures 13-2 and 13-3). As

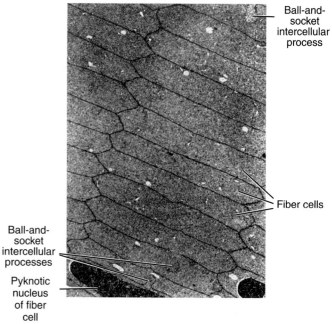

Figure 13-7. Fiber cells of the lens cortex with their typical interdigitating pattern (transmission electron microscope; ×6000). (From Krause WJ, Cutts JH [1981]: Concise Text of Histology. Williams & Wilkins, Baltimore.)

the older cells become more tightly packed, the nucleus becomes denser and harder. In dogs, after about 6 years of age this greater nuclear density becomes visible as a grayish blue haze known as *nuclear sclerosis* (Figure 13-10). This haze is probably associated with increased insoluble proteins and decreased soluble crystallins (γ-crystallin) in the lens nucleus. Advanced nuclear sclerosis may appear similar to cataract, and in fact, the two are frequently confused by owners and practitioners. However, use of mydriatics and retroillumination (illumination of the lens by reflection of strong light from the tapetum) can help in differentiating between the two entities. The retroillumination will highlight the cataractous opacities, easily distinguishing them from the transparent nuclear sclerosis. In most animals, except for the most severe cases, the effect of nuclear sclerosis on vision is minimal, and the fundus can be readily visualized.

CONGENITAL ANOMALIES

Congenital anomalies of the lens are rarely seen in clinical practice (congenital cataract is discussed later). They include the following:

- *Aphakia:* Absence of lens
- *Microphakia:* Small lens, usually associated with other ocular malformations
- *Spherophakia:* Spherical lens
- *Lenticonus:* Anterior or posterior protrusion of the lens capsule at the pole. Posterior lenticonus may occur with persistent hyaloid artery and persistent hyperplastic primary vitreous. These disorders are discussed in detail in Chapter 14.
- *Coloboma:* Notching of the lens equator, associated with similar defects in the ciliary body and zonules

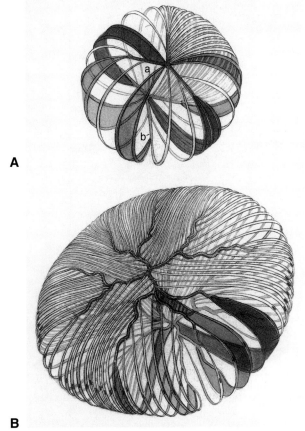

A

B

Figure 13-8. Embryonal and adult lens showing sutures and arrangement of lens cells. **A,** The embryonal nucleus. The anterior Y suture is at *a,* and the posterior at *b.* The lens cells are wide, shaded bands. Cells attaching to tips of Y sutures at one pole of the lens attach to the fork of the Y at the opposite pole. **B,** Adult lens cortex. The anterior and posterior organization of the sutures is more complex. Lens cells arising from the tip of a branch of the suture insert farther anteriorly or posteriorly into a fork at the posterior pole. This arrangement conserves the shape of the lens. This drawing shows the suture lying in a single plane for pictorial reasons, but it extends through the cortex and nucleus down to the Y sutures in the embryonal nucleus. The exact shape of the adult sutures varies in domestic species, but in young animals especially, the Y shape of the embryonal nucleus predominates and must be distinguished clinically from pathologic lens opacities (cataract). (Modified from Hogan MJ, et al. [1971]: Histology of the Human Eye. Saunders, Philadelphia.)

CATARACT

The term *cataract* comprises a common group of ocular disorders manifested as loss of transparency of the lens or its capsule. The opacities may be of varying sizes, shapes, location within the lens, etiology, age of onset, and rate of progression.

A recent large-scale retrospective study covering 40 years and 230,000 dogs has shown that the prevalence of canine cataracts in North America has slowly been increasing and is reportedly 2.42% in the last decade. The increased prevalence is attributed to improved training and diagnostic techniques in veterinary ophthalmology and to the increased popularity of purebred dogs during the twentieth century. The overall prevalence of cataracts in mixed breed dogs, which presumably are not affected by hereditary cataracts, is 1.61%.

Molecular and Cellular Pathogenesis of Cataracts

Lens biochemistry is complex, as are the many different causes of cataract. With the exception of diabetic, galactosemic, and experimental cataracts, the exact biochemical disorders responsible for the formation of cataracts in domestic animals are imperfectly understood. However, in general it may be stated that noxious influences affecting any of the following lens functions may result in opacity:

- Lens nutrition
- Energy metabolism
- Protein metabolism
- Osmotic balance

Once these disturbances occur, they will cause irreversible changes in lens protein contents, metabolic pumps, ionic concentrations, and antioxidant activity. The proportion of nonsoluble (albuminoid) proteins in the lens increases at the expense of the soluble (crystallin) protein fraction. Epithelial Na^+/K^+ adenosine triphosphate pump activity decreases, resulting in a shift in the ionic balance within the lens, and antioxidant activity in the lens likewise diminishes. At the same time, proteolytic enzyme activity increases in the lens, causing breakdown of cell membranes and degradation of lens protein. All of these events amplify and cascade as the cataract progresses, causing visible changes in the lens. These changes are caused by morphologic changes in the lens capsule, epithelium, and fibers that accompany the molecular events. The end result is loss of transparency due to lens fibers rupture, cell death, and water-cleft formation. The clinical picture is determined by the nature and position of these opacities. They seldom appear simultaneously throughout the whole lens cortex. Sometimes they remain stationary for a long time and interfere little with vision. At other times, when they are associated with considerable imbibition of fluid into the cortex, complete opacification may be rapid. Degeneration of all the cortical cells then may occur with rapid liquefaction of the fibers.

Classification

Cataract refers to a group of lens disorders of varying age of onset, speed and extent of progression, appearance, and etiology. Because of the variable nature and appearance of cataracts, numerous methods of classification are commonly used (Table 13-1).

Table 13-1 | **Summary of Cataract Classification**

FEATURE	SUBCLASSIFICATION OF TERMS
Stage of development (maturity)	Incipient, immature, mature, hypermature, morgagnian
Position within the lens	Anterior capsular, anterior subcapsular, cortical, equatorial, nuclear, posterior subcapsular, posterior capsular
Age of development	Congenital, developmental, juvenile, senile, acquired
Etiology or pathogenesis	Primary: inherited Secondary: traumatic, intraocular disease (uveitis, infection), nutritional, radiation, diabetic, toxic, congenital abnormalities, senile
Consistency	Fluid, soft, hard

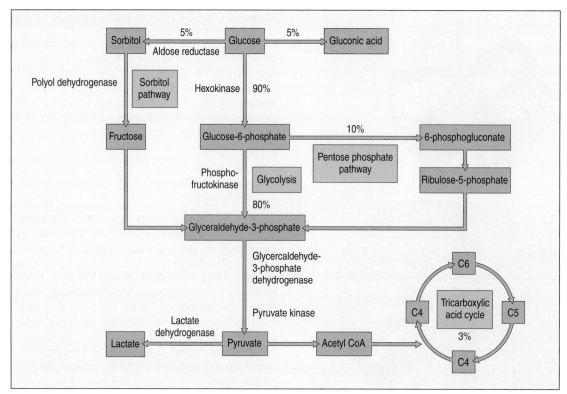

Figure 13-9. Overview of the major pathways of glucose metabolism in the lens. Percentages represent the estimated amounts of glucose used in the different pathways. (From Yanoff M, Duker JS [2004]: Ophthalmology, 2nd ed. Mosby, St Louis.)

Cataracts may be classified according to cause. In many canine breeds, inheritance is the most common cause of cataracts. Additional causes are metabolic, traumatic, toxic, and developmental disorders of the eye. Cataracts also may be caused by nutritional deficiencies or may be secondary to other ocular diseases. Causes of cataracts are discussed in detail in a later section.

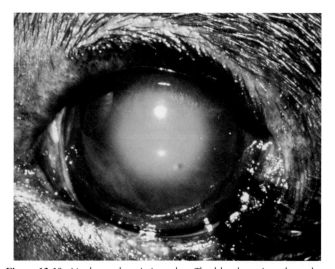

Figure 13-10. Nuclear sclerosis in a dog. The blue haze is a dense lens nucleus, containing lens fibers that have been pushed and compacted at the lens center throughout life. Although seemingly dense, the nucleus is usually transparent, and it rarely affects vision. (Courtesy University of Missouri Veterinary Ophthalmology Case Photo Collection.)

Cataracts may also be classified according to the location of the initial opacity (e.g., nuclear, cortical, anterior/posterior subcapsular). Many inherited canine cataracts are characterized by a typical initial location (see later), and therefore an opacity in a characteristic location in the lens of a susceptible breed should be suspected to be hereditary. Metabolic cataracts may also be classified according to typical location, with the vacuoles that characterize diabetic cataracts initially appearing in the equatorial cortex. Cataracts may also be classified according to age of onset. Some cataracts, usually developmental, toxic, or inherited, may be congenital. Others may appear in juvenile, adult, or elderly patients. Once again, in many dog breeds inherited cataracts are characterized by a typical age of onset (see later).

However, in many ways, the most relevant method of classifying cataracts is according to their stage of development (maturation), which determines the extent of visual deficits, the onset of lens-induced uveitis, and the time of surgical intervention.

Stages of Cataract Development

- *Incipient* (Figure 13-11): There is early, focal opacity with sight unaffected.
- *Immature* (Figure 13-12): The opacity is more extensive, and most of the lens is involved in the pathologic process. The transparency of the lens is reduced but not totally lost. Therefore the tapetal reflection is still visible, although the fundus may be partially obscured ophthalmoscopically. Vision is affected (just as it is affected by a dirty car windshield or by unclean glasses), but the animal is still visual.

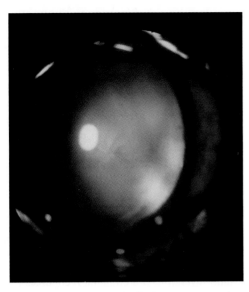

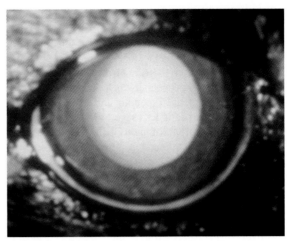

Figure 13-13. A mature cataract. The lens is totally opaque, and no fundus reflection can be seen. This eye is functionally blind, although it is possible to elicit a pupillary light reaction.

Figure 13-11. Incipient cataract. A focal white opacity can be seen in the center (to the right of the flash reflection), against the reddish reflection of the tapetum.

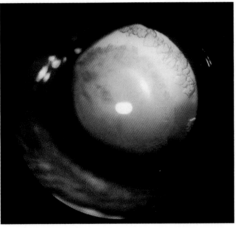

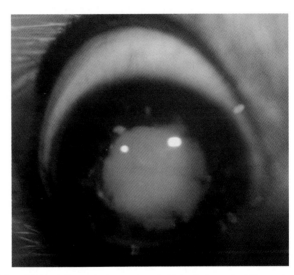

Figure 13-14. A hypermature cataract. Note that most of the cortex has resorbed, except for a few scattered remnants. Only a nuclear cataract remains.

Figure 13-12. Immature cataract. Though most of the lens is involved, it is still mostly transparent, and the animal still has vision. Note the vacuoles in the periphery, which indicate that this cataract is secondary to diabetes. These vacuoles will not be seen unless the pupil is dilated.

- *Mature* (Figure 13-13): The lens is totally opaque, and therefore the eye is functionally blind. There is no tapetal reflection, and the fundus can no longer be examined ophthalmoscopically.
- *Hypermature* (Figure 13-14): Some mature cataracts progress to hypermaturity, whereby they begin to liquefy owing to proteolysis *(lens resorption)*. This process usually begins in the cortex and spreads to the nucleus at later stages as disintegration of the cortex proceeds much more rapidly than autolysis of the nucleus. In advanced stages of resorption, the nuclear remains may be freely movable in the milky cortical fluid in which they are suspended. The degraded lens proteins leak through the lens capsule into the anterior chamber. This results in reduction in the volume of the lens, imparting a characteristic wrinkled appearance to the capsule. The nucleus may remain with a shrunken capsule around it, after the cortex has escaped, and may sink to the bottom of a lens whose cortex has

liquefied *(Morgagnian cataract).* As the lens shrinks, the anterior chamber deepens. Small glistening particles may be present from degraded lens fibers.

It should be noted that in young dogs the resorption can be extensive enough to involve most (or all) of the cataractous lens, thus allowing the animal to regain vision. Once again, however, the resulting secondary inflammation must be treated aggressively. Some lens resorption also occurs in elderly dogs affected by mature cataracts. However, in these patients its extent is limited. The resorption will trigger LIU but will rarely lead to regaining of vision.

Lens-Induced Uveitis

LIU is an inflammation of the eye caused by a reaction to the presence of lens antigens in the aqueous humor. The antigens usually leak from the lens into the anterior chamber following the degradation of lens protein in cataracts, thus causing *phacolytic uveitis.* The degradation and resulting LIU are limited in mature cataracts and more extensive in hypermature cataracts. Phacolytic uveitis is a humoral and cell-mediated immune reaction of the uvea to the released lens protein. The inflammation is a result of the fact that lens proteins are separated from the immune system before birth and are regarded as foreign. These antigens—especially the α-crystallins—are organ specific rather than species specific and cross species lines. Reaction to their presence is less severe in younger animals. A more severe form of granulomatous LIU may occur in older dogs with hypermature cataracts.

Clinical signs of uveitis include photophobia, blepharospasm, corneal edema, ciliary injection, aqueous flare (reduced transparency of aqueous humor due to leakage of inflammatory cells and mediators to the anterior chamber), miosis, a dark iris, and hypotony (reduced intraocular pressure [IOP]).

This inflammation must be treated medically (see Chapter 11) because it may gravely affect the prognosis of cataract surgery. Furthermore, the inflammation may cause secondary complications, including glaucoma and posterior synechia.

LIU may also occur after traumatic rupture of the lens capsule with subsequent exposure of lens protein to the aqueous humor. This inflammation is known as *phacoclastic uveitis*. The difference between phacolytic uveitis and phacoclastic uveitis has been proposed to be that in phacolytic uveitis (via leakage), only recrystallized lens proteins are presented to the immune system; in phacoclastic uveitis (with capsule rupture), intact lens antigens including membrane-associated antigens are released and are able to interact with Class II major histocompatibility T cells and macrophages, resulting in a cell-mediated or delayed-type hypersensitivity reaction, sustained by massive and long-term antigen release.

Causes of Cataracts

Hereditary Cataracts

In many pure breed dogs, inheritance is probably the most common cause of cataracts. The large-scale study cited earlier found 59 dog breeds that have a prevalence of cataracts higher than the "baseline" prevalence of 1.61% reported in mixed breed dogs. Seven breeds, including the toy and miniature poodle, had a cataract prevalence greater than 10%. Obviously, any breed in which the prevalence of a disease is higher than that of the general population should be suspected of being genetically susceptible to the disease. However, just as with any other disease, the inheritance of cataracts can be proven conclusively only through identification of a responsible gene, or by rigorous inheritance testing, including repeat breedings and cross-matings, over several generations. Such testing has demonstrated the inheritance of cataracts in several equine and bovine breeds and in approximately 20 canine breeds, including the Afghan hound, American cocker spaniel, bichon frise, Boston terrier, Chesapeake Bay retriever, German shepherd, golden retriever, Labrador retriever, miniature schnauzer, Old English sheepdog, toy and miniature poodle, Sealyham terrier, Staffordshire bull terrier, and wirehaired fox terrier (Table 13-2). Hereditary (and acquired) cataracts are very rare in cats.

In each of these 20 breeds the cataract is characterized by a typical age of appearance, initial opacity location within the lens, and rate of progression (or lack thereof) (see Table 13-2).

Careful examination of young animals with inherited cataracts often demonstrates early, minute changes, but behavioral signs of visual impairment may not become evident until much later. Hereditary cataracts can be either recessive or dominant genetic traits. However, determining the genetics of a particular cataract in one breed does not exclude another genetic factor from causing a different type of cataract in the same breed. For example, there is evidence that both dominant and recessive cataracts are present in the golden retriever.

It is likely that the list in Table 13-2 is by no means final. On the basis of a very high cataract incidence and the same criteria (typical age, location, and progression), it is likely that cataracts are inherited in many additional canine breeds that have a cataract prevalence greater than 1.61%, including numerous terriers, spaniels, sheepdogs, and retrievers (see the Appendix).

Although a detailed discussion of the characteristic pathogenesis of cataracts in each breed is beyond the scope of this book, their early recognition has significant implications for prognosis and prevention. If a clinician recognizes a lenticular opacity in a characteristic location in a purebred dog of the right age, it may be assumed that the cataract is inherited in origin. Client education about cataract progression in this breed, as well as recommendations concerning neutering, should be provided. Such counseling is not required if there is evidence that the cataract is secondary to some nonhereditary cause.

Congenital Cataracts

Congenital cataracts begin during fetal life, are present at birth, and may be stationary or progressive. They may be inherited, secondary to other ocular developmental abnormality, or the result of maternal influences.

Not all congenital cataracts are inherited, and in fact, the majority are not genetic. It is important to breeders to determine whether genetic factors are involved. A thorough history is needed to better determine inheritance.

When questioning the breeder, the clinician should ask the following questions:

1. Did the same dogs mate previously?
2. Were previous litters normal?
3. How many of the litter were affected?
4. What was the survival rate of the litter?
5. Were the parents normal?
6. Have cataracts been diagnosed in the bloodline?
7. Was the dam ill during pregnancy?
8. What was the dam's diet?
9. Was the dam given drugs during pregnancy?
10. Was the dam exposed to chemicals or toxins?

A thorough ocular and physical examination should be performed. If a genetic cause cannot be eliminated, repeat breeding of the parents may be necessary to determine whether a genetic influence is involved.

Congenital cataracts are observed secondary to, or associated with, other ocular developmental abnormalities, such as the following:

- Persistent pupillary membrane
- Persistent hyaloid artery and persistent hyperplastic primary vitreous

Table 13-2 | **Inherited Cataract Syndromes***

SPECIES AND BREED	INHERITANCE	AGE OF ONSET	INITIAL LOCATION
DOG			
Afghan hound	Autosomal recessive	6-12 mos	Equatorial/posterior cortex
American cocker spaniel	Autosomal recessive/polygenic	6 mos	Anterior/posterior cortex
Bichon frise	Autosomal recessive	2 yrs	Anterior/posterior cortex
Boston terrier	Autosomal recessive	Congenital	Nuclear/posterior sutures
	?	3-4 yrs	Equator, anterior cortex
Chesapeake Bay retriever	Incomplete dominant	6 mos–6 yrs	Cortex/nuclear
English cocker spaniel	?	Congenital	Bilateral anterior capsular
Entlebucher mountain dog	Autosomal recessive	1-2 yrs	Posterior cortex
German shepherd	Incomplete dominant	8 yrs	Cortex/posterior sutures
	Autosomal recessive	8 wks	Posterior sutures progressing to nuclear/ cortical cataract by 2 yrs
Golden retriever	Incomplete dominant[†]	6 mos Congenital	Posterior subcapsular (triangular)
Labrador retriever	Incomplete dominant	6 mos Congenital	Posterior subcapsular (triangular)
Miniature poodle	?	2-6 yrs	Cortical
Miniature schnauzer	Autosomal recessive	Congenital	Nuclear/posterior cortex
	Autosomal recessive	6 mos	Posterior cortex
Norwegian buhund	Autosomal dominant	Congenital	Nuclear/cortical over 4-5 yrs
Old English sheepdog	Autosomal recessive	Congenital–2 yrs	Cortex/nuclear
Rottweiler	Unknown	>10 mos	Posterior/anterior polar, cortical
Staffordshire bull terrier	Autosomal recessive	6 mos	Posterior sutures/cortex
Standard poodle	Autosomal recessive	1 yr	Equatorial cortex
Welsh springer spaniel	Autosomal recessive	Congenital	Nuclear/posterior cortex
West Highland white terrier	Autosomal recessive	Congenital	Nuclear/posterior sutures
CAT			
Himalayan	Autosomal recessive	Congenital	Posterior cortex (triangular)
CATTLE			
Friesian	Probably nonhereditary	Congenital	Bilateral spherical nuclear cataract
Holstein-Friesian	Autosomal recessive	Congenital	—
Hereford	Autosomal recessive	Congenital	—
Jersey	Dominant	Congenital	—
	Autosomal recessive	Congenital	—
White shorthorn	Dominant (?)	Congenital	Associated with multiple ocular anomalies
All breeds	Infectious (maternal bovine viral diarrhea)	Congenital	Cortical cataract
HORSE			
Belgian	Dominant	Congenital	—
Morgan	—	Congenital	Nuclear, nonprogressive
Thoroughbred	Dominant	Congenital	—
Various	—	Congenital	—

Modified from Davidson MG, Nelms SR (1999), in Gelatt KN (editor): Veterinary Ophthalmology, 3rd ed. Lippincott Williams & Wilkins, Philadelphia.
*See also the Appendix, Breed Predisposition to Eye Disorders.
†It has been suggested that this cataract is recessively inherited, with heterozygotes also expressing the condition.

- Microphthalmia
- Multiple ocular anomalies (an inherited syndrome in the Australian shepherd, characterized by multiple anomalies of both the anterior and posterior segments)

Persistent pupillary membrane (PPM) (see Chapter 11) is inherited in the basenji, but familial and noninherited PPMs may be found in any dog breed and in numerous species. PPM may cause cataracts or corneal endothelial dystrophy, or both. Stationary anterior capsular cataracts develop if a strand of membrane adheres to the lens. The strand may or may not be absorbed before maturity; in either case, it will leave a permanent capsular opacity that may interfere with vision. Adhesion of a strand of pupillary membrane to the corneal endothelium results in permanent corneal endothelial dystrophy, which will similarly affect vision. Strands are not clinically significant if both ends attach to the iris or if one end is free in the anterior chamber. Some clinicians advocate surgical treatment of severe cases through corneal transplantation or cataract extraction. Others argue against surgery due to the stationary character of the cataract and corneal lesions, and because the PPM may be patent and ocular hemorrhage could occur during surgery. Medical treatment, using topical 1% atropine applied every 2 or 3 days to dilate the pupil and help vision, has also been suggested. However, many cases receive no medical or surgical treatment.

Persistent hyaloid artery and *persistent hyperplastic primary vitreous* are discussed in detail in Chapters 2 and 14. When the remnants of the embryonic blood supply contact the lens, cataracts of the posterior capsule and/or cortex result. The extent of visual interference depends on the size of the opacity. The remnants may persist as any of the following:

- A single blood vessel attached to the posterior pole of the lens

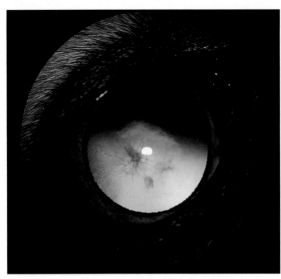

Figure 13-15. Persistent hyperplastic primary vitreous in a golden retriever. Note the fibrovascular opacity with patent vessels near the posterior lens capsule. The lesion is viewed in reflected light from the tapetum.

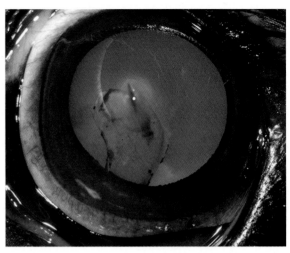

Figure 13-16. A cat claw injury caused perforation of this cornea and anterior lens capsule. Some blood from the resulting uveitis may be seen. (Courtesy Veterinary Ophthalmology Service, University of California, Davis.)

- An artery with a capsular, vascular tunic and posterior polar cataract
- A vascularized area in the posterior axial cortex. Cortical vascularization will appear as a dark area.

The most common clinical lesion resulting is a small, stationary posterior polar cataract involving the capsule and sometimes the subcapsular cortex (Figure 13-15). As in the case of opacities resulting from PPM, some clinicians advocate surgery (subject to the vessel's patency) or topical 1% atropine applied every 2 to 3 days to improve the patient's vision. Many cases, however, receive no surgical or medical treatment.

Most cataracts in foals are congenital. Occasionally a foal's history suggests an acquired cataract, but the cataract has probably been present since birth and is now becoming clinically visible. Inheritance should be considered in foals with congenital cataracts.

In cases of congenital cataracts early surgical intervention should be considered. The reason is that in experimental animals, including chickens, cats, and monkeys, reduction of light stimuli reaching central visual pathways during the period of light susceptibility—namely, from the time the eyelids open to approximately 12 weeks of age—can result in severe neurophysiologic anomalies. Experimental evidence indicates that lack of adequate light or pattern stimulation (visual stimulation) to the central nervous system produces irreversible functional and structural abnormalities in the lateral geniculate nuclei and visual cortex. Therefore *amblyopia* ("lazy eye," or dimness of vision) can develop in very young animals with dense congenital cataracts, corneal opacities, or lid occlusion. Additionally, third eyelid flaps or tarsorrhaphies placed over the globe of young animals (for 3 to 12 weeks) may, depending on the length of time the cornea is occluded, predispose to amblyopia. In considering whether an animal with congenital cataracts is a candidate for cataract surgery, one must recognize the phenomenon of amblyopia. If the animal is already several months old, it is possible that its postoperative visual performance will be affected. Furthermore, visual deprivation during the developmental period may cause elongation of the vitreous body,

resulting in severe myopia. However, studies on these subjects are lacking in veterinary ophthalmology. Another complicating factor in the decision-making process is that in young animals, cataracts may undergo significant resorption, thus allowing them to regain vision without surgical intervention.

Acquired Cataracts

There are numerous causes for acquired cataracts, including trauma, other ocular disease, nutrition, metabolic diseases, and toxicity.

Penetrating foreign bodies, such as cat claws, thorns, or firearm ammunition, cause traumatic cataracts in dogs and cats (Figure 13-16). Once the capsule is perforated the hole usually remains and aqueous enters. Lens fibers imbibe fluid, swell, and become opaque within a few hours. The main concern in these cases is the secondary (phacoclastic) LIU caused by lens material leaking through the torn lens capsule. Small holes (less than 1.5 mm) in the anterior polar region may heal with residual opacity in dogs. Usually the swollen lens material undergoes proteolytic digestion, exposing further lens substance to attack and finally rendering the lens opaque and swollen (*intumescent*). Removal of lenses with traumatic ruptures larger than 1.5 mm has been recommended. Such cases should be closely monitored for signs of LIU and should receive aggressive treatment, either medical or surgical. Metallic foreign bodies also incite an inflammatory reaction depending on the metal involved—lead pellets can be well tolerated, whereas iron and copper cause an intense inflammatory reaction. Intraocular infection, due to contamination of the penetrating foreign body, is also possible.

Cataracts may also result from other ocular disease, most notably anterior uveitis. The reason is that the avascular lens depends totally on the aqueous humor for its metabolic needs, and any change in the constitution of the latter can have grave consequences for lens metabolism and transparency. Furthermore, inflammatory material present in the aqueous humor during the course of uveitis (e.g., fibrin) may adhere to the anterior lens capsule and reduce its transparency. Posterior synechia (adherence of the iris to the anterior lens capsule) is a further complication of the anterior uveitis. It may lead to secondary glaucoma, and even if the adhesions resolve, residual iris pigment will usually be left on the anterior lens capsule.

Nutritional cataracts are caused by use of inappropriate milk-replacement formulas in young animals. In dogs and cats, such cataracts are due to a deficiency in essential amino acids in the formula. They do not progress to maturity and in fact may even regress. Most nutritional cataracts have a minimal effect on vision and do not require surgery. The opacities are located in the equatorial and posterior subcapsular regions. Similar cataracts have been observed in wolf cubs. Because the cataracts are thought to be most common if the pup is totally deprived of the dam's milk or is fed replacement milk during the first week of life, it has been proposed that these cataracts can be controlled by limiting feeding of replacements and increasing the use of the dam's milk during this first week of life.

Nutritional cataracts also develop in orphaned kangaroos and wallabies fed cow's milk (Figure 13-17). These *galactosemic cataracts* form because of the animal's inability to break down the galactose and lactose in the replacement cow's milk. These molecules are therefore diverted into the sorbitol pathway (see later discussion of diabetic cataracts). Unlike the nutritional cataracts in dogs and cats, the resulting galactosemic cataracts progress to maturity, causing loss of vision. Furthermore, the surgical prognosis for these cataracts is poor owing to severe postoperative uveitis and opacification of the vitreous in affected animals.

Nutrition has also been implicated in cataracts that develop in fish raised in hatcheries, although other husbandry conditions (e.g., oxygen and light levels, excessive handling and agression) may also play a role in the pathogenesis. Another common cause of cataracts (in wild and farmed fish) is parasitic infection. Numerous species of fish throughout the world are affected by different species of trematode larvae that enter the lens and cause cataract. The fish is an integral part of the life cycle and is usually eaten by a bird in the next phase, so presumably the blindness increases the likelihood of the fish's being caught and eaten by a bird. Infections have also been implicated in the pathogenesis of cataracts in poultry; spontaneous cataracts have been observed in turkeys and in chickens with avian encephalomyelitis and Marek's disease. *Encephalitozoa cuniculi* infection has been implicated in the pathogenesis of cataract, and lens capsule rupture, in rabbits.

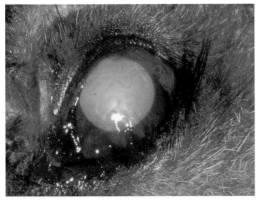

Figure 13-17. Cataract in a young kangaroo that had been fed cow's milk.

Radiated energy may cause cataracts by affecting dividing cells in the equatorial area. Use of megavoltage x-radiation to treat tumors of the nasal cavity caused cataracts in 28% of canine patients, whereas β-radiation radiotherapy treatment of intraocular tumors resulted in a 3% incidence of cataracts. Use of laser to treat glaucoma (cyclophotocoagulation) may also cause cataract in some patients.

Cataracts may also be caused by other insults to the dividing cells in the equator. These are usually due to toxicity, and numerous compounds and drugs have been shown (in toxicology studies) to cause cataracts in animals. However, most of these agents were used in high, nontherapeutic doses. An exception may be ketoconazole, which causes bilateral, progressive cataracts after long-term administration in dogs. Another type of possible "toxic" cataract is one that may result from concomitant retinal dystrophy. It has been postulated that toxic substances released by the degenerating retina cause cataracts in dogs, thus accounting for the common presentation of progressive retinal atrophy and cataract in the same patient. However, this pathogenesis, and the association between these two diseases, remains unproven and controversial in the dog, and it is possible that such eyes are affected by two separate diseases.

Senile Cataracts

Senile cataracts are part of the aging process and occur in both animals and humans. These lesions are frequently preceded by the formation of a dense nuclear sclerosis. Opaque streaks extend from the nucleus toward the cortical equator like spokes of a wheel. Opacification progresses to involve the entire lens, resulting in a mature cataract (see Figure 13-13). However, progression of senile cataracts is extremely slow, and it may take years for the cataract to reach total maturity.

A recent study reported that by age 13.5 years, all dogs examined had some degree of cataract. According to the authors, the age at which half the animals are affected by cataracts is 9.4 years in the dog, compared with 12.7 years in the cat and 28.3 years in the horse, thus demonstrating a correlation between prevalence of cataracts and longevity. However, it should be noted that senile cataracts are a controversial subject in veterinary ophthalmology, with some authorities claiming that they are in fact late-onset inherited cataracts. Other writers counter that the initial location of the opacity and the differences in the rate of progression distinguish these two entities. Large-scale studies of elderly canine populations are needed to resolve the issue.

Diabetic Cataracts

The most prevalent ocular sign of diabetes mellitus in the dog is bilateral cataracts that may mature in a very short time course (days to weeks). In fact, any dog with rapidly developing cataracts should be screened for diabetes mellitus. Though control of hyperglycemia (through diet and insulin) may delay cataract onset or progression, owners of diabetic dogs should be advised that despite treatment, the animals will most likely develop cataracts.

Hexokinase is saturated in hyperglycemia, and more glucose enters the sorbitol pathway, where it is metabolized by aldose reductase (see Figure 13-9). Therefore the development of a diabetic cataract depends on the activity of aldose reductase in lenticular cells, which leads to the formation and accumulation of sorbitol, fructose, and dulcitol in the lens. The resulting hyperosmolarity of the lens leads to fluid ingress. Initial changes include vacuole formation along the equatorial cortex that progresses to the anterior and posterior cortex (see Figure 13-12). As more fluid enters the lens and the cataract matures, it may swell dramatically, a phenomenon known as an *intumescent cataract*. The swollen lens may push the iris forward, resulting in a shallow anterior chamber and a narrowed iridocorneal angle, thus predisposing the animal to glaucoma. Because of the role of aldose reductase in the formation of diabetic cataracts, studies are underway to reduce their incidence and severity using aldose reductase inhibitors.

Diabetes is not an impediment to cataract surgery as long as the animal can withstand the anesthesia. Results of surgery in diabetic dogs are good, though postoperative medications (which usually include glucocorticosteroids) have to be replaced by nonsteroidal antiinflammatory drugs (NSAIDs).

Diabetic cataracts are rare in cats. This is because aldose reductase activity is significantly higher in cats younger than 4 years than in older cats. Because diabetes mellitus occurs primarily in older cats, the relatively low aldose reductase activity protects the lens of the elderly diabetic cat from cataract formation. Instead, diabetic cats may frequently suffer from retinal hemorrhages. However, these should not be confused with diabetic retinopathy, a complication of diabetes that leads to loss of vision in humans. The pathogenesis of the human disease involves retinal neovascularization that is not observed in cats.

Diagnosis

History

The extent of the visual deficits caused by cataract depends on the location and severity of the opacity. Small cataracts in the center of the visual axis interfere with vision through a small pupil but have less effect with a dilated pupil. Therefore owners of patients with centrally located cataracts often observe that the patient sees better under diminished light conditions (cloudy days, evenings, or inside buildings) than in bright sunshine. In diminished light the pupil dilates and the patient sees around the cataract.

The severity of the lens opacity also determines the effect on vision: Small vacuoles and opacities have minor effects. When the lens is diffusely opaque (immature cataract), sight is reduced. However, some vision is often maintained until both eyes are affected by mature cataracts. In most cases the patient is presented because the owner noted a change in behavior due to failing vision or total blindness (e.g., bumping into objects in unfamiliar surroundings, timidity or change in personality, inability to catch a ball). Such changes are more prominent when both eyes are affected (e.g., hereditary cataracts). In cases of unilateral disease (e.g., traumatic cataracts), behavioral visual deficits may be less obvious. Such patients may be presented due to a change in appearance of the eye itself (e.g., a white appearance that is more noticeable at night when the pupil is dilated).

It is also important to determine from the owner whether the animal has had poor night vision during cataract development. This feature may indicate that the patient is also suffering from progressive rod-cone degeneration. As noted previously, there is still a debate about whether such patients are suffering from two distinct hereditary diseases, or whether the cataract is caused by noxious substances secreted by the degenerating retina. Breeds commonly affected by both cataracts and progressive rod-cone degeneration are the miniature poodle, Labrador retriever, and toy poodle. However, because the two diseases can occur in any breed, an assessment of retinal health cannot be made based on signalment and history. The retina must be examined ophthalmoscopically or electrophysiologically (see following sections) before cataract surgery. As mentioned, an "opposite history" (of poor daylight vision) occurs with an axial cataract and healthy retinas: The pupil becomes miotic in bright light, restricting light entrance through the small pupil to the opaque area of the lens.

Clinical Signs

Lens examination is part of a complete ophthalmic examination. The pupil must be dilated to enable adequate evaluation of the lens; if this is not done, peripheral cortical changes and capsular opacities near the equator may be overlooked. Pupil dilation also helps distinguish between nuclear sclerosis and "true" cataracts. Topical tropicamide (1%) administered immediately after the initial examination and repeated once in 5 to 10 minutes produces adequate mydriasis in most patients in 20 minutes. Both eyes must be examined, as each may be affected differently.

Routine evaluation can be adequately performed in a dark room using a focal examining light and binocular loupe. Light reflected back from the tapetum (retroillumination) is also most helpful, as any lens opacity will appear darker than the surrounding. In some dogs, slit-lamp examination reveals early and subtle changes that cannot be seen by a binocular loupe (see Table 13-2). Common sites for initial opacity development are at the equator, at anterior and posterior subcapsular areas, and along Y sutures (Figure 13-18). As noted, hereditary cataracts in each breed have a characteristic initial location as well as characteristic progression (e.g., from subcapsular opacities to nuclear involvement, or from equatorial vacuolation to cortical opacification). However, regardless of the location of the initial lesion, the opacity (with the exception of traumatic and secondary cataracts) most frequently will progress to immature and mature cataract (see Figures 13-11 to 13-13).

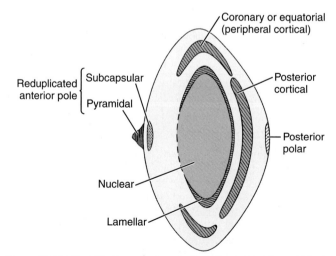

Figure 13-18. Classification of cataracts according to position within the lens. (Modified from Trevor-Roper PD [1984]: The Eye and Its Disorders. Blackwell Scientific, Oxford, England.)

Table 13-3 | Cataract Prognosis in the Miniature Schnauzer Based on Position of the Initial Opacity

POSITION	PROGNOSIS
Anterior capsular polar	Usually nonprogressive
Anterior cortical	Variable progression
Equatorial	Usually progressive
Nuclear	Usually static or reduced in size
Posterior cortical	Variable progression
Posterior capsular and axial	Usually nonprogressive

Modified from Gelatt KN, et al. (1983): Biometry and clinical characteristics of congenital cataracts and microphthalmia in the miniature schnauzer. J Am Vet Med Assoc 183:99.

Owners often ask how long it will take for the cataract to become mature and for total blindness to occur. With the exception of diabetic cataracts, which may progress rapidly to maturity (i.e., days to several weeks), this issue is most difficult to predict, although a rough estimate can sometimes be provided in breeds that have been thoroughly investigated (Table 13-3). This process may take months or longer.

As noted, breakdown and leakage of lens protein begins in mature cataracts but its extent is limited. The process is accelerated in hypermature cataracts. Signs of resorption are as follows:

- Small, shiny crystals and multifocal white plaques, resulting from protein breakdown, are visible in the lens.
- Deepening of the anterior chamber and a concave iris surface as the lens volume decreases; conversely, swelling of the lens in early cataract formation causes a shallow anterior chamber and a convex iris surface
- Decrease in lens diameter and thickness
- Corrugation of the anterior capsule
- Signs of LIU

The extent of the resorption varies with age. It will be limited in elderly patients and will rarely improve the patient's vision. In young subjects it can be more extensive. As the lens becomes small, vision can be aided with mydriatics (1% atropine every 2 to 3 days). Complete resorption allows vision comparable to that after successful surgical lens removal (without IOL implantation). Lens removal is not performed in the presence of active uveitis or resorption.

LIU is a major cause of complications in cataract surgery. It can be assumed to be present in all patients with mature or hypermature cataract until proven otherwise. Early therapy for this uveitis and referral for treatment of the cataract are essential if optimal results are to be obtained.

Treatment

Medical Therapy

In the early stages of cataract, especially when the opacity lies on the visual axis, or in advanced stages of resorption, vision can be improved with the use of a mydriatic when required. Diabetic cataracts may be amenable to therapy with aldose reductase inhibitors. Studies have shown that both systemic and topical inhibitors can slow, halt, and perhaps reverse the progression of cataracts in diabetic patients. However, such drugs are still considered experimental.

As oxidation plays a role in the pathogenesis of cataracts, it has been proposed that antioxidants may halt and reverse progression of cataracts in dogs. Various systemic and topical agents, including selenium–vitamin E, orgotein (superoxide dismutase), zinc ascorbate, and carnosine, have been studied and marketed as "anticataract drugs," most recently through Internet distributors. Many of these agents are marketed without supporting clinical and experimental data, whereas others have been evaluated only in vitro. The only clinical trial conducted to date in dogs has found a "marginal reduction" in lens opacity, which was clinically insignificant. Owners should not be misled into thinking that they can use drugs to cure their pet's cataracts. On the contrary, such attempts at treatment will only delay professional care, thereby worsening any existing LIU and impacting gravely the prognosis of the inevitable surgery. While it is hoped that one day an effective medical treatment for cataracts will be discovered, at the time of writing all cataract patients should be referred for treatment of LIU and possible surgery.

Surgical Case Selection

Not all animals with cataract are suitable candidates for surgery. The following prerequisites should be fulfilled before cataract extraction is recommended:

1. The affected eye should have a significant visual deficit. Obviously the eye shown in Figure 13-11 does not require surgery. There is some debate among veterinary ophthalmologists regarding the stage (of maturity) at which surgery should be performed. Surgery in early stages of immaturity is technically easier, and there is less preoperative uveitis. However, if there are no significant visual deficits it is difficult to justify a complex and expensive surgical procedure that does not guarantee 100% success. On the other hand, it is inadvisable to wait until the cataract reaches advanced stages of maturity, as the concomitant development of LIU will affect the surgical prognosis. The success rate is higher for surgical removal of immature cataracts than for removal of mature cataracts.

2. Obviously, for the patient to regain vision, its retina must be healthy and functional. Ideally, the fundus should be examined by the surgeon early in the disease, when the cataract is not yet advanced and the retinal details are still visible. Alternatively, if the fundus cannot be examined thoroughly (because of the cataract), retinal function should be evaluated with electroretinography (ERG) to ensure that retinal degeneration is not present. ERG is described in Chapter 15. Because retinal degeneration can occur in any breed, an ERG evaluation is mandatory in bilaterally affected dogs in which the fundus cannot be examined. The owner must be carefully questioned about the relative onset of visual difficulty, cataract, and nyctalopia. However, patient history, signalment, and the speed of pupil contraction in response to light are not reliable indicators of the presence or absence of progressive rod-cone degeneration.

3. Any incipient LIU—indicated by ciliary injection, hypotony, miosis, aqueous flare, change in iris color, or resistance to mydriasis—must first be controlled by topical corticosteroids and/or NSAIDs under the supervision of the person who will perform the surgery. The incidence of short- and long-term complications is greater when uveitis is present preoperatively.

4. No other ocular pathologic process should be present. The eye must be examined by an experienced veterinary ophthalmologist. Any concurrent disease, such as keratitis or glaucoma, must be controlled before surgery. Older dogs or dogs affected with hypermature cataracts may have zonular instability. In many practices an ultrasound examination is performed before surgery to rule out vitreal/retinal detachment. In patients that are susceptible to postoperative retinal detachment (due to vitreous disease or breed susceptibility) some clinicians advocate prophylactic retinopexy ("fixating" the retina in its place), by either cryopexy or laser photocoagulation, at the time of cataract surgery.

5. The patient should be in good general health, should not suffer from any systemic diseases, and should undergo tests to ensure it is a suitable candidate for anesthesia.

6. The patient must be amenable to intensive handling, because frequent topical applications of medication are required in both the preoperative and postoperative periods. One cannot overemphasize the importance of postoperative treatment and its effect on the outcome. An excitable or fractious dog that cannot be handled and medicated is usually an unsuitable candidate. If there is doubt regarding the owner's ability to medicate the dog postoperatively, topical medication should be provided preoperatively to determine the feasibility of drug application.

7. The owner must be prepared to sustain the cost and effort required to perform preoperative and postoperative treatment and to return for rechecks. Willingness to pay the bill is not enough. Long-term treatment to avoid uveitis, IOP monitoring for glaucoma, and frequent rechecks are mandatory for long-term visual success. An owner who cannot provide the required postoperative therapy and care should be counseled against surgery.

8. For an older dog, the owner must be counseled that senility, cognitive dysfunction, motor problems, and other aspects of old age may be as important in the dog's behavior as the cataract, and that cataract removal, although technically successful, may not result in the improvement sought (the expectation often is that the dog will see and behave like a young dog again).

Surgical Correction

Once preexisting uveitis has been controlled, retinal function determined, and other tests completed, the patient is scheduled for surgery. Many surgeons prefer to perform bilateral surgery (assuming that both eyes are similarly affected), although some prefer to operate on one eye at a time.

The four methods of surgical correction commonly used are (1) discission and aspiration, (2) extracapsular extraction, (3) phacoemulsification, and (4) intracapsular extraction.

Discission and Aspiration. Discission and aspiration consists of opening the cornea and anterior lens capsule and using irrigation and aspiration to remove the contents from within the capsule (Figure 13-19). This method is restricted to young animals with liquid cataracts and animals with very small eyes (usually exotic pets) that will not accommodate regular ophthalmic instrumentation.

Extracapsular Extraction. In extracapsular extraction, a wide (180-degree) incision is made in the limbus and the anterior lens capsule, nucleus, and cortex are extracted manually, followed

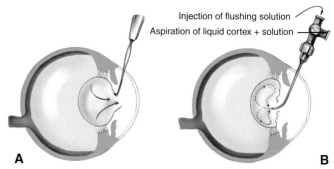

Figure 13-19. Cataract extraction using dissection and aspiration. **A,** Rupture of lens capsule. **B,** Aspiration of contents via two-way cannula.

by rigorous flushing to remove any remaining lens particles (Figure 13-20). The posterior lens capsule, which is attached to the vitreous, remains intact. This method has largely been replaced by phacoemulsification.

Phacoemulsification. Surgery begins with a small incision at the limbus and tearing of the anterior lens capsule. A special probe is then used to shatter the lens with high-frequency ultrasonic waves, and the debris is removed via automated irrigation and aspiration (Figure 13-21). In fact, the technique for phacoemulsification is similar to that for discission, with the exception that a phacoemulsifier is used instead of cannulae. Phacoemulsification has the advantages of requiring a smaller limbal incision than extracapsular extraction (the incision has to accomodate only the probe) and allowing more complete removal of lens cortical material because the smaller incision results in faster surgery and healing, and because of the automated flushing system. The method has achieved widespread use because the smaller incision results in faster surgery and healing, and because the postoperative inflammation is more moderate, in comparison with extracapsular extraction. This results in fewer postoperative complications and less patient discomfort.

Intracapsular Extraction. Removal of the entire lens without opening or tearing the lens capsule is called intracapsular extraction. This method is restricted to the removal of luxated lenses, following tearing of the zonules (see following section). Because the capsular bag is not opened during surgery there is no leakage of lens protein, and the postoperative inflammation is minimal. However, surgery may lead to anterior movement of the vitreous body (and possible secondary retinal detachment or glaucoma), as the lens that normally separates the vitreous from the anterior chamber has been removed. Therefore some surgeons will combine this surgery with prophylactic vitrectomy (removal of the vitreous body). Others will implant a synthetic IOL fixed by sutures in the ciliary sulcus as a barrier against vitreous movement and to improve postoperative vision (see later).

Postoperative Vision and Intraocular Lens Implantation

After cataract extraction surgery the patient is severely hyperopic (farsighted) owing to the loss of the refractive power of the lens. This visual deficit can be corrected by implantation of an artificial lens (an IOL), which thus helps the patient achieve postoperative emmetropia (focused vision). With this aim in mind, veterinary ophthalmologists began implanting IOLs in their canine patients in the late 1980s (Figure 13-22). Subsequent studies have shown that the optical power of canine IOLs should be approximately 41 D, and such lenses are now regularly implanted by veterinary ophthalmologists, with significant improvement in postoperative visual performance.

As stated earlier, however, the cornea is the major refractive organ of the eye, and the lens plays a less significant role in refraction and accommodation in animals. This means that contrary to popular belief, and to the owners' puzzlement, vision

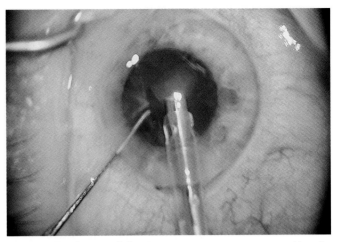

Figure 13-21. Phacoemulsification surgery to remove a cataract. Note the small incision (6 o'clock position) required to insert the tip of the phacoemulsifier into the eye. The instrument shatters the lens with ultrasound waves, and performs irrigation and aspiration. The second instrument (8 o'clock position) is used to rotate the lens pieces toward the phacoemulsification tip. (From Yanoff M, Duker JS [2004]: Ophthalmology, 2nd ed. Mosby, St Louis.)

is possible postoperatively even without an IOL. Aphakic patients (in which IOLs have not been implanted during surgery) are visual because the opaque lens has been removed and light can once more reach the retina. Indeed, for decades veterinary ophthalmologists did not implant IOLs in their canine patients, and even today implantation of IOLs in feline and equine patients is in its infancy. As in the dog, if the surgery was successful, an aphakic cat or horse will regain vision although it will be hyperopic.

Complications, Postoperative Care, and Prognosis

The two major intraoperative complications of cataract surgery are damage to the corneal endothelium and rupture of the posterior lens capsule. Damage to the endothelium may be

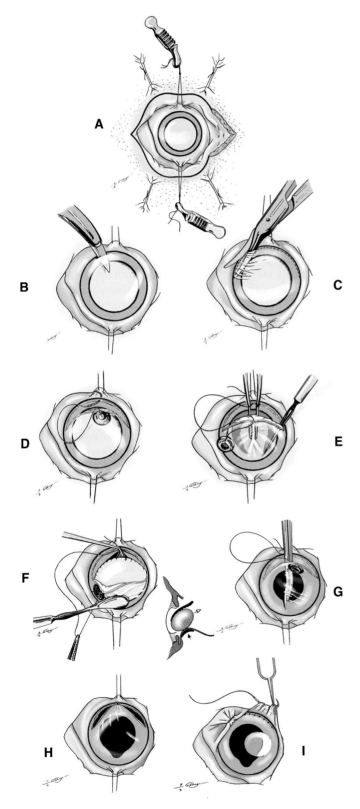

Figure 13-20. Extracapsular cataract extraction via limbal incision. **A,** A canthotomy is performed and the lids are retracted with sutures of 4/0 silk. Two fixation sutures of 6/0 silk are placed in the conjunctiva to allow manipulation of the globe. **B,** A corneal incision is made adjacent to the limbus. **C,** The incision is extended with left and right corneal scissors. **D,** A suture with a porcelain bead attached is preplaced at the 12 o'clock position. The suture (8/0 to 9/0 polyglactin 910 [Vicryl]) is used to prevent instrument damage to the endothelium. **E,** The anterior lens capsule is grasped with lens capsule forceps, and the edge of the capsule is incised. The capsule is removed. **F,** An irrigator is placed between the lens cortex and the posterior capsule, and the cortex is gently irrigated forward with balanced salt solution. A lens loop is placed behind the lens to remove it. Alternatively, the lens may be removed by careful pressure from the ventral limbus, without placement of a loop or irrigator in the eye. Care is taken to avoid the corneal endothelium. **G,** If miosis occurs during the surgery, a sphincterotomy may be performed at the 6 o'clock position to allow access to the lens. Alternatively, an iridectomy may be performed if necessary, at 12 o'clock, with electrocautery. **H,** The preplaced suture is tied and the incision is closed with simple interrupted sutures at 1-mm intervals under magnification. **I,** A modified conjunctival flap may be placed over the corneal wound to seal it. The anterior chamber may be reconstructed with an air bubble. (Modified from Severin GA [2000]: Severin's Veterinary Ophthalmology Notes, 3rd ed. Severin, Ft. Collins, CO.)

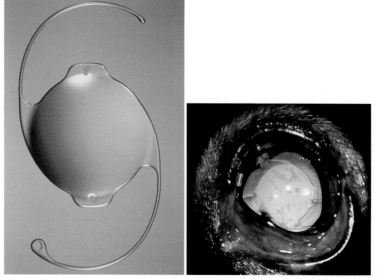

Figure 13-22. A, Intraocular canine lens for placement after cataract removal. **B,** An intraocular lens has been implanted in a dog after cataract removal. The pupil has been dilated. Margins of the lens are not normally visible in the nondilated, resting pupil. (Courtesy Dr. J Gaiddon.)

caused by improper handling of the cornea leading to trauma, or by exposure to the energy emitted by the phacoemulsifier. Endothelial cell loss can be decreased by filling the anterior chamber with viscoelastic substances (sodium hyaluronate, methyl cellulose and its derivatives), which physically shield and protect the cells, and by keeping the duration of phacoemulsification to a minimum.

In both phacoemulsification and extracapsular extraction, the surgeon will try to avoid perforating the posterior lens capsule. Such perforation may allow vitreous to enter into the anterior chamber and cause secondary glaucoma. If the posterior lens capsule is torn during cataract surgery, the surgeon may perform vitrectomy to reduce the risk of glaucoma.

The major postoperative surgical complication is LIU. Because of the immunogenicity of the lens proteins, cataract surgery (which involves opening the lens capsule) inevitably results in uveitis. The inflammation is treated aggressively with mydriatics and various combinations of topical and systemic antiinflammatory drugs. Many surgeons begin treating their patients several days before surgery to ensure a dilated pupil during the operation (because the lens is removed through the pupil) and as prophylactic treatment for the uveitis. The treatment is intensified on the day of surgery, with many animals receiving intravenous, intramuscular, and/or subconjunctival antiinflammatory drugs, and the treatment is continued postoperatively according to the surgeon's preference. Topical and/or systemic antibiotics are usually provided, and some surgeons may add prophylactic glaucoma treatment because postoperative spikes of IOP (often temporary but blinding) have been reported. Frequent rechecks to monitor IOP and LIU are mandatory in the immediate postoperative period, and some surgeons may even hospitalize their patients for 1 to 2 days for evaluation. With time, the frequency of treatments and rechecks decreases, although occasional rechecks (once every 6 to 12 months) are warranted due to the insidious nature of LIU.

With improvement in surgical techniques and instrumentation, and with better understanding and treatment of the postoperative complications, the immediate postoperative

results of cataract surgery are excellent, and more than 95% of the patients regain useful vision. However, with time some of these patients may lose vision in one or both eyes. The reasons are the insidious nature of the uveitis, secondary complications, and failure of the owners to adhere to a long-term treatment and recheck schedule. Possible complications resulting from uveitis include secondary glaucoma, posterior synechia, and lens epithelial fibrous metaplasia and postoperative opacification. Retinal detachment, intraocular hemorrhage, infection, and suture failure are possible, though less common, complications.

Cataracts in Horses

Cataracts are less common in horses than in dogs. In some breeds, including Belgian and thoroughbred horses, cataracts have been demonstrated to be hereditary (dominant). Nonprogressive, nuclear cataracts that do not interfere with vision occur in Morgan horses. However, most cataracts of adult horses are secondary to trauma or equine recurrent uveitis. Senile cataracts causing visual impairment may occur in horses older than 20 years. Elderly horses are also affected by nuclear sclerosis, which, like the condition in the dog, does not affect vision. Cataracts (both hereditary and secondary) are a relatively common ocular defect in foals.

Foals and adult horses with visual impairment are suitable candidates for lens extraction, provided the horses are tractable and can be medicated postoperatively. In foals, early return of vision is important to development of higher visual centers. The workup, techniques, and complications of cataract removal are similar to those in the dog.

LENS LUXATION

Luxation occurs when all of the lens zonules are torn, leading to displacement of the lens from the hylaoid (patellar) fossa. Following the luxation, the lens may move anteriorly, posteriorly, or in the vertical plane of the eye. Lens luxation may be preceded by *subluxation,* resulting from tearing of some (but not all) of the zonules, and leading to partial displacement of the lens from the hyaloid fossa.

Etiology

Lens luxation may be classified as primary (hereditary) or secondary. Primary lens luxation is most commonly seen in dogs. The luxation is due to weakened lens zonules that rupture early in life (up to 5 years of age). This condition is inherited in wirehaired fox, Sealyham, Manchester, Cairn, Jack Russell, Tibetan, and miniature bull terriers and miniature schnauzers. It is also common in poodles, but the hereditary nature is unconfirmed in this breed. Electron microscopy studies in the Tibetan terrier have shown that the insertions of the lens zonules into the lens capsule are abnormal. In such cases, luxation may follow minor trauma, which ruptures the weakened zonules. Primary congenital luxation, seen in multiple ocular anomalies, is rare in clinical practice.

Secondary luxation may be due to any of the following conditions:

- Blunt traumas (e.g., a violent strike to the orbital region) may cause secondary lens luxation *(traumatic luxation)*. Trauma violent enough to cause lens luxation may also cause other severe ocular lesions (e.g., hyphema, retinal detachment, scleral rupture). Perforating traumas, such as cat claws, do not cause lens luxation, as they do not generate the mechanical forces needed to tear the zonules.
- Glaucoma: When the globe enlarges in chronic glaucoma the zonules may break, leading to lens subluxation and luxation. It is noteworthy that glaucoma may also be *caused by* lens luxation (see later), and when both diseases are present in an eye it may be difficult to determine which is the cause and which the effect.
- Uveitis: Alterations in the aqueous humor, and the presence of inflammatory mediators in the posterior chamber, may weaken the zonules.
- Intraocular tumors: As a tumor enlarges, it may displace the lens, creating a luxation or subluxation.
- Cataract: If a cataractous lens swells *(intumescence)*, the zonules may break.

Clinical Signs and Diagnosis

In a normal eye, the iris rests on the anterior lens surface, which gives it its slightly convex curvature. If the zonules deteriorate or pull free from the lens, rapid eye movement causes the lens to oscillate back and forth in the hyaloid fossa. This oscillation causes iris vibration *(iridodonesis)*. Iridodonesis is an early sign of impending lens displacement and becomes more evident as the lens continues to loosen from the zonules.

Increased lens movement causes the vitreous touching the posterior lens to separate from deeper vitreous, allowing more movement of the lens. Eventually the damaged vitreous liquefies and is replaced by aqueous. This process of liquefaction of the vitreous is referred to as *syneresis* (Figure 13-23). Therefore vitreous fibrils floating through the pupil in the aqueous are also a sign of zonule disruption and potential future luxation.

If the lens is subluxated in the equatorial plane, the iris is convex where it touches the lens and flat in the area of dislocation (compare the dorsal and ventral iris in Figure 13-23, *B*). As the subluxation progresses to luxation, the luxated lens usually sinks ventrally owing to the effect of gravity. The dorsal

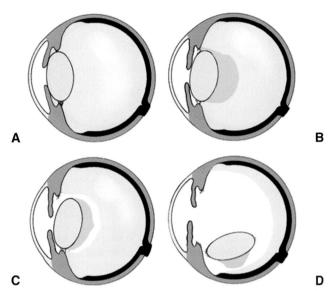

Figure 13-23. Lens luxation and vitreous syneresis. **A,** Normal lens position. **B,** Zonules are ruptured dorsally but lens is held in place by the vitreous. **C,** Early liquefaction of the vitreous, which allows more lens movement. **D,** Lens motion accelerates syneresis, and the lens may sink ventrally. (Courtesy Dr. G.A. Severin.)

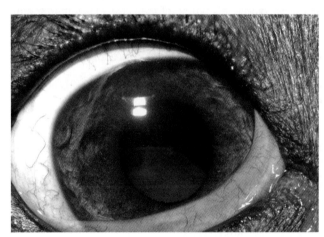

Figure 13-24. An aphakic crescent due to posterior lens luxation. The white lens is visible from the 4 to 9 o'clock positions because it luxated in a ventronasal direction (while maintaining its vertical orientation). Only the dorsotemporal part of the lens is visible; the rest of the lens is obscured by the iris. An aphakic crescent is visible between 9 o'clock and 4 o'clock, in the part of the pupil that has been vacated by the lens. (Courtesy University of California, Davis, Veterinary Ophthalmology Service Collection.)

edge of the lens becomes visible in the pupil. The dorsal area of the pupil where the lens is missing is called an *aphakic crescent* (Figure 13-24).

Syneresis may continue until most of the vitreous disappears. When this occurs, the lens may settle ventrally at the "bottom" of the eye and may disappear from the pupil (see Figure 13-23, *D*). This condition is called *posterior luxation*. In such cases, it is possible to observe the retinal blood vessels and optic disc without an ophthalmoscope, through the use of only a basic source of light.

Lens luxation causes changes in anterior chamber depth and iris (Figure 13-25). The clinician can best evaluate anterior chamber depth and iris position by observing the eye from the side rather than the front. The normal iris rests on the anterior surface of the lens and therefore is slightly convex (see Figure

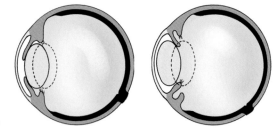

Figure 13-25. A, Lens luxation with anterior displacement of the iris (and possible pupillary blockage of aqueous passage): Anterior chamber is shallow. **B,** Luxation into the anterior chamber, which appears deep. Endothelial damage causes corneal edema where the lens capsule touches it. (Courtesy Dr. G.A. Severin.)

13-23, *A*). Initially the vitreous may swell, forcing the lens forward and resulting in a shallow anterior chamber and a more convex iris (see Figure 13-25, *A*). If the pupil dilates, the lens may luxate through the pupil into the anterior chamber (Figure 13-26). The luxation may be partial or complete.

When the lens is luxated, the depth of the anterior chamber will usually increase, regardless of the direction of the luxation (an exception is seen in Figure 13-25, *A*). In cases of anterior luxation the lens fills the anterior chamber, and therefore it physically pushes the iris posteriorly (see Figure 13-25, *B*). In cases of posterior luxation, the iris loses its posterior support and moves posteriorly (see Figure 13-23, *D*). In both cases the increase in anterior chamber depth is accompanied by a more concave position of the iris.

Anterior lens luxation is considered an ophthalmic emergency for the following reasons:

- *Edema:* Luxation into the anterior chamber brings the lens in contact with the corneal endothelium. This impairs the endothelial function, resulting in corneal edema. Furthermore, as the head of the animal moves the lens repeatedly strikes the corneal endothelium. This may cause permanent endothelial damage and irreversible corneal edema.
- *Pain:* Pain is caused by the striking of the inner cornea by the lens.

- *Glaucoma:* As the lens is luxated anteriorly, it may "pull" the vitreous behind it. The presence of vitreous in the pupil or in the anterior chamber impedes the flow of aqueous humor and causes an elevation in IOP. The presence of the lens in the anterior chamber further obstructs drainage of aqueous humor (see Figure 13-25, *B*). Glaucoma may also occur as a result of posterior lens luxation, because the "barrier" between the vitreous and the pupil disappears. As with anterior luxation, this may result in anterior movement of the vitreous, provided that it has liquefied or has become detached from its posterior attachment to the retina.

A clinician should suspect anterior lens luxation in cases of acute onset of severe pain, corneal edema, and/or glaucoma, especially when presented unilaterally and in susceptible breeds. The severe corneal edema, blepharospasm, and possible hyphema (in cases of traumatic luxation) that can accompany lens luxation may make it difficult to visualize the luxated lens or the changes in the depth of the anterior chamber and iris position. In these cases, ultrasound may be used to demonstrate the location of the lens in the eye (Figure 13-27).

Treatment

Some controversy exists regarding the treatment of subluxated lenses or posteriorly displaced lenses. Some surgeons prefer to remove them using intracapsular lens extraction techniques (in combination with vitrectomy) to prevent glaucoma. Others provide long-term miotic treatment to ensure that the luxated lens does not move anteriorly and educate the clients about signs of anterior luxation and glaucoma.

Because of the complications described in the previous section, there is no controversy surrounding the need to remove anteriorly luxated lens. These may be removed by intracapsular extraction or phacoemulsification. The major complication with extraction of luxated lenses (regardless of whether they luxated anteriorly or posteriorly) is glaucoma. Therefore many clinicians combine this procedure with vitrectomy, thus

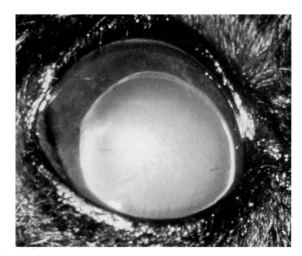

Figure 13-26. Anterior lens luxation. Note that the entire lens equator can be seen and that the lens partially obscures the iris. (Courtesy University of Missouri Veterinary Ophthalmology Case Photo Collection.)

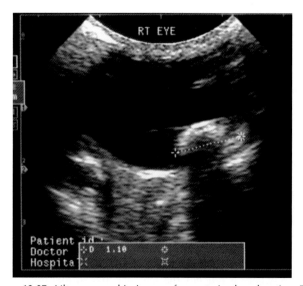

Figure 13-27. Ultrasonographic image of a posterior lens luxation. The lens, which could not be seen because of corneal edema, is visible as a hyperechoic mass in the posterior part of the eye *(dashed line connecting the two asterisks)*. (Courtesy Dr. I. Aizenberg.)

reducing the risk of anterior vitreous movement. If glaucoma is present before the lens is removed, a lower success rate is achieved than if the lens is removed before glaucoma occurs. Placement of an IOL fixed by sutures has also been advocated after removal of luxated lenses in dogs. The IOL serves as a barrier to prevent anterior vitreal movement and improves postoperative vision.

In cases of anterior luxation where surgical removal is not feasible, the lens may be pushed from the anterior chamber back to the posterior part of the eye (reclination). This is a noninvasive procedure that may be facilitated by anesthesia (to reduce globe tension caused by the extraocular muscles) and by administration of hyperosmotic agents (to decrease the volume of the vitreous body). Following the procedure, permanent miotic therapy is instituted to ensure that the lens remains in the posterior part of the eye.

BIBLIOGRAPHY

Alpar JJ (1987): Use of Healon in different cataract surgery techniques: endothelial cell count study. Ophthalmic Surg 18:529.

Barnett KC (1985): Hereditary cataract in the miniature schnauzer. J Small Anim Pract 26:635.

Barnett KC (1980): Cataract in the golden retriever. Vet Rec 111:315.

Barnett KC (1980): Hereditary cataract in the Welsh springer spaniel. J Small Anim Pract 21:621.

Barros PS, et al. (2004): Blood and aqueous humour antioxidants in cataractous poodles. Can J Ophthalmol 39:19.

Barros PS, et al. (1999): Antioxidant profile of cataractous English cocker spaniels. Vet Ophthalmol 2:83.

Basher AW, Roberts SM (1995): Ocular manifestations of diabetes mellitus: diabetic cataracts in dogs. Vet Clin North Am Small Anim Pract 25:661.

Bayon A, et al. (2001): Ocular complications of persistent hyperplasia primary vitreous in three dogs. Vet Ophthalmol 4:35.

Beach J, Irby N (1985): Inherited nuclear cataracts in the Morgan horse. J Hered 76:371.

Bernays ME, Peiffer RL (2000): Morphologic alterations in the anterior lens capsule of canine eyes with cataracts. Am J Vet Res 61:1517.

Biros DJ, et al. (2000): Development of glaucoma after cataract surgery in dogs: 220 cases (1987-1998). J Am Vet Med Assoc 216:1780.

Bjerkas E, Haaland MB (1995): Pulverulent nuclear cataract in the Norwegian buhund. J Small Anim Pract 36:471.

Brainard J, et al. (1982): Evaluation of superoxide dismutase (Orgotein) in medical treatment of canine cataract. Arch Ophthalmol 100:1832.

Brightman AH (1986): Buyer beware—another medical "cure" for cataracts. J Am Vet Med Assoc 188:5.

Brightman AH, et al. (1981): Effect of aspirin on aqueous protein values in the dog. J Am Vet Med Assoc 178:572.

Buschmann W, et al. (1987): Microsurgical treatment of lens capsule perforations. Part I: experimental research. Ophthalmic Surg 18:731.

Colitz CM, et al. (2000): Histologic and immunohistochemical characterization of lens capsular plaques in dogs with cataracts. Am J Vet Res 61:139.

Colitz CM, et al. (1999): Telomerase activity in lens epithelial cells of normal and cataractous lenses. Exp Eye Res 69:641.

Curtis RC (1983): Aetiopathological aspects of inherited lens dislocation in the Tibetan terrier. J Comp Pathol 93:151.

Curtis RC, et al. (1983): Clinical and pathological observations concerning the aetiology of primary lens luxation in the dog. Vet Rec 112:238.

Davidson MG, et al. (2000): Effect of surgical technique on in vitro posterior capsule opacification. J Cataract Refract Surg 26:1550.

Davidson MG, et al. (2000): Ex vivo canine lens capsular sac explants. Graefes Arch Clin Exp Ophthalmol 238:708.

Davidson MG, et al. (1991): Phacoemulsification and intraocular lens implantation: a study of surgical results in 182 dogs. Prog Vet Comp Ophthalmol 1:4.

Davidson MG, et al. (1991): Traumatic anterior lens capsule disruption. J Am Anim Hosp Assoc 27:411.

DeCosta P, et al. (1996): Cataracts in dogs after long-term ketoconazole therapy. Vet Comp Ophthalmol 6:176.

Denis HM, et al. (2003): Detection of anti-lens crystallin antibody in dogs with and without cataracts. Vet Ophthalmol 6:321.

Dwyer WP, Smith CE (1988): Metacercariae of Diplostomum spathaceum in the eyes of fishes from Yellowstone Lake, Wyoming. J Wildl Dis 25:126.

Dziezyc J, et al. (1991): Use of phacofragmentation for cataract removal in horses: 12 cases (1985-1989). J Am Vet Med Assoc 198:1774.

Garcia-Sanchez GA, et al. (2005): Ahmed valve implantation to control intractable glaucoma after phacoemulsification and intraocular lens implantation in a dog. Vet Ophthalmol 8:139.

Gelatt KN, et al. (2003): Cataracts in the bichon frise. Vet Ophthalmol 6:3.

Gelatt KN, Mackay EO (2005): Prevalence of primary breed-related cataracts in the dog in North America. Vet Ophthalmol 8:101.

Gelatt KN, MacKay EO (2004): Secondary glaucomas in the dog in North America. Vet Ophthalmol 7:245.

Gemensky-Metzler AJ, Wilkie DA (2004): Surgical management and histologic and immunohistochemical features of a cataract and retrolental plaque secondary to persistent hyperplastic tunica vasculosa lentis/persistent hyperplastic primary vitreous (PHTVL/PHPV) in a bloodhound puppy. Vet Ophthalmol 7:369.

Gilger BC, et al. (1998): Experimental implantation of posterior chamber prototype intraocular lenses for the feline eye. Am J Vet Res 59:1339.

Glaze M, Blanchard G (1983): Nutritional cataracts in a Samoyed litter. J Am Anim Hosp Assoc 19:951.

Glover TL, et al. (1995): The intracapsular extraction of displaced lenses in dogs: a retrospective study of 57 cases (1984-1990). J Am Anim Hosp Assoc 31:77.

Grahn BH, Cullen CL (2004): Iris to lens persistent pupillary membranes. Can Vet J 45:613.

Grahn BH, Cullen CL (2000): Equine phacoclastic uveitis: the clinical manifestations, light microscopic findings, and therapy of 7 cases. Can Vet J 41:376.

Gwin RM, et al. (1983): Effects of phacoemulsification and extracapsular lens removal on cornea thickness and endothelial cell density in the dog. Invest Ophthalmol Vis Sci 24:227.

Harding JJ (1992): Physiology, biochemistry, and epidemiology of cataract. Curr Opin Ophthalmol 3:3.

Hardman C, et al. (2001): Phacofragmentation for morgagnian cataract in a horse. Vet Ophthalmol 4:221.

Jamieson V, et al. (1991): Ocular complications following cobalt 60 radiotherapy of neoplasms in the canine head region. J Am Anim Hosp Assoc 27:51.

Johnstone N, Ward DA (2005): The incidence of posterior capsule disruption during phacoemulsification and associated postoperative complication rates in dogs: 244 eyes (1995-2002): Vet Ophthalmol 8:47.

Kenny D, et al. (2003): Intracapsular lens removal in a Przewalski's wild horse (Equus caballus przewalskii). J Zoo Wildl Med 34:284.

Lannek EB, Miller PE (2001): Development of glaucoma after phacoemulsification for removal of cataracts in dogs: 22 cases (1987-1997). J Am Vet Med Assoc 218:70.

Lazarus JA, et al. (1998): Primary lens luxation in the Chinese shar-pei: clinical and hereditary characteristics. Vet Ophthalmol 1:101.

Leasure J, et al. (2001): The relationship of cataract maturity to intraocular pressure in dogs. Vet Ophthalmol 4:273.

Ledbetter EC, et al. (2004): Microbial contamination of the anterior chamber during cataract phacoemulsification and intraocular lens implantation in dogs. Vet Ophthalmol 7:327.

Magrane WG (1969): Cataract extraction: a follow-up study (429 cases). J Small Anim Pract 10:545.

Magrane WG (1961): Cataract extraction: an evaluation of 104 cases. J Small Anim Pract 1:163.

Martin CL (1978): Zonular defects in the dog: a clinical and scanning electron microscopic study. J Am Anim Hosp Assoc 14:571.

Martin CL, Chambreau T (1982): Cataract production in experimentally orphaned puppies fed a commercial replacement for bitch's milk. J Am Anim Hosp Assoc 18:115.

Matthews AG (2004): The lens and cataracts. Vet Clin North Am Equine Pract 20:393.

Matthews AG (2000): Lens opacities in the horse: a clinical classification. Vet Ophthalmol 3:65.

Miller PE, et al. (1997): Mechanisms of acute intraocular pressure increases after phacoemulsification lens extraction in dogs. Am J Vet Res 58:1159.

Miller TR, et al. (1987): Phacofragmentation and aspiration for cataract extraction in dogs: 56 cases (1980-1984). J Am Vet Med Assoc 190:1577.

Millichamp NJ, Dziezyc J (2000): Cataract phacofragmentation in horses. Vet Ophthalmol 3:157.

Moore DL, et al. (2003): A study of the morphology of canine eyes enucleated or eviscerated due to complications following phacoemulsification. Vet Ophthalmol 6:219.

Murphy JM, et al. (1980): Sequelae of extracapsular lens extraction in the normal dog. J Am Anim Hosp Assoc 16:17.

Narfstrom K (1999): Hereditary and congenital ocular disease in the cat. J Feline Med Surg 1:135.

Narfstrom K, Dubielzig R (1984): Posterior lenticonus, cataracts and microphthalmia: congenital ocular defects in the Cavalier King Charles spaniel. J Small Anim Pract 25:669.

Nasisse MP, et al. (1995): Lens capsule opacification in aphakic and pseudophakic eyes. Graefes Arch Clin Exp Ophthalmol 233:63.

Nasisse MP, et al. (1995): Technique for suture fixation of intraocular lenses in dogs. Vet Comp Ophthalmol 5:146.

Nasisse MP, Davidson MG (1999): Surgery of the lens, in Gelatt KN (editor): Veterinary Ophthalmology, 3rd ed. Lippincott Williams & Wilkins, Philadelphia.

Nasisse MP, Glover TL (1997): Surgery for lens instability. Vet Clin North Am Small Anim Pract 27:1175.

Norton JH (1980): Cataracts in sows. Aust Vet J 56:408.

Ofri R, Horowitz I (1995): Spontaneous cataract resorption in an ostrich. Vet Rec 136:276.

Olivero DK, et al. (1991): Feline lens displacement—a retrospective analysis of 345 cases. Prog Vet Comp Ophthalmol 1:239.

O'Reilly A, et al. (2003): The use of transscleral cyclophotocoagulation with a diode laser for the treatment of glaucoma occurring post intracapsular extraction of displaced lenses: a retrospective study of 15 dogs (1995-2000). Vet Ophthalmol 6:113.

Ori JI, et al. (2000): Posterior lenticonus with congenital cataract in a shih tzu dog. J Vet Med Sci 62:1201.

Oz HH, et al. (1986): Bilateral cataract surgery in a Suffolk ewe. Vet Rec 118:512.

Paulsen ME (1986): The effect of lens-induced uveitis on the success of extracapsular cataract extraction—a retrospective study of 65 lens removals in the dog. J Am Anim Hosp Assoc 22:49.

Peiffer RL, Weintraub BA (1979): Clinical and histopathologic effects of lensectomy and anterior vitrectomy in the canine eye. J Am Anim Hosp Assoc 15:421.

Pollet L (1982): Refraction of normal and aphakic canine eyes. J Am Anim Hosp Assoc 18:323.

Ranz D, et al. (2002): Nutritional lens opacities in two litters of Newfoundland dogs. J Nutr 132:1688S.

Remillard R, et al. (1993): Comparison of kittens fed queen's milk with those fed milk replacers. Am J Vet Res 52:901.

Richter M, et al. (2002): Aldose reductase activity and glucose-related opacities in incubated lenses from dogs and cats. Am J Vet Res 63:1591.

Rooks RL, et al. (1985): Extracapsular cataract extractions: an analysis of 240 operations in dogs. J Am Vet Med Assoc 190:1580.

Sanford SE, Dukes TW (1978): Acquired bilateral cortical cataracts in mature sows. J Am Vet Med Assoc 173:852.

Sato S, et al. (1998): Dose-dependent prevention of sugar cataracts in galactose-fed dogs by the aldose reductase inhibitor M79175. Exp Eye Res 66:217.

Sato S, et al. (1991): Progression of sugar cataract in the dog. Invest Ophthalmol Vis Sci 32:1925.

Sigle KJ, Nasisse MP (2006): Long-term complications after phacoemulsification for cataract removal in dogs: 172 cases (1995-2002). J Am Vet Med Assoc 228:74.

Slatter DH, et al. (1983): Hereditary cataracts in canaries. J Am Vet Med Assoc 183:872.

Slatter DH, et al. (1980): Cataracts and depressed galactose-1-phosphate uridyl transferase deficiency in a cus cus (Phalanger maculatus). Aust Vet J 56:141.

Smith PJ, et al. (1996): Ocular hypertension following cataract surgery in dogs: 139 cases (1992-1993). J Am Vet Med Assoc 209:105.

Stephens T, et al. (1974): Deficiency of two enzymes of galactose metabolism in kangaroos. Nature 248:524.

van der Woerdt A, et al. (1993): Ultrasonographic abnormalities in the eyes of dogs with cataracts. 147 cases (1986-1992). J Am Vet Med Assoc 203:838.

van der Woerdt A, et al. (1992): Lens induced uveitis in dogs: 151 cases (1985-1992). J Am Vet Med Assoc 120:921.

Warren C (2004): Phaco chop technique for cataract surgery in the dog. Vet Ophthalmol 7:348.

Williams DL, et al. (2004): Prevalence of canine cataract: preliminary results of a cross-sectional study. Vet Ophthalmol 7:29.

Williams DL, et al. (1996): Current concepts in the management of canine cataract: a survey of techniques used by surgeons in Britain, Europe and the USA and a review of recent literature. Vet Rec 138:347.

Williams DL, Munday P (2006): The effect of a topical antioxidant formulation including N-acetyl carnosine on canine cataract: a preliminary study. Vet Ophthalmol 9:311.

VITREOUS

Ron Ofri

ANATOMY AND PHYSIOLOGY
PATHOLOGIC REACTIONS
CONGENITAL AND DEVELOPMENTAL
    ABNORMALITIES

ACQUIRED DISORDERS
ROLE OF THE VITREOUS IN THE
    PATHOGENESIS OF OCULAR DISEASES

SURGICAL AND DIAGNOSTIC
    PROCEDURES

ANATOMY AND PHYSIOLOGY

Anatomy

The *vitreous* is a transparent elastic hydrogel (Figure 14-1). It occupies about 80% of the volume of the eye (Figure 14-2). During embryonic development, *primary, secondary,* and *tertiary vitreous* are formed and laid down (Figure 14-3). Their genesis is described in detail in Chapter 2. Briefly, the primary vitreous is associated with the hyaloid vascular supply system, which nourishes the lens during development. The secondary vitreous is laid down around the primary vitreous and forms the definitive (adult) vitreous, whereas the tertiary vitreous contributes to the formation of the lens zonules.

The vitreous body is divided into the following zones (Figure 14-4):

1. Anterior vitreous, located anterior to the ora ciliaris retinae (see Figure 14-4, area 5)
2. Posterior vitreous, located posterior to the ora ciliaris retinae (see Figure 14-4, area 7)
3. Cortex, which comprises the peripheral vitreous (see Figure 14-4, area 12), including:
   a. Vitreous base, which is the attachment of the vitreous at the ora ciliaris retinae (see Figure 14-4, area 6)
   b. Peripapillary vitreous, located adjacent to the optic disc (see Figure 14-4, area 10)
4. Central vitreous, including Cloquet's canal (see Figures 14-3 and 14-4, area 13). Cloquet's canal, which is a cleft in the vitreous where the hyaloid vasculature passed during embryonic development, is visible with the biomicroscope (see Figure 14-3, *B* and *C*).

Composition

Vitreous is a complex gel with the following constituents:

- Water (99%)
- Collagen fibers, which serve as a skeleton for the gel
- Cells *(hyalocytes)*
- Hyaluronic acid

Collagen fibrils form a meshwork internal to the retina (the *vitreous cortex*) and intermingle with the fibers of the internal limiting membrane of the retina, thus forming a firm attachment between the vitreous cortex and the retina (Figure 14-5).

Therefore anterior movement of the vitreous (such as occurs after lens luxation) may pull the retina off the retinal pigment epithelium (RPE) and cause traction retinal detachment. A potential space exists between the vitreous and the inner surface of the retina. Blood and exudates may accumulate in this space if the vitreous and retina separate, resulting in *subhyaloid hemorrhage.*

The collagen fibrils are also responsible for the numerous attachments of the vitreous to the adjacent structures—the posterior lens capsule, the ora ciliaris retinae (the vitreous base), and the optic nerve head (see Figure 14-4). Collagen fibrils are present in greater concentrations at the vitreous bases and around the optic disc, where attachment is the strongest.

The lens sits in a depression in the anterior face of the vitreous cortex, the *hyaloid fossa (patella fossa).* Collagen fibrils form attachments between the posterior lens capsule and the anterior vitreous. These attachments are especially significant in dogs. Removal of the posterior lens capsule, as in intracapsular lens extraction, results in loss of vitreous.

Hyalocytes are numerous within the vitreous and are more numerous near the cortex. The functions of these cells are unclear, but they may possess secretory and phagocytic capabilities as well as the potential for reversion to primitive fibroblasts able to form scar tissue. Mucopolysaccharides, containing a high proportion of hyaluronic acid, are intimately related to the collagen fibrils and hyalocytes and are present in higher concentration where hyalocytes are common. Hyaluronic acid provides the viscoelasticity of the vitreous body.

With the exception of collagen and hyaluronic acid, aqueous humor and vitreous are similar in composition, with free movement of many substances between them. The principles that govern entry of substances, including drugs, from the vascular circulation into the aqueous humor generally apply to the vitreous as well.

Function

The vitreous does not have a specific and clearly defined role in ocular physiology of the adult. It contributes to maintaining ocular volume and possibly the shape of the globe. It also helps maintain some ocular structures, notably the lens and retina, in their correct anatomic locations. Also, it forms part of the optical pathway that light must pass on its way to the retina. However, the vitreous does not have a significant role in refraction of this light, because its refractive index is similar to that of the lens.

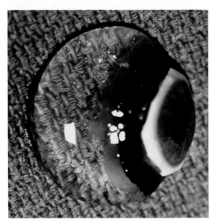

Figure 14-1. Vitreous after dissection of the sclera, choroid, and retina. A band of dark tissue can be seen posterior to the ora ciliaris retinae, circling the dorsal two thirds of the vitreous. This is neural retina that was firmly adherent to the vitreous base and could not be dissected. The vitreous also remains attached to the anterior segment (ciliary body, iris, and lens). The vitreous is almost entirely gel and thus is solid, maintaining its shape even though situated on a surgical towel exposed to room air. (From Yanoff M, Duker JS [2004]: Ophthalmology, 2nd ed. Mosby, St. Louis).

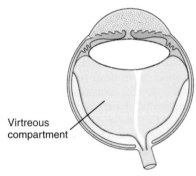

Virtreous compartment

Figure 14-2. The vitreous body *(shaded area)* occupies the posterior compartment of the eye. (Modified from Fine BS, Yanoff M [1979]: Ocular Histology. Harper & Row, New York.)

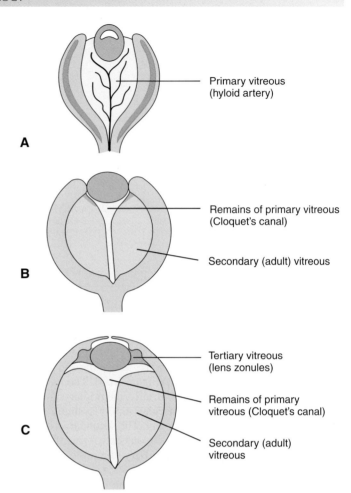

Primary vitreous (hyloid artery)

Remains of primary vitreous (Cloquet's canal)

Secondary (adult) vitreous

Tertiary vitreous (lens zonules)

Remains of primary vitreous (Cloquet's canal)

Secondary (adult) vitreous

Figure 14-3. Stages of vitreous development. **A,** Primary vitreous and hyaloid vessels nourishing the embryonic lens. **B,** The secondary vitreous laid down around the primary vitreous, which condenses into Cloquet's canal. The secondary vitreous will become the adult vitreous. **C,** Tertiary vitreous (lens zonules or ligaments) at the lens periphery. (Courtesy Dr. G.A. Severin.)

PATHOLOGIC REACTIONS

Because of its simple structure and lack of vascular and lymphatic supply, the vitreous has a limited range of pathologic reactions, as follows:

- *Liquefaction:* Because of its high water content, the vitreous gel may liquefy *(syneresis)* in response to many stimuli (e.g., infection, trauma, uveitis, senile changes). After liquefaction, the vitreous separates from the retina, encouraging retinal detachment from the underlying RPE. Liquified vitreous may also enter the subretinal space through retinal holes, predisposing to *rhegmatogenous retinal detachment.*
- *Cicatrization:* After inflammation of surrounding tissues or infection, scar tissue may form in the vitreous. These vitreous bands may contract and detach the retina *(traction detachment).*
- *Proliferative vitreoretinopathy:* This reaction occurs in association with retinal disease. In response to retinal disease, glial or RPE cells proliferate on the innermost retina or in the vitreous and form scars. Subsequently, these

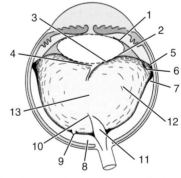

Figure 14-4. Relations and attachments of the vitreous body: *1,* attachment of anterior zonular fibers to the lens; *2,* attachment of posterior zonular fibers to the lens; *3,* attachment of anterior vitreous face to posterior lens capsule; *4,* anterior extremity of Cloquet's canal (Mittendorf's dot); *5,* anteriormost attachment of vitreous base to mid pars plana; *6,* region of vitreous "base"; *7,* region of diminishing adherence of vitreous base to retinal surface; *8,* vitreous-retinal attachment; *9,* vitreous-retinal attachment at margin of fovea centralis *(absent in domestic animals); 10,* attachment of posterior vitreous around optic disc; *11,* posterior extremity of Cloquet's canal (Bergmeister's papilla); *12,* cortical vitreous; *13,* central vitreous. Density of lines indicates approximate relative degrees of strength of attachment. (Modified from Fine BS, Yanoff M [1979]: Ocular Histology. Harper & Row, New York.)

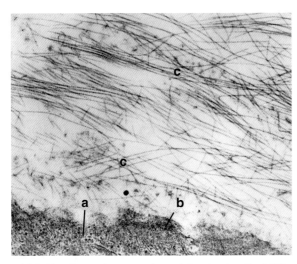

Figure 14-5. The vitreous base near the peripheral retina. The Müller cells *(a)* have a basement membrane *(b)* that forms the inner limiting membrane of the retina. The collagen fibrils *(c)* of the vitreous base form a meshwork internal to the retina. These fibrils join the internal limiting membrane. (From Hogan MJ, et al. [1971]: Histology of the Human Eye. Saunders, Philadelphia.)

fibrotic membranes may form that pull on the retina, causing it to tear and detach.
- *Vascularization:* The vitreous has no blood supply, but blood vessels may grow into it from an inflamed or malformed retina *(neovascularization)*. These vessels often are incomplete or fragile and are a source of vitreous hemorrhage (e.g., in the collie eye anomaly).
- *Infection and inflammation:* These reactions are discussed later.
- *Elongation:* Elongation of the vitreous body causes elongation of the axial length of the eye and, consequently, of the pathway that light must pass on its way to the retina. As a result, light that was previously focused on the retina is now focused in front of the retina, thereby causing shortsightedness (myopia). Such elongation occurs as a result of visual deprivation during the neonatal period. It may be induced by lid suturing and other deprivation techniques during the critical developmental period in animal models of myopia. It may also occur naturally, as a result of neonatal cataracts or corneal opacities that cause visual deprivation, resulting in neonatal myopia (as well as abnormalities in the visual cortex). This is another reason why congenital ocular opacities should be corrected as soon as possible, before irreparable changes occur in the eye, and why third eyelid flaps and tarsorrhaphies should be carefully considered in neonates.

CONGENITAL AND DEVELOPMENTAL ABNORMALITIES

Persistent Hyaloid Artery

The hyaloid artery is part of the embryonic vascular supply of the lens, which is described in Chapter 2. In most species, the hyaloid artery atrophies within a few weeks after birth (see Figure 14-3). An exception is ruminants, in which remains of the artery may be observed in a significant number of adults. However, persistent remnants of varying extent may be found in any species. The remnants of the artery origins on the surface

of optic disc, which are surrounded by glial tissue, are called *Bergmeister's papilla* (see Figure 14-4, area 11). These appear ophthalmoscopically, end-on, as red to white tufts originating from the optic disc and extending anteriorly a variable distance into the vitreous (see Figure 2-10, *B*, in Chapter 2). Similarly, at the distal end of the artery, remains of its attachment to the posterior lens capsule may be seen. The remains are known as *Mittendorf's dot* (see Figure 14-4, area 4). It does not interfere with vision, except for rare occasions when it induces focal, posterior cataracts. A persistent artery, however, may extend from the disc all the way to the posterior lens. Persistence of the hyaloid artery may be hereditary in the Doberman pinscher and Sussex spaniel. In rats, the hyaloid artery may bleed into the vitreous during normal atrophy.

A persistent hyaloid artery and its attachment to the posterior lens capsule must be differentiated from the following conditions by the following means:

- *Posterior capsular and subcapsular cataracts:* By accurate localization of the opacity. In the golden retriever and Labrador retriever, Mittendorf's dot is differentiated from a cataract on the basis of its smaller size and location on the posterior lens capsule. The cataract is much larger and is usually triangular, and careful examination may determine that it is located in the posterior lens cortex, rather than capsule. Mittendorf's dot usually has the anterior remnant of the hyaloid artery attached as a small white "tail" visible biomicroscopically.
- *Normal lens sutures (especially in cattle and horses):* By familiarity with the normal appearance
- *Vitreous bands:* By the linear appearance of the bands, which are usually located outside Cloquet's canal as well as by the presence of other signs of injury or inflammation (see Acquired Disorders)
- *Persistent tunica vasculosa lentis* and *persistent hyperplastic primary vitreous:* By the more extensive nature of the opacity on the posterior lens capsule (see following sections)

Persistent Tunica Vasculosa Lentis

This condition is similar to persistent hyaloid artery, the difference being that it is the tunica vasculosa lentis (TVL), rather than the hyaloid artery, that has also failed to regress postnatally. The TVL is visible as a netlike opacity on the posterior surface of the lens. Because the opacity is usually a very fine matrix, it does not interfere with vision.

Persistent Hyperplastic Primary Vitreous

Unlike the former two disorders, which involve failure of the hyaloid artery and TVL to regress postnatally, this disorder involves fetal and postnatal hyperplasia of the hyaloid system, TVL, and primary vitreous. Therefore the resulting opacity (which varies in size) is usually more severe. The disorder may occur in cats and in most dog breeds, and it has been demonstrated to be hereditary in the Bouvier des Flandres, Staffordshire bull terrier, and Doberman pinscher. Extensive studies of PHPV in the Doberman pinscher in The Netherlands have shown it to be an autosomal incompletely dominant trait with variable expression.

Clinically PHPV appears as a white or fibrovascular plaque in the posterior pupil near the posterior lens capsule and anterior vitreous (Figure 14-6). Vessel ingrowth and frank hemorrhage

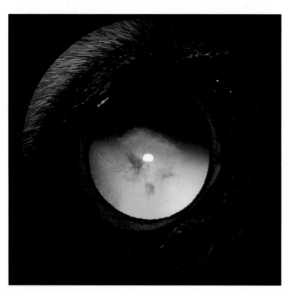

Figure 14-6. Persistent hyperplastic primary vitreous in a golden retriever. Note the fibrovascular opacity with patent vessels near the posterior lens capsule. The lesion is viewed in reflected light from the tapetum.

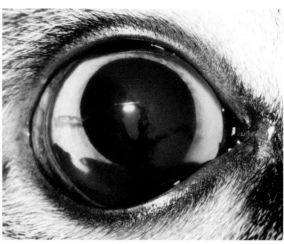

Figure 14-7. Hyphema and vitreal hemorrhage. The latter may be observed as a dark opacity in the posterior segment. (Courtesy David J. Maggs.)

into the vitreous and lens substance, calcium deposits, posterior lenticonus, microphakia, lens coloboma, intralental pigmentation, progressive cataracts, and elongated ciliary processes may also be present. Surgery of cataracts associated with PHPV carries a guarded prognosis due to opacification of the posterior lens capsule, the possibility of a patent blood vessel, and the need to combine the surgery with anterior vitrectomy.

ACQUIRED DISORDERS

Vitreous Degeneration

Vitreous degeneration is separation of the fluid and solid constituents of the vitreous into segregate fractions, resulting in vitreal liquefaction (synersis). The degeneration may occur naturally in elderly patients, or following inflammation, and may predispose the eye to retinal detachment. Degeneration of the vitreous is commonly demonstrated by ultrasonography in dogs with cataract as part of the preoperative screening of surgical candidates. In one study of 124 eyes degeneration was found in 50% of subjects with incipient cataract, 57% with immature cataract, 89% with mature cataract, and 100% with hypermature cataract. Eighty-six percent of eyes with lens-induced uveitis had vitreous degeneration, whereas 67% of those with cataracts but without uveitis were affected. The higher incidence of rhegmatogenous retinal detachments in eyes with hypermature cataracts may be associated with this increased incidence of vitreal degeneration.

Vitreous Hemorrhage

Because the vitreous does not have a vascular supply, vitreal hemorrhage is a relatively uncommon presentation (Figure 14-7). The source of the blood may be leakage from abnormally proliferating vessels, but it usually originates in retinal or uveal blood vessels due to the following:

- Hypertensive retinopathy in dogs and cats
- Clotting disorders (e.g., thrombocytopenia) and coagulopathies
- Ocular trauma

- Severe retinitis and retinochoroiditis (e.g., canine ehrlichiosis, Rocky Mountain spotted fever, brucellosis, feline infectious peritonitis, feline leukemia virus; also—depending on geographic location—intraocular mycotic disease, including blastomycosis, coccidiomycosis, cryptococcosis, histoplasmosis)
- Collie eye anomaly
- As a sequel to intraocular surgery
- Severe anterior uveitis of many different causes

Small amounts of vitreal hemorrhage may resorb, but larger amounts may cause long-term visual disturbances. Whether a vitreous hemorrhage resorbs depends on the associated pathologic changes in adjacent tissues and on the location of the hemorrhage within the vitreous body. Resorption is infrequent in collie eye anomaly because neovascularization of the vitreous near the retina has occurred with rupture of some of the vessels. In hypertensive retinopathy, resorption may occur if the hypertension is controlled, but recurrent hemorrhage is common owing to the nature of the lesions, especially if the hypertension is not well controlled. In retinitis, retinochoroiditis, ocular trauma, and anterior uveitis, resorption is more likely if the underlying inflammation and vascular damage resolve.

Conservative treatment, consisting of antiinflammatory and mydriatic drugs, is recommended for recent hemorrhages. Vitreal membranes and traction bands may develop; these abnormalities may also cause secondary traction retinal detachments months after the primary cause of the hemorrhage has resolved (Figure 14-8). Therefore, if membranes and bands are seen, an intraocular injection of tissue plasminogen activator (TPA) may be advocated. The aim of the injection is to break down fibrin traction bands and thereby prevent vitreoretinal detachment. The ideal "time window" for such an injection is 3 to 4 days after the primary event. If the TPA is injected too early, the hemorrhage may recur (because the clots that sealed the vessels are also dissolved). The injection is ineffective if enough time has passed to allow fibrin organization.

Infection and Inflammation

Inflammation of the vitreous is called hyalitis or vitritis. Because of its lack of vasculature, primary inflammation per se

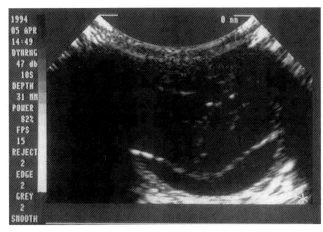

Figure 14-8. Ultrasound image of retinal detachment in a 6-year-old Samoyed with uveitis. The image shows the classic "seagull wings" sign, which is the detached retina adherent to the globe at the optic nerve head and the ora ciliaris retinae. The hyperechoic opacities anterior to the detached retina are fibrin strands that caused the detachment. (Courtesy Dr. I. Aizenberg.)

does not occur in the vitreous as in other tissues. However, the vitreous may be affected by inflammatory disorders of surrounding tissues (e.g., chorioretinitis, optic neuritis, anterior uveitis). The inflammation may cause opacification, hemorrhages, syneresis, and cellular exudation. Vitreous haze is common in inflammatory disorders of the posterior globe, and its disappearance is a valuable indicator of the efficacy of treatment. Reduction of this haze often improves vision. The treatment is similar to that of vitreal hemorrhage. The primary cause of the inflammation must be diagnosed and treated; the eye is treated symptomatically with cycloplegic and antiinflammatory drugs.

Infection of the vitreous by a variety of microorganisms is seen in penetrating injuries, systemic bacteremias, and ocular fungal infections. After the initial infection the surrounding vitreous liquefies and the infection spreads rapidly. Infections of the vitreous are associated with endophthalmitis (inflammation of all tissues of the eye except the sclera) and may progress to vitreous abscess. These infections must be treated aggressively with topical and systemic antibiotics or antifungal drugs. Severe cases are treated by intraocular injection of antimicrobial drugs, or surgically, by vitrectomy (see relevant section). Hyalocentesis (tapping of the vitreous) may be conducted for diagnostic purposes in cases that do not respond to medical therapy, with samples submitted for cytology, culture, serology, and pathology. The prognosis for these infections is usually very guarded.

The vitreous has also been implicated as a repository site for the antigens that cause the recurrent inflammation associated with equine recurrent uveitis (ERU). In particular, antigens of *Leptospira,* which are commonly associated with ERU, have been detected in the vitreous of affected horses. The involvement of the vitreous in the pathogenesis of ERU has led to the development of two novel treatment strategies. One consists of surgical removal of the vitreous (vitrectomy, discussed later). The other is based on the use of suprachoroidal implants for long-term release of cyclosporine, thereby suppressing the inflammatory reaction.

Vitreous Opacities (Floaters)

Floaters are small, mobile flakes that are seen in the vitreous. In most cases they are a benign finding in elderly patients and

probably represent degenerative changes in the vitreous. They may also appear following vitritis, especially in horses, in which case they usually contain blood or exudate. A focal light source with a binocular loupe or direct ophthalmoscope is adequate to demonstrate these opacities. Vitreous floaters are not responsible for the "fly-biting syndrome," in which an affected animal appears to be biting at moving objects in the air. This syndrome is now believed to be due to seizures of the temporal or occipital lobe and responds to appropriate medication. Surgical treatment of vitreous floaters is not required.

Asteroid Hyalosis (Asteroid Hyalitis) and Synchysis Scintillans

These are two pathologic conditions with a very similar presentation. Both are characterized by the appearance of numerous, small, refractile bodies scattered through the vitreous. Vision is not affected. The two conditions may occur spontaneously in older animals and also in association with chronic inflammatory and degenerative ocular disorders. In *asteroid hyalosis* the particles consist of calcium and phospholipids complexes (Figure 14-9). In *synchysis scintillans* the particles are composed of cholesterol. The two conditions can be distinguished clinically based on the mobility of the particles. In asteroid hyalosis the particles are attached to the collagen framework of the vitreous (Figure 14-10). Therefore they are fixed in the vitreous and move only with head or globe movements. In

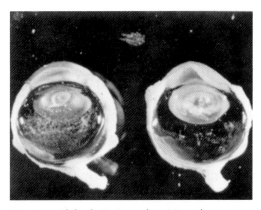

Figure 14-9. Asteroid hyalosis in a dog. Note the numerous white particles scattered in the patient's vitreous body. (From Rubin LF [1974]: Atlas of Veterinary Ophthalmoscopy. Lea & Febiger, Philadelphia.)

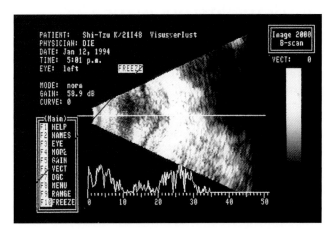

Figure 14-10. Subretinal hematoma, vitreous hemorrhage, and asteroid hyalosis in a shih tzu. (Courtesy Dr. Ursula Dietrich.)

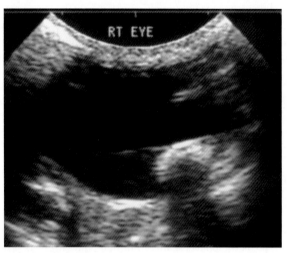

Figure 14-11. Ultrasound image of a vitreal mass, in this case a posterior luxated lens. (Courtesy Dr. I. Aizenberg.)

synchysis scintillans the bodies are mobile within the liquified vitreous. If the head is moved, the particles can be seen whirling like snowflakes in the vitreous, and then they slowly settle ventrally.

Vitreous Mass

The differential diagnosis of a mass in the vitreous includes the following entities:

- Retinal detachment (see Figure 14-8)
- Cataractous or normal, luxated lens (Figure 14-11)
- Intraocular neoplasm (usually by extension from the urea)
- Hemorrhage (acute or chronic) (see Figures 14-7 and 14-10)
- Foreign body
- PHPV
- Persistent hyaloid artery
- Traction band or fibrous tissue
- Vitreous abscess or endophthalmitis
- Parasites (e.g., *Dirofilaria immitis*, *Toxocara canis* larvae in dogs, *Echinococcus* spp., ophthalmomyiasis interna [fly larvae])
- Cyst (from the pigmented epithelial layer of the ciliary body)

ROLE OF THE VITREOUS IN THE PATHOGENESIS OF OCULAR DISEASES

Vitreous and Lens Luxation

If lens zonules break, the lens may be partially or totally luxated. In the early stages, when small numbers of lens zonules rupture, vitreous may escape into the anterior chamber and may be visible as fine strands in the anterior chamber or near the pupillary margin. Pigment may be seen in this prolapsed vitreous and is a possible indicator of the presence of uveitis. As the number of ruptured lens zonules rises, the stability of the lens decreases, and it may be subluxated within the hyaloid fossa, in the plane of the iris. Due to gravity the lens settles ventrally; the part of the pupil that is no longer occupied by the lens is visible as an aphakic crescent dorsal to the visible lens border. As the lens becomes fully luxated, more vitreous may prolapse into the pupil or iridocorneal angle, obstruct the flow of aqueous, and

cause secondary glaucoma. Lens luxation is illustrated and discussed in detail in Chapter 13.

Aqueous Humor Misdirection Syndrome

Also known as "malignant glaucoma," aqueous humor misdirection syndrome occurs in approximately 1% of cats older than 6 years presented to private practitioners for routine health care. In this disorder, aqueous humor is misdirected into the vitreous via minute breaks in the hyaloid membrane (perhaps during blinking or upon eyelid squeezing) rather than entering the posterior chamber. These breaks are suggested to act as one-way valves, trapping pools of aqueous humor in the vitreous, displacing the lens anteriorly (with intact lens zonules), dilating the pupil, and uniformly shallowing the anterior chamber. As the vitreal elements are compressed anteriorly it becomes much more difficult for aqueous humor to cross the hyaloid membrane. In some animals glaucoma may result. Therapy consists of suppressing aqueous humor production with topical carbonic anhydrase inhibitors or, in intractable cases, removal of the lens and anterior vitreous. Glaucoma is discussed in detail in Chapter 12.

Retinal Detachment

As noted, lens luxation may facilitate anterior prolapse (or movement) of the vitreous. Because of the attachment of the posterior vitreous to the inner retina, anterior movement of the vitreous may pull the retina off the choroid and cause *traction retinal detachment*. It is important to note that anterior vitreous prolapse may occur as a result of either anterior lens luxation (the lens pulls the vitreous forward) or posterior lens luxation (the lens being a "barrier" against vitreous movement, its posterior luxation may facilitate such prolapse). Traction retinal detachment may also occur following the formation of vitreal membranes or bands in the course of vitritis, infection, or hemorrhage. As the membranes and bands contract, they may pull the neuroretina off the RPE (see Figure 14-8).

The vitreous is also involved in the pathogenesis of *rhegmatogenous retinal detachment*. This kind of detachment is usually observed in elderly patients. Liquefied vitreous enters spontaneously occurring retinal holes and percolates into the subretinal space, causing detachment of the neuroretina from the RPE. Retinal detachment is discussed in detail in Chapter 15.

SURGICAL AND DIAGNOSTIC PROCEDURES

Hyalocentesis

Hyalocentesis is the removal of a small amount of liquefied vitreous for cytologic or microbiologic analysis. Indications for hyalocentesis include diagnosis of vitreous opacities suspected to be infectious or neoplastic in origin. The procedure is performed with the use of general anesthesia, after thorough preoperative preparation of the eye (see Chapter 5), and usually by an experienced veterinary ophthalmologist. Punctures must be accurately located in the pars plana ciliaris because more anterior punctures can strike the lens and result in cataract, or else they may penetrate the pars plicata ciliaris and result in severe intraocular hemorrhage (Figure 14-12 and Table 14-1). On the other hand, punctures made too posteriorly perforate the retina. A 22- to 26-gauge needle is directed into the material of interest, while pointing toward the posterior pole to avoid the lens. An equal volume of balanced salt or lactated Ringer's solution is used to replace the liquefied vitreous removed.

Hyalocentesis is performed by an experienced veterinary ophthalmologist for the diagnosis of serious intraocular disorders. It carries the risk of intraocular hemorrhage.

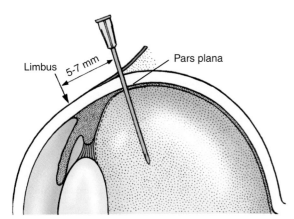

Figure 14-12. Hyalocentesis. Precise location of the point of insertion of a 22- to 26-gauge (0.70 to 0.45 mm) needle 5 to 7 mm posterior to the limbus, depending on the ocular quadrant and globe size as determined by calipers or ultrasonography, is of utmost importance to avoid intraocular trauma. (Modified from Boeve MH, Stades FC [1999]: Diseases and surgery of the canine vitreous, in Gelatt KN [editor]: Veterinary Ophthalmology, 3rd ed. Lippincott Williams & Wilkins, Philadelphia.)

Table 14-1 | **Location of the Pars Plana Ciliaris in the Dog**

QUADRANT	SITE (DISTANCE POSTERIOR TO THE LIMBUS)
Superotemporal	7 mm
Superonasal	5-6 mm
Inferotemporal	5-6 mm
Inferonasal	5 mm

Modified from Smith PJ, et al. (1997): Identification of sclerotomy sites for posterior segment surgery in the dog. Vet Comp Ophthalmol 7:180.

Vitrectomy

Vitrectomy is the removal of a portion of the vitreous body. Indications for vitrectomy include the following:

- Severe intraocular infection
- Prophylactic treatment of glaucoma, in cases where the vitreous presents in the anterior chamber following lens luxation or cataract surgery
- Surgical reattachment of a detached retina
- Recently vitrectomy has been advocated as surgical treatment for ERU, because the antigens that trigger the recurrent inflammation are postulated to be located in the vitreous.

In the course of anterior segment surgery (removal of cataracts and luxated lenses), small amounts of vitreous may present in the anterior chamber. These may be removed easily using sponges and scissors (Figure 14-13). When vitreous is removed it must not remain between wound edges, where it would interfere with wound healing, or in the anterior chamber, where it may lead to glaucoma. After lens luxation, syneresis is usually present. When syneresis or loss of vitreous is anticipated, use of hyperosmotic agents is advised to reduce the size of the vitreous body and risk of its subsequent loss.

More extensive vitrectomy is required in the treatment of ocular injuries and for treatment of retinal detachments and vitreal traction bands. The procedure requires more sophisticated instrumentation and surgical approaches to the posterior segment of the eye (see Figure 14-13, C and *D*). The incidence of postoperative complications is relatively high. Because of the intimate associations among the collagen framework of the vitreous body, lens capsule, and inner limiting membrane of the retina, removal of large amounts of vitreous carries a significant risk of postoperative retinal detachment.

Vitreous Replacement

If larger amounts of vitreous are removed, the physical deficit must be replaced. Vitreous replacements are especially useful in canine patients for maintaining retinal position after surgical correction of retinal detachment, because head shaking tends to disrupt the delicate retinal reattachments. Vitreous substitutes are also used to roll out folded retina before reattachment and to

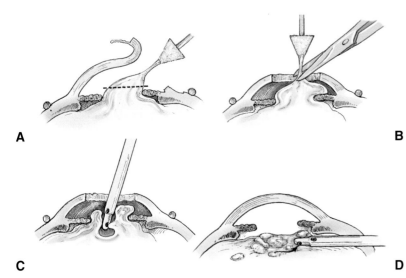

A   **B**

C   **D**

Figure 14-13. Vitrectomy can be performed manually or using automated instruments. If small amounts of vitreous are present in the anterior chamber (e.g., following lens luxation or cataract surgery), these can be removed manually. The vitreous is pulled out with a sponge (**A**) and cut with scissors (**B**). Removal of large amounts of vitreous (e.g., during surgical reattachment of the retina or as glaucoma prophylaxis) is performed using a vitrector. The instrument may be inserted through the anterior chamber (**C**) or using a scleral port (**D**). Note that in all cases, the lens has been removed. (Modified from Deustch TA, Feller DB [1985]: Paton and Goldberg's Management of Ocular Injuries. Saunders, Philadelphia.)

float pieces of dropped lens into the anterior chamber for removal during cataract extraction. Many different substances, including perfluorocarbons, silicone, and fluorosilicone, have been used. Complications from the toxicity of these substances include cataract formation, keratopathy, and glaucoma.

Advanced Vitreoretinal Surgical Techniques

Many surgical techniques have been developed for the reattachment and prevention of retinal detachments. Examples are laser and cryosurgical retinopexy, pneumatic retinopexy, scleral buckling procedures, and pars plana vitrectomy; most of these are applicable to the canine eye. For details of these methods, which are beyond the scope of this text, the reader is referred to a recent review (Vainisi and Wolfer, 2004). The scope and complexity of the surgery depends on the extent of the retinal detachment. Laser retinopexy and cryoretinopexy are used to "weld" the retina to the choroid in cases of retinal holes or partial detachment, in order to stop progression to full retinal detachment. More advanced techniques and specialized equipment are required to reattach a fully detached retina. Prognosis depends, to a large extent, on the duration of the detachment before reattachment, and it is accepted that retinas reattached within 4 weeks may regain some useful vision. A recent retrospective study of 500 canine cases reported restoration of some vision in 76% of patients.

BIBLIOGRAPHY

Allgoewer I, Pfefferkorn B (2001): Persistent hyperplastic tunica vasculosa lentis and persistent hyperplastic primary vitreous (PHTVL/PHPV) in two cats. Vet Ophthalmol 4:161.

Bayon A, et al. (2001): Ocular complications of persistent hyperplastic primary vitreous in three dogs. Vet Ophthalmol 4:35.

Blair NP, et al. (1985): Rhegmatogenous retinal detachment in Labrador retrievers. II: proliferative vitreoretinopathy. Arch Ophthalmol 103:848.

Boeve MH, Stades FC (1999): Diseases and surgery of the canine vitreous, in Gelatt KN (editor): Veterinary Ophthalmology, 3rd ed. Lippincott Williams & Wilkins, Philadelphia.

Boroffka SA (2005): Ultrasonographic evaluation of pre- and postnatal development of the eyes in beagles. Vet Radiol Ultrasound 46:72.

Boroffka SA, et al. (1998): Ultrasonographic diagnosis of persistent hyperplastic tunica vasculosa lentis/persistent hyperplastic primary vitreous in two dogs. Vet Radiol Ultrasound 39:440.

Chrisman CL (1991): Problems in Small Animal Neurology, 2nd ed. Lea & Febiger, Philadelphia.

Colitz CM, et al. (2000): Persistent hyperplastic tunica vasculosa lentis and persistent hyperplastic primary vitreous in transgenic line TgN3261Rpw. Vet Pathol 37:422.

Cullen CL, Grahn BH (2004): Diagnostic ophthalmology: persistent hyperplastic tunica vasculosa lentis and primary vitreous. Can Vet J 45:433.

Deeg CA, et al. (2001): Immune responses to retinal autoantigens and peptides in equine recurrent uveitis. Invest Ophthalmol Vis Sci 42:393.

Dietrich U (1996): Ultrasonographic examination of the eyes of dogs with cataracts using the combined B-mode/vector A-scan system, dissertation, Ludwig-Maximilians-Universitat, Munich.

Duddy JA, et al. (1983): Hyaloid patency in neonatal beagles. Am J Vet Res 44:2344.

Epstein DL, et al. (1979): Experimental perfusions through the anterior and vitreous chambers with possible relationships to malignant glaucoma. Am J Ophthalmol 88:1078.

Fruhauf B, et al. (1998): Surgical management of equine recurrent uveitis with single port pars plana vitrectomy. Vet Ophthalmol 1:137.

Gemensky-Metzler AJ, Wilkie DA (2004): Surgical management and histologic and immunohistochemical features of a cataract and retrolental plaque secondary to persistent hyperplastic tunica vasculosa lentis/persistent hyperplastic primary vitreous (PHTVL/PHPV) in a bloodhound puppy. Vet Ophthalmol 7:369.

Gilger BC, et al. (2005): Ocular parameters related to drug delivery in the canine and equine eye: aqueous and vitreous humor volume and scleral surface area and thickness. Vet Ophthalmol 8:265.

Gilger BC, et al. (2001): Use of an intravitreal sustained-release cyclosporine delivery device for treatment of equine recurrent uveitis. Am J Vet Res 62:1892.

Gilger BC, et al. (2000): Effect of an intravitreal cyclosporine implant on experimental uveitis in horses. Vet Immunol Immunopathol 76:239.

Gilger BC, et al. (2000): Long-term effect on the equine eye of an intravitreal device used for sustained release of cyclosporine A. Vet Ophthalmol 3:105.

Gorig C, et al. (2006): Evaluation of acoustic wave propagation velocities in the ocular lens and vitreous tissues of pigs, dogs, and rabbits. Am J Vet Res 67:288.

Grahn BH, et al. (2004): Inherited retinal dysplasia and persistent hyperplastic primary vitreous in miniature schnauzer dogs. Vet Ophthalmol 7:151.

Kroll MM, et al. (2001): Intraocular pressure measurements obtained as part of a comprehensive geriatric health examination from cats seven years of age and older. J Am Vet Med Assoc 219:1406.

Leon A (1988): Diseases of the vitreous in the dog and cat. J Small Anim Pract 29:448.

Leon A, et al. (1986): Hereditary persistent hyperplastic primary vitreous in the Staffordshire bull terrier. J Am Anim Hosp Assoc 22:765.

Martin CL (1978): Zonular defects in the dog: a clinical and scanning electron microscopic study. J Am Anim Hosp Assoc 14:571.

Ori J, et al. (1998): Persistent hyperplastic primary vitreous (PHPV) in two Siberian husky dogs. J Vet Med Sci 60:263.

Peiffer RL, Weintraub BA (1979): Clinical and histopathologic effects of lensectomy and anterior vitrectomy in the canine eye. J Am Anim Hosp Assoc 15:421.

Rubin LF (1963): Asteroid hyalosis in the dog. Am J Vet Res 24:1256.

Smith PJ (1999): Surgery of the canine posterior segment, in Gelatt KN (editor): Veterinary Ophthalmology, 3rd ed. Lippincott Williams & Wilkins, Philadelphia, p. 935.

Smith PJ, et al. (1997): Identification of sclerotomy sites for posterior segment surgery in the dog. Vet Comp Ophthalmol 7:180.

Stades FC (1980): Persistent hyperplastic tunica vasculosa lentis and persistent hyperplastic primary vitreous in Doberman pinschers: pathological aspects. J Am Anim Hosp Assoc 16:791.

Stades FC (1980): Persistent hyperplastic tunica vasculosa lentis and persistent hyperplastic primary vitreous in Doberman pinschers: techniques and results of surgery. J Am Anim Hosp Assoc 16:393.

Stades FC (1980): Persistent hyperplastic tunica vasculosa lentis and persistent hyperplastic primary vitreous (PHTVL/PHPV) in 90 closely related Doberman pinschers: clinical aspects. J Am Anim Hosp Assoc 16:739.

Tolentino FI, et al. (1965): Biomicroscopy of the vitreous in collie dogs with vitreous abnormalities. Arch Ophthalmol 73:700.

Vainisi SJ, Wolfer JC (2004): Canine retinal surgery. Vet Ophthalmol 7:291.

van der Woerdt A, et al. (1993): Ultrasonographic abnormalities in the eyes of dogs with cataracts: 147 cases (1986-1992). J Am Vet Med Assoc 203:838.

Wollanke B, et al. (2001): Serum and vitreous humor antibody titers in and isolation of Leptospira interrogans from horses with recurrent uveitis. J Am Vet Med Assoc 219:795.

Zeiss CJ, Dubielzig RR (2004): A morphologic study of intravitreal membranes associated with intraocular hemorrhage in the dog. Vet Ophthalmol 7:239.

CELLULAR ANATOMY
PHYSIOLOGY AND BIOCHEMISTRY
APPLIED ANATOMY (OPHTHALMOSCOPIC
   VARIATIONS)

PATHOLOGIC MECHANISMS
CONGENITAL RETINAL DISORDERS

RETINOPATHY
RETINAL DETACHMENT

The retina is the organ responsible for transducing light into neuronal signals that are eventually perceived as a visual image. One might say that the entire purpose of the eye is to enable focused light to strike a functional retina.

More specifically, the light strikes the *photoreceptors,* a complex layer of specialized cells—the *rods* and *cones*—which contain photopigments that produce chemical energy on exposure to light. This energy is converted (transduced) into electrical energy, which is processed by the retina and transmitted by the optic nerve, via the optic chiasm, optic tracts, lateral geniculate body, and optic radiations, to the visual cortex.

The retina is a unique organ in that it can be studied non-invasively with the ophthalmoscope to show in vivo intricate details of pathologic processes that in most other organs are only visible histopathologically, or during invasive surgery. This enables the clinician to correlate clinical findings with histopathologic findings and may frequently allow specific, accurate diagnosis.

CELLULAR ANATOMY

Broadly speaking, the retina can be regarded as a three-neuron sensory unit, because photoreceptors relay the visual signal through bipolar cells and onto the ganglion cells (Figure 15-1). However, this is a gross simplification, and traditionally the retina is described as having 10 layers. The structure of these layers is summarized in Table 15-1, and their function is detailed below. From the outside (facing the choroid and sclera) to the inside (facing the vitreous) these layers are as follows (Figure 15-2):

1. Retinal pigment epithelium
2. Photoreceptor layer
3. External limiting membrane
4. Outer nuclear layer
5. Outer plexiform layer
6. Inner nuclear layer
7. Inner plexiform layer
8. Ganglion cell layer
9. Optic nerve fiber layer
10. Internal limiting membrane

The *retinal pigment epithelium* (RPE) (layer 1) is the outermost layer of the retina, facing the choroid. It is pigmented in the nontapetal part of the fundus of domestic animals and gives a homogenous brown-black color to this area. It is normally unpigmented in the tapetal fundus and cannot be seen clinically; therefore it could be argued that the name *RPE* in this area is a misnomer, because the cells are nonpigmented retinal pigment epithelium. The lack of RPE pigment in the tapetal area allows incoming light that has not been absorbed by the photoreceptors to reach the tapetum. The tapetum acts as a mirror that reflects this light back toward the photoreceptor layer, thus increasing the probability that it will be absorbed by the photopigment and contribute to visual sensation in dim light (Figure 15-3).

Normal function of the pigment epithelium is essential to retinal integrity and function.

The RPE has two main functions. The first is to serve as metabolic interface between the photoreceptors and their choroidal blood supply, supplying metabolites and removing waste from the outer retina. The second function is to recycle the "used" (or *bleached*) photopigment of the photoreceptors. Discs containing the photopigment are continually synthesized and move from the base of the photoreceptor outer segment toward its distal end. After the photopigment absorbs the energy of the incoming light and transduces it into a neuronal signal, the disc is shed and phagocytized by the engulfing RPE (Figure 15-4). The recycling of the pigment by the RPE and the production of new discs by the photoreceptor outer segments are essential for the retina's sensitive response to light. The RPE also has a phagocytic role in retinal inflammations (see later).

Layers 2 through 10 are collectively called the *sensory retina* or the *neuroretina* because they process the neuronal signal, or visual sensation (as opposed to the RPE, which has only a supporting role). It may be remembered from Chapter 2 that the neuroretina and the RPE originate from two different embryonic layers.

The *photoreceptor layer* (layer 2) is composed of the outer segments of the rods and cones, which contain the visual photopigments within discs stacked like a pile of coins (Figure 15-5). This is the site where vision is "initiated," because it is here that the process of phototransduction, or the conversion of a visual stimulus into an initial neuronal signal, occurs (see Visual Photopigments). Therefore the previous statement, that the purpose of the eye is to enable focused light to strike the retina, could be refined—light should be focused precisely on the photoreceptor layer. As noted, a result of the phototransduction process is the bleaching and shedding of the photopigment by the outer segments, and its subsequent phagocytosis and recycling by the RPE.

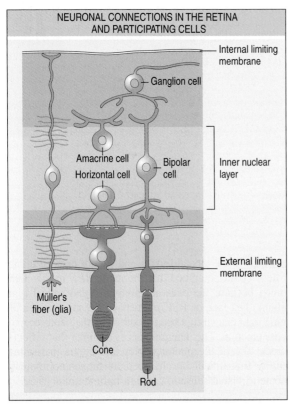

Figure 15-1. Rods and cones relay a visual signal through bipolar cells onto ganglion cells. Amacrine and horizontal cells contribute to processing of the signal, while Müller's cells provide structural support. (From Yanoff M, Duker JS [2004]: Ophthalmology, 2nd ed. Mosby, St. Louis.)

The *external limiting membrane* (layer 3) is formed by terminal processes joining the cell membranes of rods, cones, and Müller's cells. Müller's cells extend across the entire retina, from the external limiting membrane to the internal limiting membrane, and therefore serve as its structural "skeleton." Small Müller's cell processes pass between the outer limbs of rods and cones contributing to the formation of the outer limiting membrane

Table 15-1 | Summary of Retinal Structure

LAYER	CONSTITUENTS
1. Retinal pigment epithelium	Pigment epithelial cells
2. Photoreceptor layer	Outer segments of photoreceptors; processes of Müller's cells
3. External limiting membrane	Terminal processes joining rods, cones, and Müller's cells
4. Outer nuclear layer	Nuclei of rods and cones
5. Outer plexiform layer	Axons of rods and cones synapse with dendrites of bipolar and horizontal cells and with other photoreceptors
6. Inner nuclear layer	Nuclei of bipolar, Müller's, horizontal, and amacrine cells
7. Inner plexiform layer	Axons of bipolar and amacrine cells synapse with dendrites of ganglion cells
8. Ganglion cell layer	Cell bodies of ganglion cells
9. Nerve fiber layer	Axons of ganglion cells
10. Internal limiting membrane	Basement membrane and footplates of Müller's cells

(see Figures 15-5, *A,* and 15-6). The cells also perform important metabolic functions, such as energy storage and ionic regulation.

The *outer nuclear layer* (layer 4) consists of the nuclei of the rods and cones. The *outer plexiform layer* (layer 5) is a synaptic layer. Here, axonal extensions of the photoreceptors dilate to form *synaptic expansions,* which synapse with dendrites of bipolar cells as well as with adjacent photoreceptors. This is the site of the first synapse, which the neuronal visual signal must pass, and hence a potential site for its initial processing.

The *inner nuclear layer* (layer 6) contains the following four types of nuclei: (1) bipolar cells, (2) Müller's cells, (3) horizontal cells, and (4) amacrine cells. Bipolar cells synapse with photoreceptor cells in the outer plexiform layer. Horizontal and amacrine cells are lateral communicating cells that modulate the neuronal activity and the visual signal.

The *inner plexiform layer* (layer 7) is the second synaptic layer, consisting of axons of bipolar, horizontal, and amacrine cells and dendrites of ganglion cells. Numerous synapses occur

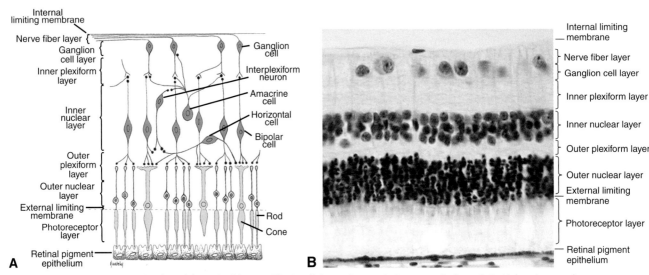

Figure 15-2. A, Plan of the retinal layers. All 10 cellular and synaptic layers are indicated. **B,** Light micrograph of full-thickness view of the retina, with the architecture corresponding to the layers indicated in **A.** (From Remington LA [2005]: Clinical Anatomy of the Visual System, 2nd ed. Butterworth-Heinemann, St. Louis.)

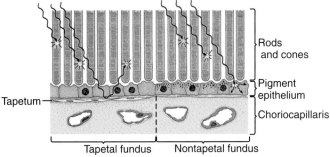

Figure 15-3. Function of the tapetum. Three incoming photons are shown. Two are absorbed by the photoreceptors and contribute to a visual sensation, and the third passes through the retina without being absorbed. In the nontapetal fundus *(right)* this photon's energy dissipates in the pigment epithelium and is therefore wasted. In the tapetal fundus *(left)* the photon is reflected back onto the photoreceptors. In this case it is absorbed and contributes to vision, thus increasing sensitivity to low levels of light. Because the photon is eventually absorbed by a photoreceptor that is not in its original trajectory, the resulting image is blurred. This blurring affects the acuity of daytime vision but has less impact at night, when the cones are not active. Note that the overlying retinal pigment epithelium is pigmented where there is no tapetum and nonpigmented over the tapetum.

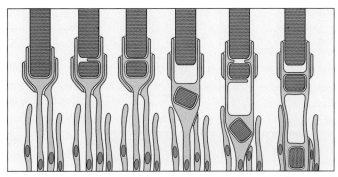

Figure 15-4. Retinal pigment epithelium (RPE, *blue*) phagocytosis of photoreceptor outer segments *(brown)*. The phagosome, containing the ingested material consisting of bleached photopigment, enters the RPE cytoplasm, where it merges with lysosomes to facilitate digestion of the outdated membranes. (Adapted from Steinberg RH, et al. [1977]: Pigment epithelial ensheathment and phagocytosis of extrafoveal cones in human retina. Philos Trans R Soc Lond 277:459.)

in the inner plexiform layer between bipolar and ganglion cells, and laterally between horizontal and amacrine cells and bipolar and ganglion cells. These lateral connections between cells coordinate and integrate retinal function.

The *ganglion cell layer* (layer 8) consists of cell bodies of the ganglion cells. Except in the central retina, the ganglion cell layer is usually one cell thick. Axons of ganglion cells form the *nerve fiber layer* (layer 9). They run parallel to the retinal surface and converge onto the *optic disc*. Here they form bundles of nerve fibers that constitute the *optic nerve*, which exits the eye through the *lamina cribrosa* (a sievelike opening in the sclera). These ganglion cell axons will reach their first synapse in the *lateral geniculate body* (although those axons contributing to the pupillary light response (PLR) will synapse in the *pretectal nucleus*).

The innermost layer, facing the vitreous, is the *internal limiting membrane* (layer 10). It is a basement membrane to which the inner ends of Müller's cells are closely attached (see Figure 15-1).

Nuclei of axons in the optic nerve lie in the ganglion cell layer of the retina.

Intuitively, it may seem that the orientation of the retina, with the photoreceptors being the outermost layer facing the choroid and the ganglion cells the innermost layer facing the vitreous, is illogical. Indeed, this anatomic arrangement is called an *inverted retina*—incoming light must transverse the entire retina to be absorbed by the outer photoreceptors, and the generated signal must again transverse the entire retina to exit the eye through the axons of the inner ganglion cells. The reason for this anatomic arrangement is the high metabolic requirements of the photoreceptors, which necessitate placing these cells next to their "private" blood supply, that is, the choroid (see next section).

Blood Supply

The retina is the most metabolically active tissue in the body, as indicated by its high oxygen consumption. Therefore in most species it has a dual blood supply. The outer retina (i.e., the photoreceptors) is supplied by the choroid, and the inner retina and midretina are supplied by inner retinal vessels, which are usually visible ophthalmoscopically on the inner retinal surface. Arterioles, capillaries, and venules originating in these inner vessels penetrate the retina to supply the midretina. Interruption of either choroidal or retinal vasculature quickly results in ischemia and severe, irreversible loss of function, despite reserves of glycogen within Müller's cells. (The clinical implication of this feature is that retinal detachment must be treated early to avoid irreversible loss of function.) The blood-retina barrier therefore has two components. The first is the RPE, which separates the retina from the choroid. The second component is formed by the endothelial cells of the inner retinal capillaries and their basement membrane. Both of these barriers limit the passage of substances into the retina. There is little extracellular space in the retina, and transport of solutes from capillaries occurs via Müller's cells and astrocytes.

In animals, the inner retina is supplied by vessels arising from the short posterior ciliary arteries (which are therefore called *cilioretinal* arteries) that penetrate the sclera in a circle around the optic disc. A notable exception is in primates, whose retinas are supplied by a single *central retinal artery*, making them susceptible to ischemia due to occlusion. Retinas of domestic animals are classified according to the pattern of their inner retinal vasculature (Table 15-2). The most common pattern is holangiotic, whereby most of the inner retinal surface is transversed by blood vessels (Figure 15-7). In merangiotic retinas, the vessels extend from the optic disc laterally and medially but other regions of the retina are uncovered (Figure 15-8), whereas in paurangiotic retinas only the area around the optic disc is supplied by short, peripapillary inner retinal vessels (Figure 15-9). In species with paurangiotic supply, such as the horse, the retina therefore depends more on choroidal supply; thus the consequences of interruption to choroidal supply by trauma or anemia are more serious for the equine retina. The avian fundus is characterized by the presence of a *pecten*—a pigmented vascular structure protruding into the vitreous from the retina (Figure 15-10). The avian retina is usually avascular, and the pecten may have a nutritional role. A similar structure, a *conus papillaris,* is found in many reptilian and amphibian species (Figure 15-11).

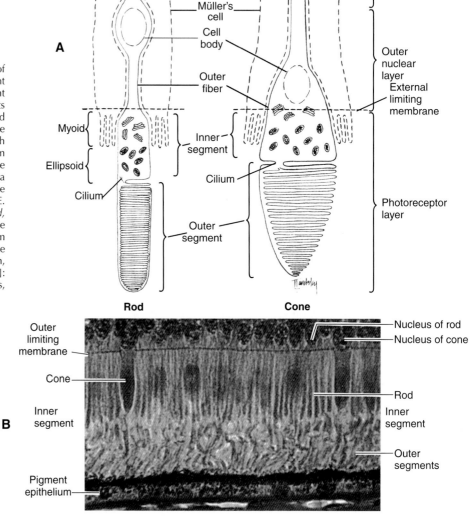

Figure 15-5. A, Photoreceptor cells. The discs of the outer segments (facing the retinal pigment epithelium [RPE]) contain the photopigment required for vision. The cells' inner segments contain the mitochondria. The rod spherule and cone pedicle are the synaptic expansions of the photoreceptors where their axons synapse with dendrites of bipolar cells in the outer plexiform layer. Portions of Müller's cells *(dotted lines)* are shown adjoining the rods and cones. **B,** Retina (×1000). Rod and cone outer segments are shown in close contact with the underlying RPE. Above them, the inner segments are visible *(Rod, Cone)*. Photoreceptor nuclei are located at the top, in the outer nuclear layer. (**A** from Remington LA [2005]: Clinical Anatomy of the Visual System, 2nd ed. Butterworth-Heinemann, St. Louis; **B** from Krause WJ, Cutts JH [1981]: Concise Text of Histology. Williams & Wilkins, Baltimore.)

Table 15-2 | **Classification of Retinal Vascular Patterns**

TYPE	FEATURES	EXAMPLES
Holangiotic	The whole inner retina receives a direct blood supply, either from a central artery (in primates) or from cilioretinal arteries that emerge as several branches from or around the optic disc (in most other mammals)	Most mammals, including the dog, cat, cow, sheep, rat, mouse, and primates
Merangiotic	Blood supply localized to the nasal and temporal parts of the inner retina	Rabbit
Paurangiotic	The vessels are minute and extend only a short distance from the optic disc, leaving most of the retina avascular	Horse, rhinoceros, elephant, marsupials
Anangiotic	Inner retinal surface is devoid of blood vessels	Most nonmammalians, including birds, reptiles, and amphibians; some mammals, including beaver, chinchilla, porcupine, armadillo, sloth, guinea pig, and bats

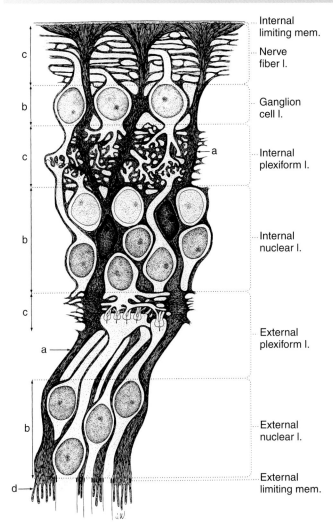

Internal limiting mem.

Nerve fiber l.

Ganglion cell l.

Internal plexiform l.

Internal nuclear l.

External plexiform l.

External nuclear l.

External limiting mem.

Figure 15-6. Structure of Müller's cells. Note how the (dark colored) cell transverses 9 of the 10 retinal layers, thus leading structural support to the entire retina and forming the outer and inner limiting membranes. *a,* Radial processes; *b,* honeycomb meshwork; *c,* horizontal fibers; *d,* fiber baskets; *l.,* layer; *mem.,* membrane. (From Hogan MJ, et al. [1971]: Histology of the Human Eye. Saunders, Philadelphia.)

PHYSIOLOGY AND BIOCHEMISTRY

Rods and Cones

As mentioned earlier, the outer segments of the rods and cones contain light-sensitive photopigments that absorb the energy of incoming light particles (photons). Because rods and cones have differing functions (Table 15-3), the pigments in each are different, and they also vary with species. Rods are much more sensitive than cones to low levels of light and to small changes in illumination. Therefore they function in dim environments and at night *(scotopic vision).* Rods are also responsible for processing motion. Cones are less sensitive to small fluctuations in light levels, functioning predominately at high levels of illumination *(photopic vision).* On the other hand, cones are capable of greater visual discrimination than rods, thus providing for high-resolution vision; in many species, cones also contain pigments for color vision.

Some of the difference in sensitivity between rods and cones is accounted for by *retinal summation.* For instance, there are approximately 130 million photoreceptors in the human retina but only 1.2 million axons in the optic nerve. This means that

Table 15-3 | **Characteristics of Rods and Cones**

RODS	CONES
Function in low light levels (scotopic)	Function in high light levels (photopic)
Sensitive to small change in light intensity	Insensitive to small change in light intensity
Low visual discrimination (low acuity)	High visual discrimination (high acuity)
Responsive to blue light	Responsive to red light
No color differentiation: monochromatic absorbance	Color differentiation: dichromatic, trichromatic, or tetrachromatic
Sensitive to motion	Sensitive to contrast
Detect light flashing at low frequency (low FFF)	Detect light flashing at high frequency (high FFF)
More in peripheral retina	More in central retina

FFF, Flicker fusion frequency.

inevitably some axons have more than one photoreceptor (typically rods) associated with them. By converging large numbers of rods in a particular area onto a single bipolar cell, and by converging several bipolar cells onto a ganglion cell, the rod pathway can amplify the response to low levels of light (Figure 15-12). This is because just a single photon falling anywhere in a large area can activate the regional ganglion cell (see Figure 15-12, left panel). However, this amplification occurs at the expense of fine discrimination—if this regional ganglion cell fires, there is no way of knowing which of its associated rods was hyperpolarized by a photon. Maximum visual discrimination occurs when one photoreceptor is connected to one bipolar cell and to one ganglion cell, which is the typical synaptic cone pathway (see Figure 15-12, right panel). This is because the firing of any given ganglion cell can be triggered only by hyperpolarization of a single, specific cone that is associated with this ganglion cell. However, more photons are required for the activation of this system, making it active only at high intensities of light. The effect of retinal anatomy and function on vision is described in detail in Chapter 1.

The retinas of birds and primates possess a specialized area called the *fovea.* This region is populated only by cones (and their associated bipolars and ganglion cells) and provides these species with their high resolution and rich color vision. In most (nonprimate) mammalian species, this function is served by a region called the *area centralis,* which has a relatively high cone concentration. In these species, however, rods outnumber cones even in the area centralis, accounting for the lower visual resolution and greater light sensitivity of most domestic species. In all animals, including those that possess a fovea, the rod-to-cone ratio rises towards the peripheral retina, which is typically characterized by low-resolution, light-sensitive vision (Figure 15-13). Some nocturnal animals have a pure rod retina with no cones, whereas some raptor species have two foveas, giving these birds very high visual resolution.

Visual Photopigments

Molecules that absorb light are termed *photopigments.* Visual photopigments in the photoreceptors can absorb a range of wavelengths, with each class of photopigment having peak absorption at a particular wavelength. The molecule is also capable of absorbing other wavelengths with decreasing efficiency, thus forming a bell-shaped curve of absorption

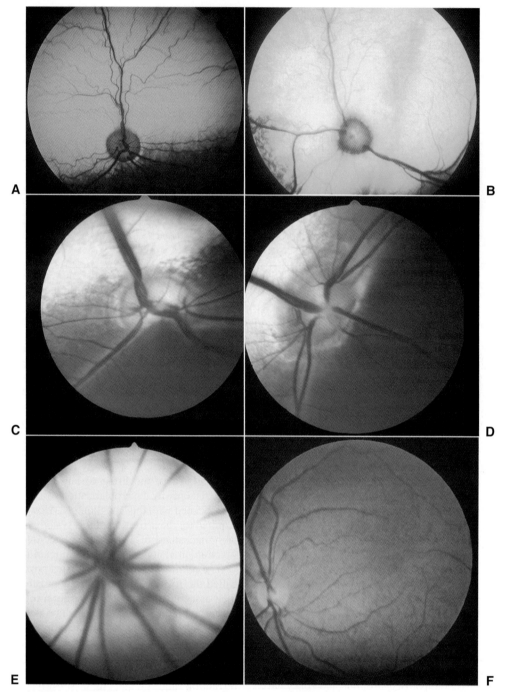

Figure 15-7. Holangiotic vascular supply of the retina in various species. **A,** Dog. Note the color and shape of disc, caused by myelination of the optic nerve fibers, and the fact that the veins form a venous circle on the surface of the optic disc. **B,** Cat. The disc is darker and rounder than the canine optic disc, owing to lack of myelination. The veins stop at the disc margin and do not cross its surface. The arteries of the feline retina are fewer and less torturous compared with those of the canine retina. **C,** Sheep. Major arteries and veins are paired and intertwined, and the optic disc is kidney shaped. **D,** Cow. The general appearance is similar to that of a sheep fundus, except that the optic disc is oval. **E,** Albino rat. A round optic disc, with vessels radiating outward like sun rays. **F,** Owl monkey. In primates, the vessels cross over the surface of the unmyelinated optic disc. (**A** and **C** to **F** courtesy University of California, Davis, Veterinary Ophthalmology Service Collection.)

versus wavelength, with its peak is known as the *absorption maximum*, or λ_{max} (Figure 15-14).

Visual photopigment molecules consist of two parts, a *chromophore* (which is a derivative of vitamin A) and a protein, or *opsin*. The chromophore is the part of the molecule that transduces the energy of the light photon into a chemical reaction, which generates a neuronal signal, as detailed in the next section (Photochemistry). The opsin is the part of the molecule that determines the wavelength the photopigment will absorb, thus allowing the eye to perceive color in that spectrum. Therefore species possessing *trichromatic vision*, such as primates, have three cone populations as defined by their respective

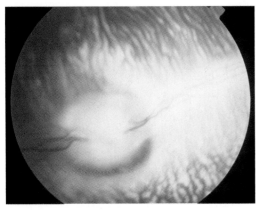

Figure 15-8. A merangiotic blood supply of the inner retina in an albino rabbit. Only the nasal and temporal retinas are supplied by vessels that can be seen at the optic disc at the 3 o'clock and 9 o'clock positions. The thick red bands elsewhere in the fundus are choroidal blood vessels. (Courtesy University of California, Davis, Veterinary Ophthalmology Service Collection.)

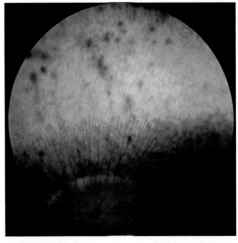

Figure 15-9. A paurangiotic blood supply of the inner retina in an 8-year-old Welsh pony. Note that vessels are restricted to the area around the optic disc. (From Rubin LF [1974]: Atlas of Veterinary Ophthalmology. Lea & Febiger, Philadelphia.)

opsins. These three opsin populations enable the cones to absorb light in three primary colors (typically red, green, and blue). The richness of the human color vision, and the number of shades we can see, is made possible by the overlapping absorption curves of these three primary colors. Species with dichromatic vision have two classes of cones (possessing two types of opsins). Contrary to popular belief that animals see in black-and-white, most domestic species, including dogs, horses, and ruminants, are *dichromatic,* enabling these animals limited color vision consisting of two primary colors and their intermediate shades; cats may even possess trichromatic vision. Tetrachromatic species, such as birds, have a fourth class of cones, with an extra opsin absorbing ultraviolet light and allowing for color vision that is richer than that of humans.

The photopigment that has been studied most extensively is *rhodopsin.* This photopigment, found in rods, also consists of a chromophore and an opsin. The rod chromophore is a vitamin A_1 derivative (11-*cis* retinal aldehyde). The rod opsin has an absorption maximum of approximately 495 nm (see Figure 15-14). Much of what we know of visual photochemistry comes from the study of rhodopsin, although it is assumed that cone photopigments function similarly.

Photochemistry

When a photon of light is absorbed by a rhodopsin molecule, it initiates a chemical process that results in *phototransduction* of its energy into a neuronal signal: The opsin breaks off the chromophore (i.e., 11-*cis* retinal aldehyde) and the chromophore is isomerized into the more stable all-*trans* retinal aldehyde. The isomerization triggers a complex chain reaction involving numerous enzymes. The final step in this cascade is hydrolysis of cyclic guanosine monophosphate (cGMP) into GMP by phosphodiesterase. The resulting decrease in cGMP levels closes sodium channels in the outer segments, leading to hyperpolarization of the photoreceptor; that is, a neuronal signal. (Photoreceptors are exceptional neurons in that they are depolarized in their resting state [at darkness] and are hyperpolarized following excitation [by light].) Mutations in the genes encoding for any of the enzymes involved in this cascade cause inherited retinal degeneration in a number of species, notably dogs and humans (see Inherited Retinopathies).

One of the by-products of the phototransduction process is the isomerized chromophore, all-*trans* retinal aldehyde. This

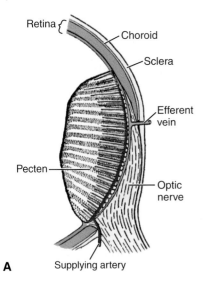

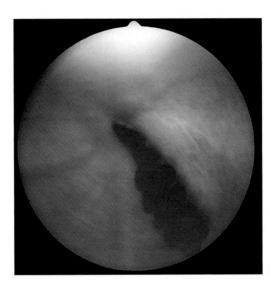

A Supplying artery

Figure 15-10. A, Structure of the pecten, showing its relationship to the entrance of the optic nerve and its vascular connections. The supplying artery sends a branch to each fold. The efferent vein receives a branch from each angle of the fold. **B,** Ophthalmoscopic view of the fundus of a barn owl *(Strix flammea).* Note that no vessels can be seen on the surface of the retina. (**A** modified from Duke-Elder S [1958]: System of Ophthalmology, Vol I. Mosby, St. Louis; **B** courtesy University of California, Davis, Veterinary Ophthalmology Service Collection.)

B

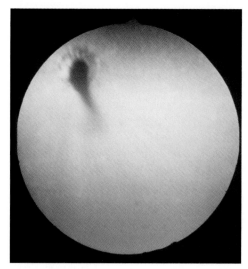

Figure 15-11. A gecko fundus, typical of the anangiotic blood supply of the reptilian retina. No vessels can be seen, and the optic disc is obscured by a conus papillaris. (Courtesy University of California, Davis, Veterinary Ophthalmology Service Collection.)

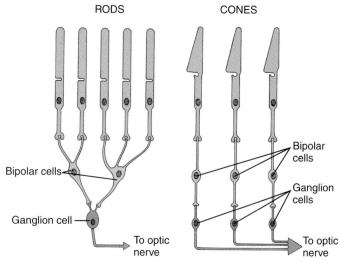

Figure 15-12. Retinal summation. The rod pathway is converging, as large numbers of rods are connected to a bipolar cell (although only two to three converging rods are shown here) and several bipolar cells are connected to a ganglion cell. In the cone pathway there is little or no summation, because one cone synapses to one bipolar cell that synapses with one ganglion cell. This arrangement allows cones faster conduction and high visual resolution at the price of low sensitivity to light levels.

molecule, representing *bleached* photopigment, is shed by the photoreceptor and phagocytized by the RPE for "recycling" (see Figure 15-4). In the RPE, the all-*trans* retinal aldehyde can be isomerized back to the 11-*cis* retinal aldehyde and re-form rhodopsin (Figure 15-15), or it can be reduced to all-*trans* retinol and esterified. The esters are stored in the pigment epithelium until required for dark adaptation (see later). After all-*trans* ester has been deesterified, oxidized, and isomerized, it is available for spontaneous regeneration of rhodopsin in the dark.

Vitamin A in the eye turns over very slowly with other body stores of vitamin A, and only a small proportion of ingested vitamin A reaches the eye to form the chromophore of the visual photopigment. Vitamin A deficiency does not affect the eye until other body stores are depleted. Hypovitaminosis A causes loss of rod function (owing to depletion of the rhodopsin) and, when chronic, leads to complete retinal degeneration and

blindness. In young animals it may also cause bone remodeling, leading to stenosis of the optic foramen and blindness due to the resulting optic nerve atrophy.

Vitamin A deficiency causes night blindness *(nyctalopia)*, retinal and optic nerve atrophy, and convulsions in cattle, and microphthalmia and nyctalopia in the offspring of deficient sows.

Dark Adaptation

Dark adaptation is the transition of the retina from the light-adapted (photopic) to the dark-adapted (scotopic) state. *Visual*

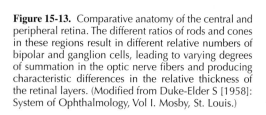

Figure 15-13. Comparative anatomy of the central and peripheral retina. The different ratios of rods and cones in these regions result in different relative numbers of bipolar and ganglion cells, leading to varying degrees of summation in the optic nerve fibers and producing characteristic differences in the relative thickness of the retinal layers. (Modified from Duke-Elder S [1958]: System of Ophthalmology, Vol I. Mosby, St. Louis.)

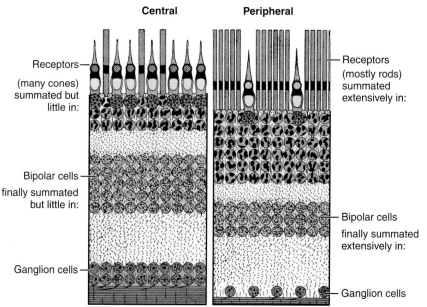

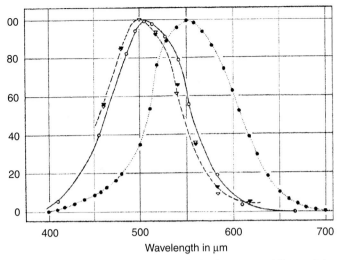

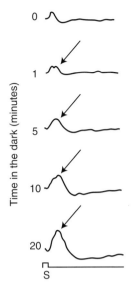

Figure 15-14. Absorption spectrum of rhodopsin (at different light intensities) as a function of wavelength. As can be seen, wavelength sensitivity is not all-or-nothing. Rhodopsin has *absorption maximum*, or λ_{max}, values of 495 and 525 nm (depending on light intensity) but can absorb shorter and longer wavelengths with decreased effectiveness. (From Moses RA [1970]: Adler's Physiology of the Eye, 5th ed. Saunders, Philadelphia. Modified from Hecht.)

Figure 15-16. Increasing amplitude of the b wave *(arrow)* in response to flashes of light during dark adaptation in a normal dog during electroretinography. Note that as the animal spends more time in the dark (indicated in minutes in the left column), the amplitude of the response increases. *S,* The timing of the light flash stimulus that elicits the retinal response. (Modified from Aguirre GD, Rubin L [1971]: The early diagnosis of rod dysplasia in the Norwegian elkhound. Am Vet Med Assoc 159:429.)

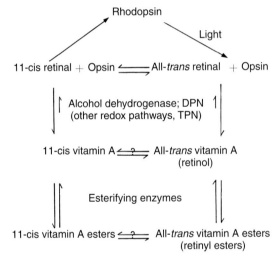

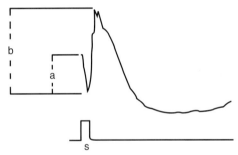

Figure 15-15. Rhodopsin (containing II-*cis,* retinal) is isomerized by light into all-*trans* retinal. All-*trans* retinal may be either isomerized to re-form rhodopsin or reduced to all-*trans* retinol. After esterification it can be stored in the retinal pigment epithelium until needed for dark adaptation. *DPN,* Diphosphopyridine nucleotide; *TPN,* triphosphopyridine nucleotide. (From Wald G [1968]: Molecular basis of visual excitation. Science 162:230.)

Figure 15-17. Electroretinogram of a normal dark-adapted canine in response to a white light flash, 0.02 second in duration (denoted as *s*). The downward deflection, the a wave, is composed mostly of photoreceptor activity. It is followed by an upward (positive) deflection, the b wave, representing bipolar and Müller's cell activity. (From Rubin LF [1974]: Atlas of Veterinary Ophthalmoscopy. Lea & Febiger, Philadelphia.)

acuity is greatest in the photopic state, whereas light *sensitivity* is maximal in the scotopic state. The three physiologic processes contributing to the increased light sensitivity of the retina in darkness are dilatation of the pupil, synaptic adaptation of retinal neurons, and increase in the concentration of rhodopsin available in the outer segments. Together, these three processes may increase the sensitivity of the eye by 5 to 8 log units (i.e., by up to 100 million). Maximal sensitivity is reached after 30 minutes or more in the darkness, depending on the species and light level before adaptation began. In making the transition from light to dark, the brighter the preexisting light level, the longer the eye takes to reach maximal

sensitivity, presumably because rhodopsin stores are lower after exposure to bright light and have to be reconstituted from stores in the pigment epithelium.

Dark adaptation in domestic animals is measured by (1) increase in amplitude of the electroretinogram (ERG) with time spent in the dark (Figure 15-16) and (2) the ability to detect dimmer lights with time spent in the dark. The latter may be measured electrophysiologically as a decrease in the stimulus intensity required to produce a given ERG amplitude in the dark.

Electroretinography

The ERG is the electrical response recorded when the retina is stimulated by flashes of light (Figure 15-17). Although it is possible to relate different parts of the ERG wave to different structures within the retina (e.g., the *a wave* to the rods and cones, the *b wave* to the bipolar and Müller's cells, and the

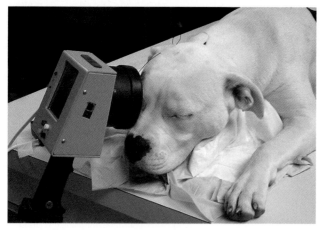

Figure 15-18. Electroretinography (ERG) performed in 6-month-old American Bulldog using the handheld multispecies ERG device (HMsERG). For the purpose of the recording, the dog is anesthetized, its pupil is dilated, and the lids are retracted with an eyelid speculum. The flash stimulus is delivered by the HMsERG, and the electrical response of the retina to the stimulus is recorded by means of a contact lens electrode placed on the cornea (visible as a red wire). (Courtesy Kristina N. Narfström.)

c wave to the pigment epithelium), such attempts are an oversimplification of a complex process that is incompletely understood. For clinical purposes the ERG is best considered a mass response of the entire outer retina to flashes of light. Therefore the ERG is usually used to assess outer retinal function in animals affected with disorders of the rods and cones. Although electroretinography requires sophisticated equipment (Figure 15-18) and specialized training in its operation and interpretation of results, it is an extremely valuable diagnostic tool for the veterinary ophthalmologist.

Electroretinography is useful in the following circumstances:

- *Routine preoperative evaluation of retinal function before cataract surgery:* Unfortunately, many dogs may be simultaneously affected with both retinal dystrophy and cataract. Regardless of whether these two diseases are related or independent, it is obvious that cataract surgery will not restore vision if the retina is not functioning. Because the cataract prevents a thorough ophthalmoscopic evaluation of the retina, an ERG is required to determine the prognosis of the surgery. It is important to note that

even in the presence of cataracts (or a corneal opacity) that affect vision, sufficient light reaches the retina to elicit an electrophysiologic response, provided that the retina is functional. This is also the reason why PLR can be elicited in cataractous patients.

- *Diagnosis of retinal disorders in which no ophthalmoscopic abnormalities are evident:* These include early stages of retinal dysplasia, day blindness (hemeralopia) in Alaskan malamutes and German short-haired pointers, congenital stationary night blindness (CSNB) in dogs and horses, and sudden acquired retinal degeneration (SARD). In all of these diseases, ERG abnormalities may be recorded even though the fundus may seem normal.
- *Differentiating between retinal and postretinal causes of blindness:* For example, cases of SARD and retrobulbar optic neuritis may manifest similarly as acute loss of vision, a normal-looking fundus, and fixed, dilated pupils. An ERG may be used to differentiate between the two, because the response will be extinguished in SARD (which is a retinal disease) but normal in optic neuritis (which is a postretinal disease).
- *Early diagnosis of inherited photoreceptor atrophies:* In many dog breeds and in some cat breeds, the ERG may detect changes in retinal function long before ophthalmoscopic or behavioral signs are observed. This early detection is invaluable to breeders wishing to screen their animals for inherited retinal diseases (Figure 15-19).

Flash electroretinography is a summed response of the outer retina. Focal retinal lesions (e.g., scars), or inner retinal disease (e.g., glaucoma) may not affect the flash ERG.

Based on the clinical indication for the ERG, two recording protocols have evolved for performing the test in dogs. The first is the rapid, "yes-no" protocol used to demonstrate retinal function. It is conducted to rule out SARD or to determine whether the patient is a suitable candidate for cataract surgery. For early detection and evaluation of inherited photoreceptor diseases, a more exhaustive recording protocol is required. This protocol involves extensive testing of rod and cone function, based on their different physiologic properties (see Table 15-3). It includes testing the process of dark and light adaptation (see Figure 15-16), responses to dim and bright light (see Figure 15-19), responses to red, blue, and white

Figure 15-19. Electroretinography (ERG) responses recorded with the handheld multispecies ERG device in a normal Abyssinian cat *(1)* and in an Abyssinian cat affected with hereditary rod cone degeneration *(2)*. The a wave (negative deflection), representing photoreceptor function, is attenuated by 80% in the affected cat. The b wave (positive deflection), representing bipolar activity, is unaffected by the disease process. (Courtesy Kristina N. Narfström.)

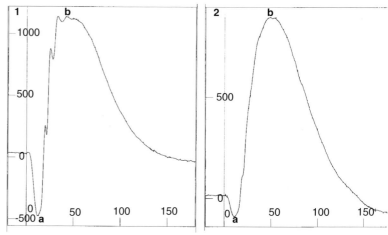

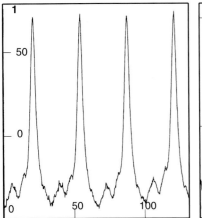
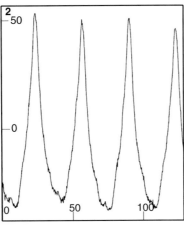

Figure 15-20. Flicker fusion responses recorded in the same cats as in Figure 15-19. The signals are recorded in response to light flashes presented at a high frequency. In the normal cat *(1)*, there is a normal signal in response to each flash, whereas in the affected cat *(2)*, the responses are diminished and delayed, because the diseased photoreceptors do not fully recover before subsequent flashes (note that the two recordings appear similar but their scales differ). If the frequency of the flashes is increased further, the normal photoreceptors will not be able to recover fully either. At a threshold frequency, the flashes are so rapid that the photoreceptors do not recover at all, and their responses "fuse." Rods and cones are characterized by different fusion threshold frequencies. (Courtesy Kristina N. Narfström.)

lights, and *flicker fusion frequency* (FFF) recorded in response to rapid flashes of light (Figure 15-20). FFF is the frequency of stimulation beyond which individual ERG responses are not recorded, and it depends on whether the rods and cones are functioning under the prevailing levels of illumination. ERG results are typically reported as a- and b-wave amplitudes and implicit times in response to the various stimuli used (Figure 15-21). A summary of electroretinographic alterations in various ocular disorders is given in Table 15-4.

The ERG is a test of retinal function, not of vision. Therefore it may be normal in some cases of blindness. For example, the ERG is normal in cases of postretinal blindness such as optic neuritis or cortical disease, even though the patient is blind.

APPLIED ANATOMY (OPHTHALMOSCOPIC VARIATIONS)

Before pathologic processes can be recognized, common variations in fundus appearance must be appreciated. Detailed fundus diagnosis is the province of the veterinary ophthalmologist, but familiarity with common, normal fundus variations is essential so that the general practitioner can recognize and distinguish them from pathologic processes. Students and clinicians are encouraged to examine the fundus of *every* patient (including

those presented for nonophthalmic reasons) as part of a comprehensive examination and in order to familiarize themselves with its normal appearance.

Tapetum

The *tapetum* is a reflective layer located in the choroid. It can be found in many mammalian species (with the notable exceptions of primates, pigs, and rodents) as well as in nocturnal nonmammalian species. Although the structure of the tapetum differs among different species (i.e., it may be fibrous or cellular), its role is similar. The tapetum acts as a mirror that reflects the light back toward the photoreceptor layer, thus increasing the probability that the light will be absorbed by the photopigment and contribute to visual sensation in dim light (see Figure 15-3). Because melanin absorbs light and would prevent it from reaching the tapetum, the RPE overlying the tapetum is nonpigmented, thereby allowing it to fulfill its physiologic role.

Color variations in the tapetum occur in all species. They are most frequent in dogs, where various shades of yellow-orange and green-blue are commonly observed, although other colors may also be seen. In newborn pups the fundus is dark at birth; the tapetal area gradually changes shades into gray and blue before adult colors appear (Figure 15-22).

ERG CALCULATIONS

b-wave peak amplitude
0 line
a-wave peak amplitude

a-wave peak implicit time   b-wave peak implicit time

Figure 15-21. Electroretinography parameters. (From Howard DR, et al. [1973]: Clinical electroretinography: a protocol for testing the retina. J Am Anim Hosp Assoc 9:219.)

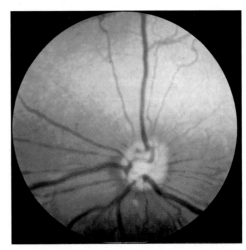

Figure 15-22. Fundus of a 13-week-old Alaskan malamute. The area of the future tapetum is blue at this age. (From Rubin LF [1974]: Atlas of Veterinary Ophthalmology. Lea & Febiger, Philadelphia.)

Table 15-4 | **Electroretinogram (ERG) Findings in Selected Ocular and Vision Disorders**

DISEASE	ERG FINDINGS	COMMENTS
Cataract	ERG indicates retinal function or lack thereof	ERG very important in determining whether retina is normal, as it can't be examined ophthalmoscopically. Therefore ERG is used to determine prognosis or severely diseased before cataract surgery.
Retinal detachment	ERG response may be present or absent, depending on duration of detachment; ERG cannot be used to determine prognosis of surgical reattachment surgery	Ultrasound may be of greater diagnostic value
Cortical blindness	ERG response normal	ERG useful in differentiating retinal and cortical blindness
Optic neuritis and optic atrophy	ERG response normal	ERG useful in cases of retrobulbar neuritis in which no ophthalmoscopic lesions can be observed
Glaucoma*	Flash ERG response normal in early cases if pressure not markedly elevated; it is absent in advanced stages of disease or in acute, high IOP spikes	In early cases of glaucoma there is ganglion cell loss with no change in flash ERG response. In advanced stages the damage spreads to the outer retina, affecting the ERG response. The flash ERG is not diagnostic for glaucoma.
Hemeralopia (day blindness)	Rod ERG response normal; cone ERG response absent	ERG essential for definitive diagnosis of hemeralopia, as fundus looks normal
Feline central retinal degeneration (taurine deficiency)	Initially, cone responses are affected. Disease affects rod function in advanced stages.	ERG may be abnormal 10 wks before onset of ophthalmoscopic signs
Congenital stationary night blindness (CSNB)	Decreased b-wave and increased a-wave amplitudes	ERG essential for definitive diagnosis of CSNB, as fundus looks normal
Inherited photoreceptor dysplasia *(rcd)*	Decreased rod/cone function, depending on type of disease	In some breeds (Irish setter, miniature schnauzer) the ERG can be diagnostic before 2 months of age
Inherited rod-cone degeneration *(prcd,* PRA)	Decreased rod function (abnormal dark adaptation, scotopic responses, and flicker fusion frequency) progressing to attenuation of all ERG responses	The ERG can be diagnostic months or years before the onset of behavioral and ophthalmoscopic signs
Retinal pigment epithelial dystrophy (RPED)	ERG response may be normal until advanced stages	Ophthalmoscopy sufficient for diagnosis; ERG is of no value
Retinal dystrophy in Briard	ERG indicates congenital abnormalities in rod function	Distinguishes the disease from RPED, although both are caused by RPE abnormality
Sudden acquired retinal degeneration	ERG response extinguished	ERG essential for diagnosis, as fundus looks normal

IOP, Intraocular pressure; *PRA,* progressive retinal atrophy; *prcd,* progressive rod-cone degeneration; *rcd,* rod-cone dysplasia.
*Describes ERG results recorded in response to a flash stimulus, which is commonly used in veterinary medicine. ERG results recorded in response to a shifting pattern stimulus are used for diagnosing glaucoma in human patients.

Pigment is occasionally observed in the normally unpigmented pigment epithelium in the tapetal area and should be differentiated from pathologic pigmentation. The pigmented areas are more common at the tapetal-nontapetal junction (Figure 15-23). The transition between tapetum and nontapetum may be gradual or sharply demarcated.

Absence of the tapetum occurs in all species, although it is most prevalent in subalbinotic and color-dilute eyes. Absence of the tapetum may be total (Figure 15-24) or focal (Figure 15-25). The RPE is often unpigmented in association with tapetal agenesis. In these regions, where there is no tapetum and the RPE is nonpigmented, the underlying wide choroidal vessels are visible through the retina as numerous thick, parallel red stripes, the so-called tigroid fundus (see Figures 15-24, *B,* and 15-25). Note that the much finer retinal vessels are visible overlying the choroidal vasculature. This type of fundus causes a red funduscopic reflection (through the pupil or ophthalmoscope), and although it is a normal variation, it is sometimes mistaken for hemorrhage.

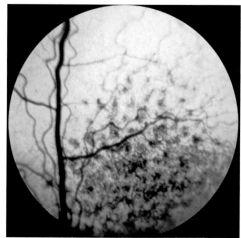

Figure 15-23. Multifocal areas of pigmentation of the retinal pigment epithelium overlying the tapetum in a dog. This is a normal variation. (From Rubin LF [1974]: Atlas of Veterinary Ophthalmoscopy. Lea & Febiger, Philadelphia.)

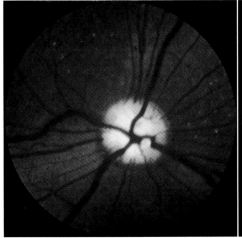
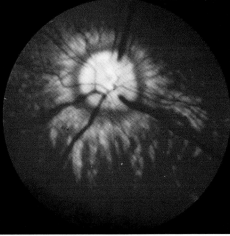

A

B

Figure 15-24. Fundus pictures of two dogs with tapetal aplasia. **A,** The retinal pigment epithelium (RPE) throughout the retina is pigmented, providing for a dark fundus. **B,** There is no pigment in the choroid and the RPE throughout the fundus, allowing for visualization of the choroidal blood vessels. Both pictures are normal variations. (From Rubin LF [1974]: Atlas of Veterinary Ophthalmoscopy. Lea & Febiger, Philadelphia.)

In some animals only small tapetum "islands" may be seen (Figure 15-26). In canine toy breeds the tapetum is frequently small. Primates (see Figure 15-7, *F*), pigs, most rodents (see Figure 15-7, *E*), and many nonmammalian species (see Figures 15-10, *B,* and 15-11) lack a tapetum all together.

Nontapetum

In most mammals, the tapetum covers approximately the dorsal third of the fundus. The rest of the fundus is called the *nontapetum.* Here the underlying RPE is pigmented, giving this area its characteristic dark appearance (see Figure 15-7, *A, C,* and *D*). However, the amount of the pigmentation may vary. Moderate amounts of RPE pigment in the nontapetal area give this region a light brown (chocolate) shade rather than the characteristic black appearance. Lack of pigment in the pigment epithelial cells of the nontapetal retina is a common variation (see Figures 15-24, *B,* and 15-27) and is frequently seen in subalbinotic or color-dilute animals (e.g., Siamese cat,

appaloosa, merle collie). If there is no pigment in the RPE, the underlying choroid and sclera may be visualized in the nontapetal area (tigroid fundus).

Optic Disc

The location of the optic disc in the eye is fixed because it is determined by the location of the underlying optic foramen through which the optic nerve exits the orbit. However, the size of the tapetal and the nontapetal regions may vary, so the disc may be visualized in the tapetal area (if the tapetum is large), in the nontapetum (if the tapetum is small), or in their junction.

The presence of myelin determines the size and shape of the optic disc. In the cat, myelination of the optic nerve fibers begins posterior to the disc, and therefore the disc is round and dark (similar to an atrophied canine disc) (see Figure 15-7, *B*). In dogs, myelination of the fibers usually begins at the level of the disc, giving it a characteristic triangular shape and pink shade (see Figure 15-7, *A*). However, variations in size, shape,

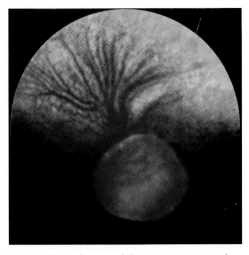

Figure 15-25. Localized absence of the tapetum in a yearling. Although the retinal pigment epithelium (RPE) in the nontapetum is pigmented, the RPE overlying the region of tapetal aplasia is unpigmented, allowing visualization of the underlying choroidal vessels, which can be seen as broad red bands. This is a normal variation. (From Rubin LF [1974]: Atlas of Veterinary Ophthalmoscopy. Lea & Febiger, Philadelphia.)

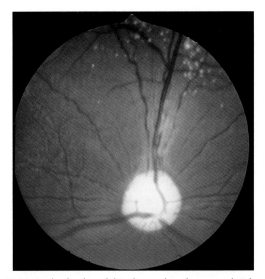

Figure 15-26. In the fundus of this dog, only a few tapetal "islands" are visible through the pigmented retinal pigment epithelium. Myelination of the nerve fibers can be seen as white streaks radiating from the disc. This is a normal variation.

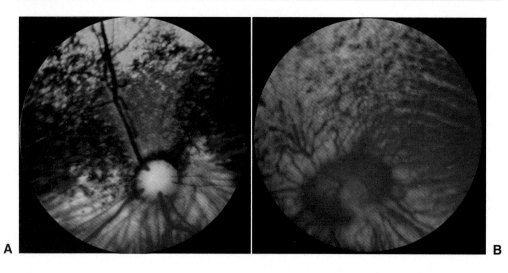

Figure 15-27. Fundus pictures of two animals in which the retinal pigment epithelium in the non-tapetum does not contain melanin. Its absence allows visualization of the underlying choroidal vessels, which can be seen as broad red bands. In both cases, the tapetal area is normal. **A,** A domestic shorthair cat; **B,** a horse. (From Rubin LF [1974]: Atlas of Veterinary Ophthalmoscopy. Lea & Febiger, Philadelphia.)

and color of the optic disc, based on the extent of myelination, are common in the dog. The disc may also be surrounded by a ring of pigment or hyperreflectivity, both of which are considered normal variations. A dark spot may be seen in the center of the disc, the physiologic cup representing the origin of the embryonic hyaloid vascualture.

Blood Vessels

As noted previously, the blood vessels seen ophthalmoscopically are those supplying the inner retina and midretina. The large, straight vessels are the veins. There are usually three veins, although it is not uncommon to see four or more large veins. In the cat the veins stop at the edge of the disc, but in dogs they cross over its surface and usually form a vascular ring (see Figure 15-7, *A* and *B*). In dogs in which the veins stop abruptly on the disc surface, a coloboma or glaucomatous cupping should be suspected.

Arteries are the smaller vessels. They are more numerous (10 to 20) and usually more tortuous than veins. In dogs arteries usually stop at the disc rim and do not cross the disc surface as do the veins. It is important to learn to distinguish arteries from veins, because arteries are the first vessels to undergo attenuation in cases of inherited retinal atrophies.

Myelination of Nerve Fiber Layer

Myelination of canine optic nerve fibers usually begins at the optic disc. Occasionally myelination spreads into the nerve fiber layer of the retina, appearing as white fan-shaped streaks radiating from the optic disc (see Figure 15-26). These are differentiated clinically from papilledema and optic neuritis (see Table 16-10 in Chapter 16).

PATHOLOGIC MECHANISMS

Ischemia

The retina has a bipartite blood supply, because the choroid supplies the outer retina, and the inner retinal vessels (visible ophthalmoscopically radiating from the disc) supply the inner retina and midretina. Owing to its high metabolic rate, the retina is particularly susceptible to interruptions in blood supply. After hypoxia begins, death of retinal cells follows rapidly, intracellular and extracellular edema occurs, neural elements disintegrate, and atrophy and gliosis of the retina result. Many disease processes

(e.g., anemia, inflammation, retinal detachment, increased intra-ocular pressure, decreased orbital circulation after trauma) may result in decreased retinal circulation and tissue hypoxia.

Repair Processes

Like other neural tissues, the retina has limited or no regenerative capacity. Changes in photoreceptor and neural elements are almost always irreversible, limiting the scope of treatment for many disorders to prevention of further damage. Repetitive or chronic stimuli thus result in cumulative damage until vision is affected.

Retina–Optic Nerve Interaction

Diseases that result in severe and widespread retinal lesions, especially of the ganglion cell layer, eventually also cause lesions of the axons of these cells in the optic nerve—the clinical disorder of *optic atrophy*. Similarly, lesions to the optic nerve fibers (e.g., in chronic optic neuritis) eventually cause death of the ganglion cell body. This is believed to be due to interruptions of *axoplasmic flow*—the flow of solutes along the axon both toward and away from the cell body.

A process of transsynaptic atrophy also takes place across the various layers of the retina. Lesions of the photoreceptors in the outer retina eventually result in damage to the intermediate layers and loss of ganglion cells with optic atrophy. Conversely, although glaucoma is primarily a ganglion cell and optic nerve disease, damage to the outer retina may be observed in chronic cases.

Interactions with Choroid

Because of their proximity, inflammation of the choroid frequently extends to involve the retina, and vice versa. Common examples are hematogenous bacterial and viral infections of the choroid (feline infectious peritonitis [FIP]), bovine malignant catarrhal fever) that extend to the retina, thereby causing *chorioretinitis*. Neurotrophic viral retinitis (e.g., canine distemper) may proceed from retina to choroid, thereby causing *retinochoroiditis*. However, the distinction between retino-choroiditis and chorioretinitis is somewhat semantic, as clinically it is impossible to distinguish between the two. The inflammation invariably results in a breakdown of the blood-ocular barrier and spreads to both the retina and choroid. The consequences of many of these disorders are often much more devastating to the retina than to the tissue from which they arose.

Primary Photoreceptor Disease

Many disorders in the group of "retinal atrophies" primarily affect the photoreceptors. In most cases the disease process begins in the more peripheral retina and in its early stages may be visualized as discoloration of the peripheral tapetum. However, with time the disease progresses to involve the entire retina. As the retina atrophies, it becomes thinner, resulting in increased tapetal reflectivity. If the tapetum and transparent retina are compared to a mirror (tapetum) and curtain (retina), when the curtain is removed (retinal atrophy), reflectivity is increased (Figure 15-28). This increased reflectivity is visible ophthalmoscopically (Figure 15-29; compare it with Figure 15-7, *B*).

The second ophthalmoscopic sign associated with retinal atrophy is gradual vascular attenuation. Vascular attenuation is *secondary* to the atrophy, rather than its cause. Blood supply diminishes as the atrophic retina has fewer metabolic requirements (see Figures 15-29, *B,* and 15-30; compare them with Figure 15-7, *B* and *A,* respectively). The attenuation may be observed as a decrease in both the diameter and number of vessels. Arteries are affected before veins, and small vessels are affected before larger vessels are affected.

Reactions of Pigment Epithelium

Besides its roles in metabolic support and photopigment recycling, the RPE has potential phagocytic activity. Therefore inflammation or infection of the retina is frequently accompanied by a phagocytic reaction of the RPE, with cells undergoing hypertrophy, proliferation, and migration to the diseased area where they phagocytose inflammatory debris. Subsequently, the RPE may also undergo atrophy.

Reactions of pigment epithelium are frequently visible ophthalmoscopically. If atrophy of the pigment epithelium occurs over the tapetum, it is not readily apparent because it is nonpigment (and hence invisible ophthalmoscopically) in this region. However, if it occurs in the nontapetal area, the affected region is visible as a depigmented or pale area, giving the nontapetal fundus a mottled appearance (Figures 15-31 and

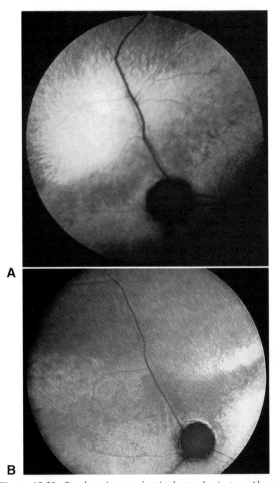

A

B

Figure 15-29. Fundus picture of retinal atrophy in two Abyssinian cats. Compare these pictures with the normal feline fundus in Figure 15-7, *B.* **A,** A moderately advanced case. Note the hyperreflectivity of the tapetal fundus, observed most clearly in the upper midperipheral area. See also Figure 15-47, which shows the histopathologic changes in this retina. **B,** Advanced stage. Note the hyperreflectivity next to the optic disc, and the further attenuation of the blood vessels. (Courtesy Kristina N. Narfström.)

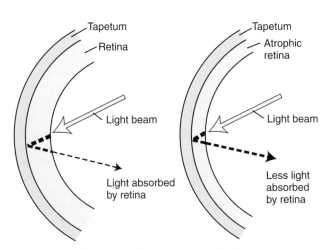

Figure 15-28. Pathogenesis of increased tapetal reflectivity in cases of retinal atrophy. A thinner (atrophied) retina absorbs less light; hence more light reaches the tapetum and is reflected toward the observer.

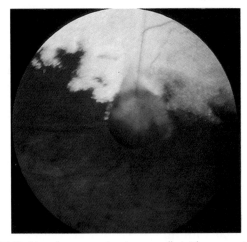

Figure 15-30. Vascular attenuation in a poodle with progressive retinal degeneration. Compare diameter of blood vessels with those seen in Figure 15-7, *A.*

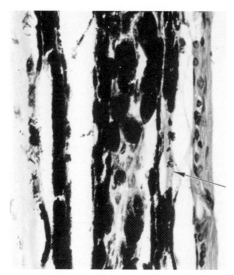

Figure 15-31. Focal loss of pigment *(arrow)* from pigment epithelial cells in the nontapetal area in a dog with progressive retinal degeneration.

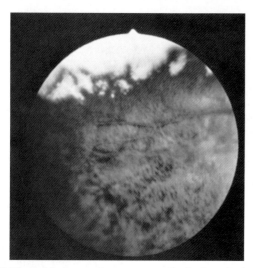

Figure 15-32. Ophthalmoscopic appearance of paler "punched-out" area of depigmentation of the pigment epithelium in the nontapetal fundus in progressive retinal degeneration.

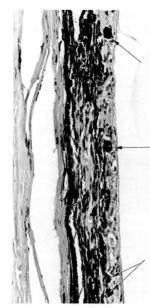

Figure 15-33. Hypertrophy of pigment epithelial cells *(arrows)* and atrophy of the underlying retina as a result of chorioretinitis in a dog.

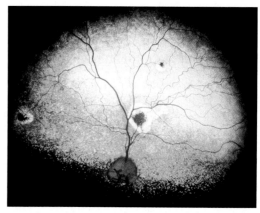

Figure 15-34. Three areas of inactive retinitis in the tapetal dog fundus. In each area, the atrophied retina is visible as a hyperreflective region, the center of which is occupied by a pigment clump. This clump is retinal pigment epithelium that migrated to this region to phagocytose inflammatory debris. (Courtesy University of California, Davis, Veterinary Ophthalmology Service Collection.)

15-32). When proliferation of pigment epithelial cells occurs, with either hyperplasia or hypertrophy, the results are visible ophthalmoscopically as focal areas of increased pigmentation, or pigment clumps. These areas are most readily visible in the tapetal fundus (Figures 15-33 and 15-34). If the primary cause is an inflammation of the retina, the hypertrophy and hyperplasia of pigment epithelial cells are often accompanied by loss of adjacent rods and cones. In such cases, areas of pigment clumping may be surrounded by focal regions of tapetal hyperreflectivity, similar to the hyperreflectivity seen in inherited photoreceptor diseases.

Perivascular Cuffing

In inflammatory and neoplastic diseases, inflammatory cells frequently accumulate around retinal vessels, as they do in any other tissue. However, in the eye, unlike any other organ, this reaction can be visualized in vivo using an ophthalmoscope (Figure 15-35). The vasculitis, or "perivascular cuffing," is visible as a white or gray sheath around vessels that sometimes obscures their color (Figure 15-36).

Retinal Hemorrhages

Hemorrhages into and around the retina occur in many diseases and conditions, such as anemia, coagulopathy, systemic hypertension, hyperviscosity, and systemic infectious diseases such as canine ehrlichiosis and bovine thromboembolic meningoencephalitis (see also Chapter 18). Based on their ophthalmoscopic appearance, it is possible to localize the position of these hemorrhages to the layer involved, that is, subretinal (between the retina and choroid), intraretinal, nerve fiber layer, or preretinal (between the retina and vitreous) (Figure 15-37). The localization helps in identifying the source of the blood because subretinal hemorrhages originate in the choroidal vessels, whereas preretinal hemorrhages originate in the ophthalmoscopically visible vessels of the inner retina.

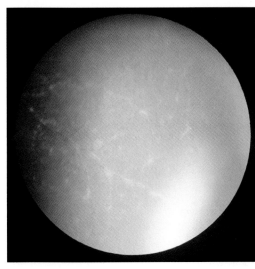

Figure 15-35. Perivascular cuffing of inflammatory cells around retinal vessels in a cat diagnosed with feline infectious peritonitis. (Courtesy University of California, Davis, Veterinary Ophthalmology Service Collection.)

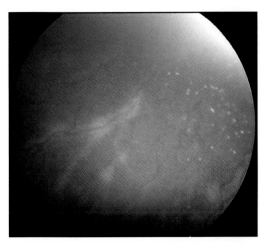

Figure 15-36. Perivascular cuffing forming a gray-white sheath around retina vessels of a dog with systemic mycosis. (Courtesy University of Wisconsin–Madison Veterinary Ophthalmology Service Collection.)

Gliosis

In many acute, severe insults, neural elements of the retina may be lost early, but the more resistant glial Müller's cells survive and may proliferate to fill spaces left by neural cells. The end stage of many chronic retinal disorders is often a glial scar replacing the retina (Figure 15-38).

CONGENITAL RETINAL DISORDERS

Retinal Dysplasia

Primary retinal dysplasia is a congenital, developmental abnormality of the retina. It occurs in all species but is of greatest clinical significance in dogs, being of lesser importance in cats and cattle. It has been defined as an anomalous differentiation, characterized histologically by linear folding of the sensory retina and formation of rosettes containing variable numbers of neuronal retinal cells around a central lumen (Figure 15-39). The most significant forms of canine retinal dysplasia are hereditary, although dysplasia may also be found with maternal viral infections (e.g., canine herpes, feline panleukopenia, ovine blue tongue, bovine viral diarrhea), toxicities in utero, and multiple ocular anomalies. Cases of noninherited retinal dysplasia are frequently accompanied by other developmental neurologic abnormalities, notably cerebellar hypoplasia.

Inherited canine retinal dysplasia occurs most commonly in American cocker spaniels, English springer spaniels, beagles, Labrador retrievers, miniature schnauzers, Australian shepherd dogs, Rottweilers, and Bedlington, Sealyham, and Yorkshire terriers, but it can occur in any breed. It can be subdivided into the following three forms:

- *Focal or multifocal retinal dysplasia:* Retinal folds and rosettes are seen as areas of reduced tapetal reflectivity, as gray streaks in the tapetal area, and as gray or white streaks in the nontapetal area (Figure 15-40). The streaks may be linear or Y- or V-shaped. They are most commonly found in the central fundus, in the tapetal area. Vision is usually normal. This form is seen in spaniels, beagles, Rottweilers, and Labrador retrievers.
- *Geographic retinal dysplasia:* Irregular or U-shaped areas are seen in the tapetal fundus. Elevated and thinned parts of the retina may be present, with gray or black areas delineating the affected retina (Figure 15-41). Areas of hyperreflectivity may also be present. Retinal pigment epithelial hypertrophy may be indicated by areas of increasing pigmentation. Vision may be severely affected, depending on the size of the lesion. The commonly affected breeds include the spaniels and Labrador retriever.
- *Complete retinal dysplasia with detachment:* A completely detached neural retina attached at the optic nerve head is seen. Vitreous dysplasia, leukocoria, rotatory nystagmus, and hemorrhages may be seen in affected animals. Blindness or severe visual impairment is usual. This form is seen in Bedlington and Sealyham terriers, English springer spaniels, and also in Labrador retrievers and Samoyeds when combined with skeletal chondrodysplasia. In the retinal dysplasia with associated chondrodysplasia in Labrador retrievers and Samoyeds, ocular lesions include cataracts, vitreous strands, persistent hyaloid remnants, retinal folds, retinal dysplasia, peripapillary hyperreflectivity, and rhegmatogenous retinal detachments. Skeletal effects include short forelimbs and abnormal morphology of the radius and ulna. The condition is due to one abnormal gene, which has recessive skeletal effects and incompletely dominant ocular effects.

The most common reasons for presentation of animals with inherited retinal dysplasia are blindness and intraocular hemorrhage in puppies, although these occur only in a small proportion of affected dogs. Milder forms of dysplasia and folds may be seen during routine screening programs for hereditary ocular defects in puppies and older dogs. Because the mild forms of the disease have minimal effect on vision, owners will frequently breed them even though the offspring may be affected with severe forms of the disease. Dysplasia is usually transmitted as a simple recessive trait, although dominant inheritance with incomplete penetrance may afflict the Labrador retriever.

Animals with retinal dysplasia should not be bred.

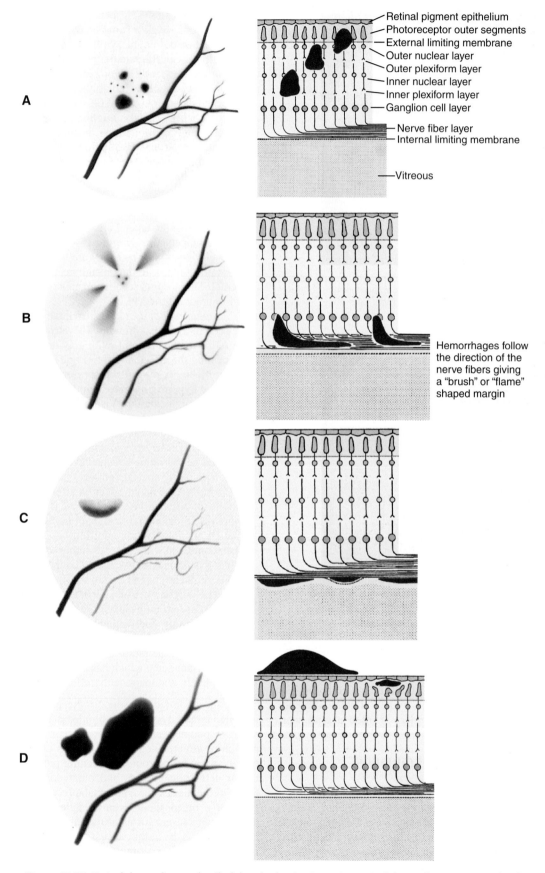

Figure 15-37. Retinal hemorrhages classified by depth. **A,** Deep intraretinal hemorrhage. **B,** Superficial intraretinal hemorrhage. **C,** Preretinal (subvitreal) hemorrhage. **D,** Subretinal hemorrhage, between the retina and choroid.

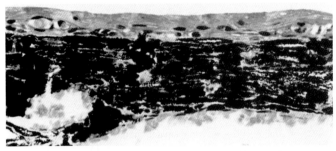

Figure 15-38. Glial band replacing the retina in chronic glaucoma.

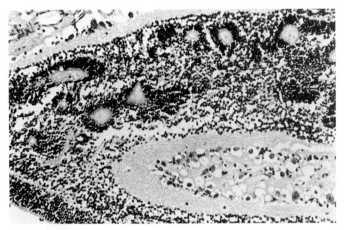

Figure 15-39. Retinal folds and rosettes in a kitten whose dam was affected with panleukopenia during pregnancy. Cerebellar hypoplasia was also present. (Courtesy Drs. G.A. Severin and Julie Gionfriddo, Colorado State University.)

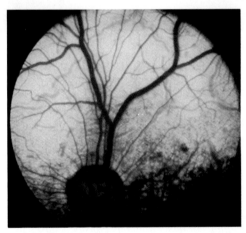

Figure 15-40. Foci of retinal dysplasia in a 7-month-old American cocker spaniel. Areas overlying the tapetum appear as dark streaks, surrounded by a narrow zone of hyperreflectivity. (Courtesy Dr. A. MacMillan.)

Collie Eye Anomaly

Collie eye anomaly (CEA) is an inherited, congenital disorder that affects collies, Shetland sheepdogs, Lancashire heelers, and Australian shepherds. It has also been reported in several non-shepherd breeds, including long-haired whippets and Nova Scotia duck-tolling retrievers. The disease has worldwide distribution, with prevalence of 30% to 85% reported in various countries. Its defining feature is choroidal hypoplasia in the region temporal to the disc. Within this area, focal absence of tapetum and RPE

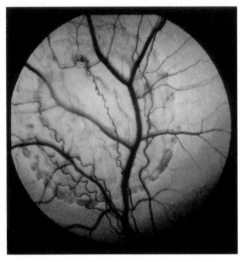

Figure 15-41. Geographic retinal dysplasia in the German shepherd. (From Geographical retinal dysplasia in the dog. American College of Veterinary Ophthalmologists, 1999.)

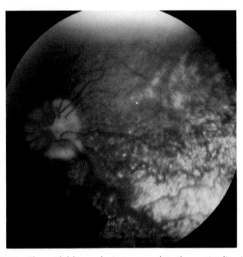

Figure 15-42. Choroidal hypoplasia temporal to the optic disc in a collie with collie eye anomaly. Owing to the hypoplasia, choroidal vessels may be visualized as thick red bands. These vessels are abnormal in number and shape (compare them with the choroidal vessels in Figure 15-27, *A*).

pigment allows visualization of abnormal choroidal blood vessels (Figure 15-42). The vessels appear wider, fewer in number, and irregularly oriented. Up to 35% of CEA cases may also be affected by optic nerve head colobomas (Figure 15-43). A coloboma can be seen as a gray indentation of variable depth in the optic disc and is further described in the following section. Other clinically significant features are intraocular hemorrhages and retinal detachments, which may be partial or complete, although these are far less frequent and occur in less than 10% of affected dogs. Tortuous blood vessels, retinal dysplasia, and microphthalmia may also be present. Dogs with complete retinal detachment are blind, whereas those with optic nerve coloboma or partial detachment have visual deficits. However, choroidal hypoplasia by itself does not cause any visual deficits, leading some breeders to downplay the significance of CEA.

The inheritance mode of CEA is still being studied. Simple autosomal recessive transmission has long been suspected, but recent evidence suggests that the disease is polygenic, thus

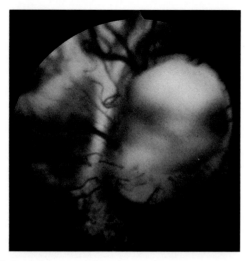

Figure 15-43. Coloboma of the sclera and optic nerve in a collie with collie eye anomaly. Retinal vessels reaching the edge of the disc coloboma disappear from view as they "dive" into the coloboma.

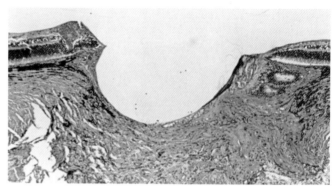

Figure 15-44. Coloboma in a basenji pup with persistent pupillary membrane. Note the retinal rosettes on the right side of the coloboma beneath the retina.

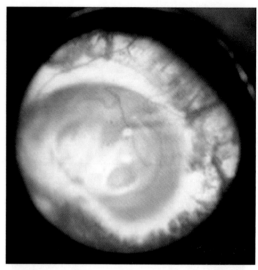

Figure 15-45. Giant coloboma of the optic nerve head in a cat. The patient also suffered from a coloboma (agenesis) in the lateral aspect of both upper eyelids. (Courtesy University of Wisconsin–Madison Veterinary Ophthalmology Service Collection.)

hindering attempts to reduce the prevalence of CEA through selective breeding. Another complicating factor in the control of the disease is the "go normal" phenomenon. In maturing puppies, the characteristic choroidal hypoplasia may be covered by RPE pigment, which masks the underlying lesion (thus making the eye appear to "go normal"). In Norway it has been shown that approximately half the CEA cases may be masked after 3 months of age. Therefore it is recommended that puppies be screened for the disease at 7 to 8 weeks of age. The advent of genetic testing for CEA may help in the control of the disease, although large-scale studies of its accuracy are still lacking.

Coloboma

Colobomas are congenital malformations caused by incomplete closure of the embryonic optic fissure (see Chapter 2). As a result, a section of the uvea, retina, choroid, sclera, and/or optic nerve may be missing. Colobomas of the iris or lens appear as actual notches in these organs. Colobomas of the retina and choroid appear as focal areas of hypopigmentation. Colobomas of the optic nerve appear as gray indentation in the optic disc. Their depth is variable and may be estimated using a direct ophthalmoscope. Blood vessels may be seen disappearing over the coloboma as they "dive" into the pit. Colobomas of the optic nerve are seen in CEA (see Figure 15-43), in basenjis in association with persistent pupillary membranes (Figure 15-44), and in Charolais cattle. Isolated colobomas are uncommon but are seen occasionally in all species (Figure 15-45). Scleral colobomas appear as actual indentation in the wall of the globe.

RETINOPATHY

Retinopathies can be divided into the following four major classes:

- *Inherited dystrophies, dysplasias, degenerations and atrophies:* For example, progressive rod-cone degeneration *(prcd)* in the poodle and American cocker spaniel, rod dysplasia in the Norwegian elkhound, etc. (discussed next)
- *Acquired retinopathies*: These retinopathies are secondary to systemic diseases, such as infectious diseases of the

choroid and/or retina (e.g., canine distemper, fungal disease, FIP) and cardiovascular diseases (e.g., systemic hypertension, anemia, hyperviscosity) (see Acquired Retinopathies in this chapter and Chapter 18).
- *Specific retinopathies:* Atrophy secondary to glaucoma (see Chapter 12), uveodermatologic syndrome (see Chapter 11), and SARD (see later).
- *Retinopathies of miscellaneous causes:* Causes may be nutritional deficiency (e.g., taurine deficiency in cats, hypovitaminosis A in cattle), storage diseases (e.g., ceroid lipofuscinosis in dogs, cats, and sheep, or mannosidosis in Aberdeen Angus cattle and cats), or drug or plant toxicity (e.g., bracken fern poisoning in sheep, oxygen toxicity in premature human infants and in animal models, including kittens and puppies).

Inherited Retinopathies

Historically, all inherited retinopathies were given the collective name *retinal atrophy*. However, this broad definition encompasses a large group of diseases that differ in the age of onset, the breed and cells they primarily affect, mode of inheritance, and genetic and molecular pathogenesis (Table 15-5). The situation is further complicated by the fact that classification and subdivision of retinal disorders in dogs continue to evolve as detailed genetic, electron microscopic, and electroretinographic studies are performed on specific disorders in different breeds. Therefore the list in Table 15-5 should by no means be regarded as final. Based on clinical examinations, many other dog breeds are suspected of being affected by inherited retinopathies, and it is possible that future studies will lead to their inclusion in this list (see the Appendix). Furthermore, inbreeding in existing breeds and "development" of new breeds may cause the disease to appear in additional breeds.

Classification of Inherited Retinopathies

AGE OF ONSET. Broadly speaking, inherited retinopathies can be classified as dysplasia or degenerative. *Rod-cone dysplasia (rcd)* (which *should not be confused* with retinal dysplasia, the abnormal differentiation and folding of the retina described previously in the section on congenital diseases) is defined as atrophy of the photoreceptors that occurs before they have completed their development. Examples of photoreceptor dysplasia are the *rcd type 1* in the Irish setter, *rcd type 2* in the collie, rod dysplasia in the Norwegian elkhound, and *photoreceptor dysplasia* in the miniature schnauzer.

Table 15-5 | **Classification of Inherited Retinopathies**

BREED	CONDITION NAME	SYMBOL	INHERITANCE
EARLY-ONSET DISEASE			
Alaskan malamute	Cone degeneration (hemeralopia)	*cd*	Autosomal recessive
Belgian shepherd	Photoreceptor dysplasia	—	?
Bernese mountain dog	Progressive retinal atrophy	PRA	Autosomal recessive
Briard	Retinal dystrophy	—	Autosomal recessive
Bull mastiff	Canine multifocal retinopathy	CMR	Autosomal recessive
Cardigan Welsh corgi	Rod-cone dysplasia 3	*rcd3*	Autosomal recessive
Collie (rough and smooth)	Rod-cone dysplasia 2	*rcd2*	Autosomal recessive
Coton de Tulear	Canine multifocal retinopathy	CMR	Autosomal recessive
Dachshund (miniature long haired)	Cone-rod degeneration 1	*crd1*	Autosomal recessive
Dachshund (standard wirehaired)	Cone-rod degeneration	*crd*	Autosomal recessive
Douge de Bourdeaux	Canine multifocal retinopathy	CMR	Autosomal recessive
French mastiff	Canine multifocal retinopathy	CMR	Autosomal recessive
German shorthaired pointer	Cone degeneration (hemeralopia)	*cd*	Autosomal recessive
Great Pyrenees	Canine multifocal retinopathy	CMR	Autosomal recessive
Irish setter* (red and white)	Rod-cone dysplasia 1	*rcd1*	Autosomal recessive
Mastiff (old English)	Canine multifocal retinopathy	CMR	Autosomal recessive
Norwegian elkhound	Rod dysplasia	*rd*	Autosomal recessive
	Early rod degeneration	*erd*	Autosomal recessive
Pit bull terrier	Cone-rod degeneration 2	*crd2*	Autosomal recessive
Schnauzer* (miniature)	Type A–progressive retinal atrophy	Type A–PRA	Partially dominant
LATE-ONSET DISEASE			
Akita	Progressive retinal atrophy	PRA	Autosomal recessive
American cocker spaniel	Progressive rod-cone degeneration	*prcd*	Autosomal recessive
American Eskimo	Progressive rod-cone degeneration	*prcd*	Autosomal recessive
Australian cattle dog*	Progressive rod-cone degeneration	*prcd*	Autosomal recessive
Australian shepherd	Progressive rod-cone degeneration	*prcd*	Autosomal recessive
Australian stumpy tail cattle dog*	Progressive rod-cone degeneration	*prcd*	Autosomal recessive
Bull mastiff	Progressive retinal atrophy	PRA	Dominant
Chesapeake Bay retriever	Progressive rod-cone degeneration	*prcd*	Autosomal recessive
Chinese crested*	Progressive rod-cone degeneration	*prcd*	Autosomal recessive
Cockapoo	Progressive rod-cone degeneration	*prcd*	Autosomal recessive
English cocker spaniel	Progressive rod-cone degeneration	*prcd*	Autosomal recessive
Entlebucher mountain dog	Progressive rod-cone degeneration	*prcd*	Autosomal recessive
Finnish Lapphund*	Progressive rod-cone degeneration	*prcd*	Autosomal recessive
Golden retriever	Progressive rod-cone degeneration	*prcd*	Autosomal recessive
Kuvasz	Progressive rod-cone degeneration	*prcd*	Autosomal recessive
Labrador retriever	Progressive rod-cone degeneration	*prcd*	Autosomal recessive
Lapponian herder*	Progressive rod-cone degeneration	*prcd*	Autosomal recessive
Mastiff (old English)	Progressive retinal atrophy	PRA	Dominant
Nova Scotia duck-tolling retriever	Progressive rod-cone degeneration	*prcd*	Autosomal recessive
Papillon	Progressive retinal atrophy	PRA	Autosomal recessive
Poodle* (miniature and toy)	Progressive rod-cone degeneration	*prcd*	Autosomal recessive
Portuguese water dog	Progressive rod-cone degeneration	*prcd*	Autosomal recessive
Samoyed	X-linked progressive retinal atrophy	XLPRA	X-linked
Schapendoe	Progressive retinal atrophy	PRA	Autosomal recessive
Siberian husky	X-linked progressive retinal atrophy	XLPRA	X-linked
Sloughi	Rod-cone degeneration 1a	*rcd1a*	Autosomal recessive
Spanish water dog	Progressive rod-cone degeneration	*prcd*	Autosomal recessive
Swedish Lapphund*	Progressive rod-cone degeneration	*prcd*	Autosomal recessive
Tibetan spaniel	Progressive retinal atrophy	PRA	Autosomal recessive
Tibetan terrier	Progressive retinal atrophy	PRA	Autosomal recessive

*Breed is probably affected by more than one form of inherited retinopathy.

Table 15-6 | **Onset of Ophthalmoscopic, Behavioral, and Electroretinogram (ERG) Signs of Progressive Retinal Degeneration (Atrophy)**

BREED	OPHTHALMOSCOPIC SIGNS	BEHAVIORAL SIGNS	ERG ABNORMALITIES
Irish setter	12-16 wks	6-8 wks	3-6 wks
Collie	12-16 wks	6 wks	2-6 wks
Norwegian elkhound (early rod degeneration)	6-12 mos	6 wks	5-6 wks
Miniature longhaired dachshund	6-12 mos	6 mos	4-9 mos
Tibetan terrier	10-18 mos	6-12 mos	10 mos
Akita	1.5-2.0 yrs	1-3 yrs	1.5-2.0 yrs
Miniature schnauzer	1-2 yrs	6-12 mos	6-8 wks
Siberian husky	1.5-2.0 yrs	2-4 yrs	1 yr
Poodle	3-5 yrs	3-5 yrs	6-9 mos
American cocker spaniel	3-5 yrs	3-5 yrs	9 mos
Portuguese water dog	3-6 yrs	3-5 yrs	1.5 yrs
Labrador retriever	4-6 yrs	3-5 yrs	3 yrs
English cocker spaniel	4-8 yrs	3-5 yrs	12 mos

Modified from Curtis R, et al. (1991): Diseases of the canine posterior segment, in Gelatt KN (editor): Veterinary Ophthalmology, 2nd ed. Lea & Febiger, Philadelphia.

Degenerative retinopathy, on the other hand, is defined as an inherited atrophy of the photoreceptor that takes place after the cells have completed their development. Therefore it is a late-onset disease, although the age of onset may vary greatly among breeds. For example, *cone-rod degeneration (crd)* may be diagnosed by age 4 to 6 months in the miniature longhaired dachshund, and *early retinal degeneration (erd)* may be observed before 1 year of age in the Norwegian elkhound (Table 15-6). On the other hand, *progressive rod-cone degeneration (prcd),* which is probably the most common form of inherited retinal degeneration, is typically diagnosed in dogs older than 3 years, although it may also be diagnosed in elderly dogs. The disease affects at least 20 breeds, including popular breeds such as the toy and miniature poodles, Labrador retriever, and American and English cocker spaniels.

AFFECTED CELLS. Inherited retinopathies may initially affect the rods, cones, or RPE. The name of the disease is commonly indicative of the cell that is primarily affected. Thus in both *rcd* and *prcd* the disease process initially involves the rods and then spreads to the cones. Cone degeneration *(cd)* in the Alaskan malamute and German shorthaired pointer is a nonprogressive disease that affects only the cones, whereas *crd* in the dachshund and pit bull terrier spreads from cones to rods. RPE dystrophy (RPED) is a disease that affects primarily the RPE.

MODE OF INHERITANCE. The great majority of the inherited retinopathies are autosomal recessive diseases, with some exceptions. RPED may be a dominant disease with variable penetrance in the Labrador retriever. PRA is inherited as a dominant disease in the mastiff and the bullmastiff, and it is X-linked in the Siberian husky and Samoyed. Sometimes the same breed may be afflicted with two different forms of the disease. The Abyssinian cat, for example, is afflicted with both early-onset *rcd,* which is inherited as an autosomal dominant disease, and a late-onset rod-cone degeneration, which is inherited as an autosomal recessive disease.

GENETIC AND MOLECULAR PATHOGENESIS. The list of breeds in which retinal atrophy is suspected to be a hereditary disease is very long (see the Appendix). During the last decade the genetic, molecular, and biochemical abnormalities that cause inherited retinopathies have been the subject of intensive research in scores of dog breeds. Obviously, the great variation in the phenotypic appearance of inherited retinopathies reflects a wide variety in the genotype of the disease. At least seven forms of PRA have been identified, based on the mutated gene or the mutation locus. Thus, for example, *rcd1* in the Irish setter and *rcd2* in the collie present with similar clinical, ERG, and histopathologic findings, but they differ as to which gene is mutated. Mating of affected dogs from the two breeds therefore produces normal offspring that are carriers of both diseases. Generally speaking, however, all of the inherited rod-cone retinopathies are caused by mutations in one of the enzymes responsible for the phototransduction process. The mutation causes disruption of the biochemical cascade that takes place in the outer segment of the photoreceptor. The disruption results in accumulation of one of the substrates (e.g., a mutation in cGMP phosphodiesterase causes elevation of cGMP), eventually leading to cell death.

Clinical Signs

A comprehensive discussion of the clinical signs associated with each form of inherited retinopathy is beyond the scope of this book. As noted previously, one of the largest variables is the age at which clinical signs appear. However, regardless of the age of onset or the exact genetic mutation and mode of inheritance, most inherited retinopathies (with some notable exceptions, such as *cd* and RPED, which are discussed later under Specific Forms of Inherited Retinopathy) give rise to similar clinical signs, as listed here. The disease *invariably* affects both eyes.

PROGRESSIVE LOSS OF VISION. Early stages of inherited retinopathy are characterized by loss of night vision *(nyctalopia)* due to early degeneration or dysplasia of rods (Figures 15-46 and 15-47). Affected animals often have difficulty seeing moving objects. As the disease progresses cones are also affected and day vision is also lost, making the animal blind. At the time of the initial diagnosis it is difficult to estimate how long it will take for the dog to become totally blind. Patients frequently have severe visual defects before any change is noticed by the owner, which often happens when the dog is taken out of its familiar environment—for example, on vacation or for grooming or boarding. Therefore owners complaining of "acute vision loss" should be carefully questioned about events surrounding the onset of blindness. Further inquiries may sometimes disclose that the loss of vision is associated with a change in the dog's surroundings, and ophthalmoscopic examination will reveal signs of long-standing, progressive disease. On the other hand, many owners will have noticed the gradual progression from

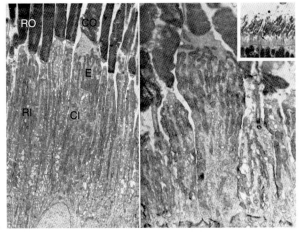

A **B**

Figure 15-46. **A,** Electron microscope image of the photoreceptor layer of a 60-day-old normal dog's eye. Rod and cone inner segments *(RI* and *CI,* respectively) are approximately the same length, although cones are broader and have a very distinct mitochondria-rich ellipsoid region *(E)* near the apex. The outer segments of rods *(RO)* and cones *(CO)* contain parallel membranous discs in a "coin stack" configuration. **B,** Photoreceptor layer from a 12-week-old Norwegian elkhound with rod dysplasia. Cone inner and outer segments are normal, but rod inner segments are small, and outer segments are disorganized and disoriented. (From Aguirre GD [1978]: Retinal degenerations in the dog. I: rod dysplasia. Exp Eye Res 26:233.)

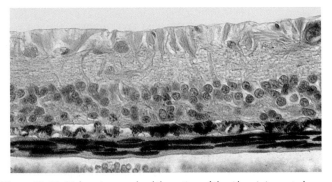

Figure 15-47. Light micrograph of the retina of the Abyssinian cat shown in Figure 15-29, *A.* Note the severe atrophy of the outer retina with only some sparse nuclei remaining of the photoreceptor cells, whereas the inner retina appears normal. Compare it with the anatomy of a normal retina, shown in Figure 15-2, *B.* (Hematoxylin & eosin stain.) (Courtesy Kristina N. Narfström.)

nyctalopia to total blindness. Owners should be carefully questioned (without being "led") about whether blindness was preceded by preferential loss of night vision.

Early loss of night vision is due to rod degeneration.

TAPETAL HYPERREFLECTIVITY. As the retina thins it absorbs less light and more light is reflected back to the observer. The granular appearance of the tapetum changes to a homogeneous sheen (see Figures 15-28 and 15-29).

PUPILS. As a result of the disease, the pupils are more mydriatic than usual, and their reaction to light is slower. However, except in the most severe cases, some degree of PLR will be present. Therefore presence of PLR should *not* be used to rule out PRA. If the tapetal hyperreflectivity is severe, it may be observed through the dilated pupil, although in most cases ophthalmoscopy is required to appreciate increased reflectivity.

RETINAL BLOOD VESSELS. The disease is characterized by progressive attenuation and thinning of retinal blood vessels. Arterioles are the first to be affected, and their appearance (at the disc margin) should be carefully examined. As the disease progresses the arteries decrease in number and the large veins become noticeably thinner (compare Figure 15-29, *B,* with Figure 15-7, *B;* and Figure 15-30 with Figure 15-7, *A*).

OPTIC DISC. The optic disc becomes pale dark brown owing to loss of capillaries on its surface and demyelination and atrophy of the nerve fibers caused by extensive degeneration of the retina (compare Figure 15-30 with Figure 15-7, *A*).

NONTAPETAL FUNDUS. Focal depigmented areas in the nontapetal fundus are seen relatively early and may enlarge to affect the entire nontapetal fundus (see Figure 15-32).

CATARACTS. Many dogs suffer from both cataracts and inherited retinopathy. The cataracts appear as radial, spokelike opacities from the equator to the center of the lens. They usually progress to maturity and are easily noticed by the owners. Because the two diseases are frequently diagnosed in the same animal, *every* patient with cataract must be screened electroretinographically before cataract surgery to determine whether its retina is functional. There is still considerable debate about whether such cases represent two separate diseases or whether the cataracts are secondary to release of toxic substances from the degenerating retina. Regardless of this debate, if inherited retinopathy is diagnosed, surgical removal of the cataract is contraindicated because it will not restore vision. An exception to this rule is the removal of an anteriorly luxated cataractous lens, which should be removed to avoid the complications discussed in Chapter 13.

Additional Diagnostic Testing

Electroretinography is a useful, noninvasive tool to assess photoreceptor function (see previous section, and Figures 15-16 through 15-21). Stimulus parameters such as light intensity and wavelength, dark adaptation, and FFF can be used to separate rod and cone function, thereby diagnosing various forms of inherited retinopathies or different stages of the disease (see Tables 15-4 and 15-6). The test is particularly important in cases of inherited retinopathies for the following reasons:

- In most dog breeds, ERG abnormalities may be detected long before the onset of behavioral signs (i.e., nyctalopia) and funduscopic abnormalities (see Table 15-6). The ERG may provide a very early diagnostic tool and is therefore particularly useful to breeders who want to begin breeding their dogs as soon as possible.
- In some inherited retinopathies, such as *cd* in the Alaskan malamute and German shorthaired pointer or CSNB in the collie dog and appaloosa horse, the animal presents with a normal-looking fundus. A definitive diagnosis can be made only with the ERG.
- As noted, electroretinography must be performed on every dog that is a candidate for cataract surgery to rule out concurrent inherited retinopathy.

With the advances in the genetics of inherited retinopathies, commercial companies now offer DNA testing for various forms of inherited retinopathies in more than 30 dog breeds. These tests have several important advantages, including the fact that they can be conducted on an animal of any age, and their ability to detect carriers (who are heterozygous for the mutated gene). This means breeders can avoid breeding two carrier dogs that are phenotipically normal but that will give birth to affected dogs. Most importantly, a DNA test that has identified the actual mutation is 100% accurate. In this context, however, it is important to note that in a number of diseases the companies test not for the actual gene but for a genetic marker of the disease. Such tests contain an unknown margin of error. Furthermore, some breeds (e.g., toy and miniature poodles) may be affected by more than one genetic form of the disease (see Table 15-5). Therefore a test targeting one form of the disease will not diagnose its other forms, in contrast to electroretinography or clinical examination, which are genetically insensitive.

Treatment

Currently there is no treatment for inherited retinopathy. Owners should be educated about the progressive nature of the disease and the inevitable blindness. Despite the initial dismay of many owners at the news that their pets are (or will become) irreversibly blind, they should be counseled that the disease is not painful and is not associated with any ocular or systemic complications. Therefore the pets can continue living happy lives while owners take the necessary precautions of living with blind animals. Websites such as www.blinddogs.com offer valuable advice to owners of such dogs.

Currently, there is no treatment for retinal dystrophy.

Although there is no treatment for inherited retinopathy, steps can be taken to decrease its prevalence. Owners of affected dogs should be made aware of the hereditary nature of the disease. They should be encouraged to neuter affected animals and should be strongly cautioned against mating them with dogs of the same breed. Another important element in preventing the spread of the disease is screening programs for inherited eye diseases. The screening, which is conducted by board-certified specialists, is mandated by many kennel clubs and encouraged by others. Results are kept in a central registry. Owners of purebred dogs of susceptible breeds should be encouraged to breed their dogs only with animals that were screened for inherited eye disease.

Humans also suffer from inherited retinopathies, some of which are very similar to the canine forms of the disease.

Intensive research is under way to restore vision to humans blinded by retinal dystrophies, with experimental studies conducted using gene therapy, retinal transplantation, stem cell therapy, neuroprotective treatments, nutritional supplementation, and even retinal prostheses. Indeed, some of the research has been conducted in dogs and cats suffering from hereditary retinal dystrophies, several of which regained long-term vision following experimental treatments. Even though these animals are sometimes just an experimental model and not the intended beneficiaries of the research, it is to be hoped that, if effective therapy is found for humans suffering from inherited retinopathy, it can also be used in canine and feline patients.

Specific Forms of Inherited Retinopathy

HEMERALOPIA. The Alaskan malamute and German shorthaired pointer are affected by a cone disorder that causes day blindness. The age at onset of clinical signs is at 8 to 10 weeks, but the disease is nonprogressive and night vision is not affected. Ophthalmoscopic examination reveals no funduscopic abnormalities, but an ERG will show lack of cone function. Dachshunds and pit bull terriers are affected by *crd*. This means that the disease starts as hemeralopia due to cone damage in the initial stages. However, unlike *cd* in the Alaskan malamute and the German shorthaired pointer, eventually rod function is also affected, and funduscopic abnormalities may be seen.

RETINAL PIGMENT EPITHELIUM DYSTROPHY. Retinal pigment epithelium dystrophy (RPED), which has been described in a number of breeds, was formerly called central PRA. The name was altered when it became clear that unlike in PRA, the primary problem in RPED is not in the photoreceptors. Rather, as the new name indicates, the disease affects the RPE, with the photoreceptors undergoing secondary atrophy as a result of losing the metabolic support of the RPE. The disease probably has both a genetic component, because it is more prevalent in some breeds, and a nutritional basis, in that low levels of vitamin E have been associated with its pathogenesis. Hypercholesterolemia and neurologic deficits have also been noted in some affected dogs.

Clinical features of *prcd* and RPED are compared in Table 15-7. Initial behavioral signs, which are compatible with central retinal dysfunction, include diminished daytime vision and poor perception of nearby or stationary objects. Peripheral

Table 15-7 | **Comparison of Clinical Features of Progressive Rod-Cone Degeneration (PRCD) and Retinal Pigment Epithelial Dystrophy (RPED)**

FEATURE	PRCD	RPED
Effect on vision:		
Night vision	Affected in early stages	Affected in advanced stages
Day vision	Affected in advanced stages	Affected in early stages
Peripheral vision	Affected in early stages	Affected in advanced stages
Central vision	Affected in advanced stages	Affected in early stages
Detecting motion	Affected in early stages	Affected in advanced stages
Detecting stationary objects	Affected in advanced stages	Affected in early stages
Blindness	Inevitable	Rare
Pupillary reflex	Diminished in advanced stages	Diminished in advanced stages
Retinal vessels	Arterioles attenuated in early stages	Normal until late in course
	Veins attenuated in advanced stages	
Tapetal fundus	Hyperreflectivity	Multifocal clumps of brown pigment, with some hyperreflectivity later
Optic disc	Pale as disease progresses	Normal until very late in course
Nontapetal fundus	Focal depigmentation and mottling later	No significant changes until very advanced stages
Electroretinography	Useful in diagnosis	No use in diagnosis as changes are seen in advanced stages

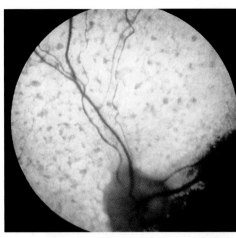

Figure 15-48. Retinal pigment epithelium dystrophy (RPED) in a dog. The brown spots represent accumulation of lipofuscin material in the RPE, impairing its function and eventually affecting vision.

vision and perception of distant and moving objects are retained until advanced stages of the disease. Ophthalmoscopically, focal areas of brown pigmentation are present in the central fundus overlying the tapetum (Figure 15-48). These represent accumulation of lipofuscin in the RPE, possibly due to anti-oxidant (vitamin E) deficiency. The size and shape of affected areas vary. With time, tapetal hyperreflectivity occurs between coalescing pigment spots. Late in the disease the fundus resembles that of end stage *prcd* as the optic disc may become pale, the vessels attenuated, and the nontapetal fundus pale and gray-brown. The ERG is often normal until late in the disease and is not used for early diagnosis.

CONGENITAL STATIONARY NIGHT BLINDNESS. This is an inherited, congenital disease affecting horses (particularly appaloosas) and dogs (particularly collies). As the name implies, affected animals are night blind, but the disease does not progress to affect day vision. Ophthalmoscopic examination shows no funduscopic abnormalities, but an ERG examination demonstrates impaired midretinal (bipolar cell) activity.

CANINE MULTIFOCAL RETINOPATHY (CMR). This disease was first reported in 1998 in Great Pyrenees in Canada but has since been reported in additional breeds, including mastiffs, bull mastiffs, Dogue de Bordeaux, and Coton de Tulear. This is an early onset disease, usually affecting dogs 3 to 6 months of age. Puppies are presented with acute, multifocal, serous retinal and RPE detachments. The lesions are circular and gray-tan. They may regress, remain, or progress into areas of multifocal retinal degeneration, but changes usually are not seen beyond 1 year of age. It is suspected that the detachments are due to secretion and absorption defects in the RPE, and therefore the disease may be regarded as a form of RPE dysplasia.

RETINAL DYSTROPHY IN BRIARDS. Affected dogs are congenitally night blind. However, unlike CSNB, the disease is progressive and day vision is impaired in advanced cases, and funduscopic changes may be seen. The disease is probably due to RPE abnormalities and therefore was initially confused with RPED, although the clinical presentation of the two differs.

INHERITED RETINAL DEGENERATIONS IN CATS. Inherited retinopathies are rarely reported in the cat. Abyssinians seem to be susceptible, with two forms of inherited diseases reported. Rod-cone dysplasia is a dominant disease. Signs of retinal degeneration are evident ophthalmoscopically at 8 to 12 weeks

and are preceded by mydriasis, nystagmus, and impairment of the PLR. The disease progresses rapidly, and by 1 year of age signs compatible with advanced canine *prcd* are observed. Rod-cone degeneration is a recessive disease of later onset in the Abyssinian, with signs beginning at 1.5 to 2.0 years of age, progressing to complete atrophy by 4 to 6 years of age. Ophthalmoscopic and clinical signs in cats are similar to those in dogs, although cataracts occur infrequently (thus casting doubts on the hypothesis suggesting a role for *prcd* in the genesis of canine cataracts). Once again, affected Abyssinian kittens can be diagnosed with electroretinography earlier than with ophthalmoscopy (see Figures 15-19 and 15-20).

Acquired Retinopathies

Acquired retinopathies are almost invariably ocular manifestations of systemic diseases and are therefore discussed in detail in Chapter 18. Only the general principles and clinical signs are discussed in this section.

Retinopathy Secondary to Cardiovascular Diseases

The eye is a unique organ in that it allows the clinician, using an ophthalmoscope, to visualize blood vessels in vivo. Therefore disorders affecting systemic blood flow can be readily diagnosed in the retina with noninvasive methods. Ophthalmoscopy can be used to detect changes in the diameter of blood vessels (which may be thinner or engorged), the tortuosity of the vessels, and the color of the blood flow (which may change in anemia, hyperlipidemia, polycythemia, and other diseases). Hemorrhages, which may be preretinal, intraretinal, or subretinal in location, can also be observed (see Figure 15-37). These are usually associated with either clotting disorders (e.g., thrombocytopenia, coagulopathies) or systemic hypertension (Figure 15-49). The latter is frequently secondary to renal disease and is more common in the cat than in the dog. Severe subretinal hemorrhage may also lead to retinal detachment (see later). In many cases, the bleeding is not restricted to the retina, and vitreal hemorrhage and/or hyphema may also be observed.

It is important to note, however, that with rare exceptions, these hemorrhages are *invariably* caused by vascular and/or cardiac diseases. Therefore changes in retinal vasculature should be regarded as ophthalmic manifestations of systemic diseases rather than a primary ophthalmic problem—despite the fact that in some cases, notably retinal detachment or severe hyphema, the animal may be presented with an ocular complaint. Thus, detection of retinal hemorrhage, changes in retinal blood vessels, and so on, should direct the clinician to perform further diagnostic evaluation, such as measurement of blood pressure, complete blood counts, serum biochemistry, and clotting profiles. Similarly, treatment should be aimed at the primary cause; ocular treatment is not required except in cases of hemorrhage, for which symptomatic treatment is provided. The various cardiac and vascular diseases that may affect the eye are discussed in detail in Chapter 18.

Retinopathy Secondary to Infectious/Inflammatory Diseases

Because of the close proximity of the retina and the choroid, the retina rarely shows isolated inflammation; the choroid is usually involved as well. In fact, in a majority of cases the

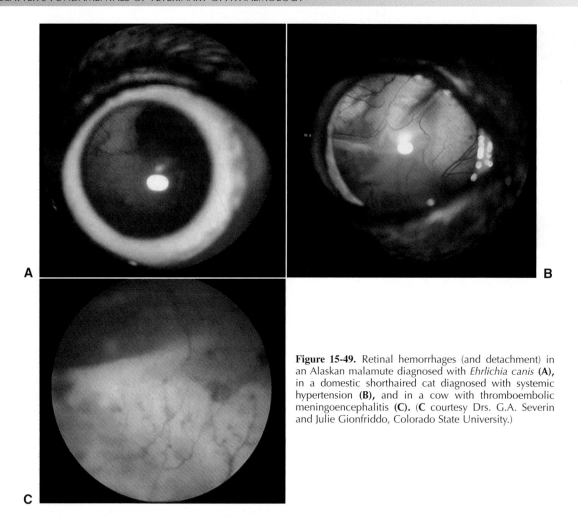

Figure 15-49. Retinal hemorrhages (and detachment) in an Alaskan malamute diagnosed with *Ehrlichia canis* **(A)**, in a domestic shorthaired cat diagnosed with systemic hypertension **(B)**, and in a cow with thromboembolic meningoencephalitis **(C)**. (**C** courtesy Drs. G.A. Severin and Julie Gionfriddo, Colorado State University.)

primary ocular manifestation of the disease is an inflammation of the choroid—choroiditis or posterior uveitis. As a result of the breakdown of the blood-retinal barrier, the inflammation spreads from the choroid to the retina, resulting in *chorioretinitis*. In rare cases, notably canine distemper and *Neospora caninum* infection, the primary infection is in the retina, with the choroid being secondarily affected (i.e., *retinochoroiditis*).

Clinically, however, it is impossible to distinguish between ophthalmic signs of retinochoroiditis and chorioretinitis. Rather, signs of posterior segment inflammation are classified as being either *active* or *inactive*. Distinguishing clinical signs of the two stages are described here.

ACTIVE RETINITIS (Figure 15-50). Clinical signs of active retinitis are similar to those of inflammation in any other organ. Edema, exudate, and cellular infiltration may be seen as white or blurry sheaths around retinal blood vessels (see Figures 15-35 and 15-36). In affected areas, the retina appears dull. This appearance is more easily observed in the tapetal region, as the edema and infiltration reduce tapetal reflectivity. The borders of the inflamed areas are indistinct. Massive cellular infiltration may lead to the formation of granulomas, which may be seen as focal white or gray spots in both the tapetum and nontapetum. The inflammation may also spread to the adjacent vitreous, causing it to appear hazy.

Active retinitis may also be accompanied by retinal hemorrhage, the appearance of which depends on its depth within the retina (see Figures 15-37 and 15-49). Significant

subretinal hemorrhage or exudation may cause retinal detachment. A retina that underwent total detachment may be seen through the pupil (without an ophthalmoscope) as a large "curtain" with blood vessels located behind the lens (see Figure 15-49). The curtain will be transparent, white, or bloody, depending on the fluid (serous, exudative, or hemorrhagic, respectively) that caused the detachment, and the eye will be blind. Partial retinal detachments may also occur but may be harder to detect and cause only partial loss of vision in the eye.

The retinitis may frequently be accompanied by anterior uveitis and its associated clinical signs. Secondary complications of the uveitis, such as synechia or glaucoma, may also be observed.

As was noted previously for the cardiac and vascular diseases, these signs of posterior segment inflammation should not be regarded as a primary problem but rather as ocular manifestations of a systemic disease. Therefore systemic diagnostic evaluation is warranted. In the case of chorioretinitis the primary cause of the inflammation is usually an infectious agent. Therefore complete blood counts, serologic evaluation, and other diagnostic tests (e.g., urinalysis, radiography) should be undertaken. If a diagnosis is not reached through systemic workup, the anterior chamber (or vitreous) may be tapped and a sample of fluid submitted to cytologic or serologic evaluation.

However, it is important to note that in cases of infective retinitis the primary infectious agent does not always enter the

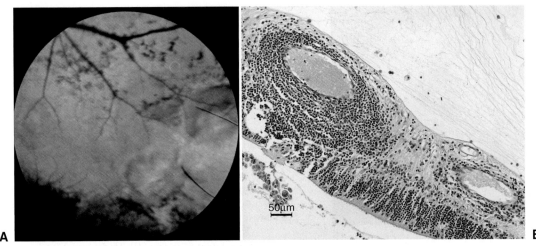

Figure 15-50. A, Peripheral retina of a cow with active retinitis. Pigmentation is evident dorsally, with several areas of active retinitis surrounded by pale edema and cellular infiltration. A hyperreflective margin *(yellow)* is present around the upper lesion. **B,** Histopathology micrograph showing a case of chronic retinitis in a dog. Note the extensive perivascular infiltration by lymphocytes and plasma cells. Retinal detachment also occurred. (Hematoxylin & eosin stain.) (**A** courtesy Dr. L. Klein; **B** courtesy Dr. Emmanuel Loeb.)

eye. Although some organisms (e.g., fungal agents) may enter the eye, others (e.g., *Ehrlichia canis*) do not. In these cases, the choroid and retina are not infected. Rather, they are inflamed owing to the presence of sensitized immunocytes and antibodies. Consequently, unless contraindicated by the systemic (or ocular) condition of the patient, the treatment of the primary cause should be augmented with systemic and topical anti-inflammatory drugs as well as mydriatic agents to treat the inflammation of the posterior segment of the eye.

INACTIVE RETINITIS. Following the inflammation, affected areas of the retina undergo atrophy. In the tapetal region, the atrophy may be seen as distinct foci of hyperreflectivity with well-defined borders alongside areas of normal retina (see Figures 15-28 and 15-34). In the nontapetal region, pale, light brown areas of depigmentation may be seen (see Figure 15-32, which is of similar clinical appearance, although the cause is different). Retinal vessels decrease in size and number in affected areas (see Figures 15-29, *B,* and 15-30, which are of similar clinical appearance, although the cause is different). On occasion, sclerotic choroidal vessels appear as radiating thin white lines through a depigmented retina and choroid.

Because the RPE has a phagocytic role during inflammation, it undergoes hypertrophy, hyperplasia, and migration. Following the inflammation, multifocal clumps of RPE may be seen in both the tapetum and nontapetum, usually within the areas of the atrophied retina (see Figures 15-33 and 15-34).

Specific Retinopathies

Glaucomatous Retinopathy

See Chapter 12.

Uveodermatologic Syndrome

See Chapter 11.

Sudden Acquired Retinal Degeneration

SARD is a disease that has been reported only in dogs. As the name implies, it is a retinal degeneration of sudden onset.

Numerous apoptotic nuclei have been recorded in the outer nuclear layer of the diseased retinas, with both cones and rods affected. The typical presentation is of acute blindness, with dilated, nonresponsive pupils. Initially the fundus looks normal, although ophthalmoscopic signs of progressive retinal degeneration may appear over the next few months. Because an animal with retrobulbar optic neuritis may also be presented with similar signs of acute blindness, dilated and nonresponsive pupils, and a normal-looking fundus, the ERG is particularly useful in distinguishing between the two diseases. The signal is normal in optic neuritis but extinguished in SARD.

Although SARD is defined as an acquired disease, intensive research has not succeeded in identifying the primary cause. For many years, the most commonly accepted theory was that SARD is the result of an endocrinologic disorder. The disease is most common in middle-aged adult dogs, especially obese, spayed females, and may be more common in winter. A history of recent polyuria, polydypsia, weight gain, and lethargy is typical. A significant percentage of patients have a blood profile suggestive of hyperadrenocorticism, with lymphopenia, elevated alkaline phosphatase, hypercholesterolemia, and an abnormal adrenocorticotropic hormone stimulation test result. Recently, however, other causes have been proposed for SARD, including autoimmune inflammation (resulting from production of anti-retinal antibodies) and toxicity. Unfortunately, because the primary cause has yet to be identified, there is currently no treatment for SARD, and the blindness is irreversible.

Miscellaneous Causes of Retinopathy

Nutritional Causes

FELINE CENTRAL RETINAL DEGENERATION. Taurine is an essential amino acid for cats, which lack the enzyme cysteine sulfinic acid decarboxylase needed to synthesize taurine. Therefore felines depend on dietary intake to meet their taurine requirements, and a deficiency in taurine may lead to progressive retinal degeneration as well as dilated cardiomyopathy. The initial lesion a small, rounded lesion temporal to and slightly above the disc in the *area centralis*. Because of its location, the syndrome has been called feline central retinal

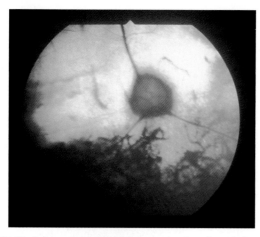

Figure 15-51. Feline central retinal degeneration in a cheetah that was fed a taurine-deficient diet. The hyperreflective band around the disc is characteristic of the disease.

degeneration (FCRD). The lesion becomes progressively ellipsoid, extending in a band from the temporal fundus across the top of the optic disc to the nasal fundus (Figure 15-51). The area within the lesion is hyperreflective. ERG has shown initial cone dysfunction starting in the *area centralis,* with rod function affected in later stages of the disease, and the animal is irreversibly blind. Administration of taurine may prevent further lesions from developing and will reverse the cardiomyopathy but has not been proved to restore vision that has been lost.

The prevalence of FCRD has been dramatically reduced after recognition of the role of taurine in its pathogenesis, because the amino acid is now added to commercial cat diets. FCRD may still be observed in cats that are fed commercial dog diets, although some manufacturers add taurine to canine diets to prevent this complication. FRCD has also been reported in captive feline wildlife species, including tigers and cheetahs, that were fed inadequate diets. Therefore the diets of all felines that do not eat commercial cat food should be supplemented with taurine. The amino acid can be supplemented in solution, powder, or tablet form, with a suggested dose of 400 ppm daily.

Cats should not be fed commercial dog food.

Feline cardiomyopathy patients should undergo ophthalmoscopic examination to detect retinopathy due to taurine deficiency.

HYPOVITAMINOSIS A. Vitamin A deficiency has been demonstrated to cause vision impairment in a number of species. The visual deficits occur via two different pathophysiologic mechanisms. First, because vitamin A (retinol) is a component of rhodopsin, the visual photopigment of rods, hypovitaminosis A causes impaired rod function. This impairment is expressed behaviorally as nyctalopia (night blindness). If the deficiency is chronic, progressive retinal degeneration and complete blindness may occur. The condition has been reported in young horses, cattle, and pigs. In cattle, nyctalopia is an important sign of hypovitaminosis A. In addition, poor reproductive efficiency, skin and central nervous system (CNS) lesions, and conjunctivitis are encountered. Plasma levels of vitamin A fall

only after depletion of hepatic reserves. Diagnosis can be made if liver vitamin A levels are less than 2.0 µg/g of liver or if plasma vitamin A levels fall below 20 µg/dL. Steers have been reported more susceptible to vitamin A deficiency than heifers. In pigs, deficiency in pregnant sows causes microphthalmia and blind piglets. Deficiency in adults can also cause nyctalopia late in the disease.

Hypovitaminosis A also causes abnormal thickening of growing bones, including those of the skull and around the optic canal, leading to compression of the optic nerve. Fundic examination reveals pale tapetum, papilledema, indistinct disc margins and tortuous retinal blood vessels. Retinal detachment, subretinal hemorrhages, and optic nerve ischemia may also occur. The condition has recently been reported in lions but is most commonly seen in calves.

Ocular signs of hypovitaminosis A are given in Box 15-1 and are depicted in Figures 15-52 and 15-53.

Storage Diseases

The large group of storage diseases is characterized by accumulation of metabolic substrates within cells. They are rare genetic disorders, in which an enzyme deficiency causes accumulation of that enzyme's substrate within neurons and glial cells as well as in other cells in the body. Accumulation in the retina causes blindness and has been reported to occur in mucopolysaccharidosis, neuronal ceroid lipofuscinosis, and gangliosidosis. In some storage diseases retinal lesions are present and are of diagnostic value. Blindness and other neuroophthalmic signs may also be the result of storage diseases affecting the postretinal visual pathways and other parts of the CNS.

Storage diseases have been reported in various breeds of dogs, cats, cattle, pigs, and sheep but not in horses. Animals usually are normal at birth but show the first clinical signs of CNS dysfunction early in life. The diseases are slowly progressive and result in the death of the affected animal. Therefore storage diseases should be considered among the differential diagnoses in cases of neonatal death or in young animals presented with nonspecific neurologic signs (e.g., ataxia, seizures), especially in purebred patients. Definitive

Box 15-1	**Ocular signs of hypovitaminosis A in cattle**

Apparent exophthalmia
Epiphora
Reduced corneal sensitivity
Nystagmus
Papilledema—in calves may be due to constriction of optic nerve by bone malformation; in calves and adults due to malasborption of cerebrospinal fluid
Retinal venous congestion
Focal superficial retinal and papillary hemorrhages
Subretinal hemorrhages and retinal detachment
Tapetal pallor
Fixed, dialted pupils
Optic atrophy
Retinal degeneration (both outer and inner retina)
Nyctalopia—night blindness may be responsive to treatment
Complete blindness—nonresponsive to treatment

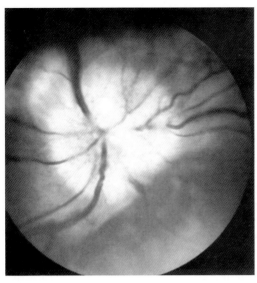

Figure 15-52. Papilledema and pigment disruption in the nontapetal region of a blind steer with vitamin A deficiency. (From Divers TJ, et al. [1986]: Blindness and convulsion associated with vitamin A deficiency in feedlot steers. J Am Vet Med Assoc 189:1579.)

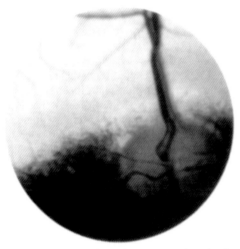

Figure 15-53. Optic atrophy with a pale gray optic disc after longstanding vitamin A deficiency in a calf. (From Rubin LF [1974]: Atlas of Veterinary Ophthalmoscopy. Lea & Febiger, Philadelphia.)

diagnosis can be made, depending on the disease process, by demonstration of either deficient enzyme activity or substrate accumulation.

Drug and Plant Toxicities

Numerous plants and chemical agents induce retinopathy in different species. However, many of these agents are experimental and only those of immediate clinical interest are discussed here.

PLANT POISONINGS IN FOOD ANIMALS. Ingestion of various plants was shown to cause blindness in grazing cattle and sheep:

- "Bright blindness" has been reported in cattle and sheep in the United Kingdom due to long-term ingestion of bracken fern *(Pteris aquilina)*. This disease causes dilated pupils,

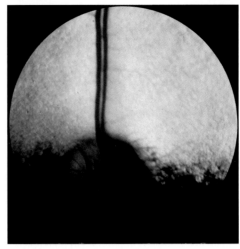

Figure 15-54. Bright blindness in a sheep. Note increased tapetal reflectivity and vascular attenuation. Compare with normal ovine fundus in Figure 15-7, C. (Courtesy Keith C. Barnett.)

depressed PLRs, tapetal hyperreflectivity (Figure 15-54), pale optic disc, and narrowing of retinal blood vessels. Outer retinal layers are destroyed, and inner layers are spared.

- "Blindgrass" *(Stypandra* sp.) toxicity occurs in Western Australia and affects sheep and goats. Most animals are affected with posterior paresis and some die, but survivors become blinded by lesions in the photoreceptor layer, optic nerve, and optic tracts.
- Male fern *(Dryopteris filix mas)* causes demyelination of the optic nerve. Blindness, fixed and dilated pupils, papilledema, and retinal hemorrhages have been described in affected cattle.
- *Helichrysum argyrosphaerum* poisonings cause gliosis and demyelination of the optic nerve, as well as outer retinal degeneration, in grazing ruminants.

PLANT POISONINGS IN HORSES. Cortical blindness was reported in hoses following ingestion of fiddleneck *(Amsinckia* sp.) and horsetail *(Equisetum arvense)*. Grazing on blindgrass causes retinal and optic nerve degeneration similar to that observed in ruminants.

DRUG TOXICITIES IN SMALL ANIMALS. In dogs, retinal toxicity has been reported after the use of ethambutol, quinine, rafoxanide, chloroquine, azalide, and diphenylthiocarbazone. The drugs cause retinal degeneration and blindness. In cats, retinal degeneration and blindness have been reported due to griseofulvin, megesterol acetate, and ethylene glycol.

OXYGEN TOXICITY IN CATS AND DOGS. Newborn and young puppies and kittens (less than 3 weeks of age) that are exposed to high oxygen concentrations demonstrate an abnormality of retinal vasculature and consequent retinopathy termed *retrolental fibroplasia* or *proliferative retinopathy*. A similar disease, known as *retinopathy of prematurity*, occurs in human infants. Clinical signs include dilated and tortuous retinal vessels, vitreous hemorrhage, altered fundus pigmentation, incomplete vascularization of peripheral retina, and massive intravitreal neovascularization. Changes in vessel diameter are seen after as little as 1 hour of a high-oxygen environment.

Severe retinal lesions are caused by exposure of neonatal dogs and cats to a high-oxygen atmosphere.

Additional Retinopathies and Neuropathies of Horses

Horses suffer from several retinopathies and neuropathies that have not been described in other species. *Proliferative optic neuropathy* is characterized by a progressive white mass enlarging on the surface of the optic nerve (see Figure 16-35 in Chapter 16). It does not affect vision and is regarded as an incidental finding. A similar white mass, however, is also seen in *exudative optic neuritis*, an acute edema of the optic disc in which the animal is blinded (see Figure 16-34 in Chapter 16). The cause of both diseases is unknown, and there is no treatment. *Ischemic optic neuropathy* is an iatrogenic disease: Ligation of the internal and external carotid arteries (to treat epistaxis caused by guttural pouch mycosis) causes ischemia of the optic nerve and irreversible blindness. Although initially the affected optic nerve appears normal, edema, hyperemia, and hemorrhages may be observed after 24 hours. A similar presentation may also be seen in cases of *traumatic optic neuropathy,* in which a blunt trauma causes acute blindness (Figure 15-55).

Equine motor neuron disease is a disorder of mature horses characterized by degeneration of motor neurons in the ventral horn of the spinal cord and selected brainstem nuclei causing muscoskeletal and neurologic deficits, including generalized weakness and muscle tremors. Equine motor neuron disease also causes ophthalmoscopically visible pigment aberrations similar to those seen in canine RPED (see Figure 15-48). The yellow-brown pigmentation is due to accumulation of ceroid lipofuscin in the RPE. As in the case of canine RPED, chronic dietary vitamin E deficiency is implicated in the pathogenesis of the disease. The effect on vision is inconsistent, but diminished b-wave amplitudes on ERG have been reported.

Equine recurrent uveitis is a common cause of blindness in adult horses worldwide. Loss of vision results from chorioretinopathy caused by posterior uveitis. The disease is discussed in detail in Chapter 11.

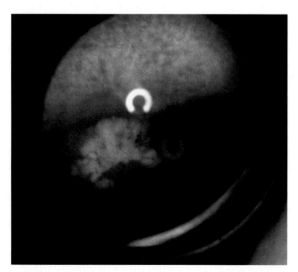

Figure 15-55. Traumatic optic neuropathy in a horse. The trauma was caused when the horse flipped over during a colic attack. (Courtesy University of Wisconsin–Madison Veterinary Ophthalmology Service Collection.)

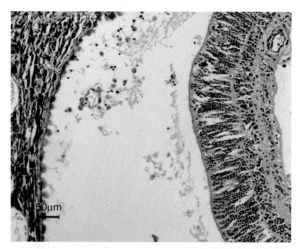

Figure 15-56. Histopathology micrograph showing a case of retinal detachment in a dog. Note that the detachment occurred between the sensory neuroretina (i.e., the outer segments of the photoreceptors) and the retinal pigment epithelium (RPE). As a result, the RPE underwent hypertrophy, giving it the classic "tombstone" appearance. There is also evidence of inflammation in the retina. (Hematoxylin & eosin stain.) (Courtesy Dr. Emmanuel Loeb.)

RETINAL DETACHMENT

Retinal detachment is the separation of the retina from the underlying choroid. More precisely, separation of the retina usually occurs between the photoreceptor layer and the pigment epithelium (Figure 15-56). This is because the RPE and the sensory neuroretina are two embryologically distinct layers, with a potential space between them (see Chapter 2). The intimate contact between the photoreceptors and pigment epithelial cells is disrupted, and metabolites are no longer available from the choroid, nor can end products of metabolism be removed. Because of the retina's high metabolic rate, severe and irreversible changes may occur soon after separation.

Etiology

Possible causes of retinal detachment/separation are as follows:

- *Congenital disorders:* Including retinal dysplasia, CEA, and multiple congenital anomalies
- *Serous detachments:* Accumulation of fluid beneath the retina pushes it away from underlying tissues. Two types of serous detachments are recognized, on the basis of the type of fluid causing the separation. Exudative detachments are due to infectious diseases caused by viral (e.g., distemper, FIP), fungal (e.g., blastomycosis) or protozoal (e.g., leishmania) disease. Hemorrhagic detachments are caused by systemic hypertension, by vascular diseases such as coagulopathy, thrombocytopenia, anemia, and hyperviscosity (see Figure 15-49), or by trauma (Figure 15-57). Specific causes are discussed in Chapter 18.
- *Traction detachments:* After uveitis (e.g., in equine recurrent uveitis), contraction of scar tissue or fibrin within the vitreous pulls the retina off the RPE. Anterior displacement of the vitreous (for example after lens luxation) may also pull the retina off the RPE.

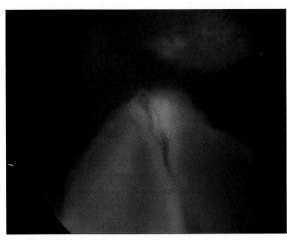

Figure 15-57. Complete retinal detachment in a dog caused by a nearby bomb blast. The detached dorsal (tapetal) retina detached at the ora ciliaris retinae and "fell" ventrally. It may be seen as a gray sheet overlying the disc and obscuring its details.

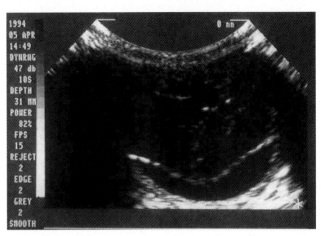

Figure 15-58. Ultrasound image of retinal detachment in a 6-year-old Samoyed with uveitis. The image shows the classic "seagull wings" sign, which is the detached retina adherent to the globe at the optic nerve head and the ora ciliaris retinae. The hyperechoic opacities anterior to the detached retina are fibrin strands that caused the detachment. (Courtesy Dr. I. Aizenberg.)

- *Vitreous degeneration:* Liquefaction of the vitreous is important in the pathogenesis of human retinal detachment. The exact role of liquefaction in spontaneous retinal detachment in aged animals is poorly understood. The liquefied vitreous enters the subretinal space through retinal holes, causing *rhegmatogenous detachment.* This type of detachment is more common in elderly patients, which are more susceptible to retinal hole formation and vitreous liquefaction (see Chapter 14).
- *Iatrogenic:* Retinal detachment may occur after cataract extraction. Tears near the ora ciliaris retinae are thought to be the cause of postoperative retinal detachment.

Signs

Signs of retinal detachment are as follows:

- Acute loss of vision. Blindness is noted in cases of complete detachment. Focal detachments are usually innocuous, and their effect on the visual field is not noticed by the owner.
- Dilated pupil that is nonresponsive to light. However, if the other eye is unaffected, a consensual light response *to* the affected eye will be present.
- Appearance of a floating sheet (i.e., the detached retina) may be seen behind the lens without the use of an ophthalmoscope (see Figure 15-49). The sheet may be transparent, white, or bloody depending on the type of fluid (serous, exudative, or hemorrhagic, respectively) involved in the pathogenesis of the detachment. Retinal vessels are clearly visible on the retina as it moves up against the lens (see Figure 15-49).
- If the posterior segment of the eye cannot be visualized (due to hyphema, for example), an ultrasound examination may be used to demonstrate the condition. The classic appearance of a detached retina is the "seagull sign"—a detached retina that remains fixed to the posterior wall of the eye at the optic nerve head and at the ora ciliaris retinae (Figure 15-58). Causes of the detachment, such as subretinal fluid and vitreal inflammation, may also be seen on ultrasound.

Therapy

In patients presented for sudden loss of vision due to serous retinal detachments, vision can sometimes be restored by medical therapy. Initial diagnostic attempts are directed at determining the cause of the detachment. Patients with retinal detachment should receive complete ophthalmic and physical examinations, a complete blood count for infectious and vascular diseases, serum chemistry profile to evaluate renal function, systolic blood pressure measurement, and serologic evaluation for possible responsible infectious causes (see Chapter 18).

Treatment consists of treating the primary cause and symptomatic treatment of the detachment itself. If hypertension is confirmed at the initial examination, antihypertensive therapy is indicated. Appropriate antimicrobial (i.e., antibiotic, antifungal) therapy should be administered systemically if the cause is infectious. Depending on the patient's systemic condition, oral diuretics and corticosteroids should be administered, with the aim of draining the subretinal fluid. Excessive amounts of fibrin, which may predispose the eye to traction retinal detachment, can be treated with an intraocular injection of tissue plasminogen activator.

Partial retinal detachments after cataract extraction may be successfully prevented from progressing to a full detachment by laser retinopexy along the edge of the separation. Similar treatment may be used to prevent progression of rhegmatogenous detachments. In some referral practices, the veterinary ophthalmologist may be able to offer additional surgical options for complete retinal detachments. See Chapter 14 for additional discussion.

BIBLIOGRAPHY

Acland GM, Aguirre GD (1987): Retinal degeneration in the dog. IV: early retinal degeneration (erd) in Norwegian elkhounds. Exp Eye Res 44:491.

Acland GM, et al. (2005): Long-term restoration of rod and cone vision by single dose rAAV-mediated gene transfer to the retina in a canine model of childhood blindness. Mol Ther 12:1072.

Acland GM, et al. (1995): Exclusion of the cyclic GMP-PDE beta subunit gene as a candidate in the pcrd dog. Invest Ophthalmology 36:S891.

Acland GM, et al. (1994): XLPRA: a canine retinal degeneration inherited as an X-linked trait. Am J Med Genet 52:27.

Acland GM, et al. (1989): Non-allelism of three genes (rcd1, rcd2, and erd) for early-onset hereditary retinal degeneration. Exp Eye Res 49:983.

Aguirre GD, Acland GM (1988): Variation in retinal degeneration phenotype inherited at the prcd locus. Exp Eye Res 46:663.

Aguirre GD, et al. (1998): Congenital stationary night blindness in the dog: common mutation in the RPE65 gene indicates founder effect. Mol Vis 4:23.

Aguirre GD, et al. (1982): Pathogenesis of rod-cone degeneration in miniature poodles. Invest Ophthalmol Vis Sci 23:610.

Aguirre GD, et al. (1982): Retinal degeneration in the dog. III: abnormal cyclic nucleotide metabolism in rod-cone dysplasia. Exp Eye Res 35:625.

Aguirre GD, et al. (1978): Rod-cone dysplasia in Irish setters: a cyclic GMP metabolic defect of visual cells. Science 201:1133.

Aguirre GD, Rubin LF (1975): Rod-cone dysplasia (progressive retinal atrophy) in Irish setters. J Am Vet Med Assoc 166:157.

Aguirre GD, Rubin LF (1975): The electroretinogram in dogs with inherited cone degeneration. Invest Ophthalmol Vis Sci 14:840.

Aguirre GD, Rubin LF (1974): Pathology of hemeralopia in the Alaskan malamute dog. Invest Ophthalmol Vis Sci 13:231.

Aguirre GD, Rubin LF (1972): Progressive retinal atrophy in the miniature poodle: an electrophysiologic study. J Am Vet Med Assoc 160:191.

Aguirre GD, Schmidt SY (1978): Retinal degeneration associated with the feeding of dog food to cats. J Am Vet Med Assoc 172:791.

Aroch I, et al. (1996): Haematologic, ocular and skeletal abnormalities in a family of Samoyeds. J Small Anim Pract 37:333.

Anderson PA, et al. (1979): Biochemical lesions associated with taurine deficiency in the cat. J Anim Sci 49:1227.

Bainbridge JW, et al. (2003): Stable rAAV-mediated transduction of rod and cone photoreceptors in the canine retina. Gene Ther 10:1336.

Barlow RM, et al. (1981): Mannosidosis in Aberdeen Angus cattle in Britain. Vet Rec 109:441.

Barnett KC, et al. (1970): Ocular changes associated with hypovitaminosis A in cattle. Br Vet J 126:561.

Barnett KC, Watson WA (1970): Bright blindness in sheep: a primary retinopathy due to feeding bracken (Pteris aquilina). Res Vet Sci 11:289.

Bedford PGC (1984): Retinal pigment epithelial dystrophy (CPRA): a study of the disease in the Briard. J Small Anim Pract 25:129.

Bedford PGC (1982): Multifocal retinal dysplasia in the Rottweiler. Vet Rec 111:304.

Bellhorn RW, et al. (1974): Feline central retinal degeneration. Invest Ophthalmol Vis Sci 13:608.

Bellhorn RW, Fischer CA (1970): Feline central retinal degeneration. J Am Vet Med Assoc 157:842.

Bergsjo T, et al. (1984): Congenital blindness with ocular developmental anomalies, including retinal dysplasia, in Doberman pinscher dogs. J Am Vet Med Assoc 184:1383.

Berson EL, Watson G (1980): Electroretinograms in English setters with neuronal ceroid lipofuscinosis. Invest Ophthalmol Vis Sci 19:87.

Bildfell R, et al. (1995): Neuronal ceroid lipofuscinosis in a cat. Vet Pathol 32:485.

Bjerkas E, Narfstrom K (1994): Progressive retinal atrophy in the Tibetan spaniel in Norway and Sweden. Vet Rec 134:377.

Blair NP, et al. (1985): Rhegmatogenous retinal detachment in Labrador retrievers. I: development of retinal tears and detachment. Arch Ophthalmol 103:842.

Bradley R, et al. (1982): The pathology of a retinal degeneration in Friesian cows. J Comp Pathol 92:69.

Burns MS, et al. (1988): Development of hereditary tapetal degeneration in the beagle dog. Curr Eye Res 7:103.

Buyukmihci N, et al. (1982): Retinal degenerations in the dog. II: development of the retina in rod-cone dysplasia. Exp Eye Res 30:575.

Carrig CB, et al. (1988): Inheritance of associated ocular and skeletal dysplasia in Labrador retrievers. J Am Vet Med Assoc 193:1269.

Cideciyan AV, et al. (2005): In vivo dynamics of retinal injury and repair in the rhodopsin mutant dog model of human retinitis pigmentosa. Proc Natl Acad Sci U S A 102:5233.

Clegg FG, et al. (1981): Blindness in dairy cows. Vet Rec 109:101.

Collier LC, et al. (1985): Tapetal degeneration in cats with Chediak-Higashi syndrome. Curr Eye Res 4:767.

Collins BK, et al. (1992): Familial cataracts and concurrent ocular anomalies in chow chows. J Am Vet Med Assoc 200:1485.

Cullen CL, Grahn BH (2002): Acute prechiasmal blindness due to sudden acquired retinal degeneration syndrome. Can Vet J 43:729.

Curtis R, Barnett KC (1994): Progressive retinal atrophy in miniature long-haired dachshund dogs. Br Vet J 149:71.

Curtis R, et al. (1987): An early onset retinal dystrophy with dominant inheritance in the Abyssinian cat: clinical and pathological findings. Invest Ophthalmol Vis Sci 28:62.

Davidson MG et al. (1998): Retinal degeneration associated with vitamin E deficiency in hunting dogs. J Am Vet Med Assoc 213:645.

Dekomien G, Epplen JT (2003): Analysis of PDE6D and PDE6G genes for generalised progressive retinal atrophy (gPRA) mutations in dogs. Genet Sel Evol 35:445.

Dekomien G, Epplen JT (2002): Screening of the arrestin gene in dogs afflicted with generalized progressive retinal atrophy. BMC Genet 3:12.

Dekomien G, Epplen JT (2002): The canine phosducin gene: characterization of the exon-intron structure and exclusion as a candidate gene for generalized progressive retinal atrophy in 11 dog breeds. Mol Vis 8:138.

Dice PF (1980): Progressive retinal atrophy in the Samoyed. Mod Vet Pract 61:59.

Divers TJ, et al. (1986): Blindness and convulsion associated with vitamin A deficiency in feedlot steers. J Am Vet Med Assoc 189:1579.

Edwards JF, et al. (1994): Juvenile-onset neuronal ceroid lipofuscinosis in Rambouillet sheep. Vet Pathol 31:48.

Ehrenhofer MC, et al. (2002): Normal structure and age-related changes of the equine retina. Vet Ophthalmol 5:39.

Evans J, et al. (2005): A variant form of neuronal ceroid lipofuscinosis in American bulldogs. J Vet Intern Med 19:44

Fischer CA (1970): Retinopathy in anemic cats. J Am Med Assoc 156:1415.

Ford M, et al. (2003): Gene transfer in the RPE65 null mutation dog: relationship between construct volume, visual behavior and electroretinographic (ERG) results. Doc Ophthalmol 107:79.

Gelatt KN, McGill LD (1973): Clinical characteristics of microphthalmia with colobomas of the Australian shepherd dog. J Am Vet Med Assoc 162:393.

Giuliano E, van der Woerdt A (1999): Feline retinal degeneration: clinical experience and new findings (1994-1997). J Am Anim Hosp Assoc 35:511.

Goebel HH, Dahme E (1986): Ultrastructure of retinal pigment epithelial and neural cells in the neuronal ceroid-lipofuscinosis affected Dalmatian dog. Retina 6:179.

Graydon RJ, Jolly RD (1984): Ceroid-lipofuscinosis (Batten's disease): sequential electrophysiologic and pathologic changes in the retina of the ovine model. Invest Ophthalmol Vis Sci 25:294.

Guven D, et al. (2006): Implantation of an inactive epiretinal poly(dimethyl siloxane) electrode array in dogs. Exp Eye Res 82:81.

Guven D, et al. (2005): Long-term stimulation by active epiretinal implants in normal and RCD1 dogs. J Neural Eng 2:S65.

Hakanson N, Narfstrom K (1995): Progressive retinal atrophy in papillon dogs in Sweden: a clinical survey. Vet Comp Ophthalmol 5:83.

Harper PA, et al. (1988): Neurovisceral ceroid-lipofuscinosis in blind Devon cattle. Acta Neuropathol 75:632.

Jolly R, et al. (1987): Mannosidosis: ocular lesions in the bovine model. Curr Eye Res 6:1073.

Katz ML, et al. (2005): Assessment of retinal function and characterization of lysosomal storage body accumulation in the retinas and brains of Tibetan terriers with ceroid-lipofuscinosis. Am J Vet Res 66:67.

Katz ML, et al. (2002): Assessment of plasma carnitine concentrations in relation to ceroid lipofuscinosis in Tibetan terriers. Am J Vet Res 63:890.

Koch SA, Rubin LF (1972): Distribution of cones in retina of the normal dog. Am J Vet Res 33:361.

Komaromy AM, et al. (2003): Flash electroretinography in standing horses using the DTL microfiber electrode. Vet Ophthalmol 6:27.

Kommonen B, et al. (1997): Impaired retinal function in young Labrador retriever dogs heterozygous for late onset rod cone degeneration. Vision Res 37:365.

Kommonen B, et al. (1994): Early morphometry of a retinal dystrophy in Labrador retrievers. Acta Ophthalmol 72:203.

Komnenou AA, et al (2007): Ocular manifestations of natural canine monocytic ehrlichiosis (Ehrlichia canis): a retrospective study of 90 cases. Vet Ophthalmol 10:137.

Kukekova AV, et al. (2006): Linkage mapping of canine rod cone dysplasia type 2 (rcd2) to CFA7, the canine orthologue of human 1q32. Invest Ophthalmol Vis Sci 47:1210.

Laratta LJ, et al. (1985): Multiple congenital ocular defects in the Akita dog. Cornell Vet 75:381.

Lavach JD, et al. (1978): Retinal dysplasia in the English springer spaniel. J Am Anim Hosp Assoc 14:192.

Le Meur G, et al. (2005): Postsurgical assessment and long-term safety of recombinant adeno-associated virus-mediated gene transfer into the retinas of dogs and primates. Arch Ophthalmol 123:500.

Leiva M, et al. (2005): Therapy of ocular and visceral leishmaniasis in a cat. Vet Ophthalmol 8:71.

Lewis DG, et al. (1986): Congenital microphthalmia and other developmental ocular anomalies in the Doberman. J Small Anim Pract 27:559.

Lightfoot RM, et al. (1996): Retinal pigment epithelial dystrophy in Briard dogs. Res Vet Sci 60:17.

MacMillan AD, Lipton DE (1978): Heritability of multifocal retinal dysplasia in American cocker spaniels. J Am Vet Med Assoc 172:568.

Matz-Rensing K, et al. (1996): Retinal detachment in horses. Equine Vet J 28:111.

McLeod DS, et al. (1998): Clinical and histopathologic features of canine oxygen-induced proliferative retinopathy. Invest Ophthalmol Vis Sci 39:1918.

McLeod DS, et al. (1996): Vaso-obliteration in the canine model of oxygen-induced retinopathy. Invest Ophthalmol Vis Sci 37:300.

McLeod DS, et al. (1996): Vasoproliferation in the neonatal dog model of oxygen-induced retinopathy. Invest Ophthalmol Vis Sci 37:1322.

Meyers VN, et al. (1983): Short-linked dwarfism and ocular defects in the Samoyed dog. J Am Vet Med Assoc 183:975.

Miller PE, et al. (1998): Photoreceptor cell death by apoptosis in dogs with sudden acquired retinal degeneration syndrome. Am J Vet Res 59:149.

Millichamp NJ (1988): Progressive retinal atrophy in Tibetan terriers. J Am Vet Med Assoc 192:769.

Munroe G (2000): Survey of retinal haemorrhages in neonatal thoroughbred foals. Mol Ther 12:1072.

Narfström K, Ekesten B (1999): Diseases of the canine ocular fundus, in Gelatt KN (editor): Veterinary Ophthalmology, 3rd ed. Lippincott Williams & Wilkins, Philadelphia.

Narfström K, Ekesten B (1998): Electroretinographic evaluation of papillons with and without hereditary retinal degeneration. Am J Vet Res 59:221.

Narfström K, et al. (2003): Functional and structural recovery of the retina after gene therapy in the RPE65 null mutation dog. Invest Ophthalmol Vis Sci 44:1663.

Narfström K, et al. (2002): Guidelines for clinical electroretinography in the dog. Doc Ophthalmol 105:83.

Narfström K, et al. (1995): Clinical electroretinography in the dog with Ganzfeld stimulation: a practical method of examining rod and cone function. Doc Ophthalmol 90:279.

Narfström K, et al. (1994): Hereditary retinal dystrophy in the Briard dog: clinical and hereditary characteristics. Vet Comp Ophthalmol 4:85.

Narfström K, et al. (1989): The Briard dog: a new animal model of congenital stationery night blindness. Br J Ophthalmol 73:750.

Narfström K, et al. (1988): Hereditary retinal degeneration in the Abyssinian cat: developmental studies using clinical electroretinography. Doc Ophthalmol 69:111.

Narfström K, et al. (1985): Progressive retinal atrophy in the Abyssinian cat: studies of the DC-recorded electroretinogram and the standing potential of the eye. Br J Ophthalmol 69:618.

Narfström K, Nilsson SE (1985): Hereditary retinal degeneration in the Abyssinian cat: correlation of ophthalmoscopic and electroretinographic findings. Doc Ophthalmol 60:183.

Nelson DL, Macmillan AD (1983): Multifocal retinal dysplasia in field trial Labrador retrievers. J Am Anim Hosp Assoc 19:388.

Nilsson SEG, et al. (1992): Changes in the DC electroretinogram in Briard dogs with hereditary congenital stationery night blindness and partial day blindness. Exp Eye Res 54:291.

Nunnery C, et al. (2005): Congenital stationary night blindness in a thoroughbred and a paso fino. Vet Ophthalmol 8:415.

Ofri R, Narfstrom K (2007): Light at the end of the tunnel? Advances in the understanding and treatment of glaucoma and inherited retinal degeneration. Vet J (E-pub ahead of print).

Ofri R, et al. (1996): Feline central retinal degeneration in captive cheetahs (Acinonyx jubatus). J Zoo Wildl Med 27:101.

O'Toole DO, et al. (1983): Retinal dysplasia of English springer spaniel dogs: light microscopy of the postnatal lesions. Vet Pathol 20:298.

Parshall C, et al. (1991): Photoreceptor dysplasia: an inherited progressive retinal atrophy of miniature schnauzer dogs. Prog Vet Comp Ophthalmol 1:187.

Paulsen ME, et al. (1989): Blindness and sexual dimorphism associated with vitamin A deficiency in cattle. J Am Vet Med Assoc 194:933.

Peiffer RL, Fischer CA (1983): Microphthalmia, retinal dysplasia and anterior segment dysgenesis in a litter of Doberman pinschers. J Am Vet Med Assoc 183:875.

Petersen-Jones S (2005): Advances in the molecular understanding of canine retinal diseases. J Small Anim Pract 46:371.

Petersen-Jones SM, Zhu FX (2000): Development and use of a polymerase chain reaction-based diagnostic test for the causal mutation of progressive retinal atrophy in Cardigan Welsh corgis. Am J Vet Res 61:844.

Pion PD, et al. (1987): Myocardial failure in cats associated with low plasma taurine: a reversible cardiomyopathy. Science 237:764.

Pizzirani S (2003): Transpupillary diode laser retinopexy in dogs: ophthalmoscopic, fluorescein angiographic and histopathologic study. Vet Ophthalmol 6:227.

Rabin AR, et al. (1973): Cone and rod responses in nutritionally induced retinal degeneration in the cat. Invest Ophthalmol Vis Sci 12:694.

Rampazzo A, et al. (2005): Collie eye anomaly in a mixed-breed dog. Vet Ophthalmol 8:357.

Reppas GP, et al. (1995): Trauma-induced blindness in two horses. Aust Vet J 72:270.

Riis R, et al. (1999): Ocular manifestations of equine motor neuron disease. Equine Vet J 31:99.

Rubin LF (1971): Hemeralopia in Alaskan malamute pups. J Am Vet Med Assoc 158:1699.

Rubin LF (1968): Heredity of retinal dysplasia in Bedlington terriers. J Am Vet Med Assoc 152:260.

Rubin LF (1963): Atrophy of rods and cones in the cat retina. J Am Vet Med Assoc 142:1415.

Sandberg MA, et al. (1986): Full field electroretinograms in miniature poodles with progressive rod-cone degeneration. Invest Ophthalmol 27:1179.

Santo-Anderson R, et al. (1980): An inherited retinopathy in collies: a light microscopic study. Invest Ophthalmol Vis Sci 19:1281.

Schaffer EH, Wallow IHL (1975): Rhegmatogenous bilateral retinal detachment in a poodle dog. J Comp Pathol 85:195.

Schmidt GM, et al. (1979): Inheritance of retinal dysplasia in the English springer spaniel. J Am Vet Med Assoc 174:1989.

Shelah M, et al. (2007): Acute blindness in a dog caused by an explosive blast. Vet Ophthalmol 10:196.

Slatter D, et al. (1980): Progressive retinal degeneration in the greyhound. Aust Vet J 56:106.

Slatter D, et al. (1980): Stypandra spp. ("blindgrass") poisoning in ruminants—ocular and neurological findings in spontaneous cases. Aust Vet J 57:132.

Slater JD, et al. (1992): Chorioretinopathy associated with neuropathology following infection with equine herpesvirus-1. Vet Rec 131:237.

Storey ES, et al. (2005): Multifocal chorioretinal lesions in borzoi dogs. Vet Ophthalmol 8:337.

Tao W, et al. (2002): Encapsulated cell-based delivery of CNTF reduces photoreceptor degeneration in animal models of retinitis pigmentosa. Invest Ophthalmol Vis Sci 43:3292.

Taylor RM, Farrow BR (1992): Ceroid lipofuscinosis in the border collie dog: retinal lesions in an animal model of juvenile batten disease. Am J Med Genet 42:622.

Url A, et al. (2001): Equine neuronal ceroid lipofuscinosis. Acta Neuropathol (Berl) 101:410.

Vainisi SJ, Packo KH (1995): Management of giant retinal tears in dogs. J Am Vet Med Assoc 206:491.

Watson P, Bedford PGC (1992): The pigments of retinal pigment epithelial dystrophy in dogs. Vet Pathol 29:5.

Watson WA, et al. (1972): Progressive retinal degeneration (bright blindness) in sheep: a review. Vet Rec 91:665.

Witzel DA, et al. (1977): Night blindness in the appaloosa: sibling occurrence. J Equine Med Surg 1:383.

Witzel ED, et al. (1977): Electroretinography of congenital night blindness in an appaloosa filly. J Equine Med Surg 1:266.

Wolf ED, et al. (1978): Rod-cone dysplasia in the collie. J Am Vet Med Assoc 173:1331.

Woodford BJ, et al. (1982): Cyclic nucleotide metabolism in inherited retinopathy in collies. Exp Eye Res 34:703.

Wrigstad A, et al. (1995): Neuronal ceroid lipofuscinosis in the Polish owczarek nizinny (PON) dog: a retinal study. Doc Ophthalmol 91:33.

Wrigstad A, et al. (1994): Slowly progressive changes of the retina and the retinal pigment epithelium in Briard dogs with hereditary retinal dystrophy. Doc Ophthalmol 87:337.

Wyman M, et al. (2005): Ophthalmomyiasis (interna posterior) of the posterior segment and central nervous system myiasis: Cuterebra spp. in a cat. Vet Ophthalmol 8:77.

Yanoff M, et al. (1970): Oxygen poisoning of the eyes: comparison in cyanotic and acyanotic dogs. Arch Ophthalmol 84:627.

Zeiss CJ, et al. (2006): CNTF induces dose-dependent alterations in retinal morphology in normal and rcd-1 canine retina. Exp Eye Res 82:395

Zeiss CJ, et al. (2000): Mapping of X-linked progressive retinal atrophy (XLPRA), the canine homolog of retinitis pigmentosa 3 (RP3). Hum Mol Genet 9:531.

Zhang Q, et al. (1999): Photoreceptor dysplasia (pd) in miniature schnauzer dogs: evaluation of candidate genes by molecular genetic analysis. J Hered 90:57.

NEUROOPHTHALMOLOGY

Ron Ofri

ASSESSING VISION AND PUPILLARY
  LIGHT RELFEXES
LESIONS IN PATIENTS WITH VISUAL AND
  PUPILLARY LIGHT REFLEX DEFICITS
LESIONS CAUSING STRABISMUS

LESIONS CAUSING EYELID
  ABNORMALITIES
LESIONS OF ADDITIONAL CRANIAL
  NERVES

AUTONOMIC INNERVATION AND
  ABNORMALITIES
VESTIBULAR SYSTEM
CENTRAL VISUAL PATHWAYS

Neuroophthalmology should not be a daunting study. If anatomy, physiology, and pathology of the ocular and visual innervation are understood, a diagnosis can be reached through deduction and elimination rather than from memory.

The following cranial nerves are significant in relation to ocular functions:

- Optic nerve: Cranial nerve (CN) II—relays the visual signal from the retina to the central nervous system (CNS)
- Oculomotor nerve: CN III—innervates four extraocular muscles (dorsal, medial, and ventral recti and the ventral oblique) and the levator palpebral muscle (elevating the upper eyelid); also provides parasympathetic innervation to the iris sphincter
- Trochlear nerve: CN IV—innervates the dorsal oblique muscle
- Trigeminal nerve: CN V—its *ophthalmic* and *maxillary* branches provide sensory innervation to the eye and its accessory organs, including the cornea, conjunctiva, lacrimal gland, and periocular skin
- Abducens nerve: CN VI—innervates the lateral rectus and retractor bulbi muscles
- Facial nerve: CN VII—innervates the various muscles controlling the blink response

In addition, significant parts of the CNS are devoted to vision processing and ocular control. Therefore the workup of the neuroophthalmologic patient requires comprehensive neurologic and systemic examinations, in addition to a thorough neuroophthalmologic examination (Table 16-1). This chapter reviews the examination, clinical signs, and diseases of the neuroophthalmologic patient.

ASSESSING VISION AND PUPILLARY LIGHT REFLEXES

Vision and the Menace Response

Vision is initially evaluated as the patient walks into the clinic or examination room. The ability to navigate in these unfamiliar surroundings may reveal visual deficits. A more direct assessment is made by testing the animal's response to a menacing gesture. The *menace response* is evoked by making a threatening gesture with the hand at each eye while the other hand covers the opposite eye. If the other eye is not covered, an alert animal that is unilaterally blind in the eye being tested may observe the threat with its normal eye and respond by blinking bilaterally, thus creating a false positive response (i.e., a blink "response" in a blind eye). It is crucial to the validity of this test that the threatening hand does not touch the patient or create enough air currents to be felt by the patient, which may also generate a false positive response (Figure 16-1).

The normal response to this threat is a rapid blink and closure of the palpebral fissure. The anatomic pathways of the afferent and efferent components are depicted in Figure 16-2. The afferent component of the response is relayed by the optic nerve, through the optic chiasm, optic tract, lateral geniculate nucleus (LGN), and optic radiation to the visual cortex located in the occipital lobe. It is assumed that the visual cortex projects to the motor cortex, which in turn projects via the internal capsule and crus cerebri to the facial nuclei in the medulla, and from there the facial nerve (CN VII) relays the efferent signal to the eyelid muscles. The complexity of this pathway implies that the resulting blinking is not a reflex but a learned response. Therefore this response may not become fully developed until 10 to 12 weeks of age in some small animals. It is usually present by 5 to 7 days in foals and calves. As a result, menace testing in young patients may result in a false negative result, as the animal does not blink even though it can see.

Crossover of optic nerve fibers occurs at the optic chiasm (Figure 16-3). Consequently, the left occipital cortex receives the axons of the lateral retina of the left eye (inputting from the right visual field) as well as the axons of the medial retina of the right eye (inputting, again, from the right visual field) (see orange pathways in Figure 16-3). The right occipital cortex inputs from the left visual fields of both eyes (see green pathways in Figure 16-3). In humans, where 50% of the axons cross over in the chiasm, the left occipital cortex inputs the right visual hemifield of both eyes, and the right occipital cortex inputs the left visual hemifield (orange and green pathways, respectively, in Figure 16-3). In animals, where a greater percentage of fibers cross over, the left occipital cortex will input a greater proportion of the right visual field of the right eye and a smaller proportion of the right visual field of the left eye. Therefore, in humans, a lesion in the left optic radiation or occipital cortex, for example, will cause a loss of the right visual hemifield, with symmetric deficits in both eyes *(homonymous hemianopia)*. In animals, however, such a lesion will cause greater deficits in the visual field of the right eye than those of the left eye. In the dog, where 25% of the fibers

Table 16-1 | **Summary of the Neuroophthalmologic Examination**

TEST OR OBSERVATION	NEUROLOGIC COMPONENTS
Menace response	CN II, optic chiasm, optic tract, lateral geniculate nucleus, optic radiation, visual and motor cortex, facial nucleus and nerve cerebellum
Size of pupils and reaction to light	CN II, optic chiasm, proximal optic tract, CN III, sympathetic nerves, diencephalon-mesencephalon (pretectal and oculomotor nuclei)
Eyelids (size of fissure)	CNs III, VII, sympathetic nerves
Third eyelid	Sympathetic nerves
Position of eyes	CNs III, IV, VI, vestibular system, brainstem
Normal and abnormal nystagmus	CN VIII—brainstem and vestibular system—CNs III, IV, VI
Palpebral reflex	CNs V, VII

CN, Cranial nerve.

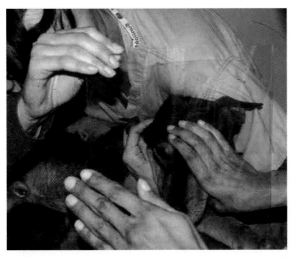

Figure 16-1. The menace response of the right eye is tested while the left eye is being covered. This eliminates the possibility of a blinking response generated by the visual, untested eye. To eliminate stimulation due to air movement or touching of hair, the menacing gesture may be made behind a transparent glass or plastic sheet.

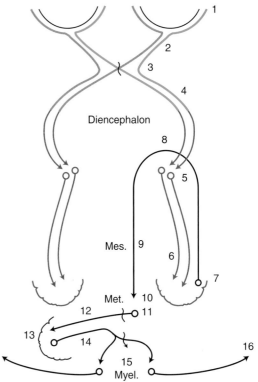

Figure 16-2. Anatomic pathway of the menace response: The afferent component of the response is relayed from the retina *(1)* by the optic nerve *(2)*, through the optic chiasm *(3)*, optic tract *(4)*, lateral geniculate nucleus *(5)* and optic radiation *(6)* to the visual cortex *(7)* located in the occipital lobe. Note that the afferent pathways common to the pupillary light reflex and menace response (up to the level of the proximal optic tract) are colored in lighter shades. Afferent pathways that serve only the menace pathways (from the distal optic tract onward) are depicted in darker shades. It is assumed that the visual cortex projects to the motor cortex, which in turn projects via the internal capsule *(8)* and crus cerebri *(9)* to the facial nuclei *(15)* in the medulla, and from there the facial nerve (cranial nerve VII) relays the efferent signal to the eyelid muscles *(16)*. The cerebellum participates in modulating the menace response and integrating function of the motor cortex, using pathways that include: *10*, longitudinal fibers of pons; *11*, pontine nucleus; *12*, transverse fibers of pons and middle cerebellar peduncle; *13*, cerebellar cortex; *14*, efferent cerebellar pathway; *15*, facial nuclei; *16*, facial muscles—orbicularis oculi. The wiggling line *(~)* indicates axons crossing the midline of the brain. (Modified from de Lahunta A [1983]: Veterinary Neuroanatomy and Clinical Neurology, 2nd ed. Saunders, Philadelphia.)

remain on the ipsilateral side and 75% of the fibers cross over in the chiasm, a unilateral lesion will cause deficits of 25% and 75% in the visual fields of the ipsilateral and contralateral eye, respectively. In the cat, the respective figures are 33% and 67%. In dogs and cats such visual deficits are difficult to detect as an animal moves in its surroundings. Occasionally, the animal may bump into an object on the side opposite the lesion, but often there is *no evidence* of visual deficit because 25% to 33% of the visual field is relayed to the unaffected lobe. In horses, sheep, and cattle with 80% to 90% decussation of optic nerve axons there is a greater tendency to walk into objects on the side of the visual deficit, contralateral to the lesion. Theoretically, these deficits could be tested separately by threats from the lateral and medial visual fields. However, this approach is unreliable, and in all domestic animals menace reflex is poor or absent on the side contralateral to the lesion.

If the menace response does not occur, the examiner should rule out another potential cause of false negative responses by checking the facial nerve innervation of the orbicularis oculi. It

is possible that the patient is visual but cannot blink due to facial nerve paralysis. This is checked by touching the lateral and medial canthi of the eyelids to test the *palpebral reflex,* which is expressed as a blink in response to the tactile stimulation. Another way to rule out a false negative response caused by facial nerve paralysis is to carefully watch the eye while performing the menace test. If a facial nerve paralysis exists, forehead or eye retraction is observed when that eye is threatened, but no blinking is observed. With slight retraction of the eye, the third eyelid passively protrudes. A patient with a facial nerve paralysis may therefore have "flashing third eyelid," which is an indication that vision is intact. If there is no facial nerve paralysis and no menace response occurs, the animal should be lightly struck two or three times with the threatening hand, and then the threat should be repeated without touching the patient. This procedure often arouses and directs the attention of the patient and is then followed by a normal response. Significant cerebellar disease may also cause

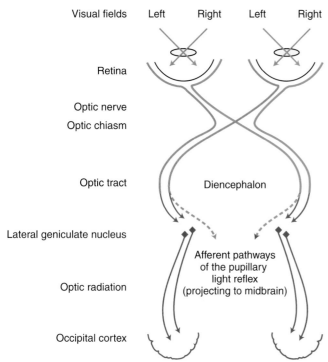

Figure 16-3. Central visual pathway for conscious perception includes the retina, optic nerve, optic chiasm, optic tract, lateral geniculate nucleus, optic radiation, and occipital cortex. Note that the afferent pathways common to the pupillary light reflex and menace response (up to the level of the proximal optic tract) are colored in lighter shades. Afferent pathways that serve only the menace pathways (from the distal optic tract onward) are depicted in darker shades. Because of the crossover in the chiasm, the left occipital cortex receives the axons of the lateral retina of the left eye (inputting from the right visual field) as well as the axons of the medial retina of the right eye (inputting, again, from the right visual field). In humans, where 50% of the axons cross over in the chiasm, the left occipital cortex therefore inputs the right visual hemifield of both eyes. In animals, where a greater percentage of fibers cross over, the left occipital cortex will input a greater proportion of the right visual field of the right eye and a smaller proportion of the right visual field of the left eye. Therefore, in humans, a lesion in the left optic radiation or occipital cortex will cause a loss of the right visual hemifield, with symmetric deficits in both eyes. In animals, the resulting deficits from the right eye will be greater than those from the left eye. (Modified from de Lahunta A [1973]: Small animal neuro-ophthalmology. Vet Clin North Am 3:491.)

lack of menace response in a visual animal, as pathways from the visual cortex to the facial nucleus likely run through the cerebellum (see Figure 16-2).

In patients in which results of the menace testing are equivocal, vision can be assessed using any of the three following tests:

Tracking Moving Objects

Vision can be assessed in young small animals that may not yet have learned the menace response, and occasionally in stoic older animals, by throwing cotton balls in the air in front of the animal. A normal, alert animal that may not readily respond to a menace gesture will follow the cotton ball. Avoid throwing heavier objects that cause significant air movement or noise, because the animal may respond to these stimuli. Some animals, especially cats, will follow the red light emitted by a laser pointer. Young, hungry calves and foals often follow a moving hand or a nursing bottle.

Maze Test

This test assesses the patient's ability to navigate through an obstacle course. The test may be conducted with one eye covered to assess unilateral vision. It can also be conducted both in light and dim environments (to test for early signs of inherited retinopathies). The patient's performance in the course should always be compared with that of normal animals.

Visual Placing Postural Reaction

In the visual placing postural reaction test, the animal is held off the ground and brought to a table edge. If it sees the table, it elevates its limbs to place them on the table's surface before the limbs touch the table. A blind animal does not elevate the limbs until they touch the table's edge (Figure 16-4).

Pupillary Light Reflex

The Anatomic Basis of the Pupillary Light Reflex

The afferent and efferent pathways controlling pupil size and reaction are depicted in Figure 16-5. The size of the pupil at rest represents a balance between two anatagonistic forces: (1) the amount of incident light stimulating the retina and influencing the oculomotor neurons to constrict the pupil (parasympathetic innervation through CN III), and (2) the emotional status of the patient (e.g., fear, anger, or excitement), which influences the sympathetic system and causes pupillary dilation. In the resting pupil, both pupillary dilator (sympathetic) and the antagonistic pupillary sphincter (parasympathetic) muscles are active. The relative resting parasympathetic and sympathetic innervation and resulting muscle tone determine the size of the pupil (see Figure 16-5, efferent pathways *A* and *B*, respectively). The pupillary sphincter (or constrictor) is *the more powerful* of the two muscles.

As noted, pupillary constriction and pupillary light reflex (PLR) are controlled by the parasympathetic system. The afferent pathway to the parasympathetic oculomotor nucleus is via the optic nerve to the optic chiasm (where some crossing occurs), through both optic tracts, over the LGNs without forming a synapse, and ventrally into the region between the thalamus and the rostral colliculus, called the pretectal area.

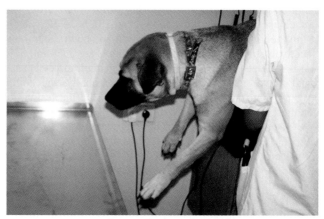

Figure 16-4. The placement reflex is evaluated in cases in which the menace response is inconclusive. The animal is suspended in the air and led toward a table. A visual animal will extend its forelimbs toward the approaching surface. This reflex is composed of an afferent visual response and an efferent motor response.

Synapse takes place in the *pretectal nuclei* in the mesencephalon (see Figure 16-5). Crossing *between sides* occurs between the pretectal nuclei via the caudal commissure. Axons of the pretectal cell bodies pass to the Edinger-Westphal (parasympathetic oculomotor) nucleus of both sides. The parasympathetic axons leave the mesencephalon with the motor axons of CN III (that control four of the extraocular muscles and the levator palpebral muscle), and enter the orbit through the orbital fissure. The ciliary ganglion is located at the rostral end of the oculomotor nerve, ventral to the optic nerve (see Figures 16-5 and 16-6). Preganglionic parasympathetic axons of the oculomotor nerve synapse here with the cell bodies of the postganglionic axons. The postganglionic axons pass via short ciliary nerves, enter the globe adjacent to the optic nerve, and innervate the ciliary body and pupillary constrictor muscles. The feline eye has

only two short ciliary nerves, each serving half of the iris. A partial parasympathetic lesion may therefore cause a hemidilated pupil (partial internal ophthalmoplegia) in the cat.

The anatomy of the sympathetic pathway, responsible for pupil dilatation, is discussed later in this chapter (see Sympathetic Lower Motor Neuron Innervation).

Testing the Pupillary Light Reflex

The size and response of pupils to light are assessed after the menace test. If there is a visual deficit, localization of the lesion depends on a careful examination of the eyes and the pupils.

First, the size of the pupils at rest (without stimulation) should be evaluated both in normal room light and in dim light. If the pupils cannot be seen without extra light, a dim penlight is held in front of the nose of the patient and at a distance that will just allow the pupillary margins to be seen, without stimulating them. The size of the pupils is assessed and compared with each other to determine if there is *anisocoria* (unequal pupils).

Next, the reaction to strong light is tested. Because of the crossover in the optic chiasm and mesencephalon (see Figure 16-5), stimulation of the retina of one eye with a bright source of light causes constriction of both pupils. First the examiner evaluates the *direct* PLR by shining a bright light into one eye while observing the reaction of its pupil. To evaluate the *indirect* PLR, the examiner shines a bright light into one eye while observing the reaction of the contralateral pupil. The patient should be relaxed for this part of the examination, because circulating epinephrines and sympathetic stimulation may interfere with the PLR.

It is important to remember that PLR, as well as the following four tests described next, evaluate subcortical reflexes. Therefore they are *not* indicators of vision and may be normal in a blind animal (e.g., in cases of cortical disease). Furthermore, the PLR is remarkably resistant to serious ocular diseases that substantially reduce its afferent input. Animals with extensive retinal disease (e.g., progressive rod-cone degeneration) or mature cataracts can be functionally blind and yet their pupils may still respond to bright light. However, these animals have pupils that are dilated more than normal in the room light because they do not react to incident light in the room. This helps distinguish them from cases of central blindness, where pupils constrict in response to incident light. If the clinician is not aware of this possibility, he or she may erroneously diagnose a lesion in the central visual pathways in that patient (based on the presence of PLR in a blind animal).

Swinging Flashlight Test

A *swinging flashlight test* is used by some clinicians. In a normal animal, a quick redirection of a flashlight from one eye to the other (by swinging it from side to side) should reveal semiconstriction of the second pupil. The second pupil initially underwent limited constriction owing to the consensual stimulus from the first eye; swinging the flashlight causes further constriction, because now the second eye is stimulated directly. On the other hand, if a retinal or optic nerve disease is present in the second eye, swinging the flashlight to this eye will result in a dilatation of its pupil. This is because the second pupil initially underwent limited constriction owing to the consensual stimulation from the first eye; however, when the light

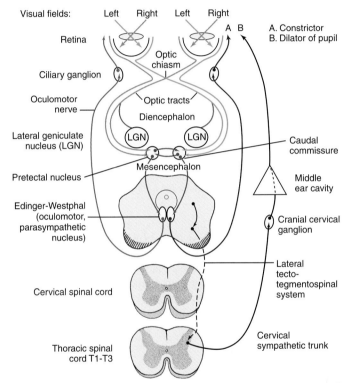

Figure 16-5. Neuroanatomic tracts controlling the pupil size and response include parasympathetic *(A)* and sympathetic *(B)* pathways. The afferent pathway to the parasympathetic oculomotor nucleus is via the optic nerve to the optic chiasm (where some crossing occurs), through both optic tracts, over the lateral geniculate nucleus (without forming a synapse) to synapse in the pretectal nuclei in the mesencephalon. Note that fibers inputting to the lateral geniculate nucleus and visual cortex diverge in the middle of the optic tract; these are depicted in darker shades of green and orange. Crossing of the afferent PLR fibers *between sides* occurs between the pretectal nuclei via the caudal commissure. Axons of the pretectal cell bodies pass to the Edinger-Westphal (parasympathetic oculomotor) nucleus of both sides. The parasympathetic axons leave the mesencephalon with the motor axons of cranial nerve III, enter the orbit through the orbital fissure, and synapse in the *ciliary ganglion*. The postganglionic axons pass via short ciliary nerves, enter the globe adjacent to the optic nerve, and innervate the pupillary constrictor muscles. Preganglionic sympathetic cell bodies are located in the first three segments of the thoracic spinal cord (T1-T3). These preganglionic axons join the thoracic sympathetic trunk inside the thorax and terminate in the *cranial cervical ganglion*. The postganglionic fibers pass between the tympanic bulla and the petrosal bone into the middle ear cavity and continue to the eye, where they innervate the iris dilator muscle. (Modified from de Lahunta A [1983]: Veterinary Neuroanatomy and Clinical Neurology, 2nd ed. Saunders, Philadelphia.)

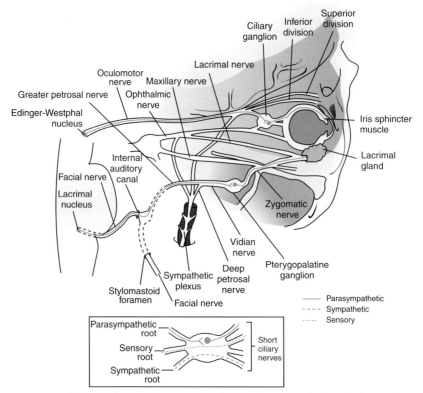

Figure 16-6. Parasympathetic (oculomotor) innervation to the iris sphincter and ciliary body muscle. Inset shows sensory, sympathetic, and parasympathetic fibers into ciliary ganglion; only parasympathetic fibers synapse. Each short ciliary nerve carries all three types of fibers. (From Remington LA [2005]: Clinical Anatomy of the Visual System, 2nd ed. Butterworth-Heinemann, St. Louis.)

is moved to the diseased eye, it dilates as it receives no direct stimulation. This quick dilation of the second pupil, called a *positive swinging flashlight test* result or presence of the *Marcus Gunn sign*, is considered pathognomonic for a prechiasmal lesion.

Pupillary Escape

Another phenomenon often seen with pupil assessment is *pupillary escape*. When a light is applied to the eye the pupil constricts and then immediately dilates slightly. This is due to light adaptation of the photoreceptors and is more common with weak light sources.

Dazzle Reflex

If the PLR cannot be evaluated (e.g., due to severe corneal edema or hyphema), the *dazzle reflex* is also often helpful in lesion localization. Shining a bright light into the eye elicits a subcortically mediated, reflex rapid eye blink (Figure 16-7). Because this is a subcortical reflex, it may be present in a blind animal. This response involves CN II, the rostral colliculus, and CN VII. Therefore it will be present in an animal blinded by a cerebrocortical lesion but absent in a patient blinded by subcortical diseases.

Electrophysiology

Retinal function can also be evaluated electrophysiologically, using electroretinography to record the responses of the retina

to light stimulation. The test is described in detail in Chapter 15. It may be used to determine whether blindness is caused by retinal or postretinal disease. Placing the active electrode over the visual cortex, rather than on the cornea, allows for the recording of *visual evoked potentials*, which are useful in determining cortical function and vision.

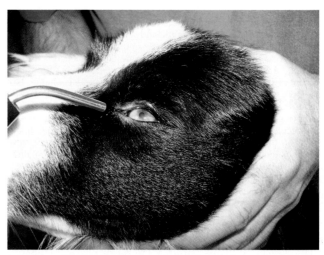

Figure 16-7. The dazzle reflex is evoked with use of a strong light source. The efferent arm of the reflex causes the patient to squint. This is a subcortical reflex, and the squinting does not necessarily mean that the animal is visual.

Table 16-2 | **Clinical Signs of Visual Deficit**

	LESIONS				
	RIGHT OPTIC NERVE*	RIGHT CRANIAL NERVE III†	RIGHT RETROBULBAR‡	RIGHT OPTIC TRACT§	RIGHT VISUAL CORTEX
FEATURES					
Left Eye (OS)					
Pupil at rest	Normal size	Normal size	Normal size	Normal size	Normal size
Response to light in OS	Both pupils constrict	Only OS constricts	Only OS constricts	Both pupils constrict	Both pupils constrict
Menace response	Present	Present	Present	Mostly absent	Mostly absent
Right Eye (OD)					
Pupil at rest	Partial dilation‖	Complete dilation	Complete dilation	Normal size	Normal size
Response to light in OD	Neither pupil constricts	Only OS constricts	Neither pupil constricts	Both pupils constrict	Both pupils constrict
Menace response	Absent	Present	Absent	Mostly present	Mostly present

Adapted from de Lahunta A (1983): Veterinary Neuroanatomy and Clinical Neurology, 2nd ed. Saunders, Philadelphia.
*See also Figure 16-8.
†See also Figure 16-11.
‡Both cranial nerve II and cranial nerve III affected.
§See also Figure 16-10.
‖Pupil not fully dilated as consensual input from OS causes some constriction.

LESIONS IN PATIENTS WITH VISUAL AND PUPILLARY LIGHT REFLEX DEFICITS

Based on the results of the visual performance and PLR tests, patients with deficits may be divided into one of three categories:

- Blind patients with normal PLRs
- Blind patients with abnormal PLRs
- Visual patients with abnormal PLRs

This simple categorization is the first step in localizing the pathologic lesion (Table 16-2 and Figures 16-8 to 16-12). It assumes that ophthalmic examination did not reveal any pathology that would prevent light from reaching the retina (e.g., hyphema, cataract).

Lesions in Blind Patients with Normal Pupillary Light Reflexes

Based on the anatomy of the PLR pathway, the size of the pupils and their response to light are normal in blind animals with disease limited to the distal optic tract (after the afferent PLR fibers have diverged), LGN, optic radiations, and/or visual cortex (see dark green and dark orange pathways, Figures 16-2 and 16-3).

Bilateral cerebral lesions that cause blindness include prosencephalic hypoplasia with no cerebral hemispheres (calves), hydranencephaly (calves, lambs), cerebral contusion, cerebral edema (following trauma, postictal, or due to space-occupying lesions), viral encephalitis, thrombotic meningo-encephalitis (*Haemophilus somnus* in cattle), inflammatory diseases such as granulomatous meningoencephalitis (GME) in dogs and horses, metabolic disorders (hypoglycemia, hepatic encephalopathy), poisonings, and nutritional and storage diseases. These diseases are discussed at the end of the chapter (see Diseases of the Central Visual Pathways).

The most common causes of a *unilateral* cerebral lesion with contralateral visual deficit are neoplasms in small animals and abscesses in large animals. Others are cerebral infarction (most common in cats), protozoan encephalitis in horses, chronic canine distemper encephalitis, *Toxoplasma* granulomas,

GME in dogs, thrombotic meningoencephalitis in cattle, and parasitic cysts (coenurosis in sheep) or migrations. These diseases are discussed at the end of this chapter (see Diseases of the Central Visual Pathways).

Lesions in Blind Patients with Abnormal Pupillary Light Reflexes

As can be seen in Figures 16-2, 16-3, and 16-5, the afferent fibers of the PLR and visual signal run together from the retina through the optic nerve, optic chiasm, and proximal optic tract, diverging just before the LGN (see light green and light orange pathways in these figures). Minor lesions in this common pathway (e.g., early retinal degeneration) may cause visual deficits without affecting the PLR. This is because, as noted earlier, the PLR is resistant to deficits in afferent input. Therefore if a lesion in this common pathway is significant enough to cause a pupillary abnormality, it usually also causes blindness. Conversely, if the eye is blind due to an afferent lesion, the PLR is almost always abnormal (though not necessarily absent). As a rule, afferent lesions that interrupt this pathway occur in the retina, optic nerve, or optic chiasm (see Figures 16-8 and 16-9). Rarely both proximal optic tracts are affected sufficiently to cause pupillary abnormalities, because the tracts are spread out over a relatively large area. A single optic tract lesion is rare and may cause no PLR abnormality (due to the crossover in the pretectal and oculomotor nuclei) (see Figure 16-10).

A patient with a *unilateral* lesion in the retina or optic nerve has no menace response in that eye. The pupil in that eye may be slightly larger (because it receives no direct parasympathetic stimulation from incident light), although it is not fully dilated (due to the indirect stimulation from the unaffected eye) (Figure 16-13). Light directed into the affected eye causes no response in either eye. Light directed into the unaffected eye elicits a bilateral response (see Figure 16-8). To assess direct and indirect responses, the examiner moves the light back and forth between the eyes. In an animal with a unilateral lesion, as the light is directed from the unaffected eye to the affected eye, the pupil in the affected eye dilates back to the resting

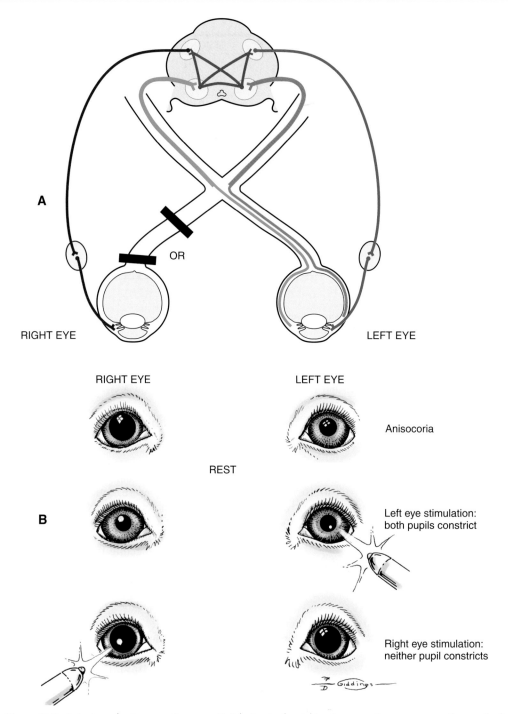

Figure 16-8. A, Lesion of retina or optic nerve. **B,** A lesion in the right retina or optic nerve causes the pupil of the right eye to be partially dilated. The pupil is not fully dilated due to consensual input from the left eye. Light stimulation of the left eye induces constriction of both pupils due to crossover in the chiasm and mesencephalon. Light stimulation of the right eye produces no change in either pupil because of the interference with the afferent (sensory) limb of the pupillary reflex in the right optic nerve.

state created by the room light (indirectly, through the unaffected eye). This is because the strong light source was taken away from the unaffected eye (thereby removing the indirect stimulation) and the lesion in the affected eye has interrupted the direct afferent pathway for this reflex. This phenomenon is readily apparent as the light is repeatedly moved between the eyes. Further confirmation of a unilateral lesion is made by covering the normal eye and observing further dilation of the pupil in the affected eye which is no

longer stimulated indirectly by room light through the normal, covered eye.

Common causes of *unilateral* lesions resulting in PLR and visual deficits include retinal detachment, glaucoma, and retrobulbar abscess or neoplasia. Trauma to the optic nerve is another common cause of unilateral lesions. The trauma may cause direct avulsion of the axons at the level of the optic canals or interference with the vascular supply of the intracanalicular part of the optic nerve. This problem may be

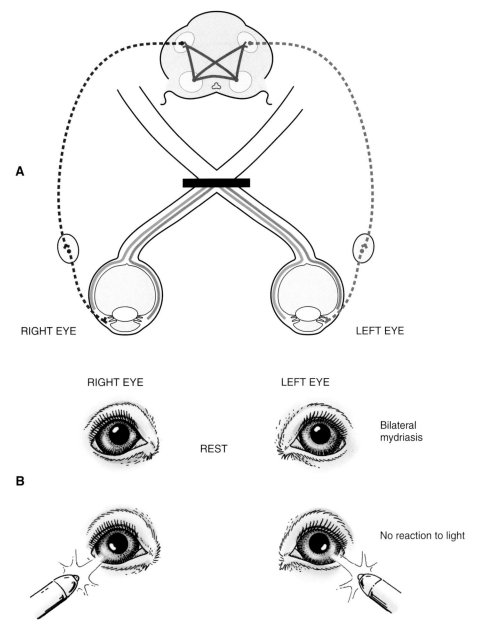

Figure 16-9. A, Lesion of the optic chiasm. **B,** A lesion of the optic chiasm causes resting bilateral mydriasis. Both pupils are unresponsive, as denoted by the dashed red and blue lines of the efferent limb of the PLR.

more common in horses and in brachycephalic dogs. Ophthalmoscopic examination often shows optic disc atrophy, with secondary retinal degeneration.

Severe *bilateral* retinal, optic nerve, or optic chiasm lesions cause blindness with dilated pupils that are unresponsive to light (see Figure 16-9). Bilateral retinal diseases include retinal detachment, end-stage retinal degeneration, SARD, and glaucoma. The most common optic nerve disease to affect vision and PLR is optic neuritis. The disease may be infective (e.g., distemper, cryptococcosis, toxoplasmosis) or inflammatory (GME) though it is frequently idiopathic in nature. It can affect both optic nerves and the optic chiasm, and the patient presents with blindness and fixed, dilated pupils (optic neuritis is discussed under Diseases of the Optic Nerve). In young cattle, vitamin A deficiency may cause optic nerve

compression from stenosis of the optic canals. Rarely in cats does ischemic encephalopathy syndrome result in infarction of the optic chiasm.

The optic chiasm may be compressed by extramedullary space-occupying lesions near the hypophyseal fossa. Pituitary neoplasms are the most common tumor in this site, although meningiomas and germ cell neoplasms (teratomas) have also been reported. The latter are more common in dogs younger than 5 years. Diseases of the optic nerve and chiasm are discussed further at the end of the chapter (see Diseases of the Central Visual Pathways).

A retrobulbar or intracranial lesion that affects both the optic nerve and the parasympathetic part of the oculomotor nerve causes a widely dilated pupil in the ipsilateral eye at rest (see Figures 16-8 and 16-11). Because of CN II involvement there

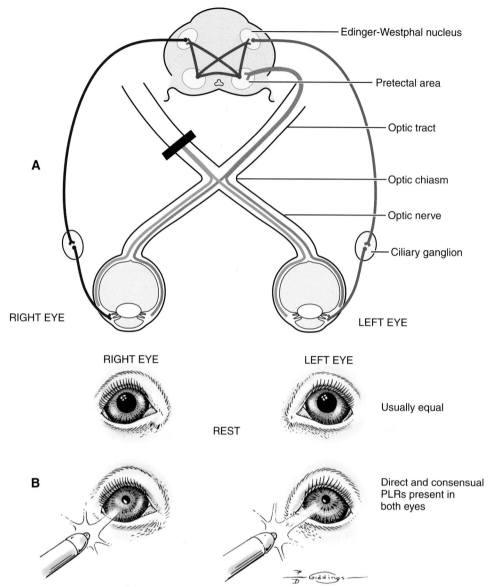

RIGHT EYE — Edinger-Westphal nucleus

LEFT EYE — Pretectal area

— Optic tract

— Optic chiasm

— Optic nerve

— Ciliary ganglion

A

RIGHT EYE

LEFT EYE

RIGHT EYE

LEFT EYE

Usually equal

REST

B

Direct and consensual
PLRs present in
both eyes

Figure 16-10. A, Lesion of the optic tract. **B,** A lesion of the right optic tract causes equal resting pupils, and light directed into either eye will cause constriction of both pupils. This is because crossover of fibers in both the optic chiasm and mesencephalon provides efferent innervation to both pupils.

is no menace response from this affected eye, and light directed into the affected eye elicits no response in either eye. Light directed into the unaffected eye causes pupillary constriction only in that eye (due to CN III lesion in the affected eye). In addition to loss of PLR, a complete oculomotor nerve deficit will also cause ventrolateral strabismus and ptosis due to denervation of four extraocular muscles and the levator palpebral muscle. However, lesions that involve only the oculomotor nerve, and do not affect vision, may also occur. These are discussed later (see Lesions Causing Pupillary Light Reflex Abnormalities in Visual Patients).

Pupils in Patients with Intracranial Injury

Pupillary abnormalities are common after intracranial trauma. They may also accompany severe acute brain lesions such as those found in polioencephalomalacia and lead poisoning in ruminants. Evaluation of the size of the pupils is important to the assessment both of the location and extent of brain

damage from intracranial injury and to evaluate the response to therapy. Pupil size and prognosis in intracranial injury are shown in Table 16-3.

Brainstem contusion with hemorrhage and laceration of the midbrain and pons is a common sequel of trauma. The parenchymal components of the oculomotor neurons are interrupted, causing both pupils to be widely dilated and unresponsive, a grave sign. Affected animals are also recumbent and semicomatose or comatose. Severe caudal brainstem lesions that are life threatening also result in partly dilated, fixed, unresponsive pupils.

Injuries that predominately involve the prosencephalon often result in very miotic pupils. Severe bilateral miosis is a sign of acute, extensive brain disturbance that by itself is not necessarily of any localizing value. The return of the pupils to normal size and response to light is a favorable prognostic sign and indicates recovery from the brain disturbance, especially following trauma. However, progression from bilateral miosis to bilateral mydriasis with fixed pupils that are unresponsive to

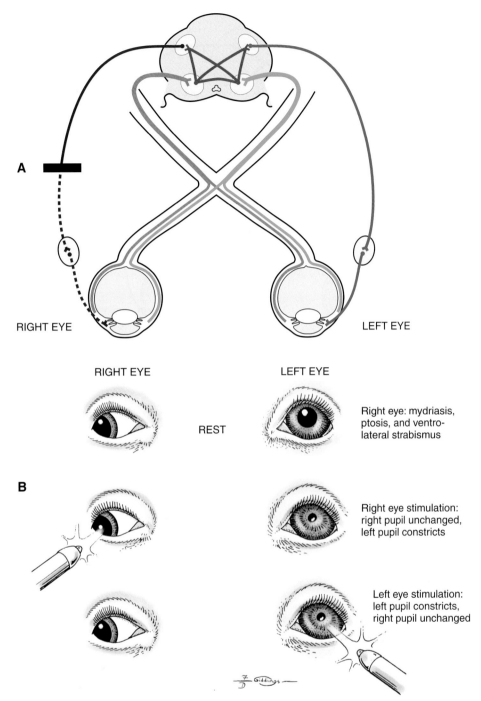

RIGHT EYE   **LEFT EYE**

REST

Right eye: mydriasis, ptosis, and ventro-lateral strabismus

Right eye stimulation: right pupil unchanged, left pupil constricts

Left eye stimulation: left pupil constricts, right pupil unchanged

Figure 16-11. A, Lesion of the oculomotor nerve. **B,** A lesion of the right oculomotor nerve causes ipsilateral mydriasis because of denervation of the iris sphincter (denoted by dashed red line). There is ptosis of the upper eyelid (note smaller palpebral fissure compared with left eye) due to denervation of the levator palpebral muscle. Ventrolateral strabismus (exotropia) owing to denervation of the dorsal, ventral, and medial recti muscles and the ventral oblique muscle is also evident. There is no direct pupillary reflex, but the consensual reflex to the left eye is normal. When the light is directed into the left eye, the direct pupillary reflex is normal, but the consensual reflex to the right eye is absent.

light in trauma cases indicates that the brain disturbance (e.g., hemorrhage, edema) is advancing and the oculomotor neurons in the midbrain are nonfunctional (Figure 16-14). This progression often accompanies severe contusion of the midbrain with hemorrhage, usually along the midline, which may cause brain swelling and herniation of the occipital lobes ventral to the tentorium cerebelli, accompanied by compression and displacement of the midbrain or oculomotor nerve (or both).

The cause of unilateral or bilateral miotic pupils in acute brain disease is not known. It probably represents facilitation of the oculomotor parasympathetic neurons released from higher-center inhibition owing to its functional disturbance. Pupillary changes may take place hourly after head trauma. Unilateral mydriasis that in some cases may be accompanied by miosis of the other pupil is probably brought about by compression of the ipsilateral oculomotor nerve; the pupils, though anisocoric, may be slightly reactive.

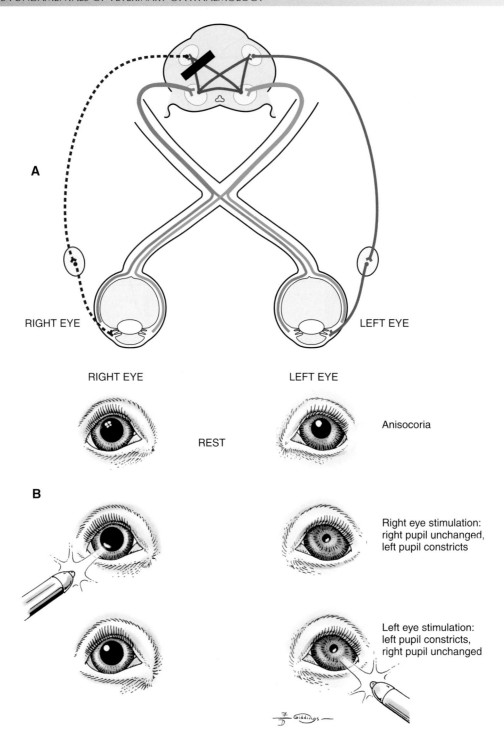

Figure 16-12. A, Lesion of the oculomotor (Edinger-Westphal) nucleus. **B,** A lesion in the right Edinger-Westphal nucleus causes a widely dilated, resting right pupil. There is no direct pupillary reflex in the right eye (as denoted by dashed red line), but the consensual pupillary reflex to the left eye is normal. In the left eye, the direct pupillary reflex is normal, but the consensual pupillary reflex to the right eye is absent.

Experiments in dogs have shown that compression of the brainstem tectum at the level of the rostral colliculus causes miosis. Compression of CN III produces mydriasis.

Lesions Causing Pupillary Light Reflex Abnormalities in Visual Patients

Abnormalities in pupillary constriction that are not accompanied by visual deficits localize the lesion to the oculomotor nerve after it has exited the mesencephalon. As noted previously, the oculomotor nerve provides (1) somatic efferent innervation to the dorsal, medial, and ventral recti muscles, the ventral oblique muscle, and the levator palpebral muscles and (2) parasympathetic innervation to the iridal sphincter. Both functions may be affected by lesions to the nerve. Therefore such a patient will present with three clinical signs (see Figure 16-11):

- A fixed, dilated pupil, due to loss of parasympathetic innervation to the iris sphincter. This sign is also called *internal ophthalmoplegia.*
- Ventrolateral strabismus, due to loss of innervation to the dorsal, medial and ventral recti and the ventral oblique muscles. This sign is also called *external ophthalmoplegia.*
- Ptosis of the upper eyelid, due to loss of innervation to the levator palpebral muscle

Common sites for lesions of the oculomotor nerve are the cavernous sinus or orbital fissure. Therefore tumors or inflammations at these sites cause *cavernous sinus syndrome* and *orbital fissure syndrome*, respectively. Because CNs IV, V, and VI also pass through these sites, both syndromes are also characterized by deficits in the function of these nerves.

It is possible for patients with oculomotor nerve lesions to present with internal ophthalmoplegia, indicating loss of parasympathetic oculomotor function, without loss of innervation to the eyelid and extraocular muscles. In other words, these patients will present with fixed, dilated pupils but no strabismus or ptosis. This presentation is possible because of the topographical arrangement of the fibers in CN III: The parasympathetic fibers are superficial and medial to the motor fibers. Therefore compression during midbrain swelling or displacement may affect the former but not the latter.

Fixed, dilated pupils caused by parasympathetic denervation are also a characteristic sign of dysautonomia. Because patients also suffer from concomitant sympathetic denervaiton, the disease is discussed later in this chapter.

Additional Causes of Pupillary Light Reflex Abnormalities
PLR abnormalities and anisocoria may also be caused by several processes that are unrelated to neurologic disease:

- Iris degeneration with atrophy causes ipsilateral mydriasis with a variable response to light (sometimes none). This is more common in older animals.
- Glaucoma causes ipsilateral mydriasis as increased intraocular pressure paralyzes the pupillary sphincter.

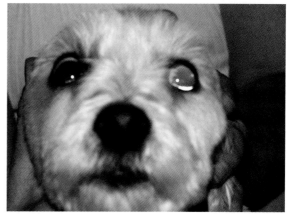

Figure 16-13. Unilateral mydriasis due to an old trauma that caused sectioning of the left optic nerve.

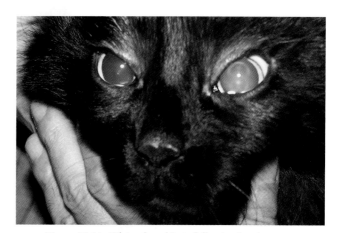

Figure 16-14. Bilateral mydriasis following head trauma.

Table 16-3 | **Pupillary Reactions in Intracerebral Injury**

CONDITION	PUPIL SIZE	PROGNOSIS
Unilateral oculomotor nuclear or nerve contusion or compression*	Anisocoria	Guarded
Compression of midbrain tectum†	Bilateral miosis	Guarded
Bilateral oculomotor nuclear or nerve contusion or compression	Bilateral mydriasis	Grave

*Asymmetric interference with cerebral control of oculomotor neurons or the sympathetic upper motor neuron system, or both.
†Bilateral sympathetic upper motor neuron deficiency or release of oculomotor parasympathetic neurons from cerebral inhibition.

Therefore there is no direct or indirect PLR in the affected eye. The consensual reflex to the contralateral eye is often lacking, because sustained elevation of intraocular pressure also damages retinal function.

- Anterior uveitis causes stimulation and spasms of the pupillary constrictor and ciliary muscles, resulting in miosis. Alternatively, anterior uveitis may cause posterior synechia, thus affecting pupil motility.
- Ocular disorders causing pain (e.g., keratitis) induce activation of the oculopupillary reflex. Therefore ocular pain leads to ipsilateral miosis due to spasms of the ciliary and iridal muscles.

- Feline leukemia virus infection occasionally results in static anisocoria. An RNA virus has been found in the short ciliary nerves and ciliary ganglia of some cats with this condition.

LESIONS CAUSING STRABISMUS

Function of the Extraocular Muscles

Innervation and action of the extraocular muscles are summarized in Figure 16-15 and Table 16-4. The globe has three axes of rotation, and the muscles are grouped into three opposing pairs. Each muscle in the pair acts in a reciprocal manner with its partner, similar to flexor and extensor muscles in the limbs.

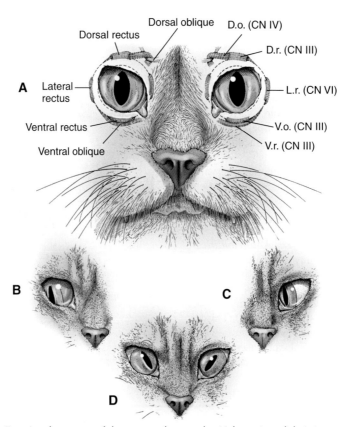

Figure 16-15. A, Functional anatomy of the extraocular muscles (right eye), and their innervation (left eye). **B,** Paralysis of the oculomotor nerve results in ventrolateral strabismus (exotropia) due to denervation of the ventral, medial, and dorsal recti muscles and the ventral oblique muscle. Upper lid and pupillary constriction are also affected (not shown). **C,** Paralysis of the abducent nerve causes denervation of the lateral rectus muscle (as well as the retractor bulbi muscle), causing medial strabismus (esotropia). **D,** Paralysis of the trochlear nerve causes denervation of the dorsal oblique muscle, resulting in dorsolateral strabismus which is especially noticeable in cats (that have a vertical pupil) and large animals (that have a horizontal pupil). (Modified from de Lahunta A [1983]: Veterinary Neuroanatomy and Clinical Neurology, 2nd ed. Saunders, Philadelphia.)

Table 16-4 | **Extraocular Muscles: Innervations and Actions**

MUSCLE	INNERVATION	ACTION
Superior (dorsal) rectus	Oculomotor (CN III)	Elevates globe (rotates upward)
Inferior (ventral) rectus	Oculomotor (CN III)	Depresses globe (rotates downward)
Medial rectus	Oculomotor (CN III)	Turns globe nasally (adduction)
Lateral rectus	Abducens (CN VI)	Turns globe temporally (abduction)
Superior (dorsal) oblique	Trochlear (CN IV)	Intorts globe (rotates 12 o'clock position nasally)
Inferior (ventral) oblique	Oculomotor (CN III)	Extorts globe (rotates 12 o'clock position temporally)
Retractor bulbi	Abducens (CN VI)	Retracts globe

CN, Cranial nerve.

Such a pair of extraocular muscles is termed *yoke muscles*. When the two eyes move in the same direction the movement is called *conjugate*. Around a horizontal axis, passing transversely through the center of the globe, the medial rectus muscle *adducts* and the lateral rectus muscle *abducts* the globe. Around the anterior-posterior axis, through the center of the globe, the dorsal oblique *intorts* the globe (rotates the dorsal portion medially toward the midline), and the ventral oblique *extorts* the globe (moves the same point laterally away from the midline). The dorsal and ventral rectus muscles rotate the globe dorsally and ventrally, respectively.

The extraocular muscles of both eyes do not function independently. Rather, they act together in a synergistic or antagonistic manner to provide conjugate movements of the two eyes in the same direction at the same time. This is demonstrated, for example, by the action of the medial and lateral rectus muscles in horizontal conjugate movement. When the eyes move conjugately to the right, facilitation of abducent neurons to the lateral rectus of the right eye and inhibition to those of the left eye are required in conjunction with inhibition of the oculomotor neurons to the medial rectus of the right eye and facilitation to those of the left eye. The *medial longitudinal fasciculus* (MLF) functions in coordinating this activity.

Functions of the extraocular muscles in domestic animals do not compare exactly with those in humans because of anatomic differences in the position of the eye with respect to the muscle insertion. Another difference between humans and animals is the presence of a retractor bulbi muscle, which is present in many mammalian species (but absent in birds and reptiles). As the name implies, this muscle, innervated by CN VI, is responsible for retracting the globe in response to pain or threats.

Lesions Causing Strabismus

Strabismus, an abnormal position of the eye, results from lesions of the nuclei or cranial nerves that innervate the striated extraocular muscles (CNs III, IV, and VI). It may also occur in some head positions with lesions in the vestibular system. When a strabismus is suspected, the eye movements are tested to verify the paralysis of the extraocular muscles. The head of the patient is moved vertically or horizontally while symmetry of ocular movements is evaluated. Movements of the head require a simultaneous conjugate response by both eyes to maintain fixation on objects in the visual field. The vestibular and cervical proprioceptive systems exert considerable influence on the nuclei of the cranial nerves that innervate the extraocular muscles in order to move the eyes so that they remain fixated on the visual target. One of the major pathways involved in connecting the vestibular system to these nuclei is the MLF.

Lesions of the vestibular system or MLF may cause an abnormal ocular position when the head is in certain positions. This appears as strabismus but usually can be corrected by repositioning of the head (see following section). Strabismus resulting from faulty extraocular muscle innervation persists in *all* positions of the head.

It should be remembered that strabismus may be also be caused mechanical and muscular disorders within the orbit that restrict movement of the globe. Common causes include tearing of extraocular muscles following traumatic proptosis, and orbital fractures that cause incarceration of muscles.

Strabismus due to Disorders of the Vestibular System

Strabismus that occurs only in certain positions of the head indicates lesions in the vestibular system. It can occur peripherally with lesions in the inner ear and vestibulocochlear nerve (CN VIII) or centrally with lesions in the vestibular nuclei of the medulla or vestibular pathways in the cerebellum. The strabismus involves the eye on the same side as the vestibular abnormality, is usually a ventrolateral strabismus, and is present with only some positions of the head. It is most evident when the head and neck are extended. Normally, in small animals, both eyes elevate and remain in the center of the fissures so that no sclera is visible. This normal ocular elevation is less obvious in horses and least in cattle. In vestibular disease the eye on the affected side fails to elevate normally in the palpebral fissure. Sclera is evident dorsally in the "drooped" eye. The ventrolateral strabismus associated with vestibular disease can be differentiated from the strabismus of an oculomotor nerve lesion based on of the presence of abnormal nystagmus and signs of vestibular system disturbance in the former. Furthermore, in oculomotor nerve lesions there is inability to adduct the eye normally on testing of normal nystagmus, as well as ptosis and mydriasis. (Nystagmus and lesions to the vestibular system are further discussed later, under Vestibular System.)

Strabismus due to Lesions in Innervation of the Extraocular Muscles

OCULOMOTOR PARALYSIS. Lesions of the oculomotor nucleus, or oculomotor nerve lesions, cause a lateral and slightly ventral strabismus— *exotropia*—primarily from loss of innervation of the medial rectus and secondarily from the denervation of the dorsal and ventral recti muscles and the ventral oblique muscle (see Figures 16-11 and 16-15, *B*). There is experimental evidence to support the direction of this strabismus, although it is difficult to explain the ventral deviation on the basis of the anatomy of the oblique muscle. Due to the lesion, eye adduction is deficient due to denervation of the medial rectus muscle. This can be observed on testing of normal vestibular nystagmus: As the head is moved in a dorsal plane, side to side, the eyes normally develop a jerk nystagmus with the quick phase in the direction of the head movement. The jerklike movement toward the nose is adduction resulting from contraction of the medial rectus innervated by the oculomotor nerve (CN III). This adduction, as well as lid opening and pupillary constriction, will be reduced by lesions to CN III.

Ptosis, ventrolateral strabismus, and a dilated, unresponsive pupil accompany a complete loss of oculomotor nerve function.

Causes of oculomotor nerve dysfunction were discussed in previous sections (see Pupils in Patients with Intracranial Injury and Lesions Causing Pupillary Light Reflex Abnormalities in Visual Patients). Depending on the location of the lesion, patients may present with or without other CNS and visual deficits.

Exotropia may also be seen in hydrocephalic animals that have an enlarged cranial cavity. Both eyes often deviate ventrolaterally, and therefore the syndrome is called *sunset eyes*. This abnormality is thought to result from a malformation of the orbit that occurs when the cranial cavity is distorted by the early development of the brain abnormality. The eyes adduct and abduct normally on testing of normal vestibular nystagmus, and no ptosis or pupillary abnormality is present. Therefore this exotropia is not related to oculomotor dysfunction.

ABDUCENT PARALYSIS. Lesions of the abducent nucleus or nerve cause paralysis (palsy) of the lateral rectus and retractor bulbi muscles. Paralysis of the *retractor bulbi* muscle prevents the eye from retracting in response to a threatening gesture. This can be tested by performing the menace test while holding the upper eyelid open. Globe retraction and the resulting third eyelid elevation may be observed in a normal animal. Paralysis of the *lateral rectus* muscle causes unilateral *esotropia* (medial strabismus), resulting in asymmetry (see Figure 16-15, *C*). Compared with the normal eye, the affected eye cannot be abducted fully. The clinician can detect this difference by moving the patient's head from side to side in a horizontal plane and observing the extent of abduction and adduction of each eye.

TROCHLEAR PARALYSIS. Lesions of the trochlear nucleus or nerve paralyze the dorsal oblique muscle, causing dorsolateral strabismus. In species with a round pupil, such as the dog, it is difficult to detect this type of strabismus; however, ophthalmoscopic examination may show that the superior retinal vein is deviated laterally from its normal vertical position because of the abnormal rotation caused by the tone in the unopposed ventral oblique muscle. In cats, which have vertical pupils, the dorsal aspect of the pupil deviates laterally with a lesion of the trochlear neurons (see Figure 16-15, *D*). In cattle and sheep, which have horizontal pupils, the medial portion of the pupil is deviated dorsally (Figure 16-16). Trochlear nerve (CN IV) lesions are rare. This abnormality is seen in polioencephalomalacia in ruminants and is thought to represent a unique susceptibility of the trochlear neurons to this metabolic encephalopathy.

LESIONS CAUSING EYELID ABNORMALITIES
Third Eyelid Abnormalities

Normally the mammalian third eyelid is kept in its position ventromedial to the eye by the tone in its smooth muscle, which keeps it retracted. This is a function of its sympathetic innervation. The normally protruded position of the eye in the orbit also contributes to the normal position of the third eyelid.

The third eyelid may protrude for a number of reasons. Except possibly in the cat, this protrusion is a passive event. The third eyelid protrudes passively when the globe is retracted actively by the retractor bulbi (CN VI). In the cat, slips of

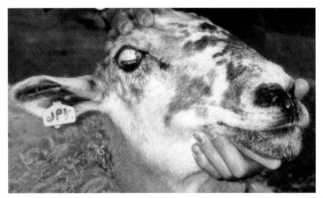

Figure 16-16. Infection with *Listeria monocytogenes* caused ventrolateral strabismus in this sheep. (Courtesy Merav H. Shamir.)

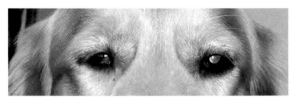

Figure 16-17. Horner's syndrome in this golden retriever presents with third eyelid prolapse, miosis, and ptosis of the upper lid in the right eye. No primary cause was diagnosed, and the syndrome was defined as idiopathic, which is a common condition in this breed.

striated muscle from the lateral rectus and levator palpebrae superioris attach to the two extremities of the membrane and may contract and contribute actively to this protrusion.

Protrusion of the Third Eyelid

Protrusion of the third eyelid is a typical feature of the following diseases:

HORNER'S SYNDROME. A constant partial protrusion of the third eyelid occurs in Horner's syndrome because of loss of the sympathetic innervation of the smooth muscle that normally keeps it retracted (Figure 16-17). The syndrome is discussed separately later in this chapter.

TETANUS. Brief, rapid, passive protrusions ("flashing") of the third eyelid occur in tetanus owing to the effect of tetanus toxin on neurons that innervate the extraocular muscles. This effect causes brief contractions of the muscles, especially if the animal is startled. Contraction of the retractor bulbi muscle causes passive flashing of the third eyelid. The reaction is most noticeable in horses but also occurs in other species.

FACIAL PARALYSIS. In an animal with facial paralysis the orbicularis oculi is paralyzed and the efferent branch of the menace response is interrupted, preventing the blinking response to a threatening gesture. However, in response to the menace the globe is retracted, causing a brief rapid protrusion of the third eyelid. Facial paralysis is discussed separately later in this section. Paralysis of the orbicularis oculi with ventral relaxation of the lower lid may also make the third eyelid appear protruded in cases of CN VII paralysis even though it is actually in its normal position.

"HAWS SYNDROME." The so-called haws syndrome in cats consists of bilateral protrusion of the third eyelid. The condition is sometimes associated with diarrhea and loose stools, but in most cases the cause is unknown and the syndrome is classified as idiopathic. It has been proposed that haws syndrome is due to an imbalance in sympathetic and parasympathetic tone—that is, a decrease in sympathetic tone, causing the protrusion of the third eyelid, and an increase in parasympathetic tone. In some cases, the latter may cause greater intestinal motility, shorter fecal passage time, and diarrhea. A torovirus-like agent has also been proposed. The syndrome may persist for 4 to 6 weeks but is usually self-limiting. Protrusion of the third eyelid may be treated symptomatically with topical sympathomimetics (1% phenylephrine solution) though this is usually not required. If diarrhea is present, it also is treated symptomatically.

DYSAUTONOMIA. Bilateral protrusion of the third eyelids occurs in dysautonomia because of sympathetic denervation. However, the patient's pupils are dilated in dysautonomia (due to parasympathetic denervation), thus distinguishing the disease from Horner's syndrome, in which the patient presents with third eyelid protrusion and pupillary constriction. The syndrome is discussed separately later in this chapter.

CONGENITAL MYOTONIA. This is an inherited disease of dogs and cats, characterized by persistence of active muscle contraction after the stimulation or voluntary movement has stopped. Bilateral protrusion of the third eyelids is one of the clinical signs associated with the disease.

NONNEUROGENIC CAUSES. Several nonneurogenic processes may cause prolapse of the third eyelid. Severe dehydration or emaciation are common causes of bilateral prolapse; decrease in the amount of orbital tissue causes enophthalmos, resulting in passive prolapse of both third eyelids. Enophthalmos and secondary third eyelid prolapse may also be caused by atrophy of the orbital fat or the temporal and pterygoid muscles after trauma or inflammation, and in senility. Paradoxically, an increase in the volume of orbital tissue (e.g., retrobulbar abscess, retrobulbar tumor) may cause protrusion of the third eyelid as the mass pushes the nictitating membrane. The resulting protrusion is usually unilateral.

Lesions Causing Abnormalities of the Palpebral Fissure

Innervation of the Upper Eyelid

In small animals, the size of the palpebral fissure primarily depends on normal tone in the levator palpebrae superioris muscle. This muscle is innervated by somatic efferent fibers of the oculomotor nerve (CN III), providing for elevation of the upper eyelid. Sympathetic tone to Müller's muscles of the eyelid helps maintain eyelid elevation. In large animals superficial facial muscles (e.g., the frontalis muscle) innervated by the facial nerve (CN VII) insert in the upper eyelid and help keep the fissure open.

Eyelid closure (blinking) is mediated by the orbicularis oculi muscle. It is innervated by the facial nerve, and its function is observed when the menace response is tested.

Lesions Increasing the Size of the Palpebral Opening

In small animals, the size of the palpebral fissure is basically unaffected by facial nerve paralysis, although it may be slightly larger because of loss of tone in the orbicularis oculi. Facial paralysis is discussed separately later in this chapter.

Occasionally in animals with serious cerebellar disease that involves the cerebellar nuclei, one palpebral fissure is slightly wider or one third eyelid is mildly elevated. These signs have also been produced experimentally with lesions in the nuclei of the cerebellum.

Lesions Decreasing the Size of the Palpebral Opening

A decrease in the size of the palpebral fissure is usually caused by *ptosis*, or drooping of the upper eyelid. Neurogenic causes include the following:

- A lesion in the oculomotor nucleus or nerve causes denervation of the levator palpebral superioris muscle, leading to ptosis. With complete oculomotor paralysis the ipsilateral pupil is dilated and is unresponsive to light directed into either eye (due to loss of parasympathetic innervation of the sphincter). There is also a lateral and slightly ventral

strabismus with decreased ability to adduct the eye normally because of denervation of the extraocular muscles (see Figure 16-11). Lesions were discussed previously under Oculomotor Paralysis.
- Horner's syndrome—sympathetic denervation causes loss of sympathetic tone to the levator palpebrae muscle, leading to ptosis. A lesion in the sympathetic innervation also produces enophthalmos, an elevated third eyelid, and miosis (see Figure 16-17). The syndrome is discussed separately later in this chapter.
- Facial nerve paralysis or paresis causes drooping of the upper eyelid in horses due to denervation of superficial facial muscles. Therefore the ptosis will be accompanied by inability to blink. Otitis media can affect facial neurons in all large animals, and rarely guttural pouch mycosis can involve such neurons in horses. Facial nerve paralysis is discussed in the next section.
- Hemifacial spasm—A narrowed palpebral fissure occurs with spasm of the facial muscles on one side.
- Tetanus
- A small palpebral fissure occurs following extensive atrophy of the muscles of mastication, as the eye retracts into the orbit. This atrophy can result from an extensive myositis of these muscles or from their denervation due to lesions of the mandibular nerve component of the trigeminal nerve.

Facial Nerve Paralysis

Lesions of the facial nucleus or the nerve up to the level of its termination into branches that supply the different muscle groups result in complete facial palsy or paralysis. Clinical signs of facial paralysis are as follows (Figure 16-18):

- *Facial asymmetry:* Paralysis is evident in the asymmetric position of the eyelids, lips, and nose. The palpebral fissure in affected small animals may be slightly wider than normal owing to paralysis of the orbicularis oculi. In large animals, the loss of tone in the frontalis muscle—which contributes fibers that elevate the upper eyelid—causes slight ptosis.

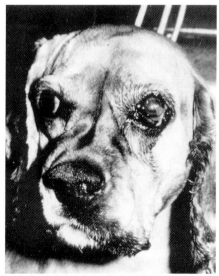

Figure 16-18. Unilateral facial paralysis (idiopathic) in a dog. Note the widened palpebral fissure, dry cornea, and drooping jaw. (Courtesy Dr. G.A. Severin.)

The ears may droop in those animals with normally erect ears, although if the ear cartilage is stiff, as in most cats and some dogs, it may keep the ear erect despite paralysis.

- *Drooling of saliva:* The lip may droop on the affected side, allowing saliva to drip from the corner of the mouth. It is helpful to extend the head with a finger between the mandibles and examine the corner of the lips for asymmetry. On the paralyzed side more mucosa is exposed, and drooling may be apparent.
- *Displacement of the nasal philtrum:* Acutely, the nose may be pulled toward the normal side, owing to the unopposed nasal muscles, especially in horses. In dogs there is slight deviation of the philtrum from its normal vertical position. During inspiration the nostril may not be opened as wide as usual on the affected side.
- *Lack of blinking:* In facial paralysis, eyelid closure is weak or absent. Lack of normal blinking, as well as absence of the menace response and the palpebral and corneal reflexes, is observed. In cases of suspected unilateral facial nerve paralysis, the eyelids of both sides are palpated simultaneously for strength of closure.
- *Corneal desiccation and ulceration:* Parasympathetic innervation to the lacrimal gland originates in the parasympathetic nucleus of the facial nerve (see Figure 16-6). These fibers run together with the motor fibers of the facial nerve till the genu. Therefore lesions to the facial nerve may also affect parasympathetic innervation to the lacrimal gland if they are located before the genu. In such cases, the patient will present with both facial paralysis and reduced tear production. Furthermore, as blinking is required to spread the tearfilm on the cornea, facial paralysis will cause desiccation of the cornea even if tear production is normal. In animals with chronic facial paralysis, dry eye and corneal ulceration may be the major clinical difficulty in management. These cases are not responsive to conventional dry eye therapy. If tear production is reduced because of lacrimal gland denervation, the patient may be treated with cholingergic drugs such as pilocarpine. Third eyelid flaps should be considered to prevent exposure of the cornea.

Lesions of individual branches of the facial nerve along their course produces paralysis restricted to the muscle groups innervated by those branches. Injury to the buccal branches of the facial nerve on the side of the masseter muscle causes the lips to droop and the nose to be pulled toward the normal side. This pattern is seen in horses that have been kept recumbent for surgery for prolonged periods without padding of the head. Eyelid and ear function is normal. On the other hand, injury to the auriculopalpebral nerve at the zygomatic arch causes paresis of the ear and eyelid muscles.

The facial and vestibulocochlear nerves are closely associated and may be affected by the same lesion in the medulla or in the petrosal bone. Both a medullary neoplasm and otitis media or interna can affect the function of these two cranial nerves at these two locations, respectively. It is important to distinguish between the two locations because of the poor prognosis for medullary lesions. Medullary lesions usually affect other brainstem structures, resulting in additional CNS signs that aid in localization of the lesion. Structures that may be affected by medullary neoplasms include the upper motor neuron, causing tetraparesis or hemiparesis; the ascending

Table 16-5 | **Frequency of Signs and Causes of Facial Paralysis**

FEATURE	% OF DOGS (79 CASES)	% OF CATS (16 CASES)
CAUSES		
Idiopathic	25	25
Surgery	9	13
Trauma	5	31
Neoplasia	2	25
Otitis media	—	6
Unknown	59	—
SIGNS*		
Neuropathy as the only sign	39	50
Associated signs:		
Hypothyroidism	25	—
Keratoconjunctivitis sicca	19	13
Otitis media	15	38
Horner's syndrome	15	25
Other cranial nerve neuropathies	8	—
Vestibular signs	7	88

Data from Kern TJ, Erb N (1987): Facial neuropathy in dogs and cats: 95 cases (1975-1985). J Am Vet Med Assoc 191:1604.
*Total of signs greater than 100% as some animals presented with more than one sign.

reticular activating system, resulting in signs ranging from depression to coma; and the abducent nucleus, causing esotropia. General proprioception may also be affected, resulting in ataxia. On the other hand, otitis may cause sympathetic denervation, in which case the clinical signs of facial and vestibulocochlear nerve dysfunction will be accompanied by signs of Horner's syndrome.

CAUSES OF FACIAL NERVE PARALYSIS. Frequency of the causes of facial nerve paralysis and associated disorders is shown in Table 16-5. In cats and horses, facial nerve paralysis is more commonly traumatic. In all species, otitis media involves the facial nerve as it passes through the facial canal in the petrosal bone, close to the tympanic bulla. The entire area of distribution of the facial nerve is usually affected by the resulting paresis or paralysis. Signs of vestibular ataxia and nystagmus are usually present, because the vestibulocochlear nerve in the inner ear is also involved. Lesions to the sympathetic fibers that pass near the middle ear will also cause concomitant signs of Horner's syndrome.

Injury to the petrosal bone may cause hemorrhage in the middle and inner ears and bleeding from the external ear canal through a ruptured tympanum, usually in association with fracture of the basioccipital or petrosal bone. Facial and vestibulocochlear nerve function may be affected. In guttural pouch mycosis in horses, extensive inflammation may cause paralysis of the adjacent facial nerve in addition to Horner's syndrome.

In dogs (and less commonly in cats) *permanent* or *temporary spontaneous facial paralysis* of unknown etiology occurs. Cocker spaniels, Pembroke corgis, boxers, and English setters are at greater risk, with dogs older than 5 years being predisposed. Temporary cases resolve within 4 to 6 weeks. Tarsorrhaphy, use of a third eyelid flap, and topical therapy may be necessary to prevent corneal dessication. An association with hypothyroidism *in some cases* has been confirmed in dogs.

LESIONS OF ADDITIONAL CRANIAL NERVES

Trigeminal Nerve Dysfunction

Sensory innervation to the eye, adnexa, and periocular region is via branches of the ophthalmic and maxillary nerves from the trigeminal nerve (CN V). Although the ophthalmic nerve branches are predominately medial and the maxillary are lateral, there is extensive overlap in the areas they innervate. The only autonomous zone of ophthalmic nerve innervation is a small area of skin dorsomedial to the medial angle of the eyelids. The only autonomous zone of the maxillary nerve innervation is ventrolateral to the lateral angle of the eyelids. Sensory deficits in the periocular skin will cause loss of the palpebral reflex, which is elicited by touching the medial and lateral canthi. Sensory deficits are uncommon compared with facial nerve paralysis and can be mistaken for it. However, animals with only a trigeminal nerve lesion blink spontaneously and when the eye is menaced, helping in the diagnosis.

The trigeminal nerve also provides sensory innervation to the cornea through long ciliary nerves originating in the ophthalmic branch. Loss of sensory innervation may cause corneal insensitivity, with resulting ulceration from local persistent minor trauma, or neurotrophic keratitis (see Chapter 10).

The most common cause of trigeminal nerve dysfunction is trauma. Bilateral mild injury (neurapraxia) of the mandibular branch has been seen in dogs after prehension of large objects. Bilateral disease of the trigeminal nerve motor neurons causes a drooped jaw that cannot be closed. The patient has difficulty grasping food or retaining it in the oral cavity. Manipulation of the jaw reveals muscle atonia, and neurogenic atrophy of the temporal muscles follows if paralysis persists. Unilateral disease may be difficult to discover until muscle atrophy appears. The lower jaw may be directed toward the side of the lesion by the unopposed tone in the normal pterygoids, and chewing may be asymmetric, although this abnormality is difficult to detect. The condition resolves spontaneously in 4 to 5 weeks if the dog is fed soft foods and the mandible is fastened to the maxilla. Recovery of the corneal reflex is slower than return of mandibular control. Lesions to the trigeminal nerve may also occur in conditions that affect multiple cranial nerves (see following section).

Multiple Cranial Nerve Disorders

Numerous conditions result in disorders of one or more of the nerves associated with the eye and adnexa. As mentioned previously (see Oculomotor Paralysis), neoplasms or inflammations in the orbital fissure or cavernous sinus may affect CNs III, IV, V, and VI. In cases of retrobulbar neoplasia or abscess, both CNs II and III may be affected. Numerous systemic diseases, including *Cryptococcus neoformans* infection, pseudorabies, GME, myasthenia gravis, listeriosis, equine focal protozoal encephalitis, and polioencephalomalacia in ruminants, may also cause multiple cranial nerve dysfunction. Some of these diseases are discussed in Chapter 18.

AUTONOMIC INNERVATION AND ABNORMALITIES

The autonomic nervous system is a physiologic and anatomic system with central and peripheral components. It consists of higher centers situated in the hypothalamus, midbrain, pons, and medulla. The hypothalamus is the primary integrating center for the autonomic nervous system. Nuclei in its rostral portion subserve the parasympathetic division of the autonomic system. These hypothalamic nuclei receive afferent input from the cerebrum (by numerous pathways), thalamic nuclei, and ascending general visceral afferent pathways. The hypothalamus influences the activity of the metabolic centers in the reticular formation of the midbrain, pons, and medulla.

In general, autonomic innervation is composed of two neurons interposed between the CNS and the organ innervated. The cell body of the first neuron is located in the gray matter of the CNS, and its axon passes through a cranial or spinal nerve to the peripheral ganglion, where it synapses with the cell body of the second neuron. The first neuron is therefore called the *preganglionic neuron.* The cell body and dendritic zone of the second neuron are in a peripheral ganglion, and its axon, the *postganglionic axon,* terminates in the innervated structure.

Anatomically and physiologically the autonomic system is grouped into two divisions. The *sympathetic system* (thoracolumbar) has cell bodies of preganglionic neurons in the intermediate gray column of the spinal cord from approximately the first thoracic to the fifth lumbar spinal cord segment. With few exceptions, the neurotransmitter released at the postganglionic axon in the sympathetic system is *norepinephrine* (Figure 16-19). The *parasympathetic system* (craniosacral) has cell bodies of preganglionic neurons in sacral segments of the spinal cord and in the nuclei of the brainstem associated with CNs III, VII, IX, and XI. The neurotransmitter released at the postganglionic axon in the parasympathetic system is *acetylcholine* (Figure 16-20).

Parasympathetic Lower Motor Neuron Innervation

The anatomy and diseases of the parasympathetic parts of the autonomic nervous system that pertain to the eye were discussed at the beginning of the chapter (see Pupillary Light Reflex and Lesions Causing Pupillary Light Reflex Abnormalities in Visual Patients).

Sympathetic Lower Motor Neuron Innervation

Preganglionic cell bodies are located in the first three segments of the thoracic spinal cord (see Figures 16-5 and 16-21). Their axons join the thoracic sympathetic trunk inside the thorax and pass *through* the cervicothoracic and middle cervical ganglia and forward in the cervical sympathetic trunk, as part of the vagosympathetic trunk. Ventromedial to the tympanic bulla, the cervical sympathetic trunk separates from the vagus and terminates in the *cranial cervical ganglion,* where the preganglionic axons synapse. The cell body of the postganglionic axon is in the cranial cervical ganglion.

The postganglionic axons for sympathetic ocular innervation in dogs and cats pass rostrally through the tympanooccipital fissure with the internal carotid artery and then between the tympanic bulla and the petrosal bone into the middle ear cavity, closely associated with the ventral surface of the petrosal bone. The axons continue rostrally between the petrosal and basisphenoid bones to join the trigeminal ganglion and ophthalmic nerve. The ophthalmic nerve enters the periorbita through the orbital fissure.

Postganglionic sympathetic axons are distributed together with ophthalmic nerve branches to smooth muscles of the orbit, Müller's muscle of the upper lid (and analogous sympathetically

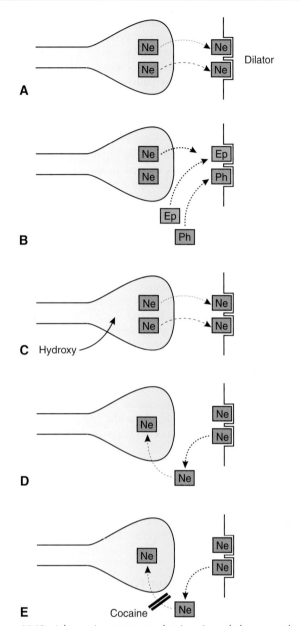

Figure 16-19. Adrenergic neuromuscular junction of the sympathetic system and actions of adrenergic agonists on the iris dilator. **A,** Norepinephrine *(Ne)* is released by axon terminal and binds to sites on iris dilator muscle, causing contraction. **B,** Epinephrine *(Ep)* and phenylephrine *(Ph)* are direct-acting adrenergic agonists that bind to those same sites on the iris dilator muscle, causing contraction. **C,** Hydroxyamphetamine *(Hydroxy)* is an indirect-acting adrenergic agonist that acts on nerve fiber, causing release of Ne. **D,** Once released from effector site, Ne is taken back up by nerve ending. **E,** Cocaine, an indirect-acting adrenergic agonist, prevents reuptake of Ne, allowing it to remain in the neuromuscular junction and rebind to the effector site. (From Remington LA [2005]: Clinical Anatomy of the Visual System, 2nd ed. Butterworth-Heinemann, St. Louis.)

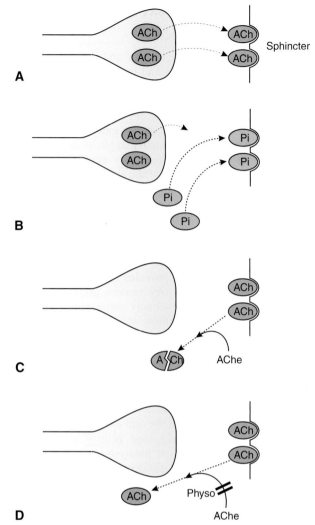

Figure 16-20. Cholinergic neuromuscular junction of the parasympathetic system and actions of cholinergic agonists on the iris sphincter. **A,** Acetylcholine *(ACh)* is released by the axon terminal and binds to sites on the iris sphincter muscle, causing contraction. **B,** Pilocarpine *(Pi)* is a direct-acting cholinergic agonist that binds to those sites on iris sphincter muscle, causing contraction. **C,** Once released from the effector site, ACh is broken down by acetylcholinesterase *(AChe)*, which prevents ACh from rebinding to site. **D,** Physostigmine *(Physo)* is an indirect-acting cholinergic agonist that inhibits AChe, allowing ACh to remain active in the neuromuscular junction. (From Remington LA [2005]: Clinical Anatomy of the Visual System, 2nd ed. Butterworth-Heinemann, St. Louis.)

Diseases of the Sympathetic System

HORNER'S SYNDROME

Clinical Signs. Loss of sympathetic innervation causes a lack of tone in the orbital smooth muscle and the eye retracts slightly, producing *enophthalmos.* Loss of tone in Müller's muscle in the upper eyelid causes slight narrowing of the palpebral fissure resulting from incomplete elevation of the upper lid *(ptosis).* As sympathetic tone contributes to maintaining the third eyelid in retracted position, denervation (combined with retraction of the eye) causes *protrusion of the third eyelid.* Lack of normal sympathetic tone in the pupillary dilator causes *miosis* and anisocoria (see Figure 16-17). These four signs, collectively called *Horner's syndrome,* are associated with lesions in any portion of the sympathetic pathway from the hypothalamus to the first three thoracic

innervated tissue in the lower lid), third eyelid, ciliary muscle, pupillary dilator, and receptors in the iridocorneal (drainage) angle (see Figures 16-6 and 16-21). The exact function of autonomic innervation in control of aqueous outflow facility in the drainage angle is unknown. Normal tone of sympathetically innervated ocular structures keeps the eye protruded, the palpebral fissure widened, the third eyelid retracted, and the pupil partially dilated.

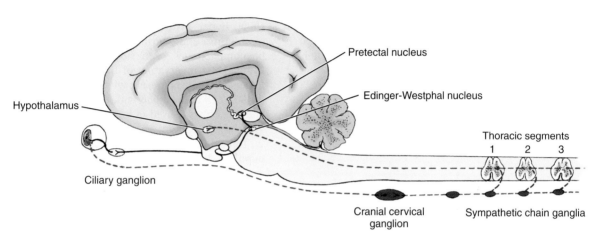

AUTONOMIC INNERVATION

SYMPATHETIC — Cranial nerve ganglion → Dilator pupillae muscle / Lacrimal gland

PARASYMPATHETIC — Ciliary ganglion via oculomotor nerve → Sphincter pupillae muscle / Ciliary muscle

Pterygopalatine ganglion via facial nerve → Lacrimal gland

Figure 16-21. The motor pathways to the iris: parasympathetic constrictor and sympathetic dilator. Preganglionic sympathetic cell bodies are located in the first three segments of the thoracic spinal cord (T1-T3). These preganglionic axons terminate in the *cranial cervical ganglion*. The postganglionic fibers pass between the tympanic bulla and the petrosal bone into the middle ear cavity, and continue to the eye, where they innervate the iris dilator muscle. Parasympathetic innervation of the eye originates in the pretectal cell bodies, which pass to the Edinger-Westphal (parasympathetic oculomotor) nucleus of both sides. Additional postganglionic sympathetic fibers synapse in the pterygopalatine ganglion and are distributed to the lacrimal acinar glands. The parasympathetic axons leave the mesencephalon with the motor axons of cranial nerve III, enter the orbit through the orbital fissure, and synapse in the ciliary ganglion. The postganglionic axons enter the globe adjacent to the optic nerve and innervate the pupillary constrictor and ciliary body muscles. (Modified from Hoerlein BF [1978]: Canine Neurology, 3rd ed. Saunders, Philadelphia.)

spinal cord segments to the effector muscle in the eye or orbit (see Figures 16-5 and 16-21).

In addition to signs of denervation of the iris dilator and orbital smooth muscle, *peripheral vasodilation* occurs and may cause increased warmth, pinkness of the skin best observed in the ear, and congestion of ipsilateral nasal mucosa. These signs may be difficult to detect, especially in small animals.

Preganglionic or postganglionic destruction of sympathetic innervation of the head in horses causes profuse sweating of the ipsilateral half of the face and cranial neck. The same area is hyperthermic, and the nasal and conjunctival mucosae are congested. Hyperthermia is determined by palpating the ears. There is a prominent ptosis of the upper eyelid, but only slight protrusion of the third eyelid and slight miosis. In cattle, sheep, and goats the most constant signs are hyperthermia detected on ear palpation, and ptosis. Miosis and third eyelid protrusion are subtle. In cattle *less sweating* is visible on the surface of the nose on the denervated side.

Etiology. Most cases of Horner's syndrome in dogs and cats are idiopathic. Golden retrievers are especially susceptible to idiopathic Horner's syndrome. Cases of idiopathic Horner's syndrome are usually postganglionic, and they resolve spontaneously within 6 to 8 weeks. Other causes should not be

Table 16-6 | **Frequency of Causes of Horner's Syndrome**

CAUSE	% OF DOGS (18 CASES)	% OF CATS (8 CASES)
Idiopathic	44	25.0
Car accidents	22	25.0
Bites	11	12.5
Cervical disc protrusion	11	—
Otitis media	6	—
Foreign body	—	12.5
Spinal neoplasia	—	12.5
Iatrogenic	6	12.5

Modified from van den Brock AHM (1987): Horner's syndrome in cats and dogs: a review. J Small Anim Pract 28:929.

dismissed, however. Based on the anatomic location of the lesion, the possible causes of Horner's syndrome are as follows (the frequency of the various causes in dogs and cats is listed in Table 16-6):

• Injury, infarction, or neoplastic involvement of the cranial thoracic spinal cord causes signs of paresis or paralysis of the pelvic limbs and deficits in the thoracic limbs, in addition to ipsilateral Horner's syndrome. Unilateral infarction of the lateral funiculus of the cervical spinal cord from fibrocartilaginous emboli may cause a persistent Horner's syndrome, along with hemiplegia, in dogs.

- Avulsion of the brachial plexus roots in dogs and cats, with resultant thoracic limb paralysis, occurs after car accidents. Ipsilateral Horner's syndrome indicates that the injury to the nerves innervating the thoracic limb is in or adjacent to the cranial thoracic spinal cord.
- Thoracic inlet or cranial mediastinal lesions (such as lymphosarcoma) involving the cranial thoracic sympathetic trunk, the caudal cervical sympathetic trunk, or both, may cause Horner's syndrome without additions CNS signs (unless the tumor invaded the spinal cord).
- Injury to the cervical sympathetic trunk from a dog bite or from surgical exposure causes an ipsilateral Horner's syndrome that is usually transient (Figure 16-22). Neoplasms involving the cervical sympathetic trunk, such as thyroid adenocarcinoma, are another cause.
- Mycosis of the guttural pouch in horses may involve the cranial cervical ganglion or internal carotid nerve and produce ipsilateral Horner's syndrome.
- Otitis media may produce Horner's syndrome often accompanied by signs of peripheral vestibular disturbance,

facial paresis, or both. There is a higher incidence of the syndrome after ear cleaning.

- Retrobulbar injury, neoplasia, and abscess are common causes of Horner's syndrome. Involvement of additional cranial nerves may cause blindness and strabismus.

Neurologic lesions causing Horner's syndrome, their location, and associated neurologic deficits are summarized in Table 16-7.

Diagnosis. *Denervation hypersensitivity* is a phenomenon peculiar to smooth muscle innervated by the general visceral efferent system. Following denervation there is increased sensitivity of the muscle to neurotransmitters. This is evident in smooth muscle innervated by sympathetic neurons when the postganglionic axon is affected. Such denervated muscle shows hypersensitivity to the application of epinephrine or to circulating epinephrine released during excitement. This phenomenon has been studied in dogs with lesions of the sympathetic innervation of the ocular smooth muscles. *Great hypersensitivity* is present with lesions of postganglionic axons or their cell bodies than with lesions of preganglionic neurons, and this effect is used in localizing the site of the lesion to the sympathetic system.

Topical application of 0.1 mL of 0.001% epinephrine causes pupillary dilation in 20 minutes with lesions of postganglionic axons or their cell bodies, and in 30 to 40 minutes with lesions of preganglionic neurons (see Figures 16-19 and 16-22).

Treatment. The most important task is to determine the site of the lesion in an animal with Horner's syndrome. In general, preganglionic lesions have a less favorable prognosis than postganglionic lesions. With postganglionic Horner's syndrome, in which an exact cause cannot be determined, symptomatic treatment may be instituted with phenylephrine drops (0.125% or 10%) as necessary to relieve the clinical signs. Most cases of postganglionic Horner's syndrome resolve spontaneously within 6 weeks. If the lesion is preganglionic, additional diagnostic procedures are undertaken to determine the site and cause, including neurologic examination and imaging (cervical and thoracic radiography; computed tomography or magnetic resonance imaging of the neck) (see Table 16-7). Because of the frequency of lymphosarcoma with cranial mediastinal lesions, thoracic radiographs are routinely taken in cats affected with Horner's syndrome.

DYSAUTONOMIA (KEY-GASKELL SYNDROME). Synonyms: Dilated pupil syndrome, feline autonomic polyganglionopathy.

Dysautonomia is an idiopathic disturbance of systemic autonomic innervation with a marked reduction in the number of neurons in autonomic ganglia, resulting in complete sympathetic and parasympathetic denervation of the eye (and other organs). The majority of affected animals are younger than 3 years. The disease was initially regarded as a feline syndrome, and it is still most common in the cat, but lately it has also been reported in clusters of dogs living in the American Midwest. The disease is of acute onset, with signs developing within 2 days in cats and 14 days in dogs.

Clinical Signs. Clinical signs of dysautonomia are as follows:

- Dilated unresponsive pupils
- Protrusion of the third eyelids
- Blepharospasm
- Keratoconjunctivitis sicca
- Dry, crusted nose

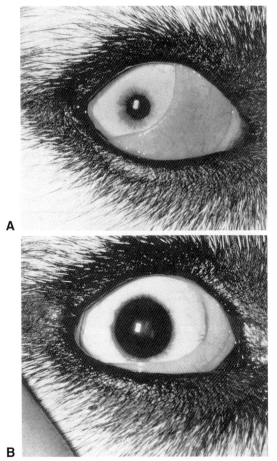

Figure 16-22. Preganglionic Horner's syndrome in the left eye of an Alaskan malamute. **A,** Before instillation of epinephrine. **B,** Mydriasis 35 minutes after application of 0.1 mL of 0.0001% epinephrine solution. The lesion was preganglionic and associated with trauma resulting from vigorous lunging on a chain. It resolved spontaneously in 5 to 6 weeks.

Table 16-7 | **Horner's Syndrome: Summary of Neurologic Lesions**

LOCATION	LESION	ASSOCIATED NEUROLOGIC DEFICIT
Cervical spinal cord	External injury Focal leukomyelomalacia (ischemic)	Tetraplegia—spastic Hemiplegia—ipsilateral, spastic
T1-T3 spinal cord	External injury Neoplasia Focal poliomyelomalacia (ischemic) Diffuse myelomalacia	Pelvic and thoracic limb paresis or paralysis with lower motor neuron deficit in thoracic limbs and upper motor neuron deficit in pelvic limbs Lower motor neuron deficit and analgesia of tail, anus, pelvic limbs, (ascending and descending) abdomen, and thorax with paretic thoracic limbs
T1-T3 ventral roots, proximal spinal nerves	Avulsion of roots of brachial plexus	Brachial plexus paresis or paralysis of the ipsilateral thoracic limb
Cranial thoracic sympathetic trunk	Lymphosarcoma Neurofibroma	None if confined to the trunk
Cervical sympathetic trunk	Injury from surgical intervention in the area, or from dog bites Neoplasm (thyroid adenocarcinoma)	None if unilateral; bilateral lesions interfere with laryngeal and esophageal function because of vagal involvement
Middle ear cavity	Otitis media	Signs of peripheral vestibular disturbance: ipsilateral ataxia, head tilt, nystagmus, and sometimes facial palsy or hemifacial spasm
Retrobulbar	Contusion Neoplasia	Varies with degree of contusion to the optic and oculomotor nerves, which also influences pupillary size

From de Lahunta A (1983): Veterinary Neuroanatomy and Clinical Neurology, 2nd ed. Saunders, Philadelphia.

- Dry oral mucous membranes and oral cavity
- Anorexia and lethargy
- Megaesophagus and difficulty in swallowing
- Vomiting/regurgitation
- Slow gastric emptying
- Fecal and urinary incontinence
- Bradycardia
- Distended bladder

Diagnosis. Dysautonomia is diagnosed from its clinical signs, especially *protrusion of the third eyelids with fixed, dilated pupils*. Together with the other signs, these two findings differentiate the disorder from Horner's syndrome, in which the denervation is limited to the sympathetic system, is usually unilateral and presents with miosis. Lack of the normal flare response in intradermal histamine injection has also been used for diagnosis of dysautonomia.

Pharmacologic testing can be used to demonstrate *denervation hypersensitivity* of both sympathetic and parasympathetic systems (see Figures 16-19 and 16-20). The principles are similar to the testing described for Horner's syndrome. The procedure consists of the following steps:

Demonstration of Parasympathetic Denervation. Parasympathetic denervation, which is also called Adie's pupil and pupillatonia, can be demonstrated as follows:

1. Instill a drop of 0.1% pilocarpine and measure pupillary diameter every 5 minutes. If denervation is present, the resulting miosis will occur much faster compared with a normal animal.
2. Instill a drop of 0.06% echothiophate iodide (phospholine iodide). The denervated eye will show no change in pupillary diameter, but miosis will occur in a normal eye.

Demonstration of Sympathetic Denervation. Instill one drop of 1:10000 epinephrine into the eye. The third eyelid will

retract in a denervated eye because of hypersensitivity of the orbital smooth muscle to the epinephrine.

Treatment. The prognosis is poor, and in cats the reported survival rate is only 25% to 50%. Many patients are euthanized owing to systemic complications. Treatment consists of the following approaches:

1. General supportive therapy, including subcutaneous and oral fluids.
2. Routine topical agents for keratoconjunctivitis sicca (KCS), including compound KCS drops and artificial tears.
3. Laxatives and prokinetic gastrointestinal drugs.

VESTIBULAR SYSTEM

The vestibular system maintains the position of the eyes, trunk, and limbs in reference to head position or movement. It consists of receptors and cell bodies in the vestibular ganglion in the petrosal bone (inner ear), axons in CN VIII, neurons in the vestibular nuclei of the cerebellum, and axons in the MLF. The MLF connects vestibular neurons with neurons in the brainstem nuclei that innervate extraocular muscles (CNs III, IV, and VI). Figure 16-23 illustrates prominent anatomic features of the system.

Nystagmus (Box 16-1)

Normal Vestibular Nystagmus

Nystagmus is an involuntary, rhythmic ocular movement, the aim of which is to keep the eyes fixated on a visual target as the head moves. The head movement induces impulses in the vestibular component of CN VIII by stimulating the receptors in the semicircular ducts of the inner ear. The afferent neuronal pathway that results in nystagmus continues through the vestibular nuclei in the medulla and via the MLF to the brainstem nuclei of CNs

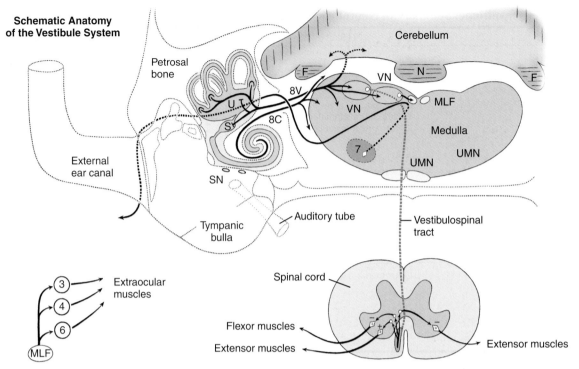

Figure 16-23. Anatomy of the vestibular system. *F,* Flocculus; *MLF,* medial longitudinal fasciculus; *N,* nodulus; *S,* saccule; *SN,* sympathetic neurons; *U,* utricle; *UMN,* upper motor neuron; *VN,* vestibular nucleus; *3,* oculomotor nucleus; *4,* trochlear nucleus; *6,* abducens nucleus; *7,* facial nucleus; *8C,* cranial nerve VIII, cochlear portion; *8V,* cranial nerve VIII, vestibular portion. The vestibular system consists of receptors and cell bodies in the vestibular ganglion in the *petrosal bone* (inner ear), axons in cranial nerve VIII, neurons in the vestibular nuclei of the cerebellum, and axons in the MLF. The MLF (located on both sides of the brainstem) connects vestibular neurons with neurons in the brainstem nuclei that innervate extraocular muscles (cranial nerves III, IV, and VI). (Modified from de Lahunta A [1983]: Veterinary Neuroanatomy and Clinical Neurology, 2nd ed. Saunders, Philadelphia.)

Box 16-1 | Characteristics of nystagmus

Normal

- Occurs with head movement
- Quick phase in same direction as head movement
- Horizontal plane → horizontal nystagmus
- Vertical plane → vertical nystagmus

Abnormal

- Occurs *spontaneously* or with head held flexed laterally or extended *(positional nystagmus)*
- *Peripheral receptor disease:* The nystagmus is either horizontal or rotatory (direction from 12 o'clock point on globe). Its quick phase is constantly to side opposite from lesion. The direction of the nystagmus does not alter when the head position changes.
- *Central vestibular disease* (pons, medulla, cerebellum): The nystagmus may be horizontal, rotary, or vertical. The quick phase may be in any direction, opposite from or toward side of lesion, or vertical. The quick phase varies in direction with different positions of the head.
- Quick phase varying in direction with different positions of the head
- *Lack* of any response to head movements or rapid rotation indicates severe bilateral receptor or severe brainstem disease.
- *Lack* of any response to cold water irrigation of *one* of the external auditory canals (caloric test) indicates a severe lesion in the receptor of that side.

III, IV, and VI, whose axons provide efferent innervation to the extraocular muscles (see Figure 16-23). Normal vestibular nystagmus is tested by slowly moving the patient's head from side to side and observing the limbus to note the resulting eye movement. This form of nystagmus has a *rapid phase in one direction and a slow phase in the other direction.*

The direction of nystagmus is defined by the direction of the rapid phase.

The rapid phase of the normal (physiologic) nystagmus is in the same direction as the movement of the head: Left movement causes left nystagmus, and ventral movement causes ventral nystagmus. Normal vestibular nystagmus occurs only as the head is being moved. Both eyes are affected and move simultaneously in conjugate fashion. Testing normal vestibular nystagmus evaluates the patient's ability to abduct and adduct each eye. The result is abnormal if nystagmus persists after the head movement is stopped or if the head is extended or flexed laterally and nystagmus develops in that position.

Lesions that destroy the vestibular system, the MLF, or neurons of CNs III, IV, and VI cause loss of normal vestibular nystagmus.

In neurologic evaluation after intracranial injury it is important to distinguish between signs of diffuse cerebral edema and of brainstem contusion. Loss of vestibular nystagmus indicates a severe lesion in the brainstem affecting the vestibular nuclei, MLF, or the nuclei of CNs III, IV, and VI.

Observation of ocular movements in normal nystagmus also allows evaluation of specific extraocular muscles. For example, signs of right abducent nerve paralysis are esotropia of the right eye and failure of the eye to abduct fully when the head is moved to the right.

Abnormal Nystagmus

When the head is flexed laterally to either side or extended fully, no nystagmus is normally found. In *vestibular disease,* nystagmus may be observed as follows:

- *Spontaneous nystagmus*: Present when the head is at rest
- *Positional nystagmus*: Present when an abnormal head position is induced

In *peripheral vestibular receptor disease* the nystagmus is either *horizontal* or *rotary,* and always in a direction (quick phase) away from the side of the lesion. The direction of rotary nystagmus is defined by the change in the dorsal limbus during the quick phase. This direction does not change when the position of the head is changed.

With *disease of the vestibular nuclei or vestibular pathways* in the cerebellum, the nystagmus may be *horizontal, rotary,* or *vertical* and may change in direction with position of the head; any of these types of nystagmus suggests central involvement of the vestibular system. However, in most cases it is impossible to further localize of the lesion based only on the nystagmus.

Peripheral receptor disease is suggested if the direction of nystagmus does not change when the position of the head is changed. Vertical nystagmus or nystagmus that changes direction when the position of the head is changed suggests a central disorder of the vestibular system.

Eye Position in Vestibular Disease

In vestibular disease, most postural reactions remain intact except for the righting response. Usually the patient experiences difficulty righting itself, with an exaggerated response toward the side of the lesion. When the head is extended in the tonic neck reaction, the eyes should remain in the center of the palpebral fissure in the dog and cat. This often fails to occur on the side of the vestibular disturbance, and resulting in a drooped or ventrally deviated eye.

In ruminants it is normal for the eyes to deviate ventrally with neck extension. In horses there is normally a slight ventral deviation, which is more pronounced in the eye ipsilateral to a vestibular system lesion. Occasionally in vestibular disease, an eye is deviated ventrally *(hypotropia)* or ventrolaterally without extension of the head and neck. This deviation appears as a lower motor neuron strabismus but can be corrected with movement of the head into a different position or with induction of the patient to move the eyes to gaze in different directions. It is referred to as a *vestibular strabismus.* The cranial nerves that innervate the extraocular muscles are not paralyzed. The ventrally deviated eye is on the side of the lesion in the vestibular system. Sometimes the other eye may appear to be deviated dorsally *(hypertropia).*

Disorders of the Vestibular System

Otitis Media and Otitis Interna

Otitis is the most common cause of pathologic nystagmus in animals. Vestibular signs occur in animals when middle ear inflammation indirectly or directly affects the function of the membranous labyrinth. Varying levels of unilateral vestibular disturbance appear, which consist of asymmetric ataxia with strength preservation. Sometimes only a head tilt and positional nystagmus are evident. If the inflammation spreads to the inner ear, these signs may be accompanied by an ipsilateral facial paresis or palsy, Horner's syndrome, or both. This is because of concurrent involvement of the facial and/or sympathetic nerves, which pass adjacent to or through the inner ear in the dog and cat (see Figures 16-5 and 16-6). Unilateral deafness may occur but is difficult to determine clinically.

Idiopathic Vestibular Disease (Feline Vestibular Syndrome, Idiopathic Benign Vestibular Disease, Old Dog Vestibular Disease)

This is a disease affecting dogs, cats, and horses. Patients present with head tilt and spontaneous nystagmus, with the fast phase opposite to the head tilt. The nystagmus is usually horizontal and occasionally rotatory. At onset a head oscillation may occur simultaneously with nystagmus. The disease is self-limiting, and after 3 or 4 days spontaneous nystagmus disappears, but abnormal positional nystagmus may still be elicited on altering the position of the head. The direction remains opposite to the head tilt.

Central Disorders

Signs of vestibular system disturbance referable to disease of the vestibular nuclei or their pathways are similar to those seen in diseases of the peripheral vestibular system.

Vestibular signs usually seen only with diseases of the central pathways are as follows:

- Vertical nystagmus
- Nystagmus that changes direction with different positions of the head
- Disconjugate nystagmus

The lesion is localized to the central pathways mostly because of the presence of signs that accompany the brainstem involvement of other functional systems.

The most common cause of central vestibular system pathology is GME. Infectious diseases affecting the central vestibular system include canine distemper, toxoplasmosis, monocytic ehrlichiosis, Rocky Mountain spotted fever, feline infectious peritonitis, and fungal diseases. In ruminants, *Listeria monocytogenes* causes inflammation of the brainstem with signs referable to this location, including vestibular disturbance.

Intracranial injury may also affect the central vestibular pathways in addition to other systems in the brainstem. The degree of vestibular disturbance manifested depends on the severity of disturbance to other systems, which may mask the vestibular disturbance. Abnormal nystagmus may be the only sign of vestibular disturbance evident in the tetraplegic, semicomatose patient.

Compression of the central vestibular system by tumors, toxicity (e.g., metronidzole overdose in dogs and cats) and thiamin deficiency may also cause pathologic nystagmus.

Congenital Nystagmus

Congenital nystagmus occurs in humans as an inherited functional abnormality or secondary to congenital lesions in the visual system of the infant. The nystagmus is usually pendular. Similar nystagmus has been described in dogs. In cattle *pendular nystagmus* occurs in the Holstein-Friesian, Jersey, Guernsey, and Ayrshire. It is significant for diagnostic purposes only and does not affect vision.

Congenital pendular nystagmus has also been reported in Siamese and albino cats. It is due to an abnormal crossover pattern of optic nerve fibers at the optic chiasm. The nystagmus and concurrent medial strabismus are believed to be an attempt by the cat to correct for the resulting abnormal projections to the visual cortex.

Congenital nystagmus occurs in young animals with severe visual deficits during the early postnatal period. These occur in animals born with significant corneal opacities or cataracts, in cases of neonatal retinal detachment or intraocular hemorrhage, or following lid suturing (third eyelid flaps or tarsorrhaphy) in young patients.

CENTRAL VISUAL PATHWAYS

Anatomy of the central visual pathways is discussed in Chapter 1 and was summarized at the beginning of this chapter (see Vision and the Menace Reponse and Figure 16-3)

Clinical Signs of Diseases of the Central Visual Pathways

The effects of diseases of the central visual pathways on the menace response and PLR have been discussed in detail in the beginning of the chapter (see Figures 16-8 to 16-12 and Table 16-2). Briefly, lesions that destroy the retina or optic nerve in one eye cause blindness and a partially dilated pupil in that eye (see Figures 16-8 and 16-13). The pupil is not fully dilated due to consensual input from the unaffected eye. The menace response and direct PLR are lost in the affected eye but are retained in the contralateral eye. The consensual PLR to the affected eye is normal, but the consensual PLR from the affected eye is absent. There are no other CNS signs. Total bilateral retinal, optic nerve, optic chiasm, or proximal optic tract destruction causes complete blindness, with both pupils widely dilated and unresponsive to light directed into either eye (see Figure 16-9). Retinal degeneration is the most common cause of this deficit.

Unilateral lesions in the distal optic tract, LGN, optic radiation, or visual cortex cause a visual deficit in the contralateral visual field (see Figure 16-10). As noted at the beginning of the chapter, in humans, where 50% of the optic nerve fibers cross over at the chiasm, the visual deficit affects 50% of the visual field in each eye. In domestic animals, where a larger percentage of fibers cross over at the chiasm, a unilateral lesion will cause a significant visual deficit in the eye contralateral to the lesion and a lesser deficit in the ipsilateral eye (see Figure 16-3). The deficit is pronounced from the temporal side (visual field) when there are contralateral lesions in the central visual pathway. In all postchiasmal unilateral lesions the PLR responses are usually normal because of decussation at the chiasm, pretectal area, and Edinger-Westphal nuclei.

Complete bilateral lesions in the optic tracts (after the afferent fibers of the PLR have diverged), LGN, optic radiations, or visual cortex produce total blindness with normal PLR. More often, however, the lesions are partial and clinical signs are difficult to determine. For example, canine distemper encephalitis often produces extensive lesions in the optic tracts without obvious clinical deficit of vision or pupillary functions.

The magnitude of visual deficit depends on location and extent of the lesion in the visual pathway.

Histopathologic Reactions of Visual Pathways to Disease

Nervous tissue is composed of three elements: neurons, neuroglia (astrocytes, oligodendrocytes, microglia), and vascular connective tissue (Figure 16-24). Neurons—for example, retinal ganglion cells (RGCs)—have large cell bodies with huge nuclei and prominent nucleoli. Dendrites conduct impulses toward the cell body—for example, RGC dendrites receive synaptic input from the midretina in the inner plexiform layer. Axons transmit impulses away from the cell body—for example, RGC axons constitute the fibers of the optic nerve, relaying the visual signal to the LGN. RGC axons in the nerve fiber layer of the retina have no myelin sheath as they converge on the optic disc. However, they are myelinated in the optic nerve by oligodendrocytes. Myelin in the optic nerve differs from that in peripheral nerves, in which Schwann cells (lemmocytes) form the myelin. Diseases affecting Schwann cells do not influence the optic nerve, and diseases that affect oligodendrocytes of the optic nerve do not affect peripheral nerve myelin.

Axoplasmic flow of metabolites and cell organelles occurs in both directions in the axon, to and from the cell body. Interruption of this flow in the optic nerve is significant in the pathogenesis of *papilledema* (see later).

Acute Neuronal Degeneration

Because neurons are specialized cells that have little ability to regenerate or proliferate, alterations seen are the result of degene-

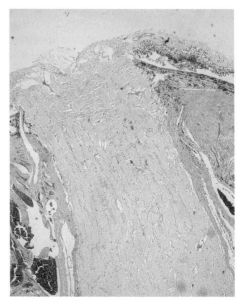

Figure 16-24. A histologic micrograph of the normal canine optic nerve in the lamina cribrosa region. The optic nerve is composed of axons of retinal ganglion cells and microglial and macroglial cells. (Hematoxylin & eosin stain.) (Courtesy Dr. Emmanuel Loeb.)

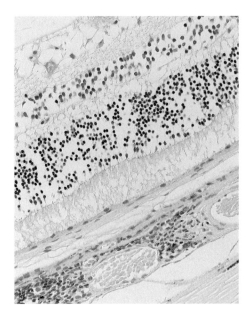

Figure 16-25. Histopathology micrograph showing inner retinal atrophy secondary to glaucoma in a dog. Note that except for a few degenerative nuclei, no ganglion cells can be observed in the inner retina *(right side)*. A marked, diffuse edema is also noted. (Hematoxylin & eosin stain stain.) (Courtesy Dr. Emmanuel Loeb.)

ration or necrosis (Figure 16-25). Severe, acute insults cause immediate damage and destroy the cell. The duration of the insult is more important than the cause. The sequence is as follows:

Acute insult → Swelling, fragmentation, and dissolution of cell bodies → Necrosis

Tissues become edematous or cystic and later collapse and shrink. There is minimal reactive proliferation, and remnants of disintegrating RGCs are phagocytized by microglia. Neuroglial cells may fill in the defect ("gliosis") (see Figure 15-38 in Chapter 15).

Chronic Neuronal Degeneration

More stages are identifiable in this process than in acute degeneration. Neurons may swell and accumulate cytoplasmic lipoidal vacuoles. Others may shrink, losing cell bodies and processes, to leave only a pyknotic nucleus.

Axonal Degeneration

Lesions and degenerative processes may occur in axons distant from the cell body. Indeed, numerous degenerative conditions affect the optic nerve, which is a collection of axons, before the RGCs are affected. Segments distal to the injury shrink rapidly, but proximal segments attached to the cell body survive longer, and bulblike swellings develop at the site of injury. However, the bubbles do not persist, and eventually both proximal and distal portions of the neuron, including the cell body, degenerate due to interruption of the axoplasmic flow. Therefore chronic atrophy of the optic nerve ultimately leads to *retrograde* atrophy of the nerve fiber and RGC layers of the retina. Similarly, loss of RGCs causes *anterograde* atrophy of the corresponding axons in toptic nerve.

Myelin Degeneration

Destruction of the optic nerve causes alterations in the myelin sheath. The complex lipids in myelin turn into simple lipids. These simple lipids are lost during routine histologic processing, leaving spaces (Figure 16-26). Macrophages phagocytize the lipid (Figure 16-27).

Pathologic Reactions of the Neuroglia

Neuroglial cells are the supporting cells of the CNS and are classified by characteristics of their cytoplasmic processes. *Astrocytes* proliferate when stimulated, although severe acute degenerations of the retina may destroy both neurons and neuroglia. In the retina the astrocytes become larger, proliferate,

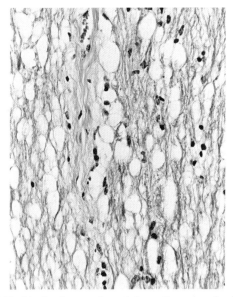

Figure 16-26. Myelin degeneration of the optic nerve of a horse with equine recurrent uveitis.

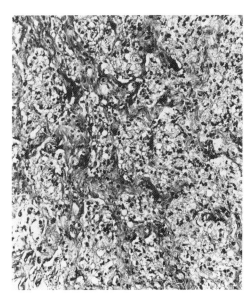

Figure 16-27. Severe acute toxic optic neuropathy in a sheep poisoned with *Stypandra imbricata* ("blindgrass"). Note the loss of normal architecture, loss and disorganization of axons, and presence of gitter (fat-laden macrophages).

and fill in defects caused by disappearance of other neuronal tissues, forming "glial scars" or areas of "gliosis." Histiocytes or fixed macrophages of the CNS are termed *microglia*. They phagocytize fatty materials released during degeneration of nervous tissue and become large and rounded with a vacuolated cytoplasm (gitter cells).

Diseases of the Central Visual Pathways

Diseases of the Optic Nerve

PAPILLEDEMA. *Papilledema* ("choked disc") is not a disease but edema of the optic nerve head caused by elevation in intracranial pressure. As the subarachnoid space of the brain is continuous with the optic nerve sheath, elevation in cerebrospinal fluid (CSF) pressure is transmitted to the optic nerve. The result is disruption of the axoplasmic flow between the RGC body and the axonal terminal. The most common cause of papilledema is brain tumors, with one study reporting a 48% incidence of papilledema in 21 dogs with brain tumor (Table 16-8). Of the 21 dogs, 11 were boxers. In addition to intracranial neoplasia, papilledema occurs in orbital inflammations and neoplasms (including optic nerve neoplasms), in vitamin A deficiency in cattle, and in some forms of toxic optic neuropathy (e.g., male fern and lead poisonings in cattle).

Clinical Signs. The clinical signs of papilledema are as follows:

- The disc is swollen and elevated above the surrounding retina.
- Disc margins are indistinct and fluffy.
- Retinal arterioles and veins show a distinct kink as they pass down over the edge of the disc into the retina.
- The disc has a "watery pink" appearance.
- Retinal veins are congested, dilated, and tortuous, and many more fine veins are visible.
- Small flame-shaped hemorrhages may be present on or near the disc margin.

The main differential diagnosis for papilledema is optic neuritis, which presents with similar clinical signs (see following section). The two are distinguished by the fact that the former causes no functional deficits, whereas the latter causes loss of vision and PLR.

Papilledema itself does not cause visual deficit.

Table 16-8 | **Clinical Signs in 21 Cases of Canine Brain Tumor**

CLINICAL SIGN	% AFFECTED
Papilledema	48
Visual defect (including pupils)	71
Hemianopia	33
Nystagmus	29
Ocular deviation and cranial nerve paralysis	33
Change of temperament	81
Locomotor deficiency	81
Circling	43
Hemiplegia	38
Convulsions	38
Head turn or tilt	33
Sensory deficit	19
Pituitary signs	14

Modified from Palmer AC, et al. (1974): Clinical signs including papilledema associated with brain tumors in twenty-one dogs. J Small Anim Pract 15:359.

Although papilledema does not cause primary loss of vision, chronic papilledema may lead to progressive visual deficits due to optic nerve atrophy. Furthermore, in cases where papilledema is caused by brain tumors, cortical lesions may cause visual deficits, as well as other neurologic deficits (see Table 16-8).

Locomotor deficiency and change in temperament in a dog with visual dysfunction and papilledema is highly suggestive of an intracranial space-occupying lesion.

CONGENITAL ANOMALIES

Aplasia and Hypoplasia. Aplasia of the optic nerve is complete absence of the nerve, an extremely rare condition. Hypoplasia of the nerve is defined as significant reduction in the number of optic nerve axons. The primary developmental abnormality is thought to be in the number or differentiation of the RGCs whose axons form the optic nerve. Therefore in optic nerve hypoplasia the number of RGCs is usually also decreased, and the nerve fiber layer is thin. Hypoplasia of the optic nerve occur infrequently in dogs, cats, horses, and cattle, and may be unilateral or bilateral. The condition is believed to be hereditary in a number of dog breeds, although it may also be acquired (see the section on vitamin A deficiency in cattle and pigs). Prenatal infection with bovine viral diarrhea–mucosal disease may cause congenital optic nerve atrophy.

In aplasia the optic disc is entirely lacking. If retinal vessels are present, hypoplasia is more likely, with a small remnant of the optic disc present. In horses few if any retinal vessels are present in either hypoplasia or aplasia. In hypoplasia the disc is gray and may be heavily pigmented (Figure 16-28). Secondary retinal degeneration may be present.

In optic nerve aplasia, the eyes are congenitally blind; pupils are dilated and unresponsive to light (Figure 16-29). In optic nerve hypoplasia there are significant visual deficits and PLR abnormalities. Their extent, however, varies with the number of functional RGCs and optic nerve axons.

Aplasia-hypoplasia should be differentiated from atrophy, which is usually not present in young animals. Histologically, the presence of retinal gliosis, inflammatory cells, or degenerative changes in retinal ganglion cells indicates atrophy rather than aplasia-hypoplasia. Another differential diagnosis (for hypoplasia) is *micropapilla*, a normal variation in which an animal has a smaller-than-usual optic nerve, but no visual or PLR deficits.

Colobomas. Colobomas are pits or excavations in the optic disc and peripapillary area, caused by incomplete closure of the embryonic fissure (see Chapter 2). They are typical if seen in the inferior medial portion of the disc, and atypical if located elsewhere. In dogs, colobomas occur most commonly in the collie eye anomaly in collies and Shetland sheepdogs (Figure 16-30), although they may also be inherited as separate distinct entities (e.g., in basenjis). Colobomas are also inherited (as an autosomal dominant trait with incomplete penetrance) in Charolais cattle but may occur sporadically in any species. The lesions are congenital and nonprogressive, varying in size from small pits to excavations several times the size of the normal optic disc. If a coloboma is large enough, vision and PLR are affected because the nerve fiber layer is disrupted as it enters the optic nerve head. Small colobomas have minimal effect on vision and PLR.

The clinical appearance of a coloboma is a white-gray indentation in the optic nerve. Blood vessels reaching the margin of the coloboma disappear from view as they "dive" into the excavation. The depth of the coloboma may be estimated by focusing on it using a direct ophthalmoscope, and

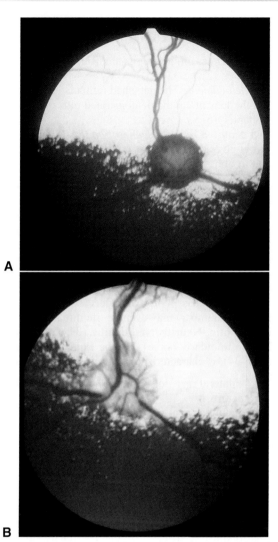

Figure 16-28. Hypoplastic **(A)** and normal **(B)** optic nerves of the left and right eyes, respectively, of a 4-year-old golden retriever. Note obvious differences in color, size, and shape of the optic discs. This was an incidental finding, and the owner was unaware that the left eye was blind.

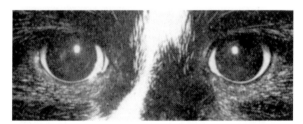

Figure 16-29. Mydriasis in a cat with bilateral aplasia of the optic discs. The two eyes are similar, are normal in size, and have dilated pupils. (From Barnett KC, Grimes TD [1974]: Bilateral aplasia of the optic nerve in a cat. Br J Ophthalmol 57:663.)

comparing the refractive power to that required to focus on the adjacent disc or surrounding retina. Colobomas must be distinguished from glaucomatous cupping, which is an indentation in the optic nerve head (centered in the center of the optic disc) caused by elevation in intraocular pressure.

INFLAMMATORY DISORDERS

Optic Neuritis. Optic neuritis is an inflammation of the optic nerve. The inflammation may be unilateral, though it is usually bilateral; it may affect the entire nerve or parts of it.

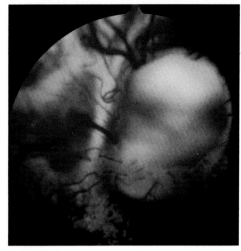

Figure 16-30. Optic nerve (and scleral) coloboma in a collie with collie eye anomaly. Note the "disappearance" of the blood vessels at the edge of the optic disc as they "dive" into the large coloboma.

Etiology. Causes of optic neuritis are as follows:

- Infectious diseases affecting other nervous tissues (e.g., canine distemper, cryptococcosis, hog cholera, toxoplasmosis, feline infectious peritonitis) (Figure 16-31)
- Inflammatory diseases, most commonly GME or meningitis
- Trauma, especially after proptosis of the globe
- Orbital diseases (e.g., orbital cellulitis and orbital abscess)
- Neoplastic disorders. These may be primary optic nerve tumors (e.g., meningioma) or orbital tumors affecting the nerve.
- Exogenous toxins (e.g., optic neuropathy in cattle from the ingestion of male fern and in sheep from the ingestion of *Stypandra imbricata* ["blindgrass"]) (see Figure 16-27). In humans, numerous drugs (e.g., chloramphenicol, alcohol, nicotine) cause optic neuropathy, and drugs are often suspected but unproven causes in sporadic cases in animals.
- Vitamin A deficiency causing abnormal bone growth that constricts the optic canal
- Many cases, especially in dogs, are of unknown etiology, and in fact most cases are classified as idiopathic.

Clinical Signs. The clinical signs of optic neuritis are as follows (in retrobulbar neuritis, the ophthalmoscopic signs marked with an *asterisk* [*] may be absent, because the more distal part of the nerve is affected; in these cases, the fundus may look normal):

- Acute loss of vision
- The pupil is dilated and unresponsive. In unilateral cases, there is a consensual PLR from the unaffected eye, but not from the affected eye.
- The optic disc is swollen and raised. It appears to be congested, and its margins are blurry (Figure 16-32).*
- Hemorrhages on or around the optic disc*
- The retina around the disc may be edematous or detached. With time, peripapillary retinochoroidal degeneration may appear.*
- Exudation and haze in the adjacent vitreous*
- Concurrent signs of CNS disease may be present, depending on the primary cause.
- Optic neuritis, if untreated or uncontrolled, frequently leads to optic atrophy, with a pale, grayish, shrunken optic disc and attenuation of blood vessels (see Optic Neuropathy later).

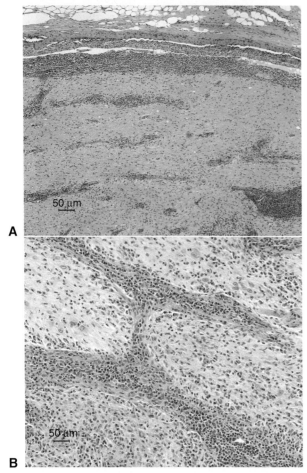

Figure 16-31. Histopathologic micrograph showing a case of canine optic neuritis secondary to viral meningoencephalitis. **A,** Note the extensive, diffuse infiltration of inflammatory cells around the nerve. There is also multifocal infiltration of the optic nerve by inflammatory cells. **B,** A higher-magnification view of the same case, showing the nonsuppurative nature of the perivascular infiltrate. (Hematoxylin & eosin stain.) (Courtesy Dr. Emmanuel Loeb.)

Differential Diagnosis. Acute blindness with fixed, dilated pupils may also be caused by the following conditions:

- *Glaucoma:* Other clinical signs are usually present (see Chapter 12).
- *Retinal detachment:* The detached retina is usually visible behind the lens or can be demonstrated ultrasonographically (see Chapter 15).
- *Sudden acquired retinal degeneration (SARD):* The electroretinogram response is extinguished in SARD but normal in optic neuritis (see Chapter 15).

The appearance of an inflamed disc should be distinguished from papilledema and from myelination of the nerve fiber layer of the retina surrounding the optic disc (Figure 16-33; Table 16-9).

Treatment. Comprehensive ophthalmic, neurologic, and physical examinations should be performed in order to identify the primary cause (if present), and appropriate therapy should be instituted. The inflammation itself is treated symptomatically with high doses of systemic steroids. However, the prognosis for return of vision is poor, and indeed some of the primary causes (e.g., distemper) may even be life threatening.

Equine Optic Neuritis/Neuropathy. These diseases are usually seen in elderly horses. Equine exudative optic neuritis (Figure 16-34), is characterized by the following signs:

- Sudden, bilateral onset of blindness, accompanied by signs of optic neuritis
- Multiple round or oval yellowish bodies protruding from the borders of the optic disc and extending into the vitreous
- Pupillary dilation and loss or depression of PLRs
- Hemorrhages on or around the optic disc that may precede or accompany the appearance of the yellow bodies

Because the condition is uncommon, cumulative experience in its treatment is lacking, and optic atrophy is the usual sequel.

An important differential diagnosis is *equine proliferative optic neuropathy*, a disease of elderly horses that is also characterized by papillary or peripapillary white masses (Table 16-10, Figure 16-35). However, this disease causes no visual disturbance and the condition is usually found incidentally

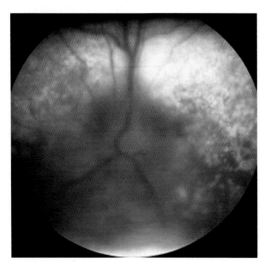

Figure 16-32. Optic neuritis in a dog. Note the blurry disc margins and the loss of detail on the disc surface, caused by edema of the nerve head. (Courtesy University of Wisconsin–Madison Veterinary Ophthalmology Service Collection.)

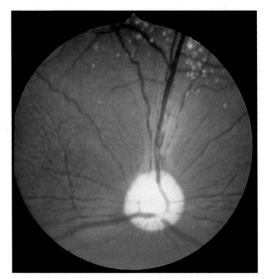

Figure 16-33. Myelination of the nerve fiber layer of the retina in a dog, seen as white streaks extending from the disc. This must be distinguished from papilledema and optic neuritis. Clinical signs are lacking, and vision is normal.

Table 16-9 | Differentiation of Optic Neuritis, Papilledema, and Excessive Nerve Myelination

FEATURE	OPTIC NEURITIS	PAPILLEDEMA	EXCESSIVE MYELINATION OF THE NERVE
Age	Middle-aged dogs	No specific age group unless associated with cerebral neoplasia, which is more common in older dogs	Present from birth, nonprogressive, and not pathologic
Vision	Severely affected or absent	No effect	No effect
Direct pupillary light reflex	Depressed or absent	Present	Present
Disc hemorrhages	Usually present	Rarely present	Absent
Peripapillary chorioretinitis	Often present	Absent (edema may be present)	Absent
"Kink" in vessels at disc margin	Often present	Often present	Absent
Vitreous haze	Often present	Absent	Absent

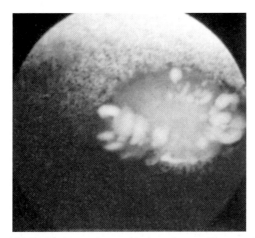

Figure 16-34. Exudative optic neuritis in a horse. (Courtesy Dr. G.A. Severin.)

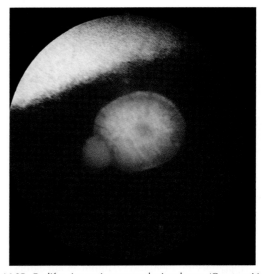

Figure 16-35. Proliferative optic neuropathy in a horse. (Courtesy University of California, Davis, Veterinary Ophthalmology Service Collection.)

during fundus examination. Lesions are unilateral, are nonprogresive, do not affect vision or PLR, and are not preceded or accompanied by hemorrhages around the disc. Proliferative optic neuropathy was formerly reported as astrocytoma, but histologic studies indicate that it is a lipid storage disorder.

Optic neuropathy in horses may also be ischemic, due to trauma or following ligation of the internal and external carotid arteries (to treat epistaxis caused by guttural pouch mycosis) (see Figure 15-55 in Chapter 15). Although initially the affected optic nerve appears normal, edema, hyperemia, and hemorrhages may be observed after 24 hours, and irreversible blindness is a common sequel.

NEOPLASMS. Primary neoplasms affecting the optic nerve include meningioma, glioma, and astrocytoma. They are uncommon in all species. Secondary metastatic neoplasms may also occur.

Clinical Signs. The clinical signs of neoplasms of the optic nerve are as follows:

- Mydriasis and abolition of the direct PLR in the affected eye, and the consensual PLR to the unaffected eye. With a large infiltrating orbital mass, the consensual reflex from the contralateral eye to the affected eye may be abnormal because of destruction of efferent nerves of CN III. In such cases, strabismus and ptosis will also be noted.
- Orbital neoplasms may cause papilledema and/or optic neuritis that will eventually progress to optic neuropathy (see following section).

- The optic nerve head or posterior section of the globe may be indented by the retrobulbar mass. Retinal edema and folds resulting from pressure exerted by orbital masses on the posterior of the globe may also be observed ophthalmoscopically.
- Progressive exophthalmous that may even lead to ptosis of the globe. Position of the globe and direction of the visual axis may assist in determining the position of the mass. Exophthalmous caused by retrobulbar neoplasia can be differentiated from that caused by a retrobulbar abscess as the latter is painful and of acute onset, whereas the former is nonpainful and slowly progressive.

Treatment. Imaging techniques, including radiography, computed tomography and magnetic resonance imaging, may be used to delineate the extent of the tumor. In cases of retrobulbar tumors, cytology samples may be obtained using ultraound-guided fine needle aspiration. Treatment of optic neoplasms consists of anterior or lateral orbitotomy if the globe is to be saved, or orbital exenteration if the neoplasm is too extensive or infiltrates the globe or secondary lesions are present in the globe.

OPTIC NEUROPATHY

Etiology. Optic neuropathy is atrophy of the optic nerve. The condition has numerous causes and is the end stage of

Table 16-10 | **Differential Diagnosis of Equine Exudative Optic Neuritis and Proliferative Optic Neuropathy**

FEATURE	EXUDATIVE OPTIC NEURITIS	PROLIFERATIVE OPTIC NEUROPATHY
Vision	Severe disturbance	No disturbance
Age	Elderly	Elderly
Symmetry	Bilateral (unless traumatic)	Unilateral
Course	Progressive, often leading to optic atrophy	Stationary
Appearance	1. Multiple bodies protruding from disc	1. Single body on disc surface
	2. Hemorrhages often present	2. No hemorrhages
	3. Vitreous haze may be present	3. No vitreous haze
Pupil	Mydriasis	Normal
Direct pupillary light reflex	Depressed or absent	Normal

From de Lahunta A (1983): Veterinary Neuroanatomy and Clinical Neurology, 2nd ed. Saunders, Philadelphia.

numerous pathologic processes. Some of the more common processes are as follows:

- Advanced retinal degeneration of any type, as the degeneration eventually spreads to the RGCs and their axons
- Glaucoma, as the RGCs and their axons are damaged by the elevation in intraocular pressure
- Orbital disorders (e.g., retrobulbar abscess, orbital cellulitis, canine extraocular myositis)
- Intraorbital nerve damage secondary to traumatic proptosis in dogs and cats
- Sequel to optic neuritis
- Prolonged papilledema
- Intraorbital and intracranial neoplasia

Clinical Signs. The clinical signs of optic atrophy are as follows:

- Pale, grayish white, shrunken disc with extensive papillary and peripapillary pigmentation (similar in appearance to Figure 16-28, *A*)
- Slight depression of the disc surface
- Exposure and increased visibility of the lamina cribrosa
- Attenuation of retinal vessels

Treatment. Except to prevent further damage to the nerve by the original cause, treatment of optic neuropathy has no effect.

Diseases of the Optic Chiasm

The most common disease of the optic chiasm is pituitary neoplasia. In domestic animals, unlike in humans, the pituitary gland is located caudal to the optic chiasm. Therefore most pituitary neoplasms expand into the hypothalamus, and the chiasm is affected only in advanced stages of growth. The result is bilateral visual and PLR deficits. Occasionally, the cerebral infarction syndrome in cats causes ischemic encephalopathy and necrosis of the optic chiasm, with blindness and dilated, unresponsive pupils (see Diseases of the Optic Radiation and Visual Cortex).

In severe proptosis or traction during enucleation, the optic chiasm may be traumatized, thus causing optic neuropathy and blindness in the contralateral eye that was not affected initially. This condition is most commonly seen in cats, as the retrobulbar optic nerve is particularly short in this species.

Diseases of the Optic Tracts

BILATERAL DISEASE. Incomplete bilateral optic tract lesions may produce partial bilateral visual deficit with variable pupillary responses. The most common histopathologic finding in optic tract disease is demyelination. It may be caused by canine distemper, which has a predilection for the optic tracts. As noted previously, the virus may also cause optic neuritis, and the dog will present with signs of optic nerve inflammation. However, often no clinical visual deficit is observed, and optic tract demyelination may be the only pathology. The diagnosis is confirmed by PCR testing of various tissues, notably conjunctival swabs and blood samples. The disease is discussed in detail in Chapter 18. Demyelination of the optic tracts may also be seen in some storage diseases (see later). Occasionally, canine pituitary neoplasms affect the optic tracts when the hypothalamus is invaded or compressed by the neoplasm.

UNILATERAL DISEASE. Neoplasms in the hypothalamus and thalamus may encroach on one optic tract, causing a visual deficit in the contralateral eye, but PLRs are unaffected.

Because of close approximation of the internal capsule and rostral crus cerebri to the optic tract, space-occupying lesions in the lateral hypothalamus or thalamus (or both) that affect the optic tract usually also affect the internal capsule and rostral crus cerebri. The result is mild contralateral hemiparesis, which often is not evident in the gait but is demonstrable as asymmetry with postural testing.

Traumatic or ischemic lesions that cause necrosis of these tissues on one side can result in the same residual neurologic signs, that is, contralateral visual deficit and postural reaction deficit ("hemiparesis").

Diseases of the Lateral Geniculate Nucleus

Destruction of the LGN produces signs similar to those observed with distal optic tract lesions. It may be caused by any multifocal or diffuse brain disease that involves the thalamus and LGN, or by inflammatory, neoplastic, or storage diseases. An abnormality in the retinogeniculate projections and neuronal organization in this nucleus occurs in albinotic cats of all sizes, from Siamese cats to tigers, and in minks. In some animals it is associated with congenital esotropia and nystagmus.

Diseases of the Optic Radiation and Visual Cortex

UNILATERAL DISEASE. Unilateral lesions of the optic radiation and visual cortex produce hemianopia in the contralateral visual field. Pupillary size and response to light are normal. Common lesions of these structures and their clinical signs are as follows:

Neoplastic Lesions. Neoplasms produce progressive signs of neurologic deficit. Convulsions or changes in behavior may accompany the visual deficit.

Traumatic Lesions. Traumatic lesions causing necrosis may leave a residual neurologic defect limited to a contralateral visual deficit. If the entire hemisphere is involved, a contralateral postural reaction deficiency may be seen on neurologic examination. Immediately after an injury the neurologic signs may be more extensive, suggesting diffuse cerebral disturbance. As hemorrhage and edema subside, the residual neurologic deficits relate to areas of necrotic tissue.

Feline Ischemic Encephalopathy. This is a syndrome consisting of peracute signs of unilateral cerebral disturbance in adult cats of all ages and both sexes, believed to be caused by aberrant migration of *Cuterebra*. CNS signs are variable, with some animals showing only severe depression with mild ataxia, circling, or both, whereas others circle continuously. Other cases begin with seizures and consist of tonic or clonic activity of the muscles on one side of the head, trunk, and limbs. Changes in attitude and behavior are common and may involve severe aggression. Pupils are often dilated, and blindness may be apparent. For the first 1 to 2 days, observable hemiparesis may be present. Acute signs usually resolve in a few days, leaving signs of a nonprogressive unilateral cerebral lesion. The loss of neurons in the visual cerebral cortex or optic radiation causes contralateral loss of the menace reflex, with normal pupillary reflexes.

Unilateral cerebral lesions are usually in the frontal lobe. Examination may demonstrate a unilateral facial hypalgesia contralateral to the cerebral lesion. No other cranial nerve deficits have been observed. Ischemic necrosis of the cerebral hemisphere is variable and is usually unilateral but occasionally bilateral. The necrosis may be multifocal or the infarction may involve up to two thirds of one entire cerebrum. Vascular occlusion occurs most commonly in the middle cerebral artery. Most cats with cerebral vascular disease survive, but behavioral changes and uncontrollable seizures may persist.

Unilateral Cerebral Abscess. In horses, abscesses caused by *Streptococcus equi* or by *Sarcocystis neurona* may affect the optic radiation and cause a contralateral visual deficit with normal pupillary reflexes. Expansion of the lesion with accompanying cerebral edema raises intracranial pressure and causes the occipital lobes to herniate ventral to the tentorium cerebelli. The herniation further compromises function of the visual cortex bilaterally, and total blindness results if both sides are affected. Similar signs occur in ruminants with *Corynebacterium pyogenes* abscess.

Encephalitis. In encephalitis caused by *Toxoplasma gondii*, a space-occupying granuloma may be produced in the optic radiation and cause a contralateral visual deficit. CSF contains inflammatory cells, often with neutrophils and increased amounts of protein.

BILATERAL DISEASE. Total blindness with normal PLRs is characteristic of bilateral visual cortex lesions. Common lesions and their findings are as follows:

Canine Distemper. Chronic encephalitis due to canine distemper may result in demyelination and astrocytosis of the optic radiation. This is a sclerosing encephalitis that may produce a unilateral or bilateral visual deficit with normal pupillary function. Chorioretinitis may be visible ophthalmoscopically. The disease is discussed in detail in Chapter 18.

Thromboembolic Meningoencephalitis. Infarction of the cerebral white matter by septic emboli occurs in cattle afflicted with thromboembolic meningoencephalitis caused by *H. somnus*. Visual deficits may result. Severe ophthalmoscopically visible retinal lesions are the probable cause of visual deficits and are

of considerable use in diagnosis (see Figure 15-49, *C* in Chapter 15).

Metabolic Diseases. Cortical blidness may also be caused by a number of metabolic diseases, notably hepatic and uremic encephalopathy, and hypoglycemia. The diseases may also affect the brainstem, resulting in subsequent PLR and eye movement abnormalities.

Inflammations. Cortical blindness may be caused by GME, an idiopathic inflammation characterized by formation of granulomas in the visual pathways, including the visual cortex. Immunosuppresive treatment is recommended, though prognosis is grave. The treatment and prognosis are similar in necrotizing meningoencephalitis, a disease of the cerebral hemispheres in small breed dogs.

Ischemic Necrosis of Cerebrum. Anesthetic overdose leading to prolonged apnea and cardiac arrest may cause diffuse ischemic necrosis of the cerebrum. Animals may recover, the only residual deficit being blindness with intact pupillary reflexes.

Poisonings in Cattle and Sheep. Severe cerebral disturbance, including frequent blindness, is seen in cattle and sheep with polioencephalomalacia, or thiamine (vitamin B_1) deficiency. The visual deficit is due to necrosis of the visual cortex caused by elevation in thiaminase levels following ingestion of bracken fern or excess thiaminase production in the rumen. Lead poisoning causes similar acute necrosis of the cerebral cortex and associated blindness. Similarly, severe water intoxication with cerebral disturbance may cause blindness.

Intoxication by wheat seed fungicide containing mercury has been reported in cattle and pigs. The metal causes chronic degeneration of neurons in the cerebral cortex and replacement of astrocytes. Convulsions and blindness may appear in the chronic stages. Mercury toxicity also occurs in dogs and cats.

Tentorial Herniation. As noted in the previous section, space-occupying granulomas caused by a number of infective agents may cause cerebral edema, leading to elevation in intracranial pressure, bilateral ventral occipital lobe herniation, and blindness. The same explanation for bilateral signs of visual deficit from tentorial herniation can be offered for any space-occupying cerebral lesion or cerebral swelling after injury. Head injury that causes progressive cerebral edema causes blindness. The pupillary activity varies with the extent of brainstem involvement (see Pupils in Patients with Intracranial Injury).

Hypoplasia of the Prosencephalon in Calves. In calves with hypoplasia of the prosencephalon, the rostral portion of the malformed diencephalon protrudes through a defect in the calvaria and is attached to the adjacent skin. The skull is flatter than normal to conform to the malformed brain, which consists of a brainstem with a small cerebellum and no cerebral hemispheres. The lack of cerebral tissue causes visual deficit despite a functional brainstem. Affected animals may be able to stand and usually live for a few days.

Hydranencephaly. In hydranencephaly the cerebral hemispheres are reduced to a membranous sac filled with CSF, which may cause a "dummy" syndrome in calves and lambs with ataxia and visual deficit. This disorder may be caused by Akabane virus in cattle and bluetongue virus in sheep.

Obstructive Hydrocephalus. Obstructive hydrocephalus is caused by obstructions in CSF flow and drainage, leading to accumulation of fluid in the lateral ventricles or subarachnoid space. The elevation in pressure compromises the optic radiation in the internal capsule, in which it forms the lateral wall of the dilated lateral ventricle. Bilateral visual deficits and ataxia are common signs, reflecting attenuation of the cerebral white matter, optic radiation, and visual cortex.

Additional Neuroophthalmic Diseases

Vitamin A Deficiency

Vitamin A deficiency is of clinical, ophthalmic, and economic significance in cattle, pigs, and sheep. The disease affects the visual system through two mechanisms. In young animals, it causes abnormal thickening of growing bones, including the bones around the optic canal. This thickening leads to constriction and compressions of the optic nerve. Clinical signs are as follows (see Figures 15-52 and 15-53 in Chapter 15):

- Papilledema. As the deficiency progresses, papilledema worsens, the optic disc enlarges and becomes pink and pale, and details of the central optic disc are obscured. In the later stages or if treatment is not given, irreversible optic nerve atrophy occurs and the optic disc becomes gray, flat, and shrunken.
- Tortuous retinal blood vessels, which later become attenuated
- Retinal detachment and hemorrhage
- Retrograde degeneration of the retina, especially in the peripapillary region
- Anterograde degeneration of the optic chiasm and tracts
- Mottling of the tapetum and pallor of the nontapetum
- Reduced CSF absorption, leading to increased CSF pressure, ataxia, tetraparesis, and seizures

As vitamin A is used in the synthesis of visual photopigments in the rods (see Chapter 15), hypovitaminosis A will also impair rod function, leading to night blindness. In chronic deficiencies, progressive loss of vision and complete retinal degeneration will occur.

Clinical signs become apparent when vitamin A levels have dropped to about 20 µg/dL of blood or 2 µg/g of liver. For diagnosis of vitamin A deficiency, liver levels are more reliable than blood levels. Affected animals should be treated as follows:

1. Vitamin A (water-soluble preparation) at 440 IU/kg intramuscularly
2. Provision of rations containing vitamin A, 65 IU/kg body weight per day

Storage Diseases

Inherited storage diseases of the nervous system occur in most domestic species and are models of comparable diseases in humans. All are progressive, degenerative disorders of the nervous system, usually of a recessive nature. The onset is usually some time after weaning. Signs represent diffuse involvement of the nervous system but often begin with pelvic limb ataxia and paresis. In the advanced stages of many of these diseases blindness is common because the retina or visual pathways are affected.

Storage diseases are usually caused by an absence or severe deficiency of a specific degradative enzyme, which leads to abnormal accumulation of the sub-strate normally metabolized by that enzyme. These metabolic disorders may be expressed in neurons by the accumulation of complex lipids in neuronal cytoplasm *(lipodystrophy)* or in the myelin by demyelination and accumulation of complex lipids in macrophages *(leukodystrophy)*. Leukodystrophy involves an abnormal metabolism of myelin and its subsequent degeneration, whereas lipodystrophy consists of abnormal neuronal metabolism associated with accumulations of complex lipids in neurons and their subsequent degeneration.

Meningitis

Canine meningitis may cause various neurologic and neuroophthalmologic deficits, depending on the cause (Table 16-11).

Cerebellar Disease

It is assumed that the pathway between the visual cortex and the facial nucleus passes through the cerebellum (see Figure 16-2). Therefore significant cerebellar disease will interrupt the efferent pathway of the menace response. Patients will have no menace response, even though they are visual. Animals with this condition also have significant signs of cerebellar ataxia. A unilateral cerebellar lesion causes an ipsilateral menace deficit with normal vision. This occurs because of the crossing of the visual pathway in the optic chiasm and the reciprocal interaction between the cerebrum on one side and the opposite cerebellar hemisphere.

Involvement of the cerebellum may also cause vestibular disturbance, with loss of equilibrium, nystagmus, bizarre postures, and a broad-based staggering gait with jerky movements as well as a tendency to fall to the side or back, especially if the thoracic limbs are elevated. Abnormal nystagmus is observed only occasionally.

Occasionally in animals with significant cerebellar disease that involves the cerebellar nuclei, one palpebral fissure is slightly wider or one third eyelid is mildly elevated. The pathogenesis of these signs in poorly understood, even though they have also been reproduced experimentally.

Table 16-11 | **Clinical Signs of Meningitis**

DISORDER	NEUROOPHTHALMIC SIGNS	OTHER SIGNS
Necrotizing vasculitis	Blindness	Cervical rigidity and pain, paralysis, seizures, neutrophilia
Pyogranulomatous meningoencephalitis	Cranial nerve deficits	Ataxia, stiff gait, cervical rigidity, hyperesthesia
Granulomatous meningoencephalitis	Blindness, facial paresis, trigeminal paralysis, nystagmus	Cervical pain, fever, ataxia, seizure circling, head tilt
Bacterial meningitis	Nystagmus, blindness	Cervical rigidity, hyperesthesia, fever, vomiting, bradycardia, seizures, hyperreflexia, paralysis, paresis, head tilt

Modified from Meric SM (1988): Canine meningitis: a review. J Vet Intern Med 2:26.

BIBLIOGRAPHY

Aguirre GD, et al. (1983): Feline mucopolysaccharidosis. VI: general ocular and pigment epithelial pathology. Invest Ophthalmol Vis Sci 24:991.

Allgoewer I, et al. (2000): Extraocular muscle myositis and restrictive strabismus in 10 dogs. Vet Ophthalmol 3:21.

Baker HJ, et al. (1971): Neuronal GM gangliosidosis in a Siamese cat with beta galactosidase deficiency. Science 174:838.

Barnhart KF, et al. (2001): Symptomatic granular cell tumor involving the pituitary gland in a dog: a case report and review of the literature. Vet Pathol 38:332.

Berghaus RD, et al. (2001): Risk factors for development of dysautonomia in dogs. J Am Vet Med Assoc 218:1285.

Bichsel P, et al. (1988): Neurologic manifestations associated with hypothyroidism in four dogs. J Am Vet Med Assoc 192:1745.

Bistner S, et al. (1970): Pharmacologic diagnosis of Horner's syndrome in the dog. J Am Vet Med Assoc 157:1220.

Boydell P (1995): Idiopathic Horner's syndrome in the golden retriever. J Small Anim Pract 36:382.

Brouwer GJ (1987): Feline dysautonomia—pharmacological studies. J Small Anim Pract 28:350.

Chrisman CL (1991): Visual dysfunction, in Chrisman CL (editor): Problems in Small Animal Neurology, 2nd ed. Lea & Febiger, Philadelphia, p. 207.

Cumming SJF, de Lahunta A (1977): An adult case of canine neuronal ceroid-lipofuscinosis. Acta Neuropathol 39:43.

Davidson MG, et al. (1991): Acute blindness associated with intracranial tumors in dogs and cats: eight cases (1984-1989). J Am Vet Med Assoc 199:755.

de Lahunta A (1983): Visual system—special somatic afferent system, in de Lahunta A (editor): Veterinary Neuroanatomy and Clinical Neurology. Saunders, Philadelphia, p. 279.

de Lahunta A, Alexander JW (1976): Ischemic myelopathy secondary to presumed fibrocartilaginous embolism in nine dogs. J Am Anim Hosp Assoc 12:37.

Dewey CW (2003): Encephalopathies: disorders of the brain, in Dewey CE (editor): A Practical Guide to Canine and Feline Neurology. Iowa State Press, Ames, p. 99.

Dewey CW (2002): External hydrocephalus in a dog with suspected bacterial meningoencephalitis. J Am Anim Hosp Assoc 38:563.

Dyce KM, et al. (1996): The sense organs, in Dyce KM, et al. (editors): Textbook of Veterinary Anatomy, 2nd ed. Saunders, Philadelphia, p. 325.

Enzerink E (1998): The menace response and pupillary light reflex in neonatal foals. Equine Vet J 30:546.

Evans HE (1993): Miller's Anatomy of the Dog, 3rd ed. Saunders, Philadelphia.

Gancz AY, et al. (2005): Horner's syndrome in a red-bellied parrot (Poicephalus rufiventris). J Av Med Surg 19:30.

Garosi LS, et al. (2003): Thiamine deficiency in a dog: clinical, clinicopathologic, and magnetic resonance imaging findings. J Vet Intern Med 17:719.

Gaskell CJ (1987): Feline dysautonomia—introduction and background. J Small Anim Pract 28:337.

Godinho HP, Getty R (1975): Peripheral nervous system, in Getty R (editor): Sisson and Grossman's the Anatomy of the Domestic Animals, 5th ed. Saunders, Philadelphia, p. 650.

Greet TRC (1986): Outcome of treatment in 35 cases of guttural pouch mycosis. Equine Vet J 18:294.

Griffiths IR (1987): Feline dysautonomia—pathology. J Small Anim Pract 28:347.

Griffiths IR, et al. (1985): Feline dysautonomia (the Key-Gaskell syndrome): an ultrastructural study of autonomic ganglia and nerves. Neuropathol Appl Neurobiol 11:17.

Guillery RW, Kaas JH (1973): Genetic abnormality of the visual pathways in a "white" tiger. Science 180:1287.

Harkin KR, et al. (2002): Dysautonomia in dogs: 65 cases (1993-2000). J Am Vet Med Assoc 220:633.

Harper PA, et al. (1988): Neurovisceral ceroid-lipofuscinosis in blind Devon cattle. Acta Neuropathol 75:632.

Hartley WJ (1963): Polioencephalomalacia in dogs. Acta Neuropathol 2:271.

Hayes KC, et al. (1968): Pathogenesis of the optic nerve lesion in vitamin A–deficient calves. Arch Ophthalmol 80:777.

Hogg DA (1987): Topographical anatomy of the central nervous system, in King AS (editor): Physiological and Clinical Anatomy of the Domestic Mammals, Vol 1: The Central Nervous System. Blackwell Science, Oxford, England, p. 256.

Hubel DH, Wiesel TN (1971): Aberrant visual projections in the Siamese cat. Physiology 218:33.

Jeffery G, Erskine L (2005): Variations in the architecture and development of the vertebrate optic chiasm. Prog Retin Eye Res 24:721.

Jolly R, et al. (1987): Mannosidosis: ocular lesions in the bovine model. Curr Eye Res 6:1073.

Kalil RE, et al. (1971): Anomalous retinal pathways in the Siamese cat: an inadequate substrate for normal binocular vision. Science 174:302.

Kay TJA, Gaskell CJ (1982): Puzzling syndrome in cats associated with pupillary dilation. Vet Rec 110:160.

Kern TJ, Erb N (1987): Facial neuropathy in dogs and cats: 95 cases (1975-1985). J Am Vet Med Assoc 191:1604.

Kern TJ, et al. (1989): Horner's syndrome in dogs and cats: 100 cases (1975-1985). J Am Vet Med Assoc 195:369.

Kern TJ, Riis RC (1981): Optic nerve hypoplasia in three miniature poodles. J Am Vet Med Assoc 178:49.

Kinde H, et al. (2000): Halicephalobus gingivalis (H. deletrix) infection in two horses in southern California. J Vet Diagn Invest 12:162.

Lorenz MD, Kornegay JN (2004): Stupor and coma, in Lorenz MD, Kornegay JN (editors): Handbook of Veterinary Neurology, 4th ed. Saunders, St. Louis, p. 297.

Martin CL, et al. (1986): Four cases of traumatic optic nerve blindness in the horse. Equine Vet J 18:133.

Mayhew IG (1989): Neurologic evaluation, in Mayhew IG (editor): Large Animal Neurology: A Handbook for Veterinary Clinicians. Lea & Febiger, Philadelphia, p. 15.

Mayhew IG, et al. (1986): Ceroid-lipofuscinosis (Batten's disease): pathogenesis of blindness in the ovine model. J Comp Pathol 254:543.

Meric SM (1988): Canine meningitis: a review. J Vet Int Med 2:26.

Miller PE, Murphy CJ (2005): Equine vision: normal and abnormal, in Gilger B (editor): Equine Ophthalmology. Saunders, St. Louis, p. 371.

Morgan RV, Zanotti SW (1989): Horner's syndrome in dogs and cats: 49 cases (1980-1986). J Am Vet Med Assoc 194:1096.

Muir P, et al. (1990): A clinical and microbiological study of cats with protruding nictitating membranes and diarrhea: isolation of a novel virus. Vet Rec 29:127.

Narfstrom K, Ekesten B (1999): Diseases of the canine ocular fundus, in Gelatt KN (editor): Veterinary Ophthalmology, 3rd ed. Lippincott Williams & Wilkins, Philadelphia, p. 869.

Nash AS (1987): Feline dysautonomia—clinical features and management. J Small Anim Pract 28:339.

O'Neill EJ, et al. (2005): Granulomatous meningencephalomyelitis in dogs: a review. Irish Vet J 58:86.

Palmer AC, et al. (1974): Clinical signs including papilloedema associated with brain tumors in twenty-one dogs. J Small Anim Pract 15:359.

Peterson BW (2004): Current approaches and future directions to understanding control of head movement. Prog Brain Res 143:369.

Pettersson LG, Perfiliev S (2002): Descending pathways controlling visually guided updating of reaching in cats. Eur J Neurosci 16:1349.

Polin M, Sullivan M (1986): A canine dysautonomia resembling Key-Gaskell syndrome. Vet Rec 118:402.

Ryan K, et al. (2001): Granulomatous meningoencephalomyelitis in dogs. Comp Cont Ed Vet Pract 23:644.

Shamir MH, Ofri R (2006): Comparative neuro-ophthalmology, in Gelatt KN (editor): Veterinary Ophthalmology, 4th ed. Blackwell Science, Philadelphia.

Singh M, et al. (2005): Thiamine deficiency in dogs due to the feeding of sulphite preserved meat. Aust Vet J 83:412.

Stadtbaumer K, et al. (2004): Tick-borne encephalitis virus as a possible cause of optic neuritis in a dog. Vet Ophthalmol 7:271.

Stalis IH, et al. (1995): Necrotizing meningoencephalitis of Maltese dogs. Vet Pathol 32:230.

Summers BA, et al. (1995): Inflammatory diseases of the central nervous system, in Summers BA, et al. (editors): Veterinary Neuropathology. Mosby, St. Louis, p. 95.

Taylor RM, et al. (1987): Canine fucosidosis: clinical findings. J Small Anim Pract 28:291.

Theissen SK, et al. (1996): A retrospective study of cavernous sinus syndrome in 4 dogs and 8 cats. J Vet Intern Med 10:65.

Thomas WB (2000): Vestibular dysfunction. Vet Clin North Am Small Anim Pract 30:227.

Troxel MT, et al. (2005): Signs of neurologic dysfunction in dogs with central versus peripheral vestibular disease. J Am Vet Med Assoc 227:570.

Vandevelde M, Zurbriggen A (2005): Demyelination in canine distemper virus infection: a review. Acta Neuropathol 109:56.

Wenger DA, et al. (1999): Globoid cell leukodystrophy in cairn and West Highland white terriers. J Hered 90:138.

Yoshitomi T, Ito Y (1986): Double reciprocal innervations in dog iris sphincter and dilator muscles. Invest Ophthalmol Vis Sci 27:83.

ORBIT

Paul E. Miller

ANATOMY
PATHOLOGIC MECHANISMS
DIAGNOSTIC METHODS

ORBITAL DISEASES
OPHTHALMIC MANIFESTATIONS OF
    DENTAL DISEASE

SURGICAL PROCEDURES
OCULAR PROSTHESES
ORBITOTOMY AND ORBITECTOMY

ANATOMY

The *orbit* is the cavity that encloses the eye. The two orbital patterns in domestic animals are as follows:

- Incomplete bony orbit, found in dogs and cats (Figures 17-1 to 17-3)
- Complete bony orbit, found in horses, oxen, sheep, and pigs (Figures 17-4 and 17-5)

The orbit separates the eye from the cranial cavity, and the *foramina* and *fissures* in its walls determine the path of blood vessels and nerves from the brain to the eye. The walls of the equine orbit are formed by the frontal, lacrimal, zygomatic, temporal, presphenoid, palatine, and maxillary bones, which are similar in other species. In the dog and cat the dorsolateral portion of the orbit is spanned by the dense collagenous *orbital ligament,* which passes from the zygomatic process of the frontal bone to the frontal process of the zygomatic bone. The basic foramina and fissures of the orbit are the orbital, rostral and caudal alar, oval, supraorbital, ethmoidal, lacrimal, maxillary, sphenopalatine, round, and palatine. In cattle, the orbital foramen and the foramen rotundum fuse to form the foramen orbitorotundum. The vessels and nerves that pass through these foramina and fissures in the dog are shown in Figures 1-16, 1-17, and 1-19 to 1-22 in Chapter 1 and Figure 17-6.

The position of the orbit within the skull varies with species. In cattle, sheep, and horses the eyes are situated laterally, giving panoramic vision, whereas in dogs and cats the eyes are located more anteriorly, which emphasizes binocular overlap between the two eyes. The visual, orbital, and optic axes, defined as follows, do not coincide (Figure 17-7):

- *Visual axis:* Line from the center of the most sensitive area of the retina to the object viewed
- *Orbital axis:* Line from the apex of the orbit to the center of the external opening
- *Optic axis:* Line from the center of the posterior pole of the eye through the center of the cornea

The angle formed by the optic axes, a measure of binocular overlap, is shown in different species in Figures 17-8 to 17-10.

The relationships of the orbit to the *paranasal sinuses, teeth, zygomatic gland,* and *ramus of the mandible* are important, because they affect incidence, diagnosis, and pathogenesis of clinical diseases of the eye and orbit, as follows:

- *Infections of the sinuses or nasal cavity* may enter the orbit in all domestic species (Figure 17-11). The junction of the frontal, lacrimal, and palatine bones in the medial wall of the canine orbit (see Figures 17-2 and 17-11) is often thin and may be eroded by disease processes in the nasal cavity, which then enter the orbit. The bone is thicker in horses (Figure 17-12).
- *Fractures of walls of the sinuses* can cause emphysema, with gas visible beneath the conjunctiva or palpable under the skin.
- *Infections of the roots of the molar teeth* can affect the orbit, uvea, and periocular area in dogs and cats.
- *Enlargement of the canine and feline zygomatic salivary gland* may cause increased pressure within the orbit or protrusion of the gland into the ventral conjunctival fornix (Figure 17-13). When the mouth is opened, especially in dogs and cats with greater mobility of the mandible, the vertical ramus of the mandible moves forward, exerting pressure on the orbital contents. This is painful if orbital contents are inflamed.

The orbital contents are completely enclosed in a sheet of connective tissue—the *periorbita*—that lies next to the bone in the bony parts of the orbital wall and that is thicker laterally where the wall is incomplete (in carnivores). The periorbita is reflected over the extraocular muscles and forward over the globe to become *Tenon's capsule,* lying beneath the conjunctiva (Figure 17-14). The periorbita is continuous with the periosteum of the facial bones at the orbital rim, with the orbital septum anteriorly, and with the dura mater of the optic nerve. The orbital fat pad lies between the periorbita and the extraocular muscles. Intraorbital fat lies between the muscles and fascial layers (Figure 17-15). In animals with an incomplete bony orbit, the masticatory muscles play a critical role in providing posterior support for the orbital contents. Orbital disease processes may thus be located in one of the following three planes:

- Within the muscle cone
- Outside the muscle cone but within the periorbita
- Within the orbit but outside the periorbita (e.g., posterior to the periorbita laterally where there is no bony wall, as occurs in myositis of the temporal muscle)

The lacrimal gland lies beneath the orbital ligament on the dorsolateral surface of the globe (see Figure 17-14). The base of the third eyelid and gland is held down by the *orbital retinaculum,* which are poorly defined sheets of collagenous

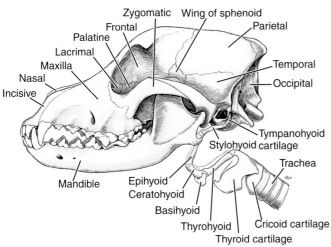

Figure 17-1. Bones of the skull, hyoid apparatus, and laryngeal cartilages, lateral aspect. (Modified from Evans HE [1993]: Miller's Anatomy of the Dog, 3rd ed. Saunders, Philadelphia.)

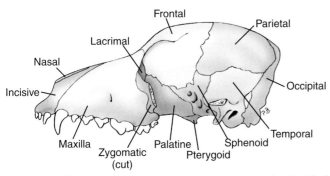

Figure 17-2. Skull, lateral aspect (zygomatic arch removed). (Modified from Evans HE [1993]: Miller's Anatomy of the Dog, 3rd ed. Saunders, Philadelphia.)

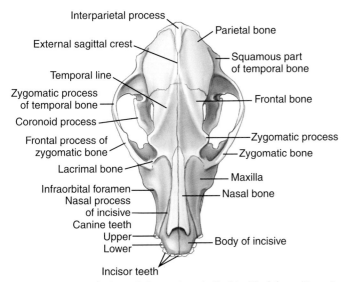

Figure 17-3. Dorsal view of the canine skull. (Modified from Getty R [1975]: Sisson and Grossman's the Anatomy of the Domestic Animals, 5th ed. Saunders, Philadelphia.)

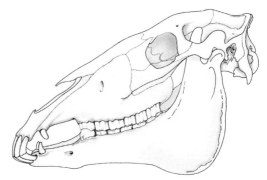

Figure 17-4. Left lateral view of the equine skull. Note the enclosed dorsolateral surface of the orbit. (Modified from Dyce KM, et al. [2002]: Textbook of Veterinary Anatomy, 3rd ed. Saunders, Philadelphia.)

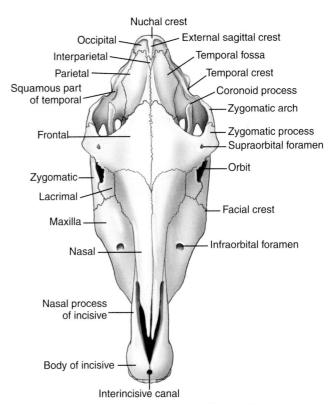

Figure 17-5. Dorsal view of the equine skull. (Modified from Getty R [1975]: Sisson and Grossman's the Anatomy of the Domestic Animals, 5th ed. Saunders, Philadelphia.)

tissue continuous with the periorbita but that contain smooth muscle with sympathetic innervation.

Extraocular Muscles

Seven extraocular muscles control movements of the globe (Figure 17-16; Table 17-1). The extraocular muscles arise from the annulus of Zinn, which circles the optic foramen and orbital fissure, and insert onto the globe. Neurologic abnormalities in their function are discussed in Chapter 16.

PATHOLOGIC MECHANISMS

Because the orbit forms a semiclosed space, increases and decreases in the volume of its contents affect the position of the

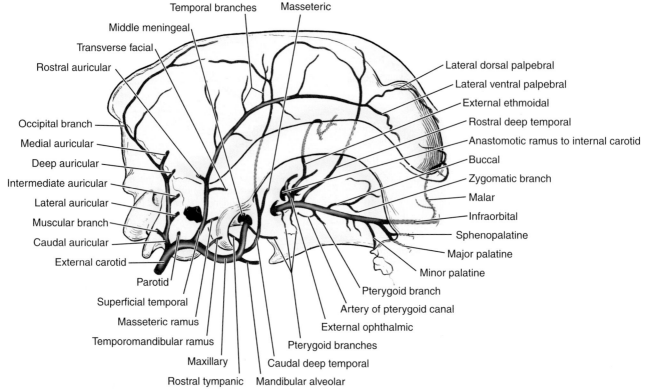

Figure 17-6. Arteries of the head in relation to lateral aspect of the skull. (Modified from Evans HE [1993]: Miller's Anatomy of the Dog, 3rd ed. Saunders, Philadelphia.)

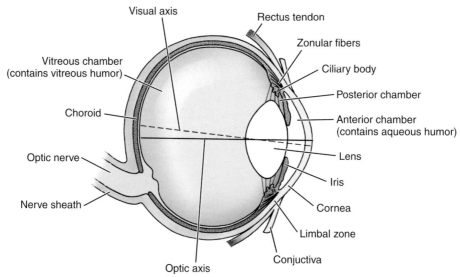

Figure 17-7. The visual and optic axes of the eye. (Modified from Getty R [1975]: Sisson and Grossman's the Anatomy of the Domestic Animals, 5th ed. Saunders, Philadelphia.)

Table 17-1 | **Extraocular Muscles: Actions and Innervations**

MUSCLE	INNERVATION	ACTION
Superior (dorsal) rectus	Oculomotor (CN III)	Elevates globe
Inferior (ventral) rectus	Oculomotor (CN III)	Depresses globe
Medial rectus	Oculomotor (CN III)	Turns globe nasally
Lateral rectus	Abducens (CN VI)	Turns globe temporally
Superior (dorsal) oblique	Trochlear (CN IV)	Intorts globe (rotates 12 o'clock position nasally)
Inferior (ventral) oblique	Oculomotor (CN III)	Extorts globe (rotates 12 o'clock position temporally)
Retractor bulbi	Abducens (CN VI)	Retracts globe
Levator superioris	Oculomotor (CN III)	Elevates upper lid

CN, Cranial nerve.

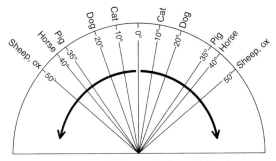

Figure 17-8. Comparison of the angle formed by the optic axes of different species of domestic animals. (From Getty R [1975]: Sisson and Grossman's the Anatomy of the Domestic Animals, 5th ed. Saunders, Philadelphia.)

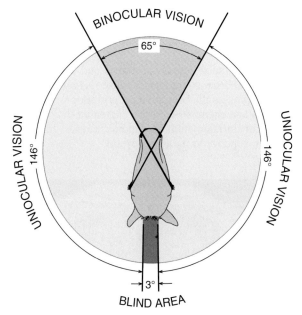

Figure 17-10. Visual field of the horse, showing a smaller binocular field, large panoramic uniocular areas, and a minute blind area.

eye in relation to the orbital rim and to the other eye. Space-occupying lesions (Figure 17-17) push the eye forward, causing *exophthalmos*, and often the third eyelid also protrudes as it is passively forced out of the orbit. In dogs and cats orbital masses usually result in swelling of the tissues caudal to the last upper molar tooth, because the orbital floor is only soft tissue in this area. With decreased volume of the orbital contents (e.g., dehydration or atrophy of fat or muscle), the eye sinks further into the orbit—*enophthalmos*—and the third eyelid protrudes. Osteomyelitis of the bones forming the orbit due to organisms such as *Cryptococcus* and *Actinomyces* spp. may also cause exophthalmos.

Exophthalmos must be distinguished from apparent exophthalmos due to shallow orbits (occurring in brachycephaly, hydrocephalus), euryblepharon, glaucoma, and facial paralysis.

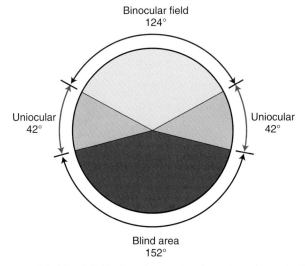

Figure 17-9. Visual field of a primate, showing a large binocular field, small uniocular areas, and a large blind area. (Modified from Duke-Elder S [1958]: System of Ophthalmology, Vol I: The Eye in Evolution. H. Compton, London.)

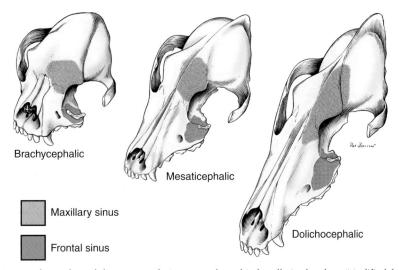

Figure 17-11. Relationship of the paranasal sinuses to the orbital walls in the dog. (Modified from Evans HE [1993]: Miller's Anatomy of the Dog, 3rd ed. Saunders, Philadelphia.)

The position of space-occupying lesions alters the direction of displacement of the globe and is used to determine the site of the offending mass (Figure 17-18) and the optimal route of surgical exploration.

Because the subconjunctival tissues and the orbit are connected, orbital diseases frequently cause *chemosis*. If the orbital lesion compresses the orbital veins, posterior venous drainage diminishes and chemosis is further increased. In horses, orbital swelling or inflammation commonly causes filling of the depression superior to the upper eyelid.

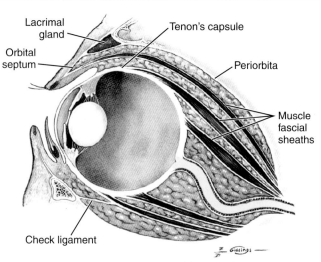

Figure 17-14. Divisions of the periorbita.

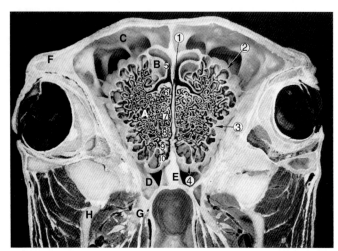

Figure 17-12. Transverse section through head of horse at level of orbital cavities; rostral surface of section. *A,* Ethmoidal labyrinth; *B,* dorsal nasal conchal sinus; *C,* frontal sinus; *D,* sphenopalatine sinus; *E,* vomer bone; *F,* zygomatic process of frontal bone; *G,* palatine bone; *H,* mandible; *1,* perpendicular plate (lamina); *2,* tectorial plate; *3,* orbital plate; *4,* basal plate; *2-4,* papyraceous plate; *5,* dorsal nasal concha (endoturbinate I); *6,* middle nasal concha (endoturbinate II); *7-10,* endoturbinates II-VI, respectively. (Modified from Getty R [1975]: Sisson and Grossman's the Anatomy of the Domestic Animals, 5th ed. Saunders, Philadelphia.)

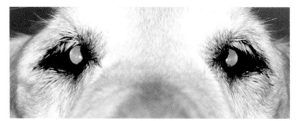

Figure 17-15. Loss of orbital fat and masticatory muscle mass, as in this aged golden retriever, can result in profound enophthalmia. (Courtesy University of Wisconsin–Madison Veterinary Ophthalmology Service Collection.)

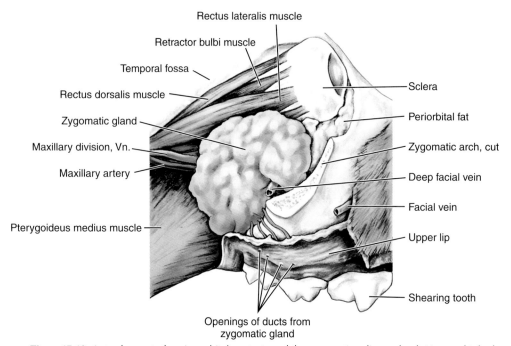

Figure 17-13. Lateral aspect of canine orbital contents and the zygomatic salivary gland. Note multiple ducts of the zygomatic gland entering the oral cavity. (Modified from Evans HE [1993]: Miller's Anatomy of the Dog, 3rd ed. Saunders, Philadelphia.)

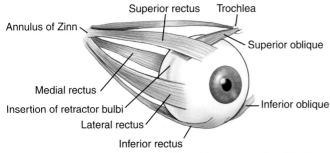

Figure 17-16. General arrangement of the orbital muscles. (Modified from Prince JH, et al. [1960]: Anatomy and Histology of the Eye and Orbit in Domestic Animals. Charles C. Thomas, Springfield, IL.)

Exophthalmos frequently causes greater evaporation of the precorneal tear film and exposure keratitis.

Because of the many tissue types present, numerous kinds of neoplasms may affect the orbit. The most common causes of exophthalmos in one case series of dogs and cats were neoplasia (52%), orbital abscesses/cellulitis (30%), hematoma (9%), zygomatic mucocele (5%), arteriovenous fistula (2%), and eosinophilic myositis (2%).

DIAGNOSTIC METHODS

The diagnosis of orbital disorders requires a complete ophthalmic examination and perhaps additional special diagnostic techniques, as follows (Figure 17-19).

- Determination of globe and optic axis displacement helps localize the lesion.

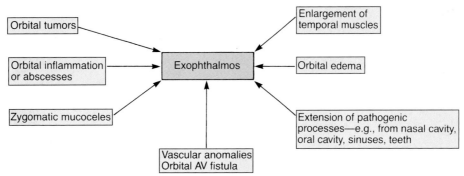

Figure 17-17. Mechanisms of exophthalmos. *AV,* Arteriovenous.

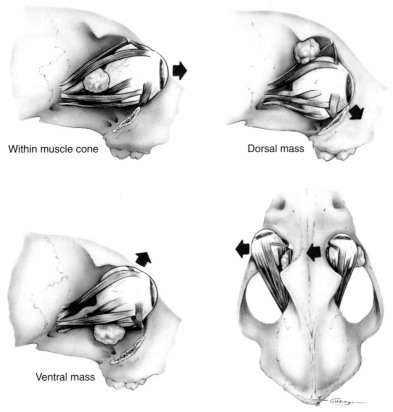

Figure 17-18. Effects of space-occupying lesions on the direction of globe displacement (as indicated by *arrows*).

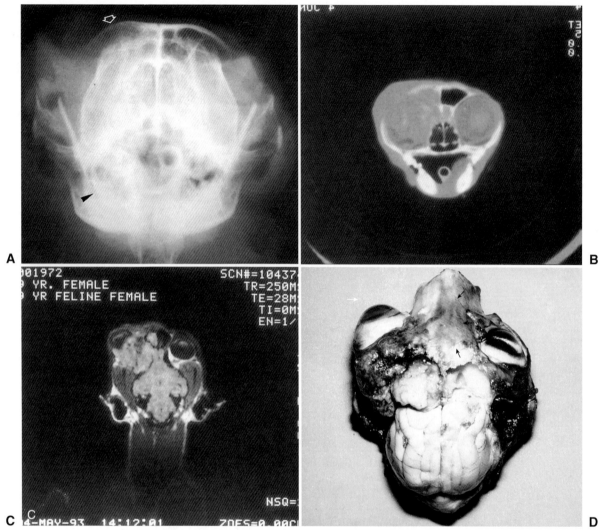

Figure 17-19. A, Rostrocaudal radiographic view of the skull of a cat with a frontal sinus/orbital mass. Lysis of cortical bone of the right frontal sinus is present *(open arrow)*. Fluid density is present in the right tympanic bulla *(arrowhead)*. **B,** Transverse computed tomographic scan of the orbit of the same cat. A large soft tissue mass with central areas of mineral opacity is present. Lysis of the cribriform plate and cortical bone of the right frontal sinus are present dorsally, ventrally, and laterally. **C,** Coronal T1-weighted magnetic resonance image of the orbit of the same cat. A large mass of uniform isointensity to peripheral brain parenchyma is displacing and compressing the dorsal medial quadrant of the globe and the parenchyma of the right rostral cerebral hemisphere and olfactory bulb. Focal areas of signal void within the mass represent mineralization or necrosis. **D,** Postmortem photograph of the skull of the same cat. The dorsal calvarium has been removed. A large orbital mass *(arrows)* is present, causing exophthalmos of the right eye and compression of the frontal lobe of the brain. Lysis of cortical bone is present dorsal and caudal to the mass. (From Ramsey DT, et al. [1994]: Comparative value of diagnostic imaging techniques in a cat with exophthalmos. Vet Comp Ophthalmol 4:198.)

- Orbital palpation. The consistency and position of orbital contents can often be determined by placing pressure on the globe itself, through the eyelids (retropulsion of the globe). Additionally, careful orbital palpation along the rim and inside the orbit with a lubricated fingertip can be useful in localizing lesions.
- Opening of the mouth. Inability to fully open the mouth with enophthalmia is consistent with a restrictive myopathy of the masticatory muscles. If the globe is exophthalmic, substantial pain on opening the mouth suggests an inflammatory process, whereas the absence of pain is more consistent with neoplasia. In dogs and cats the soft tissue posterior to the last upper molar should be carefully inspected and palpated if possible.

- B-scan ultrasonography (see Chapter 5) is very useful for evaluation of soft tissue masses within the orbit and may guide further diagnostic procedures, such as fine-needle aspiration.
- Magnetic resonance imaging (MRI) and computed tomography (CT) (Figures 17-19 through 17-21) yield superior definition in localizing orbital lesions. They allow the extent of disease to be better estimated and enable more accurate surgical planning. CT may be used to guide fine-needle aspiration or biopsy, thus avoiding exploratory orbitotomy.
- Contrast radiographic techniques have been largely supplanted by ultrasound and CT/MRI but may be useful in select cases. The techniques consist of contrast orbital

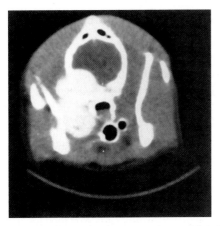

Figure 17-20. Computed tomographic scan of a multilobular ossifying fibroma (sarcoma, chondroma rodens) originating from the right petrous temporal bone and extending rostrally to invade the orbit and nasal cavity, and medially into the middle cerebral fossa, via the frontal, temporal, and parietal bones. The eye was displaced anteriorly. The patient was a 12-year-old Brittany spaniel. (Courtesy Dr. R. Bellhorn.)

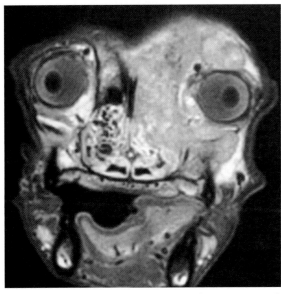

Figure 17-21. Magnetic resonance image of nasal carcinoma invading the orbit of a dog and causing exophthalmos.

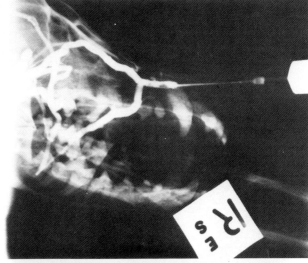

A

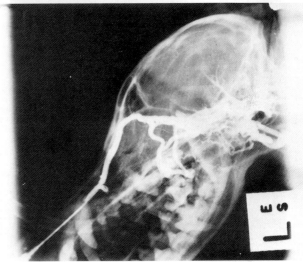

B

Figure 17-22. A, Normal lateral orbital venogram in a 5-year-old poodle (right eye). **B,** Venogram of left orbit of same dog showing a lymphoid pseudotumor in the inferonasal orbit. The inferior ophthalmic vein is obliterated. (Courtesy Dr. R. Dixon.)

venography (Figure 17-22), contrast orbitography (Figures 17-23 and 17-24), and orbital arteriography (Figures 17-25 and 17-26).

- Fine-needle aspiration or biopsy of orbital contents for cytologic analysis or culture. Guiding these procedures with ultrasound or CT imaging has allowed many orbital lesions to be characterized without resorting to surgical exploration.
- Surgical orbital exploration with or without preservation of the globe

Localization of Foreign Bodies

Depending on the type of foreign body, ultrasonography or radiography can be used to localize a foreign body. For radiography a reference ring of wire may be placed at the limbus (see Figure 17-23); radiographs are taken at four different angles (lateral, ventrodorsal, oblique, frontal) in an attempt to

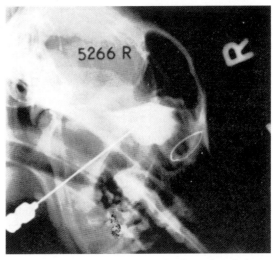

Figure 17-23. Contrast orbitography. Lateral radiograph with the needle in position in the orbital cone after injection of 4 mL of contrast medium. The cone is well filled, with leakage ventrally. A wire marker ring is placed at the limbus. (From Munger RJ, Ackerman N [1978]: Retrobulbar injections in the dog: a comparison of three techniques. J Am Anim Hosp Assoc 14:490.)

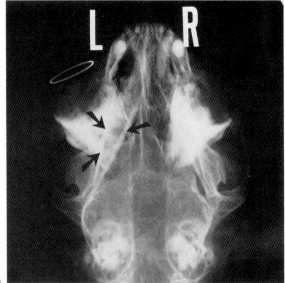

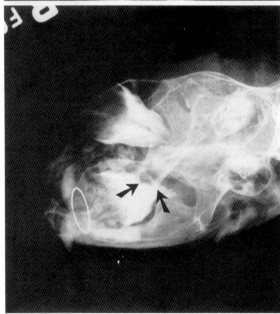

Figure 17-24. Contrast orbitography. **A,** Ventrodorsal radiograph of a cat after injection of contrast medium. The cat was blind and exhibited ophthalmoplegia and exophthalmos (orbital fissure syndrome). A filling defect *(arrows)*, present at the left orbital apex, is due to orbital extension of an intracranial lymphosarcoma involving the optic chiasm. **B,** A lateral oblique view of the skull showing a filling defect *(arrows)* at the apex of the orbit. (Courtesy Dr. R. Munger.)

differentiate ocular and orbital foreign bodies and determine their location. Nonmetallic foreign bodies tend to be better visualized ultrasonographically. Porcupine quills, which are common orbital foreign bodies in dogs in certain geographic areas, have a characteristic double-banded, linear hyperechoic appearance useful in identifying, localizing, and establishing a prognosis. Wooden slivers, however, are not easily visualized with either technique.

ORBITAL DISEASES

A summary of orbital diseases, classified by type, is given in Table 17-2.

Orbital Cellulitis and Retrobulbar Abscess

Orbital cellulitis and retrobulbar abscess occur most commonly in dogs and cats.

ETIOLOGY. Although retrobulbar abscess is common, its etiology is poorly understood and is not always confirmed. It is assumed to be a bacterial infection, either of hematogenous origin or due to penetrating injury from the oral cavity in association with a foreign body. Mixed flora or no growth is a common finding on aerobic bacterial culture, and in many cases anaerobic culture testing methods are required in order to demonstrate the organisms. *Aspergillus* spp. and *Penicillium* spp. have been isolated from orbital cellulitis in cats, and *Pasteurella* spp. have been isolated from both dogs and cats. The process begins as *orbital cellulitis;* then localization occurs and an abscess may form. At the stage of cellulitis, the clinical signs are less extreme; that is, pain may be less, oral signs nonexistent, and diagnosis more difficult.

CLINICAL SIGNS. The most important clinical signs of retrobulbar abscess/cellulitis are as follows:

- Exophthalmos (Figure 17-27)
- Periorbital swelling
- Pain on opening the mouth (often extreme)
- Fluctuating red swelling in the oral mucous membrane behind last upper molar (Figure 17-28)
- Protrusion of the third eyelid
- Chemosis, which is usually unilateral
- Pyrexia
- Anorexia
- Leukocytosis
- Acute onset (usual)

DIFFERENTIAL DIAGNOSIS. Retrobulbar abscess must be distinguished from orbital cellulitis (a generalized diffuse inflammation of orbital tissues), which has similar but less marked clinical signs. In orbital cellulitis pain is less evident, pyrexia and anorexia are not as pronounced, and less exudate or no exudate is present on orbital drainage. Orbital cellulitis may progress to retrobulbar abscess. Retrobulbar abscess may be distinguished from other causes of exophthalmos on the basis of its acute onset, pain, and, often, pyrexia. Leukocytosis with neutrophilia may be present.

Clinical signs of retrobulbar abscess are often pathognomonic.

TREATMENT. Orbital cellulitis and retrobulbar abscess are treated similarly, as follows:

1. Drainage via an incision behind the last upper molar (Figure 17-29). A small incision is made through only the oral mucosa. A pair of curved Crile hemostats or a blunt probe (Figure 17-30) is inserted and opened in small steps until the orbit is reached. Orbital tissues should not be crushed or cut during this process so as to avoid damage to the optic nerve or orbital vasculature. This technique allows pockets of exudate to be drained while limiting damage to the orbit. Considerable amounts of exudate under pressure may be released, and dependent drainage to the oral cavity is established. Although exudate is frequently *not* obtained, drainage is an important *prerequisite* step in treatment. Failure to locate exudate indicates that the process is still at

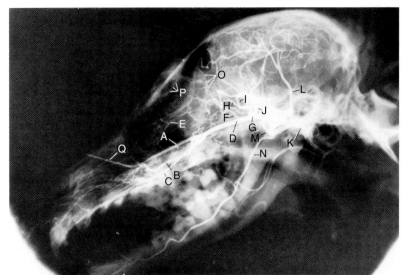

Figure 17-25. Lateral canine orbital arteriogram produced after a retrograde injection of 5 to 10 mL of contrast medium into the infraorbital artery. The arteries of the eye and orbit are outlined. *A,* Infraorbital artery; *B,* sphenopalatine artery; *C,* major palatine artery; *D,* maxillary artery; *E,* malar artery; *F,* anterior deep temporal artery; *G,* orbital artery; *H,* ventral muscular branch; *I,* external ethmoid artery; *J,* external ophthalmic artery; *K,* external carotid artery; *L,* superficial temporal artery; *M,* posterior deep temporal artery; *N,* mandibular alveolar artery; *O,* choroid; *P,* ciliary body; *Q,* cannula. (From Ticer JW [1984]: Radiographic Technique in Small Animal Practice. Saunders, Philadelphia.)

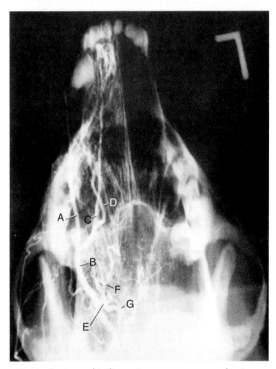

Figure 17-26. Canine orbital arteriogram, open-mouth view, produced after a retrograde injection of contrast medium into the infraorbital artery. Displacement, filling defects, and increased vascularity indicate the position of orbital lesions. *A,* Infraorbital artery; *B,* maxillary artery; *C,* major palatine artery; *D,* sphenopalatine artery; *E,* orbital artery; *F,* external ethmoid artery; *G,* external ophthalmic artery. (From Ticer JW [1984]: Radiographic Technique in Small Animal Practice. Saunders, Philadelphia.)

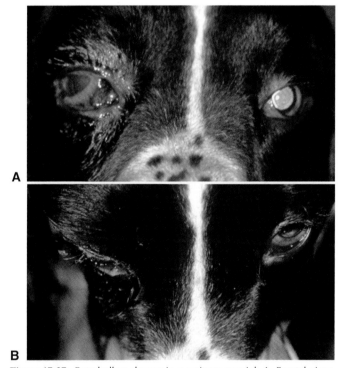

Figure 17-27. Retrobulbar abscess in a springer spaniel. **A,** Frontal view. **B,** Dorsal view. Note the exophthalmia of the right globe.

the cellulitis stage. Ultrasonographic imaging may facilitate draining an orbital abscess.

2. Exudate, if present, is collected for cytologic analysis and possibly aerobic/anaerobic culture.
3. The orbit is gently flushed with sterile saline via the oral incision and the use of a blunt cannula. The wound in the mouth is left open.
4. Systemic antibiotics (e.g., amoxicillin/clavulanic acid, clindamycin, metronidazole) are administered for 7 to 14 days.
5. Soft foods are fed during the recovery period.

Clinical improvement is usually rapid, occurring within 24 hours of treatment. In resistant cases or cases in which a retained foreign body is suspected, exploratory orbitotomy may be necessary.

Cystic Orbital and Periocular Lesions

Orbital and periocular cysts are uncommon. Numerous lesions and tissues may cause cystic swellings, including dacryops (cyst of the lacrimal sac), zygomatic and lacrimal mucoceles in both dogs and cats, retained glandular tissue from the lacrimal or third eyelid gland after enucleation or trauma, sialocele after transplantation of the parotid ducts, and mucocele of the nasal and frontal sinuses, especially in association with neoplasia. Abscesses of the

Table 17-2 | **Summary of Orbital Diseases**

TYPE OF DISORDER	CONDITION	CLINICAL SIGNS
Developmental abnormalities	1. Shallow orbit (brachycephalic breeds)	1. Exophthalmos, exposure keratitis, corneal ulceration, pigmentation
	2. Microphthalmia, anophthalmia	2. Small or no globe, narrow palpebral fissure, prominent third eyelid, epiphora, blindness
	3. Hydrocephalus with orbital malformation	3. Exotropia, hypotropia, poor vision
	4. Euryblepharon	4. Long palpebral fissure resulting in apparent exophthalmos
	5. Orbital arteriovenous fistula	5. Exophthalmos, fremitus, pulse detectable ("exophthalmos pulsans")
Trauma	1. Hemorrhages	1. Subconjunctival and episcleral hemorrhages; retrobulbar hemorrhage with exophthalmos or proptosis
	2. Penetrating foreign bodies (grass awns, needles, and so on from mouth)	2. Discharging sinus fluid through the conjunctiva, periocular skin, buccal mucosa; pain on opening mouth
	3. Orbital fractures	3. Pain, crepitus, skin abrasions, displacement of globe
Infections	1. Bacteria, fungi	1. Ocular discharge usually secondary to penetrating foreign bodies from conjunctiva or oral cavity; sinusitis, rhinitis, or infections of roots of teeth
	2. Parasites (*Dirofilaria immitis; Pneumonyssus caninum*)	2. Granulomatous lesions due to wandering larvae, e.g., *Dirofilaria* (rare), or extension of infection from nasal cavity (*Pneumonyssus*)
Neoplasia	1. Primary orbital neoplasms—sarcoma, meningioma, adenocarcinoma from nasal cavity, lymphosarcoma in cattle	1. Exophthalmos, exposure keratitis, strabismus, displacement of globe
	2. Metastatic or invasive neoplasms	2. As for (1), plus nasal or neurologic signs
Miscellaneous conditions	1. Zygomatic mucocele	1. Exophthalmos, strabismus, swelling in any part of orbit, or behind upper last molar tooth
	2. Infections of roots of teeth (especially carnassial)	2. Discharging fistula beneath eye in dogs
	3. Dehydration	3. Enophthalmos, passive protrusion of third eyelid
	4. Eosinophilic myositis	4. Exophthalmos, pain with dysphagia in acute stage; enophthalmos potentiated by opening mouth in chronic stage when temporal muscles have atrophied
	5. Horner's syndrome	5. Enophthalmos, miosis, ptosis, protrusion of third eyelid, ipsilateral sweating in horses, dermal vasodilation, and hyperthermia
	6. Orbital emphysema	6. Crepitus beneath the conjunctiva

Modified from Smith JS (1977): Diseases of the orbit, in Kirk RW (editor): Current Veterinary Therapy VI. Saunders, Philadelphia.

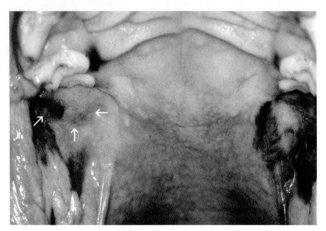

Figure 17-28. A fluctuating swelling caudal to the last upper molar in a dog with a retrobulbar abscess is indicated by arrows.

lacrimal sac and protrusion of orbital fat must be distinguished from cysts because their appearances may be similar.

Frontal Sinus Mucocele

Obstruction of drainage of the frontal sinus into the nasal cavity, combined with creation of an opening from the frontal sinus into the orbit either by trauma, malformation, or other disease processes such as neoplasia, may result in passage of sinus secretions into the orbit via the medial orbital wall. This often results in orbital swelling and orbital pain; if the tract reaches the conjunctiva or periocular skin, there may be a profuse intermittent ocular discharge. The condition often responds temporarily to antibiotic therapy. Diagnosis is made via radiography, CT, or MRI of the frontal sinus, although in select cases a blunt instrument can be passed from the conjunctival fistula into the sinus. It is imperative to rule out frontal sinus neoplasia or fungal infection in patients with mucoceles. Treatment is aimed at establishing drainage from the frontal sinus to the nasal cavity via frontal sinusotomy. Communications between the frontal sinus and the orbit secondary to osteomyelitis may be repaired with a temporalis muscle flap.

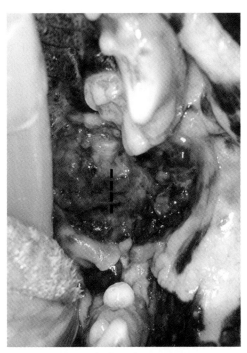

Figure 17-29. To drain a retrobulbar abscess, an incision approximately 1 cm long (indicated by *dotted line*) is made through the oral mucosa with a scalpel blade caudal to the last molar.

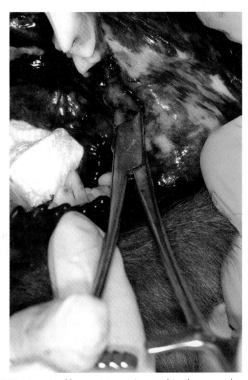

Figure 17-30. A pair of hemostats are inserted in the wound and opened in small steps to establish drainage from the orbit into the oral cavity. (Courtesy Dr. Ellison Bentley.)

Zygomatic Mucocele

A mucocele is caused by leakage of saliva from a gland or duct, with consequent inflammation and fibrous tissue reaction to the saliva. The condition is most commonly seen in dogs, occurring both spontaneously and after head trauma. Zygomatic mucoceles are uncommon but must be considered in the differential diagnosis of exophthalmos and space-occupying orbital lesions.

CLINICAL SIGNS. The clinical signs of zygomatic mucocele are as follows:

- Orbital swelling
- Exophthalmos
- Protrusion of the third eyelid
- Protrusion of the oral mucous membrane behind the last upper molar tooth
- Protrusion of a mass beneath the conjunctiva in the inferior temporal or nasal conjunctival fornix

Position of the mucocele within the orbit is variable, with the clinical signs varying accordingly. Aspiration of fluid from within the sac may reveal tenacious, straw-colored, honey-like liquid. Zygomatic mucoceles are usually painless. A zygomatic sialogram may be used to outline the mucocele for planning of surgical removal. Prior to removal, the gland may be outlined by injection of methylene blue up a zygomatic duct.

TREATMENT. Zygomatic mucoceles are best removed by localized orbitotomy depending on the location of the mass, as follows:

1. For masses protruding beneath the conjunctiva behind the lower lid: transconjunctival approach via the inferior conjunctival cul de sac behind the lower eyelid
2. For masses protruding beneath the conjunctiva laterally: an approach posterior to the orbital ligament and dorsal to the zygomatic arch. If necessary the orbital ligament may be transected and resutured.
3. For bulging of the oral mucous membrane, an oral approach behind the last upper molar tooth. If feasible, the mass may be marsupialized into the oral cavity.

Neoplasms and Space-Occupying Lesions

Numerous orbital neoplasms have been described in domestic species, including meningioma, lymphosarcoma, adenocarcinoma, fibrosarcoma, multilobular osteosarcoma, glioma, myxoma, squamous cell carcinoma, rhabdomyosarcoma, and canine lymphoid pseudotumor (Figure 17-31). Retrobulbar neoplasms are uncommon and, in the early stages, present a diagnostic challenge. The most common primary orbital neoplasm in the dog, meningioma is usually a benign solitary neoplasm that grows slowly and produces pressure atrophy. Correct diagnosis is essential to effective treatment.

CLINICAL SIGNS. The clinical signs of orbital neoplasms are as follows:

- Exophthalmos; usually unilateral, slowly progressive, and *painless*
- Intraconal deviation, displacement, or reduced motility of the globe (see Figure 17-18)
- Periocular swelling
- Prominent or protruding third eyelid
- Blindness in some cases; useful to differentiate from ocular enlargement due to glaucoma, for which blindness is the rule
- Secondary exposure keratitis
- Retinal folds or detachment on ophthalmoscopic examination, due to indentation of the globe by the neoplasm

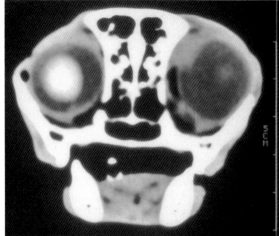

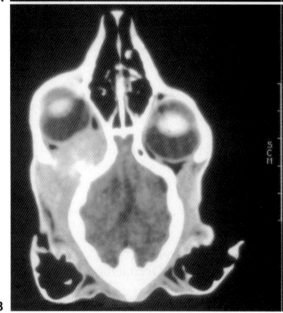

Figure 17-31. A, Transverse computed tomographic scan of a cat with a orbital tumor. The left orbit is "full," and the globe is deviated anteriorly. **B,** Reconstructed view of the same image set from above. The retrobulbar mass is clearly visible. (Courtesy University of Wisconsin–Madison Veterinary Ophthalmology Service Collection.)

- Dilated or eccentric pupil
- Papilledema
- Nasal discharge

TREATMENT. Thorough surgical removal is the treatment of choice. In dogs, approximately 90% of orbital tumors are malignant, and complete surgical excision is required. If specialized surgical assistance is available, an exploratory orbitotomy via zygomatic arch resection is recommended. This technique allows exploration and removal of the tumor mass, if possible, with retention of the globe. If the neoplasm is invasive, exenteration of the orbit may be required. In advanced cases with invasion into the bony orbital boundaries, radical orbitectomy may be considered. Orbitotomy allows removal of benign and nonneoplastic lesions (e.g., zygomatic salivary gland mucocele) without loss of the eye. If the lesion is small or well localized by diagnostic procedures, a transconjunctival approach or less radical orbitotomy is useful. Depending on

tumor type, chemotherapy, immunotherapy, and radiation may be combined with surgery to control the neoplastic tissue but are ineffective alone. If radiation therapy is used, the ocular complications must be considered (see Chapter 3).

Multilobular Osteoma

Synonyms: Chondroma rodens, calcifying aponeurotic fibroma.

Multilobular osteoma occurs in dogs, cats, and horses, in which it arises from the flat bones of the skull. Exophthalmos is the most common sign in the orbit. Diagnosis is made by either histopathology or recognition of the radiographic signs (homogenous stippling, evenly undulating well-demarcated borders with a highly radiodense granular appearance). These lesions are generally benign but are occasionally aggressive; a localized multilobular osteoma can be removed surgically. Growth is slow, metastasis is late, and local recurrence can be expected if removal is incomplete. The clinical signs and behavior of multilobular osteoma are similar to those of parosteal osteosarcoma, a rare tumor of the periosteum that has the potential to metastasize, usually later in its course.

Periorbital Fractures

Periorbital contusions and fractures, which occur most commonly in horses, are caused by trauma, uncontrolled or unrestrained behavior, or violent recovery from anesthesia. Diagnosis is more accurate through physical examination performed before and during surgical exploration than with radiography. Clinical signs include pain, crepitus, exophthalmos, periorbital swelling, abrasions, corneal ulceration, uveitis, blepharospasm, ocular entrapment, and facial asymmetry. Fracture of the supraorbital process with extension nasally to the supraorbital foramen and fractures of the lacrimal bone at the nasal canthus may damage the nasal mucosa, causing epistaxis. Bony fragments projecting into the orbit and causing pain, ocular entrapment, and exophthalmos have been observed with fractures near the medial canthus. The nasolacrimal duct may also be damaged.

If fractures are demonstrated on oblique radiographs or on surgical exploration, small pieces of bone may be removed. The conjunctival fornices are palpated, and any bony fragments palpable in the orbit are removed or surgically replaced. Larger fragments may be wired in place, pinned, or treated conservatively by restriction of the horse for 4 to 6 weeks. Early surgical treatment prevents fixation of fragments in abnormal positions by formation of fibrous tissue. Solid synthetic polymers (e.g., silicone or polytetrafluoroethylene [Teflon] sheets) may be inserted and contoured to restore facial profiles for cosmesis. Associated ocular injuries, including corneal ulceration and traumatic uveitis, are common and must be addressed. Contusions and associated edema are treated prophylactically with systemic penicillin/gentamicin and allowed to resolve spontaneously. If necessary, tetanus antiserum should be given.

Early surgical intervention in equine periorbital fractures yields superior cosmetic results.

Eosinophilic Myositis

Eosinophilic myositis occurs most commonly in German shepherds and Weimaraners but is a rare disorder. It usually can be differentiated from orbital neoplasia, orbital cellulitis, and retrobulbar abscess because it is bilateral.

The clinical signs of eosinophilic myositis are as follows:

- Typically bilaterally symmetrical swelling of masseter, temporal, and pterygoid muscles
- Exophthalmos (variable in extent)
- Chemosis/eyelid edema
- Protrusion of the third eyelid
- Pain on opening the jaws fully

Some animals die during acute attacks; in others the disease resolves, but recurrences are common. Attacks may last 10 to 21 days. Eosinophilia is not a constant sign. The disease may be diagnosed from clinical signs, electromyography, and temporal muscle biopsy. The etiology of eosinophilic myositis is unknown. High doses of systemic steroids and azathioprine have been recommended for treatment. After recovery, temporal and masseter muscle atrophy may occur, together with atrophy of orbital fat and enophthalmos. Affected animals often have difficulty opening the mouth as a result of scarring of the muscles of mastication.

Extraocular Muscle Myositis

An uncommon, presumably immune-mediated disorder, myositis of extraocular muscles affects young (usually less than 1 year) dogs of many breeds, but especially golden retrievers. It is characterized by chemosis and bilateral exophthalmia in which the globes are deviated directly along the direction of the orbital axis (Figure 17-32). Occasionally vision loss occurs if massively swollen extraocular muscles compress the optic nerve. Histologic analysis shows that extraocular muscles (with the exception of the retractor bulbi, which is spared) are infiltrated by lymphocytes and histiocytes. Therapy consists of systemic corticosteroids, with the dosage slowly tapered as the condition resolves. Azathioprine is an alternative drug for use in resistant cases. Although in most animals the disease responds rapidly, recurrence is possible.

Orbital Emphysema

Orbital emphysema uncommonly occurs in dogs and cats after trauma to the paranasal sinuses, with leakage of air into the orbit. The air is palpable as crepitus beneath the conjunctiva or periocular skin. Orbital emphysema has been described, in

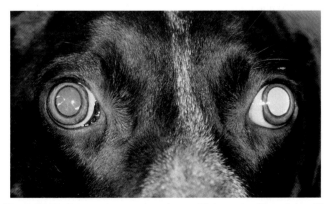

Figure 17-32. Extraocular muscle polymyositis in a mixed breed dog. The two globes are equally exophthalmic and deviated along the orbital axis.

which the air may have entered the orbit via the nasolacrimal duct during labored respirations after a routine enucleation.

If emphysema is present, a radiographic study of the sinuses is indicated. The animal is started on systemic antibiotics to prevent infection of the orbit via the paranasal sinuses. In reported cases, spontaneous resolution occurred. If the condition occurs after enucleation, the nasolacrimal duct may be ligated at its orbital exit.

Proptosis of the Globe

Proptosis constitutes an ocular emergency, and its treatment and prognosis are discussed in Chapter 19.

OPHTHALMIC MANIFESTATIONS OF DENTAL DISEASE

Because of the proximity of the roots of the teeth to the orbit, ocular manifestations and complications of dental disease are common and are frequently overlooked. The most common ocular signs are pain and swelling anterior and inferior to the globe secondary to an abscess of the upper fourth premolar in dogs. The globe may be enophthalmic, and the third eyelid may protrude. Additionally, dental disease has been associated with chronic uveitis and conjunctivitis in dogs and cats.

SURGICAL PROCEDURES

The most common orbital procedures are for removal of the whole or part of the globe or orbital contents; they are defined as follows (Figure 17-33):

- *Enucleation:* Removal of the globe, third eyelid, conjunctiva, and eyelids
- *Exenteration:* Removal of the globe, orbital contents, and eyelids
- *Evisceration:* Removal of the intraocular contents, uvea, lens, retina, vitreous, and eyelids

Enucleation

INDICATIONS. Enucleation is performed for the following reasons:

- Intraocular neoplasia
- Severe perforating ocular trauma with disruption and loss of ocular contents. An evisceration with placement of *intraocular prosthesis* can often be used instead to preserve cosmetic appearance if desired.
- Uncontrollable endophthalmitis or panophthalmitis
- Intractable ocular pain, especially in glaucomatous eyes
- Owner inability or unwillingness to give long-term treatment to a blind eye to keep it comfortable

Enucleation is an admission that therapeutic attempts to control a pathologic process have failed. It is not used in lieu of a correct diagnosis or treatment.

After enucleation, an *intraorbital prosthesis* may be used to give a superior cosmetic result. Enucleation in a young animal results in a slower rate of growth of the orbit and a decrease in the final orbital volume than in the other, normal orbit. This slower rate of growth is due to lack of orbital contents.

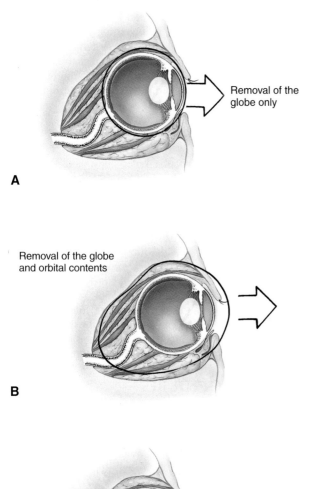

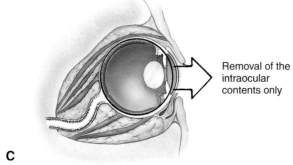

Figure 17-33. Diagrammatic representations of **(A)** enucleation, **(B)** exenteration, and **(C)** evisceration.

Replacement of orbital volume with prosthetic materials after enucleation in a young animal tends to result in an orbit that more closely approximates normal size. If a prosthesis is placed in the orbit of a young animal, a slightly larger prosthesis is chosen than would be indicated by the size of the contralateral eye, to allow for the stimulating effect of the implant on orbital growth, and for normal orbital growth.

There are numerous variations of enucleation techniques. The lateral subconjunctival and transpalpebral approaches are described here. Preoperative use of oral carprofen 12 to 24 hours before surgery in dogs, and of intramuscular morphine (dogs) or butorphanol (dogs and cats) before anesthetic induction, is recommended. Postoperative analgesia for 2 to 3 days is also advised.

Lateral Subconjunctival Enucleation Technique

The lateral subconjunctival approach to enucleation has the advantage of giving better exposure of the optic nerve and orbital vessels. It is used in dogs and cats. The technique proceeds as follows:

1. A lateral, 1- to 2-cm canthotomy is performed to improve exposure (Figure 17-34, *A*).
2. The conjunctiva is grasped near the limbus with toothed forceps, and a 360-degree perilimbal incision is made beneath it (Figure 17-34, *B*).
3. The sclera is separated from the conjunctiva, Tenon's capsule, and extraocular muscles with curved Metzenbaum or Mayo scissors around to the optic nerve (Figure 17-34, *B*). The lacrimal gland beneath the orbital ligament is left attached to the globe, if possible.
4. The optic nerve may be severed with scissors or with an electrosurgical unit equipped with a tonsil snare (Figure 17-34, *C*). *Traction must not be placed on the nerve, nor should it be twisted* because twisting or traction may damage the optic and cause blindness in the remaining eye, especially in cats. Traction on the extraocular muscles may result in a reduction in heart rate (oculocardiac reflex), especially in horses and birds. A ligature may be placed around the nerve, encircling the associated short and long posterior ciliary vessels before their entry to the sclera. Often it is unnecessary to ligate the optic nerve in dogs and cats. The globe is removed and placed in fixative.
5. An attempt is made to control arterial and venous hemorrhage from the orbital cone with ligatures. If this is impossible, one or two surgical sponges are placed temporarily (5 minutes) in the orbit (Figure 17-34, *D*).
6. The third eyelid and gland are carefully removed (Figure 17-34, *D*).
7. Two to 3 mm of the lid margins are removed from the lateral to the medial canthus (Figure 17-34, *E*).
8. Conjunctiva and Tenon's capsule are closed with a simple continuous suture of 3/0 or 4/0 absorbable material. After the conjunctiva has been almost closed, *the surgical sponges are removed* and closure is completed. Closure forms a seal to contain further hemorrhage (Figure 17-34, *F*).
9. The lid incisions are closed with simple interrupted sutures of 4/0 or 5/0 nylon or polypropylene (Prolene) (Figure 17-34, *F*). Postoperative swelling is not unusual (especially if continuing hemorrhage occurs) but resolves within 3 or 4 days. As clots within the orbit break down, bloody fluid may appear at the nostril, via the nasolacrimal duct, on the third to fifth day, and owners should be advised accordingly. Postoperative analgesia with oral carprofen and morphine is advised in dogs; carprofen is not approved for use in cats.

The emotional resistance of owners to enucleation should not be underestimated.

All enucleated globes should be submitted for histopathologic examination to rule out an unsuspected disease process, such as neoplasia (Figure 17-35) or lens capsule rupture.

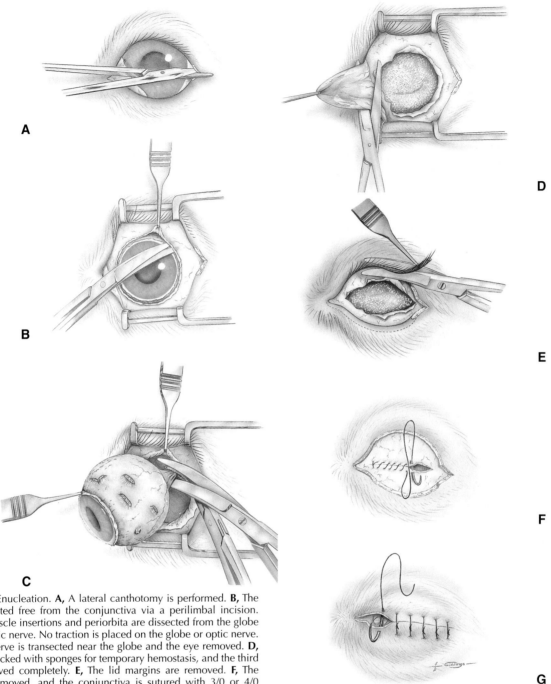

Figure 17-34. Enucleation. **A,** A lateral canthotomy is performed. **B,** The globe is dissected free from the conjunctiva via a perilimbal incision. Extraocular muscle insertions and periorbita are dissected from the globe back to the optic nerve. No traction is placed on the globe or optic nerve. **C,** The optic nerve is transected near the globe and the eye removed. **D,** The cavity is packed with sponges for temporary hemostasis, and the third eyelid is removed completely. **E,** The lid margins are removed. **F,** The sponges are removed, and the conjunctiva is sutured with 3/0 or 4/0 absorbable material. **G,** The lid incision is sutured completely with 4/0 or 5/0 nylon or polypropylene (Prolene).

Insertion of an Intraorbital Prosthesis

Silicone or methyl methacrylate spheres may be used to prevent unsightly postoperative depressions in the orbit (Figure 17-36). Insertion of an implant is a safe and inexpensive method of improving postoperative appearance. An implant should not be placed if the reason for enucleation was neoplasia outside the globe or infection inside the globe, or if the patient has foci of possible hematogenous bacterial infection elsewhere (e.g., severe periodontal or gingival disease, pyoderma, prostatitis, chronic otitis externa, or blepharitis). Bacterial invasion of the

implant can be minimized by prophylactic use of systemic bactericidal antibiotics. The size of the implant is determined by the depth and diameter of the orbit—generally 16 to 22 mm in dogs and cats, up 35 mm in horses.

In some patients the intact sphere may simply be placed in the orbit with acceptable cosmetic results. In many patients, however, shaping a silicone sphere to the contours of the orbit offers a superior cosmetic result and puts less tension on the skin incision. If a shaped sphere is to be used, the diameter of the sphere is typically chosen according to how closely it approximates the diameter of the orbit. One then determines the proper depth of the sphere by placing it within the orbit and estimating the amount of the sphere required to approximate the depth of the orbit (e.g., meet the orbital rim), allowing an additional 1 to 2 mm for postoperative contraction of orbital tissues. The excess portion of the sphere that would project beyond the orbital rim is then trimmed away with a clean horizontal slice with a No. 10 scalpel blade, and the sharp edges are smoothed and contoured with a Mayo scissors or scalpel blade. The implant is inserted with the flat side uppermost. The implant is then secured *firmly* in place by suturing of the periorbital fascia with a continuous absorbable 3/0 suture. A subcuticular suture layer and simple interrupted sutures close the incision. The success rate with orbital prostheses in dogs is high (98% to 99%), with a higher extrusion rate in cats (up to 5%).

Transpalpebral Enucleation-Exenteration Technique

Transpalpebral enucleation-exenteration, which can be used in all species, differs from the lateral conjunctival approach in that the lids are sutured closed and dissection into the orbit is made through the skin and initially *outside* the extraocular muscles. Once the orbit is entered the extraocular muscles may be cut free of the globe at their insertions on the sclera if only an enucleation is required, or the entire orbital contents may be removed if an exenteration is appropriate. This approach is preferable to a subconjunctival approach if the ocular surface is infected or if ocular neoplasia has escaped from the globe. A silicone sphere may be placed as previously described.

The transpalpebral approach is useful in the field for enucleation of bovine eyes with advanced squamous cell carcinoma. The cow is restrained in a head gate or chute, or against a strong railing fence, and tranquilized with xylazine. The recommended method of local anesthesia is to infiltrate the upper and lower lids with 10 mL of lidocaine 1 to 1.5 cm from the margin, and to perform a four-point block consisting of placing 5 to 10 mL of lidocaine into the orbit by retrobulbar injection with a 5- or 6-cm needle at each of four sites adjacent to the globe at the 12, 3, 6, and 9 o'clock positions (Figure 17-37). Gently bending the needle prior to insertion into the orbit may facilitate avoidance of the globe. An auriculopalpebral nerve block may also be useful. This produces anesthesia, akinesia, and exophthalmos, which aids in surgical exposure (Figure 17-38). As the globe is removed, additional local anesthetic may be infiltrated into orbital tissues as required. General anesthesia is

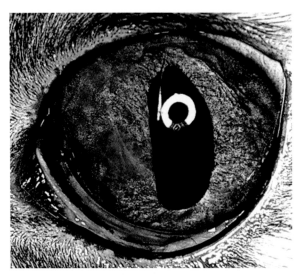

Figure 17-35. The importance of histopathologic examination of enucleated globes. Amelanotic melanoma was seen histologically in the eye of this cat, which had a history of chronic, nonresponsive anterior uveitis and secondary glaucoma. (Courtesy University of Wisconsin–Madison Veterinary Ophthalmology Service Collection.)

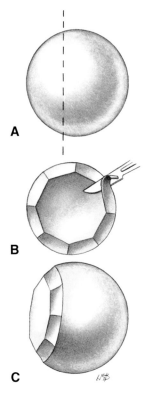

Figure 17-36. Preparation of the orbital implant. **A,** Approximately one third of the silicone sphere is removed so that the flat surface protrudes 1 to 2 mm above the level of the orbital rim when placed in the orbit. **B** and **C,** The cut edge is contoured and smoothed with Mayo scissors or a scalpel blade.

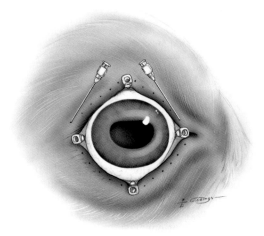

Figure 17-37. Injection sites for local anesthesia prior to transpalpebral enucleation in cattle. Five to 10 mL of lidocaine is injected at each site to produce anesthesia and proptosis. The needle may be slightly curved before injection to facilitate entry of the orbit and avoidance of the globe.

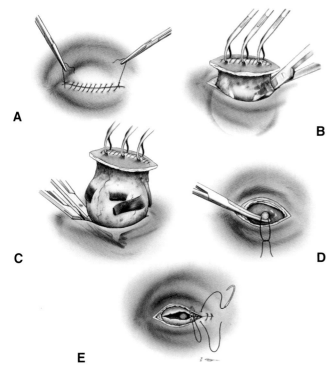

Figure 17-38. Transpalpebral enucleation/exenteration. **A,** The eyelids are sutured with a simple continuous suture tied at either end and are held with hemostats. **B,** A periocular incision is made, and dissection is performed initially outside the conjunctival sac and extraocular muscles. If an enucleation is to be performed, the extraocular muscles are severed at their insertion on the sclera. If an exenteration is to be performed, the dissection continues to the orbital apex. **C** and **D,** The optic nerve and associated vessels may be cut with scissors or clamped, ligated, and transected. **E,** The remaining periorbita and deep subcutaneous tissue are sutured with 3/0 or 4/0 absorbable suture, and the skin is closed with simple interrupted nonabsorbable sutures appropriate for the size and environment of the patient.

used in dogs, cats, and horses. The plane of dissection in this technique may be extended to perform an exenteration.

Enucleation in Birds

Techniques for removal of the eye in birds are modified because of the presence of scleral ossicles and the limited space in the avian orbit, into which the eye fits snugly. A transaural approach is suitable for owls (Figure 17-39), which allows retention of the globe for histologic analysis, and a globe-collapsing technique is suitable for all birds, although it may interfere with histologic examination (Figure 17-40). Meticulous hemostasis (including cautery, bovine thrombin, absorbable gelatin sponges, chilled saline, etc.) is also required for enucleation in a bird, because the large orbits are capable of sequestering large fractions of the animal's blood volume. Traction on the extraocular muscles is to be avoided in birds because it could invoke a lethal oculocardiac reflex.

Exenteration

Exenteration refers to removal of the globe and as much of the ocular contents as possible. It is performed in cases of orbital infection, orbital neoplasia, and ocular neoplasia that has extended beyond the globe. For orbital neoplasms, far better exposure is gained for exenteration by lateral orbitotomy. For

ocular neoplasms, an extension of the transpalpebral approach is used, with wider removal of orbital tissues. If large amounts of periocular tissues are also removed, the resulting skin defect may be repaired with a caudal auricular axial pattern flap.

Evisceration and Intrascleral Prosthesis

Evisceration (see Figure 17-33, *C*)—removal of the contents of the globe leaving only the corneoscleral shell—is appropriate for insertion of an intrascleral prosthesis in dogs and cats and, occasionally, in horses (see later).

OCULAR PROSTHESES

Ocular prostheses are of the following three types:

* *Intrascleral:* Used in the treatment of chronic glaucoma and to prevent phthisis bulbi in the early stages after severe trauma
* *Extrascleral:* Placement of porcelain shell on the surface of the globe for cosmesis
* *Intraorbital:* Used to replace an enucleated globe

Intrascleral Prosthesis

In the past, intrascleral prostheses in dogs and cats were associated with persistent infection and extrusion. Use of a silicone sphere and careful technique have greatly reduced these complications. The procedure is particularly useful in the treatment of blind glaucomatous eyes and after severe ocular trauma, in the absence of infection or severe contamination, to prevent phthisis bulbi. The diameter of the implant is equal to the horizontal corneal diameter of the contralateral normal eye *plus* 1 mm.

After thorough evisceration of the intraocular contents, a silicone sphere (Figure 17-41) is placed in the corneoscleral shell. Care should be taken to avoid trauma to the corneal endothelium if possible. After insertion into buphthalmic eyes, the sclera and cornea contract to the size of the prosthesis, the time for contraction depending on the original size of the eye. In very large eyes, contraction may take up to 6 weeks, and often the cornea has a bluish cast postoperatively. If the cornea is in better condition before surgery it may remain clear, but even then, corneal vascularization in the 2 to 3 weeks after insertion of the prosthesis is not uncommon. This vascularization resolves over the first postoperative 6 weeks but may alarm owners and therefore must be explained to them in advance. After insertion the cornea frequently pigments, usually with an improved cosmetic outcome, but the extent of pigmentation is unpredictable. The complication rate with this procedure is also low when it is performed in correctly chosen cases. Complications include corneal mineralization, ulceration, extrusion of the implant, and keratoconjunctivitis sicca. Although implants of different colors are available, the cosmetic result in cats is generally less satisfactory than that seen in dogs with dark irides because of the normal bright coloration of the feline iris and a vertically elliptical pupil. In select cases, especially in cats, "pupils" may be tattooed onto the cornea to improve cosmesis.

Extrascleral (Shell) Prosthesis

The extrascleral prosthesis, as commonly used in humans, is a porcelain shell inserted into the conjunctival sac over a

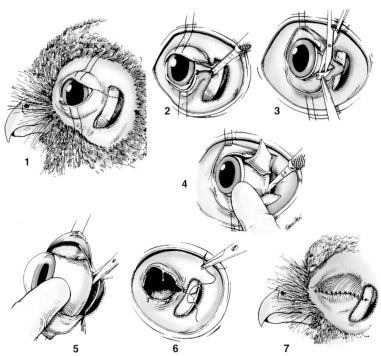

Figure 17-39. Procedure for avian enucleation. *1,* The bird is anesthetized and placed in lateral recumbency. The feathers over the orbital and auricular regions are plucked, and the area is prepared for aseptic surgery. Two stay sutures of 4/0 silk are placed in the lid margins. The anterior auricular margin is extended rostrally to visualize the posterior aspect of the globe. The incision line is indicated by the dashed line. *2,* A small scalpel blade is used to perform a lateral canthotomy that extends through the anterior auricular margin to the junction of the tubular globe with the postorbital process. A small vessel is encountered at the anterior auricular margin. Hemorrhage from this vessel can be controlled with electrocautery. The incision passes through conjunctiva and an extension of periorbital fascia, which is the equivalent of Tenon's capsule. *3,* The skin is gently dissected free, exposing the posterior limit of the tubular glove. A 360-degree subconjunctival dissection is extended posteriorly under the extension of periorbital fascia. An additional incision of this fascia at the 12 o'clock position may be necessary to mobilize the globe. *4,* A finger is placed at the limbus, and pressure is applied medially while a small scalpel blade is used to create a gap between the globe and the bony orbital elements. *5,* After a gap is created, tenotomy scissors are used to dissect the globe free of its extraocular elements and to sever the optic nerve. The globe is then delivered through the lateral aperture. Some bleeding will occur as the vessels are severed, but blood loss will be minimized if the surgeon rapidly proceeds with removal of the globe. Blood loss then can be controlled by packing of the orbit with gauze pads. The gauze is removed before closure. *6,* After hemostasis is obtained, the membrana nictitans and conjunctiva are removed, and a 2-mm strip of lid margin is resected. Closure is accomplished with the use of fine absorbable suture material (5/0 to 7/0) in a simple interrupted pattern. The fine suture is used to recreate the anterior auricular margin. The aural closure is then completed, followed by apposition of the line margins. *7,* Appearance after closure. (Modified from Murphy CJ, et al. [1983]: Enucleation in birds of prey. J Am Vet Med Assoc 183:1234.)

disfigured cornea or phthisical globe. Typically an eye (i.e., conjunctiva, cornea, and iris) is painted onto the external surface of the shell, although in some animals the dark conformer can be cosmetically acceptable in and of itself (Figure 17-42). Shell prostheses are used mainly in horses but are available for dogs. The manufacture and insertion of a shell are time consuming and expensive but the shell has gratifying results for clients prepared to bear the cost and time commitment. Each shell is individually cast to fit the affected eye, fitted over a period of several weeks, then painted to match the remaining eye. The services of a specially trained oculist are invaluable. After insertion the shell must be removed daily and washed by the owner (a relatively simple procedure in a tractable horse). A technique has also been described for insertion of a customized prosthesis into a bed of polyvinylsiloxane within the orbit of fish to improve appearance and allow public display after disfiguring eye disorders.

Intraorbital Prosthesis

See earlier discussion of intraorbital prosthesis insertion in the enucleation section.

ORBITOTOMY AND ORBITECTOMY

A detailed discussion of orbitotomy techniques is beyond the scope of this text, as the procedure is performed by veterinary ophthalmologists or specialist veterinary surgeons on an elective basis. The choice of approach to the orbit depends on the size and position of the lesion being excised, as follows:

- Superior, medial, and lateral transconjunctival approaches are used for small lesions anterior to the equator of the globe.
- Limited orbitotomy involving transection of the orbital ligament is used when limited exposure to the orbit is

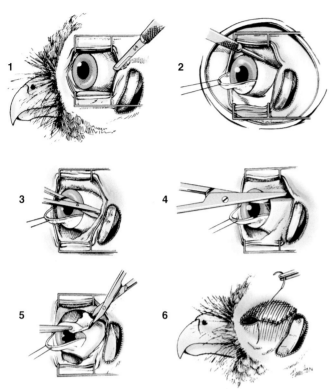

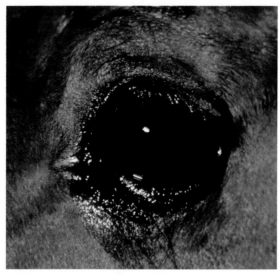

Figure 17-42. Extrascleral (shell) prosthesis in a horse. A custom-made prosthesis that fits between the conjunctival fornices may be placed over unsightly phthisical globes or after enucleation. The prosthesis may be simple, as in this case, or an oculist may paint a cosmetically convincing eye on a porcelain shell. (Courtesy University of Wisconsin–Madison Veterinary Ophthalmology Service Collection.)

Figure 17-40. Globe-collapsing procedure for enucleation. *1,* The bird is anesthetized and placed in lateral recumbency. The orbital region is plucked and prepared for aseptic surgery. A fine-wire lid speculum is placed under the membrana nictitans and lower lid. A lateral canthotomy extends dorsal to the anterior auricular margin. *2,* A 180-degree dorsal limbal incision is made, and a stay suture is placed in the incised cornea. A 360-degree subconjunctival dissection undermines the conjunctiva, membrana nictitans, and periorbital fascia. *3,* The region deep to the auricular skin is gently undermined. *4,* Mayo scissors are placed carefully between the uveal tract and sclera so that only the sclera and its associated ossicles are severed. *5,* Forceps are used to collapse the cut margins of the sclera inward, allowing access to the posterior aspect of the orbit. To prevent damage to the optic chiasm, excessive traction should be avoided. The extraocular attachments to the globe and the optic nerve are severed, and the eye is removed. *6,* The conjunctiva and membrana nictitans are removed, and a 2-mm strip of lid margin is resected. Closure is accomplished with the use of a fine (5/0 to 7/0) absorbable suture in a simple interrupted pattern. (Modified from Murphy CJ, et al. [1983]: Enucleation in birds of prey. J Am Vet Med Assoc 183:1234.)

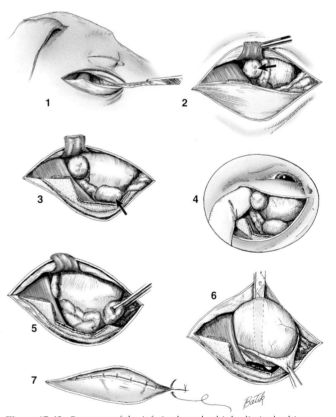

Figure 17-43. Exposure of the inferior lateral orbit by limited orbitotomy. The globe, zygomatic salivary gland, and transected orbital ligament are visible. (Modified from Bistner SI, et al. [1977]: Atlas of Veterinary Ophthalmic Surgery. Saunders, Philadelphia.)

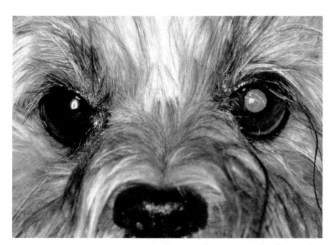

Figure 17-41. Postoperative appearance of an intrascleral prosthesis (right eye).

required (Figure 17-43), as for removal of a well-delineated zygomatic mucocele.

- Orbitotomy with zygomatic arch resection is used to completely expose the orbit, as for neoplasia (Figure 17-44).
- Extensive partial and total orbitectomy is used for invasive periorbital neoplasms, such as multilobular osteosarcomas and squamous cell carcinomas (Figure 17-45). Temporalis

muscle flaps and the medial mucosa of the lip may be used to reconstruct orbital margins, protect exposed brain, and reestablish oral, nasal, and orbital cavities. Adjuvant chemotherapy or radiation therapy may be useful for osteosarcomas, squamous cell carcinomas, and hemangiomas of the orbit because of the tendency for both local recurrence and metastasis, although protocols based on prospective studies are unavailable.

Temporalis Muscle Flap

The temporalis muscle originates from the parietal, temporal, frontal, and occipital bones and inserts onto the coronoid process of the mandible. It is the largest muscle in the head of the dog. The muscle is covered by a strong fascial sheet and supplied by the superficial temporal artery. Although the process is time consuming and technically challenging to perform, flaps from the temporalis muscle have been used to reconstruct the lateral wall of the calvarium, orbital rim, and the medial wall of the orbit. In cats, such flaps are used to obliterate the space within the frontal sinus, in combination with autogenous fat grafts.

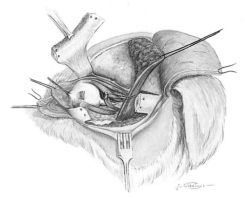

Figure 17-44. Exposure of deep orbital tissues by orbitotomy with zygomatic arch resection.

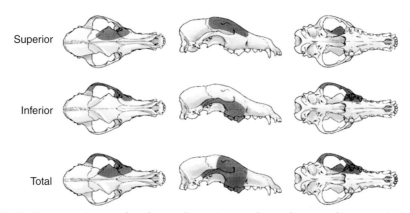

Figure 17-45. Diagrammatic examples of surgical resections used to perform an orbitectomy. As indicated, the top and middle rows illustrate superior and inferior partial orbitectomies, respectively. The bottom row illustrates total orbitectomy. (Modified from O'Brien MG, et al. [1996]: Total and partial orbitectomy for the treatment of periorbital tumors in 24 dogs and cats: a retrospective study. Vet Surg 25:471.)

BIBLIOGRAPHY

Adams WM, et al. (1998): An accelerated technique for irradiation of malignant canine nasal and paranasal sinus tumors. Vet Radiol Ultrasound 39:475.

Bellhorn RW (1972): Enucleation technique: a lateral approach. J Am Anim Hosp Assoc 8:59.

Bentley JF, et al. (1991): Use of a temporalis muscle flap in reconstruction of the calvarium and orbital rim in a dog. J Am Anim Hosp Assoc 27:463.

Calia CM, et al. (1994): The use of computed tomography scan for the evaluation of orbital disease in cats and dogs. Vet Comp Ophthalmol 4:24.

Caron JP, et al. (1986): Periorbital skull fractures in five horses. J Am Vet Med Assoc 188:280.

Carpenter JL, et al. (1989): Canine bilateral extraocular polymyositis. Vet Pathol 26:510.

Diesem C (1975), in Getty R (editor): Sisson and Grossman's the Anatomy of the Domestic Animals, 5th ed. Saunders, Philadelphia.

Duke-Elder S (1958): System of Ophthalmology, Vol I: The Eye in Evolution. H. Kimpton, London.

Evans HE (1993): Miller's Anatomy of the Dog, 3rd ed. Saunders, Philadelphia.

Gilger BC, et al. (1994): Modified lateral orbitotomy for removal of orbital neoplasms in two dogs. Vet Surg 23:53.

Gilger BC, et al. (1992): Orbital neoplasia in cats: 21 cases (1974-1990). J Am Vet Med Assoc 201:1083.

Hakanson N (1994): Frontal sinus mucocele in a dog presenting with intermittent profuse ocular discharge. Vet Comp Ophthalmol 4:34.

Hamor RE, et al. (1993): Use of orbital implants after enucleation in dogs, horses, and cats: 161 cases (1980-1990). J Am Vet Med Assoc 203:701.

Kennedy RE (1992): The effect of early enucleation on the orbit in animals and humans. Adv Ophthalmic Plast Reconstr Surg 9:1.

Kern TJ (1985): Orbital neoplasia in 23 dogs. J Am Vet Med Assoc 186:489.

Lavach JD, et al. (1984): Dacryocystitis in dogs: a review of twenty two cases. J Am Anim Hosp Assoc 20:463.

Martin CL, et al. (1987): Cystic lesions of the periorbital region. Comp Cont Ed 9:1022.

Mason DR, et al. (2001): Ultrasonographic findings in 50 dogs with retrobulbar disease. J Am Anim Hosp Assoc 37:557.

Meek LA (1988): Intraocular prosthesis in a horse. J Am Vet Med Assoc 13:343.

Morgan RV, et al. (1994): Magnetic resonance imaging of the normal eye and orbit of the dog and cat. Vet Radiol Ultrasound 35:102.

Mughannam A, Reinke JD (1994): Two cosmetic techniques for enucleation using a periorbital flap. J Am Anim Hosp Assoc 30:308.

Murphy CJ, et al. (1983): Enucleation in birds of prey. J Am Vet Med Assoc 183:1234.

Nadelstein B, et al. (1997): Orbital exenteration and placement of a prosthesis in fish. J Am Vet Med Assoc 211:603.

Nasisse MP, et al. (1988): Use of methylmethacrylate orbital prostheses in dogs and cats: 78 cases (1980-1986). J Am Vet Med Assoc 192:539.

O'Brien MG, et al. (1996): Total and partial orbitectomy for the treatment of periorbital tumors in 24 dogs and 6 cats: a retrospective study. Vet Surg 25:471.

Penninck D, et al. (2001): Cross-sectional imaging techniques in veterinary ophthalmology. Clin Tech Small Anim Pract 16:22.

Prince JH, et al. (1960): Anatomy and Histology of the Eye and Orbit in Domestic Animals. Charles C. Thomas, Springfield, IL.

Ramsey DT, et al. (1996): Ophthalmic manifestations and complications of dental disease in dogs in cats. J Am Anim Hosp Assoc 32:215.

Ramsey DT, et al. (1994): Comparative value of diagnostic imaging techniques in a cat with exophthalmos. Vet Comp Ophthalmol 4:198.

Ramsey DT, Fox DB (1997): Surgery of the orbit. Vet Clin North Am Small Anim Pract 27:1215.

Ruhli MB, Spiess BM (1995): Retrobulbar space occupying lesions in dogs and cats—symptoms and diagnosis. Tierarztl Prax 23:306.

Slatter D, Basher T (2003): Orbit, in Slatter D (editor): Textbook of Small Animal Surgery, 3rd ed. Saunders, Philadelphia.

Slatter DH (1977): Lateral orbitotomy by zygomatic arch resection. J Am Vet Med Assoc 175:1179.

Stades FC, et al. (2003): Suprascleral removal of a foreign body from the retrobulbar muscle cone in two dogs. J Small Anim Pract 44:17.

Stiles J, et al. (2003): Use of a caudal auricular axial pattern flap in three cats and one dog following orbital exenteration. Vet Ophthalmol 6:121.

Straw RC, et al. (1988): Multilobular osteosarcoma of the canine skull: 16 cases (1978-1988). J Am Vet Med Assoc 195:1764.

Turner AS (1979): Surgical management of depressed fractures of the equine skull. Vet Surg 8:29.

Valde H, Rook JS (1991): Use of fluorocarbon polymer and carbon fiber for restoration of facial contour in a horse. J Am Vet Med Assoc 188:249.

OCULAR MANIFESTATIONS OF SYSTEMIC DISEASES

Itamar Aroch, Ron Ofri, and Gila A. Sutton

Systemic diseases commonly cause associated ocular lesions and signs in all domestic species as well as in humans. Recognition of ocular signs assists both ocular and systemic diagnosis, because the eye can be examined readily. Such recognition allows earlier and more accurate diagnosis of systemic disorders as well as more effective evaluation of treatment. Ocular signs of some of the less common systemic diseases are poorly documented. Therefore this chapter focuses on the ocular manifestations of the more common systemic diseases. Ocular manifestations of neoplastic, nutritional, and dermatologic conditions as well as uncommon diseases are not discussed in this chapter; the reader is referred to standard internal medicine, oncology, and dermatology texts for discussion of these diseases.

Ocular examination is an essential part of a complete physical examination.

This chapter is divided into three sections. The first deals with ocular manifestations of systemic diseases in the dog and cat. Most of the diseases are discussed separately for these two species. For some diseases, however, the discussion of both species has been combined because the interspecies differences are minute; the heading of each subsection indicates the orientation of the discussion. The first section also includes a number of tables that provide systemic differential diagnosis for ocular signs in the two species. These tables are arranged in the anatomic order of the ocular structures to which they refer (i.e., disorders of the eyelids, conjunctiva, cornea, sclera, uvea, etc.) in order to facilitate finding the list of differential diagnosis for a given disorder. The following two sections, also containing similar tables, are devoted to ocular manifestations of systemic diseases in horses and ruminants.

It should be noted that for each systemic disease, the ocular manifestations and their treatment are described rather briefly. For detailed discussion of these manifestations, the reader is referred to the respective chapters in this book. Systemic pathogenesis, signs, diagnosis, and treatment of the diseases are discussed in greater detail. However, this discussion is not intended to replace the relevant textbooks. Rather, it is intended as a teaching and diagnostic aid to students and practitioners, who are also urged to consult the numerous tables in this

chapter for lists of systemic differential diagnosis of the various ocular disorders.

OCULAR MANIFESTATIONS OF SYSTEMIC DISEASES IN DOGS AND CATS (Tables 18-1 to 18-16)

Infectious Diseases

Canine Viral Diseases

CANINE DISTEMPER. Distemper is a disease of wo rldwide prevalence afflicting many canids, including the dog. It is caused by a paramyxovirus *(Morbillivirus)* designated canine distemper virus (CDV) that is spread by aerosol and droplet exposure.

The systemic and ocular clinical signs vary with the stages of the disease and depend on the immune status of the dog (i.e., age, vaccination status, individual variation), the virulence of the virus, and environmental conditions. Most (50% to 70%) of the infections are subclinical.

The ocular signs are the earliest manifestations of the systemic disease; they include acute, mild to severe, bilateral, serous to mucopurulent conjunctivitis, mostly with involvement of the palpebral conjunctiva. With the progression of disease, respiratory and/or gastrointestinal signs appear. CDV may also cause lacrimal gland adenitis with decreased tear production leading to blepharospasm, keratoconjunctivitis sicca (KCS), and possible corneal ulceration. Corneal ulceration may be severe and may not respond well to routine therapy. KCS may resolve after recovery from the systemic disease.

Anterior and posterior uveitis often accompany distemper encephalomyelitis and may be observed even if the dog is clinically asymptomatic for the latter. A high incidence (41%) of multifocal, nongranulomatous chorioretinitis has been found in the neurologic forms of canine distemper. Choroidal exudation may induce retinal detachment. Retinal atrophy and scarring are the chronic sequelae of chorioretinitis. In the tapetal fundus they are characteristically observed as circumscribed, hyper-reflective areas with clumps of pigment in the center, whereas the nontapetal lesions are characterized by depigmentation (see Chapter 15, Figure 15-34).

CDV has a predilection for the central nervous system (CNS), including the central visual pathways. It may cause inflammation or demyelinization of the optic nerve and tract,

Table 18-1 | **Systemic Causes of Eyelid Disorders in the Dog and Cat**

DISORDER	DOG	CAT
Infectious blepharitis*	Dermatophytosis (*Microsporum canis, Trichophyton* spp.) Leishmaniasis (*Leishmania donovani, Leishmania infantum, Leishmania chagasi*) Trypanosomiasis (*Trypanosoma brucei, Trypanosoma vivax*)	Bartonellosis (*Bartonella henselae, Bartonella* spp.) Dermatophytosis (*Microsporum canis, Trichophyton* spp.) Cryptococcosis (*Cryptococcus neoformans*)
Parasitic blepharitis*	Demodicosis (*Demodex canis*) Insect bites (spiders, fire ants, etc.)	Demodicosis (*Demodex cati, Demodex gatoi*) Mange (*Notoedres cati, Sarcoptes scabei* var. *canis*) Insect bites (spiders, fire ants, etc.)
Immune-mediated blepharitis*	Canine idiopathic granulomatous disease Pemphigus complex Systemic lupus erythematosus Juvenile pyoderma/Juvenile cellulitis	Pemphigus complex Systemic lupus erythematosus
Toxic blepharitis*	Sulfonamide/trimethoprim toxicity (in Doberman pinschers)	—
Allergic blepharitis*	Atopy Flea bite hypersensitivity	Atopy Food hypersensitivity Flea bite hypersensitivity
Miscellaneous causes of blepharitis*	Zinc responsive dermatosis	—
Eyelid masses	Canine viral papillomatosis Lymphoma Systemic histiocytosis	Larval migrans (*Cuterebra* spp.) Lymphoma
Ptosis	Pseudorabies Horner's syndrome Multifocal diseases affecting the oculomotor nucleus, including toxoplasmosis, distemper, mycosis, and granulomatous meningoencephalitis	—

*The signs of blepharitis are generalized (i.e., not cause-specific); they include dermatitis, alopecia, scales, crusts, ulcers of the skin, and conjunctivitis, chemosis, and congestion of the palpebral conjunctiva.

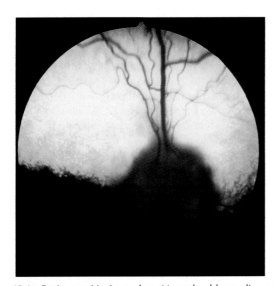

Figure 18-1. Optic neuritis in a dog. Note the blurry disc margins, hemorrhages, and loss of detail on the disc surface caused by edema of the nerve head. (Courtesy University of California, Davis, Veterinary Ophthalmology Service Collection.)

lateral geniculate nucleus, optic radiations, and visual cortex. Patients may present with actue, bilateral blindness and fixed, dilated pupils due to severe optic neuritis (Figure 18-1). The inflammation may be isolated, prodromal, or concurrent with other neurologic signs of canine distemper.

The diagnosis of canine distemper is complicated because many dogs are infected but not clinically ill. Cytoplasmic inclusion bodies may be present in conjunctival epithelial cells 5 to 21 days after exposure and may be demonstrated in cytologic smears. Immunofluorescence (IF) techniques for the detection of these inclusion bodies may be used on different cytologic smears, including conjunctival epithelial smears. Recently, CDV amplicons were detected by reverse transcriptase–polymerase chain reaction (RT-PCR) of conjunctival swabs of all dogs experimentally with CDV, from day 3 to 14 after infection. The detection rate of these amplicons in conjunctival swabs was significantly higher during most of the experimental period compared to other tissue samples. Ocular treatment, which is essentially symptomatic, consists of topical ophthalmic antibacterial preparations for conjunctivitis and corneal ulcers. Cases of KCS may be treated with artificial tears, topical antibiotics, and lacromimetics. Treatment of severe corneal ulceration may require surgical intervention. Systemic and topical steroids as well as topical atropine are indicated in cases of uveitis. However, atropine should be used with extreme caution if the animal is also suffering from KCS, and steroids may not be used if the cornea is ulcerated. Systemic administration of antiinflammatory dosages of glucocorticosteroids is indicated in an animal with acute optic neuritis following confirming diagnosis of distemper, even if there is no other sign of clinical disease.

INFECTIOUS CANINE HEPATITIS. Caused by canine adenovirus 1 (CAV-1), infectious canine hepatitis affects dogs and foxes. The virus is shed in the feces and urine of infected animals, and dogs are exposed through the oronasal route. After an incubation period of 4 to 7 days, seronegative animals infected by CAV-1 exhibit systemic clinical signs that range from those of a mild upper respiratory disease to those of a severe systemic disease, including hepatomegaly, icterus, and

Table 18-2 | **Systemic Causes of Conjunctivitis* in the Dog and Cat**

CAUSES	DOG	CAT
Viral diseases	Canine distemper virus Canine herpesvirus in neonates Canine oral papilloma virus Infectious canine hepatitis (canine adenovirus 1 [CAV-1])	Feline rhinotracheitis ([FRV], feline herpesvirus 1 [FHV-1]) Feline calicivirus (FCV) Feline immunodeficiency virus (FIV)
Bacterial and rickettsial diseases	Monocytic ehrlichiosis *(Ehrlichia canis)* Rocky Mountain spotted fever *(Rickettsia rickettsii)* Lyme borreliosis *(Borrelia burgdorferi)*	Chlamydiosis *(Chlamydophila felis,* formerly *Chlamydia psittaci)* *Neochlamydia hartmannellae* (obligate amebic host of *Hartmannella vermiformis)* Mycoplasmosis *(Mycoplasma felis, Mycoplasma gateae,* and/or *Mycoplasma arginini)* has been described as a secondary opportunistic pathogen Bartonellosis *(Bartonella henselae, Bartonella* spp.)
Protozoal diseases	Leishmaniasis *(Leishmania donovani, Leishmania infantum)* Trypanosomiasis *(Trypanosoma brucei, Trypanosoma vivax)*	—
Parasitic diseases	Ophthalmomyiasis *(Diptera* spp.)	—
Immune-mediated diseases	Canine idiopathic granulomatous disease	—
Dermal diseases	Atopy Zinc responsive dermatosis	Atopy Food hypersensitivity
Miscellaneous diseases	Ionizing radiation Sulfonamides/trimethoprim toxicity in Doberman pinschers	—

*Associated ocular signs include ocular discharge/secretion, chemosis, congestion, and follicular hyperplasia.

bleeding that may progress to disseminated intravascular coagulation. The prevalence of the disease has been dramatically reduced with the introduction of vaccination. Immunization with attenuated CAV-1 and, to a lesser extent, CAV-2 strains led to ocular signs of anterior uveitis and corneal edema in some animals. Dogs are currently vaccinated mostly with attenuated strains of CAV-2.

Ocular signs of infectious canine hepatitis are seen within 7 to 21 days of infection or vaccination. The signs are due to the presence of immune complexes in the eye and occur during convalescence. The initial signs include blepharospasm, miosis, hypotonicity, and anterior chamber flare (Figure 18-2) due to anterior uveitis. Corneal edema ("blue eye") may develop within 1 to 2 days, although it is bilateral in only 12% to 28% of cases. The edema may be severe and lead to formation of keratoconus. Such cases may progress and cause corneal scarring and pigmentation. Persistent or long-lasting corneal edema may also occur, and the Afghan hound has been described as predisposed to chronic edema and glaucoma. However, in most cases the edema is transient, and animals recover spontaneously within a few days to 2 to 3 weeks.

The diagnosis of the ocular disease is based on the signalment, history, and clinical signs. Treatment is symptomatic, including topical glucocorticoids or nonsteroidal antiinflammatory drugs (NSAIDs) and atropine. Hypertonic solutions and ointments may be used to resolve severe corneal edema.

Feline Viral Diseases

FELINE HERPESVIRUS INFECTION. Feline herpesvirus 1 (FHV-1) infection, also called feline rhinotracheitis (FRV), is caused by a member of the Alphaherpesvirinae subfamily that affects all members of the Felidae, and all isolates belong to the same serotype. The virus is widespread in the domestic cat population, especially in colonies and catteries. Cats are infected after direct and indirect contact with sick and carrier animals; the infection occurs through the oronasal and conjunctival routes. Cats that recover from the disease probably remain persistent carriers, a state characterized by latent infection and intermittent periods of virus shedding.

Secondary bacterial infections are common complications, especially with *Chlamydophila felis.* Unilateral or bilateral conjunctivitis with hyperemia, ocular discharge, chemosis, and blepharospasm are the most common lesions in adult cats with no respiratory disease. Other ocular signs are dendritic (Figure 18-3) or geographic corneal ulcers, KCS, and stromal keratitis. Symblepharon is a common sequel of infection (Figure 18-4), and FHV-1 may also play a role in the pathogenesis of corneal sequestration and eosinophilic keratitis. Vascularization of the cornea and pain may be severe or absent.

Confirmatory diagnosis of FHV-1 can be made through virus isolation in feline cell cultures. Serology is not very useful owing to the presence of antibodies from vaccination; however, immunofluorescent antibody (IFA) techniques can be used on cytologic and histologic specimens. PCR analysis has been used successfully to identify infected cats, but it is of limited use in a clinical setting because of the high prevalence of the infection in the general feline population.

In vitro sensitivity studies have identified several effective antiviral drugs—in decreasing order of potency, they are trifluridine, 5-iododeoxyuridine, and vidarabine. However, treatment is hampered by drug irritancy and availability. Trifluridine is commercially available but is topically irritating and needs to be administered at high frequency. The other two drugs are less irritating and administered less frequently but are difficult to obtain because they are not available commercially. Bromovinyldeoxyuridine and acyclovir are not effective against FHV-1, whereas valacyclovir is toxic in felines. Promising in vitro results have been reported with ganciclovir, cidofovir, and penciclovir, but large-scale clinical studies with these drugs are still lacking.

Table 18-3 | **Systemic Causes of Miscellaneous Conjunctival Disorders in the Dog**

DISORDER	CAUSES
Conjunctival hyperemia	Any cause of conjunctivitis Blastomycosis *(Blastomyces dermatitidis)* Hyperlipidemia Polycythemia Masticatory myositis
Conjunctival/subconjunctival hemorrhage	Monocytic ehrlichiosis *(Ehrlichia canis)* Rocky Mountain spotted fever *(Rickettsia rickettsii)* Thrombocytopenia Thrombopathy (including von Willebrand's disease) Anticoagulant poisoning Disseminated intravascular coagulation

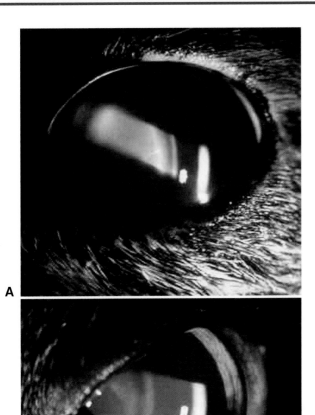

A

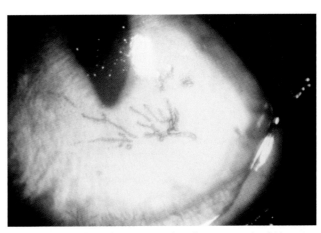

Figure 18-3. Rose bengal staining used to demonstrate dendritic corneal ulceration, typical of feline herpesvirus 1 infection. (Courtesy Mark Nasisse.)

B

Figure 18-2. Slit-lamp photography is used to illustrate aqueous flare characteristic of uveitis. **A,** Two beams of light, on the corneal and anterior lens surfaces, are visible. **B,** The aqueous humor between these two beams is translucent owing to the presence of inflammatory material. This results in light scattering similar to that observed while driving on a foggy night. (Courtesy Paul E. Miller.)

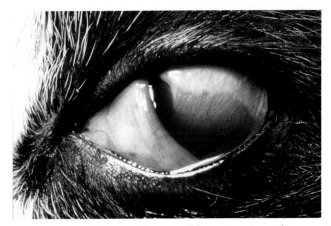

Figure 18-4. Symblepharon (adhesions of the conjunctiva to the cornea) following feline herpesvirus 1 infection in a cat. Note that the dorsotemporal part of the cornea (and inner ocular structures) is obscured by the adherent conjunctiva and its blood vessels. (Courtesy David J. Maggs.)

Use of human recombinant interferon, administered topically or orally, has shown synergism in vitro and has decreased the severity of clinical signs in experimentally infected cats when given 1 to 2 days after inoculation. L-Lysine, administered orally, may also inhibit viral replication. Treatment of deep corneal ulcers and necrosis includes surgical intervention.

The use of glucocorticoids is contraindicated, as it may induce shedding of viral particles in the latent stage. Topical tetracycline is frequently added because coinfections with *Mycoplasma* spp. and/or *Chlamydophila felis* (formerly *Chlamydia psittaci*) are common. Topical treatments are frequently continued for several weeks after resolution of clinical signs to prevent recurrence.

Table 18-4 | **Systemic Causes of Corneal Diseases in the Dog and Cat**

DISEASE	DOG	CAT
Infectious causes of keratitis*/ keratoconjunctivitis	Canine distemper virus (CDV) Canine herpesvirus (neonates only) Pseudorabies Canine oral papilloma virus Lyme borreliosis *(Borrelia burgdorferi)* Coccidioidomycosis *(Coccidioides immitis)* Leishmaniasis *(Leishmania infantum, Leishmania chagasi)* Trypanosomiasis *(Trypanosoma brucei, Trypanosoma vivax)*	Feline rhinotracheitis (feline herpesvirus 1 [FHV-1]) Bartonellosis *(Bartonella henselae, Bartonella* spp.) — —
Corneal ulcers	Hyperadrenocorticism Tyrosinemia Insect bites (spiders, fire ants, etc.)	Feline rhinotracheitis (feline herpesvirus 1 [FHV-1]) has been implicated in the pathogenesis of corneal sequestrum
Primary corneal edema†	Infectious canine hepatitis (ICH) Canine herpesvirus (puppies only) Dirofilariasis *(Dirofilaria immitis)* Tocainide toxicity	—
Nonedematous corneal opacities	Hypothyroidism Mucopolysaccharidosis Tyrosinemia Hyperlipidemia Systemic histiocytosis	Feline leukemia virus (FeLV) Mucopolysaccharidosis I, IV Gangliosidosis (GM$_1$, GM$_2$)
Keratoconjunctivitis sicca	American hepatozoonosis *(Hepatozoon americanum)* Hyperadrenocorticism Sulfonamide toxicity Phenazopyridine toxicity Ionizing radiation Systemic autoimmune secretory gland adenitis (associated with hypothyroidism, systemic lupus erythematosus, etc.) Canine distemper	Feline dysautonomia (Key-Gaskell syndrome)
Symblepharon	—	Feline rhinotracheitis (feline herpesvirus 1 [FHV-1]) Chlamydiosis *(Chlamydophila* [formerly *Chlamydia] psittaci)*

*Associated ocular signs include epiphora and discharge, blepharospasm, conjunctival congestion, corneal edema, vascularization, infiltration, ulceration, and pigmentation.
†Associated signs include corneal opacity, bullous keratopathy, keratoconus, and impairment of vision.

Stress is a very important factor in the pathogenesis of the clinical disease, and events such as the introduction of a new animal to the household or traveling to cat shows may exacerbate the symptoms. For this reason, frequent treatment with multiple drugs may sometimes aggravate the clinical signs of the disease. If worsening of signs is noted, the clinician is advised to carefully consider reducing treatment rather than increasing it.

FELINE CALICIVIRUS INFECTION. Feline calicivirus (FCV), which belongs to the family of caliciviruses, affects only members of the Felidae family. The genus consists of one serotype and many different strains varying in antigenicity and pathogenicity. It is widespread in the domestic cat population, especially in crowded conditions. The epidemiology is very similar to that of FHV-1, and despite extensive vaccinations, many cats are carriers of FCV. Some of these cats remain carriers for life and shed the virus continuously. Feline immunodeficiency virus (FIV) infection may potentiate FCV shedding from carriers. Infection by FCV occurs through the oronasal and conjunctival routes. The clinical signs may vary owing to differences in virulence and tropism of the different virus strains. They include fever, anorexia, oral and tongue ulceration, and mild respiratory signs (sneezing, nasal discharge). Certain FCV infections may manifest as shifting lameness and pyrexia for 24 to 48 hours, and

oral and respiratory signs may be absent. FCV is also involved in chronic gingivitis. Recently, highly virulent strains of FCV have emerged that are associated with high mortality and a new range of clinical signs (FCV-associated virulent systemic disease). The ocular lesions of FCV include mainly conjunctivitis, but the disease is milder than that induced by FHV-1.

The diagnosis of FCV infection is based mostly on the clinical signs. The virus can be isolated in feline cell cultures from oropharyngeal swabs. These samples may serve for PCR analysis that allows identification of the virus and its strains. Conjunctivitis should be treated symptomatically.

FELINE LEUKEMIA VIRUS INFECTION. A retrovirus with worldwide distribution, feline leukemia virus (FeLV) is transmitted primarily through the saliva, although it can be present in any body secretion. Infected cats become viremic and may be persistently infected or clear the infection. Latent infections and carrier states are common. The virus is responsible for a third of feline cancer-related deaths through cell transformation and may also lead to anemia and immunosuppression. The prevalence of FeLV-related diseases has been declining over the past 10 years owing to the introduction of a protective vaccine. The clinical signs of FeLV infection vary with the virus subtype and the body system involved.

Table 18-5 | **Systemic Causes of Scleral and Episcleral Diseases in the Dog and Cat**

DISEASE	DOG	CAT
Scleritis/episcleritis	Toxoplasmosis *(Toxoplasma gondii)* Leishmaniasis *(Leishmania infantum, Leishmania chagasi)*	—
Scleral/episcleral granulomas	Onchocerciasis *(Onchocerca stilesi, Onchocerca lienalis)* Canine idiopathic granulomatous disease	Ophthalmomyiasis *(Cuterebra* spp.)

Table 18-6 | **Systemic Causes of Uveitis in the Dog and Cat***

CAUSES	DOG	CAT
Viral diseases	Canine distemper virus (CDV) Infectious canine hepatitis ([ICH], canine adenovirus 1 [CAV-1])[†] Pseudorabies	Feline infectious peritonitis virus (FIPV) Feline immunodeficiency virus (FIV) Feline leukemia virus (FeLV) Feline sarcoma virus (FeSV) (experimental infection)
Mycotic diseases	Blastomycosis *(Blastomyces dermatitidis)*[†] Coccidioidomycosis *(Coccidioides immitis)*[†] Histoplasmosis *(Histoplasma capsulatum)* Cryptococcosis *(C. neoformans)* Opportunistic deep mycoses (e.g., aspergillosis)	Cryptococcosis *(Cryptococcus neoformans)* Blastomycosis *(B. dermatitidis)* Coccidioidomycosis *(C. immitis)* Histoplasmosis *(H. capsulatum)* Candidiasis *(Candida albicans)*
Bacterial diseases	Monocytic ehrlichiosis *(Ehrlichia canis)* Infectious cyclic thrombocytopenia *(Anaplasma platys)*[†] Lyme borreliosis *(Borrelia burgdorferi)*	—
Protozoal diseases	Toxoplasmosis *(Toxoplasma gondii)* Neosporosis *(Neospora caninum)* American hepatozoonosis *(Hepatozoon americanum)* Leishmaniasis *(Leishmania infantum, Leishmania chagasi)*[†]	Toxoplasmosis *(T. gondii)* Trypanosomiasis *(Trypanosoma brucei)*
Parasitic diseases	Dirofilariasis *(Dirofilaria immitis)* Angiostrongylosis *(Angiostrongylus vasorum)*[†] Ophthalmomyiasis interna *(Diptera* spp.) Ancylostomiasis *(Ancylosoma canium)*[†]	Larval migrans *(Metastrongylus* spp.) Ophthalmomyiasis interna *(Cuterebra* spp.)
Neoplastic diseases	Systemic histiocytosis[†] Lymphoma[†] Metastatic ocular disease[†]	Lymphoma Metastatic ocular disease
Other systemic causes	Systemic hypertension[†] Hyperlipidemia[†] Hyperviscosity syndrome[†] Uveodermatologic syndrome[†] Ionizing radiation	Periarteritis nodosa

*Associated ocular signs include corneal edema, flare, keratic precipitates, hypopyon and/or hyphema, hypotony, miosis, ciliary injection, blepharospasm, iris congestion, and photophobia. Secondary glaucoma and lens luxation are possible sequelae.
[†]Has been reported to cause secondary glaucoma.

The ocular disease in FeLV-infected cats may relate to lymphoma, and transformed lymphocytes invade the globe through the uvea, leading initially to a mild uveitis characterized by corneal precipitates. Small masses may be observed on the iris (Figure 18-5), and with progression they will lead to thickening and distortion of the iris. Secondary glaucoma is a common complication because of infiltration and obstruction of the iridocorneal angle by tumor cells.

The diagnosis of FeLV infection in cats can be made by serologic testing (enzyme-linked immunosorbent assay [ELISA], IFA) and PCR analysis. The latter can be used to detect viral material in tissues, including the cornea, when blood samples and immunohistochemistry of tissues are negative.

The treatment of lymphoma in cats usually requires a multidrug chemotherapy protocol. FeLV-positive cats with lymphoma treated chemotherapeutically were found to have significantly shorter remission and survival times compared with FeLV-negative cats with lymphoma treated with the same chemotherapeutic protocols. Other systemic conditions, including the

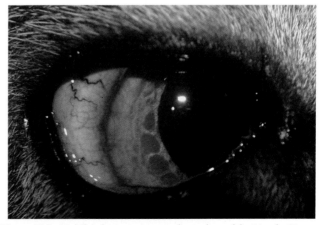

Figure 18-5. Multifocal gray masses on the surface of the iris of a 12-year-old male cat seropositive for feline leukemia virus. Histopathology confirmed the diagnosis of lymphoma.

ocular disease, are treated symptomatically. However, frequently the uveitis may be unresponsive to treatment or may cause secondary glaucoma, thus necessitating enucleation.

FELINE IMMUNODEFICIENCY VIRUS INFECTION. Feline immunodeficiency virus is a lentivirus with worldwide distribu-

tion. At least four subtypes (A to D) have been isolated in different regions of the world, and cats can be concurrently infected with more than one subtype. The seroprevalence of FIV varies among countries, approaching 30% where the free-roaming cat population is large. It is higher in sick than in healthy cats. The virus is known to infect other Felidae. The primary mode of transmission is through bite wounds, because the virus is present in the blood and saliva of infected cats. Thus, intact outdoor male cats are at the highest risk of infection. Other important modes of transmission are the in utero route and through infected queens' milk to suckling kittens.

The disease has three main phases—acute, asymptomatic, and terminal. With the beginning of the terminal phase consisting of the acquired immunodeficiency syndrome (AIDS)–related complex (ARC), cats exhibit nonspecific signs that reflect opportunistic infections (e.g., toxoplasmosis, feline infectious peritonitis virus, systemic mycoses, exacerbation of FHV-1) in different body systems.

The ocular disease manifests mainly as conjunctivitis and anterior uveitis. Pars planitis has been observed in four of nine cats with natural FIV infection. Many FIV-positive cats may exhibit a concurrent FIV- and *Toxoplasma*-induced ocular disease that manifests mainly as an anterior uveitis and chorioretinitis. Other ocular abnormalities reported are glaucoma (Figure 18-6) with or without uveitis, focal retinal degeneration, and retinal hemorrhages.

The diagnosis of an FIV infection in cats relies mostly on serologic tests for antibody detection, including ELISA (most commonly) and IFA as well as Western blot and immunoblot techniques. Cats in the acute phase of the disease may be seronegative; so if the disease is suspected in a seronegative animal, a second test should be performed after 6 to 8 weeks.

Treatment of the ocular disease in FIV- and *Toxoplasma*-positive cats should include topical glucocorticoids and atropine

Table 18-7 | Systemic Causes of Cataract in the Dog and Cat

CAUSES	DOG	CAT
Infectious diseases	Infectious canine hepatitis in neonates ([ICH] canine adenovirus 1 [CAV-1])	—
Metabolic diseases	Diabetes mellitus Hyperadrenocorticism Tyrosinemia	—
Nutritional	Vitamin E deficiency (chronic) Arginine- and methionine-deficient milk-replacement formulas (in the first week of life)	Arginine-deficient milk-replacement formulas in kittens Histidine-deficient diet in kittens
Toxic causes	Disophenol toxicity Hypercupremia Chronic toxicity of HMG-CoA reductase inhibitors Dimethylsulfoxide (DMSO) poisoning Ketoconazole toxicity	—
Other systemic causes	Uveodermatologic syndrome Ionizing radiation Electrocution/electric shock/lightning strikes	Chédiak-Higashi syndrome

Table 18-8 | Systemic Diseases Causing Posterior Uveitis* in the Dog and Cat

CAUSES	DOG	CAT
Viral diseases	Canine distemper	Feline immunodeficiency virus (FIV) Feline infectious peritonitis virus (FIPV) Feline leukemia virus (FeLV)
Bacterial diseases	Lyme borreliosis *(Borrelia burgdorferi)* Monocytic ehrlichiosis *(Ehrlichia canis)* Bartonellosis *(Bartonella vinsonii* ssp. *berkhoffi)*	Tuberculosis *(Mycobacterium bovis, Mycobacterium tuberculosis, Mycobacterium avium)* Bartonellosis *(Bartonella henselae, Bartonella* spp.*)*
Fungal diseases	Blastomycosis *(Blastomyces dermatitidis)* Coccidioidomycosis *(Coccidioides immitis)* Histoplasmosis *(Histoplasma capsulatum)* Cryptococcosis *(C. neoformans)* Opportunistic deep mycoses (e.g., aspergillosis)	Cryptococcosis *(Cryptococcus neoformans)* Blastomycosis *(B. dermatitidis)* Coccidioidomycosis *(C. immitis)* Histoplasmosis *(H. capsulatum)* Candidiasis *(Candida albicans)*
Protozoal diseases	Toxoplasmosis *(Toxoplasma gondii)* Neosporosis *(Neospora caninum)* Protothas *(Prototheca zopfii, Prototheca wickerhamii)* American hepatozoonosis *(Hepatozoon americanum)*	Toxoplasmosis *(T. gondii)*
Parasitic diseases	Ocular larval migrans *(Toxocara canis)*	Larval migrans *(Metastrongylus* spp.*)* Ophthalmomyiasis interna *(Cuterebra* spp.*)*
Neoplastic diseases	Lymphoma Systemic histiocytosis	Lymphoma
Other systemic causes	Sulfonamide/trimethoprim toxicity in Doberman pinschers Systemic hypertension	Periarteritis nodosa

*Includes chorioretinitis and choroiditis. Associated signs include diffuse or multifocal retinal edema and hemorrhage, subretinal effusion and hemorrhage, vascular cuffing, and loss of vision. Retinal detachment and retinal atrophy are possible sequelae. Retinochoroiditis, which has a similar clinical presentation, is caused by canine distemper virus.

Table 18-9 | **Systemic Noninfectious Causes of Retinal/Chorioretinal Scarring and Atrophy in the Dog and Cat***

CAUSES	DOG[†]	CAT[†]
Nutritional causes	Chronic vitamin E deficiency	Taurine deficiency
Cardiovascular diseases	Systemic hypertension Chronic severe anemia	Systemic hypertension Hyperviscosity syndrome
Toxic causes	Sulfonamide/trimethoprim toxicity in Doberman pinschers	Megestrol acetate (may induce diabetes mellitus) Griseofulvin
Other systemic causes	Sudden acquired retinal degeneration (SARD) syndrome Uveodermatologic syndrome	Chédiak-Higashi syndrome (also causes nontapetal hypopigmentation) Mucolipidosis

*Associated signs include multifocal scarring, pigment clumping, depigmentation, tapetal hyperreflectivity, and attenuation of retinal blood vessels.
[†]May be caused by any systemic disease causing posterior uveitis.

Table 18-10 | **Systemic Causes of Lipemia Retinalis in the Dog and Cat**

DOG	CAT
Hyperadrenocorticism Hypothyroidism (may also cause lipemic aqueous humor)	Primary inherited hyperchylomicronemia Idiopathic hyperchylomicronemia Idiopathic transient hyperlipidemia (and anemia) in kittens Glucocorticoid excess (iatrogenic)

In cats, it is advised to use atropine ointment rather than solution, because the latter may drain through the nasolacrimal duct and induce profound salivation due to its bitter taste. Topical tropicamide may substitute atropine. Cats may require a prolonged topical glucocorticoid therapy for control of the anterior uveitis; however, pars planitis responds poorly to such therapy. In cases of posterior uveitis, systemic clindamycin and glucocorticoids are indicated.

FELINE INFECTIOUS PERITONITIS. Feline infectious peritonitis (FIP) viruses (FIPVs) are biotypes (or strains) of feline corona virus (FCoV), along with the feline enteric corona viruses (FECV), and have a worldwide distribution. In contrast to FECV that infects and replicates only in enterocytes and leads to diarrhea, FIPV has an additional tropism to macrophages and can replicate within these cells, eventually causing

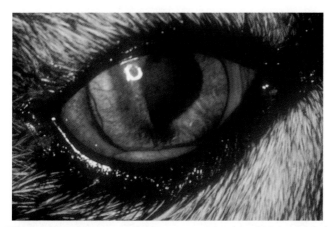

Figure 18-6. Glaucoma (secondary to posterior synechia) in domestic shorthair cat positive for feline immunodeficiency virus. Note swelling of the iris due to increased aqueous pressure in the posterior chamber, typical of the iris bombé syndrome. Color changes in the iris and ciliary congestion are indicative of uveitis.

FIP. Macrophages carry FIPV to the tissues and viscera. The exact mechanism responsible for the higher virulence of FIPV compared with FECV is currently unknown. It is postulated, however, that in immunosuppressed cats under a heavy FECV infection and replication load, mutations of FECV are more likely to occur, leading to its increased virulence and transformation to FIPV. Cats become infected with FCoV mainly through ingestion, and the virus replicates in enterocytes and is shed through the feces. It may also replicate in the tonsils, in which case it is shed in the saliva.

Kittens are more prone than adult cats to development of FIP, and 50% of the cats with FIP are younger than 2 years. The incidence of FIP is higher in cats from catteries, shelters, and multiple cat households. Stress may predispose cats to the disease. FIP is an immune complex disease resulting from interactions between the virus, or its antigens, and specific antiviral antibodies, complement, and inflammatory cells. The reaction leads to a pyogranulomatous vasculitis that affects the organs supplied by these blood vessels, including the retina (see Chapter 15, Figure 15-35). Cats with clinical FIP may exhibit an effusive (wet) or a noneffusive (dry) disease. The effusive disease is usually the more acute form. The noneffusive form develops over a longer period and is postulated to result from partial immunity to the virus.

Ocular lesions are very common in dry FIP, and the disease was found to be the most prevalent post-mortem finding in cats with uveitis. The ocular signs include iritis with color changes in the iris, bilateral anterior uveitis with aqueous flare, keratic precipitates (Figure 18-7), fibrinous exudates in the anterior chamber, hemorrhage into the anterior chamber, chorioretinitis, retinal hemorrhages and detachment, and optic neuritis. Neurologic signs may also be present due to focal, multifocal, or diffuse CNS involvement.

No single diagnostic test can confirm the presence of FIP. Rather, it is the combination of many data that leads to the final diagnosis of the disease—the history, clinical signs, hematologic and serum biochemistry abnormalities, ultrasonography findings, serologic results, cytologic and biochemical findings in effusion samples, histopathology and immunohistochemistry of biopsy and fluid samples, and RT-PCR analysis results. Each finding is given a "likelihood for FIP" grade, and a scale for the total score has been suggested, in that the higher the score the greater the likelihood of the disease.

The prognosis of cats with FIP is poor despite therapy. Treatment, which is essentially symptomatic and supportive, includes immunosuppressive drugs (i.e., glucocorticoids, cyclo-

Table 18-11 | **Systemic Causes of Retinal Hemorrhage in the Dog and Cat**

CAUSES	DOG	CAT
Infectious diseases	Canine distemper virus (CDV) Monocytic ehrlichiosis (*Ehrlichia canis*)* Rocky Mountain spotted fever (*Rickettsia rickettsii*) Lyme borreliosis (*Borrelia burgdorferi*) Blastomycosis (*Blastomyces dermatitidis*) Coccidioidomycosis (*Coccidioides immitis*)	Feline infectious peritonitis virus (FIPV) Tuberculosis (*Mycobacterium bovis, Mycobacterium tuberculosis, Mycobacterium avium*)
Parasitic diseases	Ophthalmomyiasis interna (*Diptera* spp.)	Ophthalmomyiasis interna
Cardiovascular diseases	Systemic hypertension* Hyperviscosity syndrome* Polycythemia* Thrombocytopenia Thrombopathy Severe anemia	Systemic hypertension Hyperviscosity syndrome Thrombocytopenia Thrombopathy Severe anemia
Metabolic diseases	Diabetes mellitus*	Diabetes mellitus
Toxic causes	Anticoagulant poisoning	Megestrol acetate (may induce diabetes mellitus)
Neoplastic diseases	Lymphoma Multiple myeloma Intracranial neoplasia	Lymphoma Intracranial neoplasia
Other systemic causes	Granulomatous meningoencephalitis (GME) Ionizing radiation	—

*Has also been associated with increased tortuosity and/or dilatation of retinal blood vessels.

phosphamide, melphalan, chlorambucil), human interferon-α, vitamins (A, thiamine, C), aspirin, anabolic steroids, and antibiotics. Ocular FIP is treated with glucocorticoids (topical or subconjunctival) and atropine ointment.

Canine Bacterial Diseases

BRUCELLOSIS. Brucellosis is a venereal disease of Canidae, including the dog, caused by the gram-negative intracellular coccobacillary bacterium *Brucella canis*. Transmission may occur via contact with contaminated body fluids. *B. canis* causes a long-lasting bacteremia and is spread hematogenously to the eyes, where it commonly leads to unilateral uveitis (Figure 18-8) or endophthalmitis. Owing to the insidious nature of the disease, ocular signs are sometimes the only presenting

signs of infection. Other *Brucella* species (e.g., *Brucella melitensis, Brucella abortus*) may also infect dogs and cats through contaminated milk products and infected aborted fetuses. Clinical signs of canine brucellosis may often be absent or may vary and include listlessness, fatigue, lethargy, exercise intolerance, weight loss, lymphadenopathy, back pain (due to diskospondylitis), lameness (due to arthritis), neurologic and behavioral abnormalities (due to meningoencephalitis), infertility (in both genders), painful scrotal enlargement (due to orchitis), and testicular atrophy.

Diagnosis relies mostly on serologic testing, with the rapid slide agglutination test (RSAT) as the screening test, followed by the tube agglutination test (TAT) as a confirmatory and quantifying test when the RSAT result is positive. TAT titers of 200 or higher often correlate with positive blood culture results

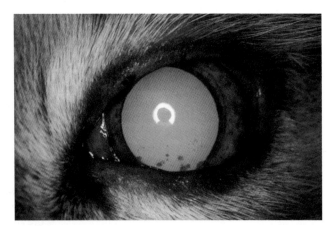

Figure 18-7. The anterior segment of a 2-year-old cat with anterior uveitis, presumably caused by feline infectious peritonitis. Inflammatory material that is prevalent in the aqueous humor is deposited on the interior (endothelial) aspect of the cornea and is seen as the ventral brown stains, a phenomenon known as keratic precipitates. Iridal congestion and fibrin deposition on the anterior lens capsule also indicate anterior uveitis.

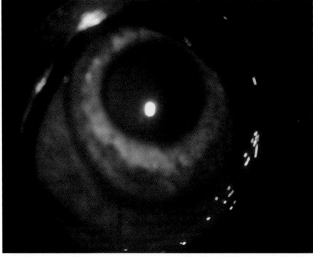

Figure 18-8. Anterior uveitis in a 3-year-old female German shepherd diagnosed with *Brucella canis*. Conjunctival and ciliary injection, corneal edema, and iridal congestion and petechiae are present.

Table 18-12 | **Systemic Causes of Retinal Detachment in the Dog and Cat***

CAUSES	DOG	CAT
Infectious diseases	Monocytic ehrlichiosis (*Ehrlichia canis*) Lyme borreliosis (*Borrelia burgdorferi*) Blastomycosis (*Blastomyces dermatitidis*) Histoplasmosis (*Histoplasma capsulatum*) Cryptococcosis (*C. neoformans*) Opportunistic deep mycoses (e.g., aspergillosis) Prototheciasis (*Prototheca zopfii, Prototheca wickerhamii*)	Feline infectious peritonitis virus (FIPV) Tuberculosis (*Mycobacterium bovis, Mycobacterium* *tuberculosis, Mycobacterium avium*) Cryptococcosis (*Cryptococcus neoformans*) Blastomycosis (*B. dermatitidis*) Coccidioidomycosis (*Coccidioides immitis*)
Parasitic diseases	Dirofilariasis (*Dirofilaria immitis*)	Ophthalmomyiasis interna
Cardiovascular diseases	Systemic hypertension Hyperviscosity syndrome	Systemic hypertension Hyperviscosity syndrome
Neoplastic diseases	Multiple myeloma Systemic histiocytosis	—
Toxic causes	—	Ethylene glycol toxicity (suspected) Megestrol acetate (may induce diabetic retinopathy)
Other systemic causes	—	Periarteritis nodosa

*Associated signs include anterior displacement of the retina and its vessels, loss of vision and pupillary light reaction, and focal/multifocal/diffuse retinal folds. Retinal detachment may also be caused by any disease causing retinal hemorrhage, as listed in Table 18-11.

and are presumptive indications of active infections. An agar gel immunodiffusion test for *B. canis* is a sensitive serodiagnostic test for the detection of infection. Recently, PCR testing of whole blood and semen samples has been shown to have equal or higher sensitivity, compared with blood culture or the RSAT, in the diagnosis of canine brucellosis.

Owners need to be aware of the zoonotic potential of the disease, and its persistent nature, before therapy is attempted. Treatment includes a long course of a systemic antibiotic of the tetracycline group, such as doxycycline or minocycline, with serologic or PCR monitoring for its efficacy. Relapses are common once antibiotic therapy is discontinued, and male dogs rarely recover from infection. Ocular treatment consists of topical glucocorticoids and atropine for uveitis. However, intractable cases of endophthalmitis may require enucleation.

BORRELIOSIS (CANINE LYME DISEASE). Lyme borreliosis is a worldwide tick-borne disease caused by the spirochete *Borrelia burgdorferi*. It is transmitted to dogs mainly by ticks of the *Ixodes ricinus* complex, including *Ixodes scapularis*. Systemic clinical signs include fever, inappetence, lymphadenopathy, and shifting lameness due to polyarthritis. Nevertheless, ocular signs can be the presenting signs. They include conjunctivitis, anterior uveitis, chorioretinitis, and retinal petechiae (Figure 18-9) and detachment.

Infection may be suspected from the clinical signs in an endemic area. Definitive diagnosis can be made through PCR analysis or by growing the spirochete in a culture from body fluids, although the latter is more challenging. Serologic testing is nonspecific because of persistence of antibodies, cross-reactivity with other bacteria, and exposure of healthy animals in endemic areas. Systemic treatment for 10 to 14 days with a variety of antibiotics (e.g., tetracyclines, ampicillin, ceftriaxone) has been shown to be effective. Uveitis is treated symptomatically with NSAIDs or glucocorticoids, and atropine.

RICKETTSIOSIS (EHRLICHIOSIS AND ROCKY MOUNTAIN SPOTTED FEVER). Rickettsiae and Ehrlichiae are two tribes within the family Rickettssiales, which include many pathogenic, obligate intracellular, gram-negative, coccobacilli bacteria.

Rocky Mountain Spotted Fever. Rocky Mountain spotted fever (RMSF) affects humans and dogs. It is caused by *Rickettsia rickettsii*, which is transmitted mainly by the wood

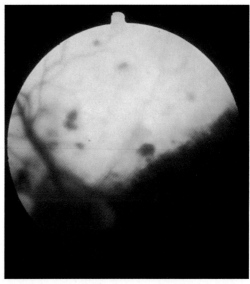

Figure 18-9. Preretinal petechiae on the fundus of a 7-year-old bloodhound diagnosed with canine Lyme disease.

tick *Dermacentor variabilis* and the American dog tick *Dermacentor andersoni*. However, the brown dog tick *Rhipicephalus sanguineus* and *Amblyomma* spp. can also transmit RMSF, and the former has recently been involved in the transmission of the disease in Arizona. The disease is seen in most parts of America, although the majority of cases in the United States occur in the Southwest. The systemic signs of RMSF are variable, resulting from endothelial damage and vasculitis. They include fever, anorexia, depression, tachypnea, coughing, and polyarthritis.

Ocular abnormalities occurred 14 to 21 days after an experimental infection, and were described in 9% to 11% of dogs in natural cases. The abnormalities include subconjunctival hemorrhage, conjunctivitis, chemosis, anterior uveitis (Figure 18-10), retinal petechiae, and focal retinal edema.

RMSF may be suspected on the basis of the seasonal occurrence, history of tick infestation, and clinical signs. Thrombocytopenia is the most consistently observed hematologic

Table 18-13 | **Systemic Causes of Optic Neuritis in the Dog and Cat***

CAUSES	DOG	CAT
Infectious diseases	Canine distemper virus (CDV) Infectious canine hepatitis ([ICH], canine adenovirus 1 [CAV-1]) American hepatozoonosis *(Hepatozoon americanum)* Blastomycosis *(Blastomyces dermatitidis)* Coccidioidomycosis *(Coccidioides immitis)* Toxoplasmosis *(Toxoplasma gondii)*	Feline infectious peritonitis virus (FIPV) Tuberculosis *(Mycobacterium bovis, Mycobacterium tuberculosis, Mycobacterium avium)* Cryptococcosis *(Cryptococcus neoformans)* Histoplasmosis *(Histoplasma capsulatum)*
Cardiovascular diseases	Systemic hypertension Hyperviscosity syndrome	Systemic hypertension Hyperviscosity syndrome
Neoplastic diseases	Intracranial neoplasia	—
Other systemic causes	Vitamin A deficiency (experimental disease only) Granulomatous meningoencephalitis (GME)	—

*Associated signs include papillary edema, optic nerve head congestion, hemorrhage of optic nerve vessels, and loss of vision and pupillary light reaction.

abnormality. Confirmation of the diagnosis is based on results of PCR analysis or serologic tests such as IFA in tissue biopsy specimens. A fourfold increase in indirect IFA antibody titer between acute and convalescent sera is also diagnostic. Culture may also be used for the confirmation of the diagnosis, although it is not readily available.

The treatment of choice for RMSF is tetracycline, 22 mg/kg q8h, or doxycycline, 5 mg/kg q12h, for 14 days. The ocular disease is treated with topical or subconjunctival glucocorticoids and topical atropine.

CANINE MONOCYTIC EHRLICHIOSIS. A worldwide tick-borne disease of dogs, canine monocytic ehrlichiosis (CME) is most prevalent in tropical and subtropical regions. It is caused by *Ehrlichia canis*, and is transmitted by *R. sanguineus*. A clinically and serologically indistinguishable disease is caused by *Ehrlichia chaffeensis*; however, its pathogenic importance and mode of transmission are currently unclear.

E. canis infection leads to acute, subclinical, and chronic disease phases. The acute phase, which lasts 2 to 4 weeks, is characterized by lymphoid hyperplasia and vasculitis with subsequent thrombocytopenia. The subclinical phase follows, consisting of persistence of thrombocytopenia, neutropenia, and anemia. The chronic phase of CME is characterized by hyperglobulinemia and bone marrow suppression with resultant pancytopenia.

The ocular disease may be present in up to 50% of the dogs in the acute phase of experimental infections. Under natural conditions, ocular signs were reported in 10% to 15% of dogs. Resulting from thrombocytopenia and vasculitis, ocular signs include hemorrhagic uveitis, hyphema, retinal hemorrhages leading to retinal detachment (Figure 18-11), and optic neuritis. Blindness may occur from ocular hemorrhage, and glaucoma is not an uncommon complication.

CME can be suspected in dogs with a history of tick infestation that manifest the preceding clinical signs and hematologic abnormalities. Confirmation of the disease is based on detection of the typical morulae within monocytes in peripheral

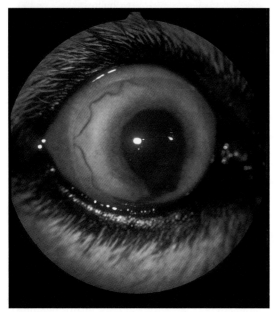

Figure 18-10. Anterior uveitis in the left eye of a 9-year-old mixed breed dog seropositive to *Rickettsia rickettsii*. Iridal congestion, blood and fibrin in the anterior chamber, and secondary glaucoma (iris bombé) can be seen.

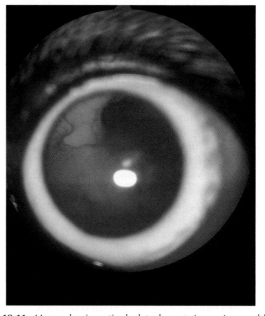

Figure 18-11. Hemorrhagic retinal detachment in a 4-year-old male Alaskan malamute diagnosed with ehrlichiosis. The retinal blood vessels as well as hemorrhage on the retinal surface may be clearly seen through the pupil without the use of an ophthalmoscope. Acute blindness was the presenting complaint in this case.

Table 18-14 | **Systemic Causes of Disorders of the Globe in the Dog and Cat**

CAUSES	DOG	CAT
Exophthalmos	Masticatory myositis Lymphoma Systemic histiocytosis Retrobulbar abscess/tumor/granuloma	Cryptococcosis (Cryptococcus neoformans) Lymphoma Retrobulbar abscess/tumor/granuloma
Enophthalmos	Masticatory myositis Dehydration Cachexia Horner's syndrome (enophthalmos associated with ptosis, third lid prolapse, and miosis)	Dehydration Cachexia Horner's syndrome (enophthalmos associated with ptosis, third lid prolapse, and miosis)

Table 18-15 | **Systemic Causes of Endophthalmitis/Panuveitis in the Dog and Cat**

CAUSES	DOG	CAT
Infectious diseases	Canine herpesvirus (puppies only) Ehrlichiosis (Ehrlichia canis) Nonspecific systemic bacterial infections Brucellosis (Brucella canis, Brucella spp.) Blastomycosis (Blastomyces dermatitidis) Histoplasmosis (Histoplasma capsulatum) Coccidioidomycosis (Coccidioides immitis) Opportunistic deep mycoses (e.g., aspergillosis) Trypanosomiasis (Trypanosoma brucei, Trypanosoma vivax) Prototothecosis (Prototheca zopfii, Prototheca wickerhamii)	Feline immunodeficiency virus (FIV) Feline infectious peritonitis virus (FIPV) Feline leukemia virus (FeLV) Cryptococcosis (Cryptococcus neoformans) Blastomycosis (B. dermatitidis) Histoplasmosis (H. capsulatum) Coccidioidomycosis (C. immitis) Candidiasis (Candida albicans)
Parasitic diseases	—	Toxoplasmosis (Toxoplasma gondii) Ophthalmomyiasis interna
Neoplastic diseases	Lymphoma Ocular metastases of distant tumors	Lymphoma Ocular metastases of distant tumors
Other systemic causes	Uveodermatologic syndrome	Periarteritis nodosa

blood smears or by PCR analysis, cell culture, or serologic antibody testing (IFA, Western blot technique, ELISA). The latter is most useful for the diagnosis in nonendemic areas.

The treatment of choice for CME is with tetracycline antibiotics (tetracycline, 22 mg/kg q8h, or doxycycline, 10 mg/kg q24h, for a minimum of 21 days). Imidocarb dipropionate may be added (5 mg/kg IM twice in 14-day interval); however, it has been associated with failure to clear the organism when used as a single agent. Systemic glucocorticoid therapy is controversial but has been suggested by some clinicians for the acute disease phase. Treatment of the ocular disease is the same as for RMSF.

Bacterial Diseases of Dogs and Cats

BARTONELLOSIS. Species of *Bartonella* are small, hemotropic, gram-negative bacteria, and they have been isolated from apparently healthy and ill dogs and cats. *Bartonella henselae*, *Bartonella clarridgeiae* (in cats), and *Bartonella vinsonii* ssp. *berkoffii* (in dogs) were established as infectious agents in companion animals. *B. henselae* is the primary cause of cat-scratch disease in people and is prevalent in most of the temperate regions of the world. The overall seroprevalence in the United States is 28%, and positive bacterial cultures have been reported in 8% to 53% of cats tested as well as in up to 89% of cats owned by *Bartonella*-infected people. Seropositivity was higher in outdoor cats and in younger cats and was associated with flea infestations. PCR studies have shown that 17% of tested cat fleas (*Ctenocephalides felis*) were positive for *B. henselae*. Prairie dogs and their fleas in Colorado were also positive for *B. henselae* when evaluated with PCR. *B. clarridgeiae* can occur in asymptomatic

cats either as a sole organism or concurrently with *B. henselae*, and has also been reported to cause cat-scratch disease in people. *B. vinsonii* ssp. *berkoffii* is transmitted by the brown dog tick (*R. sanguineus*) and has been identified as a cause of canine endocarditis and granulomatous lymphadenitis.

Despite the persistence of bacteremia in naturally *Bartonella*-infected cats, it is a subclinical infection, and a cause-and-effect relationship between infection and disease in cats has not been established. Cats may have a mild febrile disease upon infection, and a transient neurologic disease was described in a naturally infected cat. Little is known of the ocular disease in dogs and cats. It has been reported that feline bartonellosis is associated with anterior blepharitis, conjunctivitis, keratitis, corneal ulcers, uveitis, and chorioretinitis. In one study of cats chronically infected with *Toxoplasma gondii*, inoculation with *B. henselae* and later with FHV-1 failed to reactivate ocular toxoplasmosis. *B. vinsonii* ssp. *berkoffii* was implicated as a cause of canine anterior uveitis and choroiditis.

The diagnosis of bartonellosis can be made with serologic testing (IFA), blood and tissue cultures, and PCR analysis.

Feline bartonellosis can be treated with amoxicillin, amoxicillin–clavulanic acid, doxycycline, and enrofloxacin, but the doses required to suppress bacteremia are higher than recommended doses. Addition of rifampin to doxycycline has led to bacterial clearance. Infection with *B. vinsonii* ssp. *berkoffii* in dogs can be treated with doxycycline, enrofloxacin, and rifampin. The duration of therapy is controversial, but it should be at least 14 to 21 days. Culture specimens should be collected at least 3 weeks after antibiotic discontinuation to

Table 18-16 | **Systemic Disorders Causing Blindness in the Dog and Cat**

CAUSES	DOG	CAT
Acute blindness	Any cause of severe ocular opacity, retinal detachment, optic neuritis, and glaucoma Canine distemper virus (CDV) Pseudorabies Prototheosis (Prototheca zopfii, Prototheca wickerhamii) Ocular larval migrans (Toxocara canis) Uveodermatologic syndrome Masticatory myositis Intracranial neoplasia Granulomatous meningoencephalitis (GME) Ivermectin toxicity	Any cause of severe ocular opacity, retinal detachment, optic neuritis and glaucoma Systemic hypertension Ischemic encephalopathy Cerebral hypoxia Hepatic encephalopathy Intracranial neoplasia
Progressive blindness	Any cause of retinal or optic nerve atrophy Ocular larva migrans (T. canis) Diabetes mellitus Fucosidosis Globoid dystrophy Ceroid lipofuscinosis Vitamin E deficiency (chronic) Vitamin A deficiency (experimental disease only) Intracranial neoplasia GME Ionizing radiation	Any cause of retinal or optic nerve atrophy Intracranial ophthalmomyiasis (Cuterebra spp.) Cerebral coenurosis (Taenia serialis) Hepatic encephalopathy Mucolipidosis Taurine deficiency Systemic hypertension Cerebral hypoxia Intracranial neoplasia (meningioma, carcinoma)

verify treatment effectiveness. Treatment of the ocular disease in cats and dogs is essentially symptomatic.

Feline Bacterial Diseases

CHLAMYDIOSIS (CHLAMYDOPHILOSIS). Chlamydiae are obligate intracellular bacteria that also have an extracellular form during their development cycle. They are commensals of ocular, gastrointestinal, respiratory and genitourinary mucosae. *Chlamydophila felis* (formerly *Chlamydia psittaci*) is the only important chlamydial species in cats, and several strains with genetic similarity have been isolated. In the cytoplasm of susceptible cells, the organism forms an initial body that proliferates through budding and fission; later, through a phase of rapid division, these bodies form a large population of elementary bodies that are released from the cell and infect other cells. As many as 45% of healthy cats are seropositive for *Chlamydophila psittaci*; however, the organism was isolated from conjunctival swabs only in 6%. The isolation rates and seropositivity rise up to 30% and 69%, respectively, in cats with conjunctivitis, and a similar trend was observed through PCR analysis of conjunctival specimens.

Cats infected with *Chlamydophila psittaci* rarely show systemic signs, although some may have mild upper respiratory signs. The ocular signs are those of conjunctivitis, including conjunctival hyperemia, chemosis (Figure 18-12), serous to mucopurulent ocular discharge, and blepharospasm. Cats may become chronically ill. Concurrent FIV or FHV-1 infection prolongs the conjunctivitis.

The diagnosis of chlamydiosis can be made through cell culture, cytologic analysis of conjunctival swabs (Giemsa stain and IFA), serologic testing (IFA, ELISA) of patient specimens, and PCR analysis. Therapy of chlamydial infection consists of oral tetracyclines (doxycycline, tetracycline) and, in cases of multiple-cat households and catteries, should be continued for 6 weeks. Ocular infections respond well to tetracycline ophthalmic ointment. Modified live vaccines provide the best protection against the organism but do not prevent colonization

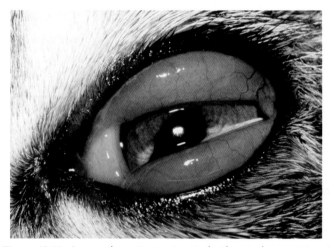

Figure 18-12. Severe chemosis (conjunctival edema) characteristic of *Chlamydia* infection in a cat. (Courtesy David J. Maggs.)

of the mucosae or shedding of the organism. Nevertheless, they lead to reduction of the clinical signs in infected cats.

MYCOPLASMOSIS. Mycoplasmas are small gram-negative bacteria. *Mycoplasma felis, Mycoplasma gateae,* and *Mycoplasma arginini* have been isolated from healthy and ill cats. Most mycoplasmas are normal inhabitants of the upper respiratory tract but do not appear in the lungs of healthy cats.

Mycoplasma organisms can be secondary opportunistic pathogens in virus infections and complicated pneumonia cases, mostly in kittens. They may also be isolated from visceral organs of seriously ill and debilitated animals. Mycoplasmosis has a controversial role in feline conjunctivitis, because the organisms have been isolated from healthy cats as well as from cats with conjunctivitis. Although *Mycoplasma* spp. lead to conjunctivitis in young cats, experimental infections in adult cats failed to induce the disease. *Mycoplasma* spp. can probably complicate cases of conjunctivitis caused by primary pathogens such as FHV-1 or *Chlamydophila psittaci*.

The diagnosis of mycoplasmosis can be made through culture and observation of the cytoplasmic inclusion bodies in epithelial cells (in cytologic preparations). PCR analysis of nasal swabs is more sensitive than culture in cats.

Mycoplasma conjunctivitis can be treated with most ocular antimicrobial preparations, although tetracycline is the drug of choice.

Mycotic Diseases of Dogs and Cats

See also Table 18-17. It should be noted that in addition to the ocular signs described here, fungal infections may also cause focal or multifocal (granulomatous) lesions in the CNS, leading to various signs of neurologic or neuroophthalmic dysfunction. Blindness due to involvement of the central visual pathways, including the optic nerve (i.e., optic neuritis) and chiasm, may also occur.

BLASTOMYCOSIS. Blastomycosis is a systemic infection caused by the dimorphic fungus *Blastomyces dermatitidis*. It affects dogs and humans most commonly, but cats are also affected. The disease is prevalent in North America and it has been reported in Africa and Central America. The endemic distribution in North America includes the Mississippi, Missouri, and Ohio River valleys, the Mid-Atlantic States, and the Canadian provinces of Manitoba, Ontario, and Quebec. The reservoir for the fungus is the soil, and proximity to water and rain facilitates the release of infectious organisms. The spores are acquired mostly by inhalation, leading to establishment of the fungus in the lung tissue, but there are rare reports of invasion through skin wounds in dogs. The organism disseminates in the body through the hematogenous route or via the lymphatics to preferred sites, including the eyes. Most dogs (85%) with blastomycosis have pulmonary lesions. Recently, cardiovascular lesions and signs such as inflammatory myocarditis endocarditis, heart block, heart base or intracardiac mass lesions, and syncope have been described in dogs from endemic areas.

Ocular signs have been reported in up to 40% of the dogs with the disease, and in 50% of cases the ocular lesions were bilateral. They include mainly granulomatous anterior (Figure 18-13) and/or posterior uveitis that may be difficult to observe owing to severe corneal edema. Obstruction of the iridocorneal angle with inflammatory material may lead to secondary glaucoma and potential loss of vision. Periorbital cellulitis also occurs. In cats, the main ocular signs are chorioretinitis, retinal detachment, and panophthalmitis.

Diagnosis of the ocular disease is based on identification of the fungus in cytologic (e.g., vitreous aspiration) or histologic (e.g., enucleated eye) preparations. Serologic testing and thoracic radiography may support the diagnosis if the history and clinical signs are compatible and when microscopic identification of the fungus has failed.

Treatment of blastomycosis includes systemic antifungals (i.e., itraconazole, amphotericin B, and ketoconazole) for at least 60 days, and for at least 1 month after all signs of the disease have resolved. Such long-term treatment may be expensive, and relapses are common. Ocular signs are treated with topical atropine and antiinflammatory therapy. Glaucoma may be treated with carbonic anhydrase inhibitors, but a nonresponsive case may require enucleation of the affected eye.

COCCIDIOIDOMYCOSIS. Caused by the geophilic, saprophytic, dimorphic fungus *Coccidioides immitis,* coccidioidomycosis is endemic in the southwest desert areas of the United States, Mexico, and South America. It affects virtually all mammalian species, including humans, dogs, and cats, as well as some reptiles; however, cats are more resistant to infection than dogs. Young (less than 4 years), medium to large dogs are most commonly affected. Rainy weather followed by dry environmental conditions promotes the spread of the arthrospores. These are inhaled into the lung and to the subpleural tissue, where spherules and subsequently endospores are formed. The disease is disseminated via the hematogenous and lymphogenous routes to many tissues, including the eyes. Almost 50% of affected dogs show no systemic signs of the disease.

The ocular disease is unilateral in 75% of the dogs, affecting mainly the posterior segment. The prevalence of ocular signs in cats is 10%. Ocular lesions include keratitis, uveitis (Figure 18-14), and chorioretinitis and may lead to retinal detachment and glaucoma.

The disease can be suspected in animals presented with the preceding clinical signs in endemic areas. Confirmation of the diagnosis can be made through identification of the organ-

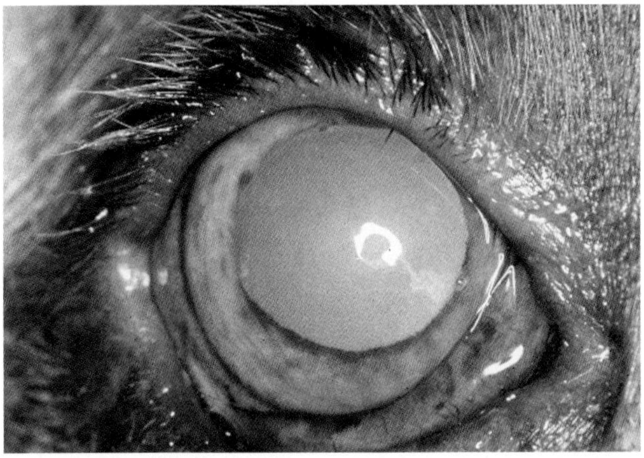

Figure 18-13. Anterior uveitis in a 1-year-old female Weimaraner diagnosed with blastomycosis. Conjunctival and ciliary injection, corneal edema, iridal congestion, and fibrin in the anterior chamber may be seen. The dog was subsequently euthanized because of progressive central nervous system signs. (Courtesy Renee Carter.)

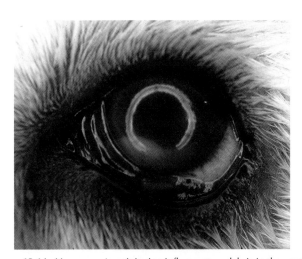

Figure 18-14. Hypopyon (precipitating inflammatory debris in the ventral aspect of the anterior chamber) in a 4-year-old mixed breed dog diagnosed with coccidioidomycosis.

Table 18-17 | Systemic and Ocular Granulomatous Diseases of Dogs and Cats

DISEASE	GEOGRAPHIC DISTRIBUTION	BREED PREDISPOSITION	SYSTEMIC SIGNS	OCULAR SIGNS	DIAGNOSTIC TESTING	SEROLOGIC TESTING	TREATMENT
Blastomycosis (*Blastomyces dermatitidis*)	North America (endemic in central Atlantic states, Mississippi, Missouri, Ohio River valleys), Canada, Central America, Africa	Young, male, large-breed dogs, hunting and sporting dogs, Doberman pinschers	*Dog:* Pulmonary involvement, skin lesions (planum nasale, face, nail beds), pyrexia, lameness (due to bone involvement), lymphadenopathy, infection of testes, kidney, bladder, brain, cardiac abnormalities (myocarditis, endocarditis), *Cat:* Dyspnea, skin lesions, weight loss	Uveitis, secondary glaucoma, corneal edema, focal granulomatous chorioretinitis, retinal detachment, vitreal hemorrhage, periorbital cellulitis	Cytology (aspirates, impression smears), Histopathology, Lymph node aspirates, Vitreocentesis, Tracheal wash, Urinalysis, Thoracic radiography	AGID, ELISA, Radioimmunoassay (experimental)	Itraconazole (drug of choice) *Dog:* 5 mg/kg bid for 2 wks, then sid (at least 60 days) *Cat:* 5 mg/kg bid Amphotericin B *Dog:* 0.5 mg/kg IV tiw Amphotericin B-lipid complex *Dog:* 1 mg/kg IV, tiw
Coccidioidomycosis (*Coccidioides immitis*)	Lower Sonoran life zone (Southwest United States, Mexico, Central and South America)	Boxers, Doberman pinschers	*Dog:* Respiratory tract infection, cough, anorexia, weight loss, skin and bone lesions, persistent pyrexia, cardiac dysfunction, CNS involvement *Cat:* Skin lesions, fever, weight loss	Keratitis, granulomatous panuveitis, chorioretinitis, orbital cellulitis, acute blindness	Cytology, Biopsy, Fungal culture, Thoracic radiography, Skin testing (coccidioidin)	Tube precipitin test (IgM antibody level), CF (IgG antibody level), Latex agglutination, AGID, ELISA	Ketoconazole *Dog:* 5-10 mg/kg bid for 8-12 mos *Cat:* 50 mg (total) sid
Cryptococcosis (*Cryptococcus neoformans*)	Worldwide	*Cats:* More susceptible than dogs (Siamese cats overrepresented) *Dogs:* Young adults (<4 yrs), Doberman pinschers, Great Danes, American cocker spaniels	*Cats/Dogs:* Neurologic symptoms (granulomatous meningoencephalitis, meningomyelitis), Upper respiratory tract disease (sneezing, chronic nasal discharge due to nasal granulomas), Cutaneous lesions (papules and nodules)	*Cats/Dogs:* Blindness with dilated, unresponsive pupils, granulomatous chorioretinitis, exudative retinal detachment, optic neuritis, papilledema, retinal hemorrhage, occasionally orbital abscess, cellulitis, rarely anterior uveitis	Cytology (nasal and skin exudates, CSF, fine needle aspirates, paracentesis, vitreocentesis), Thoracic radiography, Tissue biopsy, Urinalysis, Fungal culture, PCR (human specimens)	Latex agglutination, ELISA	Surgical removal of large masses and granulomas Amphotericin B *Cat:* 0.1-0.5 mg/kg IV or 0.5-0.8 mg/kg SC tiw *Dog:* 0.25-0.5 mg/kg IV tiw *in combination with* Flucytosine (25-50 mg/kg PO qid for 6 wks) *Cat:* 30-75 mg/kg PO bid-qid *Dog:* 50-75 mg/kg PO tid Ketoconazole *Cat:* 5-10 mg/kg PO bid or 10-20 mg/kg sid for 6-12 mos *Dog:* 5-15 mg/kg PO bid or 30 mg/kg sid for 6-12 mos Itroconazole *Cat:* 5-10 mg/kg bid or 20 mg/kg sid for 6-12 mos Fluconazole *Dog and cat:* 5-15 mg/kg PO sid-bid for 6-12 mos

AGID, Agar gel immunodiffusion; *CF*, complement fixation test; *CNS*, central nervous system; *CSF*, cerebrospinal fluid; *ELISA*, enzyme-linked immunosorbent assay; *IgG*, immunoglobulin G; *IgM*, immunoglobulin M; *PCR*, polymerase chain reaction; *tiw*, three times a week.

Table 18-17 | **Systemic and Ocular Granulomatous Diseases of Dogs and Cats—cont'd**

DISEASE	GEOGRAPHIC DISTRIBUTION	BREED PREDISPOSITION	SYSTEMIC SIGNS	OCULAR SIGNS	DIAGNOSTIC TESTING	SEROLOGIC TESTING	TREATMENT
Histoplasmosis (*Histoplasma capsulatum*)	Endemic in temperate and subtropical regions of the world	Young cats and dogs (<4 yrs), overrepresentation of pointers, Weimaraners, Brittany spaniels	*Dog:* Respiratory form: dyspnea, coughing, abnormal lung sounds Gastrointestinal form: bloody diarrhea, hepatosplenomegaly, icterus, ascites, DIC, anemia *Cat:* Weight loss, anorexia, pyrexia, pale mucous membranes, anemia, dyspnea, tachypnea, splenomegaly, hepatomegaly, visceral lymphadenopathy	*Dog:* Uveitis, chorioretinitis, granulomatous choroiditis, optic neuritis *Cat:* Conjunctivitis, granulomatous blepharitis, granulomatous chorioretinitis, retinal detachment, optic neuritis	Thoracic radiography Abdominal ultrasonography Cytology of fine needle aspirates Histopathology Endoscopy Tracheal and bronchoalveolar lavage	AGID, CF (not reliable tests)	Itroconazole 10 mg/kg PO sid-bid for 4-6 mos Fluconazole 2.5-5 mg/kg PO sid-bid Amphotericin B 0.25-0.5 mg/kg IV every second day
Aspergillosis (*Aspergillus* spp.)	Worldwide	Young to middle-aged German shepherd dogs, cats with concurrent immunosuppressive disease (FIP, FeLV)	*Dog:* Vertebral pain (lameness, paraplegia, paraparesis), anorexia, weight loss, pyrexia, muscle wasting *Cat:* Pulmonary lesions (granulomas)	*Dog:* Uveitis, endophthalmitis *Cat:* Orbital cellulitis, ocular proptosis	Cytology (urine sample) Culture Histopathology of biopsies	AGID Counterimmuno-electrophoresis ELISA FA	Amphotericin B *Dog:* 0.25 mg/kg IV every second day Itraconazole *Dog and Cat:* 2.5-5 mg/kg PO bid
Protothecosis (*Prototheca* spp.)	Ubiquitous in North America, Asia, Oceania, Europe	Dogs and cats with immunosuppression, collies, female dogs	*Dog:* Intestinal form: bloody diarrhea, melena CNS involvement: ataxia, depression, paresis Cutaneous form (rare): chronic skin lesions *Cat:* Only cutaneous form Nodules on extremities, nose, pinna	Ocular involvement in more than 50% of infected animals: granulomatous posterior uveitis, panuveitis, retinal detachment, blindness	Cytology and identification of organism in aspirates (from the vitreous, CSF, lymph nodes), rectal scrapings (Wright stained), urinalysis Histopathology of biopsy samples	—	Wide surgical removal of solitary cutaneous lesions Amphotericin B 0.25 mg/kg IV tiw in combination with Tetracycline 22 mg/kg PO tid *and either* Ketaconazole 10-15 mg/kg PO sid-bid for 28-42 days *or* Fluconazole 2.5-5 mg/kg PO bid for 28-42 days

DIC, Disseminated intravascular coagulation; *FA,* fluorescent antibodies; *FeLV,* feline leukemia virus; *FIP,* feline infectious peritonitis.

Continued

Table 18-17 | **Systemic and Ocular Granulomatous Diseases of Dogs and Cats—cont'd**

DISEASE	GEOGRAPHIC DISTRIBUTION	BREED PREDISPOSITION	SYSTEMIC SIGNS	OCULAR SIGNS	DIAGNOSTIC TESTING	SEROLOGIC TESTING	TREATMENT
Toxoplasmosis (*Toxoplasma gondii*)	Worldwide	Domestic cat and other Felidae: definitive hosts	*Dog:* Respiratory form: pneumonia Neuromuscular form: encephalitis, ataxia, paresis, paralysis, myositis Intestinal form: diarrhea, vomiting Generalized form: fever, dyspnea, diarrhea, vomiting usually in young dogs *Cat:* Pulmonary, CNS, hepatic, pancreatic and cardiac lesions, myositis	*Dog:* Anterior uveitis, retinal detachment, choroidal lesions *Cat:* Anterior uveitis, multifocal or diffuse chorioretinitis, optic neuritis	Cytology of fine needle aspirates Radiology Fecal examination Histopathology of biopsies PCR (aqueous)	Sabin-Feldman dye test Indirect FA Agglutination test ELISA Witmer-Goldman coefficient of aqueous or CSF and serum	Clindamycin *Dog:* 10-20 mg/kg PO bid for 2 wks *Cat:* 12.5 mg/kg PO bid for 2-3 wks Sulfonamides 60 mg/kg PO bid for 2 wks alone or 30 mg/kg *in combination with* Pyrimethamine 0.25-0.5 mg/kg PO bid
Tuberculosis (*Mycobacterium bovis, Mycobacterium tuberculosis, Mycobacterium avium* complex)	Worldwide	Rural cats may be infected (*M. bovis*) through ingestion of raw beef or dairy products Infection with *M. tuberculosis* mostly in urban animals in close contact with affected people	Bronchopneumonia, pulmonary nodule formation, hilar lymphadenopathy, fever, anorexia, weight loss, anemia, diarrhea, harsh nonproductive cough, dysphagia, retching, hypersalivation, tonsilar enlargement	Granulomatous uveitis (*Mycobacterium* spp.), corneal granuloma (*M. avium*)	Cytology of aspirates and impression smears (acid-fast stain) Culture Tuberculin testing Bacterial isolation Histopathology of tissue biopsy Radiology	Hemagglutination CF	Isoniazid *Dog:* 10-20 mg/kg PO sid Rifampin *Cat:* 10-20 mg/kg PO sid (euthanasia may be advisable for public health reasons) *Note:* tuberculosis in dogs and cats often comes from human infection

ism in cytologic smears from infected organs, including the vitreous, or in histopathologic specimens from biopsy. Culturing of the fungus with inoculation into animals is possible; however, because of the highly infective nature of the arthrospores and the risk to laboratory personnel, it is not performed routinely. Serologic tests include the agar gel immunodiffusion (AGID) for the detection of precipitin immunoglobulin (Ig) M antibodies, and complement fixation (CF), which detects IgG.

The treatment of coccidioidomycosis is identical to that of blastomycosis.

CRYPTOCOCCOSIS. Cryptococcosis is an opportunistic disease of worldwide distribution that affects people and animals, including the dog and the cat. It is caused by the saprophytic, round, yeastlike fungus *Cryptococcus neoformans* (var. *neoformans* and var. *gatti*). The disease is the most common systemic mycosis in the cat, in which it is much more common than in dogs. Pigeons are considered the main vectors of the organism, and high numbers of the organism are found in pigeon roosts, habitats, and droppings, where it can survive up to 2 years.

Inhalation of the organism is the most common route of infection, leading to nasal lesions. Smaller, desiccated, encapsulated organisms may reach the alveoli, where they may cause granulomas. The disease is disseminated through direct local extension or hematogenous spread and affects mainly the CNS, eyes, and skin. Natural infections in dogs and cats have been reported to worsen and accelerate owing to the immunosuppression due to glucocorticoid therapy.

Ocular lesions in cats include anterior uveitis, granulomatous chorioretinitis (Figure 18-15) frequently leading to retinal detachment, optic neuritis, and exophthalmos. In dogs, the lesions are similar; however, optic nerve leptomeningitis is common and is probably the route of ocular infection from the CNS.

The diagnosis of cryptococcosis is based on identification of the typical thickly encapsulated yeasts that show narrow base budding. These organisms can be seen in nasal and skin

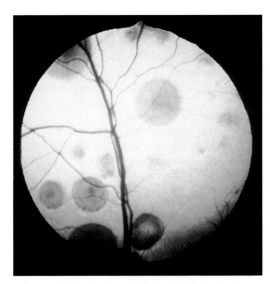

Figure 18-15. Multifocal chorioretinal granulomas, causing retinal detachments, in a cat diagnosed with cryptococcosis. The organism was identified in an aqueous humor sample. Note that the retinal blood vessels are coursing over some of the granulomas, indicating their intraretinal or subretinal nature.

exudates, cerebrospinal fluid (CSF), and in fine-needle aspirates from affected tissues, including the aqueous humor or vitreous. Gram and new methylene blue stains are superior to Romanowsky stains for their detection. Serologic tests are very rapid and useful in suspected cases in which yeasts are not detected by cytology; such tests include latex agglutination of cryptococcal capsular antigen and ELISA. Both tests detect all known serotypes and can be conducted in serum, urine, or CSF samples. Histopathologic analysis of biopsy specimens may also help if cytology has failed to reveal the organism. The organism can be cultured from exudates, body fluids, and tissues, although growth may take up to 6 weeks.

The treatment of cryptococcosis in both cats and dogs involves a long (1 to 10 months) course of a systemic antifungal drug—amphotericin B with or without flucytosine, ketoconazole, itraconazole, or fluconazole. The last has been recommended for the CNS disease because of its better distribution in the system, including the CSF. Nevertheless, itraconazole has been used successfully in cases of feline cryptococcal meningitis. Recently, the success rate of treatment of cryptococcosis in dogs and cats has been reported to be 55 and 76%, respectively. The median duration of treatment required to effect a cure at first attempt was significantly shorter for fluconazole (4 months; range 1 to 8 months) than for itraconazole (9 months; range 3 to 24 months). Cats with neurologic involvement, disseminated disease, or refractory disease treated with protocols containing amphotericin B did as well, on average, as cats with less severe disease treated with azole monotherapy. Treatment of the ocular disease is similar to that provided in cases of blastomycosis.

HISTOPLASMOSIS. Histoplasmosis is a systemic mycosis caused by the soil-borne dimorphic fungus *Histoplasma capsulatum*. The disease has been reported in North and South America. In the United States, most cases occur in the regions of the Ohio, Mississippi, and Missouri rivers. In the mycelium stage, the fungus is present in soil and produces microconidia that are infectious to mammals. Both dogs and cats can be affected; however, cats are more susceptible to infection than dogs. In both species young (less than 4 years) adults are mostly affected. The microconidia are inhaled into the lung and transformed to the yeast phase, which multiplies by budding. The disease usually starts with respiratory signs, although some cases of gastrointestinal histoplasmosis, with no respiratory involvement, have been described. Dissemination of the organism from the respiratory system occurs through hematogenous and lymphatic routes.

Ocular lesions in dogs and cats include anterior uveitis, granulomatous chorioretinitis, and optic neuritis. Blindness may result from retinal detachment or optic neuritis.

Histoplasmosis can be suspected in dogs and cats with the above clinical signs exhibiting a normocytic normochromic anemia and radiographic evidence of a linear to diffuse pulmonary interstitial pattern associated with granulomatous fungal pneumonia. A definitive diagnosis can be made with fine-needle aspiration of affected tissues and effusions, and identification of the organism within macrophages in routine Romanowsky stains. Histopathology of tissue biopsy specimens, including endoscopic samples, may be attempted when cytologic samples fail to demonstrate the organism. Culture is possible, although it is not recommended because of the potential hazard of the organism to humans. Serologic testing is unreliable owing to many false-positives and false-negative results.

Histoplasmosis is best treated with oral itraconazole, and in fulminating cases amphotericin B is added for a more rapid control of the disease. Fluconazole may be preferred in CNS or ocular disease because of its better distribution, and ketoconazole may be used. The latter is not recommended as a first-choice drug owing to its toxicity, although it may be considered when cost is a concern. The duration of treatment should be 4 to 6 months at least. Treatment of the ocular disease is similar to that provided in cases of blastomycosis.

Parasitic Diseases of Dogs and Cats

TOXOPLASMOSIS (see Table 18-17). Toxoplasmosis is a zoonotic disease of worldwide distribution that affects all mammals and is caused by the obligate intracellular coccidian *Toxoplasma gondii*. Cats, the definitive hosts, shed oocysts in their feces. Other mammals, including cats and dogs, may ingest sporulated oocysts. Cats are infected mostly by ingesting intermediate hosts infected with tissue cysts and can also be infected by ingestion of oocysts; however, only 20% of cats fed oocysts have a patent infection. Congenital infection due to transplacental infection or through the queen's milk has been reported in kittens. The incidence of congenital infection in dogs is unknown.

The brain, liver, lungs, skeletal muscle, and eyes are common sites of cyst formation, initial replication, and persistence of chronic infection.

In cats, ocular signs were observed in 81.5% of cases, most commonly consisting of bilateral anterior and/or posterior uveitis. Secondary lens luxation, glaucoma, and retinal detachment were also described. Ocular manifestations in dogs are (in decreasing order) anterior uveitis, retinitis, choroiditis, scleritis, optic neuritis, and episcleritis.

Cytologic preparations of effusions may reveal the tachyzoites, which occasionally may be observed in other samples (i.e., CSF, transtracheal or bronchoalveolar lavage, and fine-needle aspirates from tissues). There are multiple serologic tests for antibody detection; however, no one test is confirmatory, and 30% of dogs and cats in the United States are seropositive. A positive IgM titer or a fourfold increase in IgG or IgA titer can verify a recent infection; positive IgM titers can persist for months after infection, however, and high IgG titers have been detected 6 years after inoculation in cats. Serologic tests cannot be used accurately to predict the oocyst shedding period. Simultaneous measurement of *Toxoplasma*-specific antibody titers in the CSF or aqueous humor and in the serum of animals presented with a neurologic and/or an ocular disease, along with measurement of other agent-specific antibody titers in these same samples, may help discriminate between local production of *Toxoplasma*-specific antibodies and serum antibodies passively leaking through damaged endothelial barriers. High ratios of *Toxoplasma*-specific antibody titers in the CSF or aqueous humor to serum titers in comparison with other agent-specific antibody titers are evidence of local antibody production of antibodies and, thus, suggest the presence of active infection in the CNS or eye, respectively. The presence of the organism can be confirmed by inoculation of laboratory mice or cell culture, with detection of tachyzoites or specific antibodies. The presence of *T. gondii* in tissue and body fluid samples can also be confirmed by PCR analysis, although a positive result cannot confirm the presence of an active disease.

Systemic toxoplasmosis can be treated with a variety of antimicrobials. However, treatment results in suppression, rather than killing, of the organism. Clindamycin (25 mg/kg PO q12h for 21 to 30 days) is the drug of choice for treatment of clinical disease. Combinations of sulfonamides, pyrimethamine, and trimethoprim act synergistically in suppressing the parasite, although supplementation with folic acid is advisable, especially in cats. Other drugs that have shown in vitro and/or in vivo activity against *T. gondii* include doxycycline, minocycline, newer macrolides (roxithromycin, azithromycin, clarithromycin) and several other antibacterial drugs; however, these should be further evaluated in dogs and cats.

The ocular disease is treated with topical glucocorticoids and atropine, and in cases of posterior uveitis, systemic clindamycin and glucocorticoids are indicated.

Canine Parasitic Diseases

NEOSPOROSIS. Canine neosporosis has worldwide distribution. It is caused by the apicomplexan protozoan *Neospora caninum,* which has a similar morphology to *T. gondii*. Its life cycle is at present incompletely understood. The definitive host is probably a carnivore that sheds oocysts in the feces; the oocysts are ingested by herbivores, in which tissue cysts are formed. As many as 20% of dogs are seropositive, probably infected subclinically and, supposedly, transplacentally during gestation.

Ocular lesions of neosporosis include mild anterior uveitis, retinitis and retinochoroiditis.

Serologic testing (IFA) of serum and CSF is the most commonly used diagnostic method for neosporosis. Most animals with the clinical disease show an increase in IgG titers within 1 to 2 weeks of initial signs. The organism may be observed in cytologic preparations of CSF and tissue fine-needle aspirates. Biopsy specimens examined histopathologically may demonstrate the tachyzoites or the typical thick-walled cysts. PCR analysis may prove the presence of the organism and helps in its differentiation from related organisms.

Treatment of neosporosis is similar to that described for toxoplasmosis. Young affected animals have a guarded to poor prognosis, whereas adult dogs respond better to therapy.

VISCERAL LEISHMANIASIS. Leishmaniasis is a disease caused by the dimorphic protozoans of the genus *Leishmania* that affects humans and animals worldwide. The natural reservoir of the parasite, dogs have clinical disease. Visceral leishmaniasis is transmitted in the Old World by sandflies of the genus *Phlebotomus* and is caused primarily by *Leishmania infantum.* New World visceral leishmaniasis is transmitted by sandflies of the genus *Lutzomyia* and is caused by *Leishmania chagasi,* which is considered identical to *L. infantum*. In recent years, foci of leishmaniasis caused by *L. infantum* have been reported in the United States, mainly in foxhounds, and the disease has been transmitted to dogs accidentally through transfusion of contaminated blood products. In mammalian hosts the parasite is seen as the intracellular nonflagellate form, the amastigote, within macrophages. The disease incubation period before the appearance of clinical signs may last months to years, during which the parasite disseminates in the body. Some dogs develop clinical disease, whereas others remain asymptomatic carriers that are infectious to sandflies and can thus transmit the disease to other dogs and humans. Systemic signs of visceral leishmaniasis may include dermal abnormalities (e.g., exfoliative dermatitis, mainly involving the head and ears), lymphadenopathy, splenomegaly, signs of renal insufficiency, epistaxis, and musculoskeletal abnormalities.

The ocular signs include blepharitis (Figure 18-16), lid granulomas (Figure 18-17), conjunctivitis, scleritis, keratitis, anterior uveitis, panophthalmitis, and secondary glaucoma.

Serologic tests can confirm the presence of antileishmanial antibodies but cannot prove the presence of an active disease. Many highly specific and sensitive serologic tests are available, including IFA, ELISA, direct antiglobulin test, and CF. The presence of a high titer in a dog with the characteristic signs is highly suggestive of active disease. Ten percent to 20% of the seropositive dogs may eliminate the parasite spontaneously and may be apparently healthy; however, dogs may be clinically healthy and still harbor active infection. The amastigotes may be detected in cytologic and histologic preparations, within macrophages. Culture or PCR analysis of splenic or bone marrow aspirates may also confirm the presence of the organism. Recently, PCR studies have shown that conjunctival swabs were the most reliable source for parasitic DNA in dogs experimentally infected with *L. infantum*.

Treatment of infected dogs rarely achieves complete elimination of the parasite. Traditional treatment consists of daily

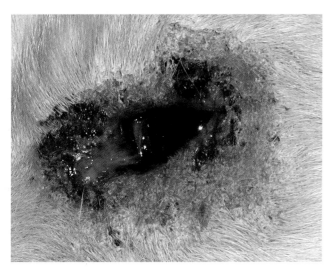

Figure 18-16. Severe blepharitis in a dog diagnosed with leishmaniasis. (Courtesy Gad Baneth.)

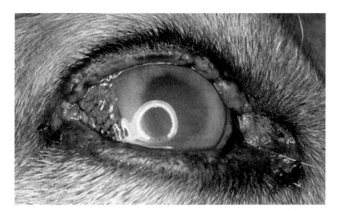

Figure 18-17. Lid granulomas (especially on the nasal aspect of the upper eyelid) and anterior uveitis (note the conjunctival and ciliary congestion and the corneal edema) in a dog diagnosed with leishmaniasis. (Courtesy Teresa M. Pena and Xavier Roura.)

injections of pentavalent antimonials (meglumine antimonate, sodium stibogluconate) for 3 to 4 weeks. Adverse effects and relapses are common. Oral allopurinol results in suppression of the parasite and clinical improvement but does not cure the disease. It has very few side effects and can be used as a sole agent or in combination with pentavalent antimonials. Lipid-associated amphotericin B has been shown to lead to clinical improvement in sick dogs but not to eliminate the infection.

Ocular treatment is directed against the inflammatory reaction and consists of topical atropine as well as glucocorticoids or NSAIDs.

Endocrine Diseases

Endocrine Diseases of Dogs and Cats

DIABETES MELLITUS. Diabetes mellitus (DM), the most common endocrine disease in dogs and cats, is similar in incidence for dogs and cats, with reported frequencies of 1:100 to 1:500. The disease is classified to two subtypes, type I (insulin-dependent diabetes mellitus [IDDM]) and type II (non–insulin-dependent diabetes mellitus [NIDDM]). IDDM, the more common form, is seen in almost all dogs and in 50% of 70% of the cats with DM. This type is characterized by loss of pancreatic beta cells and subsequent insulin deficiency, leading to hyperglycemia. In contrast, NIDDM is uncommon in dogs, is observed more commonly in cats, and is characterized by insulin resistance. Consequently, insulin concentrations are variable and can be normal, decreased, or increased; however, hyperglycemia is always present. Ketoacidosis is seen more commonly in IDDM than in NIDDM. A transient form of DM has been described in cats, and rarely in dogs, in which some factor predisposes the animals to insulin antagonism and resistance, resulting in persistent hyperglycemia. The elevated glucose concentrations may lead to beta cell refractoriness and even to glucose toxicity and irreversible lesions in beta cell functions. Treatment of the underlying disease and the diabetic state may lead to transition to subclinical DM and euglycemia, with no requirement for insulin or other oral hypoglycemic drug therapy.

The most prevalent ocular sign of DM in dogs is bilateral cataracts. Initial changes include vacuole formation along the equatorial cortex that progresses to the anterior and posterior cortex. Diabetic cataracts progress very rapidly and may reach maturity, which may develop in a short time (days to weeks), and owners may present with a complaint of relatively acute blindness (Figure 18-18). Cataract formation depends on the age of the animal as well as on the magnitude and duration of hyperglycemia. Cataracts are detected in a high proportion of diabetic dogs and lead to lens-induced uveitis. The tendency for development of a diabetic cataract depends on the activity of aldose reductase in lenticular cells. Aldose reductase is the key enzyme in the formation and accumulation of sorbitol, fructose, and dulcitol in the lens. The resulting hyperosmolarity of the lens leads to fluid ingress with subsequent swelling, fiber rupture, and eventual cataract formation. Activity of aldose reductase in dogs is high in the lens regardless of age, whereas in cats it is significantly higher in those younger than 4 years than in older cats. Because DM occurs primarily in older cats, the relatively low aldose reductase activity protects the feline lens from cataract formation. Blindness due to diabetic cataracts can be corrected only with surgical removal of the lens, although experimental work using aldose reductase inhibitors to prevent

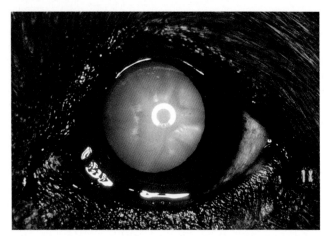

Figure 18-18. Diabetic (mature) cataract in a dog. Note the prominent anterior Y sutural clefts. (Courtesy Paul E. Miller.)

the development of diabetic cataracts has shown promising results. The prognosis for successful outcome of surgery is reportedly unaffected by the presence of DM, although perioperative medical management has to be modified to include NSAIDs instead of glucocorticoids, and the incidence of long-term complications may be higher. See Chapter 13 for additional discussion of diabetic cataracts.

Diabetic cataracts may progress to maturity within a few weeks. The disease should be considered in patients presented with rapid-onset cataracts.

DM has also been associated with retinal and vitreal hemorrhages, as well as retinal detachment. This involvement of the posterior segment is more common in the cat and rare in the dog. The presentation is similar to *diabetic retinopathy,* a blinding disease in humans. However, microaneurysms and proliferative changes in retinal vasculature, which are the hallmarks of the human disease, have not been documented in animals.

Diabetic dogs have significantly reduced corneal sensitivity compared with nondiabetic normoglycemic dogs. It has been suggested that trigeminal nerve dysfunction may be associated with recurrent or nonhealing ulcers in diabetic dogs for which no other underlying cause can be found.

The diagnosis of DM is based on detection of persistent fasting hyperglycemia (or glycosuria). In addition, ketonemia and/or ketonuria are present in ketoacidosis. Serum fructosamine or glycosylated hemoglobin concentrations may help in differentiating stress-induced hyperglycemia from DM. Some diabetic dogs and cats have concurrent hyperadrenocorticism, and diabetic cats may have concurrent hyperthyroidism. Diagnostic procedures should include specific tests to exclude these diseases in cases where there is a high index of suspicion for them. Acute pancreatitis may lead to destruction of islet cells, with subsequent DM, that may be permanent or transient; therefore screening for presence of concurrent pancreatitis is advisable. A urine culture is recommended if the urinalysis yields results consistent with urinary tract infection.

Treatment of uncomplicated DM is primarily aimed at normalizing the glucose concentration. This is achieved principally with insulin therapy, although in certain animals with NIDDM, mostly cats, oral hypoglycemic drugs (e.g., glipizide

and glyburide) can be used as sole agents or in conjunction with insulin. Oral vanadium therapy may also be useful in treatment of DM. Dietary modification should always be a part of the therapy of DM. Its aims are to minimize postprandial glucose concentration fluctuations and treat or prevent obesity. Modified diets for DM are limited in simple carbohydrates, include complex carbohydrates, and contain high fiber; some diets, mostly feline, are high in protein. Acarbose may be used in diabetic animals whose glucose concentration is poorly controlled despite insulin therapy and dietary modification. For treatment of diabetic ketoacidosis, the reader is referred to textbooks of veterinary internal medicine.

Canine Endocrine Diseases

HYPERADRENOCORTICISM. Hyperadrenocorticism (HAC, Cushing's syndrome) is a common canine endocrinopathy characterized by glucocorticoid excess. The disease can be caused by an adrenocorticotropic hormone (ACTH)–secreting hyperplastic or neoplastic pituitary gland (pituitary-dependent HAC) or a cortisol-secreting adrenocortical tumor or may be iatrogenic, due to chronic excessive glucocorticoid therapy. Dogs with HAC may have concurrent DM.

The ocular surface lesions associated with canine HAC include progressive, nonhealing corneal ulceration, corneal calcification, and KCS. Corneal ulceration is not the direct result of HAC, but the high levels of endogenous glucocorticoids may delay healing of a corneal ulcer from other mechanisms. Cataracts are usually observed in dogs that suffer from concurrent DM. Intraocular manifestations include lipid accumulation in the aqueous, lipemia retinalis, and hypertensive retinopathy. Hyperlipidemia, commonly observed in dogs with HAC, and concurrent uveitis are responsible for the development of lipemia retinalis and lipids in the aqueous. Dogs with HAC also suffer from a relatively high incidence of sudden acquired retinal degeneration (see Chapter 16).

The diagnosis of canine HAC requires endocrine tests that include urinary cortisol-to-creatinine ratio, ACTH stimulation (with measurements of cortisol, with or without 17-hydroxyprogesterone) and low-dose dexamethasone suppression. Differentiation between pituitary-dependent HAC and adrenocortical tumor may require additional testing (i.e., measurement of endogenous ACTH concentration and high-dose dexamethasone suppression).

The most commonly used drug in the treatment of canine HAC is mitotane (op′-DDD); recently, however, trilostane has been shown to be as effective as mitotane in the treatment of canine pituitary-dependent HAC. The ocular lesions are treated symptomatically. Corneal ulcers may heal once control of HAC is achieved.

HYPOTHYROIDISM. Hypothyroidism is a common canine endocrinopathy, with a prevalence of 0.2%, but is extremely rare in cats. It leads to decreased production of thyroxine (T_4) and triiodothyronine (T_3). The disease can be the result of a hypothalamic disorder leading to deficiency of thyrotropin-releasing hormone (TRH) (tertiary hypothyroidism), a pituitary disorder leading to thyrotropin deficiency (secondary hypothyroidism) or a thyroid gland disorder (primary hypothyroidism). Most canine cases are primary hypothyroidism and result from lymphocytic thyroiditis or idiopathic thyroid atrophy.

The ocular manifestations of canine hypothyroidism are primarily the result of hyperlipidemia that may lead to lipid dystrophy (corneal lipidosis) (Figure 18-19) with secondary

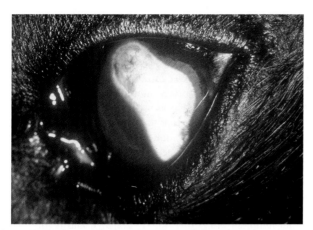

Figure 18-19. Corneal lipidosis in a dog with hypothyroidism. Extensive depositions of lipids in the cornea, such as this case, obviously affect the dog's vision and may warrant surgical removal (superficial keratectomy).

ulceration and uveitis, lipid deposition in the aqueous, and lipemia retinalis with retinal bleeding and detachment. Secondary glaucoma has been reported in canine hypothyroidism. There is an association between KCS and canine hypothyroidism, and 20% of dogs with the disease have been reported to be diagnosed with concurrent KCS. This association is probably an indirect one, likely resulting from a multiple glandular, immune-mediated inflammation.

The diagnosis of canine hypothyroidism is mainly based on evaluation of total and/or free T_4 along with canine thyroid-stimulating hormone (TSH) measurement. Other, more advanced tests are responses to TSH or TRH, measurement of anti-thyroglobulin or of anti-T_3 and anti-T_4 antibodies, scintigraphy, and thyroid biopsy. Advanced brain imaging (computed tomography, magnetic resonance imaging) may be needed to diagnose hypothalamic or pituitary lesions leading to tertiary and secondary hypothyroidism, respectively.

Treatment of canine hypothyroidism essentially comprises oral levothyroxine (L-thyroxine) supplementation (22 μg/kg q12-24h). Restriction of cholesterol and lipids in the diet is indicated. KCS should be treated, and topical glucocorticoids or NSAIDS (based on presence of corneal ulcers) should be used to treat the secondary keratitis and uveitis. Surgical removal of moderate corneal lipid plaques is contraindicated because recurrence of such plaques is often more severe than the initial lesion. Surgery is reserved for cases where significant visual deficits occur (see Figure 18-19).

Metabolic Diseases of Dogs and Cats

HYPERLIPIDEMIA. Defined as excess blood lipids, *hyperlipidemia* can result from an increase in fasting serum triglycerides, in cholesterol, or both. A serum (or plasma) that appears grossly milky or turbid, referred to as *hyperlipemic,* results from triglyceride excess; hypercholesterolemia does not lead to increased serum turbidity and hyperlipemia. The term *hyperlipoproteinemia* is sometimes used interchangeably with hyperlipidemia, because lipoproteins carry both triglycerides and cholesterol in the plasma, and often there is a concurrent increase in serum lipoproteins when hyperlipidemia is present. However, this term should be reserved to cases in which laboratory tests confirm an increase in the concentrations of serum lipoproteins. The incidence of hyperlipidemia in the canine population was approximately 14% in one study.

Hyperlipidemia may be primary (usually hereditary or familial) or secondary, and both forms have been described in dogs and cats, although secondary hyperlipidemia is much more common. In dogs secondary hyperlipidemia may result from hypothyroidism, DM, hyperadrenocorticism, glomerulonephropathy, pancreatitis, or cholestasis or may be due to a high-fat diet. Similar mechanisms lead to feline hyperlipidemia. In cats, excessive administration of megestrol acetate and glucocorticoids may lead to DM and secondary hyperlipidemia.

The ocular manifestations of hyperlipidemia include lipemia of the ocular blood vessels, corneal lipid keratopathy, lipemic aqueous, and lipid infiltration of the globe, most noticeably in the peripheral cornea and the uveal tract. When hyperlipidemia is associated with hypertriglyceridemia, visible changes may be observed in the conjunctival and retinal blood vessels, which look pink and engorged. Lipemic retinal blood vessels, *lipemia retinalis*, are more easily visualized over the nontapetal fundus (Figure 18-20). Lipids may also be observed in the anterior chamber, usually as a result of uveitis allowing leakage from vessels.

The diagnosis of hyperlipidemia relies on the demonstration of fasting hypertriglyceridemia and/or hypercholesterolemia. In secondary hyperlipidemia, depending on the primary disease, further tests include urinalysis, urine protein-to-creatinine ratio, liver function tests, serum lipase–like immunoreactivity, hormonal assays, abdominal ultrasonography, and a careful analysis of the diet. In suspected cases of primary hyperlipidemia, every effort should be made to rule out the presence of another primary disease, and additional testing includes lipoprotein profiling (e.g., electrophoresis, densitometry, precipitation techniques, and ultracentrifugation).

Treatment of secondary hyperlipidemia is directed at the primary disease, whereas primary hyperlipidemia is usually treated with low-fat diets. Treatment of the secondary ocular complications is essentially symptomatic. Anterior uveitis treatment should be provided in cases of lipemic aqueous humor. Cases of corneal lipidosis in which vision is affected

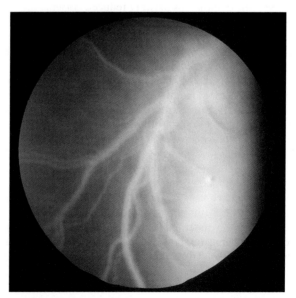

Figure 18-20. Lipemia retinalis in a cat with hyperlipidemia. The pink color of the blood vessels is easily appreciated against the dark background of the nontapetum. (Courtesy David J. Maggs.)

Table 18-18 | **Ocular Signs of Hematologic Disorders in Dogs and Cats**

DISORDER	OCULAR SIGNS
Monoclonal gammopathy and hyperviscosity	Retinal hemorrhages (small or large) Dilated tortuous retinal veins with irregular filling ("boxcar" appearance) Conjunctival hemorrhages Massive intraocular hemorrhages (rare)
Thrombocytopenia and thrombopathy	Subconjunctival, preretinal, intraretinal, and subretinal hemorrhages Hyphema Secondary retinal detachment
Severe anemia	Retinal and vitreous hemorrhages Secondary retinal detachment
Polycythemia	Dilated and tortuous dark red to brown conjunctival and retinal blood vessels, retinal hemorrhages and detachment, uveitis and chorioretinitis
von Willebrand's disease	Retinal hemorrhages Retinal detachment Conjunctival petechiae

may be treated surgically, although recurrences should be considered.

Cardiovascular Diseases of Dogs and Cats

Ocular signs associated with hematologic disorders are summarized in Table 18-18.

THROMBOCYTOPENIA AND THROMBOPATHY (THROMBASTHENIA). Thrombocytopenia is a very common hematologic disorder in the dog but is less frequent in cats. In dogs the most common causes of thrombocytopenia are infectious diseases (e.g., RMSF, monocytic ehrlichiosis, infectious cyclic thrombocytopenia, babesiosis), neoplasia (e.g., many carcinomas and sarcomas, myeloproliferative and lymphoproliferative disorders), immune-mediated disorders (e.g., immune-mediated thrombocytopenia, systemic lupus erythematosus), and toxicities due to drugs (e.g., trimethoprimsulfamethoxazole, many cytotoxic drugs) and other substances (e.g., snakebites). Vasculitis, neoplasia, protein-losing enteropathy/nephropathy, and disseminated intravascular coagulation may lead to platelet activation and consumption, and subsequently to thrombocytopenia. In cats, immune-mediated thrombocytopenia is rare; however, FeLV infection and neoplasia have been associated with thrombocytopenia.

Thrombopathy (thrombasthenia), a functional defect of platelets, can be inherited or acquired. Inherited thrombopathies have been reported mostly in dogs, and include von Willebrand's disease (vWD, also reported in cats), basset hound hereditary thrombopathia, canine thrombasthenic thrombopathy, Glanzmann's thrombasthenia, cyclic hematopoiesis, and storage pool disease. In cats the Chédiak-Higashi syndrome is associated with platelet function defects. Acquired thrombopathy may accompany thrombocytopenia and can result from drug

toxicity, paraproteinemia, immune-mediated mechanisms (e.g., antiplatelet antibodies, circulating immune complexes and vasculitis), disseminated intravascular coagulation (fibrinogen degradation products excess), uremia, neoplasia (e.g., hemangiosarcoma), and liver failure.

The ocular manifestations include both extraocular and intraocular bleeding, such as subconjunctival hemorrhage, hyphema, iridal petechias, and preretinal, intraretinal, and subretinal hemorrhages. The latter may also lead to retinal detachment and blindness. Depending on the primary cause of the platelet disease, anterior uveitis may also be present (e.g., in canine monocytic ehrlichiosis).

The diagnosis of thrombocytopenia is based on hematologic examination. Bleeding diathesis usually does not occur until platelet numbers fall below 50,000 cells/μL and is more common in acute than in chronic conditions. Very commonly, automated platelet counts in cats are falsely decreased, necessitating a manual count or a blood smear evaluation. The presence of thrombopathy can be confirmed by measurement of buccal mucosal bleeding time (provided that there is no concurrent thrombocytopenia). However, the diagnosis of the specific disorder requires special laboratory tests. Canine von Willebrand's factor assays are available (electroimmunoassay, ELISA).

Thrombocytopenia may be corrected by treatment of the primary disease but this may prove difficult. Acute life-threatening thrombocytopenia is treated with fresh whole blood or platelet-rich plasma transfusions. Von Willebrand's disease is treated with desmopressin and cryoprecipitate or fresh-frozen plasma transfusions. Intraocular hemorrhage is treated with topical steroids, and systemic glucocorticoid treatment should be considered if the animal's systemic condition allows it. Mydriatics should be considered to prevent possible posterior synechia, as should prophylactic antiglaucoma treatment.

SYSTEMIC HYPERTENSION. Systemic hypertension occurs in both dogs and cats. It is more common in cats because this species has a relatively higher incidence of chronic kidney disease. Systemic hypertension has been described in chronic kidney disease (cats, dogs) due to several renal disorders (e.g., chronic interstitial nephritis, amyloidosis, glomerulonephritis, pyelonephritis, polycystic kidney disease, renal dysplasia), HAC (dogs, 60%), pheochromocytoma (dogs, 50%), DM (dogs, 51%), hyperthyroidism (cats, 87%), primary aldosteronism (dogs) and hypothyroidism (dogs), hyperkinetic cardiac syndrome (e.g., anemia, polycythemia, fever, arteriovenous fistula), hypercalcemia (dogs), and hyperestrogenism. Physiologic hypertension is present in gazing hounds, in which it is probably a normal phenomenon. Essential (primary, idiopathic) hypertension is probably an extremely rare condition in dogs and has not been described in cats. Obesity has been described as a risk factor for systemic hypertension in dogs. Most (77%) of the hypertensive dogs are males.

The ocular lesions in systemic hypertension include retinal and papillary edema, tortuous retinal blood vessels, and preretinal, intraretinal, and subretinal hemorrhage. Secondary retinal degeneration, probably due to ischemia and/or inflammation, is a common sequel. Animals with systemic hypertension may be presented with a complaint of acute blindness (with fixed, dilated pupils) caused by bullous retinal detachment due to subretinal effusion (Figure 18-21).

The diagnosis of systemic hypertension requires measurement of systolic or, preferably, systolic and diastolic blood pressures (BPs). Fractious animals may exhibit erroneously

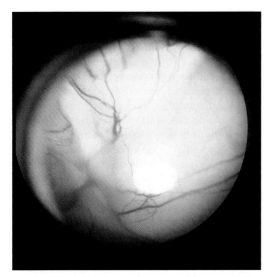

Figure 18-21. Retinal detachment in a cat with systemic hypertension. The retina is clearly visible as a vascularized membrane (note the folds of the "membrane") seen through the pupil.

Table 18-19 | **Normal Arterial Blood Pressure Values (mm Hg) in the Dog and Cat**

	DOG	CAT
Systolic	148 ± 16	171 ± 22
Diastolic	87 ± 8	123 ± 17

Data from Gordon DB, Goldblatt H (1967): Direct percutaneous determination of systemic blood pressure and production of renal hypertension in the cat. Proc Soc Exp Biol Med 125:177; and Cowgill LCD, Kallet AJ (1986): Systemic hypertension, in Kirk RW (editor): Current Veterinary Therapy IX, 9th ed. Saunders, Philadelphia.

elevated BP. Therefore acclimation and several repeated measurements in a quiet, stress-free environment are advised. BP values (systolic/diastolic) exceeding 180/100 mm Hg are considered abnormally high, and values higher than 200/110 mm Hg to have clinical significance (Table 18-19).

Treatment of systemic hypertension is primarily aimed at the underlying disorder. Commonly used drugs are listed in Table 18-20. Antihypertensive drug therapy of systemic hypertension should lower the BP to a level that is not associated with the appearance of new lesions and probably should not attempt to normalize the BP. Drug therapy may consist of one

or several agents, depending on the clinical signs and the underlying disease. These drugs include oral angiotensin-converting enzyme (ACE) inhibitors (e.g., enalapril, benazepril), calcium channel blockers (e.g., amlodipine), cardioselective adrenergic β-blockers (e.g., atenolol), vasodilators (e.g., hydralazine), and diuretics (e.g., furosemide). In emergency cases intravenous administration of nitroprusside or hydralazine may be advised; however, BP and urine production should be constantly monitored with this treatment because it may lead to a sharp drop in glomerular filtration.

Ocular treatment may be given to prevent secondary glaucoma and uveitis. Topical steroids may be prescribed, and systemic antiinflammatory treatment can be considered if the animal's systemic condition allows. Some clinicians advocate therapy with systemic carbonic anhydrase inhibitors.

POLYCYTHEMIA. *Polycythemia* is an increase in the red blood cell mass above the reference range. Relative polycythemia is also referred to as *erythrocytosis*; this term is usually reserved for milder elevations of the hematocrit, most commonly due to hemoconcentration secondary to dehydration, and is a transient condition. True polycythemia can be primary or secondary.

Table 18-20 | **Antihypertensive Drugs**

GENERIC NAME	DOSAGE DOG	DOSAGE CAT
ANGIOTENSIN-CONVERTING ENZYME INHIBITORS		
Enalapril	0.5 mg/kg PO q12-24h	0.25-0.5 mg/kg PO q12-24h
Captopril	0.5-2.0 mg/kg PO q8-12h	3.1-6.25 mg/cat PO q8-12h
Lisinopril	0.5 mg/kg PO q24h	—
Benazepril	0.25-0.5 mg/kg PO q24h	0.25-0.5 mg/kg PO q24h
CALCIUM CHANNEL BLOCKERS		
Diltiazem	0.5-1.5 mg/kg PO q8-12h to maximum of 200 mg/day	1.75-2.4 mg/kg q8h
Diltiazem sustained release	10 mg/kg PO q24h	10 mg/kg PO q24h
Amlodipine	0.1 mg/kg PO q24h or 2.5 mg/dog	0.625-1.25 mg/cat PO q24h
β-ADRENERGIC BLOCKERS		
Propranolol	0.2-1 mg/kg PO q8 to maximum of 200 mg/day	0.4-1.2 mg/kg PO q8h or 2.5-5 mg/cat PO q8-12h
Atenolol	0.2-2 mg/kg PO q12-24h or 6.25-12.5 mg/dog PO q12h	2-3 mg/kg PO q12h or 6.25-12.5 mg/cat PO q12h
β-ADRENERGIC BLOCKERS		
Prazosin	0.065 mg/kg (1 mg/15 kg) PO q8-12h	0.065 mg/kg (1 mg/15 kg) PO q8-12h
Phenoxybenzamine	0.2-1.5 mg/kg PO q8-12h	2.5-7.5 mg/cat PO q8-12h or 0.5 mg/kg PO q12h
VASODILATORS		
Hydralazine	0.5-2 mg/kg PO q12h	2.5 mg/cat PO q12-24h
Nitroprusside	1-10 µg/kg/min IV CRI	1-10 µg/kg/min IV CRI
DIURETICS		
Chlorothiazide	20-40 mg/kg PO q12-24h	20-40 mg/kg PO q12-24h
Hydrochlorothiazide	2-4 mg/kg PO q12h	2-4 mg/kg PO q12h
Furosemide	1-4 mg/kg PO, IM, IV or SC q8-12h (or as needed)	1-4 mg/kg PO, IM, IV or SC q8-24h

CRI, Constant infusion rate.

Primary polycythemia (*polycythemia rubra vera*) is a rare myeloproliferative disorder more commonly observed in cats (associated with FeLV infection) than in dogs. It is characterized by an abnormal proliferation of erythrocytes, platelets, and granulocytes; serum erythropoietin (EPO) concentrations are usually normal or mildly decreased. Secondary polycythemia may be appropriate and inappropriate and is associated with general hypoxemia or hypoxia, respectively. Chronic cardiopulmonary disorders, such as pulmonary neoplasia and right-to-left cardiac shunts, lead to hypoxemia, whereas renal neoplasia or neoplastic disorders of other abdominal organs may cause renal arterial blood flow obstruction and, consequently, renal hypoxia and a resultant increase in EPO concentrations. Hemoglobin disorders may also cause hypoxemia but are extremely rare in dogs and cats. All of these mechanisms lead to increases in production of EPO and its release from the hypoxic kidney, resulting in higher serum EPO concentrations, and, subsequently, in greater erythropoiesis and secondary polycythemia. EPO-secreting tumors have been reported rarely in humans and dogs (leiomyosarcoma, schwannoma) and were associated with secondary inappropriate polycythemia. Polycythemia leads to hyperviscosity, which reduces blood flow in the microcirculation resulting in local tissue hypoxia.

The ocular signs include dilated and tortuous dark red to brown conjunctival vessels, and the owner may complain of a "red eye." Similar changes are seen in the retinal vasculature, and retinal vessels are described as having a "boxcar appearance" (i.e., intermittent dilatation and constriction of vessels). With progression, retinal hemorrhages and detachment occur. Uveitis and chorioretinitis were observed in dogs with polycythemia vera.

Examinations to diagnose polycythemia include hematologic profile, serum biochemistry, and urinalysis to differentiate relative (erythrocytosis) from absolute polycythemia. Further tests, such as arterial blood gas measurement, thoracic radiography, abdominal ultrasonography, and serum EPO concentration measurements, should be considered. In secondary polycythemia, the serum EPO concentration will be increased, whereas in primary polycythemia it will be low normal to decreased. Bone marrow cytologic examination shows erythroid hyperplasia and a decrease in the myeloid-to-erythroid (M:E) ratio in all polycythemic patients and thus is not diagnostically useful.

Relative polycythemia is treated with fluid therapy. Severe polycythemia is treated with repeated phlebotomies (10 to 20 mL/kg per treatment, until reaching a hematocrit of 50% to 55%). The treatment of secondary absolute polycythemia is aimed at the primary disease whenever possible. In polycythemia rubra vera and in cases of secondary absolute polycythemia in which correction of the primary disease is not possible (e.g., cyanotic heart disease), repeated phlebotomies and oral hydroxyurea (30 to 50 mg/kg q24h for 7 days, and then titration of dosage to effect) are recommended. Resolution of the ocular signs has been observed in cases in which polycythemia was resolved.

HYPERVISCOSITY SYNDROME. In dogs and cats hyperviscosity syndrome is most commonly associated with malignancies such as multiple myeloma, chronic lymphocytic leukemia, lymphoma, and plasmacytoma (solitary osseous or extramedullary); however, it may also occur in certain infectious inflammatory diseases (e.g., canine ehrlichiosis and leishmaniasis). The increase of serum viscosity, which is due to the production and greater serum concentration of paraproteins, occurs more commonly with IgM class paraproteins (i.e., macroglobulinemia); however, IgA and IgG paraproteins have also been reported to lead to hyperviscosity syndrome in both dogs and cats. Clinical signs appear when serum viscosity rises to four to five times the normal level. Approximately 20% of the dogs with multiple myeloma have hyperviscosity syndrome.

The ocular signs of hyperviscosity syndrome include dilated, congested, tortuous retinal blood vessels, kinking of retinal blood vessels, papillary edema, retinal hemorrhages, intraretinal cysts, bullous retinal detachment, retinal degeneration, and blindness. Uveitis and secondary glaucoma have also been reported.

The diagnosis of hyperviscosity syndrome is based on serum viscosity measurement, although additional tests are needed to diagnose the specific causative disease. The diagnosis of multiple myeloma (and macroglobulinemia) may require serum electrophoresis and immunoelectrophoresis, skeletal survey radiographs, urinary heat precipitation test, and immunoelectrophoresis, whereas the definitive diagnosis usually requires a bone marrow aspirate or core biopsy. The diagnosis of lymphosarcoma may call for fine-needle aspirates or biopsies from lymphoid and visceral organs, thoracic radiography, and abdominal ultrasonography. The diagnosis of chronic lymphocytic leukemia is based on hematologic tests (e.g., complete blood count and peripheral blood cytology) and bone marrow cytology.

Multiple myeloma is best treated with melphalan or with other alkylating agents such as cyclophosphamide and chlorambucil. Some texts recommend the use of glucocorticoids, especially in presence of hypercalcemia and during the initial phase of treatment. Lymphoma is treated with a multidrug chemotherapeutical protocol, and chronic lymphocytic leukemia is usually treated with glucocorticoids and chlorambucil. Plasmapheresis is the preferred mode of therapy to treat hyperviscosity. Ocular treatment is symptomatic.

Immune-Mediated Diseases in Dogs

UVEODERMATOLOGIC SYNDROME (VOGT-KOYANAGI-HARADA–LIKE SYNDROME). The uveodermatologic syndrome has been described in humans as well as in several dog breeds, including Samoyed, old English sheepdog, Siberian husky, Saint Bernard, Akita, Irish setter, chow chow, Shetland sheepdog, golden retriever, and Australian shepherd. The mean reported age was 3 years, and the ocular signs most commonly preceded the dermatologic lesions. The syndrome is a combination of several dermatologic signs (i.e., poliosis, vitiligo, and sometimes ulceration) and ocular signs. Meningitis or meningoencephalitis has been reported in the human disease; however, these complications are extremely rare in dogs. The cutaneous manifestations are most commonly restricted to the head area, occurring in the planum nasale (Figure 18-22), eyelids, and lips, but the footpads and the scrotum may be affected. The immunohistochemical findings in a recent study have suggested that the skin lesions were mediated by T cells and macrophages (Th1 immunity), whereas the ocular lesions were more consistent with a B-cell and macrophage response (Th2 immunity). These immune reactions are directed against melanocytes in the skin and in the (anterior and posterior) uvea.

The ocular disease is manifested as a bilateral uveitis—anterior uveitis or both anterior and posterior uveitis (panuveitis).

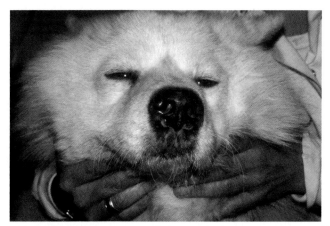

Figure 18-22. Depigmentation of the nasal planum in a 4-year-old Samoyed with uveodermatologic syndrome. Severe anterior uveitis and secondary glaucoma led to loss of vision in both eyes despite treatment with azathioprine.

Secondary ocular lesions, including cataract, posterior synechia, glaucoma, bullous retinal detachment, retinal and optic nerve atrophy, and acute blindness, are common. There is progressive depigmentation of the retinal pigment epithelium in the nontapetum, tapetal hyperreflectivity, and attenuation of the retinal blood vessels.

The diagnosis is based mainly on signalment and clinical presentation—in other words, on a combination of the ocular and dermatologic lesions. Histopathologic examination of the cutaneous lesions demonstrates a lichenoid dermatosis with dermal infiltration of histiocytes and lymphocytes and some giant cells as well as decreased melanin in the dermis and hair follicles.

Medical treatment consists of oral glucocorticoids and azathioprine for long periods (up to lifelong), combined with topical corticosteroids, NSAIDs, and atropine. In humans, an intravitreal triamcinolone-acetonide injection has led to improvement in vision and uveitis. Topical cyclosporine therapy has also been suggested. Treatment of the secondary complications of the syndrome is essentially symptomatic, and some complications (e.g., glaucoma, cataract) may require surgical intervention. Long-term prognosis for vision is usually poor. Recently, successful results were reported in a dog with use of oral and topical prednisone, along with 1% indomethacin eyedrops, methylprednisone (twice via the subconjunctival route at an interval of 15 days), and dorzolamide and timolol eyedrops, to prevent the development of secondary glaucoma due to posterior synechiae. Both dermatologic and ophthalmic signs showed good improvement, vision was preserved, and some repigmentation of the skin and hair occurred.

OCULAR MANIFESTATIONS OF SYSTEMIC DISEASES IN HORSES (Tables 18-21 to 18-32)

Infectious Diseases

Viral Respiratory Diseases

EQUINE HERPESVIRUS (RHINOTRACHEITIS OR RHINOPNEUMONITIS). Rhinotracheitis or rhinopneumonitis is a contagious viral respiratory disease caused by a member of the Alphaherpesvirinae subfamily (equine herpesvirus [EHV]-1 or EHV-4). It is difficult to differentiate clinically from signs due to other respiratory viruses. Infection is transmitted by aerosol, and the incubation period is 3 to 7 days. The disorder may also

Table 18-21 | Systemic Causes of Conjunctivitis* in Horses and Cattle

CAUSES	HORSE	COW
Viral diseases	Equine influenza Equine herpes (EHV-2) Equine adenovirus African horse sickness	Bluetongue[†] Infectious bovine rhinotracheitis (BHV-1)
Bacterial and related diseases	—	Chlamydophila (formerly Chlamydia) psittaci[‡] Mycoplasma spp.[†] Mannheimia (Pasteurella) pneumonia Leptospira pomona (experimentally induced) Septicemia Listeriosis[†]
Protozoal diseases	—	Babesiosis[†] Trypanosoma spp.[†]
Fungal diseases Parasitic diseases	Histoplasmosis[§] Habronemiasis[§] Onchocerca cervicalis	— Gedoelstiasis[†]
Immune-mediated diseases	Pemphigus foliaceus	—
Neoplastic diseases	Lymphoma/lymphosarcoma[§]	—
Toxic diseases	Generalized granulomatous disease	Vetch poisoning

*Associated ocular signs include ocular discharge/secretion, chemosis, congestion, and follicular hyperplasia.
[†]Causes disease in both bovine and ovine species.
[‡]Causes disease in ovine species.
[§]May cause ulceration of the conjunctiva and thereby lead to secondary corneal irritation.

recur from a latent phase. The virus was successfully recovered from horses experimentally treated with corticosteroids, and it has also been found in lymph nodes of horses with no clinical signs of the disease. As with other viral respiratory diseases, rhinotracheitis is characterized by a high fever (up to 41° C) that is often biphasic and a serous to mucopurulent nasal discharge. In experimentally infected pony foals, mandibular lymph nodes were more significantly enlarged and coughs were less prominent with herpesvirus infection than with influenza infection. Leukopenia is the typical hematologic response. Conjunctivitis or keratitis may be observed, and a purulent ocular discharge could develop. Experimental infection of six foals resulted in bilateral chorioretinitis with mononuclear cell infiltration in one foal. Rhinotracheitis or rhinopneumonitis is usually a self-limiting disease, but topical antibiotics may be used to control secondary bacterial infections.

EHV-1 may also cause abortions or weakness in neonatal foals within the first week of life, as well as neurologic disease, which is apparently due to an immune complex vasculitis. Horses with neurologic disease may demonstrate nystagmus or blindness, depending on the location of the CNS lesions. Exposure keratitis or KCS secondary to facial paralysis and ulcerative lesions due to prolonged recumbency have also been documented.

Table 18-22 | **Systemic Causes of Miscellaneous Conjunctival Disorders in Horses and Cattle**

DISORDER	HORSE	COW
Conjunctival/ subconjunctival hemorrhage	Equine infectious anemia African horse sickness Babesiosis Potomac horse fever Lymphoma/ lymphosarcoma Multiple myeloma Equine purpura hemorrhagica Neonatal maladjustment syndrome Neonatal isoerythrolysis Immune-mediated hemolytic anemia	Bovine viral diarrhea Septicemia *Trypanosoma* spp. Bracken fern toxicity Warfarin/coumarin toxicity
Conjunctival icterus	Equine infectious anemia Leptospirosis Babesiosis Tyzzer's disease Generalized granulomatous disease Neonatal isoerythrolysis Toxic plant ingestion	Babesiosis Toxic plant ingestion

Table 18-23 | **Systemic Causes of Keratitis/ Keratoconjunctivitis* in Horses and Cattle**

CAUSES	HORSE	COW
Viral diseases	Equine viral arteritis Equine influenza Equine herpes (EHV-2)	Bovine viral diarrhea Infectious bovine rhinotracheitis (BHV-1) Malignant catarrhal fever[†]
Bacterial and related diseases	Leptospirosis	*Chlamydophila* (formerly *Chlamydia*) *psittaci*[‡] *Mycoplasma* spp.[†] *Leptospira pomona* (experimentally induced) *Mycobacterium ovis*[‡] Listeriosis[†]
Protozoal diseases		*Trypanosoma* spp.[†]
Fungal diseases	Histoplasmosis	—
Parasitic diseases	Habronemiasis *Onchocerca cervicalis*	Gedoelstiasis[†] Elaeophorosis
Immune-mediated diseases	Combined immunodeficiency	—
Toxic diseases	Generalized granulomatous disease	Anhydrous ammonia poisoning Phenothiazine poisoning

*Associated ocular signs include epiphora and discharge, blepharospasm, conjunctival congestion, and corneal edema, vascularization, infiltration, ulceration, and pigmentation.
[†]Causes disease in both bovine and ovine species.
[‡]Causes disease in ovine species.

EQUINE VIRAL ARTERITIS. Equine viral arteritis is an *arterivirus* infection that causes vasculitis leading to abortion, respiratory disease, and even death. It can be transmitted by inhalation or venereally. There is a chronic carrier state in stallions. Clinical signs of the respiratory disease include pyrexia (up to 40.5° C) for 1 to 5 days, anorexia, depression, serous nasal discharge, lacrimation, and coughing. Edema of the limbs, eyelids, and scrotum is characteristic but is not seen in all cases. Leukopenia is found on hematologic evaluation. Neonatal foals may die acutely or may show severe respiratory signs. One ocular sign is serous to mucoid ocular discharge, as in the other respiratory viruses, but periorbital edema may also be seen. Corneal opacity and photophobia have been described.

EQUINE INFLUENZA. Equine influenza is a contagious viral respiratory disease caused by the orthomyxovirus known as *Equine influenza*, particularly subtype 2 (AE-2). Outbreaks are more common in cooler, humid weather, as in winter and spring, depending on the climate. Horses 1 to 3 years of age are more susceptible during outbreaks. Infection occurs by aerosol, and the incubation time is 1 to 3 days. The damage to respiratory epithelial cells reduces the mucociliary clearance rate, apparently leading to secondary bacterial infections. Clinical signs include elevated rectal temperatures (40° to 41° C) that may be biphasic, reduced appetite, serous to mucoid nasal discharge, enlarged mandibular lymph nodes, and a cough. The cough may be very deep and last for several weeks. Detection of viral antigen up to 3 weeks after infection within vacuoles of alveolar macrophages has been reported. Hematologic changes include lymphopenia and eosinopenia followed by monocytosis a few days later. Ocular signs include epiphora and conjunctivitis (serous and erythematous) or keratoconjunctivitis, which usually resolve with resolution of the respiratory signs and do not require local treatment.

Bacterial Diseases

STRANGLES. *Streptococcus equi* causes the disease known as "strangles" in horses. It affects primarily younger horses but may affect older horses that are immunologically naive. *S. equi* infection is transmitted by direct contact or via fomites such as water troughs, feed bunks, pastures, and stalls. The organism can survive at least 3 months in the environment. The disease usually causes fever and respiratory signs. The name is derived from the propensity of the organism to produce abscesses of lymph nodes, particularly around the head and upper neck, which can lead to suffocation through obstruction of the pharynx. Other lymph nodes, such as the mesenteric nodes, may also be involved; this condition is known as "bastard strangles." Pharyngeal lymph nodes often drain before the horse recovers. The eyes may be involved in a mild inflammatory reaction, including dacryocystitis and transient KCS. The ocular discharge is often serous initially and mucopurulent later. Intraocular manifestations include anterior uveitis, panuveitis, chorioretinitis, retinal detachment, vitreous abscess, and optic neuritis. Ocular discharge and chorioretinal depigmentation in the nontapetal fundus of several horses have been described in one report. The depigmentation resolved spontaneously. In one case, anterior uveitis developed 10 days after Strangles and subsequently progressed to corneal stromal abscesses and

Table 18-24 | **Systemic Causes of Anterior Uveitis* in Horses and Cattle**

CAUSES	HORSE	COW
Viral diseases	Equine adenovirus–microscopic panuveitis	Malignant catarrhal fever
Bacterial and related diseases	Leptospirosis[†] Strangles (Streptococcus equi) Lyme disease[‡] Salmonellosis Brucella spp.[†]	Listeriosis Leptospira pomona (experimentally induced)[‡] Mycobacterium bovis Septicemia
Protozoal diseases	Potomac horse fever[‡] Toxoplasmosis (suspected)	Trypanosoma spp. Toxoplasma gondii
Parasitic diseases	Onchocerca cervicalis[†] Setaria spp. Dirofilaria spp. Halicephalobus deletrix	Elaeophorosis
Neoplastic diseases	Lymphoma/ lymphosarcoma	—
Other systemic causes	Multiple myeloma[‡]	—
Foal diseases	Sepsis and failure of passive transfer[‡] Tyzzer's disease[‡] Immune-mediated hemolytic anemia[‡] Rhodococcus equi[‡] Neonatal isoerythrolysis[‡] Combined immunodeficiency	—

*Associated ocular signs include corneal edema, flare (hypopyon/hyphema), hypotony, miosis, ciliary injection, blepharospasm, iris congestion, and photophobia. Secondary glaucoma and lens luxation are possible sequelae. Photophobia can also be caused by equine herpesvirus 2, equine viral arteritis, Leptospira, and Onchocerca in the horse.
[†]Has been implicated as a potential cause of equine recurrent uveitis.
[‡]Has been shown to cause hyphema.

panophthalmitis. The organism was cultured from the eye. In a case of a brain abscess due to S. equi, the horse was blind.

SALMONELLOSIS. Salmonellosis typically causes an acute colitis characterized by profuse watery diarrhea, endotoxemia, and coagulopathies with many severe sequelae, such as laminitis and acute renal failure. Horses are often depressed, dehydrated, febrile, and tachycardic and may exhibit abdominal pain.

Recovered horses may shed Salmonella for months. Other manifestations of salmonella infections are chronic colitis and abortions in adult horses and respiratory infections, spinal abscesses, and septic arthritis in neonates. Signs of ocular involvement include anterior uveitis and hypopyon. The organism has been cultured from the anterior chamber.

LEPTOSPIROSIS. Leptospira interrogans serovar pomona, a spirochete, has been documented in several foals and a stallion over the past decade. Pathogenetically, infection with the bacteria primarily causes a vasculitis and endotheliitis in multiple organs, particularly the kidneys and liver. Clinical signs include fever, depression, and partial anorexia. Azotemia is common. Gross hematuria has been observed in one foal, and leptospiruria detected in one foal. Leptospirosis should be considered in cases of acute renal failure with no obvious etiology. Leptospirosis also causes abortions, although less commonly in mares than in cows. Mares may show fever, depression and anorexia, and icterus for 3 to 4 days. Abortions occur 1 to 3 weeks later. Abortions are more common from the seventh month of pregnancy to term. Placentitis via ascending infections through the cervix is the primary cause.

Uveitis has been associated with leptospirosis but primarily weeks to months after the acute disease. Uveitis was not seen until 18 to 24 months after the acute outbreak of leptospirosis in one account. In an experimental infection the uveitis appeared no earlier than 1 year after infection and as late as 2 years later. Leptospira has been implicated as causing corneal opacities, anterior uveitis, equine recurrent uveitis, peripapillary chorioretinitis (Figure 18-23), and optic neuropathies, at least in experimentally infected horses. The association with equine recurrent uveitis may be directly due to bacterial infection or secondary to an immunologic reaction to infection. Even when antigen to Leptospira was found in the eye, antibiotic treatment did not decrease the inflammation. Serum titers for leptospira organisms were similar in horses with or without uveitis, but there were significant vitreous titers in 67% of eyes with uveitis and 0% in eyes without uveitis, indicating probably intraocular synthesis of antibodies. Direct culture of Leptospira from vitreous material taken from horses affected by equine recurrent uveitis was first reported in 1998 (9% of cases). Brem et al. (1998) report that two serovars were isolated, Leptospira grippotyphosa in three cases and a serovar out of the serogroup Australis in one case.

LYME DISEASE. B. burgdorferi has been reported to cause polyarthritis in horses. One case report described organisms cultured from the anterior chamber. Spirochetes of B. burgdorferi were identified within the eye of a pony with arthritis and panuveitis.

Table 18-25 | **Systemic Diseases Causing Posterior Uveitis* in Horses and Cattle**

CAUSES	HORSE	COW
Viral diseases	Equine herpesvirus (experimental infection)	Malignant catarrhal fever
Bacterial and related diseases	Leptospirosis Strangles (Streptococcus equi) Lyme disease Tuberculosis	Thromboembolic meningoencephalitis (TEME) Mycobacterium bovis Leptospira pomona (experimentally induced)
Protozoal diseases	Toxoplasmosis	Toxoplasmosis
Parasitic diseases	Onchocerca cervicalis Halicephalobus deletrix	Elaeophorosis
Immune-mediated diseases	Combined immunodeficiency	—
Foal/calf diseases	Sepsis and failure of passive transfer	Septicemia
Toxic diseases	Generalized granulomatous disease	—

*Includes chorioretinitis and choroiditis. Associated signs include retinal edema and hemorrhage, subretinal effusion and hemorrhage, vascular cuffing, and loss of vision. Retinal detachment and retinal atrophy are possible sequelae.

Table 18-26 | **Systemic Causes of Retinal Detachment, Hemorrhage, Atrophy, and Choroidal Depigmentation in Horses and Cattle**

DISORDER	HORSE	COW
Retinal detachment	Strangles Tuberculosis Lyme disease Hydatid disease Leptospirosis Lymphoma/lymphosarcoma Multiple myeloma Failure of passive transfer and sepsis Combined immunodeficiency	Bovine viral diarrhea *Mycobacterium bovis* Scrapie Septicemia
Retinal hemorrhage	Equine infectious anemia Sepsis and failure of passive transfer Neonatal maladjustment syndrome	Bovine viral diarrhea Thromboembolic meningoencephalitis (TEME) *Leptospira pomona* (experimentally induced) Hypovitaminosis A Septicemia
Retinal atrophy	Lyme disease	Arthrogryposis-hydrencephaly Bluetongue Bovine viral diarrhea Septicemia Elaeophorosis Hypovitaminosis A
Choroidal/nontapetal depigmentation	Equine motor neuron disease *Streptococcus* spp.	—

Severe panuveitis with hyphema may occur, resulting in ocular hypotony or secondary glaucoma. Chronic inflammation may lead to rubeosis iridis (preiridal fibrovascular membranes, which appear clinically as congestion of the iris vessels), iridal hyperpigmentation, posterior synechiae, cataract, retinal atrophy and detachment, and blindness.

Protozoal Diseases

BABESIOSIS (PIROPLASMOSIS). Babesiosis (piroplasmosis) is a tick-borne protozoan parasitic disease affecting red blood cells. Horses may be infected with *Babesia caballi* or *Theileria equi* (formerly known as *Babesia equi*). Typical signs of acute babesiosis include fever (39° to 42° C), hemolytic anemia, and jaundice. Hemoglobinuria and death can occur. *B. caballi* can be recognized as large intraerythrocytic organisms on blood smears, whereas *T. equi* is smaller and is often seen as four organisms in one erythrocyte, forming a "Maltese cross."

Table 18-27 | **Systemic Causes of Optic Nerve Disease in Horses and Cattle**

DISEASE	HORSE	COW
Optic neuropathy	Leptospirosis Intracranial abscess/neoplasia	Arthrogryposis-hydrencephaly Bovine viral diarrhea Elaeophorosis Male fern poisoning
Optic neuritis	Strangles Aspergillosis Infectious meningitis Neonatal maladjustment syndrome Intracranial abscess/neoplasia	Bovine viral diarrhea *Trypanosoma* spp. Coenurosis Polioencephalomalacia Hypovitaminosis A

B. caballi can be passed vertically from one tick generation to the next, but *T. equi* is considered to be more pathogenic and tends to produce a carrier state in the horse. The ocular sign most commonly seen is icterus of the conjunctiva and sclera. Petechial hemorrhages of the conjunctiva, swelling of the periorbital fossa and eyelids as well as serous ocular discharge have also been reported with varying frequencies.

POTOMAC HORSE FEVER. *Neorickettsia risticii* (formerly *Ehrlichia risticii*) is a known cause of Potomac horse fever (PHF), a disease characterized by enterocolitis in horses. The disease causes clinical signs of acute colitis similar to those of salmonellosis. The diarrhea can be profuse and watery and may

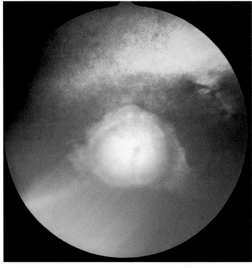

Figure 18-23. Peripapillary chorioretinal changes in a horse with chronic equine recurrent uveitis that was also seropositive for leptospirosis. The pale lesions around the optic disc, called "butterfly lesions," are pathognomonic for the chorioretinitis that characterizes the disease. (Courtesy Paul E. Miller.)

Table 18-28 | **Systemic Causes of Central Blindness in Horses and Cattle***

CAUSES	HORSE	COW
Viral diseases	Equine herpesvirus Viral encephalitis	Arthrogryposis-hydrencephaly Bovine viral diarrhea
Bacterial diseases	Strangles *(Streptococcus equi)*	Listeriosis Thromboembolic meningoencephalitis (TEME)
Protozoal diseases	Equine protozoal myeloencephalitis	—
Parasitic diseases	—	Coenurosis
Neurologic diseases	Leukoencephalomalacia Polyneuritis equi Intracranial neoplasia/abscess	—
Metabolic diseases	—	Polioencephalomacia Pregnancy toxemia/ketosis Hypovitaminosis A
Poisonings	Thiamine deficiency	Lead toxicity
Foal diseases	Neonatal maladjustment syndrome Benign epilepsy of the Arabian foal	—

*Optic nerve and retinal disorders may also cause blindness.

be accompanied by endotoxemia. Endotoxemia is characterized by fever, leukopenia, congested mucous membranes, and hypercoagulability. Complications include sequelae typical of endotoxemia, but hypoproteinemia and laminitis are more commonly seen. *N. risticii* has also been associated with abortion between 6 and 8 months of pregnancy, but the incidence is not known. The organism may directly infect the eye, or ocular complications may result from systemic reaction to the disease. Hemorrhages may occur on the ocular surfaces, and infection of the eye may result in anterior uveitis and hyphema.

Parasitic Diseases

HABRONEMIASIS. The larvae of the nematodes *Habronema muscae, Habronema majus,* and *Draschia megastoma* cause ulcerative cutaneous granulomas in horses. The adult nematodes inhabit the stomach. The eggs and larvae pass through the feces and are ingested by the maggots of the intermediate hosts (*Musca domestica* and *Stomoxys calcitrans*). The adult flies then deposit the larvae onto the mucous membranes, abraded skin, or open wounds in the horse. The disease occurs in the summer. Affected horses are predisposed to yearly recurrences. The infected area develops either proliferative, exuberant granulation tissue or ulcerative, nodular, and tumorous masses, which may have the characteristic yellow (sulfur) granules.

Lesions may be seen on limbs, ventral body, prepuce, urethral process of the penis, commissure of the lips, and any other area of traumatized skin, but also in the conjunctiva and medial canthus of the eye. The granulation tissue may be a hypersensitivity reaction to dead or dying larvae.

When 63 cases were reviewed, ocular lesions were the most common, being seen either at the medial canthus (17 cases) or in the third eyelid (8 cases). Lesions were described as raised, proliferative, nonhealing wounds or granulation tissue with sulfur granules, mucopurulent discharge, chemosis, and injection of conjunctival vessels. The lesions may be friable and pruritic and may bleed easily. Fistulous tracts and subdermal nodules may develop below the medial canthus (Figure 18-24). The sulfur granules often seen are 1 to 2 mm in size. Corneal vascularization and edema can occur as a result of irritation of the cornea and altered lid function. Occasionally, corneal ulcers (2/17 in one study) and blepharospasm have been reported. Compared with the control population, Arabian horses were overrepresented, and thoroughbreds underrepresented. Color distribution may be a confounder, however, because horses of lighter colors are overrepresented compared with those of darker color, and Arabians tend to be lighter in color than thoroughbreds. There were no cases in horses younger than 1 year.

Table 18-29 | **Systemic Causes of Neuroophthalmic Disorders in Horses and Cattle**

DISORDER	HORSE	COW

Nystagmus	Equine herpesvirus
	Equine protozoal
	   myeloencephalitis
	Viral encephalitis
	Infectious meningitis
	Intracranial abscess/neoplasia
	Unilateral vestibular disease
	Tyzzer's disease
		Listeriosis
		Thromboembolic
		   meningoencephalitis
		   (TEME)
		Polioencephalomalacia
		Hypovitaminosis A

Strabismus	Viral encephalitis
	Infectious meningitis
	Intracranial abscess/neoplasia
	Vestibular disease
		Listeriosis
		Thromboembolic
		   meningoencephalitis
		   (TEME)
		Hypovitaminosis A
		Tetanus

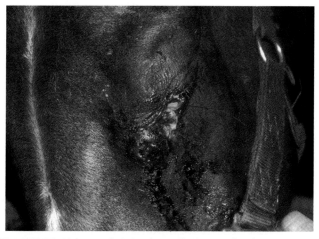

Figure 18-24. Habronemiasis in a horse. The nematode infestation caused an ulcer at the medial canthus, which drained into a fistulous tract.

Table 18-30 | **Systemic Causes of Orbital Disorders in Horses and Cattle**

DISORDER	HORSE	COW

Exophthalmos	Cryptococcosis
	Hydatid disease
	Intracranial
	  abscess/neoplasia
	Lymphoma/lymphosarcoma
		Polioencephalomalacia
		Lymphoma/
		  lymphosarcoma
		Gedoelstiasis
		Hypovitaminosis A

Periorbital
distention/
edema
	Equine viral arteritis
	African horse sickness
	Babesiosis
	Cryptococcosis
	Malignant edema
	Intracranial
	  abscess/neoplasia
	Equine purpura
	  hemorrhagica
		—

Orbital cellulitis		Actinomycosis

Table 18-31 | **Systemic Causes of Pupillary Disorders in the Horse**

DISORDER	CAUSES
Horner's syndrome	Aspergillosis Equine protozoal myeloencephalitis Intracranial abscess/neoplasia Vestibular disorders
Abnormal pupillary light reaction	Botulism Leukoencephalomalacia Viral encephalitis Infectious meningitis Intracranial abscess/neoplasia

CUTANEOUS ONCHOCERCIASIS. Cutaneous onchocerciasis, a dermatitis caused by the microfilariae of *Onchocerca cervicalis,* is seen primarily in adult horses. The adult parasites are found in the funicular part of the ligamentum nuchae. The females produce microfilariae that migrate to the superficial dermis. The larvae are ingested by the vector, *Culicoides,* and transmitted to other horses after development of the larvae within the vector. Cutaneous lesions include diffuse or patchy alopecia, erythema, and scaling. Focal cutaneous depigmentation is common. Most of the lesions are found on the ventral midline, the lower eyelid, and the lateral limbus of the eye. Some are also found at the base of the mane as well as on the dorsomedial proximal forelimbs and cranial pectoral region. A bull's-eye lesion in the center of the forehead is characteristic. The lesions are nonseasonal and nonpruritic in most cases.

Ocular involvement is common in cutaneous onchocerciasis, being seen in 10% to 50% of cases. Initially there is chemosis and hyperemia of the conjunctiva accompanied by increased lacrimation and blepharospasm. Later, conjunctivitis, keratitis, depigmentation of the lateral limbus, and intraocular lesions are observed. Small, raised, white nodules (0.5 to 2 mm in diameter) in the limbal conjunctiva and punctate, subepithelial corneal opacities of similar size are commonly present. Corneal lesions are often wedge-shaped with the base of the triangle at the limbus and are characterized by varying degrees of superficial and deep neovascularization and cellular stromal infiltrates. Lesions may progressively enlarge. With chronicity, patches of depigmentation occur. Recurrent episodes of keratoconjunctivitis are common. Both anterior and posterior uveitis are also observed. The former is characterized by photophobia, epiphora, miosis, aqueous flare, iris congestion, and hypotony. The latter is seen funduscopically as hyporeflective areas representing retinal edema. Inflammation around the optic papilla in a butterfly-shaped pattern may be present (see Figure 18-23) but is often hard to see owing to vitreous and aqueous opacification. Intraocular changes usually occur together with the eyelid lesions, suggesting that the initial invasion is in the eyelids. Intraocular filariae have been reported within the anterior chamber. *O. cervicalis* has also been implicated as a cause of equine recurrent uveitis.

***Setaria* INFECTION.** *Setaria* are primarily filarial parasites of cattle, which may aberrantly infect horses intraabdominally or in the spinal cord where they cause clinical signs of CNS disease. Reported cases included clinical signs of a hypotonic tail, bladder paralysis, ataxia, and conscious proprioceptive deficits. *Setaria digitata* and *Setaria equina* occasionally invade the eye, causing severe intraocular inflammation. They are the most common intraocular nematodes in the horse, particularly *S. digitata.* Successful surgical removal of the parasites from the anterior chamber has been reported.

Neurologic Diseases

EQUINE PROTOZOAL MYELOENCEPHALITIS. Equine protozoal myeloencephalitis (EPM) is a multifocal, progressive disease of the CNS, most commonly caused by *Sarcocystis neurona,* although there have been reports of *Neospora* spp. as a cause. Clinical signs vary with the areas of the CNS affected. Originally the disease was described as causing asymmetric ataxia and associated muscle atrophy; however, involvement of cranial nerves and lesions of the cerebrum has also been reported. Ocular changes, including exposure keratopathy secondary to facial paralysis and decreased tear production, have been reported. Ptosis, enophthalmos, and prominence of the supraorbital process due to muscle denervation atrophy, Horner's syndrome, nystagmus, and blindness have also been reported. Horner's syndrome is a neurologic condition relating to an interruption of the ocular sympathetic pathways. In horses, the signs of Horner's syndrome primarily include ptosis, sweating, and warmth on the denervated side. Other signs seen in small animals with Horner's syndrome, such as miosis and enophthalmos with elevation of the third eyelid, are not prominent in the horse.

VIRAL ENCEPHALITIS. The viruses of the Togaviridae family of arboviruses cause encephalitides in horses. The most prominent are members of the alphaviruses, which cause Eastern, Western, and Venezuelan equine encephalitides. Flaviviridae can also cause encephalitis, such as West Nile fever, and Japanese, California, St. Louis, and Murray Valley encephalitides as well as Cache Valley, Main Drain, and Borna fever. The clinical signs of all of the encephalitides are similar. Fever is often reported early in the disease. Neurologic signs related to diffuse encephalitis—depression, constant walking, head-pressing, constant chewing movements and ataxia—have been reported with Eastern and Western equine encephalitis. Additional signs, such as blindness, circling, excitement, and aggressive behavior, may also develop. As cortical damage worsens, paralysis of larynx, pharynx, and tongue may develop along with loss of brainstem function, leading to head tilt, nystagmus, strabismus, and pupil dilation. Signs of Venezuelan equine encephalitis may be similar to those of the other encephalitis viruses or may be unrelated, such as epistaxis, pulmonary hemorrhage, oral ulcers,

Table 18-32 | **Systemic Causes of Adnexal Abnormalities in Horses and Cattle**

ABNORMALITY	CAUSES IN HORSE	CAUSES IN COW
Facial nerve paralysis*	Equine herpesvirus Equine protozoal myeloencephalitis Viral encephalitis Infectious meningitis Intracranial abscess/neoplasia Polyneuritis equi	Listeriosis
Eyelid edema, infiltration, ulcers, alopecia, or crusting	African horse sickness Histoplasmosis Mycotic dermatitis Mange *Onchocerca cervicalis* Pemphigus Urticaria Generalized granulomatous disease	—
Eyelid protrusion	Tetanus Hyperkalemic periodic paralysis	—
Transient keratoconjunctivitis sicca	Strangles (*Streptococcus equi*)	—

*May lead to decreased tear production, secondary keratoconjunctivitis sicca, secondary corneal ulceration, exposure keratitis, and periorbital muscular atrophy.

and diarrhea. Horses with Venezuelan equine encephalitis occasionally appear blind. Seizures may occur with all three encephalitides.

Ocular signs are secondary to CNS disorders. They include blindness, nystagmus, strabismus, pupillary dilation, and facial nerve paralysis with secondary exposure keratopathy. Also, recumbency in horses may cause injuries to the eye or periorbital tissue owing to direct pressure, abrasion, chemical contact (e.g., urine), or foreign bodies such as shavings, dirt, and straw. These can cause conjunctivitis, keratitis, corneal ulcers, and secondary uveitis.

Clinical signs of Borna disease are similar to those of other equine encephalitides. Visual impairment and blindness may occur with CNS signs. Blindness is reportedly regularly observed in acute Borna disease. Nystagmus, strabismus, and miosis, due to involvement of the cranial nerves, have been reported.

West Nile virus meningomyeloencephalitis is a mosquito-borne virus closely related to St. Louis, Japanese, and Murray Valley encephalitides. A febrile response may occur with the onset of clinical disease. Initial signs, such as depression, listlessness, ataxia, and paresis, occur abruptly. Other signs progress over 1 to 3 days. These may include head shaking, incessant chewing, paralysis of the lower lip or tongue, severe ataxia, ascending paralysis, and terminal recumbency. Ocular signs, predominantly blindness, have been reported in horses with West Nile virus, particularly in the year 2000. This is a zoonotic disease, although horses are not a source of human infection. In humans, occlusive vasculitis, uveitis, chorioretinitis, and optic neuritis have been reported.

MENINGITIS. Meningitis occurs either by direct extension of infectious agents into the calvarium (as with skull fractures or osteomyelitis from sinusitis or otitis, or as a sequel to surgical removal of progressive ethmoidal hematomas) or from hematogenous infection. Infection may be fungal, as with *C. neoformans*, but are more commonly bacterial. Bacteria involved in equine meningitis include *Streptococcus zooepidemicus* and *Streptococcus suis* in foals and *Actinomyces* spp. in adults. Meningitis of hematogenous origin in neonates commonly involves gram-negative bacteria such as *Escherichia coli* and *Salmonella* spp. and is associated with sepsis. Signs of

meningitis include fever, anorexia, stiff neck, and hyperesthesia. It may be accompanied by diarrhea. The patient may be extremely depressed or hyperexcitable. Various other neurologic signs can be seen in addition to cranial nerve dysfunctions. Signs may progress to coma or status epilepticus. Ophthalmic signs are primarily due to cranial nerve dysfunction and include ptosis, strabismus, nystagmus, anisocoria, optic neuritis, and blindness.

PHOTIC HEAD SHAKING IN HORSES. Photic head shaking in horses is stimulated by exposure to light and is exacerbated by exercise. The onset of the condition is usually in the spring. Affected horses often seek a darkened area. The mechanism is proposed to be an optic trigeminal summation via the infraorbital or facial sensory branch of the trigeminal nerve, with nasal stimulation or, alternatively, some as yet unidentified damage to the peripheral maxillary branch of the trigeminal nerve. Some success has been reported following treatment with cyproheptadine (0.3 mg/kg bid), a histamine and serotonin blocking agent or with carbemazepine, a sodium channel blocking drug, or both. Attempts to control the signs have also included use of tinted contact lenses. Many cases do not respond to treatment.

Neuromuscular Diseases

TETANUS. Tetanus is a neuromuscular disease caused by the toxin of the bacterium *Clostridium tetani*. It is characterized by muscular rigidity and death from respiratory arrest or convulsions. Usually, isolated cases occur when wounds are contaminated with the bacterium. Signs usually appear 2 to 4 weeks from the time of the injury. Within the first 24 hours, horses may show signs of colic. Additional early signs may include stiffness or lameness in the infected limb. The signs then progress to generalized spasticity with extended head posture. The hypertonia is most evident in the extensor muscles, so that the characteristic posture resembles that of a sawhorse ("sawhorse stance"). The tail becomes elevated, and eventually the lips and ears are pulled back. The jaws are tightly shut. The rigidity can be worsened by auditory, ocular, or tactile stimulation. The mortality is high, and death is usually due to hypoxia from paralysis of the respiratory muscles. Survivors begin to improve after 2 weeks, but the disease may take a month to resolve and the signs may not disappear completely. A classic sign of the disease is called "haws"; it involves the flashing of the third eyelid due to retraction of the eye that can be induced by sudden noises or sudden movement or contact such as a menacing gesture or a sharp blow to the lower jaw or neck.

BOTULISM (SHAKER FOAL OR FORAGE POISONING). Botulism is a neuromuscular disease caused by the toxin of the bacterium *Clostridium botulinum*. Most commonly, the disease develops in adults through direct ingestion of the toxin, and in foals through ingestion of the spores or by contamination of wounds, as with tetanus. Signs of botulism are generalized muscle tremors and progressive weakness that can lead to recumbency. The animals remain bright and alert. Constipation and ileus are consistent signs that may cause colic. Dysphagia is common, and a characteristic sign is weakness of the tongue, which often appears relatively early. Death may occur from respiratory failure. In the case of recovery, the process is slow, requiring 10 to 14 days to resolve. Moderate mydriasis is an early sign of the disease and the pupillary light response may be sluggish. Ptosis has also been described.

EQUINE MOTOR NEURON DISEASE. Equine motor neuron disease is presumed to be an oxidative condition of horses deprived of adequate dietary vitamin E. Clinical signs include muscle weakness and fasciculations with prolonged recumbency. Ocular involvement is common, being identified in 40 of 42 horses in one report. The fundic changes notes consisted of a dense mosaic of brown to black discoloration in lesions that were either widespread or found primarily in the transitional zone from tapetal to nontapetal fundus. Electroretinographic recordings showed a dramatic reduction in response to light stimulation, though behavioral visual defects are inconsistent.

Neoplastic Diseases

LYMPHOMA (LYMPHOSARCOMA). Lymphoma is a sporadic but relatively common neoplasm in horses of all ages. Many organs can be involved. Leukemia is rare, although anemia is relatively common. The anemia may be due to bone marrow suppression or infiltration and therefore may be nonregenerative. Alternatively, blood loss may be the cause of the anemia or immune-mediated hemolysis may occur, particularly in the alimentary form of the disease. Lymphoma can affect horses of all ages, although the alimentary type appears to be more common in younger horses. Clinical signs include depression, weight loss, and lymphadenopathy. There may also be fever, respiratory distress, neurologic disease, mild colic, diarrhea, or ventral edema, depending on the tissues involved. Lymphadenopathy may be generalized or may involve only a few regional lymph nodes that may be internal, as occurs with the alimentary form. Splenic enlargement may be palpated rectally.

Rebhun and Del Piero (1998) describe involvement of the eye in 21 of 79 horses with lymphosarcoma seen over a 20-year period at the New York State College of Veterinary Medicine. The most common ocular manifestation was infiltration of the eyelids and palpebral conjunctivae (11 horses). Consistent findings included conjunctival thickening, hyperemia, and edema causing chemosis easily seen from a distance (Figure 18-25). Persistent serous or mucopurulent ocular discharge was observed

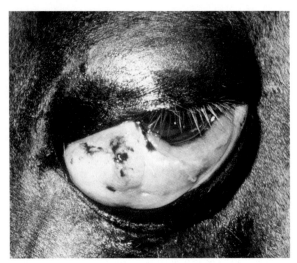

Figure 18-25. Orbital lymphoma with involvement of the bulbar and palpebral conjunctiva. (Courtesy David J. Maggs.)

in all 11 horses. Two horses had lesions limited to the third eyelid. Two horses had unilateral exophthalmos caused by diffuse orbital infiltration of lymphosarcoma, and two horses had corneoscleral masses.

Malignant lymphoma frequently also invades the uvea and induces anterior uveitis (four horses in the 1998 study). Uveitis causes corneal edema, thickening of the iris, miosis, aqueous flare, and possible intraocular hemorrhage. Intraocular pressure usually decreases but may rise if glaucoma develops. If the vitreous is invaded by neoplastic cells, hemorrhage and retinal detachment can occur, thus leading to blindness. If the conjunctivae are invaded, then conjunctival ulceration can be seen. One would expect to find pale mucous membranes or petechiae in these cases because anemia and thrombocytopenia are common findings in horses with lymphoma in general (multicentric lymphoma, intestinal or thoracic).

Neonatal Diseases

ACQUIRED ENTROPION. Entropion may be congenital or acquired in the neonate. Acquired entropion occurs with prematurity (see following section), with dehydration and the lack of periorbital fat, and with conditions associated with various disease processes, such as sepsis. Entropion leads to mechanical corneal abrasions or ulcers (Figure 18-26), which in turn cause conjunctivitis, lacrimation, and corneal edema.

PREMATURITY. Prematurity is a condition in which small or immature-appearing foals are born. A common definition is a foal born before 320 days of gestation. Signs of prematurity are small body size, short and silky haircoat, increased range of motion of joints, and immature skeletal ossification. Problems typical of premature foals include musculoskeletal problems, failure of passive transfer (see following section), and pulmonary dysfunction. Pulmonary dysfunction may be due to lung immaturity, as a primary or secondary surfactant deficiency. Retinal hemorrhages can be observed in hypoxic foals. Acquired entropion also occurs in premature foals (see Figure 18-26).

SEPSIS AND FAILURE OF PASSIVE TRANSFER. Bacterial infections are an important cause of morbidity and mortality in neonates. Infections may be acquired prenatally through the placenta, from the mare's genital tract, or from the environment

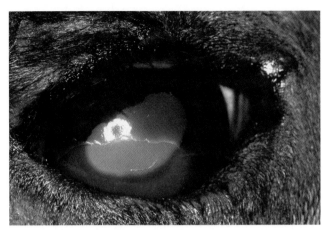

Figure 18-26. A 3-day-old Westphalian foal. Dehydration caused enophthalmia, which led to entropion of the lower eyelid. Mechanical abrasion by the inverted eyelid caused a corneal ulcer seen here stained with fluorescein. (Courtesy Paul E. Miller.)

after birth. Infections most commonly involve gram-negative organisms normally present in the genital tract, skin, or environment. *E. coli* is most commonly isolated. There seems to be a trend recently, however, to more gram-positive isolates, such as *Streptococcus, Staphylococcus, Enterococcus,* and *Clostridium* spp. Portals of entry include the respiratory and gastrointestinal tracts and the umbilicus. Failure of passive transfer of immunoglobulins is assumed to be the predisposing cause of sepsis in foals. The infection leads to septicemia, which precipitates multiple organ failure. Later, the infection localizes in various organs, causing acute sepsis. Organs such as the lung, bones, joints, CNS, gastrointestinal system, and eyes are involved. Decreased pulmonary perfusion with sepsis can lead to dyspnea, or alternatively secondary pneumonia may develop either hematogenously or because of milk aspiration due to weak suckle reflex. Infections acquired in utero can also lead to pneumonia, which can result in hypoxia. Retinal hemorrhages can be observed in hypoxic foals.

Sepsis may cause anterior uveitis (Figure 18-27), which may be due to bacterial infection in the eye or to a sterile immunologic reaction. When due to bacterial infection, vitreous abscesses may develop. Ocular signs of anterior uveitis include

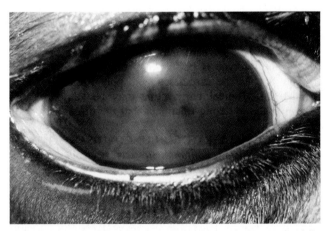

Figure 18-27. Anterior uveitis after septicemia in a foal. Note the diffuse corneal edema, the fibrin in the anterior chamber, and the miotic pupil. The large amount of fibrin in the anterior chamber is very indicative of foal septicemia. (Courtesy David J. Maggs.)

corneal edema, iris congestion, hypototony, miosis, aqueous flare with fibrin deposition, hypopyon or hyphema, and, in severe cases, panophthalmitis may be seen. Chorioretinitis, retinal detachment, blindness, and neuroophthalmologic signs due to CNS involvement may also occur.

NEONATAL MALADJUSTMENT SYNDROME. Neonatal maladjustment syndrome (NMS) is a noninfectious CNS disorder of newborn foals of normal gestational age. Synonyms for the condition include "perinatal asphyxia syndrome," "barkers," "dummies," and "wanderers." The time of onset of signs varies from immediately at birth to around 24 hours of age. Affected foals primarily have signs of cerebral dysfunction or spinal cord deficits or both. Cerebral signs include loss of suckle reflex, aimless wandering, hyperexcitability or depression, extensor spasms or clonic convulsions, excessive chewing and salivation, abnormal vocalization, abnormal respiratory patterns, and apparent central blindness. Spinal cord signs include limb weakness, ataxia, and depressed spinal reflexes. The etiology is unknown, but birth asphyxia has been proposed. Many foals diagnosed as having neonatal maladjustment syndrome make a complete recovery with no residual neurologic deficits. The prognosis is less optimistic if sepsis occurs concomitantly, or if the signs began with birth or with dystocia, or if there is a history of asphyxia.

Complete or partial blindness may be seen in neonatal maladjustment syndrome. Subconjunctival hemorrhage, anisocoria, retinal hemorrhages, and papilledema have also been reported. As with adults, however, secondary ocular findings in cases of CNS disease include keratoconjunctivitis and corneal ulcers due to trauma during recumbency and entropion, which may be caused by spasm from corneal pain but commonly results from dehydration (see Figure 18-26).

Pulmonary lesions may develop secondary to neonatal maladjustment syndrome due to sepsis or aspiration pneumonia. If lung lesions lead to hypoxia, retinal hemorrhages can be observed.

NEONATAL ISOERYTHROLYSIS. Neonatal isoerythrolysis is characterized by the destruction of red blood cells in the circulation of a foal by alloantibodies of the mother absorbed by the foal from the mare's colostrum. Because the antibodies are not naturally occurring, the disease does not appear until the mare is sensitized either by exposure during a previous pregnancy or through blood transfusion, or transplacentally during the current pregnancy, which is rare. The foals are normal at birth, developing signs 24 to 36 hours after ingesting colostrum. Early signs are those of progressive lethargy and weakness. Mucous membranes may be pale initially, but icterus develops. Hemoglobinemia and hemoglobinuria may be seen. Breathing becomes difficult, and seizures may occur as the anemia becomes more severe.

The predominant ocular sign is icterus of the conjunctiva; together with icterus of other mucous membranes, it is considered the cardinal sign of neonatal isoerythrolysis. However, conjunctival, episcleral, and intraocular hemorrhage can also occur.

***Rhodococcus equi* INFECTION.** *Rhodococcus equi* (formerly *Corynebacterium equi*) is a pleomorphic gram-positive rod that is a normal inhabitant of soil and can be cultured from horse feces. It causes a pyogranulomatous pneumonia in foals aged 2 to 6 months that are living on endemic farms. Infection is apparently transmitted through aerosolization of the bacteria and entry via the respiratory tract. Because the organism can live and multiply in alveolar macrophages, prolonged treatment with appropriate antibiotics is required. Clinical signs of *R. equi* infection are similar to those of pneumonia from other causes: fever, mucopurulent nasal discharge, tachypnea, dyspnea, and abnormal lung sounds on auscultation. Joint effusion that may be sterile, diarrhea, peritonitis, subcutaneous abscessation, and septic osteomyelitis and arthritis can also occur. Ocular signs described include hyphema and fibrin in the anterior chamber due to uveitis. The organism was cultured from the eye of one foal, indicating that the uveitis may be septic and not simply immune-mediated, as is often seen with the joint effusion. When large amounts of fibrin are found in the anterior chamber (see Figure 18-27), intracameral tissue-plasminogen activator treatment may be considered to prevent posterior synechia or traction retinal detachment.

OCULAR MANIFESTATIONS OF SYSTEMIC DISEASES IN RUMINANTS (see Tables 18-21 to 18-32)

Infectious Diseases

Bacterial Diseases

LISTERIOSIS. Listeriosis is a bacterial disease of the brain caused by *Listeria monocytogenes*. Fever, anorexia, and depression are frequently observed. The organisms have a predilection for the brainstem, producing foci of necrosis and inflammation. The multiple neurologic signs include unilateral facial nerve paresis or paralysis, abducent nerve paralysis, trigeminal nerve motor paralysis, possible paresis or paralysis of the tongue, and pharyngeal paralysis. Signs of alterations in consciousness, circling, and paresis or paralysis of the limbs indicate that the lesion is confined to the CNS. Vestibular signs often accompany the lesion because of the involvement of vestibular nuclei in the medulla. Progression of the disease is associated with decreased consciousness, coma, and convulsions. CSF is often abnormal, with changes characteristic of nonsuppurative disease (despite the fact that this is a bacterial disease).

Ophthalmic signs include exposure keratitis (Figure 18-28) and, in chronic cases, KCS, anterior uveitis, and panophthalmitis. The disease may also cause lacrimation, photophobia, conjunctival hyperemia, and corneal edema. Neuroophthalmic signs are ptosis, medial strabismus, nystagmus, amaurosis, and blindness. Medial strabismus, together with other cranial nerve dysfunctions, strongly suggests listeriosis (see Chapter 16, Figure 16-16).

Other syndromes seen with *L. monocytogenes* are abortions and neonatal septicemia. No ocular signs have been associated with listerial abortion. Infected lambs may have spinal myelitis without brainstem disease. Some animals are depressed, and some not. Clinical signs include tetraparesis, tetraplegia, paraparesis, paraplegia, conscious proprioceptive deficits, and recumbency.

OVINE CHLAMYDIAL POLYARTHRITIS AND CONJUNCTIVITIS. *Chlamydophila psittaci* (formerly *Chlamydia psittaci*) causes lameness and swollen joints in lambs. It is associated with high fever as well as with respiratory and, occasionally, neurologic disease. High morbidity and mortality are common. Up to 85% of lambs may show polyarthritis with lameness, stiff gait, and pyrexia. Ocular signs associated with keratoconjunctivitis may be an accompanying feature. Epiphora, conjunctival hyperemia, follicular hyperplasia and conjunctivitis,

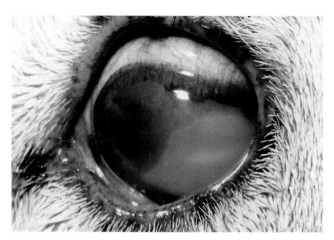

Figure 18-28. Corneal ulcer (stained with fluorescein) due to exposure keratitis in a sheep with listeriosis. The bacteria causes facial nerve paralysis, leading to this condition. Note the corneal edema and vascularization around the ulcer. (Courtesy David J. Maggs.)

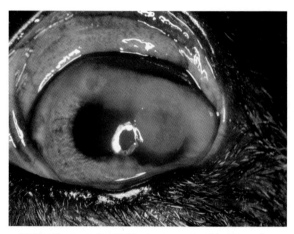

Figure 18-29. Keratoconjunctivitis in a goat with *Mycoplasma* spp. infection. Note the conjunctival congestion, severe vascular reaction, and diffuse stromal infiltration. (Courtesy University of Wisconsin–Madison Veterinary Ophthalmology Service Collection.)

keratitis with peripheral edema, especially dorsally, and neovascularization may be seen in association with the lameness and swollen joints. *C. psittaci* is also a major cause of abortion in sheep and goats. Usually abortion occurs from placentitis in the fourth or fifth month of gestation. The dam is rarely ill. Other animals in the herd may have pneumonia or arthritis, although the serotype is perhaps not the same. The abortion serotype may not be associated with polyarthritis or keratoconjunctivitis. Topical tetracycline may be administered in addition to the systemic treatment, but the disease is usually self-limiting.

MYCOPLASMAL KERATOCONJUNCTIVITIS IN GOATS AND SHEEP. *Mycoplasma conjunctivae* has been isolated from epidemics of keratoconjunctivitis, respiratory disease, and/or arthritis in goats and sheep (Figure 18-29). *Mycoplasma* and *Ureaplasma* have been isolated from cattle with conjunctivitis and mild respiratory signs. *Mycoplasma mycoides* var. *mycoides* has been isolated from an epidemic of mastitis, arthritis, and keratoconjunctivitis in goats. *Mycoplasma agalactiae* and *Mycoplasma arginini* have also been described as causing keratoconjunctivitis and systemic disease.

THROMBOEMBOLIC MENINGOENCEPHALITIS. Thrombo-embolic meningoencephalitis (TEME) in cattle is due to *Hemophilus somnus* infection. It occurs in feedlots of yearlings in North America, especially during early winter. The infection produces vasculitis with thrombosis. *H. somnus* also causes yearling calf pneumonia, vulvitis, vaginitis, endometritis, and abortion in cattle. Death may occur 36 hours after appearance of the first neurologic signs in cattle with TEME.

Clinical signs include pyrexia, holding of the head up and forward, stupor, opisthotonos, ataxia, weakness, and paralysis. Circling may also be present. The classic ophthalmic sign is retinal exudates with hemorrhages (retinitis) (Figure 18-30), although nystagmus, strabismus, and blindness may also occur.

In later stages of the disease, quadriplegia and cranial nerve deficits reflect focal brain lesions. CSF has a high protein content and neutrophilia but is usually sterile.

Thromboembolic meningoencephalitis may be tentatively diagnosed ophthalmoscopically.

Peracute deaths with neurologic and ophthalmoscopic signs are suggestive of thromboembolic meningoencephalitis. The diagnosis is confirmed by the histologic lesions. A vaccine is available. Early treatment before recumbency may be implemented, but residual joint and neurologic disease may limit long-term growth and performance.

***Mannheimia (Pasteurella)* PNEUMONIA.** Severe *Mannheimia (Pasteurella) haemolytica* pneumonia in calves may cause conjunctivitis resulting in a mucopurulent discharge. The disease also affects sheep and goats. Topical antibiotics may be indicated for treatment of the conjunctivitis.

TUBERCULOSIS. *Mycobacterium bovis* is the most common cause of tuberculosis in cattle and goats. Sheep are relatively resistant. Clinical signs are often inapparent; however, weight loss, variable appetite, and fluctuating fever may occur. Signs related to the respiratory system are relatively common, but gastrointestinal signs and reproductive disorders may also be seen. Granulomatous lesions in the eyes of cattle have been reported. The uvea is initially affected in both the anterior and posterior sections. Keratitis, anterior uveitis, chorioretinitis, and retinal detachment may be seen.

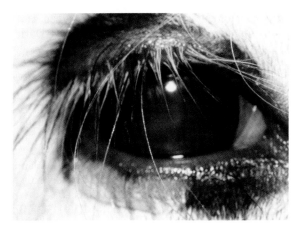

Figure 18-31. Anterior uveitis in a calf with septicemia. Note the diffuse corneal edema and miotic pupil. (Courtesy David J. Maggs.)

SEPTICEMIA. Septicemia is the most common cause of uveitis in calves. Ophthalmic signs include conjunctival and ciliary injection, miosis, iris congestion, hypotony, and fibrin or hypopyon in one or both eyes (Figure 18-31). Chorioretinitis may also occur, and panophthalmitis has been described in severe cases. Typical embolic lesions of multifocal hemorrhages, exudates, and focal retinal detachments (see Figure 18-30) may also be present but may not be observed owing to the changes in the anterior chamber. Uveitis associated with septicemia is less common in adult cattle than in calves but does occur. Adult cattle are susceptible to septic mastitis, septic metritis, peritonitis, and endocarditis. Therapy should include treatment of the uveitis. Septicemia may also result in chorioretinitis. Funduscopically, the lesions appear as focal or multifocal exudative lesions, often perivascular (see Chapter 15, Figure 15-50, *A*). Inactive retinal lesions from prior septicemia may be observed as hyperreflective areas in the tapetal region and depigmented gray areas in the nontapetal region of the retina. The scarred lesions in the tapetum may be hyperpigmented centrally. In most cases the lesions do not cause blindness. In overwhelming septicemia, thrombocytopenia can occur from the excessive consumption of platelets, which can lead to disseminated intravascular coagulation. In this situation, conjunctival hemorrhages may be seen as petechiae or ecchymoses.

Viral Diseases

ARTHROGRYPOSIS-HYDRENCEPHALY. Akabane virus is known to cause arthrogryposis (permanent joint contracture) and hydrencephaly (replacement of missing cerebral tissue) in sheep. Calves born to affected cows show arthrogryposis and hydranencephaly as well. These conditions frequently cause dystocia at birth. Those surviving can be blind and mentally deranged. Ocular lesions include attenuation of retinal vessels, tapetal hyperreflectivity, pigmentary changes, and optic atrophy. Diagnosis is confirmed by a rising titer to the virus in serum.

BLUETONGUE. Bluetongue is an arthropod-borne viral disease that infects ruminants. Clinical signs are most commonly seen in sheep, but cattle and goats occasionally show signs of the disease. Bluetongue causes a vasculitis and may cause a reproductive syndrome leading to abortion, embryonic death, and fetal anomalies. Vaccination of pregnant ewes with

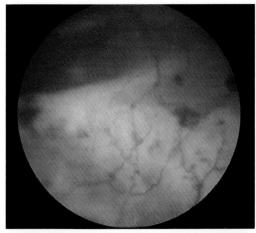

Figure 18-30. Retinal detachment and multifocal hemorrhages, characteristic of retinitis, in a cow with thromboembolic meningoencephalitis. (Courtesy Drs. G.A. Severin and Julie Gionfriddo, Colorado State University.)

attenuated bluetongue virus in the first half of pregnancy leads to necrotizing retinopathy and CNS malformations. During the last half of pregnancy the fetus is resistant.

Ewes should not be vaccinated for bluetongue in the first half of pregnancy.

In cattle infection is usually asymptomatic, although severe conjunctivitis with serous or mucopurulent discharge may be seen, particularly in chronically infected animals. Systemic signs include mucosal lesions, edema of the lips, and laminitis. Infection of a pregnant cow can lead to hydranencephaly in the fetus, abortion, arthrogryposis, and other defects.

INFECTIOUS BOVINE RHINOTRACHEITIS. Bovine herpesvirus 1 infections occur in four forms—the *conjunctival form,* in which no other signs are present, and the more common *respiratory form,* often referred to as infectious bovine rhinotracheitis or rednose. In this form, conjunctivitis is sometimes absent. *Infectious pustular vulvovaginitis* and an *abortive* form also occur, depending on the strain of virus. In the conjunctival and respiratory forms conjunctivitis is acute, erythematous, and serous with profuse lacrimation. White plaques may be present on the conjunctiva (Figure 18-32). Chemosis is sometimes present, but corneal lesions are rare. In the respiratory form, anorexia, fever, hyperemia of the nasal mucosa, nasal discharge, and salivation occur. In the *early* acute stages, ocular lesions can be distinguished from those of infectious bovine keratoconjunctivitis (pink eye) by the *lack of corneal involvement.* In later stages, nonulcerative keratitis with corneal vascularization and opacity, spreading toward the center of the cornea, may occur.

Early infectious bovine rhinotracheitis is distinguished from infectious bovine keratoconjunctivitis by lack of corneal involvement.

Goats are also susceptible to infectious bovine keratoconjunctivitis. Ocular signs include conjunctivitis and keratitis, which occur after onset of respiratory illness. Infectious bovine keratoconjunctivitis virus has been isolated from ocular and nasal discharge in goats.

MALIGNANT CATARRHAL FEVER. Malignant catarrhal fever, also known as bovine malignant catarrh, is a highly fatal viral disease of cattle that may cause sporadic outbreaks or epizootics. The disease in cattle is caused by a herpesvirus, and the sheep disease may be caused by a sheep herpesvirus. Ocular lesions are seen in the "head and eye" form of the disease, although four other syndromes have been described. The catarrhal inflammation of upper respiratory and alimentary mucous membranes aids in differentiating the disease from other fulminating bovine viral diseases. Keratoconjunctival exanthema and lymph node enlargement also occur. Ocular lesions distinguish malignant catarrhal fever from mucosal disease, rinderpest, muzzle disease, and infectious stomatitis.

The corneal lesions of malignant catarrhal fever start at the limbus and progress toward the center of the cornea, distinguishing them from infectious bovine keratoconjunctivitis, which usually begins in the center of the cornea. In addition to the classic corneal lesions, severe bilateral uveitis and panophthalmitis occur (Figure 18-33) together with the high fever (40.5° to 42° C), depression, and mucosal erosions. The disease is almost always fatal over 24 to 96 hours. Ocular manifestations include severe bilateral uveitis, leading to ciliary injection, corneal edema, hypotony, miosis, iris congestion, and fibrin or hypopyon in the anterior chamber (see Figure 18-33). The choroid is usually spared, but retinal vasculitis is often present and blindness is possible. It is difficult to observe the retinal lesions in the living animal because of the lesions in the anterior segment. Histopathologic examination shows severe vasculitis in all major organs and all parts of the eye except the choroid.

BOVINE VIRAL DIARRHEA. Bovine viral diarrhea virus is a pestivirus RNA virus of the Flaviviridae family. It causes a widespread contagious viral disease of cattle, sheep, goats, and wild ruminants, occurring in *mild, acute,* and *chronic* forms. In its mucosal disease syndrome it causes diarrhea outbreaks and can be a fatal disease in persistently infected cattle from in utero exposure. A hemorrhagic syndrome is characterized by marked thrombocytopenia, bloody diarrhea, epistaxis, hemorrhages on mucosal surfaces such as the conjunctiva, hyphema, bleeding from injection sites, pyrexia, leukopenia, and death. This syndrome is associated only with the noncytopathic isolate of bovine viral diarrhea virus. Bovine viral diarrhea also

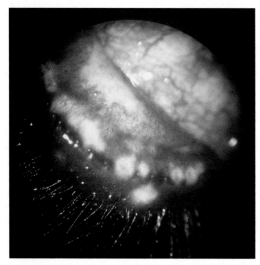

Figure 18-32. Severe conjunctivitis in a cow with infectious bovine rhinotracheitis. Note the white plaques that characterize the conjunctival form of the disease. (Courtesy Cecil Moore.)

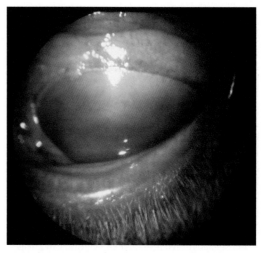

Figure 18-33. Anterior uveitis, with severe corneal edema, in a cow with malignant catarrhal fever. (Courtesy Cecil Moore.)

plays a role in the respiratory disease complex, together with *M. haemolytica* and viruses such as bovine herpesvirus 1 (BHV-1) and bovine respiratory syncytial virus (BRSV), by virtue of the immunosuppressive effects it produces. It has also been implicated in hydranencephaly, abortion and early embryonic death, and fetal anomalies.

Bovine viral diarrhea causes corneal opacity in adult cattle. Exposure of the fetus to the virus causes cataract, retinal atrophy, optic neuritis, microphthalmia with retinal dysplasia, and cerebellar hypoplasia. A gray optic disc due to optic atrophy, vascular attenuation, tapetal hyperreflectivity, pigment clumping, and multifocal depigmentation of the nontapetal fundus characterize the funduscopic lesions. Calves with ocular signs may be blind, with or without pupillary light response, and there may be ocular discharge in acute or chronic cases.

MAEDI-VISNA. Maedi-visna is a chronic progressive encephalitis of sheep caused by a retrovirus (subfamily Lentivirinae). Nervous system signs of the disease are characteristic of diffuse encephalitis. They include ataxia, twitching of the facial muscles, conscious proprioceptive deficits, staggering or stumbling when turned, circling, and blindness. PCR analysis, immunohistochemistry, and in situ PCR examination have been used to detect the virus in third eyelids of infected sheep with typical maedi-visna pulmonary lesions.

SCRAPIE. Scrapie is a transmissible form of spongiform encephalopathy that causes degenerative CNS disease in sheep and, less commonly, goats. The disease occurs in animals 1 to 5 years old. It has a slow clinical course. Nervousness, restlessness, weight loss, and pruritus have been described. In both sheep and goats scrapie causes multifocal, round retinal detachments in the tapetal fundus owing to accumulations of subretinal fluid. Finding of these lesions in association with chronic neurologic signs suggests a diagnosis of scrapie.

Protozoal Diseases

BABESIOSIS. As mentioned in the section on horses, babesiosis is a tick-borne intraerythrocytic disease. The acute disease is characterized by fever, hemolytic anemia, icterus, hemoglobinuria, and death. At least six species of *Babesia* infect cattle, and two infect sheep and goats. Cerebral babesiosis, characterized by hyperexcitability, convulsions opisthotonos, coma, and death, may be observed in cattle, particularly those infected with *Babesia bovis*. Babesiosis due to *Babesia* spp. also causes conjunctival injection and icterus in affected cattle. The signs resolve with treatment of the systemic disease. *Trypanosoma brucei* causes keratoconjunctivitis, uveitis, and optic neuritis in sheep. Other *Trypanosoma* spp. cause edema, hyperemia and petechiation of the conjunctiva in ruminants.

***Toxoplasma gondii* INFECTION.** The ubiquitous protozoan. *T. gondii* is a major abortifacient in sheep and goats. It rarely causes disease in ruminants, and infection with the protozoan is often asymptomatic. Ocular signs are rare, but *T. gondii* may infiltrate the retina and uvea, causing retinitis and chorioretinitis due to a primary posterior segment lesion. Anterior uveitis may also be present.

Parasitic Diseases

COENUROSIS. Coenurosis, also known as gid and sturdy, is a disease caused by invasion of the ovine brain by intermediate stages of *Taenia multiceps* and *Taenia serialis*. The disease is

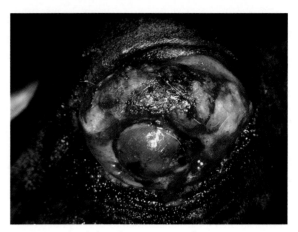

Figure 18-34. Orbital lymphosarcoma, with extensive conjunctival involvement, in a cow. The tumor also caused exposure keratitis and corneal desiccation. (Courtesy Paul E. Miller.)

most commonly seen in sheep but can occur in cattle and goats as well. The initial clinical signs include frenzy, convulsions and salivation. They are followed by dullness, head pressing, head deviation, and circling as well as by ophthalmic manifestations, including papilledema and blindness.

Neoplasia

LYMPHOSARCOMA. Lymphosarcoma should be suspected in a cow with exophthalmos, because the tumor may involve the retrobulbar lymphoid tissue. Unilateral presentation is most common. In the absence of other enlarged lymph nodes or other areas of lymphocytic infiltration, differential diagnoses include orbital cellulitis, orbital trauma, retrobulbar hemorrhage, and chronic sinusitis with orbital extension. The cornea on the affected side can be expected to undergo rapid desiccation and ulceration (Figure 18-34). A syndrome consisting of solid infiltration of the conjunctiva is also observed and must be distinguished from chemosis. Affected animals are sent to slaughter.

Metabolic Diseases

POLIOENCEPHALOMALACIA (PEM). Polioencephalomalacia, also called cerebrocortical necrosis, occurs in pigs, sheep, and cattle and may be related to thiamine deficiency. Lambs between 2 and 4 months of age and 6-month-old calves are most commonly affected. Polioencephalomalacia occurs at pasture and in feedlots.

The initial ocular sign in sheep is trochlear nerve paralysis, which causes dorsomedial strabismus. Initial clinical signs in sheep include head pressing, aimless wandering or motionless standing, and cortical blindness. These initial signs progress to recumbency, opisthotonus, hyperesthesia, tonic-clonic convulsions, and nystagmus.

Initial clinical signs in cattle include cortical blindness, muscle tremor (head especially), salivation, opisthotonus, convulsions, head pressing, depression, and anorexia. These signs are followed by recumbency, nystagmus, and papilledema.

Blindness is often the first sign to appear and the last to resolve and may be the only sign, other than depression, in adult cattle. It may take up to one week after the resolution of the other signs for vision to return. Despite the fact that the blindness is central, papilledema and decreased pupillary light reflexes may occur and bilateral dorsomedial strabismus may be present.

Toxic Diseases

TOXIC PLANTS. Various toxic plants have been described as causing ocular lesions. Among them are the following:

- Male fern (*Dryopteris* spp.), which causes blindness due to optic nerve atrophy
- Bracken fern, which can cause conjunctival hemorrhages and outer retinal degeneration
- *Helichrysum argyrosphaerum*, causing blindness with retinal lesions in sheep and cattle
- *Veratrum* in sheep, which leads to cyclopia or anophthalmia in lambs when the ewes ingest the plant during pregnancy
- Locoweed, causing blindness with various intraocular, histopathologic changes
- Many plants that cause liver damage, which manifests as jaundice of the conjunctiva and sclera

VETCH TOXICITY. Vetch (*Vicia* spp.) poisoning has been reported in cattle. The following three clinical manifestations have been described:

- An acute neurologic manifestation
- A fatal form leading to death in 12 to 15 days and causing signs of weakness and loss of appetite, alopecia, subcutaneous swellings, herpetiform eruptions of the oral mucous membranes, purulent nasal discharge, abnormal lung sounds, cough, and cyanosis of mucous membranes
- A systemic granulomatous disease, causing dermatitis, pruritus, diarrhea, dehydration, weight loss, decreased milk yield, cough, dyspnea, and conjunctivitis

A study of 10 cows with high suspicion of vetch toxicity reported moderate ocular and nasal discharge, which was usually serous but in some cases mucopurulent, in 7 animals. These researchers did not mention necropsy findings of ocular changes; however, ocular lesions in other species with vetch toxicity include conjunctivitis, ulcerative keratitis, and diffuse granulomatous inflammation of the choroid.

BIBLIOGRAPHY

Ocular Manifestations of Systemic Disease in Dogs and Cats
Canine Distemper
Gilger BC (2000): Ocular manifestations of systemic infectious diseases, in Bonagura JD (editor): Kirk's Current Veterinary Therapy XIII: Small Animal Practice, 13th ed. Saunders, Philadelphia, p. 276.
Greene CE, Appel MJ (2006): Canine distemper, in Greene CE (editor): Infectious Diseases of the Dog and Cat, 3rd ed. Saunders, St. Louis, p. 25.
Koutinas AF, et al. (2002): Relation of clinical signs to pathological changes in 19 cases of canine distemper encephalomyelitis. J Comp Pathol 126:47.
Raw ME, et al. (1992): Canine distemper infection associated with acute nervous signs in dogs. Vet Rec 130:291.
Sellon RK (2005): Canine viral disease, in Ettinger SJ, Feldman EC (editors): Textbook of Veterinary Internal Medicine, 6th ed. Saunders, St. Louis, p. 646.
Stiles J (2006): Ocular infections, in Greene CE (editor): Infectious Diseases of the Dog and Cat, 3rd ed. Saunders, St. Louis, p. 974.
Tipold A (1995): Diagnosis of inflammatory and infectious diseases of the central nervous systemic dogs: a retrospective study. J Vet Intern Med 9:304.

Willis AM (2000): Canine viral infections. Vet Clin North Am Small Anim Pract 30:1119.

Infectious Canine Hepatitis
Gilger BC (2000): Ocular manifestations of systemic infectious diseases, in Bonagura JD (editor): Kirk's Current Veterinary Therapy XIII: Small Animal Practice, 13th ed. Saunders, Philadelphia, p. 276.
Greene CE (2006): Infectious canine hepatitis and canine acidophil cell hepatitis, in Greene CE (editor): Infectious Diseases of the Dog and Cat, 3rd ed. Saunders, St. Louis, p. 41.
Sellon RK (2005): Canine viral disease, in Ettinger SJ, Feldman EC (editors): Textbook of Veterinary Internal Medicine, 6th ed. Saunders, St. Louis, p. 646.
Stiles J (2006): Ocular infections, in Greene CE (editor): Infectious Diseases of the Dog and Cat, 3rd ed. Saunders, St. Louis, p. 974.
Willis AM (2000): Canine viral infections. Vet Clin North Am Small Anim Pract 30:1119.

Feline Herpesvirus (Feline Rhinotracheitis Virus, FHV-1, FRV) Infection
Gaskell RM, Dawson S (2005): Other feline viral diseases, in Ettinger SJ, Feldman EC (editors): Textbook of Veterinary Internal Medicine, 6th ed. Saunders, St. Louis, p. 667.
Gaskell R, et al. (2006): Feline respiratory disease, in Greene CE (editor): Infectious Diseases of the Dog and Cat, 3rd ed. Saunders, St. Louis, p. 145.
Gilger BC (2000): Ocular manifestations of systemic infectious diseases, in Bonagura JD (editor): Kirk's Current Veterinary Therapy XIII: Small Animal Practice, 13th ed. Saunders, Philadelphia, p. 276.
Lappin MR, et al. (2002): Use of serologic tests to predict resistance to feline herpesvirus 1, feline calicivirus, and feline parvovirus infection in cats. J Am Vet Med Assoc 220:38.
Nasisse MP, et al. (1993): Clinical and laboratory findings in chronic conjunctivitis in cats: 91 cases (1983-1991). J Am Vet Med Assoc 203:834.
Stiles J (2006): Ocular infections, in Greene CE (editor): Infectious Diseases of the Dog and Cat, 3rd ed. Saunders, St. Louis, p. 974.
Stiles J (2003): Feline herpesvirus. Clin Tech Small Anim Pract 18:178.
Stiles J (1995): Treatment of cats with ocular disease attributable to herpesvirus infection: 17 cases (1983-1993). J Am Vet Med Assoc 207:599.
Stiles J, et al. (1997): Comparison of nested polymerase chain reaction, virus isolation, and fluorescent antibody testing for identifying feline herpesvirus in cats with conjunctivitis. Am J Vet Res 58:804.

Feline Calicivirus Infection
Dawson S, et al. (1994): Acute arthritis of cats associated with feline calicivirus infection. Res Vet Sci 56:133.
Gaskell R, et al. (2006): Feline respiratory disease, in Greene CE (editor): Infectious Diseases of the Dog and Cat, 3rd ed. Saunders, St. Louis, p. 145.
Gaskell RM, Dawson S (2005): Other feline viral diseases, in Ettinger SJ, Feldman EC (editors): Textbook of Veterinary Internal Medicine, 6th ed. Saunders, St. Louis, p. 667.
Hurley KF, Sykes JE (2003): Update on feline calicivirus: new trends. Vet Clin North Am Small Anim Pract 2003 33:759.
Knowles JO, et al. (1991): Studies on the role of feline calicivirus in chronic stomatitis in cats. Vet Microbiol 27:205.
Radford AD, et al. (2007): Feline calicivirus. Vet Res 38:319.
Ramsey DT (2000): Feline chlamydia and calicivirus infections. Vet Clin North Am Small Anim Pract 30:1015.
Stiles J (2006): Ocular infections, in Greene CE (editor): Infectious Diseases of the Dog and Cat, 3rd ed. Saunders, St. Louis, p. 974.
Sykes JE, et al. (1998): Detection and strain differentiation of feline calicivirus in conjunctival swabs by RT-PCR of the hypervariable region of the capsid protein gene. Arch Virol 143:1321.

Feline Leukemia Virus Infection
Arjona A, et al. (2000): Seroepidemiological survey of infection by feline leukemia virus and immunodeficiency virus in Madrid and correlation with some clinical aspects. J Clin Microbiol 38:3448.
Gilger BC (2000): Ocular manifestations of systemic infectious diseases, in Bonagura JD (editor): Kirk's Current Veterinary Therapy XIII: Small Animal Practice, 13th ed. Saunders, Philadelphia, p. 276.
Hartmann K (2006): Feline leukemia virus infection, in Greene CE (editor): Infectious Diseases of the Dog and Cat, 3rd ed. Saunders, St. Louis, p. 105.
Lappin MR (1995): Opportunistic infections associated with retroviral infections in cats. Semin Vet Med Surg (Small Anim) 10:244.
Levy JK, Crawford PC (2005): Feline leukemia virus, in Ettinger SJ, Feldman EC (editors): Textbook of Veterinary Internal Medicine, 6th ed. Saunders, St. Louis, p. 653.

Stiles J (2006): Ocular infections, in Greene CE (editor): Infectious Diseases of the Dog and Cat, 3rd ed. Saunders, St. Louis, p. 974.

Vail DM, et al. (1998): Feline lymphoma (145 cases): proliferation indices, cluster of differentiation 3 immunoreactivity, and their association with prognosis in 90 cats. J Vet Intern Med 12:349.

Willis AM (2000): Feline leukemia virus and feline immunodeficiency virus. Vet Clin North Am Small Anim Pract 30:971.

Feline Immunodeficiency Virus Infection

Arjona A, et al. (2000): Seroepidemiological survey of infection by feline leukemia virus and immunodeficiency virus in Madrid and correlation with some clinical aspects. J Clin Microbiol 38:3448.

Beatty JA, et al. (1998): Feline immunodeficiency virus (FIV)-associated lymphoma: a potential role for immune dysfunction in tumourigenesis. Vet Immunol Immunopathol 65:309.

Gilger BC (2000): Ocular manifestations of systemic infectious diseases, in Bonagura JD (editor): Kirk's Current Veterinary Therapy XIII: Small Animal Practice, 13th ed. Saunders, Philadelphia, p. 276.

Hartmann K (2005): Feline immunodeficiency virus infection and related diseases, in Ettinger SJ, Feldman EC (editors): Textbook of Veterinary Internal Medicine, 6th ed. Saunders, St. Louis, p. 659.

Hartmann K (1998): Feline immunodeficiency virus infection: an overview. Vet J 155:123.

Lappin MR, et al. (1996): Primary and secondary *Toxoplasma gondii* infection in normal and feline immunodeficiency virus-infected cats. J Parasitol 82:733.

Lappin MR, et al. (1992): Serologic prevalence of selected infectious diseases in cats with uveitis. J Am Vet Med Assoc 201:1005.

Malik R, et al. (1997): Prevalences of feline leukaemia virus and feline immunodeficiency virus infections in cats in Sydney. Aust Vet J 75:323.

Nasisse MP, et al. (1993): Clinical and laboratory findings in chronic conjunctivitis in cats: 91 cases (1983-1991). J Am Vet Med Assoc 203:834.

Sellon RK, Hartmann K (2006): Feline immunodeficiency virus infection, in Greene CE (editor): Infectious Diseases of the Dog and Cat, 3rd ed. Saunders, St. Louis, p. 131.

Stiles J (2006): Ocular infections, in Greene CE (editor): Infectious Diseases of the Dog and Cat, 3rd ed. Saunders, St. Louis, p. 974.

Willis AM (2000): Feline leukemia virus and feline immunodeficiency virus. Vet Clin North Am Small Anim Pract 30:971.

Feline Infectious Peritonitis Infection

Addie DD, et al. (1995): Risk of feline infectious peritonitis in cats naturally infected with feline coronavirus. Am J Vet Res 56:429.

Addie DD, Jarret O (2006): Feline coronavirus virus infection, in Greene CE (editor): Infectious Diseases of the Dog and Cat, 3rd ed. Saunders, St. Louis, p. 88.

Addie DD, Jarrett O (2001): Use of a reverse-transcriptase polymerase chain reaction for monitoring the shedding of feline coronavirus by healthy cats. Vet Rec 148:649.

Foley JE, et al. (1997): Patterns of feline coronavirus infection and fecal shedding from cats in multiple-cat environments. J Am Vet Med Assoc 210:1307.

Foley JE, et al. (1997): Risk factors for feline infectious peritonitis among cats in multiple-cat environments with endemic feline enteric coronavirus. J Am Vet Med Assoc 210:1313.

Gamble DA, et al. (1997): Development of a nested PCR assay for detection of feline infectious peritonitis virus in clinical specimens. J Clin Microbiol 35:673.

Gilger BC (2000): Ocular manifestations of systemic infectious diseases, in Bonagura JD (editor): Kirk's Current Veterinary Therapy XIII: Small Animal Practice, 13th ed. Saunders, Philadelphia, p. 276.

Legendre AM (2000): Diagnosis and prevention of feline infectious peritonitis, in Bonagura JD (editor): Kirk's Current Veterinary Therapy XIII: Small Animal Practice, 13th ed. Saunders, Philadelphia, p. 291.

Li X, Scott FW (1994): Detection of feline coronaviruses in cell cultures and in fresh and fixed feline tissues using polymerase chain reaction. Vet Microbiol 42:65.

Olsen CW (1993): A review of feline infectious peritonitis virus: molecular biology, immunopathogenesis, clinical aspects, and vaccination. Vet Microbiol 36:1.

Stiles J (2006): Ocular infections, in Greene CE (editor): Infectious Diseases of the Dog and Cat, 3rd ed. Saunders, St. Louis, p. 974.

Brucellosis (Dogs)

Carmichael LE, Greene CE (2006): Canine brucellosis, in Greene CE (editor): Infectious Diseases of the Dog and Cat, 3rd ed. Saunders, St. Louis, p. 369.

Carmichael LE, Shin SJ (1996): Canine brucellosis: a diagnostician's dilemma. Semin Vet Med Surg 11:161.

Dziezyc J (2000): Canine systemic bacterial infections. Vet Clin North Am Small Anim Pract 30:1103.

Hartmann K, Greene CE (2005): Diseases caused by systemic bacterial infections, in Ettinger SJ, Feldman EC (editors): Textbook of Veterinary Internal Medicine, 6th ed. Saunders, St. Louis, p. 616.

Hollett RB (2006): Canine brucellosis: outbreaks and compliance. Theriogenol 66:575.

Kerwin SC, et al. (1992): Diskospondylitis associated with *Brucella canis* infection in dogs: 14 cases (1980-1991). J Am Vet Med Assoc 1992 201:1253.

Mateu-de-Antonio EM, Martin M (1995): In vitro efficacy of several antimicrobial combinations against *Brucella canis* and *Brucella melitensis* strains isolated from dogs. Vet Microbiol 45:1.

Stiles J (2006): Ocular infections, in Greene CE (editor): Infectious Diseases of the Dog and Cat, 3rd ed. Saunders, Philadelphia, p. 974.

Vinayak A, et al. (2004):Clinical resolution of *Brucella canis*-induced ocular inflammation in a dog. J Am Vet Med Assoc 224:1804.

Borreliosis (Canine Lyme Disease)

Appel MJG, et al. (1995): Ocular CVT update: canine Lyme disease, in Bonagura JD (editor): Kirk's Current Veterinary Therapy XII: Small Animal Practice, 12th ed. Saunders, Philadelphia, p. 303.

Fritz CL, Kjemtrup AM (2003): Lyme borreliosis. J Am Vet Med Assoc 223:1261.

Hartmann K, Greene CE (2005): Diseases caused by systemic bacterial infections, in Ettinger SJ, Feldman EC (editors): Textbook of Veterinary Internal Medicine, 6th ed. Saunders, St. Louis, p. 616.

Littman MP (2003): Canine borreliosis. Vet Clin North Am Small Anim Pract 33:827.

Stiles J (2006): Ocular infections, in Greene CE (editor): Infectious Diseases of the Dog and Cat, 3rd ed. Saunders, St. Louis, p. 974.

Rocky Mountain Spotted Fever (Dogs) and Canine Monocytic Ehrlichiosis

Belanger M, et al. (2002): Comparison of serological detection methods for diagnosis of Ehrlichia canis infections in dogs. J Clin Microbiol 2002 40:3506.

Breitschwerdt EB (2005): Obligate intracellular bacterial pathogens, in Ettinger SJ, Feldman EC (editors): Textbook of Veterinary Internal Medicine, 6th ed. Saunders, St. Louis, p. 631.

Davidson MG, et al. (1990): Vascular permeability and coagulation during *Rickettsia rickettsii* infection in dogs. Am J Vet Res 51:165.

Gasser AM, et al. (2001): Canine Rocky Mountain spotted fever: a retrospective study of 30 cases. J Am Anim Hosp Assoc 37:41.

Gilger BC (2000): Ocular manifestations of systemic infectious diseases, in Bonagura JD (editor): Kirk's Current Veterinary Therapy XIII: Small Animal Practice, 13th ed. Saunders, Philadelphia, p. 276.

Gould DJ, et al. (2000): Canine monocytic ehrlichiosis presenting as acute blindness 36 months after importation into the UK. J Small Anim Pract 41:263-265.

Greene CE, Breitschwerdt EB (2006): Rocky Mountain spotted fever, Murine typhuslike disease, Rickettsialpox, Typhus, and Q fever, in Greene CE (editor): Infectious Diseases of the Dog and Cat, 3rd ed. Saunders, St. Louis, p. 232.

Greig B, et al. (2006): Canine granulocytotropic ehrlichiosis, in Greene CE (editor): Infectious Diseases of the Dog and Cat, 3rd ed. Saunders, St. Louis, p. 217.

Harrus S, et al. (1999): Recent advances in determining the pathogenesis of canine monocytic ehrlichiosis. J Clin Microbiol 37:2745.

Harrus S, et al. (1997): Canine monocytic ehrlichiosis: an update. Compend Contin Educ Pract Vet 19:431.

Harvey JW (2006): Thrombocytotropic anaplasmosis (A. platys [E. Platys] infection), in Greene CE (editor): Infectious Diseases of the Dog and Cat, 3rd ed. Saunders, St. Louis, p. 229.

Komnenou AA, et al. (2007): Ocular manifestations of natural canine monocytic ehrlichiosis (*Ehrlichia canis*): a retrospective study of 90 cases. Vet Ophthalmol 10:137.

Neer TM, et al. (2006): Canine monocytotropic ehrlichiosis and neorickettsiosis, in Greene CE (editor): Infectious Diseases of the Dog and Cat, 3rd ed. Saunders, St. Louis, p. 203.

Stiles J (2006): Ocular infections, in Greene CE (editor): Infectious Diseases of the Dog and Cat, 3rd ed. Saunders, St. Louis, p. 974.

Stiles J (2000): Canine rickettsial infections. Vet Clin North Am Small Anim Pract 30:1135.

Warner RD, Marsh WW (2002): Rocky Mountain spotted fever. J Am Vet Med Assoc 221:1413

Bartonellosis

Birtles RJ, et al. (2002): Prevalence of *Bartonella* species causing bacteraemia in domesticated and companion animals in the United Kingdom. Vet Rec 151:225.

Breitschwerdt EB, et al. (2003): The immunologic response of dogs to *Bartonella vinsonii* subspecies *berkhoffii* antigens: as assessed by Western immunoblot analysis. J Vet Diagn Invest 15:349.

Breitschwerdt EB, et al. (2006): Bartonellosis, in Greene CE (editor): Infectious Diseases of the Dog and Cat, 3rd ed. Saunders, St. Louis, p. 511.

Chomel BB, et al. (2001): Aortic valve endocarditis in a dog due to *Bartonella clarridgeiae*. J Clin Microbiol 39:3548.

Glaus T, et al. (1997): Seroprevalence of *Bartonella henselae* infection and correlation with disease status in cats in Switzerland. J Clin Microbiol 35:2883.

Guptill L (2003): Bartonellosis. Vet Clin North Am Small Anim Pract 33:809.

Guptill L, et al. (2004): Prevalence, risk factors, and genetic diversity of *Bartonella henselae* infections in pet cats in four regions of the United States. J Clin Microbiol 42:652-659.

Ketring KL, et al. (2004): *Bartonella*: a new etiological agent of feline ocular disease. J Am Anim Hosp Assoc 40:6.

Lappin MR, Black JC (1999): *Bartonella* spp. infection as a possible cause of uveitis in a cat. J Am Vet Med Assoc 214:1205.

Luria BJ, et al. (2004): Prevalence of infectious diseases in feral cats in Northern Florida. J Feline Med Surg 6:287.

Mexas AM, et al. (2002): *Bartonella henselae* and *Bartonella elizabethae* as potential canine pathogens. J Clin Microbiol 40:4670.

Powell CC, et al. (2002): Inoculation with *Bartonella henselae* followed by feline herpesvirus 1 fails to activate ocular toxoplasmosis in chronically infected cats. J Feline Med Surg 4:107.

Rolain JM, et al. (2004): Prevalence of *Bartonella clarridgeiae* and *Bartonella henselae* in domestic cats from France and detection of the organisms in erythrocytes by immunofluorescence. Clin Diagn Lab Immunol 11:423.

Solano-Gallego L, et al. (2004): *Bartonella henselae* IgG antibodies are prevalent in dogs from southeastern USA. Vet Res 35:585.

Chlamydiosis (Chlamydophilosis) (Cats)

Greene CE, Sikes JE (2006): Chlamydial infections, in Greene CE (editor): Infectious Diseases of the Dog and Cat, 3rd ed. Saunders, St. Louis, p. 245.

McDonald M, et al. (1998): A comparison of DNA amplification, isolation and serology for the detection of *Chlamydia psittaci* infection in cats. Vet Rec 143:97.

Nasisse MP, et al. (1993): Clinical and laboratory findings in chronic conjunctivitis in cats: 91 cases (1983-1991). J Am Vet Med Assoc 203:834.

Ramsey DT (2000): Feline chlamydia and calicivirus infections. Vet Clin North Am Small Anim Pract. 30:1015.

Sparkes AH, et al. (1999): The clinical efficacy of topical and systemic therapy for the treatment of feline ocular chlamydiosis. J Feline Med Surg 1:31.

Sykes JE, et al. (2001): Detection of feline calicivirus, feline herpesvirus 1 and *Chlamydia psittaci* mucosal swabs by multiplex RT-PCR/PCR. Vet Microbiol 81:95.

Sykes JE, et al. (1999): Comparison of the polymerase chain reaction and culture for the detection of feline *Chlamydia psittaci* in untreated and doxycycline-treated experimentally infected cats. J Vet Intern Med 13:146.

Sykes JE, et al. (1999): Prevalence of feline *Chlamydia psittaci* and feline herpesvirus 1 in cats with upper respiratory tract disease. J Vet Intern Med 13:153.

von Bomhard W, et al. (2003): Detection of novel chlamydiae in cats with ocular disease. Am J Vet Res 64:1421.

Mycoplasmosis (Cats)

Chalker VJ, et al. (2004): Development of a polymerase chain reaction for the detection of *Mycoplasma felis* in domestic cats. Vet Microbiol 100:77.

Chandler JC, et al. (2002): Mycoplasmal respiratory infections in small animals: 17 cases (1988-1999). J Am Anim Hosp Assoc 38:111.

Foster SF, et al. (2004): Lower respiratory tract infections in cats: 21 cases (1995-2000). J Feline Med Surg 6:167.

Foster SF, et al. (2004): A retrospective analysis of feline bronchoalveolar lavage cytology and microbiology (1995-2000). J Feline Med Surg 6:189.

Greene CE (2006): Mycoplasmal, ureaplasmal and L-forms infections, in Greene CE (editor): Infectious Diseases of the Dog and Cat, 3rd ed. Saunders, St. Louis, p. 260.

Rosendal S (1995): Mycoplasma infections of dogs and cats, in Bonagura JD (editor): Kirk's Current Veterinary Therapy XII: Small Animal Practice, 12th ed. Saunders, Philadelphia, p. 301.

Blastomycosis

Arceneaux KA, et al. (1998): Blastomycosis in dogs: 115 cases (1980-1995). J Am Vet Med Assoc 213:658.

Gilger BC (2000): Ocular manifestations of systemic infectious diseases, in Bonagura JD (editor): Kirk's Current Veterinary Therapy XIII: Small Animal Practice, 13th ed. Saunders, Philadelphia, p. 276.

Gionfriddo JR (2000): Feline systemic fungal infections. Vet Clin North Am Small Anim Pract 30:1029.

Hendrix DV, et al. (2004): Comparison of histologic lesions of endophthalmitis induced by *Blastomyces dermatitidis* in untreated and treated dogs: 36 cases (1986-2001). J Am Vet Med Assoc 224:1317.

Kerl ME (2003): Update on canine and feline fungal diseases. Vet Clin North Am Small Anim Pract 33:721.

Krohne SG (2000): Canine systemic fungal infections. Vet Clin North Am Small Anim Pract 30:1063.

Legendre AM (2006): Blastomycosis, in Greene CE (editor): Infectious Diseases of the Dog and Cat, 3rd ed. Saunders, St. Louis, p. 569.

Stiles J (2006): Ocular infections, in Greene CE (editor): Infectious Diseases of the Dog and Cat, 3rd ed. Saunders, St. Louis, p. 974.

Taboada J, Grooters AM (2005): Systemic mycosis, in Ettinger SJ, Feldman EC (editors): Textbook of Veterinary Internal Medicine, 6th ed. Saunders, St. Louis, p. 671.

Coccidioidomycosis

Davies C, Troy GC (1996): Deep mycotic infections in cats. J Am Anim Hosp Assoc 32:380.

Gilger BC (2000): Ocular manifestations of systemic infectious diseases, in Bonagura JD (editor): Kirk's Current Veterinary Therapy XIII: Small Animal Practice, 13th ed. Saunders, Philadelphia, p. 276.

Gionfriddo JR (2000): Feline systemic fungal infections. Vet Clin North Am Small Anim Pract 30:1029.

Greene RT (2006): Cocidioidomycosis and paracoccidioidomycosis, in Greene CE (editor): Infectious Diseases of the Dog and Cat, 3rd ed. Saunders, St. Louis, p. 598.

Greene RT, Troy GC (1995): Coccidioidomycosis in 48 cats: a retrospective study (1984-1993). J Vet Intern Med 9:86.

Johnson LR, et al. (2003): Clinical, clinicopathologic, and radiographic findings in dogs with coccidioidomycosis: 24 cases (1995-2000). J Am Vet Med Assoc 222:461.

Kerl ME (2003): Update on canine and feline fungal diseases. Vet Clin North Am Small Anim Pract 33:721.

Krohne SG (2000): Canine systemic fungal infections. Vet Clin North Am Small Anim Pract 30:1063.

Stiles J (2006): Ocular infections, in Greene CE (editor): Infectious Diseases of the Dog and Cat, 3rd ed. Saunders, St. Louis, p. 974.

Taboada J, Grooters AM (2005): Systemic mycosis, in Ettinger SJ, Feldman EC (editors): Textbook of Veterinary Internal Medicine, 6th ed. Saunders, St. Louis, p. 671.

Cryptococcosis

Gilger BC (2000): Ocular manifestations of systemic infectious diseases, in Bonagura JD (editor): Kirk's Current Veterinary Therapy XIII: Small Animal Practice, 13th ed. Saunders, Philadelphia, p. 276.

Gionfriddo JR (2000): Feline systemic fungal infections. Vet Clin North Am Small Anim Pract 30:1029.

Kerl ME (2003): Update on canine and feline fungal diseases. Vet Clin North Am Small Anim Pract 33:721.

Krohne SG (2000): Canine systemic fungal infections. Vet Clin North Am Small Anim Pract 30:1063.

Lester SJ, et al. (2004): Clinicopathologic features of an unusual outbreak of cryptococcosis in dogs, cats, ferrets, and a bird: 38 cases (January to July 2003). J Am Vet Med Assoc 225:1716.

Malik R, et al. (2006): Cryptococcosis, in Greene CE (editor): Infectious Diseases of the Dog and Cat, 3rd ed. Saunders, St. Louis, p. 584.

Malik R, et al. (1999): Serum antibody response to *Cryptococcus neoformans* in cats, dogs and koalas with and without active infection. Med Mycol 37:43.

Malik R, et al. (1997): Nasopharyngeal cryptococcosis. Aust Vet J 75:483.

O'Brien CR, et al. (2006): Long-term outcome of therapy for 59 cats and 11 dogs with cryptococcosis. Aust Vet J 84:384.

O'Brien CR, et al. (2004): Retrospective study of feline and canine cryptococcosis in Australia from 1981 to 2001: 195 cases. Med Mycol 42:449.

Stiles J (2006): Ocular infections, in Greene CE (editor): Infectious Diseases of the Dog and Cat, 3rd ed. Saunders, St. Louis, p. 974.

Taboada J, Grooters AM (2005): Systemic mycosis, in Ettinger SJ, Feldman EC (editors): Textbook of Veterinary Internal Medicine, 6th ed. Saunders, St. Louis, p. 671.

Tiches D, et al. (1998): A case of canine central nervous system cryptococcosis: management with fluconazole. J Am Anim Hosp Assoc 34:145.

Histoplasmosis

Davies C, Troy GC (1996): Deep mycotic infections in cats. J Am Anim Hosp Assoc 32:380.

Gilger BC (2000): Ocular manifestations of systemic infectious diseases, in Bonagura JD (editor): Kirk's Current Veterinary Therapy XIII: Small Animal Practice, 13th ed. Saunders, Philadelphia, p. 276.

Gionfriddo JR (2000): Feline systemic fungal infections. Vet Clin North Am Small Anim Pract 30:1029.

Greene CE (2006): Histoplasmosis, in Greene CE (editor): Infectious Diseases of the Dog and Cat, 3rd ed. Saunders, St. Louis, p. 577.

Hodges RD, et al. (1994): Itraconazole for the treatment of histoplasmosis in cats. J Vet Intern Med 8:409.

Johnson LR, et al. (2004): Histoplasmosis infection in two cats from California. J Am Anim Hosp Assoc 40:165.

Kerl ME (2003): Update on canine and feline fungal diseases. Vet Clin North Am Small Anim Pract 33:721.

Krohne SG (2000): Canine systemic fungal infections. Vet Clin North Am Small Anim Pract 30:1063.

Stiles J (2006): Ocular infections, in Greene CE (editor): Infectious Diseases of the Dog and Cat, 3rd ed. Saunders, St. Louis, p. 974.

Taboada J, Grooters AM (2005): Systemic mycosis, in Ettinger SJ, Feldman EC (editors): Textbook of Veterinary Internal Medicine, 6th ed. Saunders, St. Louis, p. 671.

Toxoplasmosis

Bresciani KD, et al. (1999): Experimental toxoplasmosis in pregnant bitches. Vet Parasitol 86:143.

Davidson MG (2000): Toxoplasmosis. Vet Clin North Am Small Anim Pract 30:1051.

Davidson MG, English RV (1998): Feline ocular toxoplasmosis. Vet Ophthalmol 1:71.

Dubey JP (2004): Toxoplasmosis—waterborne zoonosis. Vet Parasitol 126:57.

Dubey JP, Lappin MR (2006): Toxoplasmosis and neosporosis, in Greene CE (editor): Infectious Diseases of the Dog and Cat, 3rd ed. Saunders, St. Louis, p. 754.

Gilger BC (2000): Ocular manifestations of systemic infectious diseases, in Bonagura JD (editor): Kirk's Current Veterinary Therapy XIII: Small Animal Practice, 13th ed. Saunders, Philadelphia, p. 276.

Lappin MR (2005): Protozoal and miscellaneous infections, in Ettinger SJ, Feldman EC (editors): Textbook of Veterinary Internal Medicine, 6th ed. Saunders, St. Louis, p. 638.

Lappin MR (2000): Feline infectious uveitis. J Feline Med Surg 2:159.

Lappin MR (1995): CVT update: feline toxoplasmosis, in Bonagura JD (editor): Kirk's Current Veterinary Therapy XII: Small Animal Practice, 12th ed. Saunders, Philadelphia, p. 309.

Lappin MR, et al. (1992): Serologic prevalence of selected infectious diseases in cats with uveitis. J Am Vet Med Assoc 201:1005.

Powell CC, Lappin MR (2001): Clinical ocular toxoplasmosis in neonatal kittens. Vet Ophthalmol 4:87.

Schatzberg SJ, et al. (2003): Use of a multiplex polymerase chain reaction assay in the antemortem diagnosis of toxoplasmosis and neosporosis in the central nervous system of cats and dogs. Am J Vet Res 64:1507.

Stiles J (2006): Ocular infections, in Greene CE (editor): Infectious Diseases of the Dog and Cat, 3rd ed. Saunders, St. Louis, p. 974.

Neosporosis (Dogs)

Buxton D, et al. (2002): The comparative pathogenesis of neosporosis. Trends Parasitol 18:546.

Dubey JP (1999): Neosporosis—the first decade of research. Int J Parasitol 29:1485.

Dubey JP (1999): Recent advances in Neospora and neosporosis. Vet Parasitol 84:349.

Dubey JP, Lappin MR (2006): Toxoplasmosis and neosporosis, in Greene CE (editor): Infectious Diseases of the Dog and Cat, 3rd ed. Saunders, St. Louis, p. 754.

Dubey JP, Lindsay DS (1993): Neosporosis. Parasitol Today 9:452.

Lappin MR (2005): Protozoal and miscellaneous infections, in Ettinger SJ, Feldman EC (editors): Textbook of Veterinary Internal Medicine, 6th ed. Saunders, St. Louis, p. 638.

Ortuno A, et al. (2002): Seroprevalence of antibodies to Neospora caninum in dogs from Spain. J Parasitol 88:1263.

Schatzberg SJ, et al. (2003): Use of a multiplex polymerase chain reaction assay in the antemortem diagnosis of toxoplasmosis and neosporosis in the central nervous system of cats and dogs. Am J Vet Res 64:1507.

Canine Visceral Leishmaniasis

Alvar J, et al. (2004): Canine leishmaniasis. Adv Parasitol 57:1.

Baneth G, et al. (2006): Leishmaniasis, in Greene CE (editor): Infectious Diseases of the Dog and Cat, 3rd ed. Saunders, St. Louis, p. 685.

Baneth G, Shaw SE (2002): Chemotherapy of canine leishmaniosis. Vet Parasitol 106:315.

Cortadellas O (2003): Initial and long-term efficacy of a lipid emulsion of amphotericin B desoxycholate in the management of canine leishmaniasis. J Vet Intern Med 17:808.

Garcia-Alonso M, et al. (1996): Immunopathology of the uveitis in canine leishmaniasis. Parasite Immunol 18:617.

Gaskin AA, et al. (2002): Visceral leishmaniasis in a New York foxhound kennel. J Vet Intern Med 16:34.

Giger U, et al. (2002): Leishmania donovani transmission by packed RBC transfusion to anemic dogs in the United States. Transfusion 42:381.

Gilger BC (2000): Ocular manifestations of systemic infectious diseases, in Bonagura JD (editor): Kirk's Current Veterinary Therapy XIII: Small Animal Practice, 13th ed. Saunders, Philadelphia, p. 276.

Grosjean NL, et al. (2003): Seroprevalence of antibodies against Leishmania spp. among dogs in the United States. J Am Vet Med Assoc 222:603.

Lappin MR (2005): Protozoal and miscellaneous infections, in Ettinger SJ, Feldman EC (editors): Textbook of Veterinary Internal Medicine, 6th ed. Saunders, St. Louis, p. 638.

Manna L, et al. (2004): Comparison of different tissue sampling for PCR-based diagnosis and follow-up of canine visceral leishmaniosis. Vet Parasitol 125:251.

Rosypal AC, et al. (2003): Canine visceral leishmaniasis and its emergence in the United States. Vet Clin North Am Small Anim Pract 33:921.

Stiles J (2006): Ocular infections, in Greene CE (editor): Infectious Diseases of the Dog and Cat, 3rd ed. Saunders, St. Louis, p. 974.

Strauss-Ayali D, et al. (2004): Polymerase chain reaction using noninvasively obtained samples, for the detection of Leishmania infantum DNA in dogs. J Infect Dis 189:1729.

Diabetes Mellitus

Bennett N (2002): Monitoring techniques for diabetes mellitus in the dog and the cat. Clin Tech Small Anim Pract 17:65.

Cusick M, et al. (2003): Effects of aldose reductase inhibitors and galactose withdrawal on fluorescein angiographic lesions in galactose-fed dogs. Arch Ophthalmol 121:1745.

Feldman EC, Nelson RW (2004): Canine diabetes mellitus, in Feldman EC, Nelson RW (editors): Canine and Feline Endocrinology and Reproduction, 3rd ed. Saunders, St. Louis, p. 486.

Feldman EC, Nelson RW (2004): Feline diabetes mellitus, in Feldman EC, Nelson RW (editors): Canine and Feline Endocrinology and Reproduction, 3rd ed. Saunders, St. Louis, p. 539.

Fleeman LM, Rand JS (2001): Management of canine diabetes. Vet Clin North Am Small Anim Pract 31:855.

Good KL, et al. (2003): Corneal sensitivity in dogs with diabetes mellitus. Am J Vet Res 64:7.

Hess RS, et al. (2000): Concurrent disorders in dogs with diabetes mellitus: 221 cases (1993-1998). J Am Vet Med Assoc 217:1166.

Hoenig M (2002): Comparative aspects of diabetes mellitus in dogs and cats. Mol Cell Endocrinol 197:221.

Neuenschwander H, et al. (1997): Dose-dependent reduction of retinal vessel changes associated with diabetic retinopathy in galactose-fed dogs by the aldose reductase inhibitor M79175. J Ocul Pharmacol Ther 13:517.

Peikes H, et al. (2001): Dermatologic disorders in dogs with diabetes mellitus: 45 cases (1986-2000). J Am Vet Med Assoc 219:203.

Richter M, et al. (2002): Aldose reductase activity and glucose-related opacities in incubated lenses from dogs and cats. Am J Vet Res 63:1591.

Hyperlipidemia

Barrie J, Watson TDG (1995): Hyperlipidemia, in Bonagura JD (editor): Kirk's Current Veterinary Therapy XII: Small Animal Practice, 12th ed. Saunders, Philadelphia, p. 430.

Bauer JE (1995): Evaluation and dietary considerations in idiopathic hyperlipidemia in dogs. J Am Vet Med Assoc 206:1684.

Elliott DA (2005): Dietary and medical considerations in lipidemia, in Ettinger SJ, Feldman EC (editors): Textbook of Veterinary Internal Medicine, 6th ed. Saunders, St. Louis, p. 592.

Gunn-Moore DA, et al. (1997): Transient hyperlipidaemia and anaemia in kittens. Vet Rec 140:355.

Johnstone AC, et al. (1990): The pathology of an inherited hyperlipoproteinaemia of cats. J Comp Pathol 102:125.

Jones BR, et al. (1986): Peripheral neuropathy in cats with inherited primary hyperchylomicronaemia. Vet Rec 119:268.

Jones BR, et al. (1983): Occurrence of idiopathic, familial hyperchylomicronaemia in a cat. Vet Rec 112:543.

Peritz LN, et al. (1990): Characterization of a lipoprotein lipase class III type defect in hypertriglyceridemic cats. Clin Invest Med 13:259.

Sato K, et al. (2000): Hypercholesterolemia in Shetland sheepdogs. J Vet Med Sci 62:1297.

Watson P, et al. (1993): Hypercholesterolaemia in briards in the United Kingdom. Res Vet Sci 54:80.

Whitney MS (1992): Evaluation of hyperlipidemias in dogs and cats. Semin Vet Med Surg (Small Anim) 7:292.

Wisselink MA, et al. (1994): Hyperlipoproteinaemia associated with atherosclerosis and cutaneous xanthomatosis in a cat. Vet Q 16:199.

Hyperadrenocorticism (Dogs)

Behrend EN, Kemppainen RJ (2001): Diagnosis of canine hyperadrenocorticism. Vet Clin North Am Small Anim Pract 31:985.

Braddock JA, et al. (2003): Trilostane treatment in dogs with pituitary-dependent hyperadrenocorticism. Aust Vet J 81:600.

Chapman PS, et al. (2004): Adrenal necrosis in a dog receiving trilostane for the treatment of hyperadrenocorticism. J Small Anim Pract 45:307.

Feldman EC, Nelson RW (2004): Canine hyperadrenocorticism (Cushing's syndrome), in Feldman EC, Nelson RW (editors): Canine and Feline Endocrinology and Reproduction, 3rd ed. Saunders, St. Louis, p. 252.

Laus JL, et al. (2002): Combined corneal lipid and calcium degeneration in a dog with hyperadrenocorticism: a case report. Vet Ophthalmol 5:61.

Neiger R, et al. (2002): Trilostane treatment of 78 dogs with pituitary-dependent hyperadrenocorticism. Vet Rec 150:799.

Reusch CE (2005): Hyperadrenocorticism, in Ettinger SJ, Feldman EC (editors): Textbook of Veterinary Internal Medicine, 6th ed. Saunders, St. Louis, p. 1592.

Ristic JM, et al. (2002): The use of 17-hydroxyprogesterone in the diagnosis of canine hyperadrenocorticism. J Vet Intern Med 16:433.

Wenger M, et al. (2004): Effect of trilostane on serum concentrations of aldosterone, cortisol, and potassium in dogs with pituitary-dependent hyperadrenocorticism. Am J Vet Res 65:1245.

Hypothyroidism (Dogs)

Dixon RM, et al. (1999): Epidemiological, clinical, haematological and biochemical characteristics of canine hypothyroidism. Vet Rec 145:481.

Feldman EC, Nelson RW (2004): Hypothyroidism, in Feldman EC, Nelson RW (editors): Canine and Feline Endocrinology and Reproduction, 3rd ed. Saunders, St. Louis, p. 86.

Graham PA, et al. (2001): Lymphocytic thyroiditis. Vet Clin North Am Small Anim Pract 31:915.

Hess RS, et al. (2003): Association between diabetes mellitus, hypothyroidism or hyperadrenocorticism, and atherosclerosis in dogs. J Vet Intern Med 17:489.

Jaggy A (2000): Neurologic manifestation of canine hypothyroidism, in Bonagura JD (editor): Kirk's Current Veterinary Therapy XIII: Small Animal Practice, 13th ed. Saunders, Philadelphia, p. 716.

Kemppainen RJ, Behrend EN (2001): Diagnosis of canine hypothyroidism: perspectives from a testing laboratory. Vet Clin North Am Small Anim Pract 31:951.

Nachreiner RF, et al. (2002): Prevalence of serum thyroid hormone autoantibodies in dogs with clinical signs of hypothyroidism. J Am Vet Med Assoc 220:466.

Panciera D (2000): Cardiovascular complications of thyroid disease, in Bonagura JD (editor): Kirk's Current Veterinary Therapy XIII: Small Animal Practice, 13th ed. Saunders, Philadelphia, p. 716.

Panciera D (2000): Complications and concurrent conditions associated with hypothyroidism in dogs, in Bonagura JD (editor): Kirk's Current Veterinary Therapy XIII: Small Animal Practice, 13th ed. Saunders, Philadelphia, p. 327.

Panciera DL (2001): Conditions associated with canine hypothyroidism. Vet Clin North Am Small Anim Pract 31:935.

Scott-Moncrieff JC, Guptil-Yoran L (2005): Hypothyroidism, in Ettinger SJ, Feldman EC (editors): Textbook of Veterinary Internal Medicine, 6th ed. Saunders, St. Louis, p. 1535.

Thrombocytopenia and Thrombopathy (Thrombasthenia)

Boozer AL, Macintire DK (2003): Canine babesiosis. Vet Clin North Am Small Anim Pract 33:885.

Boreaux MK (2000): Acquired platelet dysfunction, in Feldman BF, et al. (editors): Schalm's Veterinary Hematology, 5th ed. Lippincott Williams & Wilkins, Philadelphia, p. 496.

Brooks MB, Catalfano JL (2005): Platelet disorders and von Willebrand disease, in Ettinger SJ, Feldman EC (editors): Textbook of Veterinary Internal Medicine, 6th ed. Saunders, St. Louis, p. 1918.

Davidson MG, et al. (1990): Vascular permeability and coagulation during Rickettsia rickettsii infection in dogs. Am J Vet Res 51:165.

Grindem CB, et al. (1991): Epidemiologic survey of thrombocytopenia in dogs: a report on 987 cases. Vet Clin Pathol 20:38.

Hackett TB, et al. (2002): Clinical findings associated with prairie rattlesnake bites in dogs: 100 cases (1989-1998). J Am Vet Med Assoc 220:1675.

Harrus S, et al. (1998): Acute blindness associated with monoclonal gammopathy induced by Ehrlichia canis infection. Vet Parasitol 78:155.

Hisasue M, et al. (2001): Hematologic abnormalities and outcome of 16 cats with myelodysplastic syndromes. J Vet Intern Med 15:471.

Kirby R, Rudolf E (2000): Acquired coagulopathy VI: disseminated intravascular coagulation, in Feldman BF, et al. (editors): Schalm's Veterinary Hematology, 5th ed. Philadelphia, Lippincott Williams & Wilkins, p. 579.

Scott MA (2000): Immune-mediated thrombocytopenia, in Feldman BF, et al. (editors): Schalm's Veterinary Hematology, 5th ed. Philadelphia, Lippincott Williams & Wilkins, p. 478.

Segev G, et al. (2004): Vipera palaestinae envenomation in 327 dogs: a retrospective cohort study and analysis of risk factors for mortality. Toxicon 43:691.

Topper MJ, Welles EG (2003): Hemostasis, in Latimer KS, et al. (editors): Duncan and Prasse's Veterinary Laboratory Medicine Clinical Pathology, 4th ed. Ames, Iowa State Press, p. 99.

Trepanier LA, et al. (2003): Clinical findings in 40 dogs with hypersensitivity associated with administration of potentiated sulfonamides. J Vet Intern Med 17:647.

Zimmerman KL (2000): Drug-induced thrombocytopenias, in Feldman BF, et al. (editors): Schalm's Veterinary Hematology, 5th ed. Philadelphia, Lippincott Williams & Wilkins, p. 472.

Systemic Hypertension

Bartges JW, et al. (1996): Hypertension and renal disease. Vet Clin North Am Small Anim Pract 26:1331.

Chetboul V, et al. (2003): Spontaneous feline hypertension: clinical and echocardiographic abnormalities, and survival rate. J Vet Intern Med 17:89.

Crispin SM, Mould JR (2001): Systemic hypertensive disease and the feline fundus. Vet Ophthalmol 4:13.

Elliott J, et al. (2001): Feline hypertension: clinical findings and response to antihypertensive treatment in 30 cases. J Small Anim Pract 42:122.

Komaromy AM, et al. (2004): Hypertensive retinopathy and choroidopathy in a cat. Vet Ophthalmol 7:3.

Maggio F, et al. (2000): Ocular lesions associated with systemic hypertension in cats: 69 cases (1985-1998). J Am Vet Med Assoc 217:695.

Mertz BP, et al. (1990): Rhegmatogenous retinal detachment in a hypertensive dog. Lens Eye Toxic Res 7:67.

Miller RH, et al. (1999): Effect of enalapril on blood pressure, renal function, and the renin-angiotensin-aldosterone system in cats with autosomal dominant polycystic kidney disease. Am J Vet Res 60:1516.

Pedersen KM, et al. (2003): Increased mean arterial pressure and aldosterone-to-renin ratio in Persian cats with polycystic kidney disease. J Vet Intern Med 17:21.

Polzin DJ, et al. (2005): Chronic kidney disease, in Ettinger SJ, Feldman EC (editors): Textbook of Veterinary Internal Medicine, 6th ed. Saunders, St. Louis, p. 1756.

Sansom J, et al. (2004): Blood pressure assessment in healthy cats and cats with hypertensive retinopathy. Am J Vet Res 65:245.

Snyder PS, et al. (2001): Effect of amlodipine on echocardiographic variables in cats with systemic hypertension. J Vet Intern Med 15:52.

Syme HM, et al. (2002): Prevalence of systolic hypertension in cats with chronic renal failure at initial evaluation. J Am Vet Med Assoc 220:1799.

Van Boxtel SA (2003): Hypertensive retinopathy in a cat. Can Vet J 44:147.

Polycythemia

Cote E, Ettinger SJ (2001): Long-term clinical management of right-to-left ("reversed") patent ductus arteriosus in 3 dogs. J Vet Intern Med 15:39.

Couto CG, et al. (1989): Tumor-associated erythrocytosis in a dog with nasal fibrosarcoma. J Vet Intern Med 3:183.

Crow SE, et al. (1995): Concurrent renal adenocarcinoma and polycythemia in a dog. J Am Anim Hosp Assoc 31:29.

Evans LM, Caylor KB (1995): Polycythemia vera in a cat and management with hydroxyurea. J Am Anim Hosp Assoc 31:434.

Foster ES, Lothrop CD Jr (1988): Polycythemia vera in a cat with cardiac hypertrophy. J Am Vet Med Assoc 192:1736.

Gorse MJ (1988): Polycythemia associated with renal fibrosarcoma in a dog. J Am Vet Med Assoc 192:793.

Gray HE, et al. (2003): Polycythemia vera in a dog presenting with uveitis. J Am Anim Hosp Assoc 39:355.

Hasler AH, Giger U (1996): Serum erythropoietin values in polycythemic cats. J Am Anim Hosp Assoc 32:294.

Henry CJ, et al. (1999): Primary renal tumours in cats: 19 cases (1992-1998). J Feline Med Surg 1:165.

Meyer HP, et al. (1993): Polycythaemia vera in a dog treated by repeated phlebotomies. Vet Q 15:108.

Moore KW, Stepien RL (2001): Hydroxyurea for treatment of polycythemia secondary to right-to-left shunting patent ductus arteriosus in 4 dogs. J Vet Intern Med 15:418.

Sato K, et al. (2002): Secondary erythrocytosis associated with high plasma erythropoietin concentrations in a dog with cecal leiomyosarcoma. J Am Vet Med Assoc 220:486.

van Vonderen IK, et al. (1997): Polyuria and polydipsia and disturbed vasopressin release in 2 dogs with secondary polycythemia. J Vet Intern Med 11:300.

Watson ADJ (2000): Erythrocytosis and polycythemia, in Feldman BF, et al. (editors): Schalm's Veterinary Hematology, 5th ed. Philadelphia, Lippincott Williams & Wilkins, p. 216.

Hyperviscosity Syndrome

Boone LI (2000): Bence-Jones proteins, in Feldman BF, et al. (editors): Schalm's Veterinary Hematology, 5th ed. Philadelphia, Lippincott Williams & Wilkins, p. 925.

Forrester SD, et al. (1992): Serum hyperviscosity syndrome associated with multiple myeloma in two cats. J Am Vet Med Assoc 200:79.

Forrester SD, Rogers KS (2000): Hyperviscosity syndromes, in Feldman BF, et al. (editors): Schalm's Veterinary Hematology, 5th ed. Philadelphia, Lippincott Williams & Wilkins, p. 929.

Fox LE (1995): The paraneoplastic disorders, in Bonagura JD (editor): Kirk's Current Veterinary Therapy XII: Small Animal Practice, 12th ed. Saunders, Philadelphia, p. 530.

Harrus S, et al. (1998): Acute blindness associated with monoclonal gammopathy induced by *Ehrlichia canis* infection. Vet Parasitol 78:155.

Hawkins EC, et al. (1986): Immunoglobulin A myeloma in a cat with pleural effusion and serum hyperviscosity. J Am Vet Med Assoc 188:876.

Hohenhaus AE (1995): Syndromes of hyperglobulinemia: diagnosis and therapy, in Kirk's Current Veterinary Therapy XII: Small Animal Practice, 12th ed. Saunders, Philadelphia, p. 523.

Hoskins JD, et al. (1983): Serum hyperviscosity syndrome associated with *Ehrlichia canis* infection in a dog. Am Vet Med Assoc 183:1011.

Ward DA, et al. (1997): Orbital plasmacytoma in a cat. J Small Anim Pract 38:576.

Weber NA, Tebeau CS (1998): An unusual presentation of multiple myeloma in two cats. J Am Anim Hosp Assoc 34:477.

Uveodermatologic Syndrome (Vogt-Koyanagi-Harada–Like Syndrome) (Dogs)

Bedford PG (1986): Uveodermatological syndrome in the Japanese Akita. Vet Rec 118:134.

Bussanich MN, et al. (1982): Granulomatous panuveitis and dermal depigmentation. J Am Anim Hosp Assoc 18:131.

Carter WJ, et al. (2005): An immunohistochemical study of uveodermatologic syndrome in two Japanese Akita dogs. Vet Ophthalmol 8:17.

Cottrell BD, Barnett KC (1986): Harada's disease in the Japanese Akita. J Small Anim Pract 28:517.

Kern TJ, et al. (1985): Uveitis associated with poliosis and vitiligo in six dogs. J Am Vet Med Assoc 187:408.

Laus JL, et al. (2004): Uveodermatologic syndrome in a Brazilian fila dog. Vet Ophthalmol 7:193.

Lindley DM, et al. (1990): Ocular histopathology of Vogt-Koyanagi-Harada–like syndrome in an Akita dog. Vet Pathol 27:294.

Muller RS, et al. (1992): The uveodermatologic syndrome in dogs. Tierarztl Prax 20:632.

Read RW (2002): Vogt-Koyanagi-Harada disease. Ophthalmol Clin North Am 15:333.

Ocular Manifestations of Systemic Disease in Horses

Aleman M, et al. (2006): Juvenile idiopathic epilepsy in Egyptian Arabian foals: 22 cases (1985-2005). J Vet Intern Med 20:1443.

Anderson CA, Divers TJ (1983): Systemic granulomatous inflammation in a horse grazing hairy vetch. J AmVet Med Assoc 183:569.

Anninger WV, et al. (2003): West Nile virus-associated optic neuritis and chorioretinitis. Am J Ophthalmol 136:1183.

Blogg JR, et al. (1983): Blindness caused by *Rhodococcus equi* in a foal. Equine Vet J Suppl 2:25.

Brem S, et al. (1998): Intraocular leptospira isolation in 4 horses suffering from equine recurrent uveitis (ERU). Berl Münch Tierärztl Wochenschr 111:415.

Browning GF, et al. (1988): Latency of equine herpesvirus-4 (equine rhinopneumonitis virus). Vet Rec 123:518.

Collinson PN, et al. (1994): Isolation of equine herpesvirus-2 (equine gammaherpesvirus-2) from foals with keratoconjunctivitis. J Am Vet Med Assoc 205:329.

Curnutte JT, (1993): Chronic granulomatous disease: the solving of a clinical riddle at the molecular level. Clin Immunol Immunopathol 67:S2.

Cutler TJ (2002): Ophthalmic findings in the geriatric horse. Vet Clin North Am Equine Pract 18:545.

Edington N, et al. (1985): Experimental reactivation of equid herpesvirus-1 (EHV-1) following the administration of corticosteroids. Equine Vet J 17:369.

Ellis PM, et al. (2000): Japanese encephalitis. Vet Clin North Am Equine Pract 16:565.

Griffith G (1987): Pemphigus foliaceus in a Welsh pony. Compend Contin Educ Pract Vet 9:347.

Heath SE, et al. (1990): Idiopathic granulomatous disease involving the skin in a horse. J Am Vet Med Assoc 197:1033.

Henry M, et al. (1989): Hemorrhagic diatheses caused by multiple myeloma in a three-month-old foal. J Am Vet Med Assoc 194:392.

Jones TC (1969): Clinical and pathologic features of equine viral arteritis. J Am Vet Med Assoc 155:35.

Kaiser PK, et al. (2003): Occlusive vasculitis in a patient with concomitant West Nile virus infection. Am J Ophthalmol 136:928.

Kuchtey RW, et al. (2003): Uveitis associated with West Nile virus infection. Arch Ophthalmol 121:1648.

Lavach JD (1992): Ocular manifestations of systemic diseases. Vet Clin North Am Equine Pract 8:627.

Leiffson PS, et al. (1997): Ocular tuberculosis in a horse. Vet Rec 141:651.

Madigan JE, et al. (1995): Photic head shaking in the horse: 7 cases. Equine Vet J 27:306.

Martin CL (1999): Ocular manifestations of systemic disease, in Gelatt KN (editor): Veterinary Ophthalmology, 3rd ed. Lippincott Williams & Wilkins, Baltimore.

McConnico RS, et al. (1991): Supportive medical care of recumbent horses. Compend Contin Educ Pract Vet 13:1287.

Miller TR, et al. (1990): Herpetic keratitis in a horse. Equine Vet J Suppl 10:15.

Newton SA, et al. (2000): Headshaking in horses: possible aetiopathogenesis suggested by the results of diagnostic tests and several treatment regimes used in 20 cases. Equine Vet J 32:208.

Ostlund EN, et al. (2001): Equine West Nile encephalitis, United States. Emerg Infect Dis 7:665.

Pusterla N, et al. (2003): Cutaneous and ocular habronemiasis in horses: 63 cases (1988-2002). J Am Vet Med Assoc 222:978.

Rames DS, et al. (1995): Ocular *Halicephalobus* (syn. *Micronema*) *deletrix* in a horse. Vet Pathol 32:540.

Rebhun WC, Del Piero F (1998): Ocular lesions of horses with lymphosarcoma: 21 cases (1977-1997). J Am Vet Med Assoc 212:852.

Richt JA, et al. (2000): Borna disease in horses. Vet Clin North Am Equine Pract 16:579.

Rico-Hesse R (2000): Venezuelan equine encephalomyelitis. Vet Clin North Am Equine Pract 16:553.

Savage CJ (1998): Lymphoproliferative and myeloproliferative disorders. Vet Clin North Am Equine Pract 14:563.

Sippel WL, et al. (1962): Equine piroplasmosis in the United States. J Am Vet Med Assoc 141:694.

Smith BP (editor) (2002): Large Animal Internal Medicine, 3rd ed. Mosby, St. Louis.

Sutton GA, et al. (1998): Pathogenesis and clinical signs of equine herpesvirus-1 in experimentally infected ponies in vivo. Can J Vet Res 62:49.

Sutton GA, et al. (1997): Study of the duration and distribution of equine influenza virus subtype 2 (H_3N_8) antigens in experimentally infected ponies in vivo. Can J Vet Res 61:113.

Wada S, et al. (2003): Nonulcerative keratouveitis as a manifestation of leptospiral infection in a horse. Vet Ophthalmol 6:191.

Woods LW, et al. (1992): Systemic granulomatous disease in a horse grazing pasture containing vetch (*Vicia* sp.). J Vet Diagn Invest 4:356.

Ocular Manifestations of Systemic Diseases in Ruminants

Abdelbaki YA, Davis RN (1972): Ophthalmoscopic findings in elaeophorosis of domestic sheep. Vet Med 67:69.

Adcock, J, Hibler CP (1969): Vascular and neuroophthalmic pathology of elaeophorosis in elk. Pathol Vet 6:185.

Bistner SI, et al. (1970): The ocular lesions of bovine viral diarrhea-mucosal disease. Pathol Vet 7:275.

Capucchio MT, et al. (2003): Maedi-visna virus detection in ovine third eyelids. J Comp Pathol 129:37.

Collier LC, et al. (1979): Ocular manifestations of the Chédiak-Higashi syndrome in four species of animals. J Am Vet Med Assoc 175:587.

Dukes TW (1971): The ocular lesions of thromboembolic meningoencephalitis in cattle. Can Vet J 12:180.

Fighera RA, Barros CSL (2004): Systemic granulomatous disease in Brazilian cattle grazing pasture containing vetch (*Cicia* spp). Vet Human Toxicol 46:62.

George L, et al. (1988): Enhancement of infectious bovine keratoconjunctivitis by modified live infectious bovine rhinotracheitis virus vaccine. Am J Vet Res 49:1800.

Hopkins JB, et al. (1973): Conjunctivitis associated with chlamydial polyarthritis in lambs. J Am Vet Med Assoc 163:1157.

Martin CL (1999): Ocular manifestations of systemic disease, in Gelatt KN (editor): Veterinary Ophthalmology, 3rd ed. Lippincott Williams & Wilkins, Baltimore.

Mushi EZ, et al. (1980): Isolation of bovine malignant catarrhal fever virus from ocular and nasal secretions of wildebeest calves. Res Vet Sci 29:168.

Pierson RE, et al. (1973): Clinical and clinicopathologic observations in induced malignant catarrhal fever of cattle. J Am Vet Med Assoc 173:833.

Pierson RE, et al. (1973): An epizootic of malignant catarrhal fever in feedlot cattle. J Am Vet Med Assoc 163:349.

Radostits O, et al. (2007): Veterinary Medicine, 10th ed. Saunders, London.

Rebhun WC (1986): Diseases of the bovine orbit and globe. J Am Vet Med Assoc 190:171.

Rebhun WC (1984): Ocular manifestations of systemic diseases in cattle. Vet Clin North Am Large Anim Pract 6:623.

Rebhun WC (1982): Orbital lymphosarcoma in cattle. J Am Vet Med Assoc 180:149.

Rebhun WC, Del Piero F (1998): Ocular lesions in horses with lymphosarcoma: 21 cases (1977-1997). J Am Vet Med Assoc 212:852.

RebhunWC, de Lahunta A (1982): Diagnosis and treatment of bovine listeriosis. J Am Vet Med Assoc 180:395.

Roeder PL, et al. (1986): Pestivirus fetopathogenicity in cattle: changing sequelae with fetal maturation. Vet Rec 118:44.

Silverstein AM, et al. (1971): An experimental virus-induced retinal dysplasia in the fetal lamb. Am J Ophthalmol 72:22.

Slatter DH, et al. (1979): Effects of experimental hyperlipoproteinemia on the canine eye. Exp Eye Res 29:437.

Smith BP (editor) (2002): Large Animal Internal Medicine, 3rd ed. Mosby, St. Louis.

Smith MO (2002): Diseases of the nervous system, in Smith BP (editor): Large Animal Internal Medicine, 3rd ed. Mosby, St. Louis, p.873.

Stephens LR, et al. (1981): Infectious thromboembolic meningoencephalitis in cattle: a review. J Am Vet Med Assoc 178:378.

van der Lugt JJ, et al. (1996): Status spongiosus, optic neuropathy, and retinal degeneration in *Helichrysum argyrosphaerum* poisoning in sheep and a goat. Vet Pathol 33:495.

Whiteley HE, et al. (1985): Ocular lesions of bovine malignant catarrhal fever. Vet Pathol 22:219.

OCULAR EMERGENCIES

Paul E. Miller

MATERIALS REQUIRED
PROPTOSIS OF THE GLOBE
GLAUCOMA
CORNEAL LACERATIONS
LID LACERATIONS

SEVERE OCULAR AND ADNEXAL
  CONTUSIONS AND CONCUSSION
PENETRATING INJURIES OF THE GLOBE
SEVERE CORNEAL ULCERATION
DESCEMETOCELE OR IRIS PROLAPSE

HYPHEMA
ACUTE ANTERIOR UVEITIS
SUDDEN BLINDNESS

The conditions discussed in this chapter are the most important disorders for which early action is necessary to prevent severe or permanent damage to the eye. Emergency treatment is outlined separately for ready clinical reference, followed by further discussion for those conditions not covered elsewhere in the text.

MATERIALS REQUIRED

Basic Diagnostic Instruments and Supplies

- Magnifying loupe 2× to 4× magnification
- Direct or indirect ophthalmoscope
- Finhoff transilluminator
- Sterile eye wash
- Schirmer tear test strips
- Fluorescein strips
- Cotton-tipped applicators or "Weck cell" cellulose sponges
- Tonometer—Schiøtz, Tono-Pen, or TonoVet
- Culture swabs and media
- No. 15 scalpel blades
- Glass microscope slides
- Needles, 20- to 27-gauge

Surgical Instruments

- Needle holders (Derf or Castroviejo)
- Tenotomy scissors
- Lacrimal cannula or 20- to 25-gauge Teflon IV catheters
- Irrigating bulb or syringe
- Fixation forceps
- No. 15 scalpel blade
- Lid retractors (Castroviejo or Vierheller)

Medications

Topical anesthetic
Tropicamide (Mydriacyl), 1%
Atropine, 1% drops and ointment
Mannitol, 20%, parenteral
Pilocarpine, 2% drops
Neomycin, polymyxin, bacitracin drops
Tear-replacement solution/cyclosporine

Always perform a thorough clinical examination before manipulating the eye.

PROPTOSIS OF THE GLOBE

At initial presentation it is often preferable to try to salvage the globe rather than to remove it.

Emergency treatment for proptosis of the globe (Figure 19-1)

1. Replace the globe as soon as possible to prevent severe corneal damage. If treatment is delayed because the animal is far away, advise that the owner keep the eye moist with saline, water, petroleum jelly (Vaseline), or antibiotic ointments and avoid additional trauma when moving the animal.
2. Carefully examine the patient for systemic injuries and provide appropriate supportive care.
3. Protect the surface of the cornea with antibiotic ointments.
4. When the patient is stable, induce anesthesia.
5. The basic procedure is to lift the lid margins over the equator of the globe while pushing the globe back into the orbit at the same time.
6. Flush the conjunctival sac free of extraneous debris with sterile lactated Ringer's solution.
7. Roll out the lid margins with hemostats or forceps and place a temporary tarsorrhaphy suture. In general, three or four simple interrupted or horizontal mattress sutures of 4/0 nylon are used as shown in Figure 19-2, *A* and *B*. Sutures should emerge from the lid margin (in line with the meibomian gland openings) rather than on the conjunctival surface so as to prevent sutures rubbing on the cornea.
8. Apply a suitable antibiotic ointment (e.g., neomycin, polymyxin B, bacitracin) to the eye.
9. Place a scalpel handle over the cornea, which is well lubricated with either an antibiotic or artificial tear ointment, and draw up on each of the sutures simultaneously, as shown in Figure 19-2, *C* and *D*. This maneuver prevents forward movement of the globe while pulling the eyelids up and over the cornea. Once the cornea

Continued

Emergency treatment for proptosis of the globe
(Figure 19-1)—cont'd

is protected, tie the sutures (Figure 19-2, *E*). If necessary (i.e., if pressure is extensive), additional sutures may be placed between the original sutures. Usually the medial canthus is left open for a few millimeters so topical medications may be applied.

10. Give dexamethasone 0.1 mg/kg IV to control secondary uveitis. Systemic steroids may then be used to treat optic neuritis if present.

Prognosis

If there is any doubt as to whether the globe can be salvaged, an attempt should be made to replace it back into the orbit. The sooner the eye is replaced, the better the prognosis, both for saving the eye and for shortening the convalescent period. Unfortunately, some eyes are inevitably lost despite early and vigorous treatment. Enucleation as the initial therapy should be considered if (1) the owner is unwilling or unable to provide what may be potentially long-term postoperative care, (2) the eye has ruptured, (3) three or more extraocular muscles are torn, or (4) the eye is completely filled with blood. The following are useful prognostic indicators.

Avulsion of Extraocular Muscles

The medial and inferior (ventral) recti and inferior (ventral) oblique muscles rupture first. Because branches of the ciliary artery to the anterior segment enter the globe with the extraocular muscles, complete avulsion of three or more muscles indicates an unfavorable prognosis. In eyes with only a few of the muscles ruptured, temporary postoperative deviations (usually lateral or superolateral) of the globe occur (Figures 19-1 and 19-3). These deviations often diminish over weeks to months (up to 6 to 9 months), or the exposed conjunctiva becomes pigmented, thereby improving the cosmetic appearance of the eye. Surgical

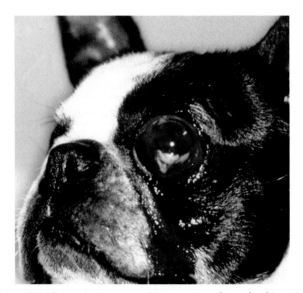

Figure 19-1. Proptosis in a young Boston terrier after a dog bite injury. (Courtesy University of Wisconsin–Madison Veterinary Ophthalmology Service Collection.)

repair of the extraocular muscle tears may be indicated in select cases.

Hyphema

Marked hyphema is an unfavorable sign, because it is usually associated with severe damage to the uveal tract or rupture of the globe, which leads to ocular hypotension and phthisis bulbi.

Pupils

The size of the pupil is not associated with the ultimate visual outcome, but the presence of an intact direct and consensual pupillary light reflex is generally a good prognostic sign. The absence of a direct or consensual pupillary light reflex, however, does not indicate that the prognosis is invariably poor. The reason is that mydriasis can result from damage to either the afferent limb of the pupillary light reflex (the retina or optic nerve) or the efferent limb (the oculomotor nerve or the iris sphincter muscle), and miosis may result from iridocyclitis attributable to the injury or loss of sympathetic innervation of the pupil. A midrange pupil may occur if the tone of both the sympathetic and parasympathetic nerves is lost, or if the optic nerve is severed only in 1 eye. The most favorable set of prognostic indicators are as follows:

- Presence of vision at initial presentation
- Minimal damage to extraocular muscles (none, one, or two injured)
- Absence of hyphema
- Normal findings on fundus examination

Skull Conformation

Proptosis occurs most frequently in brachycephalic breeds with shallow orbits (e.g., Pekingese, Boston terrier, pug). It is extremely important that excessive pressure around the neck of these breeds be avoided, especially after proptosis. Because more force is required to produce proptosis in cats and mesocephalic and dolichocephalic dogs, its presence in these animals warrants a less favorable prognosis than proptosis in brachycephalic dogs. Concurrent facial fractures also warrant a poor prognosis.

Maintenance Therapy

1. Systemic oral antibiotics for at least 7 to 14 days
2. Application of topical antibiotic ointments every 6 hours (neomycin/bacitracin/polymyxin B or gentamicin) and 1% atropine ointment every 12 hours through the medial canthus if the patient is tractable
3. Initial sutures are left in place for up to 3 weeks. If some degree of lagophthalmia is present, it may be better to remove the sutures sequentially rather than all at once. If after 3 weeks the lids still do not close well over the globe, the sutures should be replaced and maintained for an additional 2 to 3 weeks to allow residual orbital swelling to regress and to prevent corneal desiccation and ulceration. In some cases sutures may be left in place for 3 to 6 months.

Keratoconjunctivitis sicca and corneal ulceration secondary to exposure are common in the postoperative period. Supple-

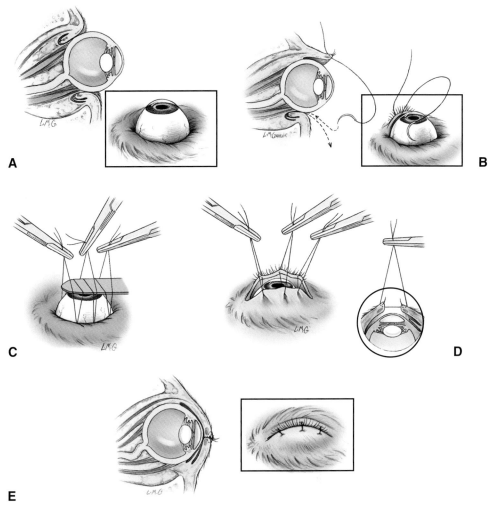

Figure 19-2. Procedure for replacement of a proptosed globe. **A,** Globe proptosis. **B,** Placement of simple interrupted traction sutures of 4/0 nylon. Alternatively, a series of modified horizontal mattress sutures may be used. Sutures should enter and exit at the lid margin and not on the conjunctival surface. **C,** Placement of scalpel handle on a cornea lubricated with an artificial tear ointment. **D,** Traction on the sutures and replacement of the globe. **E,** Completion of the sutures.

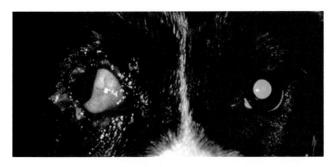

Figure 19-3. Superolateral deviation of the globe after proptosis suggests damage to the medial rectus and inferior oblique extraocular muscles.

mental artificial tears or topical antibiotic ointments are often required for several weeks or longer after proptosis to lubricate the eye and prevent infection. Additionally, many severely traumatized eyes demonstrate a deep corneal vascularization that proceeds from the limbus to the center of the cornea before gradually regressing over 4 to 8 weeks. If the cornea is not ulcerated or subject to exposure, topical corticosteroids (0.1% dexamethasone or 1% prednisolone acetate) may be used every 6 to 12 hours in an effort to moderate this vascular response.

In some patients chronic partial exophthalmos and chronic corneal exposure continue to be problems. Usually this situation results from facial nerve palsy, damage to extraocular muscles that retain the globe in the orbit, organized blood/scar tissue within the orbit, or eyelid retraction. In affected patients further surgical intervention, such as extraocular muscle repair, permanent medial or lateral tarsorrhaphy, or, in extreme cases, enucleation, should be considered. Mild cases usually do not need surgery and may be managed with supplemental artificial tear ointment to prevent corneal drying.

GLAUCOMA

The steps listed here are only for the emergency treatment of canine acute primary angle-closure glaucoma in which the eye has the potential for vision. Other forms of glaucoma (e.g., secondary to lens luxation or uveitis) are often treated quite differently (e.g., lens extraction, antiinflammatory control). Eyes that are irreversibly blind from glaucoma are often better treated surgically (evisceration and intrascleral prosthesis, enucleation, etc.). Paracentesis of the anterior chamber is usually avoided in the emergency treatment of glaucoma because of the risk of hemorrhage from the uveal tract and because sudden decompression may further damage the optic nerve.

Emergency treatment of acute primary angle closure glaucoma

Option A

1. Topical application of 0.005% latanoprost twice, 30 minutes apart
2. If intraocular pressure is not substantially reduced in 1 to 2 hours, go to Option B.

Option B

1. Intravenous mannitol 1.0 to 2.0 g/kg IV over 20 minutes
2. Oral methazolamide or dichlorphenamide at 2.2 to 4.4 mg/kg q8-12h (dogs)
3. 2% pilocarpine solution q10min for 30 min, then q6h. Monitor for bradycardia and other side effects of parasympathetic stimulation during this time.
4. Dexamethasone 0.1 mg/kg IV may be useful.

Interim Therapy

After initial lowering of pressure, the patient should be referred to a veterinary ophthalmologist for further diagnostic procedures and definitive therapy. Additionally, it should not be forgotten that the fellow eye has a 50% probability of development of glaucoma in the next 8 months. Prophylactic therapy of the fellow eye with either 0.25% demecarium bromide and a topical corticosteroid once a day at bedtime, or 0.5% betaxolol every 12 hours has been demonstrated in a clinical trial to reduce the probability of an attack by approximately fourfold. Topical pilocarpine and an oral carbonic anhydrase inhibitor should be continued until the patient can be evaluated by a veterinary ophthalmologist.

CORNEAL LACERATIONS

Emergency treatment of corneal laceration

1. Carefully examine the eye. If a laceration is suspected, either refer the patient immediately to a veterinary ophthalmologist or sedate/anesthetize the animal to prevent further damage to the eye and allow a closer examination.
2. Avoid pressure on the globe and ocular adnexa. Examine the anterior chamber with a focal light, and perform a Seidel test with fluorescein dye to determine whether the cornea has been perforated and continues to leak. "Paint" the surface of

Emergency treatment of corneal laceration—cont'd

the defect with a dry fluorescein strip. If the wound is leaking the normally orange dye mixes with the escaping aqueous humor, resulting in a green rivulet of stain exiting the wound.
3. If the wound is leaking, or if the cornea is unstable and there will be a delay until the patient is seen by a veterinary ophthalmologist, place an Elizabethan collar (or eyecup in a horse) before referral.
4. Institute systemic antibiotic therapy (e.g., cefazolin, enrofloxacin, penicillin/gentamicin).
5. Administer species-appropriate antiinflammatory therapy (systemic dexamethasone IV to dogs and cats, flunixin meglumine to horses).
6. Topical medications such as antibiotics and atropine are not usually used until the cornea is structurally intact, because solutions contain preservatives that may damage intraocular structures and some ointments may lead to the formation of intraocular granulomas.
7. If the cornea is not leaking aqueous humor, apply topical antibiotics (neomycin/bacitracin/polymyxin B) q4-6h and administer 1% atropine drops q8-24h.
8. Lacerations that are superficial, do not gape open, and do not perforate through the cornea (Seidel test result negative) are treated as described in Chapter 10. Wounds that penetrate the cornea, that are long or deep, or that gape open usually require suturing and should be treated by a veterinary ophthalmologist.

LID LACERATIONS

See also Chapter 6.

Treatment

The following four factors determine the treatment of lid lacerations:

- Time since injury, which affects extent of bacterial contamination
- Involvement of lid margin and especially lacrimal puncta and canaliculi
- Extent of lesion (plastic reconstruction may be necessary)
- Whether the laceration crosses the lid margin; if so, globe integrity should be verified

Emergency treatment of lid lacerations

1. Determine the time since injury and proceed as follows:
   a. 4 hours or less: Repair immediately.
   b. 4 to 24 hours: Repair may be immediate or delayed, depending on evaluation of injury.
   c. After 24 hours: Treat as an open wound until gross infection is controlled, then repair in an elective procedure.
2. Administer appropriate systemic antibiotics (e.g., cefazolin in dog or cat, penicillin/gentamicin in horse).
3. Induce general anesthesia.

Emergency treatment of lid lacerations—cont'd

4. If the lid margins are involved, perform reapposition accurately and suture using 6/0 nylon to prevent "notching," postoperative scarring, entropion, ectropion, and epiphora, and to generally improve the cosmetic appearance (see Chapter 6).
5. If lid margins are not involved, treat as a simple skin laceration, avoiding tension on the lid margins.
6. If the wound is extensive, requires plastic surgical repair, or involves the lacrimal canaliculi, complete initial first aid procedures and protect the wound against further damage (e.g., by use of bandage, Elizabethan collar, and systemic antibiotics) before the animal is transported to a referral center for final evaluation and treatment.

Important Facts

1. Preserve as much lid tissue as possible—minimal debridement is best.
2. Because of the excellent blood supply to the eyelids, lid lacerations usually heal well even if contaminated.
3. Because lid lacerations are often irritating during the healing phase, the following measures may be taken if necessary to prevent self-mutilation:
   - Elizabethan collar
   - Eyecup in horses
   - Sedation or tranquilization
   - Analgesics as indicated

SEVERE OCULAR AND ADNEXAL CONTUSIONS AND CONCUSSION

A *contusion* is damage from direct contact of the globe with an object. A *concussion* is damage due to trauma adjacent to the eye when forces are transmitted to the eye. The two important factors in treatment of contusions or concussions involving the eye are as follows:

1. External trauma may cause severe intraocular injuries even if the globe is not penetrated.
2. Posttraumatic uveitis is common and must be controlled.

Common Clinical Signs Associated with Ocular Trauma

- Hyphema
- Chemosis
- Subconjunctival hemorrhages
- Corneal desiccation
- Proptosis of the globe (see Figure 19-1)
- Swollen lids
- Paralysis of lids
- Absence of pupillary light reflexes
- Pain on palpation
- Fibrin in the anterior chamber
- Miosis or anisocoria (difference in the size of pupils)
- Corneal edema
- Lens luxation or subluxation
- Retinal detachment and hemorrhages
- Decreased motility or deviation of the globe
- Blindness or visual field defects
- Associated signs of central nervous system damage (e.g., coma, nystagmus)

Emergency treatment of ocular contusions and concussions (Figure 19-4)

1. After a general physical examination and treatment of life-threatening disorders, examine the eye and adnexa and record findings. If necessary, anesthetize the patient. Palpate the orbital rim and facial bones, and, if necessary, radiograph the area.
2. Evaluate for direct and consensual pupillary light reflexes.
3. Carefully examine the cornea with a magnifying loupe and, if necessary, stain with fluorescein.
4. Perform an ophthalmoscopic examination and check for the position of the lens, hemorrhages in the vitreous or retina, retinal detachment, and fibrin in the anterior chamber.
5. Administer the following agents:
   a. Antiinflammatory agents (systemic corticosteroids, e.g., dexamethasone, in dog and cat, flunixin meglumine in a horse)
   b. Systemic antibiotics (cefazolin in dog and cat, penicillin/gentamicin in horse)
   c. 1% atropine ointment or drops q8-24h
   d. Tear replacement solutions as necessary
6. Provide cage rest or stable confinement immediately, and examine the eye frequently (at least every 4 hours) thereafter.
7. If complications develop or severe intraocular lesions are suspected, refer animal for specialist treatment.

PENETRATING INJURIES OF THE GLOBE

Emergency treatment of penetrating injuries of the globe

Initial attempts are directed at preventing further injury.

1. Obtain a thorough history of the cause of the trauma and how it occurred. This is important so that preventive measures to avoid further complications may be taken if necessary (e.g., in the case of vegetable foreign bodies, which are sources of saprophytic fungal infections).
2. Administer tranquilizers or analgesics as necessary to prevent self-trauma.
3. Avoid all pressure on the eye and periorbital area until the corneasclera have been determined to be structurally stable.
4. Carefully examine the eye to evaluate the extent of injuries.
5. Administer systemic antibiotics to prevent infection (cefazolin at 20 mg/kg IM or IV in dogs and cats; penicillin/gentamicin in horses). Administer topical antibiotics (drops) frequently if the outer coat of the eye (cornea/sclera) is intact and intraocular contents are leaking through the wound.
6. Administer species-appropriate antiinflammatory agents (systemic corticosteroids in dogs and cats, flunixin meglumine in horses).
7. Protect the eye from further trauma by the following means, as necessary:
   a. Third eyelid flap or temporary tarsorrhaphy
   b. Elizabethan collar
   c. Tranquilizers and analgesics
   d. Eyecups, cross-tying, or neck brace in horses

Continued

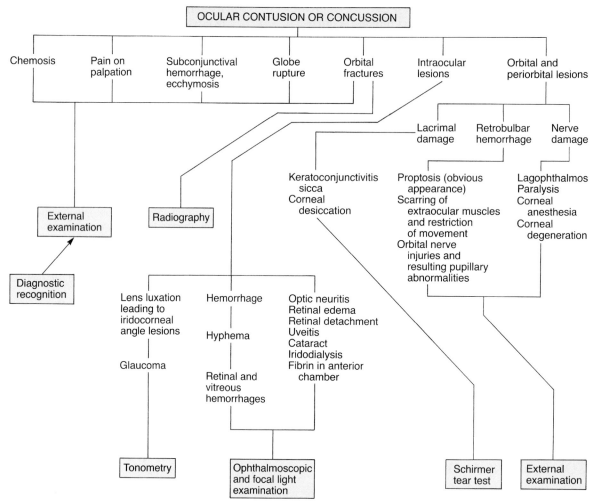

Figure 19-4. Algorithm for diagnosis and sequelae of ocular concussions and contusions.

Emergency treatment of penetrating injuries of the globe—cont'd

8. Maintain antibiotic and steroid coverage until specialist assistance can be obtained. (All penetrating or severe ocular injuries should be treated by a veterinary ophthalmologist, if possible.)

SEVERE CORNEAL ULCERATION

A thorough eye examination is performed with special attention given to the eyelids, third eyelid, and anterior chamber.

Emergency treatment of corneal ulceration

1. Perform a Schirmer tear test.
2. Perform a culture, cytologic examination, and Gram stain of a scraping from the margins of the ulcer (not the conjunctiva). Use a moistened swab to obtain the specimen.
3. Fluorescein stain: Carefully draw the extent of the defect so the efficacy of therapy can be accurately determined.

Emergency treatment of corneal ulceration—cont'd

4. Initial antibiotic therapy is based on cytology results and, ultimately, on culture and sensitivity testing results. Initial therapy usually consists of topical neomycin/polymyxin B/bacitracin, or ciprofloxacin, or a combination of cefazolin/tobramycin q2-4h. The last is prepared by reconstituting injectable cefazolin with artificial tears to a final concentration of 33 mg/mL of cefazolin. The tobramycin is fortified by adding injectable tobramycin to the commercial ophthalmic preparation so as to achieve a final concentration of 9 mg/mL.
5. In horses topical antifungal therapy consisting of miconazole or itraconazole in dimethyl sulfoxide (DMSO) should be considered. A subpalpebral lavage system may be required in some horses to effectively medicate the eye.
6. Give atropine 1% drops q6-24h if substantial pain or intraocular inflammation is present and keratoconjunctivitis sicca is *not* present.
7. If ulceration is especially severe, the patient should be referred to a specialist.
8. The patient should be closely monitored for worsening of the ulcer.

DESCEMETOCELE OR IRIS PROLAPSE

Once the diagnosis has been confirmed, immediate steps are undertaken to prevent either rupture of the cornea or further displacement of the iris before surgery. Therapy is directed toward stabilizing and supporting the cornea until definitive surgical treatment can be performed.

Emergency treatment of descemetocele or iris prolapse

1. Anesthetize or tranquilize the patient.
2. Prevent further trauma with an Elizabethan collar, eyecup, or other device.
3. If the ulcer is deep, but has not perforated the cornea, begin aggressive antibiotic therapy as for severe corneal ulceration and consider anticollagenase therapy (see Chapter 3) if examination by a specialist will be delayed.
4. Refer the patient for surgical repair by a specialist (e.g., direct suturing, a grafting procedure, corneoscleral transposition).
5. If referral is not possible and the iris has prolapsed, the protruding piece of iris (usually grayish in appearance) may be excised, the cornea sutured, and the anterior chamber reconstituted with physiologic saline or an air bubble (Figure 19-5). Surgical success requires microsurgical skills, fine suture material (7/0 or smaller), and high magnification.

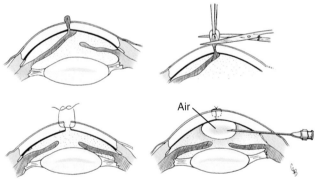

Figure 19-5. Technique for removal of incarcerated iris tissue in a corneal wound. Sutures sized 7/0 to 10/0 are placed at approximately 90% of the depth of the corneal stroma but do not enter the anterior chamber. The anterior chamber can be reformed by an air bubble delivered through a 27-gauge needle entering the eye at the limbus. Adequately closed corneal wounds are airtight and do not leak aqueous humor when stained with fluorescein stain (Seidel test). Optimal surgical success requires microsurgical skills, fine suture material, and high magnification. (Modified from Bistner SI, Aguirre GD [1972]: Management of ocular emergencies. Vet Clin North Am 2:359.)

HYPHEMA

Hyphema is the presence of blood in the anterior chamber. It most commonly results from hemorrhage from the iris and ciliary body. Less commonly blood originates from the posterior uveal tract or retina (e.g., systemic hypertension).

Emergency treatment of hyphema

1. Prevent further ocular trauma and confine the patient as soon as possible after injury. If there is no evidence of trauma, begin diagnostic testing for disorders such as immune-mediated thrombocytopenia, coagulopathy, intraocular neoplasia, and systemic hypertension.
2. Administer corticosteroid drops or ointment (0.1% dexamethasone or 1.0% prednisolone acetate) q6-8h if the cornea does not retain fluorescein stain and the hyphema is mild to moderate in severity.
3. If the hyphema is mild and is not secondary to uveitis, administer 1% to 2% pilocarpine drops 3 times daily and attempt to dilate the pupil every second day with phenylephrine (10%) to prevent synechia formation. If the glaucoma is secondary to uveitis, dilate the pupil with 1% atropine q8-12h.
4. If the hyphema is severe, administer 1% atropine drops q8h to control the presumed uveitis, and monitor intraocular pressure once or twice daily as the blood is resorbed. Rebleeding occasionally occurs within the first 5 days. Administer systemic corticosteroids (e.g., prednisolone or dexamethasone) in appropriate systemic antiinflammatory dosages for dogs and cats.
5. If glaucoma is impending, use a topical or systemic carbonic anhydrase inhibitor or topical dipivefrin.
6. If the color of the hyphema changes from bright red to bluish black ("8-ball hemorrhage") at 5 to 7 days after onset and intraocular pressure increases, surgical intervention may be indicated. If available, tissue plasminogen activator may be used to resolve the clot.
7. If the hyphema recurs and a laboratory evaluation has not already been done, obtain specimens for measurements of complete blood cell count, platelet count, buccal mucosal bleeding time, and clotting parameters. Ocular ultrasound to look for an intraocular tumor should be considered.

Note: Although uveitis is often present with hyphema, use of prostaglandin inhibitors is not advised because many agents also prolong blood clotting through their effect on platelets. Carprofen (Rimadyl) is claimed by the manufacturer to have a lesser effect on clotting than other nonsteroidal antiinflammatory agents.

ACUTE ANTERIOR UVEITIS

Acute anterior uveitis requires urgent treatment for the following reasons:

- It can be extremely painful.
- It may be associated with life-threatening systemic disorders.
- Permanent structural lesions may result in undesirable consequences (e.g., secondary glaucoma, iris bombé, cataract).

Emergency treatment of acute anterior uveitis

After diagnosis the following treatment is instituted:

1. Full ophthalmic and physical examination and laboratory evaluation to find the cause of the uveitis. Even if a specific cause is not identified, this approach allows potentially life-threatening systemic disorders to be ruled out.
2. Topical 0.1% dexamethasone or 1% prednisolone acetate q4-6h

Continued

Emergency treatment of acute anterior uveitis—cont'd

3. Species-appropriate systemic antiinflammatory drugs in moderate to severe cases. Consider IV dexamethasone or oral prednisone in dogs and cats, and flunixin meglumine or phenylbutazone in horses. See Chapters 3 and 11.

   Note: Use systemic corticosteroids at immunosuppressive doses with caution, or not at all, if an infectious cause is suspected.

4. Topical atropine 1% 3 times daily

5. Topical and systemic antibiotics typically have limited value in most forms of uveitis except those due to bacterial keratitis or systemic bacterial infections; they are useful for prophylactic application in patients undergoing immunosuppressive therapy.

SUDDEN BLINDNESS

A complete history and eye examination are necessary to diagnose the cause of sudden loss of vision. Differential diagnosis in dogs and cats includes the following conditions:

- Acute glaucoma
- Retinal detachment
- Acute uveitis with retinal detachment or optic neuritis (e.g., uveodermatologic syndrome)
- Retinal or vitreous hemorrhages (e.g., feline hypertensive retinopathy, rodenticide poisoning)
- Sudden acquired retinal degeneration syndrome (canine)
- After epileptic seizures
- Various toxicities (e.g., owner-administered marijuana in small animals, *Stypandra imbricata* toxicity in sheep, ivermectin in dogs/cats, enrofloxacin in cats)
- End-stage progressive retinal degenerations
- Acute onset of cataract (e.g., in diabetes mellitus)
- Inflammatory disorders of the central visual pathways (e.g., post-distemper encephalitis, reticulosis)
- Cerebral hypoxia after general anesthesia for routine procedures such as declawing or neutering or after cardiopulmonary resuscitation with a period of hypoxia

BIBLIOGRAPHY

Fritsche J, et al. (1996): Prolapse of the eyeball in small animals: a retrospective study of 36 cases. Tierarztl Prax 24:55.

Gilger B, et al. (1995): Traumatic ocular proptoses in dogs and cats: 84 cases (1980-1993). J Am Vet Med Assoc 206:1186.

Giuliano EA (2005): Feline ocular emergencies. Clin Tech Small Anim Pract 20:135.

Hamilton HL (1999): Pediatric ocular emergencies. Vet Clin North Am Small Anim Pract 29:1003.

Mandell DC, Holt E (2005): Ophthalmic emergencies. Vet Clin North Am Small Anim Pract 35:455.

Rebhun WC (1994): Ocular emergencies. Vet Clin North Am Equine Pract 10:591.

Severin GA (1995): Veterinary Ophthalmology Notes, 3rd ed. Severin, Fort Collins, CO.

OPHTHALMOLOGY OF EXOTIC PETS

Bradford J. Holmberg

OPHTHALMIC EXAMINATION AND
 DIAGNOSTIC TESTING
RABBITS
FERRETS

MICE AND RATS
RAPTORS AND PET BIRDS
LIZARDS, TURTLES, TORTOISES, AND
 CROCODILIANS

SNAKES
AMPHIBIANS

Ocular anatomy of the vertebrate has been remarkably conserved throughout evolution. Structures universally present in these eyes are an outer fibrous tunic (cornea and sclera), middle vascular tunic or uvea (iris, ciliary body, choroid), inner neural tunic (retina), and internal optical media (aqueous humor, lens, vitreous). This basic pattern, particularly as it applies to mammals, is outlined in Chapter 1. Familiarity with general ocular anatomy and physiology is crucial to understanding the clinical signs and pathogenesis of ophthalmic disease. The objective of this chapter is to discuss differences in ocular anatomy and provide the general practitioner with information pertaining to the ophthalmic examination and diagnostic testing, common ophthalmic diseases, and their treatments in exotic species.

OPHTHALMIC EXAMINATION AND DIAGNOSTIC TESTING

Many of the exotic animal species are not accustomed to frequent handling or the restraint necessary to perform a thorough ophthalmic examination. Knowing the appropriate technique for proper restraint not only allows a better examination but also reduces overall stress on the animal. For example, the rear limbs and spine of a rabbit should always be adequately supported. When stressed, they may struggle, possibly resulting in hyperextension of the lumbosacral spine and vertebral fractures. During the examination of raptors, the practitioner must always be cognizant of the talons, because severe injury can occur if appropriate precautions are not taken.

The techniques used in the ophthalmic examination are no different whether one is examining an exotic species or a dog or cat. A guide to these techniques is outlined in Chapter 5. However, evaluation of the tear film, intraocular pressure (IOP), and fundus may be more difficult in exotic animals owing to their smaller globes.

The most common method of evaluating the tear film is through the quantification of aqueous tear production with a Schirmer tear test (see Chapter 9). The strips used for the test are 5 mm wide, making their use difficult in eyes in which palpebral fissure length is less than 1 cm. Historically, these strips have been cut lengthwise to decrease their width, allow-ing easier placement. However, because this practice is not standardized, there is large variability between results, making interpretation of values difficult.

A phenol red thread test is more appropriate for the smaller eyes of exotic animals. The test is performed similarly to the Schirmer tear test. The thread is placed in the lateral canthus for 15 seconds, and the millimeters of wetting are measured. Normal values for the Schirmer tear test and phenol red thread test for a number of species are shown in Table 20-1. Qualitative tear film deficiencies are currently diagnosed in canine and feline ophthalmology through the use of the tear film break-up time. This technique is not yet in common usage with exotic species.

The phenol red thread test is the preferred method to evaluate tear production in exotic pets.

IOP evaluation, or tonometry, can readily be performed in conscious exotic animals. Two types of tonometers are most frequently used to evaluate IOP, an applanation tonometer (Tono-Pen) and rebound tonometer (TonoVet). Published IOP values for a number of exotic animal species are shown in Table 20-2.

The small globe (short axial length) of many exotic animals increases the difficulty of critically examining the fundus. However, performing indirect ophthalmoscopy should be a standard part of the ophthalmic examination and is facilitated through pharmacologic mydriasis and use of a highly refractive indirect lens. Lenses of 30, 40, or 60 D are particularly useful. Pupillary dilation in mammals is achieved with 1% tropicamide, usually within 20 minutes and persists for 4 to 8 hours. The pupils of birds and reptiles will not dilate with anticholinergic agents owing to the presence of striated muscle fibers in both the pupillary sphincter and dilator muscles. Achieving mydriasis in these species is more difficult and may require intracameral infusion of curariform neuromuscular blocking agents. More recently, topical application of vecuronium bromide (1 drop twice at a 15-minute interval) with or without the addition of phenylephrine and atropine has been demonstrated to cause consistent mydriasis lasting 1.5 to 4 hours in birds. Other curariform neuromuscular blocking agents used topically have been associated with severe side effects, including paralysis of

Table 20-1 | **Normal Values for Tear Quantification Tests in Exotic Species**

SPECIES	SCHIRMER TEAR TEST RESULT	PHENOL RED THREAD TEST RESULT
Rabbit	5 ± 3 mm/min	24 ± 4 mm in 15 sec
Rat	8 ± 3 mm in 5 min	14 ± 3 mm in 2 min
Mice	3 ± 0.2 mm in 2 min*	3 ± 1 mm/min
Birds (Psittaciformes)	5 ± 3 mm/min	22 ± 4 mm in 15 sec

*Modified Schirmer tear test strip.

Table 20-2 | **Normal Intraocular Pressure Values for Exotic Species**

SPECIES	TONOMETRY VALUE (mm Hg)
Rabbit	13 ± 6
Ferret	23 ± 5
Mice	15 ± 5
Rat	15 ± 5
Birds (raptors)	20 ± 4
Owls	11 ± 4

muscles outside the eye, especially those of respiration. Caution should always be exercised in the use of these agents topically or intracamerally. Their use has not yet been evaluated in reptiles. Mydriasis may also be achieved with general anesthesia, although this method has its own inherent risks and complications.

Pharmacologic mydriasis is difficult to achieve in birds and reptiles due to the presence of striated iridal muscle fibers.

Other diagnostic tests, including fluorescein and rose bengal staining, exfoliative cytology, and microbial culture, are completed as they are in the more common domestic species; they are described in detail in Chapter 5.

RABBITS

Ophthalmic Anatomy

Like many prey species, rabbits have large, laterally placed eyes. The angle between their orbits is 150 to 175 degrees, allowing a visual field of almost 360 degrees. Their stereoptic vision is poor, with only 10 to 35 degrees of binocular overlap. The orbit contains a large venous sinus, extending from the orbital apex to the globe equator and draining posteriorly to the pterygoid and cavernous sinuses. This extensive vascular network within the orbit is a common cause of significant hemorrhage during enucleation.

The nasolacrimal apparatus of the rabbit is unique. Although rabbits only blink once every 5 to 6 minutes, their tear film remains stable and they rarely have exposure keratitis secondary to evaporation. Tear film stability is likely enhanced by the presence of four orbital glands: the lacrimal gland, an accessory lacrimal gland with retrobulbar, orbital, and infraorbital lobes, superficial gland of the third eyelid, and deep gland of the third eyelid (harderian gland). Retention of the lacrimal lake may be facilitated by the lack of a superior lacrimal puncta, which would result in a slower rate of tear clearance. The nasolacrimal duct follows a tortuous route through the lacrimal and maxil-lary bones and passes in close proximity to the apices of the molar and incisor teeth before emerging through the nasal mucosa. Owing to several sharp bends and associated duct narrowing, blockage of the duct and subsequent dacryocystitis is common.

The most remarkable anatomic difference of the rabbit eye from that of other species is its retinal vascular pattern. Lagomorphs are the only species with a merangiotic fundus, in which the retinal blood vessels radiate horizontally from the optic disc, running with the myelinated nerve fiber layer. The optic disc is situated in the superior fundus and thus requires that the examiner use an upward gaze to view the optic disc. An obvious central depression in the optic disc (physiologic cup) is apparent secondary to lack of a developed lamina cribrosa and extensive myelination of optic nerve axons at that point. This appearance can be challenging to distinguish from glaucomatous cupping of the optic nerve head.

Orbital Disease

Exophthalmos is the most prevalent clinical sign associated with orbital disease. In rabbits, retrobulbar abscesses are commonly the cause of exophthalmos (Figure 20-1). *Pasteurella multocida* has frequently been implicated as the cause for these abscesses, although confirmation through culture is rarely attained. Regardless of the specific pathogen responsible, it likely gains access to the orbit either through infected molar tooth roots or from hematogenous spread. Diagnosis is made through clinical signs and ocular ultrasonography. Successful treatment is difficult. The abscess cannot be drained through the oral cavity because of the rich vascular plexus lining the rabbit orbit as well as the extremely caseous nature of the contents. Many cases require exenteration and long-term medical therapy with a broad-spectrum antibiotic. True *Pasteurella*-induced abscesses may respond favorably to parenteral penicillin therapy at a dose of 60,000 IU/kg q24h for several weeks. However, the use of penicillins in rabbits warrants extreme caution because they can cause anaphylaxis or fatal enterocolitis due to alteration of the normal gastrointestinal flora. Even with aggressive surgical and medical therapy, many of these abscesses recur and at times necessitate euthanasia. Less common causes of exophthalmos in rabbits include parasitic cysts, orbital neoplasia, and metastatic thymoma.

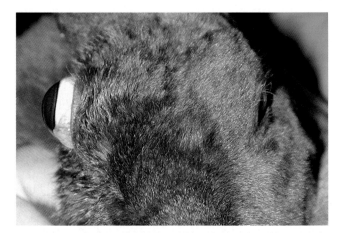

Figure 20-1. Marked exophthalmos of the right eye of a rabbit secondary to a large retrobulbar abscess. Culture of the abscess was negative for aerobic and anaerobic organisms.

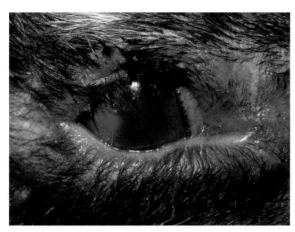

Figure 20-2. Entropion of the right upper eyelid of a rabbit with secondary ulcerative keratitis.

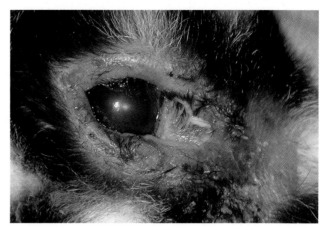

Figure 20-3. Marked blepharitis and severe mucopurulent ocular discharge in a rabbit with *Treponema cuniculi.*

The indiscriminate use of antibiotics with a gram positive spectrum in rabbits can result in severe, life-threatening complications.

Adnexal Disease

Adnexal disease is uncommon in rabbits, with entropion being the most commonly observed abnormality. Entropion may involve the upper and/or lower eyelids and may be primary or secondary. Primary (congenital) entropion has been described in the New Zealand white and French lop breeds. These breed predispositions suggest an inherited basis, but a mode of inheritance has not been determined. The lower eyelids are most commonly affected in New Zealand white rabbits, whereas the upper eyelids are affected in French lops. Clinical signs associated with primary entropion include epiphora, blepharospasm, conjunctival hyperemia, and, sometimes, ulcerative keratitis (Figure 20-2). Application of a topical anesthetic such as 1% proparacaine will facilitate ophthalmic examination by alleviating surface ocular pain. It will also remove any spastic component to the entropion, allowing appropriate surgical planning. Correction of entropion with a modified Hotz-Celsus procedure allows restoration of normal anatomic conformation, thereby preventing further ocular irritation.

Entropion may occur from cicatrix formation secondary to chronic blepharitis or blepharoconjunctivitis. Before any attempt at surgical correction, the underlying cause must be identified and treated. Otherwise entropion will likely recur. Cicatricial entropion is corrected using a Y-to-V blepharoplasty, with care taken to completely excise the offending fibrotic tissue during the procedure. Infectious blepharitis may result from exposure to *Treponema cuniculi,* or rabbit syphilis (Figure 20-3). *T. cuniculi* is a spirochete bacillus transmitted by infected dams. The most commonly affected areas are the vulva, prepuce, lips, nares, and anus. Clinical signs include thickening, crusting, and, possibly, ulceration of the eyelid. Diagnosis is confirmed through identification of spirochetes in biopsy or skin scraping samples. Darkfield microscopy enhances visualization of the organism. Three doses of parenteral benzathine penicillin G or procaine penicillin G at a dose of 42,000 IU/kg at 7-day intervals is the treatment of choice. Careful monitoring of the patient for potentially fatal enterocolitis is necessary. Blepharitis

may also be caused by self-induced trauma or maceration due to ocular discharge secondary to dacryocystitis, conjunctivitis, or keratitis (discussed later).

Neoplasia of the eyelids is rarely reported in the rabbit. The most common tumors of the eyelid are squamous cell carcinoma, fibrosarcoma, and melanoma. Squamous cell carcinoma must be differentiated from treponemal blepharoconjunctivitis, because both can have similar clinical presentations. Diagnosis is made through biopsy, preferably excisional biopsy, which may be curative in cases of squamous cell carcinoma. If diffuse disease prevents complete excision, adjunctive therapy with β-irradiation or cryotherapy may be used. If these modalities are not available, referral or enucleation is recommended. Fibrosarcoma manifesting in the eyelid may represent extension from the orbit. Careful examination, including globe retropulsion as well as advanced imaging using computed tomography (CT) or magnetic resonance imaging, may aid in distinguishing the extent of tumor involvement. Orbital involvement carries a guarded prognosis. Exenteration may be palliative and may increase survival time. Melanomas of the eyelid tend to be benign although locally invasive. Surgical excision is curative.

Conjunctival Disease

Conjunctivitis may be a primary clinical sign but is frequently associated with blepharitis or keratitis. Noninfectious causes of conjunctivitis include keratoconjunctivitis sicca, trauma (self-induced or due to foreign bodies such as straw, dust, seed husks), and environmental allergens. Keratoconjunctivitis sicca is uncommon, is diagnosed with the aid of a Schirmer tear test with accompanying clinical signs, and is frequently the result of chronic conjunctivitis. Treatment consists of artificial tear replacement therapy.

Bacteria and viruses are commonly present in infectious conjunctivitis; however, fungi are rarely encountered. Offending bacteria may represent overgrowth of the normal conjunctival flora and include *Staphylococcus aureus, P. multocida, Haemophilus* spp., *Pseudomonas* spp., and *Chlamydia* spp. Treatment should be based on results of culture and sensitivity testing but frequently includes topical chloramphenicol or ciprofloxacin used long term. Relapses are common, and the addition of systemic antimicrobial agents may be necessary.

Viral causes of ophthalmic disease are relatively uncommon in domestic rabbits in the United States. Myxoma virus is a member of the Poxviridae family and is endemic in the western United States (especially among brush rabbits in California), Europe, and Australia. The virus is transmitted by an arthropod vector, including both mosquitoes and fleas. Clinical signs are blepharoconjunctivitis with a thick mucopurulent discharge, blepharedema, and edema and nodule formation on the ears, head, body, and limbs. Myxoma virus was formally thought to have 100% mortality, but more recent data suggest that the prognosis varies according to the strain of the virus and species/breed of rabbit. Diagnosis is obtained from clinical signs, gross pathology findings, and polymerase chain reaction (PCR) analysis of tissue extracts. Treatment is supportive only.

Rabbit fibroma virus has also been responsible for the formation of flat, subcutaneous tumors of the periocular skin. Similar to myxoma virus, it is also a member of the Poxviridae family and is transmitted by an arthropod vector. Unlike with myxoma virus, lesions resolve spontaneously and treatment is usually not necessary. A predisposition of fibroma virus for cottontail rabbits is reported. Differentiation of this virus from myxoma virus is important because the prognoses for survival are significantly different.

Formation of a conjunctival membrane over the corneal surface is a condition unique to rabbits. This condition has been labeled pseudopterygium, corneal occlusion syndrome, conjunctival centripetalization, and epicorneal membrane (Figure 20-4). Progressive ingrowth of the bulbar conjunctiva occurs symmetrically and centripetally. The conjunctiva does not adhere to the corneal surface, separating this condition from true pterygium described in humans. The disease may be unilateral or bilateral. The cause has not been determined, although a collagen dysplasia has been proposed. Surgical correction is completed through a modified Arlt procedure. The conjunctival tissue is partially trimmed by sharp dissection, divided in half along the horizontal axis, and the leading edge is sutured to the conjunctival fornix. Because of the likelihood that this disease is immune mediated, application of cyclosporine, mitomycin C, or a steroid may decrease recurrence. However, topical administration of these agents may result in systemic immunosuppression and therefore they must be used with caution.

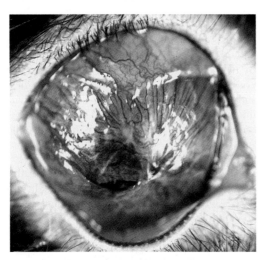

Figure 20-4. Pseudopterygium in a rabbit. The conjunctiva has grown centripetally over the corneal surface. Only a small area of cornea is noticeable (black ovoid area).

Nasolacrimal Disease

The tortuous path of the rabbit nasolacrimal duct predisposes it to recurrent dacryocystitis. Primary duct occlusion may occur with oil droplets or inspissated purulent material. Dental disease or osseous changes to the maxillary bone secondary to nutritional hyperparathyroidism may also lead to the development of duct obstruction. Of these, dental disease is alleged to be the most common cause. Malocclusion of the molars and premolars and, less frequently, the incisors results in retropulsion of the tooth and impingement on the nasolacrimal duct. Secondary infection ensues, and a wide range of organisms has been cultured, including *Neisseria, Moraxella, Bordetella, Streptococcus viridans, Oligella urethralis, Pasteurella,* and *Pseudomonas.* Clinical signs include epiphora, usually in conjunction with mucopurulent discharge. Secondary conjunctivitis may also be present. Dacryocystitis can be differentiated from primary conjunctivitis by digital pressure on the lacrimal sac. With dacryocystitis, a mucopurulent exudate can usually be expressed from the lacrimal puncta. Diagnosis is made on the basis of clinical signs and a negative fluorescein dye passage test result. A CT scan or plain radiograph of the head, sometimes augmented by dacryocystorhinography, may aid in differentiating the underlying cause and location of duct obstruction. Treatment is first aimed at correcting the underlying abnormality, especially correction of any dental disease (occlusal adjustment). The duct is then flushed with sterile saline through a 23-gauge lacrimal cannula. After flushing with saline, dilute povidone-iodine solution (1:50) is flushed through the duct. Repeated flushings may be necessary to maintain patency of the duct. If the duct cannot be flushed, long-term systemic antibiotic therapy (enrofloxacin 5 mg/kg/day) may be necessary to control infection. Recurrences are common.

Dacryocystitis is usually secondary to dental disease in rabbits.

As in dogs, prolapse of the gland of the third eyelid may occur in rabbits. This is uncommon and usually involves the harderian gland. Chronic conjunctivitis commonly persists without treatment. Surgical therapy is curative and involves performing a modified Morgan-pocket technique. The gland should not be surgically excised because there is significant vascularization of the gland, so severe hemorrhage may occur.

Corneal Disease

The large, prominent globes and decreased blink rate of rabbits may predispose them to corneal disease. Corneal ulceration is common; it may be associated with trauma, exposure after anesthesia, distichiasis, entropion, and trichiasis and may occur secondary to blepharoconjunctivitis or dacryocystitis. Thorough examination will aid in differentiating the underlying cause. If no conformational abnormality is noted, trauma can be assumed. Diagnosis is facilitated by the use of fluorescein stain as in other species. Uncomplicated defects are treated symptomatically with a broad-spectrum topical antibiotic, such as chloramphenicol, several times daily. Ulcers that do not heal, have significant stromal loss, or are infected are deemed "complicated" and require more intensive therapy. Nonhealing or indolent corneal ulcers are common and should be treated like those in dogs. Aggressive corneal débridement with a cotton-tipped applicator after topical anesthesia is recommended. A grid or multiple superficial punctate keratotomy may also be necessary to promote healing. Cytology and culture and sensitivity testing of infected corneal ulcers are recommended so that appropriate antibiotic therapy can be initiated. When there is significant stromal loss or a descemetocele is present, referral to an ophthalmologist is warranted. Placement of a conjunctival pedicle graft is the treatment of choice, although this procedure is more difficult in rabbits owing to their notably thin cornea (0.36 mm) compared with dogs (0.56 mm). After surgery, antimicrobial therapy is initiated on the basis of cytology and culture results. Reflex uveitis secondary to keratitis likely occurs in rabbits as it does in dogs, and application of atropine may help alleviate ciliary spasm associated with uveitis through cycloplegia. However, the presence of atropinase in the rabbit uvea may prevent its effectiveness. Because atropinase is not universally present and not all rabbits are immune to atropine's effects, its application is recommended. During treatment of corneal disease in rabbits, ophthalmic solutions or suspensions are preferred to ointments because of their normal grooming behaviors.

White corneal opacities are occasionally observed and may represent either mineral or lipid. Corneal dystrophy with subepithelial mineral deposition has been described as an inherited trait in American Dutch belted rabbits. Treatment is not usually necessary because the lesions do not cause visual deficits or keratitis. Corneal lipidosis occurs secondary to high cholesterol diets in most rabbit species. A hereditary hyperlipidemia has been described in the Watanabe rabbit. Lipid accumulates first at the limbus and then may proceed axially, resulting in either a subtle or marked opacity with obvious keratitis. Depending on the degree of keratitis and size of the plaque, conservative (dietary) therapy may be sufficient. However, if the plaque is large and causing visual deficits, a superficial keratectomy is recommended. Definitive diagnosis is obtained through histopathologic analysis of keratectomy specimens with appropriate stains such as oil red O.

Cataract

Cataracts may occur spontaneously or may be secondary to uveitis in rabbits. Some spontaneous cataracts (Figure 20-5) are suspected to be inherited in nature, although no genetic evidence is available because of the low incidence. Evaluation of laboratory New Zealand white rabbits revealed a 4% prevalence of spontaneous cataracts with no difference between males and females. Treatment is necessary only if secondary lens-induced uveitis or visual deficits are present. Removal of the lens via phacoemulsification is the treatment of choice. The procedure is similar to that performed in dogs, although the surgeon must take care upon entering the anterior chamber, because it is shallow and iris prolapse through the incision is more likely. Additionally, meticulous irrigation/aspiration of the peripheral lens cortex is necessary owing to the greater likelihood of lens fiber regrowth.

Uveitis was considered the most common cause of cataracts in rabbits. Rabbits were usually presented with a discrete, white, raised abscess within the iris overlying a focal cataract. Aqueous flare and hypotony were also present. Septicemia secondary to *Pasteurella* or *Staphylococcus* spp. was implicated as the cause of uveitis. Diagnosis was based solely on ophthalmic clinical signs, although many animals also had systemic disease consistent with septicemia. Diagnostic samples for culture and

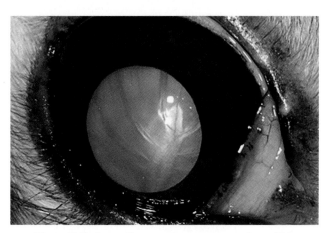

Figure 20-5. A complete, spontaneous cataract in a rabbit.

cytology via aqueocentesis were obtained infrequently due to the relative invasiveness of this procedure. When performed, organisms were rarely cultured or observed on cytologic preparations. Further evaluation of these iridal abscesses has revealed pyogranulomatous inflammation associated with lens capsule rupture (phacoclastic uveitis). Therefore the uveitis may have not been the inciting cause but the result of cataract formation with subsequent lens capsule rupture.

Intralenticular organisms have been identified in approximately 75% of rabbits with cataract formation with secondary phacoclastic uveitis. These organisms were 1 to 6 μm in size and consistent with the obligate intracellular protozoa, *Encephalitozoon cuniculi*. Rabbits are infected with *E. cuniculi* after ingestion of food contaminated with urine. Nonocular signs include neurologic disease (head tilt, torticollis, seizures, ataxia, paralysis) and renal disease. Lens infection occurs in utero owing to vertical transmission from an infected dam. Dwarf and young rabbits are predisposed. Clinical signs are usually unilateral and include spontaneous lens capsule rupture with resultant phacoclastic uveitis (including aqueous flare, hypopyon, and hypotony), iridal granuloma formation, and cataract formation (Figures 20-6 and 20-7). Diagnosis is based on clinical signs along with supportive results from serology (indirect fluorescent antibody test, enzyme-linked immunosorbent assay) or PCR analysis of lens tissue. Serology is quite

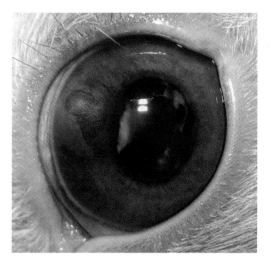

Figure 20-6. Focal lens capsule rupture, cataract, and iridal granuloma formation in a dwarf rabbit with *Encephalitozoon cuniculi*.

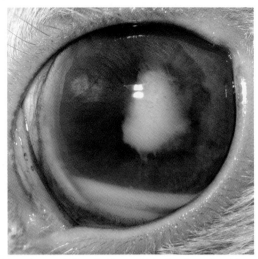

Figure 20-7. Same rabbit as in Figure 20-6, after 2 weeks without therapy. Phacoclastic uveitis is present as evidenced by lens capsule rupture, cataract formation, hyphema, and hypopyon.

sensitive, as rabbits mount a humoral response within 2 weeks, and in one study 100% of rabbits with ocular signs were seropositive.

Surgical therapy is recommended for *E. cuniculi*–induced lens capsule rupture and, when successful, is curative. The lens is removed by phacoemulsification and the iridal granuloma can be aspirated by automated irrigation/aspiration. Medical therapy alone may slow progression of the uveitis but rarely clears the infection. Medical treatment involves frequent use of topical antiinflammatory agents. Because of their relative lack of potential side effects, nonsteroidal antiinflammatory drugs (NSAIDs), such as flurbiprofen and diclofenac, are preferred over topical steroids. The antiparasitic agent albendazole has demonstrated efficacy in vitro, but its in vivo activity seems poor. The recommended dose of albendazole is 20 to 30 mg/kg once daily for 3 to 10 days, and that for fenbendazole is 20 mg/kg once daily for 28 days. However, they must be used with extreme caution because severe side effects, including death, have occurred with their use.

Encephalitozoon cuniculi is the most common cause of phacoclastic uveitis in rabbits.

Glaucoma

An inherited glaucoma is recognized in New Zealand white rabbits. Rabbits homozygous for the *bu* gene experience an increase in IOP at 1 to 3 months of age. Buphthalmos and blindness ensue, and over time the IOP returns to normal secondary to ciliary body degeneration. Histopathology demonstrates classic pectinate ligament dysplasia as the cause of glaucoma. Medical therapy is ineffective, and surgical intervention (cyclophotocoagulation, cyclocryoablation, gonioimplants) has not been reported. The *bu* gene is semilethal, and affected rabbits should not be bred. Primary glaucoma not associated with the *bu* gene is uncommon.

Most cases of glaucoma are secondary to lens-induced uveitis due to *E. cuniculi* infection. These cases may respond to topical carbonic anhydrase inhibitors applied every 8 hours (see Chapter 12). If satisfactory control of IOP is not accomplished,

a topical β-blocker, such as 0.25% timolol, can be added to the treatment protocol. Whenever using topical medications the animal must be carefully monitored for systemic side effects.

FERRETS

Ophthalmic Anatomy

Even though ferrets are carnivorous, their eyes have aspects consistent with eyes of both predator and prey species. The globes are laterally placed in a deep, open orbit approximately 32 degrees off midline, providing a visual field of about 270 degrees. Stereopsis is limited to approximately 40 degrees. The pupil is horizontally ovoid, decreasing light exposure and bleaching of the rod photopigment during daylight hours. Nocturnal vision is improved by the rod-dominated retina and a tapetum rich in zinc and cysteine, similar to that in the dog. Ferrets have a holangiotic retinal vascular pattern, and the optic disc is variably myelinated.

Orbital Disease

Like rabbits and rodents, ferrets have a well-developed retrobulbar venous plexus. This has been used as a blood collection site, with a technique similar to that described in rodents. However, this technique should not be used, especially in pet ferrets, owing to the potential for severe ocular complications, including globe rupture, corneal ulceration, hematoma formation, and exophthalmos. Exophthalmos may also be caused by retrobulbar neoplasia or zygomatic salivary gland mucocele formation. Lymphoma is the third most common neoplasia in pet ferrets as well as the most common retrobulbar neoplasia in this species. Exophthalmos is often the initial clinical sign of lymphoma. Complete blood count alterations and mediastinal masses may also be present, necessitating a thorough systemic evaluation. Because clinical progression can be rapid, early diagnosis and treatment with chemotherapy offer the best chance for remission.

The ferret's zygomatic salivary gland is located ventral and posterior to the globe. Trauma to the head has been implicated as the cause of mucocele formation. Diagnosis is based on findings of ocular ultrasonography and cytologic evaluations of fine-needle aspirates. Cytology may show mucinous debris with few red blood cells, inflammatory cells, and epithelial cells. Treatment is surgical removal via orbitotomy, which is curative.

Conjunctival Disease

Infectious conjunctivitis in ferrets is usually a manifestation of systemic disease. Commonly incriminated causes are canine distemper virus, human influenza virus, salmonellosis, and mycobacteriosis.

Canine distemper virus is a RNA virus of the morbillivirus genus. Ferrets are infected by direct contact with saliva, feces, or urine. Infection is now uncommon because of vaccination, which is recommended because mortality rates approach 100%. Clinical signs begin 7 to 10 days after infection with the onset of moderate conjunctivitis and mucopurulent ocular discharge. Additional ocular signs include blepharitis, keratoconjunctivitis sicca, ulcerative keratitis, and photophobia. With disease progression, anorexia, pyrexia, and hyperkeratosis of the foot pads occur. Death ensues within 12 to 35 days after infection, depending on the strain (canine versus ferret). Diagnosis is obtained in an animal with suspicious clinical signs by means of the indirect fluorescent antibody test on conjunctival scrapings. Cytologic examination of conjunctival scrapings may also show intracytoplasmic eosinophilic inclusions similar to those seen in the dog.

Human influenza virus types A and B have been responsible for mild conjunctivitis in ferrets. Infection occurs via aerosolized droplets from the nasal mucosa. Other clinical signs are anorexia, sneezing, pyrexia, and serous nasal discharge. Treatment is merely supportive because most adults recover. Neonates may succumb to a secondary bacterial infection, requiring systemic antibiotics. The clinical signs may mimic those of canine distemper virus infection, and differentiation of these two etiologies is important because the prognoses for survival differ significantly.

More substantial conjunctivitis has been noted with septicemia secondary to *Mycobacterium* and *Salmonella*. Disseminated mycobacteriosis caused by *Mycobacterium genavense* may cause generalized conjunctivitis or a focal lesion. Aggressive therapy with oral rifampicin, clofazimine, and clarithromycin along with topical chloramphenicol was curative. Diagnosis is obtained through PCR analysis of conjunctival biopsy samples. Systemic salmonellosis may result in conjunctivitis and is commonly accompanied by hemorrhagic diarrhea and fever.

Conjunctivitis in ferrets may be an extension of systemic disease and warrants thorough evaluation.

Cataract

Spontaneous cataracts are considered the most common ocular abnormality in ferrets. When their eyes were evaluated by slit-lamp biomicroscopy, approximately 47% of 1-year-old laboratory ferrets in one study had some form of cataract. Cataracts ranged from incipient to hypermature, and progression was common. The cause is not known, although genetic and nutritional (hypovitaminosis A) causes have been postulated. An autosomal dominant cataract has been described and is associated with microphthalmia, thickened irides, and progressive retinal degeneration. Surgical removal of spontaneous cataracts via phacoemulsification in ferrets with normal-size globes is similar to that in other species. The normal ferret is moderately hyperopic (approximately 7 D), and therefore one can assume that the aphakic eye is severely hyperopic and visual acuity is greatly impaired. However, aphakic ferrets appear to behave as if sighted but may be using olfactory cues and vibrations from the vibrissae to navigate.

MICE AND RATS
Ophthalmic Anatomy

The rodent eye is similar in structure to the rabbit eye. Posterior to the globe, an orbital venous plexus is present in rats, and an orbital venous sinus is present in mice. As in the rabbit, this collection of vessels and blood behind the globe can become a source of significant hemorrhage during enucleation. This area has been used for blood collection in laboratory animals but should not be performed in pet mice and rats owing to the potential for severe, globe-threatening complications, including exophthalmos, retinal detachment, globe puncture, and necrosis of the harderian gland. Three lacrimal glands are also located posterior to the globe: the intraorbital, extraorbital, and harderian glands. The extraorbital gland is commonly mistaken for a mass because it is located at the base of the masseter muscle. The harderian gland is located within the orbit adjacent to the third eyelid. This gland not only is important in production of the tear film but also may have a role in social interactions through the production of pheromones. Melatonin, a hormone involved in regulating circadian rhythms, is also produced by the harderian gland and has been suggested to be involved in extraretinal photoreception much like the pineal gland. However, because diurnal fluctuations in harderian gland melatonin concentration and secretion are not always present, the purpose of this tear component is not known.

The lens of mice and rats is large and spherical, resulting in a narrow anterior chamber. The size and shape of the lens suggest that the rat eye is hyperopic. However, retinoscopy of rat eyes has revealed a large variation in refractive error, ranging from near emmetropia (-0.1 D) to extreme hyperopia ($+19$ D). The large lens also distorts the image of the fundus obtained with indirect ophthalmoscopy, making the retina *appear* detached. The retina is holangiotic with blood vessels radiating from the optic disc. Because of the rat's nocturnal lifestyle, it is not surprising that its retina is dominated by rod photoreceptors. In young rats it is common to see persistent hyaloid vasculature extending from the optic disc toward the posterior pole of the lens. The patency of this vessel usually subsides over time but can occasionally cause transient vitreous hemorrhage. Common diseases of the rat and mouse eye involve the nasolacrimal system, cornea, lens, and fundus.

Nasolacrimal Disease

Chromodacryorrhea is the excessive production of "red tears." The red discoloration of the tears should not be confused with blood. Porphyrins in the tears secreted by the harderian gland are responsible for the reddish brown color seen with this condition (Figure 20-8). The harderian gland is innervated by the parasympathetic nervous system, and any increase in parasympathetic drive can result in chromodacryorrhea. Usually clinical signs are associated with nutritional deficiencies, chronic physiologic stress, chronic light exposure, or dacryoadenitis. Evidence of chromodacryorrhea should prompt the clinician to evaluate the animal for systemic disease.

Dacryoadenitis in rats is commonly secondary to sialodacryoadenitis virus (SDAV) or mycoplasmosis. SDAV is a coronavirus that is readily transmitted between rats by aerosol,

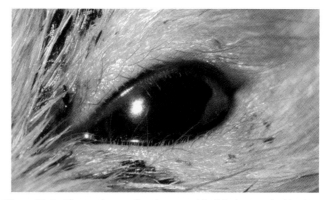

Figure 20-8. Chromodacryorrhea in a rat with sialodacryoadenitis virus.

direct contact, or fomite transmission. Early signs include blepharospasm, photophobia, and epiphora, but the most obvious finding is intermandibular swelling due to inflammation of the submandibular salivary glands. Chromodacryorrhea and exophthalmos due to inflammation of the harderian gland may occur over several days. Chronic cases may cause keratitis, ulcerative keratitis, keratoconjunctivitis, uveitis, hyphema, multifocal retinal degeneration, and secondary cataract or glaucoma formation. The virus is usually self-limiting, and the harderian gland may recover, depending on the degree of ductal squamous metaplasia and periacinar fibrosis. Mycoplasmosis is a primary cause of conjunctivitis in rats and may also cause dacryoadenitis. Other bacteria, including *Pseudomonas, Salmonella, Streptobacillus,* and *Corynebacterium,* have been implicated in conjunctivitis in rats. Treatment is based on culture and sensitivity results. Chloramphenicol (0.25 mg/mL) or oxytetracycline in the drinking water (3.5 mg/day) may be efficacious, depending on the offending agent.

Exophthalmos is not commonly observed in rats and mice. Most cases are secondary to inflammation of the harderian gland or iatrogenic trauma to orbital structures during retrobulbar blood collection. Aged rats may be presented with unilateral exophthalmos without signs of dacryoadenitis. In these cases retrobulbar neoplasia secondary to adenocarcinoma, carcinoma, and poorly differentiated sarcomas may be present.

Corneal Disease

Multifocal, punctate subepithelial white opacities are commonly observed in the interpalpebral fissure of both rat and mice corneas. Approximately 6% to 15% of rats have corneal dystrophy, with Sprague-Dawley, Wistar, and Fischer 344 breeds predisposed. The opacities are usually present shortly after birth and do not tend to progress. Corneal degeneration has been reported in mice, most likely secondary to environmental ammonia concentrations. Mice kept in clean cages or lower in racks had a much lower incidence of corneal degeneration than those kept in cages cleaned less frequently or in higher racks. Unlike dystrophy, corneal degeneration is not inherited and may progress, as evidenced by more severe corneal opacification in aged mice. Treatment is not necessary for dystrophy. Degeneration is best treated by prevention, keeping environments clean and ammonia concentrations low.

Cataract

Spontaneous cataracts occur in about 10% of rats and mice, with mice more frequently affected. These cataracts are usually focal and do not significantly interfere with vision. An interesting phenomenon has been observed in anesthetized mice. After approximately 10 minutes of anesthesia, anterior subcapsular cataracts develop and become denser over time. After anesthetic recovery, the cataracts gradually resolve over 24 hours. Theories for the formation of the transient cataracts included anesthetic type and changes in anterior chamber temperature. However, it has been demonstrated that these cataracts are secondary to tear film evaporation. With evaporation of the tear film, the aqueous osmolarity increases and fluid is lost from the anterior lens, resulting in a cataract. Prevention of these cataracts is easily accomplished by either taping the eyelids closed or applying a lubricating artificial tear preparation at the start of anesthesia.

Transient, anesthesia-induced cataracts in mice and rats are secondary to tear film evaporation.

Retinal Disease

Two retinal diseases in mice and rats warrant discussion, primary and secondary retinal degeneration. Primary or heritable retinal degeneration has been described in the Royal College of Surgeons rat. Degeneration occurs within the first 2 weeks of life secondary to impaired phagocytosis of rod outer segments by the retinal pigmented epithelium. This rat strain has been extensively used as a model for retinitis pigmentosa in humans. The most common form of secondary retinal degeneration is phototoxic retinopathy. There are two forms, determined by whether animals are exposed to extremely bright light for short durations or to low-intensity light for long periods. The first type results in damage to both the photoreceptors and retinal pigmented epithelium, and the second type primarily affects the photoreceptors. Factors associated with occurrence of phototoxic retinopathy include location of cage relative to the light source (usually animals in top cages are more severely affected), type of cage top (clear plastic versus metal), duration and intensity of light, age of the animal, and extent of ocular melanosis. Albino mice and rats are more sensitive because they lack protective melanin in the retinal pigmented epithelium. Phototoxic retinopathy most commonly occurs because of a light timer malfunction or human error.

RAPTORS AND PET BIRDS

Ophthalmic Anatomy

The structure of the avian eye is truly remarkable. The globes are very large and may outweigh the brain. The globe may have one of three shapes: flat, globose, or tubular. The flat shape is most common and has a short anteroposterior axis and a partly concave ciliary region. The posterior segment is hemispheric, increasing retinal surface area. Crows and diurnal raptors have a globose globe, in which the ciliary region protrudes farther from the posterior segment but is still somewhat concave. This shape contributes to high-resolution distance vision. Owls have a tubular globe, in which the concave intermediate zone (ciliary region) is elongated in the anteroposterior axis. The shape of the avian globe is formed and maintained by scleral hyaline cartilage along with 10 to 18 scleral ossicles. The cartilage is located in the posterior sclera, and the ossicles in the ciliary region. In addition to structural rigidity, these bones contribute to accommodation, becoming a buttress for ciliary muscle action on the lens. The globe fits snugly into the bony orbit, which is large, shallow, and incomplete. A thin bony septum separates the two eyes. The six of the extraocular muscles common to mammals are present (four recti, superior and inferior oblique) but are poorly developed, and therefore there is minimal globe movement. The retractor bulbi muscle is not present but rather is replaced by the pyramidalis and quadratus muscles, which are responsible for third eyelid movement. These two muscles are suspected to be evolutionarily derived from retractor bulbi of crocodilians.

Birds have upper and lower eyelids, of which the lower eyelid is more mobile. Meibomian glands are absent. The third eyelid is 90% transparent, arising at the dorsomedial orbit and covering the globe by extending ventrolaterally. Movement is achieved by contraction of the pyramidalis muscle as it loops through the quadratus muscle posterior to the globe. The leading edge of the third eyelid contains a marginal plait that acts much like a squeegee, collecting and distributing the tear film along the corneal surface. The tear film is produced by lacrimal and harderian glands located ventrolateral to the globe and adjacent to the base of the third eyelid, respectively. Two lacrimal puncta are present, allowing drainage of tears through the nasolacrimal duct and into the nasal cavity.

The anterior uvea of birds has a distinct role in accommodation. The iris musculature is predominantly striated, although limited amounts of smooth muscle and myoepithelium exist within the dilator muscle. Therefore pharmacologic dilation must involve the use of curariform neuromuscular blocking agents applied either intracamerally or topically. Topical use of such agents frequently does not provide sufficient mydriasis, although the inherent risk of intracameral injection limits this route. The ciliary muscles are also striated, allowing quick accommodation. Accommodation in the avian eye is accomplished through three mechanisms: change in the corneal curvature, deformation of the lens, and anterior movement of the lens. Three muscles are involved in accommodation. The muscle of Crampton is the most anterior ciliary muscle. It extends from the innermost scleral ossicles to the corneoscleral junction. With contraction, the radius of curvature of the cornea is altered. Brücke's muscle and Müller's muscle are posterior to the muscle of Crampton. Contraction of these muscles exerts force on the ciliary processes that are fused to the lens capsule equator. As these muscles act, the lens is squeezed or moved anteriorly to assist in accommodation. Similar to the muscle of Crampton, Brücke's muscle and Müller's muscle insert along the scleral ossicles and push against them during contraction. Using these three mechanisms, the avian eye has an accommodation range from 2 to 50 D.

To allow faster accommodation, the avian lens is softer and more pliable than lenses of mammals. It is relatively spherical in nocturnal species and flattened anteriorly in diurnal species. An interesting modification of the equatorial lens is the presence of the ringwulst, or annular pad located adjacent to the fused ciliary processes. It consists of hexagonal lens fiber cells arranged in a radial fashion and likely contributes to accommodation.

The avian fundus is perhaps the most interesting of all species. Indirect ophthalmoscopy reveals a nontapetal, anangiotic retina with a large, pigmented, vascular pecten extending into the vitreous. The pecten overlies the optic disc, obscuring its view. The three shapes of pecten that have been described are pleated (found in most species), vaned (present in ostriches), and conical (found in the kiwi). Although numerous functions have been proposed for the pecten, it likely serves a nutritional role and may contribute to aqueous production. Depending on the species, the distribution and ratio of rods to cones in the retina vary. A predominance of double cone photoreceptors is present that each contain an oil droplet in the chief cone. A remarkable adaptation further increasing visual acuity is the presence of a fovea. Most domestic species are afoveate, and others are monofoveate. However, many diurnal raptors and others (such as hummingbirds) are bifoveate, having a fovea centrally and another laterally. The lateral fovea is believed to be important for binocular vision, and the central fovea for monocular vision. The combination of several ocular adaptations along with a large occipital cortex (called the visual wulst) provides some birds with visual acuity several times better than that of humans.

Several ocular anatomic modifications exist in the avian eye that result in faster accommodation and possibly enhanced vision compared with mammals.

Ophthalmic Disease

Trauma

In raptors and wild passerines, blunt trauma is a common cause of ophthalmic disease. Clinical signs may be confined only to the globe, but usually other systemic signs are evident. Ophthalmic signs include periocular bruising, subconjunctival hemorrhage (Figure 20-9), conjunctivitis, hyphema, anterior uveitis, and posterior segment abnormalities. The posterior segment is most commonly affected, most likely because of the large size of the globe, its tight fit in the orbit, and its inflexibility due to scleral ossicles. A coup-contrecoup injury may cause anteroposterior shifting of the vitreous and lead to retinal detachment, retinal tears, vitreous and choroidal hemorrhage, or avulsion of the pecten.

The systemic condition of the bird should first be evaluated, and supportive care given. When only anterior segment abnormalities are present, prognosis for vision is sometimes good. If present, anterior uveitis should be treated with a topical NSAID several times daily. Topical steroids should be used with caution, because their systemic absorption may lead to generalized immunosuppression. When the posterior segment is involved, prognosis for vision is usually guarded to poor. Because vision is integral to catching prey, affected birds are frequently euthanized. Owls and other auditory hunters may be an exception to this rule and can possibly be rehabilitated and released into the wild. However, some authorities have suggested that changes in facial (and therefore aural symmetry) with altered globe size (buphthalmos or phthisis) or subsequent to enucleation may affect the birds' ability to hunt and survive using auditory cues. In pet birds or birds destined to a life in a rehabilitation facility, enucleation may be necessary if penetrating trauma or severe panophthalmitis is present. Enucleation

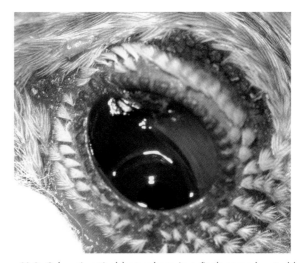

Figure 20-9. Subconjunctival hemorrhage in a finch secondary to blunt trauma. Erythema of the dorsal periocular skin is also present.

can be completed through either a transaural approach or a globe-collapsing technique.

Conjunctival Disease

Conjunctivitis is the most common ocular disease in captive birds and nonraptor species. Clinical signs usually involve a serous or seropurulent discharge, blepharospasm, conjunctival hyperemia, and increased preening activity. Causes include trauma from foreign bodies, excessive preening/pecking, environmental irritants, and infectious agents such as parasites, bacteria, virus, and fungi. Obtaining a thorough history and examining the bird in its natural environment may facilitate diagnosis. After performing a complete ophthalmic examination, the practitioner should obtain conjunctival swabs for cytologic examination and appropriate culture.

Traumatic conjunctivitis may be secondary to accumulation of foreign material in the conjunctival sac or excessive preening or pecking by cage mates. Foreign bodies can be gently removed through the use of copious lavage with balanced salt solution or manually with fine forceps. If trauma is secondary to the housing situation, separation of the affected bird is warranted. Treatment may not be necessary once the offending agent is removed. A broad-spectrum antibiotic drop, such as a triple-antibiotic formulation, may be used as needed. Topical steroids should be used with caution, because systemic toxicity can occur.

Several parasites, including *Oxyspirura*, *Thelazia*, and *Cryptosporidium* spp., have been demonstrated to cause avian conjunctivitis. Pet birds, especially budgerigars, are more commonly infested with the scaly face mite *Knemidokoptes pilae*. Clinical signs include scaly, proliferative lesions of the legs, cere, and eyelids. Diagnosis is made through identification of the organism in skin scrapings. Treatment involves systemic administration of ivermectin, diluted 1:10 in saline and given at $200\,\mu g/kg$ subcutaneously or orally. Treatment is usually curative.

Bacteria and viruses are the most commonly diagnosed infectious causes of conjunctivitis in birds. Bacterial conjunctivitis may be an extension of infection from the upper respiratory system or secondary to an opportunistic infection by the normal conjunctival flora. A thorough examination of the choanal region and periorbital sinuses is recommended. Offending bacteria include *Pseudomonas*, *Staphylococcus*, *Pasteurella*, *Citrobacter*, *Escherichia coli*, and *Klebsiella*. *Mycoplasma* spp. are not frequently isolated from the normal conjunctiva but are likely a common cause of conjunctivitis. *Mycoplasma* is contracted through inhalation or direct contact and is usually associated with an upper respiratory infection. Diagnosis is difficult and may be aided by PCR analysis of conjunctival, sinus, or tracheal swabs. Because mortality can be high, aggressive treatment with systemic tetracyclines or fluoroquinolones is recommended. For conjunctivitis not secondary to *Mycoplasma*, treatment is based on results of culture and sensitivity testing of isolates. The majority of gram-positive organisms are susceptible to triple-antibiotic preparations, and most gram-negative organisms to topical fluoroquinolones. If concurrent respiratory disease is present, additional systemic antimicrobial therapy should be initiated.

Numerous viruses have been implicated in avian conjunctivitis. Avian poxvirus is responsible for most cases of viral conjunctivitis in birds. Poxvirus is spread by infected mosquitoes.

Clinical signs, which appear approximately 10 to 14 days after infection, include unilateral or bilateral ulcerative blepharitis and secondary conjunctivitis and ocular discharge. Scabs and raised papules may develop on the eyelids. Diagnosis is made through identification of eosinophilic, intracytoplasmic inclusion bodies (Bollinger bodies) from skin or mucosal scrapings. Rhinitis commonly accompanies the blepharoconjunctivitis. Treatment is supportive, involving gentle cleaning of the eyelid margins and topical application of a broad-spectrum antibiotic for secondary bacterial infections. Other, less common viruses causing conjunctivitis in birds are adenovirus, reovirus, herpesvirus, and paramyxovirus (Newcastle's disease). Severe systemic signs, including death, are usually associated with these viruses.

LIZARDS, TURTLES, TORTOISES, AND CROCODILIANS

The class Reptilia is comprised of five orders: lizards, snakes, chelonians (turtles and tortoises), crocodilians, and the tuatara (New Zealand "lizard"). Snakes have several anatomic differences from the other reptiles and therefore are considered separately.

Ophthalmic Anatomy

Reptilian and avian eyes are remarkably similar. Except in certain geckos and the ablepharine skinks, well-developed eyelids are present, with the lower lid being more mobile than the upper. Chameleons are an exception because their palpebrae are constricted around the cornea and have limited movement. A lacrimal gland and a harderian gland are present ventromedial and dorsolateral to the globe, respectively. Tear secretions drain through an inferior punctum located in the ventromedial conjunctival sac and into the oral cavity. Chelonians do not have lacrimal puncta or a lacrimal duct, and therefore epiphora and periocular tear staining are commonly observed. A third eyelid is present and arises at the ventromedial orbit, although a true gland of the third eyelid as seen in mammals is absent. All extraocular muscles are present, but they are poorly developed, because reptiles tend to move their heads more than their eyes to scan the environment. Chameleons, however, have exceptional independent movement of each globe, permitting exact fixation on their prey. Scleral ossicles and cartilage are present, with the cartilage present from the posterior pole to the equator and the ossicles extending anteriorly. As in birds, these give shape and stability to the globe and serve as support for the ciliary muscle during accommodation. An annular or equatorial pad similar to the ringwulst of birds is present and plays a role in accommodation.

Reptilian eyes have a ciliary roll rather than the ciliary processes present in birds and mammals. The retina is avascular and receives nutrition from the choriocapillaris. The conus papillaris is an epithelium-lined, pigmented, highly vascular structure derived from the hyaloid and, like the pecten of birds, projects into the vitreous cavity (Figure 20-10) to provide nutrition for the retina. There is also a vast capillary network along its periphery. The conus regresses in crocodilians, giving the optic disc a melanotic appearance. All reptiles lack the choroidal tapetum typical of many mammals, but crocodilians have an accumulation of guanine crystals in the retinal pigmented epithelial cells (i.e., a retinal tapetum) that may aid

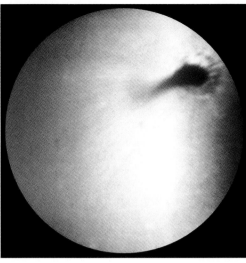

Figure 20-10. Conus papillaris of a gecko. The conus extends from the optic disc into the vitreous cavity.

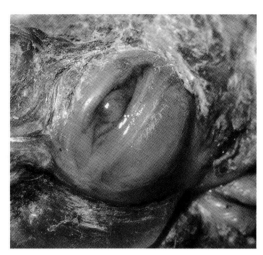

Figure 20-12. Severe blepharedema in a turtle with hypovitaminosis A.

nocturnal vision. The ratio of rods and cones in the retina varies greatly among species. Chameleons have a pure cone retina necessitated by their diurnal lifestyle and exact targeting of their prey. The ellipsoid region of the cone photoreceptors contains oil droplets, which are believed to function as light filters and to contribute to color discrimination.

Ophthalmic Disease

Suboptimal husbandry, including poor diet, inappropriate thermal gradient, overcrowding, overhandling, inappropriate humidity, poor sanitation, and environmental stressors, is the primary contributing factor to ophthalmic disease in captive reptiles. Ocular trauma from bedding material is common. Foreign material in the conjunctival fornices is frequently observed and may lead to conjunctivitis, ulcerative keratitis, or corneal perforation with resultant uveitis (Figure 20-11). After topical application of proparacaine, the foreign material can be removed either by gentle flushing or with fine forceps. Fluorescein staining will aid in evaluation of the integrity of the corneal surface. Corneal ulceration in reptilians is treated like that of mammals, with topical antibiotics and surgery if necessary. Parasympatholytic agents are ineffective and do not cause cycloplegia because of the abundance of striated iridal

muscle, as in birds. Addressing the husbandry issues is paramount to avoiding future insults.

Feeding an unbalanced diet, specifically one deficient in vitamin A, can lead to squamous metaplasia of ductal epithelium. This condition has been most commonly reported in young, fast-growing aquatic reptiles being fed primarily an insect- and/or meat-only diet. For unknown reasons, tortoises appear to be much less susceptible to hypovitaminosis A. With metaplasia, the orbital glands enlarge and the ducts become plugged with desquamated cells and debris, resulting in the ophthalmic clinical signs of palpebral edema and blepharoconjunctivitis. The palpebral fissure may be narrowed with edematous conjunctiva protruding through the fissure (Figure 20-12). Because the renal, gastrointestinal, and respiratory epithelia are also affected, early diagnosis and treatment are necessary to prevent death. In very early stages, changing the diet and adding a vitamin A supplement, such as cod liver oil, may reverse the clinical signs. However, as the disease progresses, parenteral administration of vitamin A at 1000 to 5000 IU weekly until clinical signs abate may be necessary. Parenteral administration of vitamin A must be done carefully, because oversupplementation will lead to epidermal sloughing.

The majority of ocular diseases in reptiles is secondary to poor husbandry.

Other ophthalmic diseases occur sporadically in reptiles. Congenital microphthalmos has been reported and may be associated with other craniofacial abnormalities. Abnormal environmental temperatures during gestation and/or incubation of eggs may lead to congenital abnormalities. Conjunctivitis in reptiles has been associated with three viruses: herpesvirus, iridovirus, and virus "X." Other mucosa-lined organ systems are usually involved, and stomatitis, rhinitis, and pneumonia are frequently present. Fibropapillomas in marine turtles often occur as aggregates around the eyelids and may become large enough to obscure vision and prevent normal feeding. The cause of the fibropapillomas is unknown, although replicating herpesvirus has been identified within the masses. Bacterial ocular infections are not common and when present are likely a manifestation of septicemia. Uveitis with hypopyon has been

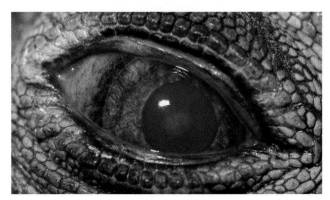

Figure 20-11. Superficial corneal ulcer secondary to trauma in a basilisk lizard.

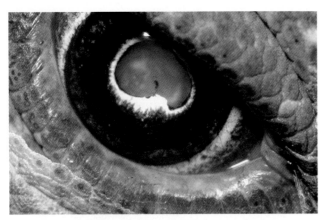

Figure 20-13. Complete cataract in a monitor lizard secondary to uveitis. Note the focal posterior synechia ventrally.

observed in septicemic reptiles. Cataracts are uncommon but may occur secondary to uveitis (Figure 20-13).

SNAKES

Ophthalmic Anatomy

Although a member of the class Reptilia, snakes have several unique anatomic alterations separating them from lizards, chelonians, and crocodilians. Like geckos and ablepharine skinks, snakes possess not eyelids but a clear, transparent spectacle. The spectacle is formed embryologically by fusion of the eyelids. Although it is transparent, there is a vast vascular network within the spectacle that has been demonstrated by microsilicone injection. The spectacle is, in essence, skin and prevents topical medications from reaching the ocular surface. The outermost layer or epidermal aspect of the scales is normally shed through a process called *ecdysis*. Ecdysis depends on food intake, humidity, air temperature, age, and presence or absence of systemic disease. Just before ecdysis the skin dulls, including the spectacle; at this point the snake is severely visually impaired and may become more aggressive. The outer skin and spectacle should be shed in one complete piece but may not do so, depending on systemic health and husbandry conditions.

Snakes do not have a lacrimal gland or third eyelid but do possess a well-developed harderian gland, located posterior to the globe. Oily secretions from the harderian gland bathe the subspectacular space and exit through the lacrimal duct into the mouth, as in lizards. This direct communication between the mouth and subspectacular space may allow ascending infections.

Unlike in other reptiles and birds, there is no cartilage present in the sclera of snakes. The cornea is relatively thin with only a single layer of epithelium. A thick corneal epithelium is not necessary because the cornea is protected by the spectacle. The anterior chamber is narrow, secondary to a large spherical lens. As in other reptiles and birds, the iridal musculature is striated. Accommodation in the snake is believed to occur via action of a muscle at the root of the iris that presses on an anterior lens pad to alter lens shape. In addition, the ciliary muscle exerts force on the vitreous, causing forward displacement of the lens. The retina is similar to that of mammals in that it contains both rods and cones; the ratio of rods to cones varies significantly between species, most likely owing to their diurnal or nocturnal lifestyle. Unlike reptiles, snakes do not

have oil droplets within their retinas. Retinal nutrition likely comes from the choroid, although a membrana vasculosa is present within the vitreous that may have some nutritive role. The optic nerve is similar to that in reptiles, but a conus papillaris is not present. Ophthalmoscopically, the central aspect of the optic disc is commonly melanotic, similar to that in crocodilians. This feature is suspected to be a remnant of the conus papillaris that regressed during ocular development. The conus may persist in the viper.

Almost all reported ophthalmic disease in snakes concerns the anterior segment, most likely owing to the difficulty examining the fundus. Not only does the small eye present a challenge, but mydriasis is difficult to achieve. Topical medications are not effective because of the presence of the spectacle. Additionally, the striated muscle in the iris would require the use of curariform neuromuscular blocking agents for paralysis. General anesthesia with injectable or inhalant anesthetics may produce sufficient mydriasis for fundus examination.

Spectacular Disease

Retained spectacles, subspectacular abscesses, and pseudo-buphthalmos are the most common ophthalmic diseases of snakes. Spectaculitis has also been reported secondary to mites of the *Ophionyssus* spp. that tend to congregate around the spectacle, where they are able to receive a blood meal. Spectacular opacification has been demonstrated after contact with aerosolized organophosphates or polyurethane solvents. Mycotic keratitis has also been described, likely secondary to penetrating injury of the spectacle and cornea.

Dysecdysis is abnormal shedding of the epidermal or superficial layer of the skin. When it occurs over the eye, the spectacle is retained and forms a cloudy, wrinkled opacification (Figure 20-14) that obscures vision. Many factors may contribute to dysecdysis, but poor husbandry, specifically insufficient humidity, is the most common cause of retained spectacles. Initial treatment is conservative, involving correction of husbandry issues. Increasing the cage humidity to at least 50% to 60% and ensuring proper hydration may be all that is necessary for dislodgement of the retained epidermal layers. If the condition persists, the snake can be soaked in water or topical acetylcysteine can be applied to help loosen the spectacle. Most times, after the husbandry issues are addressed, the retained spectacle is shed at the next ecdysis. If not, manual

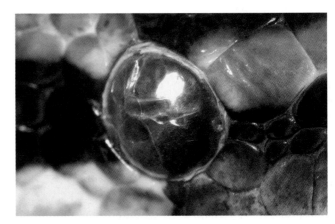

Figure 20-14. Retained spectacle in a Burmese python.

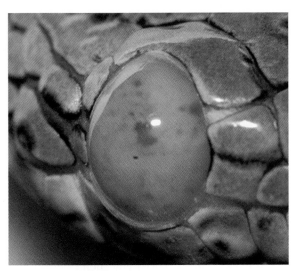

Figure 20-15. Subspectacular abscess in a green tree snake. Note the distension of the spectacle with purulent exudate.

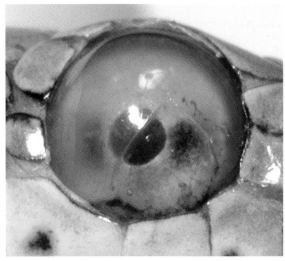

Figure 20-16. Right eye of the snake in Figure 20-15 after a wedge spectaculectomy. Note the wedge-shaped incision in the ventral spectacle that allows drainage and treatment of the subspectacular space.

removal may be necessary. This procedure usually warrants referral because it must be done with magnification, fine forceps, and extreme caution. If more than just the outer layers of the spectacle are removed, a severe exposure keratitis will ensue, potentially requiring enucleation.

Subspectacular abscesses occur when there is an accumulation of purulent debris between the spectacle and cornea within the subspectacular space (Figure 20-15). Infection arises within the subspectacular space via three potential routes: penetrating spectacular trauma, ascending infection through the lacrimal duct from the mouth, and hematogenous spread. On examination, anterior bulging of the spectacle is evident. The bulging is caused by a grossly distended subspectacular space filled with caseous purulent debris. Evaluation and treatment for septicemia and stomatitis are necessary, along with ophthalmic treatment; otherwise recurrence is likely. Treatment is surgical and is best performed by an ophthalmologist. After either injectable or inhalant anesthesia is achieved, magnification and Vannas scissors are used to resect a 30-degree spectacular wedge ventrally (Figure 20-16). Particular care must be taken not to injure the cornea. After partial spectacular resection, the purulent debris is lavaged from the subspectacular space with balanced salt solution. Aerobic, anaerobic, and fungal culture of the debris should be obtained. *Pseudomonas* spp. have been implicated as the causative agent, although other organisms may be present. Pending results of culture and sensitivity testing, a broad-spectrum antibiotic is applied topically until the next ecdysis. Fluoroquinolones and aminoglycosides have been efficacious in clinical cases. Systemic antimicrobial agents may be indicated if there are clinical signs of disease elsewhere.

Gross distention of the subspectacular space with clear fluid from the harderian gland occurs secondary to occlusion of the lacrimal duct. Because the globe appears (but is not) larger, this condition has been referred to as pseudobuphthalmos, but bullous spectaculopathy is a more appropriate term. Causes of lacrimal duct obstruction include ulcerative stomatitis, congenital atresia, cicatrization from trauma or burns, and blockage from an external granuloma or neoplastic mass. Treatment

involves creating a new drainage pathway. A spectacular wedge resection, as described previously, is efficacious although it may need to be repeated after ecdysis because of healing of the spectacular incision. Conjunctivoralostomy has been performed, although it requires significant skill and should not be attempted without proper training.

Retained spectacle, subspectacular abscess, and pseudo-buphthalmos are the most common ocular diseases observed in snakes.

AMPHIBIANS

Ophthalmic Anatomy

Amphibians are classified into three orders, tailless (Anurans such as frogs and toads), tailed (Urodelas such as salamanders and newts), and legless (Apoda). Many Apoda species live underground and have either no or rudimentary eyes. The anuran eye is the most highly developed of the three and has been extensively used in research. The structure of the adnexa depends on the animal's habitat. Larval amphibians and aquatic adults do not have eyelids. Urodelas have well-formed eyelids. Anurans have poorly developed, immobile upper eyelids and a transparent ventral conjunctival fold serving as a "false third eyelid" or lower eyelid. The conjunctival fold moves dorsally to cover the cornea when retractor bulbi muscle contraction causes enophthalmos. This contraction not only is important for corneal protection but also serves a vital role in swallowing. With retraction, the globe and associated musculature contact the oropharynx and aid in pushing the prey material into the esophagus. The globe is returned to its normal position by a levator bulbi muscle located posteriorly. The other six typical extraocular muscles are present, but their function is negligible. The tear film is derived from a lacrimal gland, a harderian gland, and superior or inferior (in the case of terrestrial salamanders) eyelid glands. The presence of lacrimal puncta and a nasolacrimal duct varies among species, but these structures are usually absent.

The uvea is quite peculiar in amphibians. The iris can be very colorful owing to carotenoid pigments and guanine crystals. A myoepithelial sphincter and dilator muscle is present, although pupil movement is minimal. The shape of the pupillary aperture varies dramatically at rest and with miosis but is circular with mydriasis. The ciliary body is triangular with numerous folds, which may continue to the pupillary margin and result in a nodule. As in elasmobranchs, a protractor lentis muscle is present. Contraction of the muscle moves the lens anteriorly, aiding in accommodation. The lens is large and spherical. Interestingly, some species are capable of regenerating the lens from either the pigmented epithelial cells of the dorsal iris or from the cornea, like tail and limb regeneration after amputation. Examination of the fundus is difficult but when accomplished demonstrates a remarkable vascular preretinal membrane within the vitreous. Urodelas that do not have a vascular preretinal membrane receive all retinal nutrition from the choroid. The retina is similar to that of reptiles, with some cone photoreceptors having oil droplets.

Ophthalmic Disease

Only sporadic cases of amphibian ocular disease are reported in the literature and are usually associated with systemic disease. *Redleg*, one of the most common systemic diseases of Anurans, is a catchall term for infection secondary to gram-negative bacteria including *Aeromonas hydrophila* and *Citrobacter freundii*. Redleg septicemia in fire-bellied toads was found to result in diffuse corneal edema, hyphema, hypopyon, iridocyclitis, cataract, chorioretinitis, and, sometimes, periocular blood-filled blisters. Experimentally induced septicemia with *Flavobacterium indologenes* caused anterior uveitis and secondary corneal edema in leopard frogs. Affected animals usually do not show response to therapy, and morbidity is high. Corneal ulceration infrequently occurs and may progress to bullous keratopathy. Because of the size of the animals, systemic toxicity after topical application of antibiotics is possible. Gentamicin diluted to 2 mg/mL has been effective and reported to be safe. Alternatively, the false third eyelid can be sutured to the upper eyelid to provide protection of the corneal surface.

The most commonly encountered and best studied ocular disorder in amphibians is lipid keratopathy. It was first reported in Cuban tree frogs and has since been identified in several other species. In hylid, leptodactylid, and ranid species, generalized xanthomatosis occurred, affecting not only the cornea but also brain, some viscera, peripheral nerves, periarticular soft tissues, and digital pads. Ophthalmic signs appear similar to those of corneal arcus, including a circumferentially progressive sparkly or creamy white anterior stromal infiltrate consisting of cholesterol and lipid-laden macrophages. Classically, excessive lipid mobilization associated with oogenesis was suspected as the cause because all affected frogs were female. A later study demonstrated that diet may be responsible, with frogs fed high-cholesterol diets demonstrating corneal lipid deposition independent of gender or stage of vitellogenesis. Nutritional therapy may slow the accumulation of lipid but is rarely curative. If lipid keratopathy is left untreated, diffuse corneal vascularization and superficial melanosis may occur (Figure 20-17).

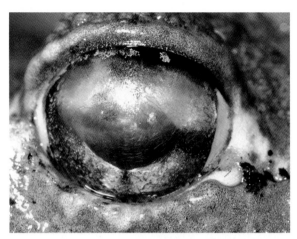

Figure 20-17. Lipid keratopathy in an African bullfrog. Corneal melanosis and superficial vascularization are also present.

BIBLIOGRAPHY

Abrams GA, et al. (2002): Conjunctivitis in birds. Vet Clin North Am Exot Anim Pract 5:287.

Andrew SE (2002): Corneal diseases of rabbits. Vet Clin North Am Exot Anim Pract 5:341.

Bagley LH, Lavach D (1995): Ophthalmic diseases in rabbits. California Vet 49:7.

Bauck L (1989): Ophthalmic conditions in pet rabbits and rodents. Comp Cont Educ 11:258.

Beaumont SL (2002): Ocular disorders of pet mice and rats. Vet Clin North Am Exot Pract 5:311.

Bellairs Ad'A (1981): Congenital and developmental diseases, in Cooper J, Jackson OF (editors): Diseases of the Reptilia. Academic Press, London, p. 469.

Burling K, et al. (1991): Anatomy of the rabbit nasolacrimal duct and its clinical implications. Vet Comp Ophthalmol 1:33.

Coke RL, Couillard NK (2002): Ocular biology and diseases of Old World chameleons. Vet Clin North Am Exot Anim Pract 5:275.

Cullen CL, et al. (2000): Diagnostic ophthalmology. Can Vet J 41:327.

Davidson MG (1986): Canine distemper virus infection in the domestic ferret. Comp Cont Ed 8:448.

Donnelly TM (1997): What's your diagnosis? Blood-caked staining around the eyes in Sprague-Dawley rats. Lab Anim 26:17.

Duke-Elder S (1958): The eyes of amphibians, in System of Ophthalmology, Vol I: The Eye in Evolution. Mosby, St. Louis, pp. 333-351.

Duke-Elder S (1958): The eyes of birds, in System of Ophthalmology, Vol I: The Eye in Evolution. Mosby, St. Louis, pp. 397-427.

Duke-Elder S (1958): Reptiles, in System of Ophthalmology, Vol I: The Eye in Evolution. Mosby, St. Louis, pp. 353-395.

Elkan E, Zwart P (1967): The ocular disease of young terrapins caused by vitamin A deficiency. Pathol Vet 4:201.

Felchle LM, Sigler RL (2002): Phacoemulsification for the management of *Encephalitozoon cuniculi*-induced phacoclastic uveitis in a rabbit. Vet Ophthalmol 5:211.

Fox JG, et al. (1979): Congenital entropion in a litter of rabbits. Lab Anim Sci 29:509.

Glorioso JC, et al. (1974): Microbiological studies on septicemic bullfrogs (*Rana catesbeiana*). Am J Vet Res 35:1241.

Good KL (2002): Ocular disorders of pet ferrets. Vet Clin North Am Exot Anim Pract 5:325.

Greenacre CB (2005): Viral diseases of companion birds. Vet Clin North Am Exot Anim Pract 8:85.

Harcourt-Brown FM, Holloway HKR (2003): Encephalitozoon cuniculi in pet rabbits. Vet Rec 152:427.

Jacobsen ER (1977): Histology, endocrinology, and husbandry of ecdysis in snakes. Vet Med Small Anim Clin 72:275.

Janssens G (2002): Ophthalmic diseases in the rabbit. Eur J Comp Anim Pract 12:61.

Kashuba C (2005): Small mammal virology. Vet Clin North Am Exot Anim Pract 8:107.

Keller CB, Shilton CM (2002): The amphibian eye. Vet Clin North Am Exot Anim Pract 5:261.

Kern TJ (1997): Rabbit and rodent ophthalmology. Semin Avian Exot Pet Med 6:138.

Krogstad AP, et al. (2005): Viral diseases of the rabbit. Vet Clin North Am Exot Anim Pract 8:123.

Langlois I (2005): Viral diseases of ferrets. Vet Clin North Am Exot Anim Pract 8:139.

Li X, et al. (1998): Neoplastic diseases in ferrets: 574 cases (1968-1997). J Am Vet Med Assoc 212:1402.

Loerzel SM, et al. (2002): Vecuronium bromide, phenylephrine and atropine combinations as mydriatics in juvenile double-crested cormorants (Phalacrocorax auritus). Vet Ophthalmol 5:149.

Lucas J, et al. (2000): Mycobacterium genavense infection in two aged ferrets with conjunctival lesions. Aust Vet J 78:685.

Marini RP, et al. (1989): Proven or potential zoonotic diseases of ferrets. J Am Vet Med Assoc 195:990.

Mauel MJ, et al. (2002): Bacterial pathogens isolated from cultured bullfrogs (Rana castesbeiana). J Vet Diagn Invest 14:431.

McCalla TL, et al. (1997): Lymphoma with orbital involvement in two ferrets. Vet Comp Ophthalmol 7:36.

Mead AW (1976): Vascularity of the reptilian spectacle. Invest Ophthalmol Vis Sci 15:587.

Mikaelian I, et al. (1994): Comparative use of various mydriatic drugs in kestrels (Falco tinnunculus). Am J Vet Res 55:270.

Miller PE (1997): Ferret ophthalmology. Semin Avian Exotic Med 6:146.

Miller PE, Dubielzig RR (1995): Autosomal dominant microphthalmia, cataract, and retinal dysplasia in a laboratory colony of ferrets. Invest Ophthalmol Vis Sci 36(Suppl):S64.

Miller PE, et al. (1993): Cataracts in a laboratory colony of ferrets. Lab Anim Sci 43:562.

Miller PE, Pickett JP (1989): Zygomatic salivary gland mucocele in a ferret. J Am Vet Med Assoc 194:1437.

Millichamp NJ (1990): Lipid keratopathy in frogs: histopathology and biochemistry. Invest Ophthalmol Vis Sci 15:587.

Millichamp NJ, et al. (1986): Conjunctivoralostomy for treatment of an occluded lacrimal duct in a blood python. J Am Vet Med Assoc 9:1136.

Millichamp NJ, et al. (1983): Diseases of the eye and ocular adnexa in reptiles. J Am Vet Med Assoc 183:1205.

Moore CP, et al. (1987): Anterior corneal dystrophy of American Dutch belted rabbits: biomicroscopic and histopathologic findings. Vet Pathol 24:28.

Munger RJ, et al. (2002): Spontaneous cataracts in laboratory rabbits. Vet Ophthalmol 5:177.

Murphy CJ (1987): Raptor ophthalmology. Comp Cont Educ 9:32.

Murphy CJ, Dubielzig RR (1993): The gross and microscopic structure of the golden eagle (Aquila chrysaetos) eye. Prog Vet Comp Ophthalmol 3:74.

Murphy CJ, et al. (1983): Enucleation in birds of prey. J Am Vet Med Assoc 11:1234.

Mutti DO, et al. (1992): Retinoscopic measurement of the refractive state of the rat. Vision Res 32:583.

Ramer JC, et al. (1996): Effects of mydriatic agents in cockatoos, African gray parrots, and blue-fronted Amazon parrots. J AmVet Med Assoc 208:227.

Ridder, WH, et al. (2002): Causes of cataract development in anesthetized mice. Exp Eye Res 75:365.

Rothwell TL, Everitt AV (1986): Exophthalmos in ageing rats with harderian gland disease. Lab Anim 20:97.

Roze M, et al. (2001): Comparative morphology of epicorneal conjunctival membranes in rabbits and human pterygium. Vet Ophthalmol 4:171.

Ryland LM, et al. (1983): A clinical guide to the pet ferret. Comp Cont Ed 5:25.

Seely JC (1987): The harderian gland. Lab Anim 16:33.

Stiles J, et al. (1997): Encephalitozoon cuniculi in the lens of a rabbit with phacoclastic uveitis: confirmation and treatment. Vet Comp Ophthalmol 7:233.

Wellehan JF, Johnson AJ (2005): Reptile virology. Vet Clin North Am Exotic Anim Pract 8:27.

Williams DL (2002): Ocular disease in rats: a review. Vet Ophthalmol 5:183.

Williams DL (2002): Rabbits, in: Petersen-Jones S, Crispin S (editors): Manual of Small Animal Ophthalmology, 2nd ed. British Small Animal Veterinary Association, Gloucester, UK, pp. 276-284.

Williams DL (1996): Ophthalmology, in Mader DR (editor): Reptile Medicine and Surgery. Saunders, Philadelphia, pp. 175-184.

Williams DL, Whitaker BR (1994): The amphibian eye—a clinical review. J Zoo Wildl Med 25:18.

BREED PREDISPOSITION TO EYE DISORDERS*

Paul E. Miller

Conditions listed are those observed or reported with higher frequency in the listed breed. Some are of breeding significance and others, such as chronic immune-mediated keratoconjunctivitis, are considered not inherited but seen more frequently in certain breeds (e.g., German shepherd).

The following list reflects recognized breed predispositions to ocular diseases. Predispositions to ocular disease may be present in breeds not covered here, but at this time there is insufficient data to include them.

DOGS

Afghan Hound

Cataract—anterior cortical
Cataract—equatorial
Cataract—recessive, equatorial/posterior cortex
Corneal dystrophy—epithelial/stromal
Deep medial canthal pockets
Eversion of the cartilage of the third eyelid
Glaucoma—goniodysgenesis with angle closure
Persistent pupillary membranes
Progressive retinal degeneration
Uveodermatologic syndrome (formerly known as Vogt-Koyanagi-Harada syndrome)

Airedale

Chronic superficial keratitis (pannus)
Corneal dystrophy
Distichiasis

Author's note: Considerable geographic variation occurs in breed disorders. Conditions are often reported in a particular breed for scientific purposes, when such conditions do not represent a common clinical problem in that breed (e.g., glaucoma in the beagle). Frequent reports in the literature of a condition in a particular breed may indicate study of the disorder in a successful experimental colony. A single report of a condition does not constitute a "breed problem."

Entropion
Progressive retinal degeneration
Retinal dysplasia

Akbash

Ciliary body cysts
Entropion

Akita

Entropion
Glaucoma—goniodysgenesis and angle closure
Multiple ocular anomalies (microphthalmia, congenital cataracts, posterior lenticonus, retinal dysplasia)
Persistent pupillary membranes
Progressive retinal degeneration
Retinal dysplasia—folds
Retinal dysplasia—geographic/detached
Uveodermatologic syndrome

Alaskan Malamute

Cataract—fibrillar nuclear
Cataract—posterior cortical
Chronic corneal erosion syndrome
Corneal dystrophy
Distichiasis
Glaucoma—goniodysgenesis with angle closure
Hemeralopia (cone dysplasia)
Persistent pupillary membranes
Progressive retinal degeneration

American Cocker Spaniel

Cataract—recessive/polygenic—anterior, posterior, or equatorial cortex
Chronic corneal erosion syndrome
Chronic superficial keratitis
Corneal dystrophy epithelial/stromal
Distichiasis
Ectopic cilia
Ectropion
Entropion
Eyelid neoplasia

Glaucoma—narrow to closed angle
Keratoconjunctivitis sicca
Lacrimal punctal atresia
Lens luxation (± secondary glaucoma)
Optic nerve colobomas
Persistent pupillary membranes
Pigmentary keratitis
Progressive retinal degeneration
Prolapse of the gland of the third eyelid
Retinal dysplasia—folds
Retinal dysplasia—geographic/detached
Staphylococcal blepharitis with hypersensitivity
Trichiasis

American Eskimo Dog

Cataract—anterior cortex
Persistent pupillary membranes
Progressive retinal degeneration

American Pit Bull Terrier

Distichiasis
Persistent pupillary membranes
Retinal dysplasia—folds
Retinal dysplasia—geographic

American Staffordshire Terrier

Distichiasis
Entropion
Persistent pupillary membranes
Progressive retinal degeneration
Retinal dysplasia—folds

American Water Spaniel

Cataract—anterior and posterior cortex
Distichiasis
Entropion
Retinal dysplasia—folds

Australian Cattle Dog (Queensland Heeler or Blue Heeler)

Cataract—anterior, posterior, or equatorial cortex

Ceroid lipofuscinosis
Chronic superficial keratitis (pannus)
Lens luxation
Persistent hyperplastic primary vitreous
Persistent pupillary membranes
Progressive retinal degeneration
Retinal dysplasia—folds
Retinal dysplasia—geographic/detached

Australian Shepherd

Cataract—anterior cortex
Cataract—nuclear fibrillar
Cataract—posterior cortex
Choroidal hypoplasia (collie eye anomaly)
Corneal dystrophy—epithelial/stromal
Distichiasis
Fundus coloboma
Heterochromia iridis
Iris coloboma
Microphthalmia with multiple congenital
    defects
Persistent hyaloid artery
Persistent pupillary membranes
Progressive retinal degeneration
Retinal detachment
Retinal dysplasia—folds
Uveodermatologic syndrome

Australian Terrier

Cataract
Persistent pupillary membranes
Progressive retinal degeneration
Retinal dysplasia—folds

Basenji

Cataract—a variety of forms
Coloboma of the optic disc
Corneal dystrophy—endothelial
Corneal dystrophy—epithelial/stromal
Persistent pupillary membranes
Progressive retinal degeneration
Spontaneous retinal detachment

Basset Hound

Distichiasis
Ectropion
Entropion
Eversion of the cartilage of the third eyelid
Glaucoma—goniodysgenesis with angle
    closure
Iris/ciliary body cysts
Lens luxation (± secondary glaucoma)
Persistent hyaloid artery
Persistent pupillary membranes
Progressive retinal degeneration
Retinal dysplasia—folds

Beagle

Cataract—anterior capsular
Cataract—posterior cortex
Corneal dystrophy
Distichiasis
Eyelid tumors
Glaucoma (primary open-angle)
Lens luxation (secondary to glaucoma)
Microphthalmia/multiple ocular defects
Optic nerve hypoplasia
Persistent pupillary membranes
Progressive retinal degeneration
Prolapse of the gland of the third eyelid
Retinal dysplasia—retinal folds
Tapetal degeneration

Bearded Collie

Cataracts
Choroidal hypoplasia (collie eye anomaly)
Corneal dystrophy epithelial/stromal
Persistent pupillary membranes
Progressive retinal degeneration
Retinal dysplasia—folds

Bedlington Terrier

Atresia of lacrimal puncta or canaliculi
Cataract—anterior, posterior, or equato-
    rial cortex
Corneal dystrophy epithelial/stromal
Distichiasis
Entropion
Microphthalmia
Nyctalopia
Persistent pupillary membranes
Progressive retinal degeneration
Retinal dysplasia—folds
Retinal geographic/detached

Belgian Malinois

Cataract—anterior or posterior cortex
Chronic superficial keratitis (pannus)
Persistent pupillary membranes
"Plasmoma"
Progressive retinal degeneration
Retinal dysplasia—folds

Belgian Sheepdog (Belgian Shepherd—Groenendael)

Cataract—anterior or posterior cortex
Chronic superficial keratitis (pannus)
Corneal dystrophy—epithelial/stromal
Micropapilla
Persistent pupillary membranes
"Plasmoma"
Progressive retinal degeneration
Retinal dysplasia—folds

Belgian Tervuren

Cataract—anterior or posterior cortex
Chronic superficial keratitis (pannus)
Corneal dystrophy—epithelial/stromal
Distichiasis
Micropapilla
Persistent pupillary membranes
"Plasmoma"
Progressive retinal degeneration
Retinal dysplasia—folds and geographic

Bernese Mountain Dog

Cataract—posterior and equatorial cortex
Distichiasis
Ectropion
Entropion
Optic nerve coloboma
Persistent pupillary membranes
Progressive retinal degeneration
Retinal detachment
Systemic histiocytosis

Bichon Frise

Cataract—anterior or posterior cortex
Corneal dystrophy—epithelial/stromal
Distichiasis
Entropion
Persistent pupillary membranes
Progressive retinal degeneration
Retinal dysplasia—folds

Black and Tan Coonhound

Cataract
Progressive retinal degeneration
Retinal dysplasia—folds
Retinal pigment epithelial dystrophy

Bloodhound

Cataract—anterior or posterior cortex
Distichiasis
Ectropion
Entropion
Eversion of the cartilage of the third
    eyelid
Keratoconjunctivitis sicca
Macroblepharon
Persistent pupillary membranes
Prolapse of the gland of the third eyelid
Retinal dysplasia—folds

Border Collie

Cataract—anterior cortex
Ceroid lipofuscinosis
Choroidal hypoplasia (collie eye anomaly)
Chronic superficial keratitis (pannus)
Corneal dystrophy—epithelial/stromal

Lens luxation
Nodular episcleritis
Optic nerve coloboma
Persistent pupillary membranes
Progressive retinal degeneration
Retinal dysplasia—folds
Retinal pigment epithelial dystrophy

Border Terrier

Cataract—anterior, posterior, or equatorial cortex
Persistent pupillary membranes
Progressive retinal degeneration
Retinal dysplasia—folds

Borzoi

Cataract—nuclear fibrillar
Cataract—posterior cortex
Microphthalmia/multiple ocular defects
Optic nerve hypoplasia/micropapilla
Persistent pupillary membranes
"Plasmoma"
Progressive retinal degeneration

Boston Terrier

Cataract—anterior, posterior, or equatorial cortex
Cataract—recessive congenital—posterior sutures/nuclear
Chronic corneal erosion syndrome
Corneal dystrophy—endothelial
Corneal dystrophy—epithelial stromal
Distichiasis
Glaucoma—closed angle
Haired medial caruncle
Iris/ciliary body cysts
Keratoconjunctivitis sicca
Medial canthal entropion/trichiasis
Persistent hyaloid artery
Persistent pupillary membranes
Pigmentary keratitis
Progressive retinal degeneration
Prolapse of the gland of the third eyelid
Strabismus
Vitreal degeneration

Bouvier de Flandres

Cataract—posterior cortex and nucleus
Ectropion
Entropion
Glaucoma—goniodysgenesis with angle closure
Persistent pupillary membranes
Retinal dysplasia—folds

Boxer

Cataract—anterior cortex

Chronic corneal erosion syndrome
Corneal dystrophy—endothelial
Corneal dystrophy epithelial/stromal
Distichiasis
Ectopic cilia
Ectropion
Entropion
Eyelid neoplasia
Macroblepharon
Progressive retinal degeneration

Boykin Spaniel

Cataract—posterior cortex
Corneal dystrophy—epithelial/stromal
Distichiasis
Persistent hyaloid artery
Persistent pupillary membranes
Progressive retinal degeneration
Retinal dysplasia—folds

Briard

Cataract—anterior or posterior cortex
Corneal dystrophy—epithelial/stromal
Persistent pupillary membranes
Progressive retinal degeneration
Retinal dystrophy (congenital stationary night blindness)
Retinal pigment epithelial dystrophy

Brittany Spaniel

Cataract—posterior cortex
Distichiasis
Glaucoma—closed angle or secondary
Lens luxation
Persistent pupillary membranes
Progressive retinal degeneration
Retinal dysplasia
Retinal dysplasia—folds
Vitreous degeneration

Brussels Griffon

Cataract—anterior, posterior, or equatorial cortex
Chronic corneal erosion syndrome
Corneal dystrophy—epithelial/stromal
Distichiasis
Exposure keratitis
Lens luxation
Optic nerve coloboma
Persistent pupillary membranes
Progressive retinal degeneration
Retinal dysplasia—folds/geographic
Ulcerative keratitis
Vitreous degeneration

Bull Mastiff

Cataract—cortical

Distichiasis
Ectropion
Entropion
Glaucoma—closed angle
Macroblepharon
Optic nerve hypoplasia
Persistent pupillary membranes
Progressive retinal degeneration
Retinal dysplasia—folds

Bull Terrier

Cataract—cortical
Corneal dystrophy—epithelial/stromal
Distichiasis
Ectropion
Entropion
Keratoconjunctivitis sicca
Lens luxation
Micropalpebral fissure
Microphthalmia
Optic nerve hypoplasia
Persistent hyperplastic primary vitreous
Persistent pupillary membranes
Progressive retinal degeneration
Prolapse of the gland of the third eyelid
Vitreal degeneration

Cairn Terrier

Cataract—anterior cortex
Cataract—posterior and equatorial cortex
Chronic corneal erosion syndrome
Ectopic cilia
Globoid cell leukodystrophy
Keratoconjunctivitis sicca
Lens luxation (± secondary glaucoma)
Ocular melanosis with and without glaucoma
Persistent pupillary membranes
Progressive retinal degeneration
Retinal dysplasia—folds

Cardigan Welsh Corgi

Cataract—anterior cortex
Chronic corneal erosion syndrome
Distichiasis
Lens luxation (± secondary glaucoma)
Persistent pupillary membranes
Progressive retinal degeneration
Retinal dysplasia—folds
Retinal pigment epithelial dystrophy

Cavalier King Charles Spaniel

Cataracts—cortical
Corneal dystrophy—epithelial/stromal
Distichiasis
Entropion
Exposure keratopathy syndrome
Keratoconjunctivitis sicca

Microphthalmia with multiple ocular defects
Prolapse of the gland of the third eyelid
Progressive retinal degeneration
Retinal dysplasia—folds
Retinal dysplasia—geographic/detached
Vitreal degeneration

Chesapeake Bay Retriever

Cataract—incomplete dominant, posterior cortex
Chronic corneal erosion syndrome
Distichiasis
Entropion
Eversion of the cartilage of the third eyelid
Iris/ciliary body cysts
Persistent pupillary membranes
Progressive retinal degeneration
Retinal dysplasia—folds
Retinal dysplasia—geographic/detached
Retinal pigment epithelial dystrophy

Chihuahua

Ceroid lipofuscinosis
Corneal dystrophy—endothelial
Distichiasis
Keratoconjunctivitis sicca
Lens luxation (± secondary glaucoma)
Persistent pupillary membranes
Progressive retinal degeneration
Senile iris atrophy
Trichiasis
Vitreal degeneration

Chinese Crested

Cataract—cortical
Entropion
Keratoconjunctivitis sicca
Persistent pupillary membranes
Progressive retinal degeneration
Retinal dysplasia—folds
Vitreal degeneration

Chow Chow

Distichiasis
Ectropion
Entropion
Glaucoma—closed angle
Persistent pupillary membranes
Pigmentary keratitis
Progressive retinal degeneration

Clumber Spaniel

Cataract—posterior cortex
Chronic superficial keratitis (pannus)
Distichiasis

Ectropion
Entropion
Macroblepharon
Persistent pupillary membranes
Progressive retinal degeneration
Prolapse of the gland of the third eyelid
Retinal dysplasia—folds

Collie (Rough and Smooth)

Blepharophimosis (micropalpebral fissure)
Collie eye anomaly:
    Choroidal hypoplasia
    Optic nerve coloboma
    Retinal detachment
Corneal dystrophy—stromal
Deep medial canthal pockets
Dermatomyositis
Distichiasis
Entropion
Eyelid neoplasia
Microphthalmia
Nodular episcleritis
Optic nerve hypoplasia
Persistent hyaloid artery
Persistent pupillary membranes
Progressive retinal degeneration—rod/cone degeneration
Progressive retinal degeneration—rod/cone dysplasia
Retinal dysplasia—folds
Retinal pigment epithelial dystrophy

Coonhound

Cataract—cortical
Chronic superficial keratitis (pannus)
Distichiasis
Persistent pupillary membranes
Prolapse of the gland of the third eyelid
Retinal dysplasia—folds

Corgi

See Cardigan Welsh Corgi, Pembroke Welsh Corgi.

Coton de Tulear

Chronic superficial keratitis (pannus)
Distichiasis
Persistent pupillary membranes
Progressive retinal degeneration
Retinal dysplasia—folds, bullae
Vitreal degeneration

Curly Coated Retriever

Cataract—anterior and posterior cortex
Choroidal hypoplasia (collie eye anomaly)
Distichiasis

Entropion
Optic nerve coloboma
Persistent pupillary membranes
Progressive retinal degeneration
Retinal dysplasia—folds

Dachshund (All Varieties)

Ceroid lipofuscinosis
Chronic corneal erosion syndrome
Chronic superficial keratitis (pannus)
Corneal dystrophy—endothelial
Corneal dystrophy—epithelial
Dermoid
Distichiasis
Entropion
Iris coloboma
Keratoconjunctivitis sicca
Microphthalmia with multiple ocular defects
Optic nerve hypoplasia/micropapillae
Persistent pupillary membranes
Progressive retinal degeneration
Punctate keratitis
Sudden acquired retinal degeneration syndrome
Uveodermatologic syndrome

Dalmatian

Cataract—cortical
Ceroid lipofuscinosis
Chronic superficial keratitis (pannus)
Corneal dystrophy—epithelial/stromal
Dermoid
Distichiasis
Entropion
Glaucoma—closed angle
Iris coloboma
Persistent pupillary membranes
Progressive retinal degeneration

Dandie Dinmont Terrier

Chronic corneal erosion syndrome
Distichiasis
Glaucoma—goniodysgenesis with angle closure
Persistent pupillary membranes

Doberman Pinscher

Cataract—posterior cortex
Deep medial canthus pockets
Dermoid
Distichiasis
Entropion
Eversion of the cartilage of the third eyelid
Eyelid melanomas, multiple
Microphakia
Microphthalmia with multiple ocular defects

Persistent hyperplastic primary vitreous
Persistent pupillary membranes
Persistent tunica vasculosa lentis
"Plasmoma"
Progressive retinal degeneration
Retinal dysplasia—folds

English Bulldog

Chronic corneal erosion syndrome
Chronic staphylococcal blepharitis
Chronic superficial keratitis
Distichiasis
Ectopic cilia
Ectropion
Entropion
Keratoconjunctivitis sicca
Macroblepharon
Nasal fold trichiasis
Persistent pupillary membranes
Prolapse of the gland of the third eyelid
Redundant forehead skin
Retinal dysplasia—folds
Trichiasis

English Cocker Spaniel

Cataract—anterior, posterior, or equatorial
Cataract—nuclear fibrillar
Corneal dystrophy—epithelial/stromal
Distichiasis
Ectropion
Entropion
Glaucoma—goniodysgenesis with angle closure
Imperforate lacrimal puncta
Keratoconjunctivitis sicca
Optic nerve coloboma
Persistent pupillary membranes
Progressive retinal degeneration
Retinal dysplasia—folds
Retinal dysplasia—geographic/detached

English Setter

Cataract—posterior cortex
Ceroid lipofuscinosis
Distichiasis
Ectropion
Entropion
Eversion of the cartilage of the third eyelid
Eyelid neoplasia
Progressive retinal degeneration
Retinal dysplasia—folds
Retinal pigment epithelial dystrophy

English Springer Spaniel

Cataract—cortical

Cataract—nuclear fibrillar
Chronic corneal erosion syndrome
Chronic superficial keratitis (pannus)
Corneal dystrophy epithelial/stromal
Distichiasis
Ectropion
Entropion
Eyelid neoplasia
Glaucoma—goniodysgenesis with angle closure
Persistent pupillary membranes
"Plasmoma"
Progressive retinal degeneration
Retinal dysplasia—folds
Retinal dysplasia—geographic/detached
Retinal pigment epithelial dystrophy

English Toy Spaniel (King Charles, Prince Charles, Ruby, Blenheim)

Cataract—anterior or posterior cortex
Corneal dystrophy epithelial/stromal
Distichiasis
Entropion
Persistent hyaloid artery
Pigmentary keratitis
Progressive retinal degeneration
Retinal dysplasia—folds
Retinal dysplasia—geographic

Entlebucher

Cataract—anterior, posterior, or equatorial cortex
Cataract—autosomal recessive—posterior cortex
Distichiasis
Persistent pupillary membranes
Progressive retinal degeneration

Field Spaniel

Cataract—anterior cortex
Distichiasis
Ectropion
Entropion
Persistent pupillary membranes
Progressive retinal degeneration
Retinal dysplasia—folds

Flat Coated Retriever

Cataract—cortical
Corneal dystrophy—epithelial/stromal
Distichiasis
Entropion
Glaucoma—goniodysgenesis with angle closure
Micropapilla
Persistent pupillary membranes
Progressive retinal degeneration
Retinal pigment epithelial cell dystrophy

Fox Terrier (Smooth)

Cataract—anterior or posterior cortical
Glaucoma—primary open angle?
Lens luxation (± secondary glaucoma)
Persistent pupillary membranes

Fox Terrier (Wirehaired)

Cataract—anterior, posterior, or equatorial cortex
Chronic corneal erosion syndrome
Corneal dystrophy (epithelial, endothelial)
Distichiasis
Glaucoma—primary open angle?
Lens luxation (± secondary glaucoma)
Persistent pupillary membranes
Progressive retinal degeneration
Superficial corneal erosion syndrome

French Bulldog

Cataract—cortical
Cataract—posterior lenticonus
Distichiasis
Entropion
Persistent pupillary membranes
Retinal dysplasia—folds

German Shepherd

Cataract—incomplete dominant—congenital—rare
Cataract—posterior cortical or nuclear
Chronic corneal erosion syndrome
Chronic superficial keratitis (pannus)
Corneal dystrophy—epithelial/stromal
Conjunctival melanoma
Distichiasis
Deep medial canthus pockets
Dermoid
Epibulbar melanoma
Eversion of the cartilage of the third eyelid
Medial canthal erosion syndrome
Myopia
Optic nerve hypoplasia/micropapilla
Persistent pupillary membranes
"Plasmoma"
Progressive retinal degeneration
Retinal dysplasia—folds
Retinal pigment epithelial dystrophy (Europe)

German Shorthaired Pointer

Cataract—posterior cortex
Cone degeneration—day blindness
Distichiasis
Entropion
Eversion of the cartilage of the third eyelid

Persistent hyperplastic primary vitreous
Persistent pupillary membranes
Persistent tunica vasculosa lentis
Progressive retinal degeneration
Retinal dysplasia—folds
Strabismus

German Wirehaired Pointer

Cataract—posterior cortex
Distichiasis
Entropion
Retinal dysplasia—folds

Giant Schnauzer

Cataract—posterior or equatorial cortex
Everted cartilage of the third eyelid
Glaucoma—goniodysgenesis with angle closure
Persistent hyperplastic primary vitreous
Persistent pupillary membranes
Progressive retinal degeneration
Retinal dysplasia—folds

Golden Retriever

Adult onset ciliary body neoplasia
Cataract—anterior cortex
Cataract—incomplete dominant—posterior cortex
Chronic corneal erosion syndrome
Congenital tumors of the iris and ciliary body
Corneal dystrophy—epithelial/stromal
Distichiasis
Entropion
Glaucoma—primary angle closure or secondary
Persistent pupillary membranes
Iris/ciliary body cysts (± secondary glaucoma)
Pigmentary uveitis
Progressive retinal degeneration
Pseudopapilledema (heavily myelinated optic disc)
Retinal pigment epithelial dystrophy
Retinal dysplasia—folds
Retinal dysplasia—geographic/detached
Uveodermatologic syndrome

Gordon Setter

Cataract—posterior cortex
Deep medial canthal pockets
Distichiasis
Ectropion
Entropion
Iris/ciliary body cysts
Persistent pupillary membranes
Progressive retinal degeneration
Retinal dysplasia—folds

Great Dane

Cataract—anterior, posterior, or equatorial cortex
Congenital nyctalopia
Deep inferior conjunctival fornix
Deep medial canthal pockets
Distichiasis
Ectropion
Entropion
Eversion of the cartilage of the third eyelid
Glaucoma—ganiodysgenesis with angle closure
Iris/ciliary body cysts (± secondary glaucoma)
Multiple ocular defects with merling
Persistent pupillary membranes
Progressive retinal degeneration

Great Pyrenees

Cataract—anterior, posterior, or equatorial cortex
Corneal dystrophy—epithelial/stromal
Deep medial canthus pockets
Distichiasis
Ectropion
Entropion
Persistent pupillary membranes
Progressive retinal degeneration
Retinal dysplasia—folds

Greater Swiss Mountain Dog

Cataract—anterior, posterior, or equatorial cortex
Distichiasis
Entropion
Optic nerve hypoplasia/micropapilla
Persistent pupillary membranes
Retinal dysplasia—folds

Greyhound

Cataract—posterior cortex
Chronic superficial keratitis (pannus)
Corneal dystrophy
Deep medial canthal pockets
Glaucoma—secondary
Lens luxation
Progressive retinal degeneration
Retinal dysplasia—folds
Retinal pigment epithelial dystrophy
Vitreal degeneration

Havanese

Cataract—posterior cortex
Distichiasis
Lens luxation
Persistent pupillary membranes
Progressive retinal degeneration

(Irish Setter area header)

Prolapse of the gland of the third eyelid
Retinal detachment
Retinal dysplasia—folds
Vitreous degeneration

Irish Setter

Cataract—anterior or posterior cortex
Chronic corneal erosion syndrome
Deep inferior conjunctival fornix
Distichiasis
Entropion
Everted cartilage of the third eyelid
Glaucoma
Optic nerve hypoplasia
Persistent hyaloid artery
Persistent hyperplastic primary vitreous
Persistent pupillary membranes
Progressive retinal degeneration—rod/cone dysplasia
Retinal pigment epithelial dystrophy
Uveodermatologic syndrome

Irish Water Spaniel

Cataract—anterior, posterior, or equatorial cortex
Distichiasis
Persistent hyaloid artery
Persistent pupillary membranes
Progressive retinal degeneration

Irish Wolfhound

Cataract—posterior cortex or nuclear
Corneal dystrophy—epithelial/stromal
Distichiasis
Entropion
Everted cartilage of the third eyelid
Iris/ciliary body cysts
Optic nerve hypoplasia/micropapilla
Progressive retinal degeneration
Retinal dysplasia—folds

Italian Greyhound

Cataract—anterior, posterior, or equatorial cortex
Glaucoma—associated with vitreal degeneration
Lens luxation
Persistent hyaloid artery
Persistent pupillary membranes
Progressive retinal degeneration
Retinal detachment
Vitreous degeneration

Jack Russell Terrier

Cataract—anterior or posterior cortex
Distichiasis

Lens luxation (± secondary glaucoma)
Persistent pupillary membranes
Progressive retinal degeneration
Vitreal degeneration

Japanese Chin

Cataract—anterior, posterior, or equatorial cortex
Chronic superficial keratitis (pannus)
Distichiasis
Entropion
Exposure/pigmentary keratitis
Persistent hyaloid artery
Persistent hyperplastic primary vitreous
Persistent pupillary membranes
Persistent tunica vasculosa lentis
Progressive retinal degeneration
Retinal dysplasia—folds/geographic
Ulcerative keratitis
Vitreal degeneration

Keeshond

Cataract—cortical
Distichiasis
Ectopic cilia
Entropion
Glaucoma—open angle
Iris/ciliary body cysts
Progressive retinal degeneration
Retinal pigment epithelial dystrophy

Kerry Blue Terrier

Cataract—posterior cortex
Corneal dystrophy—epithelial/stromal
Distichiasis
Entropion
Keratoconjunctivitis sicca
Persistent pupillary membranes
Progressive retinal degeneration
Trichiasis
Vitreal degeneration

Komondor

Cataract—posterior cortical
Distichiasis
Ectropion
Entropion
Persistent pupillary membranes
Trichiasis

Kuvasz

Distichiasis
Ectropion
Entropion
Persistent pupillary membranes
Progressive retinal degeneration

Labrador Retriever

Cataract—anterior or equatorial cortex
Cataract—incomplete dominant—posterior cortical
Ciliary body neoplasia
Corneal dystrophy—epithelial/stromal
Deep medial canthal pockets
Distichiasis
Entropion
Iris/ciliary body cysts
Persistent pupillary membranes
Progressive retinal degeneration
Pseudopapilledema (heavily myelinated optic disc)
Retinal dysplasia—detached
Retinal dysplasia—folds/geographic
Retinal dysplasia with skeletal abnormalities
Retinal pigment epithelial dystrophy

Lakeland Terrier

Cataract—posterior cortical
Distichiasis
Lens luxation (± secondary glaucoma)
Persistent pupillary membranes

Leonberger

Cataract—posterior cortex
Distichiasis
Ectropion
Entropion
Everted cartilage of the third eyelid
Glaucoma—primary angle closure
Iris/ciliary body cysts
Macroblepharon
Persistent pupillary membranes

Lhasa Apso

Cataract—anterior or posterior cortex
Chronic corneal erosion syndrome
Ciliated caruncle
Corneal dystrophy—epithelial/stromal
Distichiasis
Ectopic cilia
Entropion, medial lower lid
Euryblepharon
Keratoconjunctivitis sicca
Persistent pupillary membranes
Pigmentary keratitis/exposure keratitis
Progressive retinal degeneration
Prolapse of the gland of the third eyelid
Retinal dysplasia—folds/geographic
Vitreal degeneration

Lowchen

Cataract—anterior or posterior cortex
Distichiasis

Persistent pupillary membranes
Progressive retinal degeneration
Vitreal degeneration

Maltese Terrier

Canine allergic inhalant conjunctivitis (atopy)
Distichiasis
Ectopic cilia
Entropion (lower medial canthus)
Glaucoma—narrow to closed angle
Haired medial caruncle
Persistent pupillary membranes
Progressive retinal degeneration
Retinal dysplasia—folds
Tear-staining syndrome

Manchester Terrier

Cataract—posterior cortex
Lens luxation (± secondary glaucoma)
Progressive retinal degeneration

Mastiff

Cataract—nuclear and cortical
Distichiasis
Ectropion
Entropion
Eversion of the cartilage of the third eyelid
Glaucoma
Iris/ciliary body cysts
Macroblepharon
Persistent pupillary membranes
Progressive retinal degeneration
Prolapse of the gland of the third eyelid
Retinal dysplasia—folds/geographic

Miniature Australian Shepherd

Choroidal hypoplasia (collie eye anomaly)
Distichiasis
Fundus colobomas
Iris coloboma
Persistent pupillary membranes

Miniature Bull Terrier

Corneal dystrophy—endothelial
Entropion
Lens luxation
Optic nerve hypoplasia/micropapilla
Persistent pupillary membranes
Vitreal degeneration

Miniature Pinscher

Chronic superficial keratitis (pannus)
Corneal dystrophy—epithelial/stromal
Lens luxation
Persistent hyaloid artery

Persistent pupillary membranes
Progressive retinal degeneration
Vitreal degeneration

Miniature Schnauzer

Atresia of lacrimal puncta and canaliculi
Cataract—recessive—nuclear/posterior cortex—congenital
Cataract—recessive—posterior cortex
Ceroid lipofuscinosis
Corneal dystrophy—epithelial/stromal
Distichiasis
Entropion
Keratoconjunctivitis sicca
Lens luxation
Microphthalmia/multiple ocular defects
Optic nerve hypoplasia
Persistent hyperplastic primary vitreous
Persistent pupillary membranes
Progressive retinal degeneration—rod/cone dysplasia
Retinal dysplasia with or without persistent hyperplastic primary vitreous
Sudden acquired retinal degeneration syndrome

Newfoundland

Cataract—posterior cortex
Deep medial canthal pockets
Ectropion
Entropion
Euryblepharon
Eversion of the cartilage of the third eyelid
Glaucoma
Iris/ciliary body cysts
Persistent pupillary membranes
Progressive retinal degeneration
Prolapse of the gland of the third eyelid
Retinal dysplasia—folds

Norfolk Terrier

Cataract—posterior cortex
Lens luxation
Optic nerve coloboma
Optic nerve hypoplasia/micropapilla
Persistent pupillary membranes

Norwegian Buhund

Cataract— dominant—nuclear fibrillar

Norwegian Elkhound

Cataract—posterior or equatorial cortex
Distichiasis
Entropion
Glaucoma—primary open angle
Lens luxation (with primary open angle glaucoma)

Persistent pupillary membranes
Progressive retinal degeneration—early rod degeneration
Progressive retinal degeneration—rod dysplasia
Retinal dysplasia—folds

Norwich Terrier

Cataract—posterior or equatorial cortex
Corneal dystrophy—epithelial/stromal
Lens luxation
Persistent pupillary membranes
Prolapse of the gland of the third eyelid

Nova Scotia Duck Tolling Retriever

Cataract—posterior cortex
Corneal dystrophy—epithelial/stromal
Distichiasis
Optic nerve hypoplasia/micropapilla
Persistent hyaloid artery
Persistent pupillary membranes
Progressive retinal degeneration
Retinal dysplasia—folds/geographic

Old English Sheepdog

Cataract—autosomal recessive—nuclear/cortical—congenital
Cataract—posterior cortex—adult onset
Corneal dystrophy—epithelial stromal
Distichiasis
Entropion
Glaucoma
Microphthalmia/multiple ocular defects
Persistent pupillary membranes
Progressive retinal degeneration
Retinal detachment
Retinal dysplasia—folds
Uveodermatologic syndrome

Papillon

Cataract—cortical
Cataract—nuclear
Corneal dystrophy—epithelial/stromal
Distichiasis
Entropion
Lens luxation
Persistent pupillary membranes
Progressive retinal degeneration
Prolapse of the gland of the third eyelid
Retinal dysplasia—folds
Vitreal degeneration

Parson Russell Terrier

Cataract—posterior cortical
Corneal dystrophy—epithelial/stromal
Distichiasis

Glaucoma—primary open angle?
Lens luxation
Progressive retinal degeneration
Vitreal degeneration

Pekingese

Atresia of lacrimal puncta and canaliculi
Cataract—anterior cortex
Chronic corneal erosion syndrome
Deep corneal ulcers
Distichiasis
Ectopic cilia
Entropion/trichiasis (medial)
Exotropia
Haired medial caruncle
Keratoconjunctivitis sicca
Macroblepharon
Nasal fold trichiasis
Pigmentary keratitis
Progressive retinal degeneration
Traumatic proptosis

Pembroke Welsh Corgi

Cataract—posterior cortex
Chronic corneal erosion syndrome
Distichiasis
Lens luxation (± secondary glaucoma)
Persistent hyaloid artery
Persistent pupillary membranes
Progressive retinal degeneration
Prolapse of the gland of the third eyelid
Retinal dysplasia—folds
Retinal dysplasia—geographic/detached

Petit Basset Griffon Vendeen

Cataract—anterior or posterior cortex
Corneal dystrophy—endothelial
Distichiasis
Entropion
Glaucoma
Lens luxation
Persistent pupillary membranes
Progressive retinal degeneration
Retinal dysplasia
Vitreal degeneration

Pointer

Cataract—initially equatorial
Chronic superficial keratitis (pannus)
Corneal dystrophy—epithelial/stromal
Entropion
Progressive retinal degeneration
Retinal dysplasia

Polish Lowland Sheepdog

Corneal dystrophy—epithelial/stromal
Distichiasis

Persistent pupillary membranes
Progressive retinal degeneration
Retinal pigment epithelial dystrophy

Pomeranian

Atresia of lacrimal puncta
Canine allergic inhalant conjunctivitis (atopy)
Cataract—anterior or posterior cortex
Distichiasis
Entropion
Persistent pupillary membranes
Progressive retinal degeneration
Tear-staining syndrome
Trichiasis

Poodle (All Varieties)

Atresia of lacrimal puncta and canaliculi
Canine allergic inhalant conjunctivitis (atopy)
Cataract—anterior, posterior, or equatorial cortex
Cataract—recessive—equatorial cortex (standard)
Chronic corneal erosion syndrome
Deep medial canthal pockets (standard)
Distichiasis
Ectopic cilia
Entropion
Glaucoma—goniodysgenesis with angle closure
Glaucoma—primary open angle (rare)
Haired medial caruncle
Iris atrophy—senile
Lens luxation (± glaucoma)
Microphthalmia
Optic nerve hypoplasia/micropapilla
Persistent pupillary membranes
Progressive retinal degeneration—rod/cone degeneration
Prolapse of the gland of the third eyelid
Retinal dysplasia—folds
Tear-staining syndrome
Trichiasis

Portuguese Water Dog

Cataract—cortical
Distichaisis
Entropion
Lens luxation
Microphthalmia/multiple ocular defects
Persistent pupillary membranes
Progressive retinal degeneration

Pug

Distichiasis
Entropion (medial)
Ectopic cilia

Haired medial caruncle
Keratoconjunctivitis sicca
Macroblepharon
Nasal fold trichiasis
Persistent pupillary membranes
Pigmentary keratitis
Progressive retinal degeneration
Ulcerative keratitis

Puli

Corneal dystrophy—epithelial/stromal
Entropion
Persistent pupillary membranes
Progressive retinal degeneration
Retinal dysplasia—folds

Queensland Blue Heeler

See Australian Cattle Dog.

Rat Terrier

Cataract
Distichiasis
Lens luxation
Persistent pupillary membranes
Vitreal degeneration

Redbone Coonhound

Retinal pigment epithelial dystrophy

Rhodesian Ridgeback

Cataract—posterior cortex
Distichiasis
Entropion
Eversion of the cartilage of the third eyelid
Persistent pupillary membranes
Progressive retinal degeneration

Rottweiler

Cataract—anterior or posterior cortex
Chronic corneal erosion syndrome
Corneal dystrophy—epithelial/stromal
Deep medial canthal pockets
Distichiasis
Ectropion
Entropion
Iris/ciliary body cysts
Iris coloboma
Macroblepharon
Microphthalmia
Myopia
Persistent pupillary membranes
Progressive retinal degeneration
Retinal dysplasia—folds
Retinal dysplasia—geographic/detached

Saint Bernard

Cataract—posterior cortex
Dermoid
Distichiasis
Ectropion
Entropion
Eversion of the cartilage of the third eyelid
Macroblepharon
Microphthalmia/multiple ocular defects
Persistent pupillary membranes
Progressive retinal degeneration
Prolapse of the gland of the third eyelid
Redundant facial skin
Uveodermatologic syndrome

Saluki

Cataract—equatorial cortex
Corneal dystrophy
Deep medial canthal pockets
Entropion
Glaucoma—goniodysgenesis with angle closure
Neuronal ceroid lipofuscinosis
Persistent pupillary membranes
Progressive retinal degeneration

Samoyed

Cataract—anterior or posterior cortex
Cataract—nuclear fibrillar
Chronic corneal erosion syndrome
Corneal dystrophy—epithelial/stromal
Distichiasis
Glaucoma—goniodysgenesis with angle closure
Glaucoma—primary open angle (rare)
Keratoconjunctivitis sicca
Persistent pupillary membranes
Progressive retinal degeneration
Retinal dysplasia—folds (± skeletal dysplasia)
Retinal dysplasia—geographic/detached
Uveodermatologic syndrome

Schipperke

Cataract—anterior cortex
Distichiasis
Entropion
Persistent pupillary membranes
Progressive retinal degeneration
Retinal dysplasia—folds

Scottish Terrier

Cataract—cortical or nuclear
Corneal dystrophy—epithelial/stromal
Distichiasis
Lens luxation

Persistent pupillary membranes
Progressive retinal degeneration
Retinal dysplasia—folds

Sealyham Terrier

Atresia of the lacrimal puncta and canaliculi
Cataract—anterior or posterior cortex
Distichiasis
Lens luxation (± secondary glaucoma)
Persistent pupillary membranes
Progressive retinal degeneration
Retinal dysplasia—complete with complete retinal detachment
Retinal dysplasia—folds
Vitreal degeneration

Shar-Pei

Cataract
Entropion
Glaucoma—goniodysgenesis with angle closure
Lens luxation
Progressive retinal degeneration
Protrusion of the gland of the third eyelid
Redundant facial skin

Shetland Sheepdog (Sheltie)

Atresia of the lacrimal puncta and canaliculi
Choroidal hypoplasia (collie eye anomaly)
Colobomas (optic disc)
Corneal dystrophy epithelial/stromal (multifocal and often ulcerative)
Distichiasis
Ectopic cilia
Nodular episcleritis
Persistent pupillary membranes
Progressive retinal degeneration
Prolapse of the gland of the third eyelid
Retinal dysplasia
Retinal pigment epithelial dystrophy
Uveodermatologic syndrome

Shiba Inu

Corneal dystrophy—epithelial/stromal
Distichiasis
Ectopic cilia
Glaucoma—goniodysgenesis with angle closure
Lens luxation
Persistent pupillary membranes
Progressive retinal degeneration
Vitreal degeneration

Shih Tzu

Cataract—anterior cortex

Chronic exposure keratitis/pigmentary keratitis
Corneal dystrophy—endothelial
Corneal dystrophy—epithelial/stromal
Corneal ulceration
Distichiasis
Ectopic cilia
Entropion (medial)
Haired medial caruncle
Keratoconjunctivitis sicca
Macroblepharon
Progressive retinal degeneration
Retinal detachment
Vitreal degeneration

Siberian Husky

Cataract—posterior cortex and juvenile
Chorodial hypoplasia (collie eye anomaly)
Chronic superficial keratitis (pannus)
Corneal dystrophy—endothelial
Corneal dystrophy—epithelial/stromal
Distichiasis
Entropion
Glaucoma—goniodysgenesis with closed angles
Persistent pupillary membranes
Progressive retinal degeneration—X-linked
Retinal detachment
Uveitis
Uveodermatologic syndrome

Silky Terrier

Atopic conjunctivitis and blepharitis
Cataract—anterior, posterior, or equatorial cortex
Chronic corneal erosion syndrome
Persistent pupillary membranes
Progressive retinal degeneration
Vitreal degeneration

Skye Terrier

Lens luxation

Smooth Fox Terrier

See Fox Terrier (Smooth).

Soft Coated Wheaten Terrier

Cataract—anterior or posterior cortex
Distichiasis
Micropapilla
Microphthalmia with multiple ocular defects
Persistent hyaloid artery
Persistent pupillary membranes
Progressive retinal degeneration
Retinal dysplasia—folds

Spinone Italiano

Cataract—anterior cortex
Entropion
Eversion of the cartilage of the third eyelid
Iris coloboma
Persistent pupillary membranes
Prolapse of the gland of the third eyelid
Retinal dysplasia—folds

Spitz

Progressive retinal degeneration

Staffordshire Bull Terrier

Cataract—recessive—posterior sutures/cortex
Distichiasis
Entropion
Persistent hyaloid artery
Persistent hyperplastic primary vitreous
Persistent pupillary membranes
Progressive retinal degeneration

Standard Schnauzer

Cataract—congenital with microcornea
Cataract—posterior cortex
Corneal dystrophy—epithelial/stromal
Distichiasis
Progressive retinal degeneration
Retinal dysplasia—folds

Sussex Spaniel

Distichiasis
Ectropion
Persistent hyaloid artery
Retinal dysplasia—folds

Swedish Vallhund

Cataract
Corneal dystrophy epithelial/stromal
Distichiasis
Persistent pupillary membranes
Progressive retinal degeneration
Retinopathy
Vitreal degeneration

Tibetan Spaniel

Cataract—cortical
Ceroid lipofuscinosis
Chronic superficial keratitis (pannus)
Distichiasis
Entropion
Iris/ciliary body cysts
Keratoconjunctivitis sicca
Micropapilla

Persistent hyaloid artery
Persistent pupillary membranes
Progressive retinal degeneration
Prolapse of the gland of the third eyelid

Tibetan Terrier

Cataract—posterior cortex
Ceroid lipofuscinosis
Corneal dystrophy—epithelial/stromal
Distichiasis
Lens luxation (± secondary glaucoma)
Persistent pupillary membranes
Progressive retinal degeneration
Retinal degeneration—night blindness—
    young age
Retinal dysplasia—folds

Toy Havanese

Progressive retinal degeneration

Toy Terrier

Lens luxation (± secondary glaucoma)

Vizsla

Cataract—anterior or posterior cortex
Corneal degeneration—epithelial/stromal
Distichiasis
Entropion
Eyelid melanomas, multiple
Persistent pupillary membranes
Progressive retinal degeneration

Weimaraner

Cataract—anterior cortex
Chronic corneal erosion syndrome
Corneal dystrophy—epithelial/stromal
Deep medial canthal pockets
Distichiasis
Entropion
Eversion of the cartilage of the third eyelid
Eyelid neoplasia
Persistent pupillary membranes
Retinal dysplasia—folds

Welsh Springer Spaniel

Cataract—anterior cortex
Cataract—recessive—congenital—nuclear/
    posterior cortex
Corneal dystrophy—epithelial/stromal
Distichiasis
Entropion
Glaucoma—dominant—closed angle
Persistent pupillary membranes
Progressive retinal degeneration
Retinal dysplasia—folds

Welsh Terrier

Cataract—anterior or posterior cortex
Distichiasis
Ectopic cilia
Glaucoma—closed angle
Keratoconjunctivitis sicca
Lens luxation (± secondary glaucoma)
Persistent pupillary membranes
Progressive retinal degeneration

West Highland White Terrier

Atopic conjunctivitis and blepharitis
Cataract—adult—anterior or posterior
    cortex, nuclear
Cataract—recessive—posterior sutures
Chronic corneal erosion syndrome
Keratoconjunctivitis sicca
Lens luxation
Microphthalmia
Persistent pupillary membranes
Progressive retinal degeneration
Retinal dysplasia—folds

Whippet

Lens luxation (± secondary glaucoma)
Progressive retinal degeneration
Vitreal degeneration

Wire Fox Terrier

See Fox Terrier (Wirehaired).

Yorkshire Terrier

Atopic conjunctivitis and blepharitis
Cataract—anterior, posterior, or equato-
    rial cortex
Corneal dystrophy—epithelial/stromal
Distichiasis
Entropion
Keratoconjunctivitis sicca
Persistent pupillary membranes
Progressive retinal degeneration
Retinal dysplasia—geographic/detached

CATS

Abyssinian

Progressive retinal degeneration—domi-
    nant trait—kitten
Progressive retinal degeneration—reces-
    sive trait—2 to 4 years old

Albinotic Felidae

Esotropia

Birman

Cataract—congenital—posterior nuclear
Corneal dermoids

Burmese

Corneal dermoids
Corneal sequestrum
Eyelid hypoplasia ("coloboma")
Glaucoma—narrow to closed angles
Progressive retinal degeneration
Prolapse of the gland of the third eyelid

Domestic Shorthair

A-mannosidosis
GM^1 gangliosidosis
GM^2 gangliosidosis
Mucopolysaccharidosis I

Himalayan

Cataracts—posterior cortex
Corneal sequestrum
Epiphora
Medial lower lid entropion

Korat

GM^1 gangliosidosis
GM^2 gangliosidosis

Manx

Progressive corneal edema

Persian

A-mannosidosis
Atresia of the lacrimal puncta and canaliculi
Chédiak-Higashi syndrome
Corneal sequestrum
Epiphora
Medial lower lid entropion
Progressive retinal degeneration—recessive
    —early onset

Siamese

Congenital nystagmus
Convergent strabismus
Corneal sequestrum
Glaucoma—primary
Globoid cell leukodystrophy
Glycogen storage disease type II (Pompe's
    disease)
GM^1 gangliosidosis
Herpetic keratitis
Iris atrophy
Mucopolysaccharidosis VI
Progressive retinal degeneration

Sphingomyelin lipidosis (Niemann-Pick disease)
Tapetal degeneration (hereditary)

CATTLE

Aberdeen Angus

Mannosidosis

Ayrshire

Pendular nystagmus
Esotropia

Beef Master

Neuronal lipodystrophy

Brahman

Squamous cell carcinoma

Brown Swiss

Esotropia
Extra lacrimal drainage openings
Heterochromia with complete albinism
Multiple ocular anomalies (including cataracts)

Charolais

Colobomas (posterior pole)
Squamous cell carcinoma

Devon

Ceroid lipofuscinosis

Friesian (Holstein)

Accessory nasolacrimal duct openings
Cataract, lens luxation, glaucoma (dominant)
Cataract—congenital—recessive
Congential corneal edema
Esotropia
GM^1 gangliosidosis
Pendular nystagmus

German Spotted

Squamous cell carcinoma

Guernsey

Microphthalmia
Multiple ocular anomalies
Heterochromia with complete albinism
Pendular nystagmus

Hereford

Cataract—congenital—recessive
Chédiak-Higashi syndrome (recessive)
Dermoids (hereditary)
Heterochromia with complete albinism
Infectious bovine keratoconjunctivitis
Microphthalmia
Multiple ocular anomalies
Optic nerve coloboma (associated with incomplete albinism)
Squamous cell carcinoma

Jersey

Cataract—congenital—recessive
Convergent strabismus with exophthalmia
Esotropia and exophthalmos
Multiple ocular defects—inherited
Pendular nystagmus

Shorthorn

Congenital nystagmus
Convergent strabismus with exophthalmia
Dermoids
Esotropia and exophthalmos
Glycogen storage disease type II
Heterochromia with complete albinism
Microphthalmia
Multiple ocular anomalies
Susceptibility to infectious bovine keratoconjunctivitis
Susceptibility to squamous cell carcinoma

Simmental

Entropion
Squamous cell carcinoma

SHEEP

Corriedale

Congenital (possibly inherited) photosensitivity
Glycogen storage disease type II
Glucocerebroside storage disease type II

Hampshire Downs

Entropion

New Zealand Romney

Cataract

Piebald

Congenital upper eyelid eversion
Eyelid agenesis

Shropshire

Essential iris atrophy

Southdown

Congenital (possibly inherited) photosensitivity

South Hampshire

Neuronal ceroid lipofuscinosis

Suffolk

Essential iris atrophy

HORSES

Appaloosa

Congenital stationary night blindness
Equine recurrent uveitis (chronic form)
Squamous cell carcinoma
Strabismus

Arabian

Cataract
Melanoma

Belgian

Congenital aniridia and cataract (dominant)
Squamous cell carcinoma

Clydesdale

Squamous cell carcinoma

Lipizzaner

Melanoma

Morgan

Cataract—nuclear—congenital—possibly dominant

Quarter Horse

Aniridia—dominant?
Cataracts—nuclear and cortical—dominant
Dermoid (with cataracts and iridal hypoplasia)
Sarcoids

Rocky Mountain Horse

Anterior segment dysgenesis
Megalocornea
Uveal cysts

Shire

Squamous cell carcinoma

Thoroughbred

Cataract—congenital—dominant
Entropion—congenital

GOAT
Angora

Squamous cell carcinoma

PIGS
Miniature Swine

Entropion
Optic nerve and choroidal colobomas

Pot-Bellied

Entropion

Yorkshire

Cerebrospinal lipodystrophy
Microphthalmia

REFERENCES

American College of Veterinary Ophthalmologists (2007): Ocular Disorders Presumed to be Inherited in Dogs, 5th ed. ACVO, Urbana, IL.

Bistner SI, et al. (1977): Atlas of Veterinary Ophthalmic Surgery. Saunders, Philadelphia.

Blogg JR (1980): The Eye in Veterinary Practice, Vol. 1. Saunders, Philadelphia.

Bonagura A (1994): Current Veterinary Therapy XII. Saunders, Philadelphia.

Clark RD, Stainer JR (1983): Medical and Genetic Aspects of Purebred Dogs. Veterinary Medicine Publishing Co., Edwardsville, KS.

Helper LC (1989): Magrane's Canine Ophthalmology, 4th ed. Lea & Febiger, Philadelphia.

Rubin LF (1989): Inherited Eye Diseases in Purebred Dogs. Williams & Wilkins, Baltimore.

GLOSSARY

accommodation adjustments in focal power of the eye necessary to maintain a clearly focused image on the retina as an object moves closer to or farther from the eye; largely accomplished by changes in shape or position of the lens through action of the ciliary muscle. In some species (e.g., birds, fish) additional mechanisms are involved.

adnexa (ocular) periocular structures, consisting of orbit, orbital contents, eyelids, nasolacrimal system, conjunctiva, and third eyelid.

agenesis failure of development of an organ/tissue.

albinism congenital and inherited absence of melanin. In ocular structures, this is most striking in the iris (which is pink) and fundus (in which the choroid is easily seen).

alopecia absence of hair from an area where it is normally found.

amaurosis complete blindness without overt ocular cause (cf. *amblyopia*).

amblyopia reduced vision without overt ocular cause (cf. *amaurosis*).

angle-closure glaucoma glaucoma due to mechanical obstruction of the iridocorneal angle that prevents aqueous humor from reaching the trabecular meshwork. Also known as narrow-angle or closed-angle glaucoma (cf. *open-angle glaucoma*).

aniridia inherited congenital complete absence of iris. Aniridia is extremely rare because usually some iris root is present.

anisocoria disparity in pupil size between the two eyes.

ankyloblepharon fusion of the eyelid margins; physiologic for the first 10 days in puppies and kittens.

anophthalmos/anophthalmia complete absence of the eye. Anophthalmos is extremely rare; usually some ocular tissues are present; *microphthalmos* is more common.

anterior chamber space bounded anteriorly by the cornea and posteriorly by the iris and anterior lens. Contains aqueous humor.

anterior segment collective term for those parts of the eye anterior to the vitreous; consisting of the lens, ciliary body, iris (and pupil), anterior chamber, cornea, anterior sclera, and conjunctiva (cf. *posterior segment*).

anterior uveitis inflammation of the ciliary body (cyclitis) and iris (iritis); also called *iridocyclitis*.

aphakia absence of the lens. Occurs extremely rarely as an inherited condition; extreme microphakia is more likely.

aphakic crescent crescent-shaped space created between the equator of a dislocated (luxated or subluxated) lens and the dilated pupil. Pathognomonic for lens dislocation.

aqueous flare Tyndall effect seen when a focal beam of light passes through aqueous humor containing excessive protein and/or cells (plasmoid aqueous). Pathognomonic for disruption of the blood-aqueous barrier.

aqueous humor clear fluid made by the ciliary body epithelium; is released into the posterior chamber, fills the anterior chamber, and egresses through the iridocorneal angle. Responsible (in part) for meeting the metabolic needs of the avascular lens and cornea.

area centralis retinal region with high density of cone photoreceptors and ganglion cells that is lateral to the optic nerve head in cats. Important for visual acuity.

asteroid hyalosis fixed opacities composed of a calcium-lipid complex and occurring in an otherwise normal vitreous body. Relatively common in older animals (cf. *syneresis* and *synchysis scintillans*).

astigmatism optical condition in which light coming from a single point in the environment is not focused to a single point on the retina, usually owing to irregularities in corneal curvature. In **regular astigmatism** the cornea is shaped more like a football than like part of a sphere and the resulting image is distorted but in a somewhat predictable fashion. In **irregular astigmatism** the cornea is very irregular and light is not uniformly brought into focus on the retina; usually due to corneal disease or injury.

Bergmeister's papilla mass of glial cells surrounding the hyaloid artery in the center of the optic disc; pathologic in most species; seen commonly in ruminants.

binocular vision the ability to use the two eyes simultaneously to focus on the same object. Fusion of these two separate images by the brain allows for stereopsis and a further improvement in the ability to detect depth.

blepharitis inflammation of the upper or lower eyelids.

blepharoplasty plastic surgery of the eyelids.

blepharospasm spasm of the orbicularis oculi muscle resulting in eyelid closure.

blood-aqueous barrier physiologic barrier formed by the iris and ciliary body vascular endothelium and the ciliary epithelium that limits movement of plasma components into the aqueous humor. Part of the blood-ocular barrier.

blood-ocular barrier physiologic barrier formed by the vascular endothelium and some intraocular epithelial tissues that limits movement of plasma components into the eye. Composed of the blood-aqueous barrier anteriorly and the blood-retinal barrier posteriorly.

blood-retinal barrier physiologic barrier formed by the retinal vascular endothelium and the retinal pigment epithelium that limits movement of plasma components into the retina and vitreous. Part of the blood-ocular barrier.

bulla a large fluid-filled vesicle or blister, usually due to corneal edema.

bullous keratopathy disease of the cornea associated with bullae formation.

buphthalmos/buphthalmia enlargement of the eye due to glaucoma.

canaliculus small epithelium-lined tube at the inner aspect of the upper and lower lids, leading from the nasolacrimal punctum to the lacrimal sac (plural: canaliculi).

canthoplasty plastic surgery on the medial or lateral canthus.

canthotomy surgical incision of (usually the lateral) canthus to improve surgical visualization or access.

canthus the angle at the medial and lateral ends of the palpebral fissure where the upper and lower eyelids join.

caruncle a small piece of skin at the medial canthus from which hairs often protrude.

cataract opacity of the lens and/or lens capsule.

central progressive retinal atrophy a group of disorders in which retinal degeneration is accompanied by numerous, small, pigmentlike foci over the tapetal fundus. The primary defect is in the retinal pigment epithelium, whereas in generalized progressive retinal atrophy (PRA) the defect is in the photoreceptors. Also known as *retinal pigment epithelial dystrophy*.

chalazion lipogranuloma of a tarsal (meibomian) gland due to impaction of secretions and sometimes rupture into the surrounding eyelid tissue.

chemosis conjunctival edema.

"cherry eye" lay term for prolapsed gland of the third eyelid.

chorioretinitis inflammation of the choroid and retina in which choroiditis is the dominant and presumed initiating factor (cf. *retinochoroiditis*).

choroid the posterior aspect of the uveal tract immediately external to the retina; responsible for nutrition of the outer retinal layers.

choroiditis inflammation of the choroid; usually caused by or causing associated retinitis, resulting in *retinochoroiditis* and *chorioretinitis*, respectively.

chronic immune-mediated kerato-conjunctivitis syndrome (CIKS) characteristic immune-mediated disease of the cornea and conjunctiva of dogs also known as chronic superficial keratitis (CSK), pannus, and Uberreiter's syndrome.

chronic superficial keratitis (CSK) a general descriptive pathologic term that is sometimes used to describe a characteristic immune-mediated disease of the cornea and conjunctiva of dogs also known as pannus, chronic immune-mediated keratoconjunctivitis syndrome (CIKS), and Uberreiter's syndrome.

ciliary body part of the uveal tract between the iris and the choroid; consists of ciliary processes that produce aqueous humor and the ciliary muscle responsible for accommodation and iridocorneal angle/trabecular meshwork opening.

ciliary sulcus poorly defined transition point between the posterior surface of the iris and the anterior surface of the ciliary body.

cilium eyelash (plural: cilia).

closed-angle glaucoma glaucoma associated with apposition of the peripheral iris to the peripheral cornea (cf. *open-angle glaucoma*).

collie eye anomaly inherited developmental defect of collies and some other breeds characterized by choroidal hypoplasia, with or without colobomas, and retinal detachment.

collyrium eye wash.

coloboma congenital absence of any ocular tissue. Commonly affected tissues are eyelid, iris, choroid, and optic disc. Usually present as a gap, hole, fissure, or notch-shaped defect. Sometimes differentiated into **typical colobomas** (defects lying in or near the 6 o'clock position within the eye and due to failed closure of the fetal fissure) and **atypical colobomas** (defects occurring in areas other than the fetal fissure).

cone retinal photoreceptor adapted for vision in bright light, for color vision, and for fine visual acuity.

conjugate ocular movements movement of the eyes in the same fashion; e.g., movement of both eyes to the right, left, up, or down. These movements are known as *versions*.

conjunctiva mucus membrane lining the posterior aspect of the upper and lower eyelids *(palpebral conjunctiva)*, both surfaces of the third eyelid, and the anterior sclera *(bulbar conjunctiva)*.

conjunctival follicles hypertrophy and coalescence of conjunctival lymphoid tissue in response to conjunctival inflammation. Produces a characteristic cobblestone appearance on the conjunctival surfaces, especially within the conjunctival fornix.

conjunctival fornix region where the palpebral conjunctiva reflects to become bulbar conjunctiva or to cover the anterior face of the third eyelid. There is also a secondary fornix between the posterior aspect of the third eyelid and the globe. Also known as the *conjunctival cul-de-sac*.

conjunctivorhinostomy surgical creation of a communication between the conjunctiva and the nasal cavity performed to circumvent a dysfunctional nasolacrimal system.

contact lens thin plastic lens that fits directly on the cornea under the eyelids, thereby protecting the cornea during healing. Also known as a *therapeutic soft contact lens* (TSCL).

contralateral situated on or pertaining to the other side.

corectopia displacement of the pupil from its normal position.

corneal degeneration unilateral or bilateral keratitis characterized by corneal edema and subepithelial deposition of lipid and/or mineral, and often with corneal vascularization (cf. *corneal dystrophy*).

corneal dystrophy progressive, bilateral, approximately symmetrical hereditary corneal disease unassociated with inflammation; may affect the epithelium, stroma, or endothelium (cf. *corneal degeneration*).

corneal erosion loss of corneal epithelium. Distinguished from corneal ulcers by connotation, erosions being superficial (sometimes not even all epithelial layers) and typically recurrent.

corneal graft surgical placement of a section of donor cornea to replace a diseased region of host cornea (cf. *keratoplasty*).

corneal mummification see *corneal sequestrum*.

corneal necrosis see *corneal sequestrum*.

corneal reflex closure of the eyelids induced by light touching of the cornea with a few wisps of cotton teased off a cotton-tipped applicator.

corneal sequestrum enigmatic condition unique to the cat cornea in which a (usually axial) region of stroma becomes amber to black, undergoes degeneration, and may be slowly extruded by the surrounding normal cornea while eliciting a marked foreign body reaction. Corneal ulceration may or may not be present. Also known as *feline keratitis nigrum, corneal necrosis*, and *corneal mummification*.

corneal ulcer a break in continuity of corneal epithelium with or without loss of corneal stroma. Also known as *ulcerative keratitis* (cf. *corneal erosion*).

corpora nigra irregular cystic dilations on the pupillary margin of the iris in large herbivores. Most notable dorsally but typically also present ventrally. Also known as *granula iridica*.

cortical blindness blindness caused by a lesion in the visual (occipital) cortex.

cotton-wool spots fluffy white opacities within the nerve fiber layer of the retina due to edema secondary to microinfarcts. Seen as an early change with systemic hypertension.

cryotherapy localized tissue destruction by freezing.

cyclitic membrane organized fibrinous exudate and, subsequently, a fibrovascular membrane extending from the ciliary body over the posterior lens capsule as a result of uveitis.

cyclitis inflammation of the ciliary body; usually seen with iritis and therefore termed *iridocyclitis* (or *anterior uveitis*).

cyclo- of or pertaining to the ciliary body.

cyclocryotherapy cryodestruction of the ciliary body epithelium by application of a cryoprobe to the overlying sclera to reduce the rate of aqueous humor formation and lower intraocular pressure for the treatment of glaucoma (cf. *cyclophotoablation*).

cyclodialysis surgical procedure for glaucoma to establish a communication between the anterior chamber and the suprachoroidal space.

cyclodiathermy procedure for glaucoma to destroy a portion of the ciliary body by diathermy and reduce the quantity of aqueous humor produced.

cyclophotoablation destruction of the ciliary body epithelium by application of a laser probe to the overlying sclera to reduce the rate of aqueous humor formation and lower intraocular pressure for the treatment of glaucoma (cf. *cyclocryotherapy*).

cycloplegia paralysis of the ciliary muscle induced to reduce pain due to ciliary spasm associated with anterior uveitis.

dacryoadenitis inflammation of the lacrimal glands (orbital or third eyelid).

dacryocystitis inflammation of the lacrimal sac.

dacryocystorhinography use of contrast material for radiographic studies of the nasolacrimal drainage system.

dacryocystorhinostomy surgical procedure to construct an alternate nasolacrimal drainage system into the nasal sinuses.

dark adaptation biochemical and neurologic process by which the eye becomes more sensitive to light during a period in darkness.

dazzle reflex subcortical reflex in which a rapid eye blink is elicited by a bright light shone into an eye.

decussation crossing of nerve fibers or tracts from one side of the nervous system to the opposite side, for example as occurs at the optic chiasm.

denervation hypersensitivity increased sensitivity to neural effector substance that follows postganglionic interruption of the nerve supply of organs innervated by the autonomic nervous system.

dermoid a congenital tumor consisting of skin and its appendages.

descemetocele deep corneal ulcer characterized by sufficient stromal loss that there is exposure of Descemet's membrane.

Descemet's membrane the basement membrane of the corneal endothelium.

diopter unit of measurement of the refractive power of lenses, equal to the reciprocal of the focal length of the lens expressed in meters.

diplopia the perception of one object as two images ("double vision").

distichiasis condition in which a single cilium emerges from one or more meibomian (tarsal) gland orifices (cf. *districhiasis, ectopic cilia,* and *trichiasis*).

districhiasis condition in which multiple cilia emerge from one meibomian (tarsal) gland orifice (cf. *distichiasis, ectopic cilia,* and *trichiasis*).

drainage angle traditional outflow pathway by which aqueous humor exits the eye. It is bounded anteriorly by the peripheral cornea, posteriorly by the iris and ciliary muscles, internally by the pectinate ligaments, and externally by the sclera. The trabecular meshwork and ciliary cleft are contained within the iridocorneal angle. In some cases this term is used to refer to the geometric angle between the anterior surface of the iris and cornea (synonyms: *filtration angle, iridocorneal angle*).

dyscoria abnormally shaped pupil (adj. *dyscoric*).

dystrophy noninflammatory, developmental, nutritional, or metabolic abnormality.

ectasia dilation or expansion; may be toward the observer (e.g., corneal ectasia) or away from the observer (e.g., posterior scleral ectasia).

ectopia displacement or malposition, especially congenital (adj. *ectopic*).

ectopic cilia hair/cilia protruding through palpebral conjunctiva. The cilia usually abrade the cornea, causing pain and ulceration.

ectropion an eversion or rolling out of the eyelid.

ectropion uvea eversion of the posterior iris epithelium around the pupillary margin and into the anterior chamber; usually associated with anterior uveitis (cf. *entropion uvea*).

electroretinogram (ERG) a graphic record of the action potential that follows stimulation of the retina by light.

emmetropia condition in which no refractive error is present within the eye such that a distant point of light is properly focused onto the retina when the eye is "at rest" (i.e., not accommodating).

endophthalmitis inflammation of the intraocular contents, excluding the corneoscleral tunic (cf. *panophthalmitis*).

enophthalmos abnormal recession of the eye within the orbit (cf. *exophthalmos*).

entropion an introversion or rolling in of the eyelid.

entropion uvea posterior rolling (or inversion) of the pupillary margin into the posterior chamber; usually associated with anterior uveitis (cf. *ectropion uvea*).

enucleation surgical removal of the eye (cf. *evisceration, exenteration*).

epilation removal of hair, especially cilia.

epiphora overflow of tears due to impaired drainage, excessive production, or both.

episcleritis inflammation of the connective tissue immediately exterior to the sclera.

equine recurrent uveitis (ERU) recurrent inflammation of the anterior and/or posterior uvea in horses; the cause is unknown (older terms include "periodic ophthalmia" and "moon blindness").

esotropia form of strabismus in which there is convergent deviation of one eye toward the midline while the other fixates normally (cf. *exotropia*).

euryblepharon horizontally enlarged palpebral fissure due to excessive eyelid length (also known as *macropalpebral fissure*).

evisceration surgical removal of the intraocular contents, with retention of the corneoscleral tunic and placement of a prosthesis within the corneoscleral shell.

exenteration (orbital) surgical removal of all the orbital tissues, including the eye and its nervous, vascular, and muscular connections.

exophthalmos abnormal protrusion of the eye from the orbit (cf. *enophthalmos*). May be pulsatile when associated with an orbital arteriovenous fistula.

exotropia form of strabismus in which there is divergent or lateral deviation of one eye while the other fixates normally (cf. *esotropia*).

fascia bulbi connective tissue sheath encircling the globe posterior to the limbus (also known as *Tenon's capsule*).

filtration angle traditional outflow pathway by which aqueous humor exits the eye. It is bounded anteriorly by the peripheral cornea, posteriorly by the iris and ciliary muscles, internally by the pectinate ligaments, and externally by the sclera. The trabecular meshwork and ciliary cleft are contained within the iridocorneal angle. In some cases this term is used to refer to the geometric angle between the anterior surface of the iris and cornea (synonyms: *drainage angle; iridocorneal angle*).

fluorescein angiography serial photography of the ocular fundus after intravenous administration of fluorescein solution. Used to characterize vascular disease of the retina, choroid, and optic nerve head.

fluorescein dye/stain a vital dye that fluoresces when stimulated with blue light. Used in many ophthalmic diagnostic tests, including the identification and characterization of corneal ulcers.

focus point of convergence of light rays.

fovea retinal region of high visual acuity in primates and birds.

fundus (ocular) the posterior portion of the eye visible through an ophthalmoscope, composed of the sclera, choroid, retina, and optic nerve head.

glands of Moll apocrine glands of the upper and lower eyelid margins.

glands of Zeis sebaceous glands of the upper and lower eyelid margins.

glaucoma ocular disease that may produce a syndrome of findings but that in domestic animals is uniformly characterized by increased intraocular pressure with resulting damage to the optic nerve. Categorized as **primary glaucoma** (occurring without pre-existing ocular disease in an otherwise apparently healthy eye) or **secondary glaucoma** (glaucoma attributable to another ocular abnormality, such as lens luxation, intraocular tumor, anterior uveitis).

gonioscope specialized instrument for studying the iridocorneal angle.

gonioscopy examination of the iridocorneal angle with a goniolens, magnifying device, and light source.

granular iridica irregular cystic dilations on the pupillary margin of the iris in large herbivores. Most notable dorsally but typically also present ventrally. Also known as *corpora nigra*.

Haab's striae linear gray-blue opacities deep within the cornea caused by fractures or stretching of Descemet's membrane and development of fibrosis

and edema within the crack. Pathognomonic for glaucoma in most species; however, their significance in horses is not understood. Also called *striate keratopathy*.

haws syndrome bilateral condition in cats characterized by protrusion of the third eyelids without detectable cause.

hemeralopia visual impairment/ blindness in bright light ("day blindness").

hemianopia blindness involving one half of the visual field.

heterochromia iridis condition in which the iris is not of uniform color or in which the right and left irides of one animal differ in color from each other.

hippus spasmodic dilation and contraction of the pupil independent of stimulation with light.

hordeolum localized, purulent infection of a gland of the eyelid. May be **external** (infection of the glands of Moll or Zeis; also known as *stye*) or **internal** (infection of the meibomian [tarsal] glands).

Horner's syndrome set of ocular signs due to sympathetic denervation. May include miosis, ptosis, enophthalmos, and protrusion of the third eyelid.

hyalitis evidence of inflammation (usually white blood cells, inflammatory proteins/ debris, etc.) within the vitreous body; reflects inflammation of the surrounding tissues (ciliary body, retina, and choroid) rather than primary inflammation of the vitreous body itself (cf. *aqueous flare*).

hyalo-/hyaloid pertaining to the vitreous.

hyperopia (hypermetropia) refractive state of the eye in which the parallel rays of light would come to focus behind the retina if not intercepted by it ("farsightedness"). (See also *myopia*.)

hypertropia deviation of the eyes in which one eye is higher than the other.

hyphema blood in the anterior chamber.

hypopyon white blood cells in the anterior chamber.

hypotony reduced intraocular pressure.

image visual impression of an object formed by a lens or mirror. In optics, a **real image** is an optical image that can be received on a screen. It is formed by the meeting of convergent rays of light, whereas a **virtual image** is an optical image that cannot be received on a screen. It is formed by diverging rays of light that appear to come from the image point but do not pass through it.

intraocular lens (IOL) artificial lens placed within the eye to correct

refractive error created by lens removal for cataract or lens dislocation.

intumescent lens a swollen or enlarged lens.

ipsilateral situated on or pertaining to the same side.

iridencleisis surgical procedure for glaucoma in which an incision is made at the limbus and the iris is incarcerated into the wound to create a filtering wick between the anterior chamber and the subconjunctival space. Performed rarely in domestic animals owing to the excessive inflammatory response in these species.

iridocorneal angle traditional outflow pathway by which aqueous humor exits the eye. It is bounded anteriorly by the peripheral cornea, posteriorly by the iris and ciliary muscles, internally by the pectinate ligaments, and externally by the sclera. The trabecular meshwork and ciliary cleft are contained within the iridocorneal angle. In some cases this term is used to refer to the geometric angle between the anterior surface of the iris and cornea (synonyms: *filtration angle; drainage angle*).

iridocyclitis inflammation of the iris (iritis) and ciliary body (cyclitis). Also called *anterior uveitis*.

iridodialysis separation of the base of the iris from the ciliary body; usually posttraumatic.

iridodonesis tremor or "fluttering" of the iris that occurs after loss of support due to luxation or removal of the lens.

iridoplegia paralysis of the iris sphincter muscle (i.e., mydriasis).

iris bombé adhesions (synechiae) between the pupillary margin of the iris and the anterior lens capsule due to anterior uveitis. The condition results in accumulation of aqueous humor in the posterior chamber, ballooning forward of the iris, and obstruction of the iridocorneal angle, which induces secondary glaucoma.

iris "freckle" lay term for iris nevus; a focal region of increased pigmentation of the iris.

iris prolapse protrusion of the iris through a perforating corneal or corneoscleral wound (cf. *staphyloma*).

iritis inflammation of the iris.

keratectomy excision of part of the cornea.

keratic precipitates (KPs) clumps of leukocytes and fibrin adhering to the corneal endothelium as a result of (and pathognomonic for) anterior uveitis.

keratitis inflammation of the cornea. Typically classified as ulcerative or nonulcerative.

keratitis nigrum see *corneal sequestrum*.

kerato-/keratic pertaining to the cornea.

keratoconjunctivitis simultaneous inflammation of the cornea and conjunctiva.

keratoconjunctivitis sicca (KCS) inflammation of the cornea and conjunctiva secondary to dryness caused by impaired lacrimal gland function and decreased tear flow.

keratoconus enlargement of the cornea in which the cornea is protruded and conical.

keratoglobus enlargement of the cornea in which the cornea is protruded and globular.

keratomycosis keratitis caused by fungi.

keratoplasty transplantation of a portion of the cornea. May be **lamellar** (replacement of only the deep or superficial layers) or **penetrating** (replacement of the entire depth of a corneal region; a corneal graft).

lacrimation secretion of the precorneal tear film (tears).

lagophthalmos incomplete eyelid closure and globe coverage. Often associated with exposure keratitis.

lamina cribrosa fenestrated area of sclera approximately at the posterior pole of the globe, where optic nerve fibers exit the eye.

lens glass or other refractive material used to optically modify the path of light.

lens dislocation collective term for lens subluxation or luxation.

lens luxation disinsertion of lens zonules from the complete lens equator such that the lens luxates into the anterior chamber **(anterior lens luxation)** or into the vitreous cavity **(posterior lens luxation).**

lens subluxation disinsertion of lens zonules from the less than 100% of the lens equator such that the lens subluxates away from the region of disinsertion.

lenticonus abnormality of the lens characterized by a conical prominence on the anterior or posterior lens surface.

lentiglobus abnormality of the lens characterized by a spherical bulging of the anterior or posterior lens surface.

leukocoria literally, "white pupil." Usually a sign of cataract, nuclear sclerosis, or retinal detachment.

leukoma notable corneal opacity; a less marked opacity is called a *macula*, and the least dense opacity is termed a *nebula*. **Adherent leukoma** describes a corneal opacity in which the iris adheres to the endothelial surface.

limbus circular junction of the cornea and sclera.

macropalpebral fissure horizontally enlarged palpebral fissure due to excessive eyelid length (also known as *euryblepharon*).

macula moderate corneal opacity; a less marked opacity is called a *nebula*, and the most dense opacity is termed a *leukoma*. Alternative definition: a cone-rich area of high visual acuity in the primate retina that is devoid of blood vessels.

meibomian glands altered sebaceous glands located in the eyelids and opening onto the eyelid margin, producing the outer, oily layer of the tear film. Also known as *tarsal glands*.

menace response eyelid closure in response to a visually threatening movement.

microphakia abnormally small lens.

microphthalmos/ia congenitally small globe.

miosis constriction of the pupil (cf. *mydriasis*).

miotic pertaining to or characterized by constriction of the pupil (cf. *mydriatic*).

Mittendorf's dot opacity of the posterior lens capsule at the posterior pole marking the embryologic site of hyaloid artery insertion.

"moon blindness" see *equine recurrent uveitis (ERU)*.

morgagnian cataract a hypermature cataract in which the cortex is liquefied, permitting the lens nucleus to float or sink within the capsule.

mydriasis dilation of the pupil (cf. *miosis*).

mydriatic pertaining to or characterized by dilation of the pupil (cf. *miotic*).

myopia refractive state of the eye in which parallel rays of light come into focus in front of the retina ("nearsightedness"). (See also *hyperopia*.)

narrow-angle glaucoma glaucoma due to mechanical obstruction of the iridocorneal angle that limits aqueous humor from reaching the trabecular meshwork. Also known as *closed-angle* or *angle-closure glaucoma* (cf. *open-angle glaucoma*).

nebula minor corneal opacity; a moderate opacity is called a *macula*, and the most dense scar is termed a *leukoma*.

neovascularization formation of new blood vessels where there were previously none (as in cornea or on face of iris. (See also *rubeosis iridis*.)

neurotrophic keratitis keratitis caused by dysfunction of cranial nerve V with associated anesthesia of the cornea.

nevus region of focally increased pigmentation, usually of the iris (lay term: "iris freckle").

nodular granulomatous episclerokeratoconjunctivitis (NGE) a disease seen in many breeds but particularly rough collies and characterized by a tan-pink raised mass arising from the episclera (subconjunctiva) usually at the dorsolateral corneoscleral limbus, with adjacent conjunctival inflammation and often with corneal inflammation evident as corneal edema and corneal lipid degeneration. Suspected to be immune-mediated. Terminology is confusing but various synonyms have been used: *nodular fasciitis, proliferative keratoconjunctivitis syndrome, fibrous histiocytoma, limbal granuloma, collie granuloma.*

nyctalopia visual impairment/blindness in reduced illumination ("night blindness").

nystagmus oscillatory movement of the eye. May be physiologic (optokinetic) or pathologic due to vestibular disease. Categorized as **jerk nystagmus** (having fast and slow phases), **pendulous nystagmus** (oscillations are approximately equal in deviation and speed; occurring in individuals in whom vision in both eyes has been defective since birth), and **rotary nystagmus** (the eye partially rotates around the visual axis; seen in central vestibular disease).

oculocardiac reflex vagally mediated decrease of heartbeat caused by pressure or traction on the eye; most notable with patient under general anesthesia and especially in horses and birds.

O.D. oculus dexter; the right eye.

open-angle glaucoma glaucoma associated with a gonioscopically normal appearing drainage angle (cf. *closed-angle glaucoma, narrow-angle glaucoma*).

ophthalmia neonatorum conjunctivitis in the newborn, especially behind closed lids of neonatal kittens and puppies with physiologic ankyloblepharon.

ophthalmoplegia paralysis of the ocular muscles. Further categorized as **external** (paralysis of the extraocular muscles; with strabismus) or **internal** (paralysis of the iris and ciliary body muscles; with pupil dilation and loss of accommodation).

ophthalmoscope an instrument with a special illumination system for viewing the inner eye, particularly the retina and associated structures.

optic disc ophthalmoscopically visible portion of the optic nerve in the globe. Also called the *optic nerve head* and *optic papilla*.

optic disc cupping abnormal depression in the optic disc associated with glaucoma.

optic neuritis inflammation of the optic disc with decreased vision. Also called *papillitis* (cf. *papilledema*).

optic papilla ophthalmoscopically visible portion of the optic nerve in the globe. Also called *optic nerve head*.

O.S. oculus sinister; the left eye.

O.U. oculi uterque; both eyes.

palpebral reflex eyelid closure in reaction to stimulation of the periocular skin.

pannus classically, nonspecific vascularization of avascular connective tissue (e.g., cartilage, cornea). However, the term is used commonly in ophthalmology to describe a characteristic immune-mediated disease of the cornea and conjunctiva of dogs. Synonyms include Uberreiter's syndrome and chronic immune-mediated keratoconjunctivitis syndrome (CIKS).

panophthalmitis inflammation of all ocular and intraocular tissues, including the neural, uveal, and fibrous tunics of the eye, and often the orbital tissue as well (cf. *endophthalmitis*).

papilledema edema of the optic disc with normal vision (cf. *optic neuritis*).

papillitis inflammation of the optic disc with decreased vision. Also called *optic neuritis* (cf. *papilledema*).

pectinate ligaments thin "fingers" of anterior uveal tissue spanning from the iris root to the inner cornea/sclera across the iridocorneal angle.

"periodic ophthalmia" see *equine recurrent uveitis (ERU)*.

peripheral anterior synechiae adhesions between the iris root and the peripheral cornea. May occur after unrelieved attacks of angle-closure glaucoma or chronic anterior uveitis (often seen only with gonioscopy).

persistent pupillary membranes (PPMs) congenital defect in which persistent strands of fetal vascular tissue extend from the iris collarette to other regions of the iris **collarette (iris-to-iris PPMs),** to the anterior lens capsule **(iris-to-lens PPMs),** or to the corneal endothelium **(iris-to-cornea PPMs).**

Peter's anomaly developmental defect in which ocular components surrounding the anterior chamber fail to cleave properly, resulting in anterior segment dysgenesis. Severity varies. May include adherent corneal leukoma, corneolenticular stalk, persistent pupillary membranes, cataract, and iridocorneal angle malformations with glaucoma.

photophobia ocular discomfort induced by bright light. (Because this is a symptom, not a clinical sign, it must be inferred in domestic animals.)

photopic pertaining to vision in bright ambient light; an eye that has become light-adapted.

photoreceptor specialized outer retinal cell (rod or a cone) that converts light to an electrical stimulus through phototransduction.

phthisis bulbi A small, shrunken, and deranged globe due to scarring secondary to (usually massive or chronic) intraocular inflammation.

plasmoid (secondary) aqueous proteinaceous aqueous resulting from leakage of plasma proteins into the aqueous humor across a disrupted blood-aqueous barrier. Pathognomonic for anterior uveitis.

polycoria occurrence of more than one pupil in the iris; classified as *true polycoria* if surrounded by sphincter muscle, and as *pseudopolycoria* if not.

posterior chamber space into which the aqueous humor is first released bounded anteriorly by the posterior surface of the iris and posteriorly by the anterior lens capsule.

posterior segment collective term for those parts of the eye posterior to the lens, including the vitreous, retina, choroid, optic nerve, and sclera (cf. *anterior segment*).

presbyopia refractive condition in which there is a diminished power of accommodation arising from impaired elasticity of the crystalline lens, as occurs with aging.

progressive retinal atrophy (PRA) collective term for a series of inherited but rarely congenital progressive degenerative conditions affecting the neurosensory retina or retinal pigment epithelium and associated with impaired vision and, ultimately, blindness. Also known as *progressive retinal degeneration* (PRD).

proptosis forward displacement of the globe (exophthalmos) such that the globe equator protrudes beyond the eyelid margins as occurs during trauma, especially in brachycephalic dogs.

pseudopterygium region of bulbar conjunctiva that advances over but does not adhere to the cornea (cf. *pterygium*); seen most commonly in rabbits, in which it is also called *corneal occlusion syndrome*.

pterygium region of bulbar conjunctiva that advances onto and adheres to the cornea (cf. *pseudopterygium*).

ptosis drooping of the upper lid due to dysfunction of the oculomotor nerve (cranial nerve III), sympathetic denervation, or excessive weight of the upper eyelids.

pupil hole in the center of the iris that regulates light entering the posterior eye. Shape varies with species.

pupillary block blockage of the passage of aqueous through the pupil between the posterior and anterior chambers. Associated with some forms of glaucoma.

pupillary light reflex (PLR) constriction of the pupil when the retina of the same eye is stimulated with light **(direct PLR)** or when the retina of the opposite eye is stimulated **(consensual PLR).**

reflex involuntary, invariable, adaptive subcortical reaction to a stimulus. See also descriptions of *corneal reflex, pupillary light reflex, palpebral reflex,* and *dazzle reflex* (cf. *response*).

refraction the bending of rays of light that occurs as they pass from one transparent medium into another of different density, such as passage from air into the cornea, or from the aqueous humor into the lens.

response cortically mediated voluntary reaction to a stimulus that can be exaggerated or over-ridden and that may need to be learned so is not always present from birth. An example is the *menace response* (cf. *reflex*).

retina the innermost tunic of the eyeball, containing the neural elements for reception and transmission of visual stimuli.

retinal detachment separation of the neurosensory retina from the retinal pigment epithelium. Because this is an intraretinal breach, the term *retinal separation* is more strictly correct.

retinal dialysis tearing of the retina from its attachment at the ora ciliaris retinae or, less commonly, from the optic disc in association with retinal separation such that the retina is seen hanging from the optic nerve or ora ciliaris retinae (also called *retinal disinsertion*).

retinal disinsertion tearing and disinsertion of the retina from the ora ciliaris retinae in association with retinal separation such that the retina is seen hanging from the optic nerve or ora ciliaris retinae (also called *retinal dialysis*).

retinal dysplasia abnormal differentiation of retinal layers.

retinal pigment epithelial dystrophy collective term for a group of disorders in which retinal degeneration is accompanied by numerous, small, pigmentlike foci over the tapetal fundus. The primary defect is in the retinal pigment epithelium, whereas in generalized progressive retinal atrophy (PRA) the defect is in the photoreceptors. Also known as *central progressive retinal atrophy*.

retinal separation separation of the neurosensory retina from the retinal pigment epithelium. Sometimes less correctly called *retinal detachment*.

retinitis inflammation of the retina; usually caused by or causing associated choroiditis, resulting in the term *chorioretinitis* or *retinochoroiditis*, respectively.

retinochoroiditis inflammation of the choroid and retina in which retinitis is the dominant and presumed initiating factor (cf. *chorioretinitis*).

retinopathy any disease condition of the retina.

retinoschisis a congenital cleft of the retina; a cleavage of retinal layers.

retrobulbar optic neuritis inflammation of the optic nerve occurring without funduscopically visible involvement of the optic disc.

retroillumination use of light reflected from a deeper structure to examine a more anterior structure; for example, light reflected from the tapetum may be used to examine the clarity and position of the lens (cf. *transillumination*).

rod retinal photoreceptor adapted for vision in dim light and motion detection. Most domestic animal retinas are relatively rod-rich compared with the primate retina. (See also *cone*.)

rubeosis iridis neovascularization of the iris.

Sanson-Purkinje images series of images reflected from the surface of the cornea and the anterior and posterior lens capsules. Used to judge depth within the eye.

Schiøtz tonometer indentation tonometer for assessing intraocular pressure.

Schirmer tear test (STT) test for tear formation in which absorbent paper is folded over the lid margin for 1 minute and the amount of wetting measured.

scleritis inflammation of the sclera.

scotopic pertaining to vision in dim ambient light or to an eye that has become dark-adapted.

sector iridectomy removal of an entire sector of iris extending from the pupillary margin to the root of the iris. Usually performed for tumor removal.

sequestrum see *corneal sequestrum*.

slit-lamp biomicroscope microscope for examining the eye, consisting of a binocular microscope with a movable light source that that can be changed in size, color, and focus.

spherophakia abnormally spherical lens.

staphyloma protrusion of uveal tissue (iris or ciliary body) into a bulging area of cornea/sclera due to thinning (ectasia) or rupture of the wall of the eye.

stars of Winslow multiple dark dots seen throughout the tapetal area of the fundus, which represent an end-on view of small choroidal vessels penetrating the tapetum to reach the outer retina. Most notable in herbivores and cats.

strabismus condition in which the two eyes are not simultaneously directed at the same object in a coordinated fashion. Categorized as **concomitant strabismus,** in which the angle of deviation remains constant for all directions of gaze and with either eye fixating (typically without muscle paralysis), and **nonconcomitant strabismus,** in which the angle of deviation varies with the direction of the gaze or the eye that fixates (typically caused by paralysis or paresis of one or more extraocular muscles). Further categorized as **convergent strabismus,** in which the deviating eye turns inward ("cross-eyed"), and **divergent strabismus,** in which the deviating eye turns outward.

striate keratopathy linear gray-blue opacities deep within the cornea caused by fractures or stretching of Descemet's membrane and development of fibrosis and edema within the crack. Pathognomonic for glaucoma in most species; however, their significance in horses is not understood (also called *Haab's striae*).

stye localized, purulent infection of a gland of Zeis or Moll. Also known as an internal hordeolum. (See also *hordeolum*.)

swinging flashlight test observation of contralateral pupil size after light is directed into the opposite eye. The result is positive when the contralateral pupil dilates as the light is diverted to it and is associated with a severe prechiasmal (retinal or prechiasmal optic nerve) lesion on that side.

symblepharon permanent adhesion between adjacent conjunctival surfaces or between cornea and conjunctiva.

synchysis scintillans cholesterol crystals in a liquefied vitreous body (cf. *asteroid hyalosis*).

syndrome a group of clinical signs that occur together; a disease or definite morbid process having a characteristic sequence of signs; may affect the whole body or any of its parts. Syndromes of importance in veterinary ophthalmology are listed in alphabetical order within this glossary.

synechiae adhesions between the iris and adjacent structures occurring as a result of anterior uveitis. **Anterior synechiae** occur between the iris and cornea. **Posterior synechiae** occur between the iris and anterior lens capsule (sing. *synechia*).

syneresis liquefaction of the vitreous body. May occur as a result of pathology or normal aging.

tapetum approximately semicircular, reflective layer of the choroid occupying up to the dorsal half of the fundus in many domestic species.

tarsal glands altered sebaceous glands located in the eyelids and opening onto the eyelid margin that produce the outer, oily layer of the tear film. Also known as *meibomian glands*.

tarsorrhaphy operation in which the lids are sutured together to reduce corneal exposure. May be temporary or permanent; partial or complete.

tear film break-up time (TFBUT) an assessment of precorneal tear film stability. In the presence of a normal lipid layer of the tear film, the TFBUT is a quantitative measure of mucin quantity and quality. Decreased mucin quantity or quality causes tear film instability and a shortening of the TFBUT.

Tenon's capsule connective tissue sheath encircling the globe posterior to the limbus (also known as *fascia bulbi*).

Tenon's space episcleral space between Tenon's capsule and the globe.

therapeutic soft contact lens (TSCL) thin plastic lens that fits directly on the cornea under the eyelids, thereby providing corneal protection during healing.

tonography measurement of amount of fluid forced from the eye by constant pressure during a constant period. Used to assess the facility of aqueous outflow. Reduced in patients with glaucoma or a predisposition to glaucoma.

tonometer instrument for measuring the tone of the eye wall; used to estimate intraocular pressure. Categorized as **applanation tonometer** (instrument that estimates intraocular pressure by measuring the resistance of a specified area of cornea to being flattened or applanated; e.g., Tono-Pen), **indentation tonometer** (instrument that estimates intraocular pressure by measuring the resistance of the cornea and anterior chamber to being indented; e.g., Schiøtz tonometer), or **induction-impact (or rebound) tonometer** (instrument that estimates intraocular pressure by measuring the vibration of a plunger as it rebounds from the ocular surface; e.g., TonoVet).

transillumination examination of an ocular structure by use of a transversely directed beam of focal light; especially useful when the transilluminated structure is semitransparent and permits some light to pass through it (e.g., iris cyst) (cf. *retroillumination*).

trichiasis pathologic condition in which hairs from normal skin reach and irritate the corneoconjunctival surface (cf. *distichiasis, ectopic cilia*).

tumor a swelling or enlargement of varying size that may involve any structure; not necessarily neoplastic.

Uberreiter's syndrome characteristic immune-mediated disease of the cornea and conjunctiva of dogs. Also known as chronic immune-mediated keratoconjunctivitis syndrome (CIKS), pannus, or chronic superficial keratitis (CSK).

uvea/uveal tract middle vascular tunic of the globe; consists of the iris and ciliary body anteriorly, and the choroid (including the tapetum) posteriorly.

uveitis inflammation of the iris, ciliary body, or choroid in any combination. Termed **anterior uveitis** or *iridocyclitis* when the iris and/or ciliary body is involved; **posterior uveitis** when the choroid is involved; and **panuveitis** when all three are involved. Sometimes categorized by cause as **endogenous** (arising from causes within the body, such as neoplasia and infection) and **exogenous** (arising from causes outside the body, such as trauma).

uveodermatologic syndrome autoimmune destruction of melanocytes causing marked panuveitis, retinitis, and dermatitis seen in dogs. The human counterpart condition is Vogt-Koyanagi-Harada (VKH) syndrome.

versions simultaneous parallel movements of both eyes, such as eyes right, eyes left, eyes up, and eyes down.

viscoelastic material gel-like hyaluronic acid or methylcellulose derivative used to protect the corneal endothelium and inflate the anterior chamber during intraocular surgery.

vision faculty of seeing; sight. Requires functional eye and central nervous system, including visual (occipital) cortex. Can be further defined as **binocular vision** (image formed using both eyes synchronously), **color vision** (ability to distinguish subjectively a large variety of wavelengths of light in the visible spectrum), **photopic vision** (vision in bright illumination), and **scotopic vision** (vision in dim illumination).

visual acuity ability to distinguish shape and detail. This depends on the optical system of the eye (cornea, aqueous humor, lens, and vitreous), the sensitivity of the retina, and the interpretation of the images by the brain. Regions of higher visual acuity within the retina are usually associated with a greater density of cone photoreceptors and occur in species-dependent regions of the retina. (See also *fovea, macula,* and *area centralis.*)

visual-evoked potentials (VEPs) recording of electrical activity in the central (retrobulbar) visual pathways after visual stimulation; used to assess the integrity and function of these pathways.

visual field extent of space that can be perceived when the head and eyes are kept fixed; the field may be monocular or binocular.

vitreous body transparent, colorless, gel-like mass between lens and retina.

vitreous cavity space containing the vitreous body and bounded anteriorly by the posterior lens capsule and posteriorly by the inner limiting membrane of the retina.

vitreous veils/plicae faint curtainlike opacities seen by focal light through a dilated pupil in the normal eye. The veils move gently in the vitreous when the eye moves.

Vogt-Koyanagi-Harada (VKH) syndrome autoimmune destruction of melanocytes causing marked panuveitis, retinitis, and dermatitis seen in humans. The term *VKH-like* or *uveodermatologic syndrome* is preferred for the similar syndrome in dogs.

Wood's light light source equipped with a nickel oxide filter that produces ultraviolet light, used to stimulate fluorescence of fluorescein dye.

xeromycteria drying of the nasal mucosal surfaces as seen with neurogenic keratoconjunctivitis sicca.

xerophthalmia drying of the ocular surface tissues as seen with tear film abnormalities.

xerosis pathologic dryness of the conjunctiva, mucus membranes, or skin.

xerostomia drying of the oral mucosal surfaces, as seen with reduced salivation as in Sjögren's syndrome.

zonules the numerous fine tissue strands (ligaments) that stretch from the ciliary processes to the lens equator for a full 360 degrees and hold the lens in place.

zonulysis dissolution of the zonules, as with chymotrypsin, to facilitate intracapsular lens extraction.

A

Abducent nerve
  anatomy and function of, 14, 318
  strabismus due to lesions of, 332
  testing of, 100
Abscess
  cerebral, 349
  corneal, 191-192, 192f
  retrobulbar, 360-361, 361f, 362f, 363f
    in rabbits, 428, 428f
  subspectacular in snakes, 439, 439f
Absolute glaucoma treatment, 253-254, 253b, 254f
Absorption maximum, 290, 293f
Acariasis, 127t, 128t
Accommodation, 5, 6f, 258, 260f, 435
Acetylcholine, 53b
Acyclovir, 45, 45t, 146
Adaptation in ocular injury, 63
Adenocarcinoma
  third eyelid, 154, 155f
  uveal, 225, 225f
Adenoma
  meibomian, 125, 125f
  uveal, 225, 225f
Adenovirus, canine, 144, 375-376, 377f
Adhesion molecules
  in inflammatory process, 67
  in keratic precipitates, 79
Adhesives
  cyanoacrylate, 189
  surgical, 56
Adnexa
  disease of
    in rabbits, 429, 429f
    systemic causes of in horses and cattle, 405t
  nerve supply of, 13
Adrenaline, 53-54
Adrenergic agents, 53-54
Adrenergic antagonists, 54
Advancement conjunctival graft, 187, 187f, 188f
Advancement flap for eyelid reconstruction, 123, 124f
Age factors
  in cataract formation, 267
  in inherited retinopathies, 305-306
  in intraocular pressure, 232
Agenesis, 63
Akabane virus, 409
Albendazole, 432
Albinism, ocular, 210, 211t
Algae in uveitis, 214t
Allergic conjunctivitis, 137t, 147, 147f

Allergic disorders of eyelid skin, 130t
Allergy, food, eyelid skin disease due to, 130t
Alopecia areata, 132t
Amblyopia, 266
Amelanotic leading edge of third eyelid, 152
Amikacin, 42, 185b
Aminoglycosides, 41-42
Amoxicillin, 40
Amphibians, 439-440, 440f
Amphotericin B, 44t, 45, 192t
Ampicillin, 40
Analgesics for corneal ulcers, 186
Anaplasia in neoplasm, 78
Anemia, 396t
Anesthetics
  local, 55
  topical
    for injections, 36
    for microbiologic samplings, 83-84
Angiography, fluorescein, 104, 105f
Angiosarcoma, conjunctival, 150
Aniridia, 31, 209
Anophthalmos, 30
Anterior chamber
  anatomy of, 17, 18f
  embryonic and fetal development of, 28, 29f
  examination of, 88, 88f
  shallow, in glaucoma, 236
Anterior segment
  dysgenesis of, 210, 210f
  examination of, 85-89, 85f, 86f, 87f, 88f
Anterior uveitis, 213t
  atropine for, 51-52
  classification of, 215t
  defined, 69, 208
  emergency treatment of, 425-426
  systemic causes of, 401t
Antibiotics, 37-43, 37b. See Also specific types
  aminoglycosides, 41-42
  azithromycin, 42
  bacitracin, 42
  cephalosporins, 40
  chloramphenicol, 40
  for conjunctivitis, 141
    allergic, 147
    viral, 146
  for corneal lacerations, 424
  for corneal ulcers, 184-186, 185b, 186
  for equine recurrent uveitis, 221
  fluoroquinolones, 42-43, 43t
  for hordeolum and meibomian adenitis, 122, 122t
  for ocular contusions and concussions, 423
  penicillins, 38-40
  polymyxin B, 42
  selection and administration of, 37-38, 38t, 39t, 40t, 41t
  sulfonamides, 42
  tetracyclines, 42

Anticholinergic drugs, 51-53
Antifungals, 43-45, 44t
Antiglaucoma drugs, 215-216
Antihistamines, 50, 141
Antihypertensive drugs, 397, 397t
Antiinflammatory drugs. See Also Corticosteroids
  for corneal ulcers, 186
  for emergency treatment of ocular contusions and concussions, 423
  nonsteroidal (See Nonsteroidal antiinflammatory drugs)
Antioxidants for cataracts, 269
Antiparasitic agents, 59
Antiseptics, 58
Antivirals, 45, 45t, 145-146
Aphakic crescent, 273, 273f
Aplasia, 63
Applanation tonometry, 96-97, 96f
Aqueous
  loss of, necrosis and, 66
  physiology of, 17-19, 18f, 18t
  production and drainage of, 230-232, 231f, 232f
  surgical procedures on, for glaucoma, 250-251, 251f
Aqueous compartment, 17, 18f
Aqueous flare
  corneal inflammation and, 68
  detection of, 94-95, 94f, 95f
  histology, 79
  in uveitis, 212
Aqueous humor misdirection syndrome, 282
Aqueous layer of precorneal tear film, 157
  deficiency of, 166
Arrowhead procedure for lateral entropion, 118, 119f
Arterial blood pressure, normal, 397t
Arterial circle of iris, 12
Arterial supply, 10-12, 12f
Arteriography, orbital, 359, 361f
Arteritis, equine viral, 400
Arthrogryposis-hydrencephaly, 409
Arthropods in skin disease of eyelid, 128t-129t
Artificial tears, 56, 57t-58t
A-scan ultrasound, 103, 104f
Aspergillosis, 389t
Aspirin, 48, 49t, 219
Asteroid hyalosis, 281-282, 281f
Astigmatism, 5, 6f
Astringents, 59
Atopic dermatitis, 130t
Atresia, congenital lacrimal, 162-163
Atrophy, 63, 64f
  of iris, 63, 227-228, 228f
  optic, 298
  retinal, 304, 381t, 402t
  in uveitis, 213

Atropine, 51-53, 53b
    for emergency treatment of ocular
        contusions and concussions,
        423
    for equine recurrent uveitis, 219
    for hyphema, 224
Auriculopalpebral nerve block, 85, 85f
Autoimmune disease
    of eyelid skin, 131t-132t
    uveitis, 209
Autonomic drugs, 51-54, 51f, 52f, 53b
Autonomic nervous system
    innervation of, 15-16, 15t, 17f, 335-336,
        336f, 337f
    sympathetic system diseases of, 336-339,
        337t, 338f, 339t
Avulsion of extraocular muscles, 420, 420f,
        421f
Axonal degeneration, 343
Azalides, 42
Azathioprine, 48, 215
Azithromycin, 42
Azoles, 43, 44t

B

Babesiosis, 402, 411
Bacitracin, 42
Bacterial culturing in conjunctivitis, 138-139
Bacterial infection
    canine, 382-386, 382f, 383f, 384f
    conjunctival, 137t, 141-142
        in birds, 436
        in rabbits, 429
    equine, 400-402, 402f
    of eyelid skin, 129t
    feline, 385-387, 386f
    meningitis, 350t
    ruminant, 408-409, 408f, 409f
    uveal, 214t
Barkers, 407
Barrier function, loss of, necrosis and, 65-66,
        66f
Bartonellosis, 385-386
Basal cells in corneal epithelium, 175, 176f
Behavioral testing of vision, 101-102
Benign neoplasm, 78
Benzalkonium chloride, 58
Bergmeister's papilla, 24, 25f, 279
Beta blockers, 53b, 54
Betamethasone, 47
Betaxolol, 249b
Binocular field, 352, 355f
Binocular indirect ophthalmoscope, 90, 90f
Biomicroscope, slit-lamp, 86, 86f, 94, 95f
Biopsy, conjunctival, 139, 141f
Birds, 434-436, 435f
    normal intraocular pressure values for, 428t
    orbital enucleation in, 369, 370f, 371f
    third eyelid of, 151, 152f
β-Irradiation, 59, 59f
Blastomycosis, 129t, 387, 387f, 388t
Blepharitis
    marginal, 122-123, 122f , 122t
    in rabbit, 429, 429f
    staphylococcal, in keratoconjunctivitis sicca,
        168
    systemic causes of, 375t
Blepharoplasty, v-to-y, 120, 120f

Blepharospasm
    in cilia disorders, 113
    in entropion, 116
    in glaucoma, 235
    in keratoconjunctivitis sicca, 168
Blindgrass toxicity, 313
Blindness
    bright, in sheep, 313, 313f
    color, 7
    congenital stationary night, 309
    due to cerebral lesion
        with abnormal pupillary light reflexes,
            323-328, 329f, 329t
        with normal pupillary light reflexes,
            323
    electroretinogram in, 296t
    epidemic, 227
    in retinopathies, 306-307
    sudden, emergency treatment of, 426
    systemic disorders causing, 386t, 403t
Blinking, 107, 109f
Blood-aqueous barrier, 18, 207
Blood disorders, 396t
Blood flow, intraocular pressure and, 232
Blood-ocular barriers
    inflammation in alterations of, immune-
        mediated disease and, 71
    structure and function of, 18
    uvea and, 207-208, 208f
Blood pressure, normal, 397t
Blood-retinal barrier, 18, 207
Blood vessels, retinal, 298
"Blue eye," 199
Bluetongue, 409-410
Borreliosis, 383, 383f
Botulism, 406
Bovine keratoconjunctivitis, infectious, 145,
        145t
Bovine rhinotracheitis, infectious. See
        Infectious bovine rhinotracheitis
"Boxer" ulcer, 189-190, 189f, 190f
Brachycephalic ocular syndrome, medial
        canthoplasty for, 118-119, 119f
Bracken fern, bright blindness due to, 313
Brain injury, 326-328, 329f, 329t
Brain lesions
    in blind patients
        with abnormal pupillary light reflexes,
            323-328, 329f, 329t
        with normal pupillary light reflexes, 323
    clinical signs in, 344, 344t
    in visual patients with normal pupillary light
        reflexes, 328-330
Brainstem contusion, 326
Bridge conjunctival grafts, 187, 187f
Bright blindness in sheep, 313, 313f
Brucellosis, 382-383, 382f
B-scan ultrasound, 103, 103f
    orbital, 358
Bullous dermatosis, 131t
Bullous keratopathy, 197, 197f
Buphthalmos, 235-236, 236f
Bystander injury, inflammatory, 68
    corneal, 68, 69f
    uveal, 209

C

Calicivirus infection, 378

Calves
    arthrogryposis-hydrencephaly in, 409
    Mannheimia pneumonia in, 409
    prosencephalon hypoplasia in, 349
    septicemia in, 409, 409f
Canaliculi, lacrimal, 159-160, 159f, 160f
Canine adenovirus, 144, 375-376, 377f
Canine distemper virus, 374-376, 375f, 377f
    in conjunctivitis, 137t, 144
    in ferrets, 432-433
    in keratoconjunctivitis sicca, 167
    in optic radiation and visual cortex
        disorders, 349
Canine familial dermatomyositis, 132t
Canine monocytic ehrlichiosis, 384-385, 384f
Canine multifocal retinopathy, 309
Canthoplasty, medial, 118-119, 119f
Carbachol, 53b, 54
Carbonic anhydrase
    in aqueous humor production, 230
    inhibitors of, 54-55, 250b
Carboxymethylcellulose, 57t
Cardiovascular disease, 309, 310f, 396-398,
        397f, 397t
Carotid artery, 11
Carprofen, 48, 49t
Caspofungin, 44t
Cat
    bacterial disease in, 385-387, 386f
    cardiovascular disease in, 396-398, 397f,
        397t
    cataracts in, 265t
    chlamydial conjunctivitis in, 142, 143t
    color vision in, 8
    diabetes mellitus in, 393-394, 394f
    diffuse iris melanoma in, 226-227, 227f
    eosinophilic keratitis in, 196, 196f
    facial paralysis in, 334t
    fundus of, examination of, 92, 92f
    fungal infection in, 387-392, 388t-389t,
        391f
    glaucoma in, treatment of, 254-255
    heterochromia iridis in, 210t
    Horner's syndrome, 337t
    ischemic encephalopathy in, 349
    leprosy in, 129t
    metabolic disease in, 395-396, 395f
    nocturnal vision of, 1, 2f
    normal flora of, 39t
    normal intraocular pressure in, 97
    parasitic infection in, 390t, 392
    retinal degeneration in, 309, 311-312, 312f
    sarcomas in, 77, 77f, 226
    uveitis in, 217
    vestibular disease in, 341
    viral conjunctivitis in, 143-144, 144b, 144f,
        145t
    viral disease in, 376-382, 377f, 379f, 381f,
        382f
    visual acuity in, 7
    visual field of, 3, 4f
Cataract, 261-272
    acquired, 266-267, 266f, 267f
    after uveitis, 212
    as anomaly associated with
        microphthalmos, 31, 31t
    classification of, 261-263, 261t, 263, 263f
    congenital, 264-266, 266f

Cataract—cont'd
 diabetic, 267-268
 diagnosis of, 268-269, 268f, 269t
 disease of in mice and rats, 434
 electroretinogram in, 296t
 in ferrets, 433
 hereditary, 264, 265t
 in horses, 272
 inflammation as cause of, 69-70
 intumescent, 268
 lens-induced uveitis and, 263-264
 molecular and cellular pathogenesis of, 261
 nutritional, 267
 persistent hyaloid artery *versus,* 279
 in rabbits, 431-432, 431f, 432f
 retinopathies and, 307
 stages of development of, 262-263, 263f
 systemic causes of, 380t
 treatment of, 269-272, 270f, 271f, 272f
Catheterization, nasolacrimal, 161-162, 162f
Cattle
 cataracts in, 265t
 conjunctival squamous cell carcinoma in, 150
 fundus of, examination of, 92, 93f
 heterochromia iridis in, 210t
 hypovitaminosis A in, 312b
 infectious keratoconjunctivitis, 197-198, 198b, 198f
 infectious rhinotracheitis in, 198-199
 lymphosarcoma in, 411, 411f
 normal flora of, 39t
 ocular albinism in, 211t
 ocular manifestations of systemic disease in, 408-412
 thromboembolic meningoencephalitis in, 409, 409f
 toxic disease in, 412
 viral conjunctivitis in, 145, 145t
Cauterants, 59
Cavernous sinus syndrome, 329
CEA. *See* Collie eye anomaly
Cefazolin, 185b
Cellulitis
 juvenile, 133t
 orbital, 360-361, 361f, 362f, 363f
Central visual pathways
 disease of, 342-350, 342f, 343f, 344t, 345f, 346f, 347f
 structure and function of, 8-10, 10f, 11f
Cephalosporins, 40
Cephalothin, 185b
Cerebellar disease, 350
Cerebral abscess, 349
Cerebral cortex, 10, 11f
Cerebral lesions
 in blind patients
  with abnormal pupillary light reflexes, 323-328, 329f, 329t
  with normal pupillary light reflexes, 323
 clinical signs of, 344, 344t
 in visual patients with normal pupillary light reflexes, 328-330
Cerebral peduncle, 9
Cerebrum, ischemic necrosis of, 349
Chalazion, 72, 121-122, 121f, 122f
Chemical mediators in inflammation, 67
Chemosis, 137

"Cherry eye," 153-154, 153f, 154f
China eye, 211
Chlamydial infections, 137t, 142, 142t, 143t, 386, 386f, 408
Chloramphenicol, 40
Cholinergic agents, 54
Choriocapillaris, 26
Chorioretinitis, 209, 298
Choroid
 anatomy and physiology of, 206-207, 207f, 208f
 examination of, 92
 retinal interaction of, 298-299
Choroiditis, 208
Chromodacryorrhea, 433, 433f
Chromophore, 290, 291
Cicatricial ectropion, 119
Cicatricial nasolacrimal obstruction, 163-164, 164f
Cicatrization, vitreous, 278
Cidofovir, 45t
Cilia
 anatomy of, 107, 108f
 disorders of, 111-115, 114f, 115f
Ciliary arteries, 11-12, 12f, 27, 207
Ciliary body
 anatomy and physiology of, 203-206, 205f, 206f, 207f
 embryonic and fetal development of, 22, 27, 29f
Ciliary body–vitreous–lens block glaucoma, 247-248, 247f, 248f
Ciliary muscle
 anatomy of, 13, 15, 203-206, 207f
 fetal development of, 27
Ciliary processes, 203, 205f, 206f
Ciliary veins, 12f, 13
Ciprofloxacin, 43, 43t
Circle of Willis, 11
Cleansing agents for conjunctivitis, 141
Closed-angle glaucoma, 238b, 244f
Clotrimazole, 43
CME. *See* Canine monocytic ehrlichiosis
CMR. *See* Canine multifocal retinopathy
Cocaine, 53b
Coccidioidomycosis, 387-391, 387f, 388t
Coenurosis, 411
Colliculus, superior, 9
Collie eye anomaly, 31, 32f, 303-304, 303f, 304f
Collyria, 56
Coloboma, 31-32, 31f, 32f
 eyelid, 109, 112f
 in iris, 210, 210f
 lens, 260
 optic nerve, 344-345, 345f
 retinal, 304, 304f
  in collie eye anomaly, 303, 304f
 scleral, 199, 199f
Color of iris, changes in, 79
Color vision, 7-8, 8f, 9f
Computed tomography, 104, 104f, 358, 359f
Concussion, emergency treatment of, 423, 424f
Cone-rod degeneration, 306
Cones
 anatomy of, 286f, 288f, 289, 289t, 292f
 in central visual pathway, 8
 in color vision, 7-8
 fetal development of, 23

Conformational ectropion, 116
Congenital abnormalities, 30-32
 anophthalmos and microphthalmos, 30-31, 30f, 31t
 cataracts, 264-266, 266f
 coloboma, 31-32, 31f, 32f
 cyclopia and synophthalmus, 31, 31f
 lacrimal atresia, 162-163
 of lens, 260
 myotonia, 333
 nystagmus, 342
 optic nerve, 344-345, 345f
 retinal, 301-304
  collie eye anomaly, 303-304, 303f, 304f
  coloboma, 304, 304f
  dysplasia, 301, 303f
 stationary night blindness, 309
 subepithelial geographic corneal dystrophy, 182
 uveal, 209-211, 209f, 210t, 211f, 211t
 of vitreous, 279-280, 280f
Conjunctiva, 135-150
 anatomy and physiology of, 135, 136f
 cell types found in, 140f-141f
 disorders of
  cellular response in, 135, 137f, 137t
  clinical signs of, 135-138, 137b, 137t
  conjunctivitis (*See* Conjunctivitis)
  drug plaques, 147, 148f
  in ferrets, 432-433
  lacerations, 147, 148f
  neoplastic, 148-150, 149f
  in rabbits, 429-430, 430f
  in raptors and pet birds, 436
  systemic causes of, 377t, 400t
 edema of, 137
 emphysema of, 138
 examination of, 87
 hemorrhage from, 137
 hyperemia of, 136-137, 137t
  in cilia disorders, 113
 palpebral, 29
 wound healing in, 74
Conjunctival grafts, 187-188, 187f, 188f
Conjunctivitis, 138-147, 213t
 bacterial, 141-142
 in birds, 436
 cellular responses in, 137t
 chlamydial, 142, 142t, 143t
  ovine, 408
 classification of, 138b
 diagnosis of, 138-139, 140f, 141f
 differential diagnosis of, 138, 139f
 in ferrets, 432-433
 frictional irritants causing, 138t
 immune-mediated, 147, 147f
 ligneous, 147-148, 148f
 lipogranulomatous, 148, 148f
 mycoplasmal, 142-143
 mycotic, 146
 parasitic, 146-147, 146t
 pruritus associated with, 138
 in rabbits, 429-430, 430f
 systemic causes of, 376t, 399t
 treatment of, 139-141
 viral, 143-146, 144b, 144f, 145t
Conjunctivobuccostomy, 164, 164f
Conjunctivorhinostomy, 164, 164f

Contact dermatitis, 130t
Contact lenses, 59
Contrast radiography, 102-103, 358-359, 359f
Contusion
    brainstem, 326
    emergency treatment of, 423, 424f
Conus papillaris, 287, 292f
Corectopia, 209
Cornea
    anatomy and physiology of, 175-176, 176f, 177f
    astigmatism of, 5, 6f
    cutaneous metaplasia of, 64, 65f, 74, 75f
    disease of in mice and rats, 434
    disease of in rabbits, 430-431
    drug administration and, 33
    edema of (See Corneal edema)
    embryonic and fetal development of, 28, 29f
    epithelial inclusion cyst of, 190-191, 190f
    examination of, 87
    fibrosis in, 179-180, 180f
    foreign bodies in, removal of, 193-194, 193f
    infectious bovine keratoconjunctivitis and, 197-198, 198b, 198f
    infectious bovine rhinotracheitis and, 198-199
    infectious canine hepatitis and, 199, 199f
    inflammation of, 68-69, 69f
    inherited disease of, 181-183, 182f, 183f
    keratitis of (See Keratitis)
    lacerations of, 192-193, 193f
        emergency treatment of, 422
    lipid and/or mineral accumulation in, 181, 181f
    malignant catarrhal fever and, 199
    pannus of, 194-195, 194f
    pathologic responses in, 178
    pigmentation in, 180, 180f
        histology of, 79
        in keratoconjunctivitis sicca, 168
    reactions of to disease, 178-181
    sequestration of, 196-197, 197f
    stroma of (See Corneal stroma)
    ulceration of (See Corneal ulceration)
    vascularization in, 179, 179f
        in keratoconjunctivitis sicca, 168
    in visual acuity, 4-5
    wound healing in, 74, 176-178, 177f
Corneal edema, 178-179, 179f
    in corneal inflammation, 68
    in glaucoma, 235, 235f
    histology of, 79
    lens luxation and, 274
    systemic causes of, 378t
Corneal reflex, 16-17, 17t
Corneal stroma
    abscess in, 191-192, 192f
    anatomy of, 175, 176f
    healing in, 177, 177f
    inflammatory cell infiltration of, with white blood cells, 180, 181f
    malacia of, 181, 182f
    ulcers in, 186-189, 186f, 187f, 188f
        fluorescein staining of, 98, 99f
    wound healing and, 76
Corneal ulceration
    in cilia disorders, 113-114
    common causes of, 183-184, 184f

Corneal ulceration—cont'd
    fluorescein staining of, 98-99, 99f
    in keratoconjunctivitis sicca, 168
    in rabbits, 430-431
    simple versus complicated, 184
    systemic causes of, 378t
    treatment of, 184-190, 185b, 186f, 187f, 188f, 190f
        emergency, 424
    wound healing of, 76
Corpora nigra, cystic, in horses, 225
Corticosteroids, 45-48
    for conjunctivitis, 141
        allergic, 147
    effects of on corneal healing, 177-178
    feline herpesvirus 1 and, 195
    for hyphema, 224, 425
    long-term therapy with, 47-48
    ocular penetration of, 47
    properties of, 45-47, 46f, 47f
    for uveitis, 215
        equine recurrent, 219, 221
Cortisone concentration in topical preparation, 34t
Corynebacterium spp., 41t
Cranial nerves. See Also specific nerves
    anatomy and function of, 13-14, 14f, 15f, 16f, 318
    disorders of, 335
    strabismus due to lesions in, 331-332, 332f
    testing of, 100-102
    ventral view of, 10f
Crocodilians, 436-438
Cryoepilation, 114-115, 114f, 115f
Cryotherapy
    for eyelid tumors, 123
    for glaucoma, 251-252, 251f
Cryptococcosis, 129t, 388t, 391, 391f
CT. See Computed tomography
Cuffing, perivascular, retinal, 300, 301f
Culturing, bacterial, in conjunctivitis, 138-139
Cupping, optic disc, in glaucoma, 238-239, 239f, 240f
Cutaneous habronemiasis, 128t
Cutaneous metaplasia of cornea, 64, 65f, 74, 75f
Cutaneous onchocerciasis, 128t, 404
Cyanoacrylate, 56, 189
Cyclitic membranes in uveitis, 213
Cyclitis, 208
Cyclocryotherapy for glaucoma, 251-252, 251f, 254-255
Cyclooxygenase pathway
    corticosteroids and, 46, 46f
    nonsteroidal antiinflammatory drugs and, 48
Cyclopentolate, 53
Cyclophotocoagulation, laser, for glaucoma, 252
Cyclopia, 31, 31f
Cycloplegics for uveitis, 215
Cyclosporine, 48-49
    for allergic conjunctivitis, 147
    for keratoconjunctivitis sicca, 169, 170
    for uveitis, 215
        equine recurrent, 221
Cyst
    corneal, 190-191, 190f
    orbital, 361-363

Cyst—cont'd
    periocular, 361-363
    uveal, 224-225, 224f
Cystic corpora nigra in horses, 225
Cystic lacrimal disorders, 163
Cytokines
    in inflammatory process, 67
    in wound healing, 74

D

Dacryoadenitis in rats, 433-434
Dacryocystitis, 161-162, 161f, 162f, 163f
Dacryocystorhinography, 103, 103f
Dacryocystotomy, 162, 163f
Dark adaptation, 292-293, 293f
Dazzle reflex, 17t, 101, 322, 322f
Degeneration
    axonal, 343
    cone-rod, 306
    myelin, 343, 343f
    neuronal, 342-343, 343f
    retinal (See Retinal degeneration)
    vitreous, 280
        retinal detachment and, 315
Degenerative retinopathy, 306, 306t
Demecarium, 53b, 54, 249b
Demodicosis, 127t
Denervation hypersensitivity, 51, 53, 338, 339
Dental disease
    orbital manifestations of, 365
    uveitis associated with, 217
Deoxyribonucleic acid testing, 307
Depth perception, 4, 5f
Deracoxib, 48, 49t
Dermatitis
    atopic, 130t
    contact, 130t
    irritant, 130t
    superficial necrolytic, 132t
    zinc-responsiveness, 132t
Dermatomyositis, canine familial, 132t
Dermatopathy, vaccine-induced, 132t
Dermatophilosis, 129t
Dermatophytosis, 129t
Dermoid
    conjunctival, 148-149, 149f
    corneal, 181-182, 182f
Descemetoceles
    fluorescein staining of, 98-99, 99f
    treatment of, 186-189, 186f, 187f, 188f
        emergency, 424, 425f
Descemet's membrane, 175, 176f, 177
Descemet's streaks in glaucoma, 235-236, 236f
Deuteranopia, 7
Developmental orbital abnormalities, 362t
Dexamethasone, 34t, 47
    for glaucoma, 249b, 250b, 422
    for hyphema, 224
    for uveitis, 215
        equine recurrent, 219, 221
Diabetes mellitus, 267-268, 393-394, 394f
Diagnosis, 81-106
    anterior segment examination in, 85-89, 85f, 86f, 87f, 88f
    aqueous flare detection in, 94-95, 94f, 95f
    electroretinography and visual evoked potentials in, 102, 102f
    examination in, 81, 82b, 82f, 83f

Diagnosis—cont'd
in exotic pets, 427-428, 428t
fluorescein angiography in, 104, 105f
fundus examination in, 90-93, 91f, 92f, 93f
gonioscopy in, 97-98, 98f
imaging techniques for, 102-104, 103f, 104f, 105f
lacrimal patency testing in, 100
medical history in, 81
microbiologic sampling in, 83-84, 84f
neuroophthalmic testing in, 100-102
ophthalmoscopy in, 89-90, 89f, 90f, 91f
posterior segment examination in, 93-94
pupil assessment in, 84-85, 84f, 85f
retinoscopy in, 102
Schirmer tear test, 81-82, 84f
tonography in, 97
tonometry in, 95-97, 95f, 96f, 97f
vital dyes in, 98-100, 99f, 100f
Diarrhea, bovine viral, 410-411
Diastolic blood pressure, normal, 397t
Dichlorphenamide, 249b, 250b, 422
Dichromatic vision, 291
Differentiation in embryonic and fetal development, 20, 21
Diffusion, aqueous, 230
Diopters, 5
Dipivefrin, 53-54, 53b
Direct ophthalmoscopy, 89-90, 89f, 94, 95f
Dirofilaria immitis, 222
disaccommodation, 258, 260f
Discharge
in conjunctival disease, 137
in differential diagnosis of ocular inflammation, 213t
in keratoconjunctivitis sicca, 167-168, 167f, 168f, 170
Discission and aspiration of cataracts, 270, 270f
Distemper. See Canine distemper virus
Distichiasis, 111, 114-115, 114f
Diurnal variation in intraocular pressure, 232
DM. See Diabetes mellitus
DNA testing, 307
Dog
bacterial disease in, 382-386, 382f, 383f, 384f
canine familial dermatomyositis in, 132t
cardiovascular disease in, 396-398, 397f, 397t
cataracts in, 264, 265t
color vision in, 7-8
conjunctival papillomatosis in, 150
deep muscles of head of, 110f
endocrine disorders in, 393-395394f, 395f
eye anatomy in, 1, 2f
eyelid tumors in, 123, 123t
facial paralysis in, 334t
fundus of, examination of, 92, 92f
fungal infection in, 387-392, 388t-389t, 391f
glaucoma in, 237-238, 238b, 245t
heterochromia iridis in, 210t, 211
Horner's syndrome, 337t
immune-mediated disease in, 398-399, 399f
indolent corneal ulcer in, 189-190, 189f, 190f
infectious hepatitis in, 199, 199f
lens luxation in, 237, 237b

Dog—cont'd
metabolic disease in, 395-396, 395f
microphthalmos in, 30f, 31, 31t
motion detection in, 2
myopia in, 5
normal flora of, 38t
normal intraocular pressure in, 97
parasitic infection in, 390t, 392-393
pigmentary uveitis in, 217
retinopathies in
degenerative, 306t
inherited, 305t
multifocal, 309
tear-staining syndrome in, 164-165, 164f, 165f, 166f
vestibular disease in, 341
viral conjunctivitis in, 144
viral disease in, 374-376, 375f, 377f
visual acuity in, 7
visual field of, 3-4, 3f
Doll's eye reflex, 17t
Doxycycline, 221
Drainage angle
examination of, 97-98, 98f
obstruction of, glaucoma due to, 246-247, 247f
Draschia megastoma, 146t
Drooling of saliva due to facial paralysis, 334
Drops, 34, 34f
Drugs, 33-61
antibiotics, 37-43, 37b, 38t, 39t, 40t, 41t
antifungals, 43-45, 44t
antivirals, 45, 45t
autonomic, 51-54, 51f, 52f, 53b
carbonic anhydrase inhibitors, 54-55
corticosteroids, 45-48, 46f, 47f
effects of on intraocular pressure, 231, 232
enzymes and enzyme inhibitors, 55-56
eyelid skin disease due to hypersensitivity to, 130t
hyperosmotic, 50
immunomodulating, 48-50
keratoconjunctivitis sicca due to, 166
local anesthetics, 55
mast cell stabilizers and antihistamines, 50
nonsteroidal antiinflammatory, 48, 49t
ocular emergencies, 419
plaques due to, conjunctival, 147, 148f
prostaglandin analogues, 55
retinopathy due to toxic levels of, 313-314, 313f
routes of administration for, 33-37, 34f, 35f, 36f, 37f
tear replacement preparations, 56, 57t-58t
therapeutic formations for, 33
Dryopteris filix mas, 313
Dysautonomia, 332-333, 338-339
Dyscoria, 209
Dysecdysis, 438
Dysgenesis, anterior segment, 210, 210f
Dysplasia, 65, 65f
pectinate ligament, glaucoma and, 245-246, 245t
retinal, 301, 303f
in wound healing, 74
rod-cone, 305, 308t
Dystrophy, 65
corneal, 182, 183

Dystrophy—cont'd
retinal pigment epithelium, 308-309, 308t, 309f

E
Ecdysis, 438
Echothiophate, 53b
Ectopia lentis, 31
Ectopic cilia, 111-112, 114f, 115, 115f
Ectropion, 79, 119-120, 119f, 120f
Edema
conjunctival, 137
corneal (See Corneal edema)
Edinger-Westphal nucleus lesion, 328f
Effusion, serous, in inflammatory process, 67
Ehrlichiosis, canine monocytic, 384-385, 384f
EHV-1. See Equine herpesvirus 1
Electrical activity, loss of, necrosis and, 66
Electroepilation, 115
Electrophysiology, 322
Electroretinography, 102, 102f, 293-295, 293f, 294f, 295f, 296t, 307
Embryogenesis, 20
congenital malformation development during, 30
Embryonic and fetal development, 20-30
abnormalities of, 30-32, 30f, 31f, 31t, 32f
of ciliary body and iris, 27, 29f
of cornea and anterior chamber, 28, 29f
of eyelids and third eyelid, 28-29, 30f
of lens, 24-26, 26f, 27f, 28f
of nasolacrimal system, 29-30
of optic nerve, 23-24, 24f, 25f
of optic primordia, 20-21, 21f, 22f, 23f
of retina, 21-23, 24f
of sclera and extraocular muscles, 28
of vascular system, 26-27, 28f
of vitreous, 24, 26f
Emergencies, 419-426
acute anterior uveitis, 425-426
corneal lacerations, 422
corneal ulceration, 424
descemetocele or iris prolapse, 424, 425f
diagnostic instruments and supplies needed for, 419
glaucoma, 248-250, 249b, 250b, 422
hyphema, 425
lid lacerations, 422-423
medications for, 419
ocular adnexal contusions and concussion, 423, 424f
penetrating injuries of globe, 423-424
proptosis of globe, 419-421, 420f, 421f
sudden blindness, 426
surgical instruments needed for, 419
Emmetropia, 5, 5f
Emphysema
orbital, 365
subconjunctival, 138
Encephalitis, viral, 404-405
Encephalopathy, feline ischemic, 349
Endocrine disease, 393-395, 394f
Endophthalmitis, 69, 70f, 385t
Endothelial dystrophy, corneal, 183
Endothelium, corneal
anatomy of, 175
embryonic and fetal development of, 28
healing in, 74-75, 177

Enrofloxacin, 42-43
Enterobacter spp., antibiotics of choice for, 41t
Entropion, 79, 116-119, 116f, 117f, 118f, 119f
    neonatal equine, 406, 407f
    in rabbits, 429, 429f
Enucleation, orbital, 365-369
    in birds, 369, 370f, 371f
    for equine recurrent uveitis, 222
    lateral subconjunctival approach, 366, 367f,
        368f
    prosthesis insertion following, 367-368, 368f
    transpalpebral enucleation-extenteration
        technique, 368-369, 368f, 369f
Enzymes, 55-56
Enzyme inhibitors, 55-56
Eosinophilic exudate, 72
Eosinophilic folliculitis, 128t
Eosinophilic furunculosis, 128t
Eosinophilic keratitis, 196, 196f
Eosinophilic orbital myositis, 364-365
Eosinophils in conjunctival disease, 135
Epibulbar melanocytoma, 201, 201f
Epidemic blindness, 227
Epinephrine, 53-54, 53b
Epiphora
    in cilia disorders, 113
    in lacrimal system disorders, 161-65, 161f,
        162f, 163f, 164f, 166f
Episcleritis, 199-200, 200f, 379t
Episclerokeratoconjunctivitis, nodular
        granulomatous, 200, 200f
Epithelial cells in conjunctivitis, 140f-141f
Epithelial inclusion corneal cyst, 190-191, 190f
Epithelium
    corneal
        anatomy of, 175, 176f
        embryonic and fetal development of, 28
        healing in, 74, 177
    lens, 258, 259f
        fetal formation of, 25
    retinal pigment (*See* Retinal pigment
        epithelium)
Epitome spreading, 209
EPM. *See* Equine protozoal myeloencephalitis
Equine eosinophilic keratitis, 196, 196f
Equine herpesvirus 1, 399-400
Equine influenza, 400
Equine protozoal myeloencephalitis, 404
Equine recurrent uveitis, 217-222, 218f, 219f,
        220f, 221f
    vitreous and, 281
ERG. *See* Electroretinography
ERU. *See* Equine recurrent uveitis
Escherichia coli
    antibiotics of choice for, 41t
    fluoroquinolones for, 43t
Esotropia, 332
Etodolac, 48, 49t
    keratoconjunctivitis sicca due to, 166
Eversion of third eyelid, 153, 153f
Evisceration
    with intrascleral prosthesis, for absolute
        glaucoma, 253-254, 253b, 254f
    orbital, 369
Examination, 81, 82b, 82f, 83f
    anterior segment, 85-89, 85f, 86f, 87f, 88f
    in cataracts, 268, 268f
    of exotic pets, 427-428, 428t

Examination—cont'd
    fundus, 90-93, 91f, 92f, 93f
    in lacrimal disorders, 160-161
    neuroophthalmic, 100-102, 319t
    ophthalmoscopic, 89-90, 89f, 90f, 91f
    posterior segment, 93-94
    of third eyelid, 151-152
Examination sheet, 83f
Excision, neoplastic, eyelid, 123, 124f
    third, 155, 155f, 156f
Exenteration, orbital, 368-369, 368f, 369, 369f
Exophthalmos, 355, 357f, 428, 428f
Exotic pets, 427-441
    amphibians, 439-440, 440f
    ferrets, 432-433
    lizards, turtles, tortoises, and crocodilians,
        436-438, 437f, 438f
    mice and rats, 433-434, 433f
    ophthalmic examination and diagnostic
        testing of, 427-428, 428t
    rabbits, 428-432, 428f, 429f, 431f, 432f
    raptors and pet birds, 434-436, 435f
    snakes, 438-439, 438f, 439f
Exotropia, 331-332
External limiting membrane of retina, 286,
        286f, 286t
External ophthalmoplegia, 329
Extracapsular cataract extraction, 270, 271f,
        272
Extraocular muscles
    anatomy of, 353, 354t, 357f
    avulsion of, with proptosis of globe, 420,
        420f, 421f
    embryonic and fetal development of, 28, 29f
    function of, 330-331, 330f
    in globe movement, 353, 354t, 357f
    myositis of, 365, 365f
    nerve supply to, 13-16, 330t
        strabismus due to lesions in, 331-332,
        332f
Extrascleral prosthesis, 369-370, 371f
Exudate, inflammatory, 67, 71-73, 72f, 73f
Eye
    anatomy of, 1
        in amphibians, 439-440
        aqueous physiology in, 17-19, 18f, 18t
        arterial supply in, 10-12, 12f
        in dogs, 2f
        in ferrets, 432
        in lizards, turtles, tortoises, and
        crocodilians, 436-437, 437f
        in mice and rats, 433
        nerve supply in, 13-16, 13f, 14f, 15f, 16f
        ocular reflexes in, 16-17, 17f, 17t
        in rabbits, 428
        in raptors and pet birds, 434-435
        in snakes, 438
        venous drainage in, 12-13, 13f
        vision and, 1-8
    embryonic and fetal development of, 20-30
        (*See Also* Embryonic and fetal
        development)
    examination of, 81, 82b, 82f, 83f (*See Also*
        Diagnosis)
Eyedrops, 34, 34f
Eyelid, 107-134
    anatomy and function of, 107-108, 108f,
        109f, 110f, 111f, 112f

Eyelid—cont'd
    disorders of
        chalazion, 121-122, 121f, 122f
        cilial, 111-115, 114f, 115f
        coloboma, 109, 112f
        ectropion, 119-120, 119f, 120f
        entropion, 116-119, 116f, 117f, 118f,
        119f
        hordeolum and meibomian adenitis,
        122-123, 122f, 122t
        lesions causing, 332-334, 332f, 333f,
        334t
        prominent nasal folds, 109-111, 113f
        systemic causes of, 375t
    embryonic and fetal development of, 28-29,
        30f
    examination of, 87
    injuries of, 120-121, 121f
    innervation of upper, 333
    neonatal delayed or premature opening of,
        108-109
    neoplasia of, 123-126, 123t, 124f, 125f,
        126f, 429
    pathologic responses of, 108
    skin diseases of, 126, 127t-133t
    third (*See* Third eyelid)
Eye washes, 56

F
Facial asymmetry due to facial paralysis, 333-
    334
Facial nerve
    anatomy and function of, 15, 107, 110f, 318
    testing of, 100
Facial paralysis, 405t
    palpebral fissure abnormalities in, 333-334,
        333f, 334t
    third eyelid protrusion in, 332
Facility of outflow, 18-19, 18t
Failure of passive transfer, 406-407, 407f
Familial dermatomyositis, canine, 132t
Farsightedness, 5, 5f, 6
FCRD. *See* Feline central retinal degeneration
FCV. *See* Feline calicivirus infection
FEK. *See* Feline eosinophilic keratitis
Feline calicivirus infection, 378
Feline central retinal degeneration, 311-312,
    312f
Feline eosinophilic keratitis, 196, 196f
Feline herpesvirus 1, 376-378, 377f
    antiviral drugs used for, 45, 45t
    in conjunctivitis, 137t, 143-146, 143t, 144b,
        144f, 145t
    in eosinophilic keratoconjunctivitis, 196
    in eyelid skin disease, 130t
    in keratitis, 195, 195f
Feline immunodeficiency virus infection,
    380-381, 381f
Feline infectious peritonitis, 72, 381-382, 382f
Feline ischemic encephalopathy, 349
Feline leprosy, 129t
Feline leukemia virus infection, 378-380, 379f
Feline pox virus, 130t
FeLV. *See* Feline leukemia virus infection
Fern toxicity, 412
Ferrets, 432-433
    normal intraocular pressure values for,
        428t

Fetal development. *See* Embryonic and fetal development
FFF. *See* Flicker fusion frequency
FHV-1. *See* Feline herpesvirus 1
Fibrosarcoma, eyelid, equine, 125-126, 125f
Fibrosis
corneal, 179-180, 180f
in ocular injury, 63
Fibrovascular membranes, preiridal. *See* Preiridal fibrovascular membranes
Finoff transilluminator, 86, 86f
FIP. *See* Feline infectious peritonitis
FIV. *See* Feline immunodeficiency virus infection
Flap
temporalis muscle, 372
third eyelid for corneal ulcers, 188-189
Fleas, sticktight, 128t
Flicker fusion frequency, 295, 295f
Flies, eyelid, 128t
Floaters, 281
Florida keratopathy, 197
Fluconazole, 43, 44t, 192t
Flucytosine, 43-45, 44t
Fludrocortisone concentration in topical preparation, 34t
Flunixin, 48, 49t
for equine recurrent uveitis, 219
for glaucoma, 250b
Fluorescein angiography, 104, 105f
Fluorescein passage test, 99-100, 100f, 160-161
Fluorescein staining, 98-100, 99f, 100f
of indolent corneal ulcer, 189, 189f
Fluoroquinolones, 42-43, 43t, 185
Foal, shaker, 406
Focal folliculitis, 129t
Focal furunculosis, 129t
Folliculitis
eosinophilic, 128t
focal, 129t
Food allergy, eyelid skin disease due to, 130t
Forage poisoning, 406
Foramen and canals, optic, 9, 11f
Foramen orbitorotundum, 14
Foreign bodies
cataracts due to, 266, 266f
corneal, removal of, 193-194, 193f
orbital, localization of, 359-360
Foscarnet, 45t
Fracture, periorbital, 364
Free conjunctival grafts, 187, 187f, 188
Frontal sinus mucocele, 362-363
Fundus
of birds, 435
effects of glaucoma on, 238-241, 238f, 239f, 240f, 241f
examination of, 90-93, 91f, 92f, 93f
Fungal infection
antifungal drugs for, 43-45, 44t
canine and feline, 387-392, 388t-389t, 391f
conjunctival, 146
corneal, 191, 191f, 192t
of eyelid skin, 129t
in keratitis, 191, 191f, 192t
uveal, 214t
Furunculosis
eosinophilic, 128t
focal, 129t

G
Galactosemic cataracts, 267, 267f
γ-Irradiation, 59-60
Ganciclovir, 45t
Ganglion cells
in central visual pathway, 8
fetal development of, 23
retinal, 286f, 286t, 287
in visual acuity, 6, 7f
Geniculate body, lateral, 9
Gentamicin, 41
for corneal ulcers, 184-185, 185b
for equine recurrent uveitis, 221
Geographic corneal dystrophy, congenital subepithelial, 182
Geographic distribution of equine recurrent uveitis, 217-218
Geographic retinal dysplasia, 301, 303f
Germicides, 58
Germinal cells in wound healing, 74-75, 74f, 75f
Glands of Moll, 157
Glands of Zeis, 157
Glaucoma
aqueous production and drainage and, 230-232, 231f, 232f
associated with neoplasia, 78, 78f
ciliary body–vitreous–lens block, 247-248, 247f, 248f
classification of, 241-242, 242f, 243f, 244b, 244f
clinical signs of, 233-241, 234f
anterior chamber depth changes, 236
corneal/scleral changes, 235-236, 235f, 236f
engorged episcleral vessels, 235
fixed dilated pupil, 236, 236f
fundus changes, 238-241, 238f, 239f, 240f, 241f
increased intraocular pressure, 235
lens changes, 236-238, 237b, 237f, 238b
pain, blepharospasm, and altered behavior, 235
diagnosis of, 213t, 232-233, 233f, 234f
due to uveitis, 212
treatment of, 215-216
inflammation as cause of, 70-71, 70f, 71f
lens luxation and, 274
malignant, vitreous and, 282
primary angle-closure, 243f, 244-246, 245f, 245t, 246f
emergency treatment of, 422
primary open-angle, 242, 242f
in rabbits, 432
secondary, 241, 246-248, 247f, 248f
treatment of, 248-254, 249b, 249f, 250b, 422
in cats, 254-255
in horse, 255
Gliosis, retinal, 301, 303f
Globe proptosis, emergency management of, 419-421, 420f, 421f
Glucose metabolism in lens, 259, 260, 262f
Glycerin, 58t, 249-250
Goat
fundus of, examination of, 92, 93f
mycoplasmal keratoconjunctivitis in, 408, 408f

Goat—cont'd
ocular manifestations of systemic disease in, 408-412
tuberculosis in, 409
Goblet cells in conjunctivitis, 140f-141f
Golden retrievers, pigmentary uveitis in, 217
Gonioimplants for glaucoma, 250-251, 251f
Gonioscopy, 97-98, 98f, 232-233, 233f, 234f
Graft, conjunctival, 187-188, 187f, 188f
Granulation tissue, 76
Granulomatous inflammation, 72
Grid keratotomy for indolent corneal ulcer, 190, 190f

H
Haab's striae, 236, 236f
Habronema spp., 128t, 146t, 403, 403f
Haller-Zinn vascular circle, 27
Harderian gland protrusion in rabbit, 154
Haws syndrome, 332
Head trauma, 326-328, 329f, 329t
Heart disease. *See* Cardiovascular disease
Helichrysum argyrosphaerum poisoning, 313
Helper T cells, cyclosporine and, 48-49
Hemangiosarcoma, third eyelid, 154, 155f
Hematologic disorders, 396t
Hemeralopia, 308
Hemophilus spp., 41t
Hemorrhage
conjunctival and subconjunctival, 137, 377t
in birds, 435, 435f
retinal, 300, 302f, 382t, 402t
subhyaloid, 277
vitreous, 280, 280f
Hepatitis, infectious canine, 199, 199f, 375-376, 377f
Hepatocutaneous syndrome, 132t
Herniation, tentorial, 349
Herpesvirus 1
equine, 399-400
feline (*See* Feline herpesvirus 1)
Heterochromia, 210-211, 210t, 211f, 211t
Histiocytoma, eyelid, 126, 126f, 133t
Histoplasmosis, 129t, 389t, 391-392
History, 81
Homatropine, 53
Hood conjunctival grafts, 187, 187f
Hordeolum, 122-123, 122f, 122t, 157
Horizontal cells, retinal, 23
Horner's syndrome, 332, 332f, 336-338, 337t, 338f, 339t
Horse
bacterial disease in, 400-402, 402f
cataracts in, 265t, 272
color vision in, 8, 8f, 9f
conjunctival angiosarcoma in, 150
cystic corpora nigra in, 225
eosinophilic keratitis in, 196, 196f
eyelid sarcoid in, 125-126, 125f
fundus of, examination of, 92-93, 93f
glaucoma in, 255
heterochromia iridis in, 210t
iris prolapse in, 223
lymphoma in, 406, 406f
motor neuron disease in, 314
neonatal disease in, 406-408, 407f
neurologic disease in, 404-405
neuromuscular disease in, 405-406

Horse—cont'd
  normal flora of, 39t
  ophthalmic examination in, 85
  optic neuritis/neuropathy in, 346-347, 347f
  parasitic disease in, 403-404, 403f
  plant poisoning in, 313
  protozoal disease in, 402-403
  recurrent uveitis in, 217-222, 218f, 219f, 220f, 221f
  retinopathies and neuropathies in, 314, 314f
  viral conjunctivitis in, 144-145
  viral disease in, 399-400
  visual acuity in, 7, 9f
  visual field of, 3, 4f
Hotz-Celsus procedure, 117-118, 118f
H-plasty for eyelid reconstruction, 123, 124f
Hyalin, 58t
Hyalocentesis, 282-283, 283f, 283t
Hyaloid artery
  embryonic and fetal development of, 20-21, 23f
  persistent, 279
    cataracts and, 265-266
Hyalosis, asteroid, 281-282, 281f
Hyaluronidase, 56
Hydranencephaly, 349
Hydrocephalus, 10
  obstructive, 349-350
Hydrocortisone, 34t, 47
Hydroxyamphetamine, 53b
Hydroxypropylmethylcellulose, 57t-58t
Hyperadrenocorticism, 394
Hyperemia
  conjunctival, 136-137, 137t
    in cilia disorders, 113
    systemic causes of, 377t
  in inflammatory process, 67
Hyperlipidemia, 395-396, 395f
Hyperopia, 5, 5f
  loss of lens and, 6
Hyperosmotic drugs, 50
Hyperplasia, 63, 64f
Hyperplastic primary vitreous, persistent, 279-280, 280f
  cataracts and, 265-266
Hyperreflectivity, retinal, 90
Hypersensitivity
  arthropod, 128t-129t
  denervation, 51, 53, 338, 339
  drugs, eyelid skin disease due to, 130t
  mosquito-bite, 129t
Hypertension, systemic, 396-397, 397f, 397t
Hyperthermia, 60, 60f
Hypertrophy, 63, 63f
Hyperviscosity syndrome, 398
Hyphema
  etiology of, 223, 224f
  glaucoma associated with, 250b
  histology of, 79
  neoplasia and, 78
  with proptosis of globe, 420
  treatment of, 223-224, 425
Hypophysis, 9
Hypoplasia, 63
  iris, 227
  optic nerve, 344, 345f
  of prosencephalon in calves, 349
Hypopyon, 79

Hypothyroidism, 394-395, 395f
Hypovitaminosis A, 292, 312, 312b, 313f, 350

I

IBK. See Infectious bovine keratoconjunctivitis
IBR. See Infectious bovine rhinotracheitis
Idoxuridine, 45, 45t, 146
Imaging techniques, 102-104, 103f, 104f, 105f
Imbert-Fick law, 96
Imidazoles, 192t
Immune-mediated disease
  conjunctival, 147, 147f
  corticosteroids for, 46-47
  disruption in blood-ocular barrier and, 71
  keratoconjunctivitis sicca, 166-167
  superficial keratoconjunctivitis, 194-195, 194f
  uveitis, 214t, 216-222
  uveodermatologic syndrome, 72, 132t, 216, 398-399, 399f
Immunodeficiency virus infection, feline, 380-381, 381f
Immunofluorescent antibody test, 144, 145t
Immunomodulating drugs, 48-50
Immunostimulants, 50
Immunosuppressives for uveitis, 215
Imperforate puncta, 162-163, 163f
Implantation, lens, for cataracts, 270-271, 272f
Inclusion cyst, corneal epithelial, 190-191, 190f
Indentation tonometry, 95-96, 95f, 96f
Indirect ophthalmoscopy, 90, 90f
Indolent corneal ulcer
  in dog, 189-190, 189f, 190f
  fluorescein staining of, 99, 99f
Infection
  bacterial (See Bacterial infection)
  orbital, 362t
  parasitic (See Parasitic infection)
  protozoal (See Protozoal infection)
  retinal, 309-311, 311f
  uveal, 214t
  viral (See Viral infection)
  vitreous, 280-281
Infectious bovine keratoconjunctivitis, 145, 145t, 197-198, 198b, 198f
Infectious bovine rhinotracheitis, 198-199, 410, 410f
  in conjunctivitis, 145, 145t
  in infectious bovine keratoconjunctivitis, 197, 198b
Infectious canine hepatitis, 199, 199f
Infectious uveitis, 214t, 216
Inflammation, 66-73
  blood-ocular barrier alterations due to, immune-mediated disease and, 71
  cataracts due to, 69-70
  corneal, 68-69, 69f
  corticosteroids for, 45-48
  effects on intraocular pressure, 232
  exudate from, 71-73, 72f, 73f
  glaucoma due to, 70-71, 70f, 71f
  granulomatous, 72
  necrosis and, 66
  in ocular injury, 63
  optic nerve, 345-347, 346f, 347f, 347t
  peculiarities of, 68, 68f
  retinal detachment due to, 69, 70f
  retinopathy secondary to, 309-311, 311f

Inflammation—cont'd
  third eyelid, 155
  vitreous, 280-281
Inflammatory cell infiltration of corneal stroma, 180, 180f
Influenza, equine, 400
Injection
  for entropion in lambs, 117
  subconjunctival, subteton, and retrobulbar, 34f, 36, 36f, 37f
Injury. See Trauma
Inner retina, 23
Innervation. See Nerve supply
Instruments
  for examination, 82b
  for microbiologic sampling, 84, 84f
  for ocular emergencies, 419
Interferon for viral conjunctivitis, 146
Internal limiting membrane of retina, 286f, 286t, 287
Internal ophthalmoplegia, 329
Intracapsular cataract extraction, 270
Intracranial injury, pupils and, 326-328, 329f, 329t
Intraocular pressure, 18-19, 18t
  aqueous balance in, 231, 232f
  causes of variations in, 232
  corticosteroids and, 46, 47
  in differential diagnosis of ocular inflammation, 213t
  in glaucomas, 235 (See Also Glaucoma)
  measurement of, 95-97, 95f, 96f, 97f
  normal, 97
    in exotic species, 428t
  reduction of
    carbonic anhydrase inhibitors for, 55
    hyperosmotic agents for, 50
    in uveitis, 212, 215-216
Intraorbital prosthesis, 367-368, 368f
Intrascleral lens implantation for cataract, 270-171, 272f
Intrascleral prosthesis, 369, 371f
  for absolute glaucoma, 253-254, 253b, 254f
  evisceration for, 369
Intumescent cataract, 268
Inverted retina, 23, 287
IOP. See Intraocular pressure
Iridocorneal angle
  anatomy of, 203, 205f
  examination of, 97-98, 98f, 232-233, 233f, 234f
  obstruction of, glaucoma due to, 246-247, 247f
Iridocyclitis, 69, 208
Iridodialysis, 223
Iris
  anatomy and physiology of, 203, 204f, 205f
  arterial circle of, 12
  atrophy of, 63, 227-228, 228f
  changes in color of, 79
  coloboma in, 210, 210f
  embryonic and fetal development of, 22, 27, 29f
  examination of, 88
  feline diffuse melanoma in, 226-227, 227f
  hypoplasia of, 227
  pigmentation disorders of, 210-211, 210t, 211f, 211t

Iris—cont'd
  prolapse of, 223
    in corneal ulceration, 187
    emergency treatment of, 424, 425f
Iris bombé, 212, 247
Iris nevi, 211, 211f
Iritis, 208
Irradiation, 59-60, 59f
Irritant dermatitis, 130t
Ischemic disease of eyelid skin, 132t
Island conjunctival grafts, 187, 187f, 188
Isoerythrolysis, neonatal, 407
Isoflurophate, 53b
Itraconazole, 43, 192t
Ivermectin, 59, 222

J

Jones test, 99-100, 100f, 160-161
Jugular vein, 13
Juvenile cellulitis, 133t

K

KCS. *See* Keratoconjunctivitis sicca
Keratic precipitates, 79, 212
Keratitis
  eosinophilic, 196, 196f
  herpetic, 195, 195f
  mycotic, 191, 191f, 192t
  neurogenic, 195
  pigmentary, 194
    corneal, 180, 180f
  superficial punctate, 183, 183f
  systemic causes of, 378t, 400t
  ulcerative, of cornea (*See* Corneal
    ulceration)
Keratoconjunctivitis
  chronic immune-mediated superficial,
    194-195, 194f
  herpetic, 45, 45t
  infectious bovine, 145, 145t, 197-198, 198b,
    198f
  mycoplasmal in goats and sheep, 408, 408f
  systemic causes of, 378t, 400t
Keratoconjunctivitis sicca, 137t, 166-171, 168f,
  172f-173f, 378t
Keratoma, eyelid, 149, 149f
Keratomalacia, suppurative, 68-69
Keratopathy
  bullous, 197, 197f
  Florida, 197
  lipid in amphibians, 440, 440f
Keratotomy, grid, 190, 190f
Ketoconazole, 43, 44t
Ketoprofen, 48, 49t
Ketorolac, 48, 49t
Key-Gaskell syndrome, 338-339

L

Lacerations
  conjunctival, 147, 148f
  corneal, 192-193, 193f, 422
  eyelid, 422-423
    third, 155, 156f
Lacrimal canaliculi, 159-160, 159f, 160f
Lacrimal fossa, 159, 160f
Lacrimal glands, 157, 158f, 159f
Lacrimal lake, 160
Lacrimal nerve, 14, 110f

Lacrimal pump, 160
Lacrimal puncta
  anatomy and physiology of, 159-160, 159f,
    160f
  embryonic and fetal development of, 30
Lacrimal sac, 159
Lacrimal system, 157-174
  anatomy and physiology of, 157-160, 158f,
    159f, 160f
  disorders of, 160-171
    cicatricial nasolacrimal obstruction,
      163-164, 164f
    congenital atresia, ectopia, and
      imperforate puncta, 162-163, 163f
    cystic, 163
    dacryocystitis, 161-162, 161f, 162f, 163f
    examination in, 160-161
    keratoconjunctivitis sicca, 166-171,
      168f, 172f-173f
    precorneal tear film, 160, 165-166
    tear-staining syndrome in dogs,
      164-165, 164f, 165f, 166f
  neoplasm of, 171
Lacrimomimetic agents, 56, 57t-58t
Lamina cribrosa, 8
Lanolin ointment, 58t, 170
Laser therapy, 60
  for glaucoma, 251, 252, 255
Latanoprost for glaucoma, 249, 249b, 422
Lateral geniculate nucleus disease, 348
Lateral subconjunctival orbital enucleation
  technique, 366, 367f, 368f
Lavage system for drug administration, 35, 35f
Leishmaniasis, 130t, 392-393, 393f
Lens, 258-276
  anatomy and physiology of, 258-260, 259f,
    260f
    capsule in, 258, 260f
    epithelium in, 258
    fibers in, 258, 260f, 261f
    metabolism and composition in,
      259-260, 262f
    nuclear sclerosis in, 260, 262f
  cataract of, 261-272
    acquired, 266-267, 266f, 267f
    classification of, 261-263, 261t, 263,
      263f
    congenital, 264-266, 266f
    diabetic, 267-268
    diagnosis of, 268-269, 268f, 269t
    hereditary, 264, 265t
    in horses, 272
    lens-induced uveitis and, 263-264
    molecular and cellular pathogenesis of,
      261
    senile, 267
    stages of development of, 262-263, 263f
    treatment of, 269-272, 270f, 271f, 272f
  congenital anomalies of, 260
  effects of glaucoma on, 236-238, 237b,
    237f, 238b
  embryonic and fetal development of, 24-26,
    26f, 27f, 28f
  examination of, 88-89
  implantation, 270-171, 272f
  loss of in severe hyperopia, 6
  luxation of (*See* Lens luxation)
  opacity of, 80

Lens—cont'd
  subluxation of, 272-273
  uveitis induced by, 216-217, 217f
  in visual acuity, 5
  wound healing in, 74-75
Lens capsule, 25-26
Lens-induced uveitis, 263-264, 269
Lens luxation, 272-275, 273f, 274f
  in glaucoma, 236, 237, 237b
    treatment of, 250b, 252-253
  vitreous and, 282
Lens placode, 20, 22f, 23f, 26f
Lens suture, 25
Lens vesicle, 20, 21f, 24, 27f
Lens zonules, 24
Lenticonus, 260
Lentigo simplex, 133t
Leprosy, feline, 129t
Leptospira spp., 218, 221, 401, 402f
Leukemia virus infection, feline, 378-380, 379f
Leukocytes, 67, 68-69
Leukoma, corneal, 180, 180f
LGN. *See* Lateral geniculate nucleus disease
Lid lacerations, emergency treatment of, 422-423
Lid retractors for drug administration, 36, 36f
Light
  flickering, sensitivity to, 2-3
  sensitivity to, 1-2, 2f, 3f
Ligneous conjunctivitis, 147-148, 148f
Limbal neoplasm, 201, 201f
Limiting membrane of retina
  external, 286, 286f, 286t
  internal, 286f, 286t, 287
Lipemia retinalis, 381t, 395, 395f
Lipid
  corneal accumulation of, 181, 181f
  deficiency of, precorneal tear film and,
    165-166
Lipid dystrophy, corneal, 183, 183f
Lipid keratopathy in amphibians, 440, 440f
Lipid layer of precorneal tear film, 157
Lipogranulomatous conjunctivitis, 148, 148f
Lipoxgenase pathway, corticosteroids and, 46,
  46f
Liquefaction, vitreous, 278
Listeriosis, 408, 408f
LIU. *See* Lens-induced uveitis
Lizards, 436-438
Local anesthetics, 55
Locoweed poisoning, 167, 412
Lower motor neuron innervation, 335-336, 337f
Luxation of lens. *See* Lens luxation
Lyme disease
  canine, 383, 383f
  equine, 401-402
Lymph node, conjunctival sac and, 135, 136f
Lymphocytes in inflammatory process, 72-73
Lymphoma, 406, 406f
  third eyelid, 154, 155f
Lymphosarcoma
  equine, 406, 406f
  ruminant, 411, 411f
  uveal, 227, 227f
Lysine, 146

M

Macrophages, 72
Macula, corneal, 179, 180f

Maedi-visna, 411
Magnetic resonance imaging, 104, 104f, 358, 358f, 359f
Magnifying scope, 86f
Malacia, stromal, 181, 182f
Malaris muscle, 107
Male fern, 313
Malignant catarrhal fever, 410, 410f
    in conjunctivitis, 145, 145t
    corneal signs in, 199
Malignant glaucoma, 282
Malignant neoplasm, 78
Mannheimia pneumonia, 409
Mannitol, 50, 249, 249b, 422
Marcus Gunn pupil, 101, 322
Mast cell stabilizers, 50, 141, 147
Mast cell tumor, eyelid, 133t
Mastocytoma, eyelid, 133t
Maxillary artery, 10-11
Maxillary nerve, 14
Maxillary vein, 13
Maze test, 102, 320
MCF. See Malignant catarrhal fever
Medial canthoplasty, 118-119, 119f
Medial longitudinal fasciculus, 331
Mediators in inflammation, 67
Medical history, 81
Medications. See Drugs
Meibomian gland
    adenoma of, 125, 125f
    anatomy of, 107, 108f, 157, 159f
    chalazion of, 121-122, 121f, 122f
Meibomitis, 122-123, 122f, 122t
Melanin, congenital absence of on leading edge of third eyelid, 152
Melanocytoma
    limbal, 201, 201f
    uveal, 225-226, 226f
Melanoma
    epibulbar, 226, 226f
    eyelid, 133t
    feline diffuse iris, 226-227, 227f
    glaucoma secondary to, 253
    uveal, 225-226, 226f
Melanosis, corneal, 180, 180f
Meloxicam, 48, 49t
"Melting," stromal, 181, 182f
Menace response, 101, 318-320, 320f, 321f
Meningitis, 350, 350t, 405
Meningoencephalitis, thromboembolic, 349, 409, 409f
Metabolic disease
    of dogs and cats, 395-396, 395f
    of eyelid skin, 132t
    optic radiation and visual cortex disorders in, 349
    ruminant, 411-412
    uveitis in, 214t
Metabolism in lens, 259, 260, 262f
Metaplasia, 63-65, 64f
Metastatic neoplasm, 77-78
Methazolamide, 249b, 422
Methicillin, 38-40
Methylcellulose, 57t, 169
Mice, 433-434, 433f
    normal intraocular pressure values for, 428t
Miconazole, 43, 192t
Microbiologic sampling, 83-84, 84f

Microcornea, 181, 182f
Microphakia, 31
Microphthalmos, 30-31, 30f, 31t
Mineral oil ointment, 58t, 170
Minerals, corneal accumulation of, 181, 181f
Mittendorf's dot, 279
MLF. See Medial longitudinal fasciculus
Mobility, retinal, assessment of, 84-85
Monocular indirect ophthalmoscopy, 90, 90f, 91f
Moraxella spp., 41t, 141
Mosquito-bite hypersensitivity, 129t
Motion sensitivity, 2
Motor neuron disease, equine, 314, 406
MRI. See Magnetic resonance imaging
Mucin deficiency, 165
Mucinomimetic agents, 56
Mucocele, 362-363
Mucoid discharge in keratoconjunctivitis sicca, 167-168, 167f, 168f, 170
Mucoid layer of precorneal tear film, 157-159
Mucous threads in lacrimal system, 159
Müller's cells, 286, 288f, 289f
    fetal development of, 23
Müller's muscle, action of, 15
Multilobular osteoma, 364
Muscles
    action of with autonomic innervation, 15, 15t
    extraocular (See Extraocular muscles)
    of eyelids, 107, 111f
Mycoplasmas
    in conjunctivitis, 137t, 142-143
    feline, 386-387
    in keratoconjunctivitis
        bovine, 197, 198b
        in goats and sheep, 408, 408f
Mycotic infection. See Fungal infection
Mydriatic therapy
    atropine in, 51-52
    for corneal ulcers, 185-186
    for uveitis, 215
Myelination of optic nerve fibers, 298
Myelin degeneration, 343, 343f
Myeloencephalitis, equine protozoal, 404
Myopia, 5, 5f
Myositis, eosinophilic, orbital, 364-365
Myotonia, congenital, 333
Myxoma virus, 430

N

Nasal folds, prominent, 109-111, 113f
Nasociliary nerve, 14
Nasolacrimal system
    anatomy and physiology of, 159-160, 159f, 160f
    catheterization of, 161-162, 162f
    disease of
        in mice and rats, 433-434, 433f
        in rabbits, 430
    embryonic and fetal development of, 29-30, 30
    examination of, 87
    obstruction of
        assessment of, 100
        cicatricial, 163-164, 164f
    of rabbits, 428
Natamycin, 43, 192t

Nearsightedness, 5, 5f
Nebula, corneal, 179, 180f
Necrolytic dermatitis, superficial, 132t
Necrosis, 65-66, 66f
    of cerebrum, 349
Neisseria spp., 41t
Neomycin, 41, 184
Neonatal maladjustment syndrome, 407
Neonate
    delayed or premature eyelid opening in, 108-109
    equine, diseases of, 406-408, 407f
Neoplasm, 77-79, 77f, 78f
    cerebral, 344, 344t
    conjunctival, 148-150, 149f
    corneoscleral limbal, 201, 201f
    eyelid, 123-126, 123t, 124f, 125f, 126f, 133t
    glaucoma secondary to, 253
    lacrimal gland, 171
    lymphoma, 406, 406f
    optic nerve, 347
    optic radiation and visual cortex disorders, 348
    orbital, 362t, 363-364, 364f
    in rabbits, 429
    uveal, 214t, 225-227, 225b, 225f, 226f, 227f
Neosporosis, 391
Nerve block, auriculopalpebral, 85, 85f
Nerve fibers
    in central visual pathway, 8-10
    retinal, 286f, 286t, 287
Nerve growth factor ointment, 169
Nerve supply, 13-16, 13f, 14f, 15f, 16f
    autonomic innervation in, 15-16, 15t, 17f, 335-336, 336f, 337f
    cranial nerves in, 13-15, 13f, 14f, 15f, 16f
    to extraocular muscles, 330f, 330t
        strabismus due to lesions in, 331-332, 332f
    to eyelids, 107, 111f
    to lacrimal system, 160
Neural crest, 20
Neural groove, 20, 21f
Neural tube, 20, 21f
Neuritis, optic, 345-347, 346f, 347f, 347t, 384t
Neuroblastic layer, 23
Neurogenic keratitis, 195
Neurogenic keratoconjunctivitis, 167
Neuroglia, pathologic reactions of, 343-344
Neurologic disorders, equine, 403t, 404-405
Neuromuscular disease, 405-406
Neuronal degeneration, 342-343, 343f
Neuroophthalmologic examination, 100-102, 319t
Neuroophthalmology
    autonomic innervation and abnormalities, 335-339, 336f, 337f, 337t, 338f, 339t
    central visual pathways, 342-350, 342f, 343f, 344t, 345f, 346f, 347f, 347t
    lesions causing eyelid abnormalities, 332-334, 332f, 333f, 334t
    lesions causing strabismus, 330-332, 330f, 331t, 332f
    lesions in patients with visual and pupillary light reflexes, 323-330, 329f, 329t, 330f, 331t
    meningitis, 350, 350t

Neuroophthalmology—cont'd
  pupillary light reflex in, 320-321, 321f, 322f
  storage diseases, 350
  vestibular system, 339-342, 340b
  vision assessment in, 318-320, 320f, 321-322, 321f, 322f
  vitamin A deficiency, 350
Neuropathy, equine, 314, 314f
  optic, 346-347, 347f
Neuroretina, 285
Neutrophils
  in conjunctival disease, 135, 140f-141f
  in corneal healing, 72, 72f, 73f
  in suppurative exudate, 72
Nevi, iris, 211, 211f
"New Forest eye," 197-198, 198b, 198f
NGE. See Nodular granulomatous episclerokeratoconjunctivitis
Night blindness, congenital stationary, 309
NMS. See Neonatal maladjustment syndrome
Nodular granulomatous episclerokeratoconjunctivitis, 200, 200f
Nodular panniculitis, 132t
Nonsteroidal antiinflammatory drugs, 48, 49t
  for corneal ulcers, 186
  keratoconjunctivitis sicca due to, 166
  properties of, 46
  for uveitis, 215
    equine recurrent, 219, 220-221
    traumatic, 222
Nontapetum
  anatomy of, 297, 298f
  examination of, 91
Norepinephrine, action of, 51, 52f
Normal flora, 38t, 39t, 40t
Notch defect, scleral, 199
Notoedric acariasis, 127t
NSAIDs. See Nonsteroidal antiinflammatory drugs
Nuclear layer of retina, 286, 286f, 286t
Nuclear sclerosis in lens, 80, 260, 262f
Nutrition
  cataracts and, 267, 267f
  retinopathy and, 311-312, 312b, 312f, 313f
  wound healing and, 76
Nutritional disorders of eyelid skin, 132t
Nystagmus, 339-341, 340b
  congenital, 342
Nystatin, 192t

O

Oblique muscles, 13, 14
Obstruction
  cicatricial nasolacrimal, 163-164, 164f
  iridocorneal angle, glaucoma due to, 246-247, 247f
  lacrimal, 160
Obstructive hydrocephalus, 349-350
Ocular reflexes, 16-17, 17f, 17t
Oculomotor nerve, 10
  anatomy and function of, 13-14, 14f, 15f, 318
  lesion of, 327f, 328-329
    strabismus due to, 331-332
  testing of, 100
Oculomotor nucleus lesion, 328f
Oestrus ovis, 146t

Ofloxacin, 43
Ointments, route of administration for, 35-36
Onchocerca cervicalis, 128t, 146t, 222, 404
Opacity
  due to corneal edema, 178, 179f, 378t
  lenticular, 90
  retinal, 90
  of vitreous, 281
Ophthalmia, sympathetic, 213
Ophthalmic artery, 10, 11
Ophthalmic examination. See Examination
Ophthalmic vein, 13, 13f
Ophthalmoplegia
  external, 329
  internal, 329
Ophthalmoscopy, 89-90, 89f, 90f, 91f
  in aqueous flare detection, 94, 95f
  in glaucomas, 232
Opsin, 290-291
Optical canal, 13
Optic axis, 352, 353f, 355f
Optic chiasm
  in central visual pathway, 9
  diseases of, 325f, 348
  optic nerve anatomy and, 13
Optic cup, 20, 21-23, 21f, 22f, 24, 24f
Optic disc
  anatomy of, 297-298
  in central visual pathway, 8
  cupping of in glaucoma, 238-239, 239f, 240f
  examination of, 91
    in dogs, 92
    in horses, 93
  retinopathies and, 307
Optic foramen and canals, 9, 11f
Optic grooves or pits, 20, 21f, 22f
Optic nerve
  anatomy and function of, 13, 318
  in central visual pathway, 8-9
  disease of, 324f, 344-348, 344t, 345f, 346f, 347f, 347t
    systemic causes of, 402t
  embryonic and fetal development of, 23-24, 24f, 25f
  examination of, 91, 94, 100
    in cats, 92
    in sheep, goats, and cattle, 93, 93f
  fibers of, myelination of, 298
  retinal interaction with, 298
Optic neuritis, 345-347, 346f, 347f, 347t, 384t
Optic neuropathy, 314, 314f
Optic primordia, formation of, 20-21, 21f, 22f, 23f
Optic radiation, 10
  disease of, 348-349
Optic stalks, 20, 22f
Optic tract
  anatomy of, 9
  disease of, 326f, 348
Optic vesicle, 20, 21f, 22-23
Optivisor magnifying scope, 86f
Orbicularis oculi muscle, 107
Orbifloxacin, 42-43
Orbit, 352-373
  anatomy of, 352-353, 353f, 354f, 354t, 355f, 356f, 357f
  dental disease and, 365

Orbit—cont'd
  disease of, 357-365
    cellulitis and retrobulbar abscess, 360-361, 361f, 362f, 363f
    cysts, 361-363
    diagnosis of, 357-360, 358f, 359f, 361f
    emphysema, 365
    eosinophilic myositis, 364-365
    extraocular muscle myositis, 365, 365f
    in ferrets, 432
    fractures, 364
    neoplasm and space-occupying lesions, 356, 357f, 363-364, 364f
    systemic causes of, 385t, 404t
  extraocular muscles and, 353, 354t, 357f
  pathologic mechanisms in, 353-357, 357f
  penetrating injuries of, 423-424
  proptosis of, emergency management of, 419-421, 420f, 421f
  prosthesis for, 369-370, 371f
  surgical procedures on
    enucleation, 365-369, 367f, 368f, 369f, 370f, 371f
    orbitotomy and orbitectomy, 370-372, 371f, 372f
    prosthesis, 369-370, 371f
    temporalis muscle flap, 372
Orbital axis, 352, 353f
Orbital fissure, 14
Orbital fissure syndrome, 329
Orbital venography, 103, 358-359, 359f
Orbital venous plexus, 13, 13f
Orbitectomy, 370-372, 371f, 372f
Orbitography, contrast, 359, 359f, 360f
Orbitotomy, 370-372, 371f, 372f
Organogenesis, 20
  congenital malformation development during, 30
Organophosphates, 54
Osteoma, multilobular, 364
Otitis interna, 341
Otitis media, 341
Oxacillin, 40
Oxygen available to cornea, 175-176, 176f
Oxygen toxicity, 313-314
Oxyspirura mansoni, 146t
Oxytetracycline, 198

P

PABA. See Para-aminobenzoic acid
PACG. See Primary angle-closure glaucoma
Pain
  in differential diagnosis of ocular inflammation, 213t
  of glaucoma, 235
  of lens luxation, 274
  management of in uveitis, 216
Palpation, orbital, 358
Palpebral conjunctiva
  anatomy of, 135
  embryonic and fetal development of, 29
Palpebral fissure, lesions causing abnormalities of, 333-334, 333f, 334t
Palpebral reflex, 16-17, 17t, 101
Panniculitis, nodular, 132t
Pannus, 194-195, 194f
Panophthalmitis, 69
Panuveitis, 209, 385t

Papilledema, 344, 344t, 347t, 350
Papillomatosis
    conjunctival, canine, 150
    viral, of eyelid, 126, 126f
Para-aminobenzoic acid, 42
Parallax, 4, 86, 86f
Paralysis
    facial, 405t
        palpebral fissure abnormalities in,
            333-334, 333f, 334t
        third eyelid protrusion in, 332
    oculomotor, 331-332
Paranasal sinuses, orbit and, 352, 355f, 356f
Parasiticides, 59
Parasitic infection
    canine and feline, 390t, 392-393
    conjunctival, 146-147, 146t
        in birds, 436
    equine, 403-404, 403f
    of eyelid skin, 127t-128t
    uveal, 214t
Parasympathetic nervous system, 15t, 16, 16f,
    335
Parasympatholytic drugs, 51-53, 51f, 53b
Parasympathomimetic agents, 53b, 54
Parotid duct transposition, 171, 172f-173f
Pars plana ciliaris, 282, 283f
Passive transfer, failure of, 406-407, 407f
Pathology, 62-80
    common clinical lesions seen with, 79-80
    inflammation, 66-73
        blood-ocular barrier alterations due to,
            immune-mediated disease and, 71
        cataracts due to, 69-70
        corneal, 68-69, 69f
        exudate from, 71-73, 72f, 73f
        glaucoma due to, 70-71, 70f, 71f
        peculiarities of, 68, 68f
        retinal detachment due to, 69, 70f
    injury, 62-66
        causes of, 62
        consequences of, 62-66, 63f, 64f, 65f,
            66f
    neoplasia, 77-79, 77f, 78f
    wound healing, 73-77
        diseases resulting from defective, 76-77
        germinal cells in, 74-75, 74f, 75f
        nutrition in, 76
        tissue scaffolding in, 75-76
Pecten, 287, 291f
Pectinate ligament dysplasia, glaucoma and,
    245-246, 245t
PEM. See Polioencephalomalacia
Pemphigus erythematosus, 131t
Pemphigus foliaceus, 131t
Pemphigus vulgaris, 131t
Penciclovir, 45t
Penetrating injury
    to globe, 423-424
    to lens, uveitis due to, 217
Penicillins, 38-40
Penicillin G, 38
Periocular cyst, 361-363
Periorbita
    anatomy of, 352, 356f
    fracture of, 364
Peripheral neuroanatomy, 13-16, 13f, 14f, 15f,
    16f

Peritonitis, feline infectious, 72, 381-382, 382f
Perivascular cuffing, retinal, 300, 301f
Persistent hyaloid artery, 279
    cataracts and, 265-266
Persistent hyperplastic primary vitreous,
    279-280, 280f
    cataracts and, 265-266
Persistent pupillary membranes, 182, 182f, 209,
    209f
    cataracts and, 265
    embryonic and fetal development of, 27
Persistent tunica vasculosa lentis, 279
Phacoclastic uveitis, 72, 72f, 222, 222f, 264
Phacoemulsification, 270, 271f, 272
Phacolytic uveitis, 263-264
Pharmacology. See Drugs
Phenol red thread test, 427, 428t
Phenylbutazone, 48, 49t, 219
Phenylephrine, 53-54, 53b, 224
PHF. See Potomac horse fever
Photic head shaking in horses, 405
Photochemistry, 291-292, 293f
Photophobia in differential diagnosis of ocular
    inflammation, 213t
Photopic vision, 289
Photopigments, 287f, 289-291
Photoreceptors
    anatomy of, 285, 286t, 288f
    in central visual pathway, 8
    in color vision, 7
    dysplasia of, 305
    fetal development of, 23
    primary disease of, 299, 299f
    in visual acuity, 6
Phototoxic retinopathy in mice and rats, 434
PHPV. See Persistent hyperplastic primary
    vitreous
Physical therapy, 59-60, 59f, 60f
Physiologic optic cup, 24
Physostigmine, 53b
Pigmentary keratitis, 194
Pigmentary uveitis in golden retrievers, 217
Pigmentation
    corneal, 180, 180f
        histology of, 79
        in keratoconjunctivitis sicca, 168
    eyelid, disorders of, 133t
    iris, disorders of, 210-211, 210t, 211f, 211t
    of retinal pigment epithelium, 296, 296f
Pigment epithelium, retinal. See Retinal
    pigment epithelium
Pilocarpine, 53b, 54
    for glaucoma, 249b, 422
    for hyphema, 224
    for keratoconjunctivitis sicca, 169
Pink eye, 197-198, 198b, 198f
Piroplasmosis, 402
Pituitary fossa, 9
Placement reflex, 320, 320f
Plant toxicity
    retinopathy due to, 313-314, 313f
    in ruminants, 412
Plaque, conjunctival, 147, 148f, 149, 149f
Plasma cells, 72-73, 140f-141f
PLD. See Pectinate ligament dysplasia
Plexiform layer of retina, 8, 286-287, 286f, 286t
PLR. See Pupillary light reflex
Pneumonia, Mannheimia, 409

POAG. See Primary open-angle glaucoma
Poisoning. See Toxicity
Polioencephalomalacia, 411-412
Polyarthritis, ovine chlamydial, 408
Polycoria, 209
Polycythemia, 396t, 397-398
Polymerase chain reaction, 144, 145t
Polymyxin B, 42, 184
Polyvinyl alcohol, 57t-58t, 169
Posterior chamber anatomy, 17, 18f
Posterior segment examination, 93-94
Posterior uveitis
    defined, 69, 208
    systemic causes of, 380t, 401t
Postsphenoid bone, 9
Potomac horse fever, 402-403
Povidone-iodine solution, 58
Pox virus, 130t, 436
PPMs. See Persistent pupillary membranes
Precorneal tear film
    anatomy and physiology of, 157-159, 159f
    deficiency of, 165-166
    dysfunction of, 160
Prednisolone, 34t, 47
    for equine recurrent uveitis, 219, 221
    for hyphema, 224, 250b
Preiridal fibrovascular membranes
    glaucoma from, 70, 71f
    in uveitis, 213
    in wound healing, 76
        defective, 77
Prematurity, equine, 406
Preservatives in drugs, 33
Pretectal area, 9
Primary angle-closure glaucoma, 241, 243f,
    244-246, 245f, 245t, 246f
    in dogs, 238b
    emergency treatment of, 422
    vision loss in, 240-241
Primary open-angle glaucoma, 240-241, 242,
    242f
Prolapse
    iris, 223
        in corneal ulceration, 187
        emergency treatment of, 424, 425f
    third eyelid gland, 153-154, 153f, 154f
Prominence of third eyelid, 151-152
Proptosis of globe, 419-421, 420f, 421f
Prosencephalon
    hypoplasia of in calves, 349
    injury to, 326-327
Prostaglandin analogues, 55
Prosthesis
    extrascleral, 369-370, 371f
    insertion of intraorbital, 367-368, 368f
    intrascleral, 369, 371f
        for absolute glaucoma, 253-254, 253b,
            254f
        evisceration for, 369
Protease inhibitors, 56, 189
Proteus spp., 41t, 43t
Prototheccosis, 389t
Protozoal infection
    equine, 402-403
        neurologic, 404
    of eyelid skin, 130t
    ruminant, 411
    uveal, 214t

Protrusion
  third eyelid, 332-333, 332f
  third eyelid gland, 153-154, 153f, 154f
Pseudomonas aeruginosa, 41t, 43t
Psoroptic acariasis, 128t
Ptosis, 15, 375t
Puncta, lacrimal
  anatomy and physiology of, 159-160, 159f, 160f
  imperforate, 162-163, 163f
Punctate keratitis, superficial, 183, 183f
Pupil
  congenital abnormalities of, 209
  examination of, 84-85, 84f, 85f, 88
  fixed and dilated, in glaucoma, 236, 236f
  intracranial injury and, 326-328, 329f, 329t
  Marcus Gunn, 101, 322
  proptosis of globe and, 420
  retinopathies and, 307
  shape of
    changes in, histologic basis for, 79
    examination of, 84-85, 84f, 85f
  systemic causes of disorders in, 404t
Pupillary block, glaucoma due to, 71, 71f, 247, 247f
Pupillary escape, 322
Pupillary light reflex, 16, 17f, 17t, 320-321, 321f, 322f
  abnormal, 323-328, 329-330, 329f, 329t
    in blind patients, 323-328, 329f, 329t
    in visual patients, 328-330
  assessment of, 84, 85
  in differential diagnosis of ocular inflammation, 213t
  lesions in blind patients with normal, 323
  nerve fibers in, 10
  proptosis of globe and, 420
Pupillary membranes, persistent, 182, 182f, 209, 209f
  cataracts and, 265
  embryonic and fetal development of, 27
Pupillary sphincter muscle, 10
Pupillary zone of iris, 203, 204f
Pyriform lobe, 9

R
Rabbits, 428-432
  adnexal disease in, 429, 429f
  cataracts in, 431-432, 431f, 432f
  conjunctival disease in, 429-430, 430f
  corneal disease in, 430-431
  glaucoma in, 432
  nasolacrimal disease in, 430
  normal intraocular pressure values for, 428t
  ophthalmic anatomy of, 428
  orbital disease in, 428, 428f
  phacoclastic uveitis in, 222, 222f
  protrusion of harderian gland in, 154
Radiation therapy, 59-60, 59f
  keratoconjunctivitis sicca due to, 167
Radiography, 102-103, 103f
  orbital, 358-359, 358f, 359f
Ranitidine, 219
Raptor, 434-436, 435f
  normal intraocular pressure values for, 428t
Rat, 433-434, 433f
  normal intraocular pressure values for, 428t
Rebound tonometry, 97, 97f

Recrudescent disease, 143
Rectus muscles
  anatomy of, 13
  paralysis of, 332
Redleg, 440
Reflexes
  corneal, 16-17, 17t
  dazzle, 17t, 101, 322
  ocular, 16-17, 17f, 17t
  palpebral, 17t, 101
  pupillary light (*See* Pupillary light reflex)
Reflex uveitis, 214t
Refractive error, 5
Reptilia, 436-438, 437f, 438f
Resistance in ocular injury, 63
Retina, 285-317
  anatomy of, 295-298, 295f, 296f, 297f
    cellular, 285-289, 286f, 286t, 288f, 289f
      optic disc in, 297-298
      in rabbits, 428
    atrophy of, 63, 64f, 381t
    blood supply to, 287, 288f, 290f, 292f
  in central visual pathway, 8
  congenital disorders of, 301-304
    collie eye anomaly, 303-304, 303f, 304f
    coloboma, 304, 304f
    dysplasia, 301, 303f
  degeneration of (*See* Retinal degeneration)
  detachment of (*See* Retinal detachment)
  dystrophy of, in briards, 309
  embryonic and fetal development of, 21-23, 24f
  examination of, 91-92, 91f, 94
  hyperreflectivity of, 80
  inverted, 287
  lesions of, 324f
  opacity of, 80
  pathologic mechanisms in, 298-299, 298-301
    choroid interactions, 298-299
    gliosis, 301, 303f
    hemorrhage, 300, 302f
    ischemia, 298
    perivascular cuffing, 300, 301f
    pigment epithelium reactions, 299-300, 300f
    primary photoreceptor disease, 299, 299f
    repair, 74, 298
    retina-optic nerve interaction, 298
  physiology and biochemistry of, 289-295
    dark adaptation in, 292-293, 293f
    electroretinography, 293-295, 293f, 294f, 295f, 296t
    photochemistry in, 291-292, 293f
    rods and cones in, 289, 289f, 292f
    visual photopigments in, 289-291, 293f
  plexiform layers in, 8
  venous drainage of, 12-13, 12f, 13f
  in visual acuity, 6-7, 7f
  wound healing in, 74
Retinal artery, 287
Retinal degeneration
  feline, 309, 311-312, 312f
  in glaucoma, 239-241, 240f, 241f
  in mice and rats, 434
  sudden acquired, 311

Retinal detachment, 314-315, 314f, 315f
  electroretinogram in, 296t
  inflammatory, 69, 70f
  systemic causes of, 383t, 402t
  in uveitis, 213
  vitreous and, 280, 280f, 282
Retinal pigment epithelium
  anatomy of, 285, 286f, 286t, 287f
  degeneration of, electroretinogram in, 296t
  examination of, 91, 91f
  hypertrophy of, 63, 63f
  reactions of, 299-300, 300f
Retinal pigment epithelium dystrophy, 308-309, 308t, 309f
Retinal summation, 289, 292f
Retinitis, 310-311, 311f
Retinochoroiditis, 209, 298
Retinopathy, 304-314
  degenerative, 306, 306t
  due to drug and plant toxicities, 313-314, 313f
  due to infectious/inflammatory disease, 309-311, 311f
  in horses, 314, 314f
  inherited, 304-309
    classification of, 305-306, 305t, 306t
    clinical signs of, 306-307, 307f
    diagnosis of, 307-308
    treatment of, 308
    types of, 308-309, 308t, 309f
  nutritional causes of, 311-312, 312b, 312f, 313f
  phototoxic in mice and rats, 434
  secondary to cardiovascular disease, 309, 310f
  storage disease and, 312-313
  sudden acquired retinal degeneration, 311
Retinoscopy, 102
Retractor bulbi muscles
  anatomy of, 13
  paralysis of, 332
Retractors for drug administration, 36, 36f
Retrobulbar abscess, 360-361, 361f, 362f, 363f, 428, 428f
Retrobulbar injection
  routes of administration, 36, 36f
Retroillumination, 84, 84f, 85f
Rhegmatogenous retinal detachment, 282
Rhinopneumonitis, herpetic, 399-400
Rhinotracheitis
  equine herpetic, 399-400
  infectious bovine, 198-199, 410, 410f
    in conjunctivitis, 145, 145t
    in infectious bovine keratoconjunctivitis, 197, 198b
Rhodococcus equi infection, 407-408
Rhodopsin
  light sensitivity and, 1-2
  as photopigment, 290, 291, 293f
RMSF. *See* Rocky Mountain spotted fever
Rocky Mountain spotted fever, 383-384, 384f
Rod-cone dysplasia, 305, 308t
Rods
  anatomy of, 286f, 288f, 289, 289f, 292f
  in central visual pathway, 8
  dysplasia of, 305
  fetal development of, 23

Rods—cont'd
    sensitivity to motion and, 2
    in visual acuity, 6
Rose bengal stain, 100
Rotational pedicle conjunctival grafts, 187, 187f
Routes of administration, 33-37, 34f
    for ocular surface lavage system, 35, 35f
    for ointments, 35-36
    for solutions and suspensions, 34, 34f
    for subconjunctival, subtenons, and retrobulbar injections, 36, 36f, 37f
    systemic, 36-37
RPE. *See* Retinal pigment epithelium
RPED. *See* Retinal pigment epithelium dystrophy

S

Saliva, drooling of, due to facial paralysis, 334
Salivary gland, zygomatic, relationship to orbit, 352, 356f
Salmonellosis, 401
Sampling, microbiologic, 83-84, 84f
Sanson-Purkinje images, 86, 86f
Sarcoid, eyelid, 125-126, 125f, 133t
Sarcoma in cats, 77, 77f, 226
Sarcoptic acariasis, 127t
SARD. *See* Sudden acquired retinal degeneration
Scabies, 127t
Scaffold, tissue, in wound healing, 73, 75-76
Scarring, 73
    corneal, 179-180, 180f
    retinal, 381t
SCC. *See* Squamous cell carcinoma
Schiøtz tonometer, 95-96, 95f, 96f
Schirmer tear test, 81-82, 84f
    on exotic pets, 427, 428t
    in keratoconjunctivitis sicca, 168, 169, 170
Sclera
    anatomy and physiology of, 178
    disorders of, 199-201, 199f, 200f, 201f
    effects of glaucoma on, 235-236, 236f
    embryonic and fetal development of, 22, 28, 29f
    examination of, 87-88
Scleritis, 199-200, 200f, 379t
Sclerosis, nuclear, in lens, 80, 260, 262f
Scotopic vision, 289
Scrapie, 411
Scraping, conjunctival, 139, 140f-141f
Scrolling of third eyelid, 153, 153f
SDAV. *See* Sialodacryoadenitis virus
Seidel test, 99
Self-trauma, prevention of in corneal ulceration, 186
Senile cataract, 267
Senile iris atrophy, 228, 228f
Sensory retina, 285
Septicemia
    in cattle, 409, 409f
    neonatal equine, 406-407, 407f
Sequestration, corneal, 196-197, 197f
Serous detachment, 314
Serous effusion in inflammatory process, 67
Serous uveitis, 79
Setaria infection, 404
Shaker foal, 406

Sheep
    bright blindness in, 313, 313f
    chlamydial polyarthritis and conjunctivitis in, 142, 408
    fundus of, examination of, 92, 93f
    injection technique for entropion in, 117
    maedi-visna in, 411
    mycoplasmal keratoconjunctivitis in, 408, 408f
    ocular manifestations of systemic disease in, 408-412
    tuberculosis in, 409
Shell prosthesis, 369-370, 371f
Sialodacryoadenitis virus, 433-434
Sinuses, paranasal, orbit and, 352, 355f, 356f
Sinus mucocele, frontal, 362-363
Skin diseases of eyelid, 126, 127t-133t
    allergic, 130t
    arthropod hypersensitivity, 128t-129t
    autoimmune, 131t-132t
    bacterial, 129t
    fungal, 129t
    ischemic/vascular, 132t
    neoplastic, 133t
    nutritional/metabolic, 132t
    parasitic, 127t-128t
    pigmentary, 133t
    protozoal, 130t
    viral, 130t
Skull conformation, proptosis of globe and, 420
Slit-lamp biomicroscope, 86-87, 86f, 94, 95f
Snakes, 438-439, 438f, 439f
Snellen fraction, 7
Snip biopsy of conjunctiva, 139, 140f
Sodium chloride preparations, 50
Sodium methicillin, 38-40
Sodium oxacillin, 40
Solutions, route of administration for, 34, 34f
Spastic entropion, 116
Spectacular disease in snakes, 438-439, 438f, 439f
Spherophakia, 260
Sphincter muscle, pupillary, 10
Squamous cell carcinoma
    conjunctival, 149-150, 149f
    eyelid, 123-125, 124f, 133t
        third, 154, 154f
Squamous epithelium, corneal, 175, 176f
Staining, vital dyes, 98-100, 99f, 100f
Staphylococci
    antibiotics of choice for, 41t
    fluoroquinolones for, 43t
    in hordeolum and meibomian adenitis, 122
Staphyloma, traumatic, 200, 223
Stapling for tear-staining syndrome, 165, 165f
Stars of Winslow, 207
Stationary night blindness, congenital, 309
Stereopsis, 4
Sticktight flea, 128t
Storage disease, 312-313, 350
Strabismus, lesions causing, 331-332, 332f
Strangles, 400-401
Streptococci
    antibiotics of choice for, 41t
    in strangles, 400
Stroma, corneal. *See* Corneal stroma
STT. *See* Schirmer tear test
Stye, 122-123, 122f, 122t, 157
Stypandra, 313, 345

Subalbinism, 210
Subconjunctival emphysema, 138
Subconjunctival hemorrhage, 137, 435, 435f
Subconjunctival injection, routes of administration, 34f, 36, 36f, 37f
Subepithelial geographic corneal dystrophy, 182
Subhyaloid hemorrhage, 277
Subluxation, lens, 272-273
Subpalpebral lavage system, 35, 35f
Subtenon drug administration, 36
Sudden acquired retinal degeneration, 311
Sulfonamides, 42
Summation, retinal, 289, 292f
Sunset eyes, 331
Superficial necrolytic dermatitis, 132t
Superficial punctate keratitis, 183, 183f
Supplies for examination, 82b
Suppurative exudate, 72
Suppurative keratomalacia, 68-69
Supraorbital nerve, 14
Surgery
    cataract, 269-272, 270f, 271f, 272f
    ectropion, 120, 120f
    entropion, 117-119, 117f, 118f, 119f
    eyelid injury, 121-121, 121f
    eyelid neoplasm, 123, 124f
    glaucoma, 250-252, 251f
        feline, 254
    orbital, 365-369, 366f, 367f, 368f, 369f, 370f, 371f
    third eyelid, 153-154, 153f, 154f
        keratoconjunctivitis sicca development following, 166
    uveal, 228
    vitreous, 283, 283f
Surgical adhesives, 56
Surgical instruments needed for ocular emergencies, 419
Suspensions, route of administration for, 34, 34f
Sutures, temporary, for entropion, 117, 117f
Swinging flashlight test, 100-101, 321-322
Symblepharon, 143, 144f
Sympathetic nervous system
    anatomy of, 15t, 16, 335-336, 337f
    diseases of, 336-339, 337t, 338f, 339t
Sympathetic ophthalmia, 213
Sympatholytic agents, 52f, 53b, 54
Sympathomimetic agents, 53-54
Synchysis scintillans, 281-282, 281f
Synechiae
    in corneal ulceration, 187
    in glaucoma, 70, 70f, 71f
    in uveitis, 212
Syneresis, vitreous, 273, 273f, 278
Synophthalmus, 31
Systemic disease
    adnexal abnormalities due to, 405t
    bacterial
        canine, 382-386, 382f, 383f, 384f
        equine, 400-402, 402f
        feline, 385-387, 386f
        ruminant, 408-409, 408f, 409f
    blindness due to, 386t, 403t
    cardiovascular, 396-398, 397f, 397t
    cataracts due to, 380t
    choroidal depigmentation due to, 3402t
    conjunctival disorders due to, 376t, 377t, 399t, 400t

Systemic disease—cont'd
  corneal disease due to, 378t
  endocrine, 393-395, 393f, 394f
  endophthalmitis/paneveitis due to, 385t
  eyelid disorders due to, 375t
  fungal
    canine and feline, 387-392, 387f, 388t-390t, 391f
    equine, 403-404, 403f
    ruminant, 411
  globe disorders due to, 385t
  hematologic, 396t
  immune-mediated, 398-399, 399f
  keratitis/keratoconjunctivitis due to, 400t
  lipemia retinalis due to, 381t
  metabolic
    canine and feline, 395-396, 395f
    ruminant, 411-412
  neonatal, 406-408, 407f
  neoplastic
    equine, 406, 406f
    ruminant, 411, 411f
  neurologic, 404-405
  neuromuscular, 405-406
  neuroophthalmic disorders due to, 403t
  optic nerve disease due to, 384t, 402t
  orbital disorders due to, 404t
  parasitic, 390t, 392-393
  protozoal
    equine, 402-403
    ruminant, 411
  pupillary disorders due to, 402t
  retinal/chorioretinal scarring and atrophy due to, 381t
  retinal detachment due to, 383t, 402t
  retinal hemorrhage due to, 382t, 402t
  scleral and episcleral disease due to, 379t
  toxic, 412
  uveitis due to, 379t
    anterior, 401t
    posterior, 380t, 401t
  viral
    canine, 374-376, 375f, 377f
    equine, 399-400
    feline, 376-382, 377f, 379f, 381f, 382f
    ruminant, 409-411, 410f
Systemic drug administration, 34f, 36-37
Systemic lupus erythematosus, eyelid skin disease due to, 131t
Systolic blood pressure, normal, 397t

T

"Tacking" for entropion, 117, 117f
Tacrolimus, 50, 169, 170
Tapetum
  anatomy of, 1, 206, 207, 208f, 295-297, 295f, 296f, 297f
  examination of, 90-91, 92-93, 92f
  function of, 285, 287f
  hyperreflectivity of, retinopathies and, 307
Tarsal gland, 107, 108f
Tarsorrhaphy, temporary, for corneal ulcers, 188-189, 188f
T cells
  cyclosporine and, 48-49
  in immune-mediated disease, 71
Tear film
  conjunctiva and, 135

Tear film—cont'd
  precorneal
    anatomy and physiology of, 157-159, 159f
    deficiency of, 165-166
    dysfunction of, 160
  of rabbit, 428
Tear film break-up time, 100
Tear quantification tests in exotic pets, 427, 428t
Tear replacement preparations, 56, 57t-58t, 169-170
Tear-staining syndrome in dogs, 164-165, 164f, 165f, 166f
Technique of Morgan, 154, 154f
TEME. See Thromboembolic meningoencephalitis
Temporalis muscle flap, 372
Tenon's capsule, 352, 356f
Tentorial herniation, 349
Teratology, 30
Tetanus, 332, 405-406
Tetracycline, 42, 165, 165f, 198
TFBUT. See Tear film break-up time
Thelazia spp., 146t
Therapeutic formations, 33
Therapeutic soft contact lenses, 59
Thiamine deficiency, 349
Third eyelid, 151-156
  anatomy and physiology of, 151, 152f
  disease of, 152-154, 153f, 154f, 323
  embryonic and fetal development of, 28-29, 30f
  examination of, 87, 151-152
  gland of, 157, 158f
  inflammatory disorders of, 155
  neoplasm of, 154-155, 154f, 155f, 156f
  prominence of, 151-152
  protrusion of, 332-333, 332f
  trauma to, 155, 156f
Third eyelid flap for corneal ulcers, 188-189
360-degree conjunctival grafts, 187, 187f, 188
Thrombocytopenia, 396, 396t
Thromboembolic meningoencephalitis, 349, 409, 409f
Thrombopathy, 396
Ticarcillin, 185b
Ticks, eyelid, 128t
Tissue adhesives, 56, 189
Tissue plasminogen activator, 56, 280
Tissue scaffolding in wound healing, 75-76
Tobramycin, 42, 185, 185b
Tonography, 97
Tonometry, 95-97, 95f, 96f, 97f, 232
Tono-Pen, 96-97, 96f
Tono-Vet rebound tonometer, 97, 97f
Topical anesthetics
  for injections, 36
  for microbiologic samplings, 83-84
Topical application of drugs, 33, 34f
Tortoises, 436-438
Toxicity
  cataracts due to, 267
  cerebral disturbances due to, 349
  enrofloxacin, 42-43
  locoweed, 167, 412
  oxygen, 313-314
  retinopathy due to, 313-314, 313f

Toxicity—cont'd
  in ruminants, 412
  vetch, 412
Toxic uveitis, 214t, 222
Toxoplasmosis, 390t, 392, 411
TPA. See Tissue plasminogen activator
Traction retinal detachment, 314
Transilluminator, Finoff, 86, 86f
Transpalpebral enucleation-extenteration technique, 368-369, 368f, 369f
Trauma, 62-66
  cataracts due to, 266, 266f
  causes of, 62
  cerebral, pupils in, 326-328, 329f, 329t
  consequences of, 62-66, 63f, 64f, 65f, 66f
  eyelid, 120-121, 121f
    third, 155, 156f
  globe
    penetrating injuries of, 423-424
    proptosis of, 419-421, 420f, 421f
  lacrimal system, keratoconjunctivitis sicca due to, 167
  lens, uveitis due to, 217
  in optic radiation and visual cortex disorders, 349
  orbital, 362t
  in raptors and pet birds, 435-436, 435f
  scleral, 200, 201f
  uveal, 214t, 222-223
Treponema cuniculi, 429, 429f
Triamcinolone, 47, 215, 221
Trichiasis, 113, 114f, 115, 115f
Trichromacy, 8
Trichromatic vision, 290
Trifluorothymidine, 45
Trifluridine, 45, 45t, 145-146
Trigeminal nerve
  anatomy and function of, 14, 16f, 318
  dysfunction of, 335
  testing of, 100
Trochlear nerve
  anatomy and function of, 14, 318
  strabismus due to lesions of, 332, 332f
  testing of, 100
Tropicamide, 53, 53b
TSCLs. See Therapeutic soft contact lenses
Tuberculosis, 390t, 409
Tumor. See Neoplasm
Tunica vasculosa lentis, 20, 27, 28f
  persistent, 279
Turtles, 436-438
TVL. See Tunica vasculosa lentis

U

Uberreiter's syndrome, 194
Ulcer, corneal. See Corneal ulceration
Ultrafiltration, aqueous, 230
Ultrasonography, 103-104, 103f, 104f
Uvea, 203-229
  anatomy and physiology of, 203-208, 204f
    in blood-ocular barrier, 207-208, 208f
    choroid in, 206-207, 207f, 208f
    ciliary body in, 203-206, 205f, 206f, 207f
    iris in, 203, 204f, 205f
  congenital abnormalities of, 209-211, 209f, 210f, 211f, 211t
  cysts of, 224-225, 224f

Uvea—cont'd
glaucoma secondary to, 250b, 253
hyphema, 223-224, 224f
immune mechanisms and, 209
iris atrophy in, 227-228, 228f
iris hypoplasia in, 227
neoplasm of, 225-227, 225b, 225f, 226f, 227f
pathologic reactions in, 208-209
surgical procedures on, 228
Uveitis, 208, 211-222
anterior (*See* Anterior uveitis)
associated with neoplasia, 78-79
cataract and, 263-264, 269
clinical signs of, 211-212, 212f
diagnosis of, 213-215, 213t, 214t, 215t
immune-mediated, 216-222
dental disease and, 217
due to *Dirofilaria immitis,* 222
equine recurrent, 217-222, 218f, 219f, 220f, 221f
feline, 217
lens-induced, 216-217, 217f
phacoclastic in rabbits, 222, 222f
pigmentary in golden retrievers, 217
toxic, 222
uveodermatologic syndrome, 216
infectious, 216
phacoclastic, 264
inflammatory exudate in, 72, 72f
phacolytic, 263-264
posterior
defined, 69
systemic causes of, 380t, 401t
in rabbits, 431
sequelae of, 212-213
serous, 79
systemic causes of, 379t
traumatic, 222-223
treatment of, 215-216
Uveodermatologic syndrome, 72, 132t, 216, 398-399, 399f

V

Vaccine
for equine recurrent uveitis, 221-222
ischemic dermatopathy induced by, 132t
Valacyclovir, 45, 146
Vancomycin, 185b
Vascularization
corneal, 179, 179f
vitreous, 279
Vascular system
anatomy of
arterial supply in, 10-12, 12f
venous drainage in, 12-13, 13f
disease of, eyelid skin, 132t
embryonic and fetal development of, 26-27, 28f
hyaloid, 20
retinal, 287, 288t, 290f, 292f
Vasoactive agents, 141
Venography, orbital, 103, 358-359, 359f
Venous drainage, 12-13, 13f
Venous plexus, orbital, 13, 13f

Veratrum californium, 31, 32f
Vertebral sinuses, 13
Vestibular system, 339-342, 340f
disorders of, 341-342
eye position in, 341
strabismus due to, 331
nystagmus and, 339-341, 340b
Vestibuloocular reflex, 17t
Vetch toxicity, 412
Vidarabine, 45, 45t, 146
Viral infection
canine, 374-376, 375f, 377f
conjunctival, 143-146, 144b, 144f, 145t
in birds, 436
in rabbits, 430
equine, 399-400
in encephalitis, 404-405
feline, 376-382, 377f, 379f, 381f, 382f
ruminant, 409-411, 410f
uveal, 214t
Viral papillomatosis of eyelid, 126, 126f
Vision, 1-8
assessment of, 318-320, 320f, 321f
behavioral testing of, 101-102
color, 7-8, 8f, 9f
deficits of
clinical signs of, 323t
in glaucoma, 238, 238f
lesions in, 323-328
depth perception and, 4, 5f
dichromatic, 291
field of view and, 3-4, 3f, 4f
flickering light sensitivity and, 2-3
light sensitivity and, 1-2, 2f, 3f
loss of in retinopathies, 306-307, 307f
motion sensitivity and, 2
postoperative, cataract surgery, 270-271
scotopic, 289
trichromatic, 290
visual acuity and, 4-7, 5f, 6f, 7f
Visual acuity, 4-7, 5f, 6f, 7f
Visual axis, 352, 353f
Visual cortex
anatomy of, 10
disease of, 348-349
Visual evoked potentials, 102, 102f, 322
Visual field, 3-4, 3f, 4f
central visual pathway and, 9
Visual pathways, central, structure and function of, 8-10, 10f, 11f
Visual streak, visual acuity and, 6-7, 7f
Vitamins, 59
Vitamin A deficiency, 292, 312, 312b, 313f, 350
Vitamin B$_1$ deficiency, 349
Vitiligo, 133t
Vitrectomy, 283, 283f
Vitreoretinal surgery, advanced, 284
Vitreoretinopathy, proliferative, 278-279
Vitreous, 277-284
anatomy and physiology of, 277-278, 278f
aqueous humor misdirection syndrome of, 282
asteroid hyalosis of, 281-282, 281f
congenital and developmental abnormalities of, 279-280, 280f

Vitreous—cont'd
degeneration of, 280
retinal detachment and, 315
elongation of, 279
embryonic and fetal development of, 24, 26f
examination of, 93-94
hemorrhage of, 280, 280f
hyalocentesis of, 282-283, 283f, 283t
infection and inflammation of, 280-281
lens luxation and, 273, 282
mass in, 282, 282f
opacities of, 281
pathologic reactions in, 278-279
persistent hyperplastic primary, 279-280, 280f
cataracts and, 265-266
replacement of, 283-284
retinal detachment and, 282
surgical removal of portion of, 282-283, 283f, 283t
synchysis scintillans of, 281-282, 281f
syneresis of, 273, 273f, 278
Vogt-Koyanagi-Harada–like syndrome, 72, 132t, 216, 398-399, 399f
von Willebrand's disease, 396t
Voriconazole, 43, 44t, 192t
v-to-y blepharoplasty, 120, 120f

W

Waardenburg's syndrome, 211
Wall eye, 211
Wanderers, 407
Watch eye, 211
Wedge resection
for ectropion, 120
for entropion, 117
for eyelid coloboma, 109, 112f
Wharton-Jones blepharoplasty, 120, 120f
White blood cells, corneal stromal infiltration with, 180, 180f
White petroleum ointment, 58t
Wolves, visual streak of, 6-7, 7f
Wound healing, 73-77
conjunctival, 135
corneal, 176-178, 177f
diseases resulting from defective, 76-77
germinal cells in, 74-75, 74f, 75f
nutrition in, 76
tissue scaffolding in, 75-76

X

X-irradiation, 59-60

Y

Yeasts in uveitis, 214t

Z

Zinc-responsiveness dermatitis, 132t
Zonal fibers of ciliary body, 203, 206f
Zygomatic mucocele, 363
Zygomatic salivary gland
in ferret, 432
relationship to orbit, 352, 356f
Zygomatic sialogram, contrast, 103